CURRENT
Diagnosis & Treatment
Geriatrics

CURRENT
Diagnosis & Treatment
Geriatrics

Third Edition

Editors

Louise C. Walter, MD
Professor and Chief, Division of Geriatrics
University of California, San Francisco
San Francisco Veterans Affairs Health Care System
San Francisco, California

Anna Chang, MD
Professor, Division of Geriatrics
University of California, San Francisco
San Francisco Veterans Affairs Health Care System
San Francisco, California

Associate Editors

Pei Chen, MD
Assistant Professor, Division of Geriatrics
University of California, San Francisco
San Francisco, California

Rebecca Conant, MD
Professor, Division of Geriatrics
University of California, San Francisco
San Francisco, California

G. Michael Harper, MD
Professor, Division of Geriatrics
University of California, San Francisco
San Francisco Veterans Affairs
Health Care System
San Francisco, California

Daphne Lo, MD, MAEd
Assistant Professor, Division of Geriatrics
University of California, San Francisco
San Francisco Veterans Affairs
Health Care System
San Francisco, California

Josette Rivera, MD
Professor, Division of Geriatrics
University of California, San Francisco
San Francisco, California

Michi Yukawa, MD, MPH
Professor, Division of Geriatrics
University of California, San Francisco
San Francisco Veterans Affairs
Health Care System
San Francisco, California

New York   Chicago   San Francisco   Athens   London   Madrid
Mexico City   Milan   New Delhi   Singapore   Sydney   Toronto

Current Diagnosis & Treatment: Geriatrics, Third Edition

1 2 3 4 5 6 7 8 9   LCR   25 24 23 22 21 20

ISBN 978-1-260-45708-7
MHID 1-260-45708-7
ISSN 1549-5736

Notice

Medicine is an ever-changing science. As new research and clinical experience broaden our knowledge, changes in treatment and drug therapy are required. The authors and the publisher of this work have checked with sources believed to be reliable in their efforts to provide information that is complete and generally in accord with the standards accepted at the time of publication. However, in view of the possibility of human error or changes in medical sciences, neither the authors nor the publisher nor any other party who has been involved in the preparation or publication of this work warrants that the information contained herein is in every respect accurate or complete, and they disclaim all responsibility for any errors or omissions or for the results obtained from use of the information contained in this work. Readers are encouraged to confirm the information contained herein with other sources. For example and in particular, readers are advised to check the product information sheet included in the package of each drug they plan to administer to be certain that the information contained in this work is accurate and that changes have not been made in the recommended dose or in the contraindications for administration. This recommendation is of particular importance in connection with new or infrequently used drugs.

This book was set in Minion Pro by Cenveo® Publisher Services.
The editors were Karen Edmonson and Christie Naglieri
The production supervisor was Richard Ruzycka.
Project Management was provided by Garima Poddar, Cenveo Publisher Services.

This book is printed on acid-free paper.

McGraw Hill books are available at special quantity discounts to use as premiums and sales promotions, or for use in corporate training programs. To contact a representative, please visit the Contact Us pages at www.mhprofessional.com.

Contents

Section II. Care Settings

Section III. Common Conditions in Geriatrics

Section IV. Managing Common Symptoms and Concerns in Geriatrics

Section V. Special Populations and Health Policies for an Aging Society

Authors

Gallane Dabela Abraham, MD
Assistant Professor, Associate Director Geriatric Emergency
    Medicine Department
Department of Emergency Medicine
Icahn School of Medicine at Mount Sinai
Mount Sinai Hospital, Mount Sinai Health System
New York, New York
Emergency Department Care

Cathy Alessi, MD
Director, Geriatric Research
Education and Clinical Center and Chief, Division of
    Geriatrics
Veterans Administration Greater Los Angeles
    Healthcare System
Professor
David Geffen School of Medicine at University of
    California, Los Angeles
North Hills, California
Sleep Disorders

Márlon J.R. Aliberti, MD, PhD
Division of Geriatrics, Department of Internal Medicine
University of Sao Paulo Medical School
Professor, Medicine
Hospital das Clinicas da Faculdade de Medicina da
    Universidade de Sao Paulo
Sao Paulo, Brazil
Functional Assessment & Functional Decline

Theresa A. Allison, MD, PhD
Professor of Medicine and Family and Community
    Medicine
Division of Geriatrics, Department of Medicine
University of California, San Francisco
San Francisco, California
Nursing Home Care & Rehabilitation

Katherine Anderson, MD
Assistant Professor of Medicine
Department of Medicine, Division of Geriatrics
University of Utah School of Medicine
Physician Investigator
VA SLC Geriatric Research, Education and Clinical Center
Salt Lake City, Utah
Headaches

Sik Kim Ang, MB, BCh, BAO
Assistant Professor of Medicine
Division of Geriatrics, Palliative Care and Postacute Medicine
University of Massachusetts-Baystate Medical School
Springfield, Massachusetts
Peripheral Arterial Disease & Venous Thromboembolism

Louise Aronson, MD, MFA
Professor of Medicine
Division of Geriatrics, Department of Medicine
University of California, San Francisco
San Francisco, California
Integrative Geriatrics & Cannabis Use

Gina Ayers, PharmD, BCPS, BCGP
Center for Geriatric Medicine
Cleveland Clinic
Cleveland, Ohio
Hypertension

Amy Baca, MD
Clinical Instructor/HIV Clinical Fellow
Division of HIV, Infectious Disease, and Global Medicine
University of California, San Francisco
San Francisco, California
HIV & AIDS

Alan H. Baik, MD
Department of Medicine, Division of Cardiology
University of California, San Francisco
San Francisco, California
Coronary Artery Disease

Lisa C. Barry, PhD, MPH
Associate Professor of Psychiatry
UConn School of Medicine Farmington, Connecticut
Helping Older Persons in the Criminal Justice System

Scott R. Bauer, MD, MSc
Departments of Medicine and Urology
University of California, San Francisco
Division of General Internal Medicine
Veterans Affairs Medical Center
San Francisco, California
*Benign Prostatic Hyperplasia & Lower Urinary
    Tract Symptoms*

Michele Bellantoni, MD, CMD
Associate Professor and Clinical Director
Division of Geriatric Medicine and Gerontology
Johns Hopkins University School of Medicine
Baltimore, Maryland
Osteoporosis & Hip Fractures

Rebecca J. Beyth, MD, MSc
Professor of Medicine
University of Florida College of Medicine
Associate Director
Clinical Innovation, NF/SG Veterans Health
    System GRECC
Gainesville, Florida
Anticoagulation

Ellen F. Binder, MD
Division of Geriatrics and Nutritional Science
Washington University School of Medicine
St. Louis, Missouri
Encouraging Appropriate Exercise for Older Adults

C. Barrett Bowling, MD, MSPH
Associate Director Clinical
Durham Veterans Affairs Geriatric Research Education
    and Clinical Center
Associate Professor
Division of Geriatrics
Duke University
Durham, North Carolina
Chronic Kidney Disease

Cynthia M. Boyd, MD, MPH
Professor of Medicine
Division of Geriatric Medicine and Gerontology,
    Department of Medicine
Johns Hopkins University School of Medicine
Center for Transformative Geriatric Medicine
Baltimore, Maryland
Addressing Multimorbidity

Rebecca Brown, MD, MPH
Assistant Professor of Medicine
Division of Geriatric Medicine
Perelman School of Medicine of the University of
    Pennsylvania
Corporal Michael J. Crescenz Veterans Affairs
    Medical Center
Philadelphia, Pennsylvania
*Effects of Homelessness & Housing Instability on
    Older Adults*

Albert Bui, MD
Department of Internal Medicine, Division of
    Geriatric Medicine
UCLA David Geffen School of Medicine at UCLA
Los Angeles, California
Overview of Geriatric Assessment

Crystal Burkhardt, PharmD, MBA, BCPS, BCGP
Clinical Associate Professor
University of Kansas
Lawrence, Kansas
The Interprofessional Team

Daniel Butler, MD
Assistant Professor
Department of Dermatology
University of California, San Francisco
San Francisco, California
Common Skin Disorders

Dawn Butler, JD, MSW
Indiana University School of Medicine
Director GRACE Training & Resource Center
Indianapolis, Indiana
Caregiving & Caregiving Support

Laura K. Byerly, MD
Assistant Professor of Medicine
Division of General Internal Medicine & Geriatrics
Oregon Health & Science University
Portland, Oregon
Nursing Home Care & Rehabilitation

Brook Calton, MD, MHS
Associate Professor of Medicine
Division of Palliative Medicine, Department of Medicine
University of California, San Francisco
San Francisco, California
Persistent Pain

Teresa L. Carman, MD
University Hospitals Cleveland Medical Center
Case Western Reserve University School of Medicine
Cleveland, Ohio
Chronic Venous Insufficiency

David B. Carr, MD
Professor of Medicine and Neurology
Division of Geriatrics and Nutritional Science
Washington University School of Medicine
St. Louis, Missouri
Driving & Older Adults

Anna Chang, MD
Professor of Medicine
Division of Geriatrics, Department of Medicine
University of California, San Francisco
San Francisco Veterans Affairs Health Care System
San Francisco, California
Transforming the Care of Older Persons

Elisa M. Chávez, DDS
Associate Professor
Department of Diagnostic Sciences
University of the Pacific Arthur A. Dugoni School
 of Dentistry
San Francisco, California
Common Oral Diseases & Disorders

Helen Chen, MD
Chief Medical Officer
Hebrew SeniorLife
Assistant Professor of Medicine
Harvard Medical School
Roslindale, Massachusetts
The Social Context of Older Adults

Pei Chen, MD
Assistant Professor of Medicine
Division of Geriatrics, Department of Medicine
University of California, San Francisco
San Francisco, California
The Interprofessional Team
Unique Needs of Older Immigrants

Anna H. Chodos, MD, MPH
Assistant Professor of Medicine
Division of Geriatrics, Department of Medicine
University of California, San Francisco
Zuckerberg, San Francisco General Hospital
San Francisco, California
Optimizing Care of Older Adults with Limited Health Literacy

Audrey K. Chun, MD
Department of Geriatrics and Palliative Medicine
Icahn School of Medicine at Mount Sinai
New York, New York
Diabetes

Rebecca Conant, MD
Professor of Medicine
Division of Geriatrics, Department of Medicine
University of California, San Francisco
San Francisco, California
Residential Care & Assisted Living

Kenneth E. Covinsky, MD, MPH, BS
Professor of Medicine
Division of Geriatrics, Department of Medicine
University of California, San Francisco
San Francisco Veterans Affairs Health Care System
San Francisco, California
Functional Assessment & Functional Decline
Applying Evidence-Based Care to Older Persons

William Dale, MD, PhD
Arthur M. Coppola Family Chair in Supportive Care
 Medicine
Clinical Professor and Chair, Department of Supportive
 Care Medicine
City of Hope Comprehensive Cancer Center
Duarte, California
Common Cancers

Jeffrey de Castro Mariano, MD, AGSF
Assistant Clinical Professor
Kaiser Permanente School of Medicine
Associate Program Director
Kaiser Permanente Geriatric Medicine Fellowship
Assistant Clinical Professor
David Geffen School of Medicine at UCLA
Assistant Chief
Kaiser Permanente West Los Angeles Geriatrics and
 Palliative Medicine
Los Angeles, California
Meeting the Unique Needs of LGBT Older Adults

Sanket S. Dhruva, MD, MHS
Department of Medicine, Division of Cardiology
University of California, San Francisco
San Francisco VA Medical Center
San Francisco, California
Coronary Artery Disease

Jessica A. Eng, MD, MS
Associate Professor of Medicine
Division of Geriatrics, Department of Medicine
San Francisco Veterans Affairs Healthcare System
San Francisco, California
Transitions and Continuity of Care

Kathryn J. Eubank, MD
Professor of Medicine
Division of Geriatrics, Department of Medicine
University of California, San Francisco
San Francisco Veterans Affairs Health Care System
San Francisco, California
Hospital Care

Anne Fabiny, MD
Professor of Medicine
Division of Geriatrics, Department of Medicine
University of California, San Francisco
Associate Chief of Staff for Geriatrics, Palliative and
    Extended Care Service
San Francisco Veterans Affairs Health Care System
San Francisco, California
Cerebrovascular Disease

Ronan M. Factora, MD
Assistant Professor of Medicine
Cleveland Clinic Lerner College of Medicine at Case
    Western Reserve University
Center for Geriatric Medicine, Cleveland Clinic
Cleveland, Ohio
Hypertension

Emily Finlayson, MD, MS, FACS
Professor of Surgery
Department of Surgery
University of California, San Francisco
San Francisco, California
Perioperative Care for Older Surgical Patients

Lynn A. Flint, MD
Associate Professor of Medicine
Division of Geriatrics, Department of Medicine
University of California, San Francisco
San Francisco Veterans Affairs Health Care System
San Francisco, California
Transitions and Continuity of Care

Nicholas B. Galifianakis, MD, MPH
Associate Professor of Neurology
Director, Movement Disorders Fellowship
University of California, San Francisco
San Francisco, California
Parkinson Disease & Essential Tremor

Steven R. Gambert, MD
Professor, Department of Medicine
University of Maryland School of Medicine
Director of Geriatric Medicine
University of Maryland Medical Center and R. Adams
    Crowley Shock Trauma Center
Baltimore, Maryland
Thyroid, Parathyroid, & Adrenal Gland Disorders

Angela Gentili, MD
Professor of Internal Medicine
Associate Director, Geriatrics Fellowship Program
Internal Medicine, Division of Geriatric Medicine
McGuire VAMC and Virginia Commonwealth University
    Heath System
Richmond, Virginia
Sexual Health & Dysfunction

Samira Ghaniwala, MD
University Hospitals Cleveland Medical Center
Cleveland, Ohio
Chronic Venous Insufficiency

A. Ghazinouri, MD, CWSP
Assistant Clinical Professor
University of California, San Francisco
San Francisco Veterans Affairs Health Care System
San Francisco, California
Parkinson Disease & Essential Tremor

Meredith Gilliam, MD, MPH
Assistant Professor
Division of Geriatric Medicine
University of North Carolina School of Medicine
Chapel Hill, North Carolina
Osteoporosis & Hip Fractures

Lauren J. Gleason, MD, MPH
Assistant Professor of Medicine
The University of Chicago Medicine
Department of Medicine
Section of Geriatrics and Palliative Medicine
Chicago, Illinois
Applying Evidence-Based Care to Older Persons

Michael Godschalk, MD
Professor of Internal Medicine
Internal Medicine, Division of Geriatric Medicine
McGuire VAMC and Virginia Commonwealth University
    Heath System
Richmond, Virginia
Sexual Health & Dysfunction

Michael Goldrich, MD
Geriatric Lead Physician
Over 60 Health Center, Lifelong Medical Care
Berkeley, California
Atypical Presentations of Illness

Courtney K. Gordon, DNP, GNP-BC, MSN
Geriatrics Nurse Practitioner
University of California, San Francisco
San Francisco, California
Pressure Ulcers

Meredith Greene, MD
Assistant Professor of Medicine
Division of Geriatrics, Department of Medicine
University of California, San Francisco
San Francisco, California
HIV & AIDS

Corita R. Grudzen, MD, MSHS, FACEP
Vice Chair for Research, Associate Professor of Emergency
    Medicine and Population Health
Ronald O. Perelman Department of Emergency Medicine
NYU School of Medicine
NYU Langone Health/Bellevue Hospital Center
New York, New York
Emergency Department Care

Jean Y. Guan, MD
Division of Geriatrics and Gerontology, Department of
    Internal Medicine
University of California, San Diego
San Diego, California
Falls & Mobility Impairment

Lesca Hadley, MD
Geriatric Medicine Specialist
Fort Worth, Texas
Fluid & Electrolyte Abnormalities

Lindsay A. Hampson, MD, MAS
Department of Urology
University of California, San Francisco
San Francisco, California
*Benign Prostatic Hyperplasia & Lower Urinary Tract
    Symptoms*

Annie C. Harmon, PhD
Assistant Professor of Medicine
Division of Geriatrics and Nutritional Science
Washington University School of Medicine
St. Louis, Missouri
Driving & Older Adults

G. Michael Harper, MD, AGSF
Professor of Medicine
Division of Geriatrics, Department of Medicine
University of California, San Francisco
San Francisco Veterans Affairs Health Care System
San Francisco, California
Urinary Incontinence

Krista L. Harrison, PhD
Assistant Professor of Medicine
Division of Geriatrics, Department of Medicine
Philip R. Lee Institute for Health Policy Studies
University of California, San Francisco
San Francisco, California
Ethics & Informed Decision Making

Holly M. Holmes, MD, MS, AGSF
Associate Professor
Division of Geriatric and Palliative Medicine
McGovern Medical School, University of Texas Houston
    Health Science Center
Houston, Texas
Principles of Prescribing & Adherence

Abigail Holley Houts, MD
Medical Director for Ambulatory Services
Minnesota Department of Human Services
Direct Care and Treatment
St. Paul, Minnesota
Detecting, Assessing, & Responding to Elder Mistreatment

Annsa Huang, MD
Division of Gastroenterology and Hepatology
University of California, San Francisco
San Francisco, California
Gastrointestinal Diseases

Susan Hyde, DDS, MPH, PhD
Professor of Clinical Preventive and Restorative Dental
    Sciences
University of California, San Francisco
San Francisco, California
Common Oral Diseases & Disorders

James C. Iannuzzi, MD, MPH
Assistant Professor of Surgery
Division of Vascular and Endovascular Surgery
Department of Surgery
University of California, San Francisco
San Francisco, California
Peripheral Arterial Disease & Venous Thromboembolism

Sharon K. Inouye, MD, MPH
Professor of Medicine
Harvard Medical School
Division of Gerontology
Beth Israel Deaconess Medical Center
Milton and Shirley F. Levy Family Chair
Director, Aging Brain Center
Marcus Institute for Aging Research
Hebrew SeniorLife
Boston, Massachusetts
Delirium

Todd C. James, MD
Associate Professor of Medicine
Division of Geriatrics, Department of Medicine
University of California, San Francisco
San Francisco, California
Caregiving & Caregiving Support

Diana V. Jao, MD
Staff Physician
Ron Robinson Senior Care Center
San Mateo Medical Center
San Mateo, California
Sleep Disorders

Bree Johnston, MD, MPH
Department of Internal Medicine, Division of
    Geriatric Medicine
University of Arizona College of Medicine
Tucson, Arizona
Overview of Geriatric Assessment

Robin Jump, MD, PhD
Geriatric Research Education and Clinical Center
VA Northeast Ohio Healthcare System
Division of Infectious Diseases and HIV Medicine
Department of Medicine and Department of Population
    and Quantitative Health Sciences
Case Western Reserve University School of Medicine
Cleveland, Ohio
Common Infections

Jamie N. Justice, PhD
Assistant Professor
Division of Gerontology and Geriatrics, Department of
    Internal Medicine
Wake Forest School of Medicine
Winston-Salem, North Carolina
Geroscience: The Biology of Aging as a Therapeutic Target

Deborah M. Kado, MD, MS
Department of Family Medicine and Public Health
Division of Endocrinology, Department of Internal Medicine
Division of Geriatrics & Gerontology, Department of
    Internal Medicine
University of California, San Diego
San Diego, California
Falls & Mobility Impairment

Evie Kalmar, MD, MS
Clinical Fellow
Division of Geriatrics, Department of Medicine
University of California, San Francisco
San Francisco, California
The Social Context of Older Adults

Ravi Kant, MD
Affiliate Associate Professor
Medical University of South Carolina
Division of Endocrinology
AnMed Health
Anderson, South Carolina
Thyroid, Parathyroid, & Adrenal Gland Disorders

Priya Kathpalia, MD
Division of Gastroenterology and Hepatology
University of California, San Francisco,
San Francisco, California
Gastrointestinal Diseases

Salomeh Keyhani, MD, MPH
Professor
Department of Medicine
University of California, San Francisco
Staff Physician and Researcher
San Francisco VA
San Francisco, California
Integrative Geriatrics & Cannabis Use

Lawrence J. Kerzner, MD, FACP, AGSF
Geriatric Medicine Fellowship Director
Division of Geriatric Medicine, Department of Medicine
Hennepin Healthcare
Assistant Professor of Medicine, University of Minnesota
Minneapolis, Minnesota
Detecting, Assessing, & Responding to Elder Mistreatment

Candace J. Kim, MD
Assistant Professor of Medicine
Division of Geriatrics, Department of Medicine
University of California, San Francisco
San Francisco, California
Confusion

Tonse A. Kini, MD
Department of Ophthalmology, Blanton Eye Institute
Houston Methodist Hospital
Houston, Texas
Managing Vision Impairment

Myung Ko, MD
Clinical Fellow
Division of Gastroenterology
University of California, San Francisco
San Francisco, California
Constipation

Ashwin A. Kotwal, MD, MS
Assistant Professor of Medicine
Division of Geriatrics, Department of Medicine
University of California, San Francisco
San Francisco Veterans Affairs Health Care System
San Francisco, California
Dyspnea

Margot Kushel, MD
Professor of Medicine
Director, Center for Vulnerable Populations
Division of General Internal Medicine
University of California, San Francisco
Zuckerberg San Francisco General Hospital and
    Trauma Center
San Francisco, California
*Effects of Homelessness & Housing Instability on
    Older Adults*

C. Kent Kwoh, MD
University of Arizona Arthritis Center
Tucson, Arizona
Osteoarthritis

Bonnie Lederman, DDS
On Lok Lifeways
Adjunct Faculty
Department of Diagnostic Sciences
University of the Pacific Arthur A. Dugoni School of Dentistry
Department of Clinical Preventive and Restorative Dental
    Sciences
University of California, San Francisco
Geriatric Dentist
Veteran Hospital Administration San Francisco.
San Francisco, California
Common Oral Diseases & Disorders

Andrew G. Lee, MD
Department of Ophthalmology, Blanton Eye Institute
Houston Methodist Research Institute
Houston Methodist Hospital
Houston, Texas
Departments of Ophthalmology, Neurology, and
    Neurosurgery
Weill Cornell Medicine
New York, New York
Managing Vision Impairment

Sei Lee, MD, MAS
Professor of Medicine
Division of Geriatrics, Department of Medicine
University of California, San Francisco
San Francisco Veterans Affairs Health Care System
San Francisco, California
Diabetes

Bruce Leff, MD
Professor of Medicine
Division of Geriatrics and Gerontology
Johns Hopkins University School of Medicine
Baltimore, Maryland
Home-Based Care

Aleksandr Lewicki, MD
Faculty and Clinical Instructor
Kaiser Permanente Geriatric Medicine Fellowship
Faculty and Clinical Instructor
Kaiser Permanente Palliative Medicine Fellowship
Kaiser Permanente Los Angeles
Los Angeles, California
Meeting the Unique Needs of LGBT Older Adults

Sara Lewin, MD
Assistant Professor
Division of Gastroenterology
University of California, San Francisco
San Francisco, California
Constipation

Eleni Linos, MD, DrPH
Professor
Department of Dermatology
Stanford University
Stanford, California
Common Skin Disorders

Dandan Liu, MD
Geriatrician
Department of Medicine
Permanente Medicine—The Permanente Medical Group
    South San Francisco Medical Center
South San Francisco, California
Prevention & Health Promotion

Daphne Lo, MD, MAEd
Assistant Professor of Medicine
Division of Geriatrics, Department of Medicine
University of California, San Francisco
San Francisco Veterans Affairs Health Care System
San Francisco, California
Technology in the Care of Older Adults

Gillian Love, MD
PGY-IV, Geriatric Fellow
Department of Family and Community Medicine
Division of Geriatric Medicine and Palliative Care
Thomas Jefferson University
Philadelphia, Pennsylvania
Chronic Lung Disease

Anna Malkina, MD
Assistant Clinical Professor
Division of Nephrology
Department of Medicine
University of California, San Francisco
San Francisco, California
Fluid & Electrolyte Abnormalities

Lindsey Merrihew Haddock, MD
Clinical Fellow
Division of Geriatrics, Department of Medicine
University of California, San Francisco
San Francisco, California
Managing Hearing Impairment

Myron Miller, MD
Professor
Department of Medicine
Johns Hopkins University School of Medicine
Director
Division of Geriatric Medicine, Department of Medicine
Sinai Hospital of Baltimore
Baltimore, Maryland
Thyroid, Parathyroid, & Adrenal Gland Disorders

Meredith Mirrer, MD, MHS
Staff Physician
On Lok Lifeways
San Francisco, California
Ambulatory Care & Care Coordination

Lona Mody, MD, MSc
Division of Geriatric and Palliative Medicine
Department of Internal Medicine
University of Michigan School of Medicine
Geriatrics Research Education and Clinical Center
Veterans Affairs Ann Arbor Healthcare System
Ann Arbor, Michigan
Common Infections

Ana Montoya, MD, MPH
Division of Geriatric and Palliative Medicine
Department of Internal Medicine
University of Michigan School of Medicine
Ann Arbor, Michigan
Common Infections

John C. Newman, MD, PhD
Assistant Professor of Medicine
Buck Institute for Research on Aging
Division of Geriatrics, Department of Medicine
University of California, San Francisco
Novato, California
Geroscience: The Biology of Aging as a Therapeutic Target

Ivy Nguyen, MD
University of California, San Francisco
San Francisco, California
Cerebrovascular Disease

Mary A. Norman, MD
Medical Director
Highland Springs Retirement Community
Erickson Living
Dallas, Texas
Depression & Other Mental Health Issues

Nzube Okonkwo, MD
Geriatric Medicine Fellow
Division of Geriatric Medicine, Department of Medicine
Hennepin Healthcare
Minneapolis, Minnesota
Detecting, Assessing, & Responding to Elder Mistreatment

Bruce Ovbiagele, MD, MSc, MAS, MBA
San Francisco, California
Cerebrovascular Disease

Miguel Paniagua, MD, FACP, FAAHPM
Medical Advisor, National Board of Medical Examiners
Adjunct Professor of Medicine
Perelman School of Medicine
University of Pennsylvania
Philadelphia, Pennsylvania
Chest Pain

Asha Patnaik, MD
Assistant Professor of Clinical Medicine
Associate Rheumatology Fellowship Program Director
Rheumatology Clinic Director
Division of Rheumatology, Department of Medicine
Stony Brook University, Renaissance School of Medicine
Stony Brook, New York
Common Rheumatologic Disorders

Leslie Pelton, MPA
Director, Age-Friendly Initiative
Institute for Health Care Improvement
Boston, Massachusetts
Age-Friendly Health Systems

Laura Perry, MD
Assistant Professor of Medicine
Division of Geriatrics, Department of Medicine
University of California, San Francisco
San Francisco, California
Chronic Kidney Disease

Edgar Pierluissi, MD
Professor of Medicine
Division of Geriatrics, Department of Medicine
University of California, San Francisco
Zuckerberg San Francisco General Hospital
San Francisco, California
Hospital Care

Kah Poh Loh, MBBCh, BAO
Senior Instructor
Division of Hematology/Oncology
University of Rochester
James P. Wilmot Cancer Center
Rochester, New York
Common Cancers

YaoYao G. Pollock, MD
Clinical Fellow
Division of Hematology/Oncology
Division of Geriatrics, Department of Medicine
University of California, San Francisco
Helen Diller Family Comprehensive Cancer Center
San Francisco, California
Common Cancers

Anita Rajasekhar, MD, MS
Associate Professor, University of Florida College of
  Medicine
Division of Hematology/Oncology
Gainesville, Florida
Anticoagulation

Megan Rau, MD, MPH
Division of Geriatrics and Palliative Medicine, Department
  of Internal Medicine
New York University School of Medicine
New York, New York
Older Travelers

Thomas Reske, MD
Assistant Professor of Clinical Medicine
Section of Geriatric Medicine and Hematology and Oncology
LSU Health Science Center New Orleans
Louisiana State University
New Orleans, Louisiana
Anemia

David B. Reuben, MD
Department of Internal Medicine, Division of Geriatric
  Medicine
UCLA David Geffen School of Medicine
University of California, Los Angeles
Los Angeles, California
Overview of Geriatric Assessment

Michael W. Rich, MD
Professor of Medicine
Cardiovascular Division
Washington University School of Medicine
St. Louis, Missouri
Heart Failure & Heart Rhythm Disorders
Valvular Disease

Tessa Rife, PharmD, BCGP
Academic Detailing Program Manager, Clinical Pharmacy
  Specialist, Addiction Consult and Prescription Opioid
  Safety Team
San Francisco Veterans Affairs Health Care System
Volunteer Clinical Assistant Professor
University of California, San Francisco, School of Pharmacy
San Francisco Veterans Affairs Medical Center
San Francisco, California
Persistent Pain

Josette A. Rivera, MD
Professor of Medicine
Division of Geriatrics, Department of Medicine
University of California, San Francisco
San Francisco, California
The Interprofessional Team

Veronica Rivera, MD
Icahn School of Medicine at Mount Sinai
New York, New York
Ambulatory Care & Care Coordination

Stephanie E. Rogers, MD, MS, MPH
Assistant Professor of Medicine
Division of Geriatrics, Department of Medicine
University of California, San Francisco
San Francisco, California
Age-Friendly Health Systems

Esperanza Romero Rodríguez, MD, MSc
Research Fellow
Boston University School of Public Health
Boston, Massachusetts
Clinical Investigator
Maimonides Biomedical Research Institute of Cordoba
    (IMIBIC)/Reina Sofia University Hospital
University of Cordoba
Cordoba, Spain
Unhealthy Alcohol Use

Leah B. Rorvig, MD, MS
Assistant Professor of Medicine
Division of Geriatrics, Department of Medicine
University of California, San Francisco
San Francisco, California
*Optimizing Care of Older Adults with Limited Health
    Literacy*

Nami Safai Haeri, MD
Department of Geriatrics and Palliative Medicine
Icahn School of Medicine at Mount Sinai
New York, New York
Diabetes

Richard Saitz, MD, MPH
Chair, Department of Community Health Sciences
Professor of Community Health Sciences & Medicine
Boston University School of Public Health
Boston Medical Center
Boston, Massachusetts
Unhealthy Alcohol Use

Brooke Salzman, MD
Associate Professor
Department of Family and Community Medicine
Division of Geriatric Medicine and Palliative Care
Thomas Jefferson University
Philadelphia, Pennsylvania
Chronic Lung Disease

Alejandra Sanchez-Lopez, MD
University of California, San Francisco
San Francisco, California
Chest Pain

Natalie A. Sanders, DO, FACP
Assistant Professor
Division of Geriatrics
University of Utah
Salt Lake City, Utah
Syncope

Breck Sandvall, MD
Fellow-in-Cardiology
Barnes-Jewish Hospital and Washington University School
    of Medicine
St. Louis, Missouri
Heart Failure & Heart Rhythm Disorders

Saket Saxena, MD
Clinical Assistant Professor of Medicine
Cleveland Clinic Lerner College of Medicine at Case
    Western Reserve University
Center for Geriatric Medicine, Cleveland Clinic
Cleveland, Ohio
Hypertension

Mattan Schuchman, MD
Johns Hopkins University School of Medicine
Division of Geriatrics and Gerontology
Baltimore, Maryland
Home-Based Care

Mina S. Sedrak, MD, MS
Assistant Professor
Department of Medical Oncology and Therapeutics
    Research
City of Hope Comprehensive Cancer Center
Duarte, California
Common Cancers

Christine Seel Ritchie, MD, MSPH
Division of Palliative Care and Geriatric Medicine,
    Department of Medicine
Mongan Institute Center for Aging and Serious Illness
Massachusetts General Hospital
Boston, Massachusetts
Addressing Multimorbidity

Amit Shah, MD
Associate Dean of Faculty Affairs
Mayo Clinic Alix School of Medicine
Scottsdale, Arizona
Atypical Presentations of Illness

Kerry Sheets, MD
Geriatric Medicine Fellow
Division of Geriatric Medicine, Department of Medicine
Hennepin Healthcare
Minneapolis, Minnesota
Detecting, Assessing, & Responding to Elder Mistreatment

Meera Sheffrin, MD, MAS
Stanford University School of Medicine
Stanford, California
Defining Adequate Nutrition

Jennifer Shiroky, MD, MPH
Johns Hopkins Bayview Medical Center
Baltimore, Maryland
Home-Based Care

Bobby Singh, MD
Health Sciences Clinical Professor
University of California, San Francisco, School of Medicine
Staff Psychiatrist, San Francisco VA Health Care System
San Francisco, California
Depression & Other Mental Health Issues

Kaycee M. Sink, MD, MAS
Senior Medical Director
Genentech
South San Francisco, California
Cognitive Impairment & Dementia

Daniel Slater, MD, FAAFP
Department of Family Medicine and Public Health
University of California, San Diego
San Diego, California
Falls & Mobility Impairment

Alexander K. Smith, MD, MS, MPH
Associate Professor of Medicine
Division of Geriatrics, Department of Medicine
University of California, San Francisco
San Francisco Veterans Affairs Health Care System
San Francisco, CA
Goals of Care & Consideration of Prognosis
Ethics & Informed Decision Making

Danielle Snyderman, MD
Assistant Professor
Department of Family and Community Medicine
Division of Geriatric Medicine and Palliative Care
Thomas Jefferson University
Philadelphia, Pennsylvania
Chronic Lung Disease

Margarita M. Sotelo, MD
Clinical Professor of Medicine
University of California, San Francisco
San Francisco, California
Valvular Disease

Rebecca Starr, MD, AGSF
Assistant Professor, Tufts University School of Medicine
Medical Director, Geriatrics
Cooley Dickinson Hospital, Massachusetts General Hospital
    Affiliate
Northampton, Massachusetts
Dyspnea

Michael A. Steinman, MD
Professor of Medicine
Division of Geriatrics, Department of Medicine
University of California San Francisco
San Francisco Veterans Affairs Health Care System
San Francisco, California
Principles of Prescribing & Adherence

Caroline Stephens, PhD, GNP, FAAN
Associate Professor and the Helen Lowe Bamberger Colby
    Presidential Endowed Chair in Gerontological Nursing
University of Utah College of Nursing
Salt Lake City, Utah
Confusion

Lisa Strano-Paul, MD, FACP
Professor of Clinical Medicine
Department of Internal Medicine
Assistant Dean for Clinical Education
Director 3YMD Curriculum Track
Director of Primary Care Clerkship
Stony Brook University, Renaissance School of Medicine
Stony Brook, New York
Common Rheumatologic Disorders

Sangita Sudharshan, MD
Advanced Heart Failure Cardiologist
St. Vincent Medical Group
Indianapolis, Indiana
Heart Failure & Heart Rhythm Disorders

Rebecca L. Sudore, MD
Professor of Medicine
Division of Geriatrics, Department of Medicine
University of California, San Francisco
San Francisco Veterans Affairs Health Care System
San Francisco, California
Optimizing Care of Older Adults with Limited Health Literacy

Mark A. Supiano, MD, AGSF
D. Keith Barnes, M.D. and Dottie Barnes Presidential
  Endowed Chair in Medicine
Professor and Chief, Division of Geriatrics
University of Utah School of Medicine
Director
VA Salt Lake City Geriatric Research, Education, and
  Clinical Center
Executive Director
University of Utah Center on Aging
Salt Lake City, Utah
Syncope

Anne M. Suskind, MD, MS, FACS, FPM-RS
Associate Professor of Urology; Obstetrics, Gynecology, and
  Reproductive Sciences
Director, Neurourology, Female Pelvic Medicine, and
  Reconstructive Surgery
University of California, San Francisco
San Francisco, California
Urinary Incontinence

Victoria Tang, MD, MAS
Assistant Professor of Medicine
Division of Geriatrics, Department of Medicine
University of California, San Francisco
San Francisco Veterans Affairs Health Care System
San Francisco, California
Perioperative Care for Older Surgical Patients

David R. Thomas, MD, FACP, AGSF, GSAF
St. Louis University School of Medicine
St. Louis, Missouri
Pressure Ulcers

Tammy Ting Hshieh, MD MPH
Assistant Professor of Medicine, Harvard Medical School
Division of Aging, Department of Medicine, Brigham and
  Women's Hospital
Associate Physician, Older Adult Hematologic Malignancy
  Program
Dana-Farber Cancer Institute
Boston, Massachusetts
Delirium

Ernest R. Vina, MD, MS
University of Arizona Arthritis Center
Tucson, Arizona
Osteoarthritis

**Margaret I. Wallhagen, PhD, GNP-BC, AGSF,
  FGSA, FAAN**
Professor, Department of Physiological Nursing
Director, UCSF Hartford Center of Gerontological Nursing
  Excellence
Senior Nurse Scholar, VA Quality Scholars Program
School of Nursing
University of California, San Francisco
San Francisco, California
Managing Hearing Impairment

Louise C. Walter, MD
Professor and Chief
Division of Geriatrics, Department of Medicine
University of California, San Francisco
San Francisco Veterans Affairs Health Care System
San Francisco, California
Transforming the Care of Older Persons
Prevention & Health Promotion

Katherine Wang, MD
Assistant Professor
Department of Geriatrics and Palliative Medicine
  Icahn School of Medicine at Mount Sinai
New York, New York
Residential Care & Assisted Living

Elizabeth Waring, MD
OB/Gyn, Hospice & Palliative Medicine Fellow
Internal Medicine, Division of Hematology, Oncology, and
  Palliative Care
Virginia Commonwealth University Health System
Richmond, Virginia
Sexual Health & Dysfunction

Michael Weissberger, MD
PGY-IV, Geriatric Fellow
Department of Family and Community Medicine
Division of Geriatric Medicine and Palliative Care
Thomas Jefferson University
Philadelphia, Pennsylvania
Chronic Lung Disease

Meredith M. Whiteside, OD
Associate Clinical Professor
School of Optometry
University of California, Berkeley
Berkeley, California
Managing Vision Impairment

Eric Widera, MD
Professor of Medicine
Division of Geriatrics, Department of Medicine
University of California, San Francisco
San Francisco Veterans Affairs Health Care System
San Francisco, California
Goals of Care & Consideration of Prognosis
Geriatric Palliative Care

Kaitlin Willham, MD
Assistant Professor of Medicine
Division of Geriatrics, Department of Medicine
University of California, San Francisco
San Francisco Veterans Affairs Health Care System
San Francisco, California
Technology in the Care of Older Adults

Brie A. Williams, MD, MS
Professor of Medicine
Division of Geriatrics, Department of Medicine
University of California, San Francisco
San Francisco, California
Helping Older Persons in the Criminal Justice System

Grant R. Williams, MD
Assistant Professor
Divisions of Hematology/Oncology and Gerontology,
    Geriatrics, and Palliative Care
Institute for Cancer Outcomes and Survivorship
University of Alabama at Birmingham
Birmingham, Alabama
Common Cancers

Leah Witt, MD
Assistant Professor of Medicine
Division of Geriatrics, Department of Medicine
University of California, San Francisco
San Francisco, California
Older Travelers

Jana Wold, MD
Associate Professor of Neurology
Department of Neurology
Division of Vascular Neurology
University of Utah School of Medicine
Salt Lake City, Utah
Headaches

Melisa L. Wong, MD, MAS
Assistant Professor
Division of Hematology/Oncology
University of California, San Francisco
Helen Diller Family Comprehensive Cancer Center
San Francisco, California
Common Cancers

Kristine Yaffe, MD
Scola Endowed Chair and Vice Chair
Professor, Psychiatry, Neurology and Epidemiology/
    Biostatistics
University of California, San Francisco
San Francisco, California
Cognitive Impairment & Dementia

Natalie C. Young, MD
Assistant Professor of Medicine
Division of Geriatrics, Department of Medicine
University of California, San Francisco
San Francisco, California
Geriatric Palliative Care

Michi Yukawa, MD, MPH
Professor of Medicine
Division of Geriatrics, Department of Medicine
University of California, San Francisco
San Francisco Veterans Affairs Health Care System
San Francisco, California
Defining Adequate Nutrition

Paul D. Zito, MBBS
Hematology and Oncology Fellow
Section of Hematology and Oncology
LSU Health Science Center New Orleans
Louisiana State University
New Orleans, Louisiana
Anemia

Preface

Current Diagnosis and Treatment: Geriatrics, 3rd edition, is written for clinicians who provide care to older persons. In the context of a rapidly aging population, clinicians are continually adapting their practice to meet the needs of their older patients. *Current Diagnosis and Treatment: Geriatrics* provides a framework for using a person's functional and cognitive status, prognosis, and social context to guide diagnosis and treatment of medical conditions. In this edition, authors apply the **principles of geriatric medicine** in different **care settings** to address **common conditions and diseases** and **manage common symptoms and concerns** encountered by clinicians in the care of older persons.

In the first section, **Principles of Geriatric Care**, the authors examine how the care of older persons differs from the more disease- or organ-focused care geared toward younger persons. The introductory chapter describes the theoretical framework of geriatric care. Each subsequent chapter provides an in-depth review of fundamental components of care, including an overview of geriatric assessment and individual chapters that provide detailed information about each component of geriatric assessment. This section also includes a discussion of the intersection between geriatrics and palliative care and includes new content about caregiving, legal issues and conservatorship. This section ends with the application of evidence-based care to older adults.

Care Settings, the second section, presents the different health care system settings in which clinicians provide care to older adults. Beginning with an overview of ambulatory care and transitions of care between settings, the section focuses on the cornerstones of care for older adults in the clinic setting, in the emergency department, in the hospital, in residential and assisted living care, in nursing homes and rehabilitation facilities, and in home care settings. Also included are special situations, such as addressing the needs of older patients in the perioperative period and using technology, such as telemedicine, to enhance geriatric care.

In the third section, **Common Conditions in Geriatrics**, authors discuss approaches to managing medical conditions and diseases in older adults, applying and integrating the current knowledge base to guide decision making. Some of the clinical challenges included are evaluating delirium, cerebrovascular disease, and chronic lung disease; managing gastrointestinal disease and common skin disorders; and a new chapter on HIV and AIDS in older persons.

The **Common Clinical Scenarios in Geriatrics** section addresses some of the common symptoms and unique concerns encountered in clinical practice with older persons. Some of the common symptoms included are sleep disorders, chronic pain, lower urinary tract symptoms, and constipation. This section also includes new content on concerns such as driving safety and the use of marijuana in older persons.

The final section is **Broadening Clinical Practice**, which guides clinicians in treating vulnerable subpopulations of older persons (eg, those who are LGBTQ, those with low health literacy, those in the criminal justice system, and those who are homeless). This section also includes new content about the unique needs of older travelers and older immigrants. The section ends with a broader look at how clinical systems are responding to the aging population and strategies for all of us to advocate for more age-friendly health systems.

We thank our authors for their contributions to the third edition of *Current Diagnosis and Treatment: Geriatrics,* and we look forward to advancing the care of older persons together.

Louise C. Walter, MD, and Anna Chang, MD
and
Pei Chen, MD
Rebecca Conant, MD
G. Michael Harper, MD
Daphne Lo, MD, MAEd
Josette Rivera, MD
Michi Yukawa, MD, MPH

Acknowledgements

The editors are deeply grateful to our patients, colleagues, mentors, and learners at the University of California, San Francisco and the San Francisco Veterans Affairs Health Care System. They inspire us and teach us every day.

We thank our chapter authors, who are expert clinicians, researchers, educators, and pioneers in our field. It is because of their generosity that we are able to share this collection of the most current, evidence-based, and practical advice with our readers. It is our hope that this work improves the care of older persons globally.

Most importantly, we thank our spectacular editorial project manager, Bryony Mearns, PhD. Over the course of a year, Dr. Mearns's leadership was instrumental in assisting our team of editors and authors toward completion of this book. She did this one step at a time, with great expertise, kindness, and skill. We were fortunate to have Bryony as our partner on this journey.

Louise C. Walter, MD
Anna Chang, MD
Pei Chen, MD
Rebecca Conant, MD
G. Michael Harper, MD
Daphne Lo, MD, MAEd
Josette Rivera, MD
Michi Yukawa, MD, MPH

CHAPTER ACKNOWLEDGEMENTS

Chapter 5 We thank Susan E. Hardy, MD, PhD, who worked on this chapter in the previous edition. Her work has tremendously contributed to the content of this updated version.

Chapter 8 The authors acknowledge Dane J. Genther, MD, and Frank R. Lin, MD, PhD, who wrote the original version of this chapter that appeared in the second edition of this textbook and that was revised to create the current chapter.

Chapter 16 With acknowledgment to Carla M. Perissinotto, MD, MHS, and Christine Ritchie, MD, MSPH, who authored an earlier edition of this chapter.

Chapter 19 The authors recognize Drs. Tessa del Carmen and Mark S. Lachs for their work in producing an earlier version of this chapter that served as a foundation for the current publication.

Chapter 21 We appreciate the work of Bernard Lo, MD, who authored an earlier draft of this work.

Chapter 29 We would like to acknowledge and recognize the contribution of Lawrence Oresanya, MD, who previously co-authored the previous edition of this chapter.

Chapter 30 We would like to acknowledge and recognize the contributions of Jessica Colburn, MD, and Jennifer Hayashi, MD, who previously co-authored the previous edition of this chapter.

Chapter 38 We acknowledge the contributions of Daniel Antoniello, MD, who was a prior author of this chapter.

Chapter 39 We acknowledge Melvin Cheitlin, MD, and Michael Rich, MD, for their contributions to prior editions.

Chapter 40 We acknowledge Dr. Susan Joseph and Dr. Jane Chen for their contributions to this chapter in an earlier edition of this book.

Chapter 41 The authors of this chapter update would like to acknowledge the work of Dr. Quratulain (Annie) Syed and Dr. Barbara Messinger-Rapport, whose work on the previous version of this chapter served as the foundation for this update.

Chapter 43 The authors acknowledge input from the previous chapter author Teresa L. Carman, MD.

Chapter 48 We would like to acknowledge the work of Mariko Koya Wong, MD, and Kellie Hunter Campbell, MD, MA, the authors of this chapter in the previous edition of the book.

Chapter 51   The authors would like to thank Dr. Josette A. Rivera and Dr. Jessamyn Conell-Price for their contributions to earlier edition of this chapter.

Chapter 53   The authors thank Joanne E. Mortimer, MD, FACP, and Janet E. McElhaney, MD, for their contributions to prior editions of this chapter.

Chapter 56   The authors would like to acknowledge the prior authors of this chapter, Christine O. Urman, MD, and Daniel S. Loo, MD.

Chapter 61   The authors acknowledge Alayne Markland, DO, MSc, for work on a previous edition of this chapter.

Chapter 62   The authors would like to acknowledge Serena Chao and Ryan Chippendale for their contributions to the previous version of this chapter.

Chapter 65   We would like to acknowledge Christina Paruthi, MD, who co-authored the version of this chapter included in the previous edition of the book.

Chapter 66   We would like to acknowledge Leslie Kernisan, MD, MPH, for her work on the earlier version of this chapter.

Chapter 72   I would like to acknowledge the work of Sara J. Francois, PT, DPT, MS; Jennifer S. Brach, PhD, PT; and Stephanie Studenski, MD, MPH, the authors of the chapter in the previous edition of the book.

Chapter 73   We thank the authors of the previous edition of this chapter, Mark Simone, MD, and Manuel Eskilden, MD, MPH. We acknowledge their contribution to this current version.

Chapter 77   We gratefully acknowledge the efforts of this chapter's previous author, Gerald Charles, MD.

CURRENT
Diagnosis & Treatment
Geriatrics

Transforming the Care of Older Persons

1

Anna Chang, MD

Louise C. Walter, MD

Populations are aging worldwide. This demographic shift will dominate the health care landscape of the 21st century. As the number of older persons continues to grow, it becomes increasingly important to know how to help everyone age well, preserving independence, dignity, and purpose. As health care providers, we all have a responsibility to learn the unique aspects of medical care for older persons that will maximize their health and well-being, as defined and redefined by each individual as they age.

Many scientific discoveries, educational advances, and health system innovations have led to improvements in medical and social care for older persons. Such advances guide us today in caring for those with chronic illness, as well as their caregivers. For example, we now have best practices in managing polypharmacy, transitions across health care settings, and falls. We are increasingly aware of the impact of loneliness, iatrogenesis, and caregiver burden. Advances also guide us in optimizing the health and well-being of older persons in good health through health promotion activities. Furthermore, we have become knowledgeable about ways to avoid the hazards of medical care. For example, models such as the acute care for elders (ACE) hospital units are designed to increase mobility in the hospital and prevent delirium so that more older persons can return directly home after a hospital stay.

Yet, there remains much to be done to improve the health and well-being of older persons. Currently, there are fewer than 7000 US geriatricians, and there remain many gaps between science, practice, and what is important to patients. Across the globe, the World Health Organization has designated 10 priorities for a decade of actions on healthy aging, including supporting innovation, collecting data, promoting research, aligning health care systems, combating ageism, and developing age-friendly cities and communities. The field of geriatrics aims to support these actions and bridge the gaps, helping clinicians incorporate the fundamental principles of geriatric medicine into their care of older persons.

In this chapter, we describe guiding principles and clinical practice frameworks to assist all clinicians who care for older persons across the world in home care, ambulatory, hospital, long-term care, and end-of-life settings.

GUIDING PRINCIPLES

Three principles guide the care of older persons.

A. Complexity, Multimorbidity, and Physiologic Reserve

A holistic, interprofessional, team-based approach is necessary in caring for older persons with complex psychosocial circumstances and multiple medical conditions. In addition, older persons have lower physiologic reserve in each organ system when compared with younger adults, placing them at risk for more rapid decline when faced with acute or chronic illness. Some examples include decreases in muscle mass and strength, bone density, exercise capacity, respiratory function, thirst and nutrition, and ability to mount effective immune responses. For these reasons, older persons are often more vulnerable to periods of bedrest and inactivity, external temperature fluctuations, and complications from common infectious diseases. Although preventive measures, such as vaccinations, may be beneficial, decreased physiologic reserve may also impair older persons' ability to mount an effective immune response to vaccines. These processes can also delay or impair recovery from serious illnesses such as hip fractures or pneumonia. As a result, older persons are prone to developing complex geriatric syndromes, such as delirium and falls.

B. The Importance of Cognition & Function

In older persons, cognitive and physical function are often more accurate predictors of health, morbidity, mortality, and health care utilization than individual diseases or chronologic age. Cognitive status includes executive function, memory, orientation, and visual-spatial ability. Functional status includes the ability to perform activities of daily living (ADLs) and instrumental activities of daily living (IADLs). Cognitive impairment places older persons at risk for functional decline, medication errors, and environmental hazards, and creates a significant stress on caregivers. Functional impairment itself also strongly affects health outcomes. Losing the ability to transfer or walk in the hospital, for example, increases the likelihood of nursing home placement and death after discharge. Thus, assessments of cognitive and functional status are critical to providing comprehensive health care, and they are critical to an accurate prognosis and planning for family and social supports to optimize aging for each older person. By detecting changes early on, we can offer strategies to preserve physical function and optimize quality of life.

C. The Role of Goals & Prognosis in Clinical Decision Making

An effective clinical encounter with an older person relies heavily on an understanding of an older person's goals of care and likely prognosis. This individualized approach informs diagnostic and therapeutic plans in order to maximize benefit and minimize harm for each older person. Some older persons may prioritize decreasing pain and symptoms. Some may prioritize independent physical function. Others wish to remain close with, yet not burden, their loved ones. In addition, for older persons with a limited life expectancy, some interventions would only cause burden and not yield the desired benefit within their lifetime. Considering prognosis in the context of each patient's goals of care represents an appropriate starting place for individualized clinical decisions and treatment plans.

FOR CLINICIANS: THE GERIATRIC 5M'S FRAMEWORK

The three guiding principles above must be applied at the clinician, community, and health care system levels. For example, the Geriatric 5M's Framework aids clinicians in incorporating the guiding principles into clinical practice: (1) **Mind:** The first "M" reminds us to assess for delirium, dementia, depression, and ways to maintain mental activity, when appropriate. (2) **Mobility:** The second "M" prompts us to ask whether an older person requires assistance with ADLs and IADLs, requires ambulation aids for home or community mobility, or has fallen. (3) **Medications:** The third "M" asks us to critically examine every medication and the medication list as a whole to eliminate medications that cause more burden and harm than benefit. (4) **Multimorbidity:** The fourth "M" guides us to consider the impact of therapeutics on the whole person to avoid the situation where an intervention targeting one condition inadvertently worsens several other conditions. (5) **Matters Most:** The final "M" gives us a place to start, and end, every medical decision and encounter by aligning all actions according to what is most important to the older person.

FOR COMMUNITIES: EMBRACING OLDER PERSONS

Optimizing aging also occurs within the broader context of an older person's family, friends, and community. The social network of an older person's life plays a significant role in each individual's well-being, influences preferences, and provides resources and support in times of need. In managing a complex therapeutic plan at home (eg, one that involves multiple medications or dressing changes), effective therapy may hinge on the helping hands of family or friends. In addition, the well-being of older adults with chronic illness is often contingent upon adequate care and support for caregivers who often suffer from caregiver burden, stress, and health effects of their own. Even in the absence of chronic medical illness, loneliness is associated with poor outcomes, such as functional decline and death. An older person's health and survival may depend on routine contact with a social network. Thus, the best health care for older persons is inseparable from a thorough consideration of their social context.

FOR HEALTH CARE SYSTEMS: CARING FOR OLDER PERSONS

Health care systems caring for older persons are challenged by conflicting clinical principles, care models, and financial incentives. As a result, older persons often experience new symptoms and conditions that represent adverse effects from being cared for and moved across multiple care settings. During times of transition, such as from emergency department to hospital to nursing home, the older person is particularly at risk for poor outcomes from incomplete medication reconciliation processes or inadequate hand-off communication. Additional potential harms include pressure ulcers as a result of waiting an excessive amount of time on gurneys or immobility in hospital beds and falls related to hazards such as intravenous tubing and medical devices in an unfamiliar environment without one's sensory aids, such as eyeglasses or hearing aids. Health care systems increasingly have a responsibility to implement evidence-based best practice care models to protect older persons from harm in times of illness.

As we age, interaction with the health care system often becomes a bigger part of our lives. Unfortunately, suffering among older persons and their caregivers remains too common and is often not addressed by our current health care systems. For example, the typical medical encounter designed for younger persons with an acute illness is often insufficient for an older person with multiple medical and social complexities. Now is the time to embrace guiding principles and frameworks of geriatric medicine to transform our health care systems to optimize the health of our aging society.

Creditor MC. Hazards of hospitalization of the elderly. *Ann Intern Med.* 1993;118:219-223.

Friedman SM, Shah K, Hall WJ. Failing to focus on healthy aging: a frailty of our discipline? *J Am Geriatr Soc.* 2015;63:1459-1462.

Perissinotto CM, Stijacic Cenzer I, Covinsky KE. Loneliness in older persons: a predictor of functional decline and death. *Arch Intern Med.* 2012;172:1078-1084.

Reuben DB. Medical care for the final years of life: "when you're 83, it's not going to be 20 years." *JAMA.* 2009;302(24):2686-2694.

Tinetti M. Mainstream or extinction: can defining who we are save geriatrics? *J Am Geriatr Soc.* 2016;64:1400-1404.

Tinetti M, Huang A, Molnar F. The Geriatrics 5M's: a new way of communicating what we do. *J Am Geriatr Soc.* 2017;65:2115.

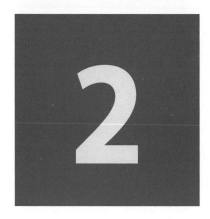

Overview of Geriatric Assessment

Albert Bui, MD
David B. Reuben, MD
Bree Johnston, MD, MPH

INTRODUCTION

Geriatric assessment is a broad term that describes a clinical approach to older patients that goes beyond a traditional medical history and physical exam to include functional, psychological, and social domains that affect well-being and quality of life. As an organizational framework, a geriatric scaffold (Figure 2–1) can help a clinician visualize how these domains are often connecting and overlapping. The scaffold is organized into three main outcomes of the geriatric assessment: prognosis, goals of care, and functional status. Functional status encompasses the effects of the core elements of the geriatric patient's health, including medical, cognitive, psychological, social, and communications barriers. This chapter will outline the geriatric assessment via the scaffold, its three main outcomes, and the core elements that contribute. We will also address how the geriatric assessment may be influenced by the clinical site of care.

TEAMS AND CLINICAL SITES OF CARE

Although geriatric assessment may be comprehensive and involve multiple team members (eg, social workers, nurses, physicians, rehabilitation therapists, pharmacists), it may also involve just a single clinician and be much simpler in approach. In general, teams that use an *interprofessional* approach, in which multiple professions work together to develop a single comprehensive treatment plan for a patient, are most common in settings that serve primarily frail, complex patients, such as inpatient units, rehabilitation units, Program for All-Inclusive Care of the Elderly (PACE) sites, and long-term care facilities. In outpatient settings, teams are less likely to be formalized and, if present, are more likely to be virtual, asynchronous, and *multidisciplinary* (teams in which each discipline develops its own assessment and treatment plan) than interprofessional. (For more information, see Chapter 3, "The Interprofessional Team.")

Regardless of team composition, the setting and functional level of the patient population being served will determine what assessment tools are most appropriate. For example, long-term care settings are likely to focus on basic activities of daily living (ADLs), such as bathing, whereas outpatient teams are more likely to focus on higher levels of functioning, such as mobility and ability to prepare meals. In inpatient settings, the focus is on preventing deconditioning; providing medical support, such as nutrition; and planning discharge, including assessing rehabilitation potential and the best setting for discharge. Regardless of the team structure, site, and tools being used, many of the principles of geriatric assessment are the same.

PROGNOSIS

An older adult's prognosis is important in determining which interventions are likely to be beneficial or burdensome for that individual. In community-dwelling older persons, prognosis can be estimated initially by using life tables that consider the patient's age, gender, and general health. When an older patient's clinical situation is dominated by a single disease process, such as lung cancer metastatic to brain, prognosis may be better estimated with a disease-specific instrument. Even when disease-specific prognostic information is available, frequently the range of survival is wide. Moreover, prognosis generally worsens with age (especially age >90 years) and with the presence of serious age-related conditions, such as dementia, malnutrition, or functional impairment. See Chapter 4, "Goals of Care & Consideration of Prognosis," for a more comprehensive approach to prognostication in the older patient.

When an older person's life expectancy is >10 years, the appropriateness of tests and treatments is generally the same as for younger persons. When life expectancy is <10 years, and especially when it is much less, choices of tests and treatments should be made on the basis of their ability to improve

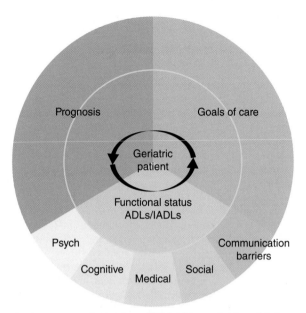

▲ **Figure 2–1.** Geriatric scaffold. ADLs, activities of daily living; IADLs, instrumental activities of daily living.

that particular patient's prognosis or quality of life in the context of that patient's life expectancy and goals of care. The relative benefits and harms of tests and treatments often change as prognosis worsens.

Palliative care services should be considered for any patient with a life-limiting illness, particularly when the prognosis is <1 year, symptom burden is high, and/or goals of care are uncertain. If the prognosis is 6 months or less, hospice should be considered, if consistent with the patient's goals of care.

PATIENT GOALS

Conducting goals of care discussions is a critical tool for all clinicians caring for older adults, especially frail older adults. Although patients vary in their values and preferences, it is reasonable to assume that most patients value living a long life free of incapacitating illness. For many older adults, not all goals are achievable and trade-offs need to be made (eg, between length and quality of life). Older persons may prioritize maintaining their independence or relieving pain or other symptoms over prolonging survival.

In assessing a patient's overarching goals of care, it is often more useful to ask about values and preferences rather than interventions lacking a context, such as asking, "Would you want pressors?" Once a clinician understands a patient's values in more detail, it is often easier to have discussions about personal goals within the context of the person's specific medical and social situation. For example, if a patient

who has recurrent falls places high value on living at home, then a goal may be to make the home safer and adapt it to accommodate the person's disabilities or hire caregivers. Knowing a person's values also facilitates making patient-specific recommendations; for example, "I don't think dialysis will help you reach your stated goals because . . . ." Patients' values may influence clinical decisions, such as continuing life-prolonging treatments based on the desire to live to see the graduation or birth of a grandchild. Conversely, knowing values may prompt recommendations for additional care, including recommending that patients purchase continued physical therapy out of pocket when Medicare coverage has been exhausted. Patients' preferences often change over time. For example, some patients find living with a disability more acceptable than they would have before experiencing it. Tools such as the Serious Illness Conversation Guide (www.ariadnelabs.org/resources/), VitalTalk (www.vitaltalk.org), and goal attainment scaling can help clinicians improve their skills in conducting these discussions.

Every older person should be encouraged to designate a surrogate decision-maker, complete advance directives for both health care (eg, prepareforyourcare.org) and finances, and discuss their values and preferences with their surrogate and with their health care clinicians. Many states honor a form that is signed by both the patient and physician and serves as an order sheet for intervention preferences that is portable across different sites of care (eg, Physicians Orders for Life-Sustaining Treatment).

Kale MS, Ornstein KA, Smith CB, Kelley AS. End-of-life discussions with older adults. *J Am Geriatr Soc.* 2016;64(10):1962-1967.

Reuben DB, Tinetti ME. Goal oriented patient care: an alternative health outcomes paradigm. *N Engl J Med.* 2012;366:777-779.

FUNCTIONAL STATUS

Functional status can be viewed as a summary measure of the overall impact of health conditions in the context of a patient's physical and psychosocial environment on the ability to perform their ADLs and instrumental ADLs (IADLs) (Table 2–1).

Functional status is important for planning care, monitoring responses to therapy, and determining prognosis. Functional impairment is common in older adults and has many potential causes, including age-related physiologic and cognitive changes, disuse, disease, social factors, and the interplay between any of these. In the next sections, we outline the components that contribute to a patient's functional status, including medical, cognitive, psychological, social, and communication domains. Functional status should be assessed initially and periodically thereafter, particularly after hospitalization, severe illness, or the loss of a spouse or caregiver. Unexpected changes in functional status should prompt a comprehensive evaluation looking for contributing

Table 2–1. List of activities of daily living and instrumental activities of daily living.

Activities of Daily Living	Instrumental Activities of Daily Living
Bathing	Using the telephone
Dressing	Shopping
Toileting	Food preparation
Transfers	Housekeeping
Continence	Laundry
Feeding	Driving
	Taking medications
	Managing money

conditions. If no reversible cause of functional decline is found after a medical search or if it cannot be fully reversed, the clinician should focus on supportive services and, when necessary, placement in a different living setting. For more information about functional ability and assessment in older persons, refer to Chapter 5, "Functional Assessment & Functional Decline."

ADLs AND IADLs

In 2016, 8% of community-dwelling adults age 65 years and older reported difficulty in self-care, and another 15% reported difficulty in living independently according to the US Census Bureau. Loss of function in ADLs or IADLs often signals a worsening disease process or the combined impact of multiple chronic conditions. Level of ADL and IADL impairment can usually be determined by self-report or proxy report but should be corroborated when possible. When accurate functional information is essential for planning for any patient assistance, such as adaptive equipment or more caregiver help, direct observation by a physical or occupational therapist can be invaluable.

For highly functional independent older adults, standard functional screening measures will not capture subtle functional impairments. One technique that may be useful for these older adults is to identify and regularly query about a patient-identified target activity, such as playing bridge, golfing, or fishing, that the patient enjoys and regularly participates in (advanced ADLs). Although many of these activities reflect patient preferences that may change over time, if the patient begins to drop the activity, it may indicate an early impairment, such as dementia, incontinence, or worsening vision or hearing loss.

If possible, it is important to distinguish whether an ADL/IADL impairment is primarily due to cognitive decline, a physical disability, or cultural or family customs because this will help guide management, including rehabilitation, adaptive devices, and additional personal assistance.

MEDICAL DOMAIN

▶ Falls and Strength, Balance, and Gait Impairment

Another important assessment is evaluating fall risk. Falls are the leading cause of nonfatal injuries and unintentional injury and death in older persons. Every older person should be asked about falls at least annually. Because strength, gait, and balance impairments commonly contribute to fall risk, it is important to evaluate each of these as well as other risk factors, including visual impairment, medications, and home safety.

Components of the strength and gait exam include observing whether the patient can get up from a chair without using hands, which tests quadriceps strength, and observing gait symmetry, stride length, step height, and width of stance. Balance can be tested by observing stability with eyes closed, with a sternal nudge, and with a 360-degree turn, and ability to maintain side-by-side, semi-tandem, and full-tandem stance for 10 seconds each. The Timed Up and Go test measures a person's ability to get up from a chair, walk 3 meters, return, and sit down. Although a variety of cutoff scores are used for this test, inability to complete the task in <15 seconds is generally considered abnormal, and longer times are associated with a greater risk of functional impairments and falls. Patients with an abnormal gait evaluation should be evaluated further for potentially reversible causes (see Chapter 6, "Falls & Mobility Impairment," and Chapter 67, "Syncope").

Guirguis-Blake JM, Michael YL, Perdue LA, et al. Interventions to prevent falls in older adults: updated evidence report and systematic review for the US Preventive Services Task Force. *JAMA*. 2018;319(16):1705-1716.

▶ Appropriate Medication Use

Although older persons may have many of the same medical problems as younger persons, including diabetes, heart failure, and chronic kidney disease, a higher percentage of older adults have multiple chronic conditions, which, in turn, results in more medications and therefore higher risks associated with adverse drug reactions and drug-drug interactions. The average older person takes four to five medications, and many older adults are prescribed medications by more than one clinician, which increases the risk for medication discrepancies and adverse drug events. Patients should be encouraged to bring all of their medications, including nonprescription drugs (the "brown bag assessment"), to every visit and review them with the primary care practitioner, pharmacist, or nurse. Regular pharmacy reviews, commercially available medication management programs, and electronic health records can help primary care providers monitor for potential inaccuracies and potential drug-drug interactions (see Chapter 14, "Principles of Prescribing &

Adherence"). Tools such as STOPP (Screening Tool of Older People's Prescriptions)/START (Screening Tool to Alert to Right Treatment) and the Beers Criteria can help guide clinicians in appropriate prescribing for older adults.

Koronkowski MJ, Semla TP, Schmader KE, Hanlon JT. Recent literature update on medication risk in older adults, 2015-2016. *J Am Geriatr Soc.* 2017;65(7):1401-1405.

Merel SE, Paauw DS. Common drug side effects and drug-drug interactions in elderly adults in primary care. *J Am Geriatr Soc.* 2017;65(7):1578-1585.

Nutrition

See Chapter 13, "Defining Adequate Nutrition." Nutritional problems among older adults include obesity, undernutrition, and specific vitamin and nutrient deficiencies. Loss of 5% of body weight in 1 month or 10% of body weight over 6 months is associated with increased morbidity and mortality and should trigger further evaluation. Evaluation includes consideration of oral health issues (eg, loss of dentures), medical issues (eg, dementia or malignancy), and social issues (eg, loss of transportation), and potentially, goals of care.

Increasingly, obesity is becoming a problem in older adults and is associated with multiple morbid conditions, including diabetes, osteoarthritis, poor mobility, and obstructive sleep apnea. Traditionally, obesity in the older adult is defined as a body mass index (BMI) of ≥ 30 kg/m^2. However, there is increasing evidence that using a lower BMI cutoff for obesity in certain ethnicities, including Asian, Hispanic, Latino, and Native Americans, may be a more accurate reflection of risk than using the traditional BMI cutoff of 30.

Preventive Services

Preventive services include counseling on healthy behaviors, screening to detect asymptomatic disease, and vaccinations. Specific preventive interventions for an individual patient should be based on evidence-based guidelines, the patient's estimated life expectancy, and the patient's values and goals. The US Preventive Services Task Force has an interactive website with specific recommendations based on the patient's age, gender, tobacco use, and sexual activity (http://epss.ahrq .gov/PDA/about.jsp) (see Chapter 20, "Prevention & Health Promotion").

Incontinence

Incontinence in older adults is common but often goes unmentioned by patients. Women are twice as likely as older men to be incontinent; overall, approximately 6% to 14% of older women experience incontinence daily. Ask a simple question, such as, "Is inability to control your urine

a problem for you?" or "Do you have to wear pads, diapers, or briefs because of urine leakage?" Positive answers should be followed up with a more complete assessment, as determined by the patient's goals and preferences. For example, different patients may prefer behavioral interventions, medication, surgery, or pads to manage their incontinence (see Chapter 10, "Urinary Incontinence"). Incontinence may contribute to falls, especially nocturnal incontinence when poor lighting combined with existing visual impairment may magnify the risk.

COGNITIVE DOMAIN AND DEMENTIA

The cognitive domain evaluation aims to differentiate normal versus abnormal brain aging. In normal brain aging, reaction time, mental processing speeds, name and word retrieval, and multitasking may become slower or more difficult but may still be considered normal age-related cognitive decline. In contrast, more severe impairment raises the suspicion for mild cognitive impairment or dementia, which are common in older adults but, in early stages, are commonly missed by primary care practitioners. Screening for dementia in primary care has not been proven to improve outcomes. However, early detection of Alzheimer disease and related disorders may help to identify potentially treatable contributors (which are uncommon) and to involve the patient in advance care planning for health care and finances. The Mini-Cog, a three-item recall and clock drawing activity, is a brief screen that is sensitive for detecting dementia. Patients who fail the Mini-Cog should be followed up with a more in-depth mental status examination, such as the Montreal Cognitive Assessment (MOCA), or more extensive neuropsychological examinations along with evaluating for decline in functional status. The Mini-Mental Status Exam (MMSE) may be useful in screening for more advanced cognitive impairment but is generally less sensitive for detecting mild cognitive impairment. The Rowland Universal Dementia Assessment Scale (RUDAS) is another cognitive assessment tool designed to minimize the effects of cultural or language diversity. Cognitive impairments that are severe enough to interfere with a patient's prior level of function raise the concern for dementia.

It is important to note that the clinical site of care in which an individual is being assessed (eg, inpatient vs outpatient) should be considered. Cognitive impairment in hospitalized patient evaluations should be interpreted cautiously to distinguish dementia from delirium. The Confusion Assessment Method (CAM) is a useful tool to screen for delirium in emergency departments, hospitals, and nursing home settings.

Patients who are diagnosed with dementia or related disorders should also have further assessment of whether or not they have advance directives, decision-making capacity, and processes in place for managing and protecting their finances (see Chapter 9, "Cognitive Impairment & Dementia," and Chapter 60, "Confusion").

Lin JS, O'Connor E, Rossom RC, Perdue LA, Eckstrom E. Screening for cognitive impairment in older adults: an evidence update for the U.S. Preventive Services Task Force. *Ann Intern Med.* 2013;159(9):601-612.

McMinn J, Steel C, Bowman A. Investigation and management of unintentional weight loss in older adults. *BMJ.* 2011;342:d1732.

PSYCHOLOGICAL DOMAIN AND DEPRESSION

Many older adults find old age to be a time of fulfillment and happiness. However, personal losses, illness, and other challenges may contribute to sadness, grief, anxiety, or depression. Therefore, questions about mood should be part of every geriatric assessment. Although major depression is no more common in older adults than in younger populations, depressive symptoms are more common in older adults. In ill and hospitalized older patients, the prevalence of depression may exceed 25%. The Patient Health Questionnaire (PHQ)-2 is a sensitive screening tool for depression. Positive responses should be followed up with more extensive screens (eg, the PHQ-9), and if positive, a comprehensive interview should be conducted (see Chapter 12, "Depression & Other Mental Health Issues").

US Preventive Services Task Force (USPSTF); Siu AL, Bibbins-Domingo K, et al. Screening for depression in adults: US Preventive Service Task Force recommendations. *JAMA.* 2016;315:380-387.

COMMUNICATION BARRIERS

▶ Vision Impairment

The prevalence of cataract, age-related macular degeneration, glaucoma, and need for corrective lenses increases with advancing age. Given this and the inability of most primary care physician's offices to perform high-quality, comprehensive eye examinations, periodic examinations should be performed by an optometrist or ophthalmologist, particularly for those who have diabetes or are at high risk of glaucoma, such as African Americans.

Vision screening in the primary care setting, with a Snellen eye chart for far vision and a Jaeger card for near vision, may provide valuable on-the-spot information for the practitioner. A vision screening question such as, "Do you have difficulty driving, watching television, reading, or doing any of your daily activities because of your eyesight, even while wearing glasses?" is helpful but may not be sensitive enough to replace a formal vision assessment (see Chapter 7, "Managing Vision Impairment").

For individuals with balance problems and fall risk factors, bifocal lenses should be discouraged because they make depth perception more difficult, particularly when navigating steps or stairs, and increase risk of falls.

▶ Hearing Impairment

More than 33% of individuals older than 65 years and 50% of those older than 85 years have some hearing loss. Hearing loss is associated with social and emotional isolation, clinical depression, accelerated cognitive decline, and limited activity.

The optimal screening method for hearing loss in older adults has yet to be determined. The whispered voice test is easy to perform, but if positive, formal follow-up testing is necessary; sensitivities and specificities range from 70% to 100%. Handheld audiometry with the Welch-Allyn audioscope can increase the accuracy of screening if performed in a quiet environment. The US Screening and Prevention Task Force recommends using screening questions about hearing loss in older adults. Structured questionnaires such as the Hearing Handicap Inventory for Elderly–Screening are most useful for assessing the degree to which hearing loss interferes with functioning (see Chapter 8, "Managing Hearing Impairment"). Technology is advancing rapidly for people with hearing loss, including smartphone apps and lower-cost alternatives to standard hearing amplification.

Goman AM, Lin FR. Prevalence of hearing loss by severity in the United States. *Am J Public Health.* 2016;106(10):1820-1822.

SOCIAL DOMAIN

▶ Caregiver Support

Providing primary care for a frail older adult requires that attention be paid to family caregivers as well as to the patient, because the health and well-being of the patient and caregivers are intricately linked. High levels of functional dependence place an enormous burden on a caregiver. Burnout, depression, and poor self-care are possible consequences of high caregiver loads. Asking the caregiver about stress, burnout, anger, and guilt is often instructive. The Modified Caregiver Strain Inventory is a 13-item validated tool used to assess severity of caregiver strain. The index targets financial, physical, psychological, and social aspects of strain. For the stressed caregiver, a social worker can often identify helpful resources such as caregiver support groups, respite programs, adult daycare, and hired home health aides.

▶ Financial, Environmental, and Social Resources

Old age can be a time of reduced social and financial resources. Older persons are at particular risk of social isolation and poverty. Screening questions about social contacts and financial resources are often helpful in guiding providers in designing realistic treatment and social service planning. Every older person should be encouraged to engage in advance financial planning when completing medical advance directives.

Assessment of the patient's environment should include asking about the ability to access needed community resources (eg, banking, grocery, pharmacy) either themselves or via proxy, the safety of their home, their level of social interaction, driving and driving safety, potentially unsafe practices (eg, tobacco use, high-risk sex) and the appropriateness of their environment for their level of function. When the safety of the home is in question, a home safety assessment by a home health care agency is appropriate.

▶ Abuse

Clues to the possibility of elder abuse include observation of behavioral changes in the presence of the caregiver, delays between injuries and seeking treatment, inconsistencies between an observed injury and an associated explanation, lack of appropriate clothing or hygiene, and unfilled prescriptions. A simple question—"Does anyone hurt you?"— is a reasonable initial screen (see Chapter 19, "Detecting, Assessing, & Responding to Elder Mistreatment"). If abuse is suspected, older adults should have the opportunity to be interviewed alone. Direct questioning about abuse and neglect may be useful, particularly under circumstances of high caregiver load.

Burnes D, Henderson CR Jr, Sheppard C, et al. Prevalence of financial fraud and scams among older adults in the United States: a systematic review and meta-analysis. *Am J Public Health*. 2017;107(8):1295.

Rosay AB, Mulford CF. Prevalence estimates and correlates of elder abuse in the United States: the National Intimate Partner and Sexual Violence Survey. *J Elder Abuse Negl*. 2017;29(1):1-14.

Thornton M, Travis SS. Analysis of the reliability of the modified caregiver strain index. *J Gerontol B Psychol Sci Soc Sci*. 2003;58: S127-S132.

GERIATRIC ASSESSMENT IN PRIMARY CARE

A number of strategies can help make the process of geriatric assessment more efficient for busy primary care practices, such as using previsit screening questionnaires, using nonphysician personnel to help perform standard geriatric assessments, and having standardized protocols for following up on positive results. A number of well-designed previsit questionnaires for older adults are available (see websites below). The Medicare Annual Wellness Visit also can facilitate the performance of many of these assessments in a separate visit that does not need to also address the patient's ongoing medical problems.

USEFUL WEBSITES

Agency for Healthcare Research and Quality. Search for recommendations. http://epss.ahrq.gov/ePSS/search.jsp. Accessed March 4, 2020.

American College of Physicians. Annual wellness visit. https://www.acponline.org/practice-resources/business-resources/payment/medicare-payment-and-regulations-resources/how-to-bill-medicares-annual-wellness-visit-awv. Accessed March 4, 2020.

Centers for Disease Control and Prevention. http://www.cdc.gov/mmwr/PDF/wk/mm753-Immunization.pdf

Centers for Medicare and Medicaid Services. Annual wellness visit. https://www.cms.gov/Outreach-and-Education/Medicare-Learning-Network-MLN/MLNProducts/MLN-Publications-Items/CMS1246474.html. Accessed March 4, 2020.

Social Security Administration. Life expectancy tables. http://www.ssa.gov/OACT/STATS/table4c6.html. Accessed March 4, 2020.

UCLA GeroNet. Healthcare office forms. http://geronet.ucla.edu/centers/acove/office_forms.htm https://www.uclahealth.org/geriatrics/workfiles/education/clinical-skills/handouts/PVQ.pdf

US Preventive Services Task Force. Home page. http://www.uspreventiveservicestaskforce.org/. Accessed March 4, 2020.

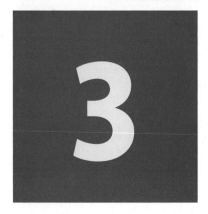

The Interprofessional Team

Pei Chen, MD

Crystal Burkhardt, PharmD, MBA, BCPS, BCGP

Josette A. Rivera, MD

INTRODUCTION

Nationally and worldwide, interprofessional teamwork is increasingly recognized as a means to address the challenges of the current health care system. Patients with complex problems and diverse needs require the expertise and collaboration of different health professionals. In the United States, a series of landmark Institute of Medicine reports recommended interprofessional collaboration and training of all health care professionals in teamwork as a key mechanism to increase health care safety and quality. Additional factors driving the need for effective teamwork include patient expectations; a primary care workforce shortage; a renewed focus on creating health care systems that demonstrate efficiency, lower cost, and improved outcomes; and national policy changes that incentivize the creation of interprofessional collaborative models. For example, the passage of the Patient Protection and Affordable Care Act (ACA) has led to the development of accountable care organizations with a focus on improving population health through interprofessional teamwork.

Older adults, with their increased prevalence of multiple chronic conditions, functional decline, geriatric syndromes, and terminal illness, are high utilizers of the health care system and its teams. The American Geriatrics Society has developed two position statements that underscore the benefits of interprofessional team care for older adults, and endorses interprofessional team training for all professions. This chapter defines the multiple types of interprofessional work in health care, describes practice-based interprofessional geriatrics innovations in the United States, reviews the evidence for interprofessional collaboration in the care of older adults, provides resources for building interprofessional skills and teams, and discusses barriers and future steps to improve interprofessional teamwork in geriatrics.

Mion L, Odegard PS, Resnick B, et al. Interdisciplinary care for older adults with complex needs: American Geriatrics Society position statement. *J Am Geriatr Soc.* 2009;57(10):1917.

Partnership for Health in Aging Workgroup on Interdisciplinary Team Training. Position Statement on interdisciplinary team training in geriatrics: an essential component of quality healthcare for older adults. *J Am Geriatr Soc.* 2014;62(5):961-965.

KEY DEFINITIONS AND CONCEPTS

The teamwork literature consists of a wide array of terms, often used interchangeably, to describe this phenomenon, including interdisciplinary, multidisciplinary, and interprofessional. In addition to this terminology uncertainty, different authors describing "teams" and "teamwork" often employ very different conceptualizations related to team composition, function, and outcome. A first distinction to clarify is discipline versus profession. "Discipline" refers to various fields of study, such as economics, anthropology, and medicine, whereas a "profession" typically refers to fields with licensing and/or regulatory requirements. Although the terms *interdisciplinary* and *multidisciplinary* have been prevalent for at least the past 40 years in US health care, including in geriatrics, scholars increasingly contend that applying these terms in a health care setting is conceptually incorrect, as the notion of "interprofessional" collaboration more accurately describes the various health care professionals who work together to deliver services. A second distinction to clarify is interprofessional versus intraprofessional. Interprofessional collaboration refers to different types of health care professionals (eg, dentistry, nursing, medicine, pharmacy) working together, whereas intraprofessional collaboration refers to persons representing different specialties within the *same* profession working together. Intraprofessional collaboration examples include surgeons and cardiologists working together, or gerontological nurse practitioners working with clinical nurse specialists in geriatrics. We focus on interprofessional work in this chapter in light of the prevalence and effectiveness of interprofessional teams in the care of older adults.

In addition to acknowledging the different professions involved, it is important to distinguish the types of interprofessional practice that exist in health care. Reeves and colleagues proposed a framework that differentiates four types of interprofessional practice (teamwork, collaboration, coordination, and networking) based on a number of factors that address a shared identity, roles, and level of interdependence and integration, among others. Interprofessional *teamwork* is a "tighter," more integrated type of work where members share a team identity, have clarity of roles, and work in an integrated and interdependent manner to provide care to patients. Examples of interprofessional teamwork include geriatrics teams, intensive care teams, and emergency department teams. This is a different arrangement to interprofessional *collaboration*, which is a "looser" type of work where membership is more fluid and shared membership less important. Examples of this type of work can occur in primary care and general medical settings where key team members might not be in the same physical location. Like collaboration, interprofessional *coordination* has less emphasis on a shared identity, but integration and interdependence are even less critical. *Networking* entails the most informal type of work. Examples include groups of professionals who share information of common interest but who are not necessarily providing joint patient care. When using these terms—teamwork, collaboration, coordination, and networking—independently without the interprofessional association, there is more focus on the activities rather than the individuals who are involved in the activities.

Finally, it is important to distinguish interprofessional education (IPE) from interprofessional practice. *IPE* is an activity that occurs when members (including students) of two or more health care professions engage in learning with, from, and about each other to improve interprofessional teamwork and the delivery of care. *Interprofessional practice* occurs when "multiple health care workers from different professional backgrounds provide comprehensive health services by working with patients, their families, caregivers, and communities to deliver the highest quality of care across settings." The National Center for Interprofessional Practice and Education in the United States is merging these two concepts into a working definition of *interprofessional practice and education* (the "new IPE"). The new IPE is a means to create a shared space between IPE and interprofessional practice that stresses the importance of education to improve health, create support systems, and test different models of practices.

Reeves S, Lewin S, Espin S, et al. *Interprofessional Teamwork for Health and Social Care.* London, United Kingdom: Blackwell-Wiley; 2010.

World Health Organization. *Framework for Action on Interprofessional Education and Collaborative Practice.* Geneva, Switzerland: WHO Press; 2010.

INTERPROFESSIONAL TEAM INNOVATIONS IN GERIATRICS

In the United States, the care of older adults has been a major impetus for innovations in interprofessional practice and education. Accordingly, there are many geriatric models of care where teamwork is fundamental (Table 3–1). These teams vary widely with respect to their goals, procedures, setting, number and type of professionals, and membership stability.

The Department of Veterans Affairs developed the earliest training initiatives, Interdisciplinary Team Training in Geriatrics, in the 1970s. This was followed by the creation of three programs administered by the Health Resources and Services Administration (HRSA) of the US Department of Health and Human Services. First, the Geriatric Education Centers (GECs), founded in the 1980s, supported collaboration between health professions schools and health care clinics, facilities, and systems to provide training in geriatrics and

Table 3–1. Examples of team care in geriatrics.

Disease specific	Dementia Diabetes Falls prevention Heart failure Post-stroke
Program specific	Annual wellness visits Geriatric assessment/consultative clinics Geriatric Resources for Assessment and Care of Elders (GRACE) Hospice Medical-legal partnership for seniors Palliative care Program of All-Inclusive Care for the Elderly (PACE) Transitional care
Site specific	Acute care for the elder (ACE) units Adult day health centers Emergency department Home care Long-term care nursing homes Short-term rehabilitation

team care to four or more professions. Second, the Geriatric Academic Career Awards (GACAs), which originated in the 1990s, support the career development of junior faculty to become academic geriatricians and to provide clinical geriatrics training to interprofessional teams. Third, in 2015, HRSA replaced the GECs with Geriatric Workforce Enhancement Programs (GWEPs) to promote the development of an interprofessional geriatric workforce through integration of geriatrics with primary care, promotion of patient and family engagement, and collaboration with community partners to address the gaps in older adult health care.

Beyond the support of the federal government, the John A. Hartford Foundation has significantly supported the development of team training and models of care for older adults. In 1997, the Hartford Geriatric Interdisciplinary Team Training (GITT) initiative funded eight institutions to develop innovative models of formal team training, resulting in a repository of teaching materials and a collectively produced curriculum and implementation guide described further in the section "Resources and Tools for Teamwork." In 2000, Hartford funded the Geriatric Interdisciplinary Teams in Practice initiative that supported the design and testing of models of interprofessional team care of older adults with chronic illnesses. Five models that transformed team care in everyday practice and demonstrated positive impact on patient outcomes and cost include: (1) the Care Transitions intervention, developed at the University of Colorado Health Sciences Center, which used a transition coach to work with patients and family caregivers on self-management skills to promote safer transitions from hospital to home; (2) the Care Management Plus model, developed by Intermountain Health Care and Oregon Health and Science University, which used a care manager and an electronic information technology system to improve communication among health care clinicians; (3) the Senior Health and Wellness Clinic model, developed by PeaceHealth Oregon Region, which provided comprehensive geriatric primary care with a focus on chronic care management; (4) the Virtual Integrated Practice model, developed at Rush University Medical Center, which improved working relationships and communication among interprofessional members by using e-mail, voicemail, and electronic medical record; and (5) the Senior Resource Team model, developed by the Group Health Cooperative Puget Sound, which embedded a geriatric consulting team in a primary care practice. Among these five models, the Care Transitions and the Care Management Plus models have demonstrated widespread dissemination.

Geriatrics has led other innovations in team-based models of care supported by Medicare and Medicaid funding. In the ambulatory care setting, the Program of All-Inclusive Care for the Elderly (PACE) is a capitated, joint Medicare-Medicaid program that provides comprehensive, team-based care for frail, nursing-home-eligible older adults living in the community. In the inpatient setting, the acute care for

elders (ACE) unit provides hospitalized older adults with an interprofessional team that aims to preserve function and to avoid unnecessary procedures and medications. As of 2019, there are 126 PACE programs in 31 states and an estimated 200 ACE units nationally. Both the PACE and ACE models have been shown to improve patient outcomes while reducing costs. Since 2013, the Centers for Medicare and Medicaid Services have recognized interprofessional teamwork and reimbursed the efforts of innovative interprofessional models of care, including annual wellness visits, transitional care management, chronic care management, dementia care, and advance care planning activities.

Coleman EA, Parry C, Chalmers S, Min SJ. The care transitions intervention: results of a randomized controlled trial. *Arch Intern Med*. 2006;166(17):1822-1828.

Fox MT, Persaud M, Maimets I, et al. Effectiveness of an acute geriatric unit care using acute care for elders components: a systematic review and meta-analysis. *J Am Geriatr Soc*. 2012: 60(12):2237-2245.

Hirth V, Baskins J, Dever-Bumba M. Program of all-inclusive care (PACE): past, present, and future. *J Am Med Dir Assoc*. 2009; 10(3):155-160.

Stock R, Mahoney ER, Reese D, Cesario L. Developing a senior healthcare practice using the chronic care model: effect on physical function and health-related quality of life. *J Am Geriatr Soc*. 2008; 56(7):1342-1348.

Wieland D, Kinosian B, Stallard E, Boland R. Does Medicaid pay more to a program of all-inclusive care for the elderly (PACE) than for fee-for-service long term care? *J Gerontol A Biol Sci Med Sci*. 2013;68(1):47-55.

EVIDENCE FOR INTERPROFESSIONAL TEAMS IN THE CARE OF OLDER ADULTS

Substantial research shows benefits of geriatric interprofessional team care for specific diseases and geriatric syndromes, across models of care, and in settings from acute care and skilled nursing facilities to rehabilitation and outpatient clinics. Team-based models of care, such as PACE and the Geriatric Resources for Assessment and Care of Elders (GRACE), have demonstrated improved quality of care and reduced utilization of services. Team care has reduced morbidity and mortality after a stroke and shown improvement in behavioral and psychological symptoms without a significant increase in medications among patients with Alzheimer disease. Team-based approaches reduce the prevalence of delirium and the incidence of falls and related injuries. Interprofessional teams also improve medication adherence and reduce adverse drug reactions.

Although there is promising evidence on interprofessional teamwork in specific areas of health care, overall results are mixed regarding the ability of interprofessional teams to reduce health services utilization and costs. Boult and colleagues offer possible explanations for the difficulty in demonstrating these reductions in older adults with multimorbidity, which include unavoidable exacerbations requiring acute care in patients with multiple chronic conditions and not knowing which patients benefit most from team care or what aspects of team care reduce utilization and costs. Moreover, quality team care may also increase utilization by high-risk patients by recognizing and addressing gaps in care that improve quality of life. Finally, clinical trial duration may be too short to capture the cost savings "downstream" that could offset the initial and operating costs of a team-based model.

Tsakitzidis and colleagues expand the outcomes of interprofessional teams that should be evaluated beyond collaboration and costs, to outcomes that are impactful at the patient level. Patient-level outcome indicators include pain, fall incidence, quality of life, independence for daily life activities, and depression and agitated behavior. When organizing and studying interprofessional collaboration and/or IPE, patient-level outcome indicators are important aspects that should be considered in addition to health services utilization and cost.

In addition to the emerging evidence on teamwork, there exists a deep and intuitive logic for why effective teamwork is necessary: patients frequently have conditions that have multiple causes and require multiple treatments from a range of health care professionals with different skills and expertise. As it is unusual for one profession to deliver a complete episode of care in isolation, good-quality care depends on professions working together in interprofessional teams. In general, when a team works "well," it does so because every member has a role. Every member not only knows and executes his or her own role with great skill and creativity, but also knows the responsibilities and activities of every other role on the team and understands the personal nuances and skills that each individual brings to his or her role. As has been shown in military training and the aviation industry, when everyone on the team understands each person's role, teamwork contributes to reducing waste, better coordination, enhanced safety, and high-quality outcomes.

Boult C, Reider L, Leff B, et al. The effect of guided care teams on the use of health services: results from a cluster-randomized controlled trial. *Arch Intern Med.* 2011;171(5):460-466.

Callahan CM, Boustani MA, Unverzagt FW, et al. Effectiveness of collaborative care for older adults with Alzheimer disease in primary care: a randomized controlled trial. *JAMA.* 2006;295(18):2148-2157.

Counsell SR, Callahan CM, Clark DO, et al. Geriatric care management for low-income seniors: a randomized controlled trial. *JAMA.* 2007;298(22):2623-2633.

Farrell TW, Luptak MK, Supiano KP, Pacala JT, Lisser R. State of the science: interprofessional approaches to aging, dementia, and mental health. *J Am Geriatr Soc.* 2018;66:S40-S47.

Tsakitzidis G, Timmermans O, Callewaert N, et al. Outcome indicators on interprofessional collaboration interventions for elderly. *Int J Integr Care.* 2016;16(2):5.

RESOURCES AND TOOLS FOR TEAMWORK

IPE and team training have received increasing recognition in recent years. In 2016, the Interprofessional Education Collaborative (IPEC), which consists of 15 national health professions education associations, updated the core competencies for interprofessional collaborative practice as a means of providing a framework to move IPE forward and achieving the Quadruple Aims of health care, which are improving the health of populations, enhancing experience of care for individuals, reducing cost of health care, and attaining joy at work. The competency domains identified were:

- Values/ethics for interprofessional practice
- Roles/responsibilities for collaborative practice
- Interprofessional communication practices
- Interprofessional teamwork and team-based practice

The competencies identify behaviors that reflect underlying attitudes, knowledge, and values essential for effective, patient-centered teamwork. The domains provide a guide for individual learning and practice improvement, for curriculum and program development, and for setting accreditation and licensing standards for schools and professionals alike.

Salas and colleagues detail principles for team training, which include using teamwork competencies to focus the training content to align with desired outcomes and local resources; concentrating on teamwork and excluding individual-level tasks; providing hands-on practice in as authentic an environment as possible; providing detailed, timely feedback by team skills experts; evaluating knowledge, behaviors, and patient-level outcomes; and sustaining teamwork through continued coaching, incentives, and performance evaluations.

Salas and colleagues also provide practical guidelines and tips for improving teamwork based on their framework of communication, coordination, and cooperation. An overarching theme is the creation of an environment that encourages open discussion and input from all members. This includes ensuring time for members to jointly reflect upon their team performance and to give "process feedback" that is descriptive and specific. Team members should also reflect upon their own and other members' behaviors, while both eliciting and providing constructive feedback along with ideas for improvement. Additionally, health care teams may improve their teamwork by focusing explicitly on creating a culture of inclusiveness and psychological safety, in which each individual feels valued and able to speak up without fear of judgment or punishment.

Two well-developed team training programs offer online practical guidelines and tools for teamwork. The Geriatric Interdisciplinary Team Training 2.0 (GITT 2.0) program is now part of an array of geriatrics educational materials offered through the ConsultGeri of the Hartford Institute for Geriatric Nursing. Unlike the first GITT, which was a paper-based curriculum with cases and videos, GITT 2.0 is a web-based curriculum that includes updated cases with videos and focuses on improving patient and caregiver-centered quality outcomes through interprofessional collaboration. Although designed for trainees, the content is relevant to practicing interprofessional members. A set of six complementary Interprofessional Education and Practice (IPEP) eBooks offer tools with guided interactive activities to teach the core domains of interprofessional competencies. The TeamSTEPPS program, developed by the Department of Defense, is not geriatrics specific but presents an evidence-based teamwork training system for health professionals. Like the GITT 2.0, it offers a curriculum and implementation guide accessible online, but the materials are more extensive and contain slide sets with speaker notes, handouts, videos, and assessment and evaluation tools. The training system provides detailed guidance on its three-step process that includes a local needs assessment, planning and training, and sustainment. Practical communication tools and strategies are a prominent part of the curriculum. TeamSTEPPS also offers webinars and in-person training sessions nationwide for master trainers.

The Health Professions Accreditor Collaborative (HPAC), founded in 2014, created a platform to share information on a board range of interprofessional topics, to formalize interactions among accreditors, and to problem solve emerging challenges in the health system. To meet the urgent needs for interprofessional collaboration necessary for quality and cost-effective care, the HPAC implemented a multiyear and multiphase process endorsed by 24 health care professional training programs to create a guide on the development, implementation, and evaluation of quality IPE.

A key resource for educators, clinicians, and administrators to bridge the gap between health professions education and health care delivery in the United States is the National Center for Interprofessional Practice and Education (The NEXUS), created by a public-private partnership. The NEXUS informs, connects, and engages educators and clinicians to advance the Quadruple Aims, and its website contains discussion boards and a digital library of diverse resources.

See Table 3–2 for a list of resources and tools discussed in this section.

Health Professions Accreditors Collaborative. *Guidance on Developing Quality Interprofessional Education for the Health Professions.* Chicago, IL: Health Professions Accreditors Collaborative; 2019.

Interprofessional Education Collaborative. *Core Competencies for Interprofessional Collaborative Practice: 2016 Update.* Washington, DC: Interprofessional Education Collaborative; 2016.

Table 3–2. Resources and tools for teamwork.

Geriatric Interdisciplinary Team Training 2.0 (GITT 2.0)	https://consultgeri.org/gitt-2.0-toolkit
Health Professions Accreditor Collaborative (HPAC)	https://healthprofessionsaccreditors.org/
Interprofessional Education and Practice (IPEP) eBooks	https://consultgeri.org/education-training/e-learning-resources/interprofessional-education-and-practice-ipep-ebooks
Interprofessional Education Collaborative (IPEC)	https://www.ipecollaborative.org/
National Center for Interprofessional Practice and Education (NEXUS)	https://nexusipe.org/
TeamSTEPPS	https://www.ahrq.gov/teamstepps/index.html

Salas E, Almeida SA, Salisbury M, et al. What are the critical success factors for team training in health care? *Jt Comm J Qual Patient Saf.* 2009;35(8):398-405.

Salas E, Wilson KA, Murphy CE, King H, Salisbury M. Communicating, coordinating, and cooperating when lives depend on it: tips for teamwork. *Jt Comm J Qual Patient Saf.* 2008;34(6):333-341.

The National Center for Interprofessional Practice and Education. https://nexusipe.org. Accessed April 11, 2019.

BARRIERS TO THE ADVANCEMENT OF TEAMWORK

While data support the benefits of interprofessional teamwork for patients and health professionals, most practicing professionals have received minimal or no relevant training, and efforts to increase interprofessional teamwork often meet attitudinal, educational, and fiscal barriers. One challenge relates to the medical profession's history of unchallenged authority and attitudes toward teams. Physician attitudes toward teamwork, in general, are particularly problematic. Reasons may include medical training that rewards autonomy and individual efforts, lack of perceived value added by teamwork, and perceived losses of power, time, and money. With a paucity of role models and strong cultural influences, it is not surprising that medical trainees have rated lower agreement on the benefits of teamwork compared with nursing, pharmacy, and social work students.

Additional barriers to improving interprofessional teamwork are systems and infrastructure based. First, despite the ubiquity of health care teams, widespread formal teamwork education of practicing clinicians has lagged in the United States. Consequently, because teams in practice do not use principles of teamwork, minimal ongoing team training occurs. Second, few incentives exist for implementing or improving IPE and practice as there are currently limited reimbursement opportunities for the implementation of innovative and collaborative educational programs or for team services provided by practicing health professionals. In addition, few medical and health professional schools or medical practices recognize teamwork skills for the purposes of individual advancement or promotion. Third, logistical barriers are a prevalent problem that often centers on finding time for teaching or participating in teamwork. At the preprofessional level, hindrances include conflicting academic calendars and locations of training sites, while tension in the practice setting centers on balancing release time for team training with staffing needs of hospitals and clinics for patient care. Finally, the current infrastructure does not support clinical workflow to facilitate communication and accountability among clinicians ascertaining and communicating patients' health priorities and concerns.

Boyd C, Smith CD, Masoudi FA, et al. Decision making for older adults with multiple chronic conditions: executive summary for the American Geriatrics Society guiding principles on the care for older adults with multimorbidity. *J Am Geriatr Soc.* 2019;65:665-674.

Leipzig, RM, Hyer K, Ek K, et al. Attitudes toward working on interdisciplinary health care teams: a comparison by discipline. *J Am Geriatr Soc.* 2002;50(6):1141-1148.

Young HM, Siegel EO, McCormick WC, Fulmer T, Harootyan LK, Dorr DA. Interdisciplinary collaboration in geriatrics: advancing health for older adults. *Nurs Outlook.* 2011;59(4):243-250.

FUTURE STEPS

As demonstrated by its historic and current state, interprofessional practice is essential to achieve the desired patient-centered outcomes of the aging population. Along with the development and dissemination of new interprofessional practice models, IPE and learning environments must be positioned to meet the challenges in developing future health care professionals. In order to transform the current standard of care, it is necessary for interprofessional practice and education to develop in tandem.

In the United States, the Centers for Medicare and Medicaid Services Innovation Center, established in 2010 as part of the ACA, tests models that improve care, lower costs, and better align payment systems to support patient-centered practices. The Innovation Center plays a critical role in implementing the Quality Payment Program, which Congress created as part of the Medicare Access and CHIP Reauthorization Act of 2015 (MACRA) to replace prior payment structures. In the Quality Payment Program, clinicians may earn incentive payments by participating to a sufficient extent in Advanced Alternative Payment Models (APMs). In Advanced APMs, clinicians accept some risk for their patients' quality and cost outcomes and must meet other specified criteria. Many of these models of care, such as Medicare Shared Savings Programs in Accountable Care Organizations (ACOs) and Comprehensive Primary Care Plus (CPC+) in Primary Care Transformation, developed through the Innovation Center, incorporate interprofessional care. These steps toward development, implementation, and testing of innovative interprofessional care models must continue in the future in order to truly transform the delivery of care to older adults.

Implementation and dissemination of innovative models of interprofessional practice and education will require continued culture evolution and investment of time and resources. Differences in professional identities and cultures must be reconciled, with the recognition that everyone, from early learners to seasoned professionals, harbors biases, stereotypes, and inadequate knowledge of other professions. Health system and academic leaders need to address the practical problems of differences in roles, priorities, service needs, structural barriers, schedules, and licensure and accreditation requirements among health professionals and students. Continued research will guide understanding of the most effective timing, teaching strategies, methods, settings, and assessment tools to develop team-ready professionals. Additionally, the impact of interprofessional practice and education on the Quadruple Aims, with a particular emphasis on patient-centered outcomes, must be demonstrated in order to ensure quality team-based health care is sustained. Professional and faculty development courses should train a cadre of health professionals who effectively teach and role model teamwork skills. Licensure, regulation, and accreditation are also powerful ways through which to promote interprofessional practice and education that advances patient-centered care of the older adult.

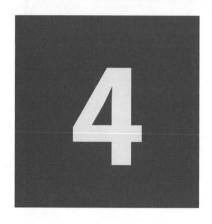

Goals of Care & Consideration of Prognosis

Eric Widera, MD

Alexander K. Smith, MD, MS, MPH

GENERAL PRINCIPLES OF GOALS OF CARE DISCUSSIONS

Goals of care discussions provide a broad framework for decision making, helping align patients' underlying values and hopes with the realistic and achievable options for care given the current medical circumstances. This is no easy task, however, as patients and their family members may simultaneously express multiple goals for their health care, which may include maintenance of independence, prevention of illness, prolongation of life, relief of suffering, and maximization of time with family and friends. The relative importance placed on each goal may change over time as new information is shared with the patient or family, such as a new diagnosis or a worsening prognosis. These goals should serve as a guide from which patients and their physicians can develop specific plans for treatment when dealing with acute or chronic illnesses.

A PRACTICAL GUIDE TO GOALS OF CARE DISCUSSIONS

Goals of care can provide a guide for various decisions, including immediate decisions regarding life-sustaining treatments and decisions regarding preferences for preventive therapies such as cancer screening, and for the completion of advance directives. There is no one right way of having these discussions; however, the following outlines seven practical steps for having a discussion (see Table 4–1 for words to use, and Table 4–2 for words to avoid).

1. *Prepare:* Clinicians should establish an appropriate setting, one that is quiet with enough space for all participants to sit down. The clinician should identify appropriate participants, including extended family, other consultants, or team members, such as social work or chaplaincy. A facilitator should be identified in advance if more than one clinician or team member will be present. Also, ensure

adequate time is set aside for the meeting and that interpreters are used if needed.

2. *Create structure:* At the start of the meeting, all participants should introduce themselves. The purpose of the meeting should be made explicit. Clinicians should also ask about patient and family preferences for information sharing and decision making.

3. *Explore understanding of medical situation and underlying values:* Effective decision making depends on both health care providers and patients having an understanding of the patient's illness and prognosis. Clinicians should determine what the patient and family members understand about the patient's illness and its expected natural course. Information should be given in small, easy-to-understand statements with frequent checks to assess for comprehension. This is also a time to explore what outcomes patients and families are hoping for and which ones they would want to avoid, as well as what is most important in their lives and what they would like most to accomplish. These discussions can elicit a variety of emotional reactions including anger, disbelief, relief, and shock. Always acknowledge patient emotions first, before you give more factual information.

4. *Define overarching goals:* Based on what was learned about the patient's and family's hopes and expectations, providers can explore or suggest overarching goals. This should also be a time to address hopes and goals that may be unreasonable or unrealistic given the current health state or future prognosis.

5. *Assist in making a decision based on the patient's beliefs and values:* Discuss how goals can be achieved by discussing treatment options consistent with the patient's goals of care. This should include the potential benefits, harms, and burdens associated with various therapies, and the likelihood that the proposed intervention will accomplish the goals that have been specified.

Table 4–1. Words that may be useful when discussing goals.

1	Prepare	"At our next visit, I would like to talk about your health and the ways we can go forward with your care. Is there someone who you think should be at this meeting?"
2	Create structure	"Some patients feel it is important to know all the details of their illness, prognosis, and treatment options; others don't and want others to make decisions for them. How do you feel?"
3	Explore understanding and values	"Tell me how things are going for you?" "What do you understand about your current health?" "Given what we know about your health and prognosis, what things are most important to you? What are your hopes? Fears?" "When you think about getting very sick, what worries you the most?"
4	Define overarching goals	"It seems to me that what is most important to you is that you remain comfortable and that we get you back to your home. Is that correct?"
5	Assist in making a decision	"Considering how important being pain free and remaining at home appears to be for you, I recommend that we...."
6	Plan for follow-up	"It sounds like you could use some more time to think about these issues and discuss them with your family. Can we talk more tomorrow afternoon?" "I am sure you will have lots of questions later. Here is how to reach me."
7	Document goals and decisions	"Considering your wishes, I think it would be important to document this in orders by using a physician order for life-sustaining treatment (POLST) form, which can help ensure that your preferences for end-of-life care are followed."

6. *Plan for follow-up:* Goals and preferences may change over time, so these discussions should be considered part of an ongoing process.

7. *Document goals and decisions:* This may include documentation in the chart, in advance directives, or if preferences for potentially life-prolonging therapies are clear, in state-authorized portable orders such as the physician orders for life-sustaining treatments (POLST). See Chapter 21, "Ethics & Informed Decision Making," for more information on advance care planning.

IMPORTANCE OF SURROGATE DECISION MAKERS

One out of four older adults may require surrogates to make or help make medical treatment decisions before death. Physicians have a responsibility to help these surrogates make decisions consistent with the preferences, values, and goals for care of the patient. However, because of the often uncertain and unanticipated nature of medical illness, even if specific preferences have been laid out in advance directives, these directives may not address the decision at hand and may still require interpretation by the surrogate. Complicating matters further, older adults may desire that future decisions be made based on the wishes and interests of family members, not just their own stated preferences for care.

Involving surrogates in advance care planning discussions with the patient prior to incapacitation may help increase the chances that the wishes of a patient are known to the surrogate and may help lessen the burden of surrogate decision making. These discussions should focus on preparing surrogates for future decisions, including appointing a health care proxy to serve as a surrogate in the event of incapacity, clarifying and articulating a patient's values and preferences, and addressing how much leeway surrogates have in decision making.

Table 4–2. Words to avoid when discussing goals.

Words to Avoid	Rationale
"There is nothing more we can do"	There is always something more that can be done, including symptomatic relief and provision of psychosocial support to patients and family members.
"We plan to withdraw care"	Care is never withdrawn. We always continue to care.
"Heroic measures"	Too vague of a term. Who would not want to be a hero?
"Your diagnosis is terminal"	Sounds cold (like the terminator), as if the patient is cut off from all options.
"Would you like us to do everything possible?"	"Everything possible" is too vague, and "everything possible" may include contradictory treatments. Hospice care and intensive care unit care may both be possible, for example.

PROGNOSTICATION

Prognostication can be divided into two parts. The first is the estimation of the patient's prognosis by the clinician. The second is communicating the prognosis to the patient and/or family. Studies have shown that older adults often care about their prognosis for remaining independent and cognitively intact as much as or more than their prognosis for survival. However, life and death predictions are often implied when individuals ask about "prognosis." Clinicians should ask patients to clarify the outcome they are concerned about.

▶ Why Prognosis in Older Adults Is Important

Estimating and communicating prognosis are both key components in clinical decision making. Prognostication provides patients and families with information to determine realistic, achievable goals of care. It targets interventions to those likely to live long enough to realize the beneficial outcomes. It establishes patients' eligibility for care programs such as hospice or advance illness management programs. It also impacts decisions outside of the health care setting, including how individuals decide to spend time and their money.

A key part of decision making based on goals of care is the need for explicit consideration of the likely outcomes of possible medical interventions. Simply asking a patient's preferences for an intervention such as cardiopulmonary resuscitation (CPR) is rather meaningless unless there is consideration of likelihood that the intervention will produce a desirable outcome consistent with the individual's goals. Furthermore, if outcomes are not explicitly discussed, patients may hold on to erroneous ideas about the likelihood of particular outcomes. However, if misconceptions are corrected and outcomes are clearly discussed, patients may change their preferences for certain interventions to those more consistent with the underlying values. For example, patients are more likely to express a preference against CPR if they are informed of the likelihood of survival after an arrest.

There are three important concepts to remember when considering prognosis in the older adults. The first is that estimating prognosis in older adults is made more complicated in that they are more likely to have more than one chronic progressive illness that impacts life expectancy. In these individuals, it would be inadequate to focus on only one problem when estimating prognosis, as it would not take into account the interaction of their medical problems. The second is that most prognostic tools in younger patients are based on specific diseases; in the oldest old, however, functional limitations are greater predictors of mortality than chronic conditions. Most disease-specific prognostic tools do not adequately account for functional

status. The third is that clinical decision making must take into account the likelihood that a patient will live long enough to survive to benefit from a proposed intervention. For example, preventative therapies, such as cancer screening, blood pressure management, and glycemic control, have all been shown to be effective in healthier, highly functional cohorts of older adults. Because the benefits of these treatments all require many years to accrue, frail older adults may not realize the benefit in the time they have left to live. They are, however, exposed to the risks and harms of the intervention, which often occur much earlier than the delayed benefits.

▶ Estimating Prognosis

The most common type of prognostication is simply using clinician judgment and experience. Prognostication based on clinician judgment is correlated with actual survival; however, it is subject to various shortcomings that limit prognostic accuracy. Clinicians are more likely to be optimistic and tend to overestimate patient survival by a factor of between three and five. Clinical predictions also tend to be more accurate for short-term prognosis than long-term prognosis. The length of doctor-patient relationships also appears to increase the physician's odds of making an erroneous prognostic prediction. Accuracy of clinician predictions may be improved by integrating clinical predictions with some other form of estimating prognosis such as life tables or prognostic indices.

Life tables estimate remaining life by comparing to national averages for individuals of similar age, sex, and race (see Chapter 20, "Prevention & Health Promotion," for an example of a life table). These estimates give information on median life expectancy, although the heterogeneity in health states and prognosis among older adults of the same age significantly decreases its value. Using clinical characteristics such as comorbidities and functional status to estimate whether a patient will live shorter or longer than the median life expectancy may help individualize prognostic estimates in the clinical setting.

Prognostic indices are a useful adjunctive in prognostication. Clinicians should select indices that predict mortality over a time frame equal to that time to benefit for the intervention. Clinicians should also select indices that have been tested in settings that resemble the patient's clinical situation, that have reasonable accuracy in predicting risk, and that use readily available data as their variables. A helpful repository of published geriatric prognostic indices can be found at www.ePrognosis.org. Prognostic indices are intended to supplement rather than replace the clinical judgment of clinicians based on their assessment of the patient's condition. When using any of these methods to estimate prognosis, it is important to know that it is not a one-time event. Rather, it is a process that involves periodic reassessment.

Non–Disease-Specific Prognosis

Many older adults do not die from a single disease; instead, they die from the interacting effects of multiple chronic conditions, functional impairment, and cognitive decline. Several non–disease-specific prognostic indices have been created in recognition of this fact. These indices were the subject of a systematic review. Here we list some of the highest-quality indices, commenting on their practical application in clinical settings.

- *Schonberg 5- and 9-year index for community-dwelling older adults:* This index was developed from a nationally representative survey of older adults. Included risk measures are general aspects of clinical care that most geriatric providers would have access to, including history of diabetes, cancer, independence in instrumental activities of daily living (IADLs), and mobility. The only exception is self-rated health. The 9-year time frame may be particularly useful for making long-term screening decisions.

- *Lee 4- and 10-year index for community-dwelling older adults:* Similar to the Schonberg index, this index was also developed from a national representative survey of older adults. Included risk measures are clinically accessible. Of note, the Lee and Schonberg indices have been combined into a single index on ePrognosis.org to help clinicians quickly get multiple prognostic estimates.

- *Walter 1-year index for hospitalized older adults:* This index was developed from the Acute Care for Elders data set from two hospitals in Cleveland, Ohio. All risk measures would be easy to locate in the patient's medical record, including admission creatinine and albumin and activities of daily living (ADL) disability at the time of discharge. For decisions about hospice eligibility at hospital discharge, the risk of death at 6 months crosses the 50% threshold in the highest-risk group.

- *Porock 6-month index for nursing home residents:* All risk measures are derived from the minimum data set and should be readily accessible to the clinician.

PROGNOSIS RELATED TO SPECIFIC DISEASES

Advanced Dementia

The long clinical course of advanced dementia makes estimating an accurate short-term prognosis difficult. Individuals with advanced disease may survive for long periods of time with severe functional and cognitive impairments. They are also at risk of sudden, life-threatening complications of advanced dementia, such as pneumonia and urinary tract infections. These complications can serve as a marker of a very poor short-term survival. In one prospective study of patients with advanced dementia residing in a nursing home, the 6-month mortality rates after the development of pneumonia, a febrile episode, or eating problems were 47%, 45%, and 39%, respectively. Short-term survival rates are similar for individuals with advanced dementia who are admitted to the hospital with either pneumonia or a hip fracture, with 6-month mortality rates exceeding 50%.

Several validated indices have been developed to predict survival in advanced dementia; however, their ability to predict the risk of death within 6 months is poor. An example of a mortality index that can be used in nursing home residents with advanced dementia is the Advanced Dementia Prognostic Tool (ADEPT), also found on ePrognosis.org. The ADEPT can help identify nursing home residents with advanced dementia who are at high risk of death within 6 months, although only marginally better than current hospice eligibility guidelines.

Congestive Heart Failure

The majority of deaths from advanced heart failure are preceded by a period of worsening symptoms, functional decline, and repeated hospitalizations as a result of progressive pump failure. Despite significant advances in the treatment of heart failure, the prognosis in patients who have been hospitalized for heart failure remains poor, with a 1-year mortality rate ranging from 20% to 47% after discharge. The prognosis only worsens for those with multiple hospitalizations. In one prospective study, the median survival times after the first, second, third, and fourth hospitalization were 2.4, 1.4, 1.0, and 0.6 years, respectively. Advanced age also worsens prognosis as the median survival decreases to 1 year for 85-year-olds after one hospitalization and to approximately 6 months after two hospitalizations.

Other indicators of a poor prognosis in heart failure include patient demographic factors, heart failure severity, comorbid diseases, physical examination findings, and laboratory values. Heart failure–specific prognostic indices often combine many of these factors to help identify patients who have a high short-term mortality. The Seattle Heart Failure Model is a well-validated index composed of 14 continuous and 10 categorical variables that provides accurate estimates on 1-, 2-, and 5-year mortality for community-dwelling heart failure patients, as well as mean life expectancy both before and after intervention. An online calculator is available at http://depts.washington.edu/shfm/. For hospitalized patients, providers can use the EFFECT Heart Failure Mortality Prediction tool, which can be found at http://www.ccort.ca/Research/CHFRiskModel.html.

Chronic Obstructive Pulmonary Disease

Severity of disease, comorbidities, and, to a lesser degree, acute exacerbations influence prognosis in chronic obstructive pulmonary disease (COPD). The most widely studied

Table 4–3. BODE index.

Variable	Points on BODE Index			
	0	1	2	3
FEV$_1$ (% predicted)	≥65	50–64	36–49	≤35
6-minute walk test (meters)	≥350	250–349	150–249	≤149
MMRC dyspnea scale	0–1	2	3	4
Body mass index	>21		≤21	
Higher BODE scores correlate with an increasing risk of death				
BODE Index Score	**Approximate 4-Year Survival**			
0–2	80%			
3–4	67%			
4–6	57%			
7–10	18%			

FEV$_1$, forced expiratory volume in 1 second; MMRC, Modified Medical Research Council.

Data from Celli BR, Cote CG, Marin JM, et al. The body-mass index, airflow obstruction, dyspnea, and exercise capacity index in chronic obstructive pulmonary disease, *N Engl J Med* 2004 Mar 4;350(10):1005-1012.

mortality index in COPD is the BODE index (Table 4–3). It includes four variables known to influence mortality in COPD: weight (body mass index [BMI]), airway obstruction (forced expiratory volume at 1 second [FEV$_1$]), dyspnea (Medical Research Council dyspnea score), and exercise capacity (6-minute walk distance). The BODE index has been shown to be more accurate than mortality prediction based solely on FEV$_1$. However, the BODE index is not useful in predicting short-term life expectancy (in weeks to months).

▶ Cancer

Prognosis for earlier stage cancer is primarily based on tumor type, disease burden, and aggressiveness suggested by clinical, imaging, laboratory, pathologic, and molecular characteristics. Tumor-specific factors tend to lose prognostic significance for patients with very advanced cancer. For these advanced cancers, patient-related factors, such as performance status and clinical symptoms, have increasing significance in regard to short-term mortality. Performance status has consistently been found to be a strong predictor of survival in cancer patients. Several different measures of performance status have been developed, including the Eastern Cooperative Oncology Group (ECOG) performance status and the Karnofsky performance status (KPS); however, these are crude measures of function compared to a geriatric assessment that includes evaluation of ADLs and IADLs. High-performance status score does not necessarily predict

long survival, although low or decreasing performance status has been shown to be reliable in predicting a poor short-term prognosis. Symptoms that are associated with a poor short-term prognosis in advanced cancer include dyspnea, dysphagia, weight loss, xerostomia, anorexia, and cognitive impairment. The Palliative Prognostic Index (PPI) is an example of a tool that predicts the short-term survival of advanced cancer patients in the palliative care setting by combining functional status with presence of symptoms of edema, delirium, dyspnea at rest, and oral intake. Nomograms can be used to predict outcomes for a variety of different common cancers. A helpful repository of cancer nomograms can be found at https://www.mskcc.org/nomograms.

COMMUNICATING PROGNOSIS TO PATIENT OR SURROGATE

Communicating bad news, such as a poor prognosis, to a patient or a patient's family is one of the most difficult tasks in medicine. Most physicians are not trained in how to communicate about prognosis, most believe their training in prognostication is deficient, and the prognosis clinicians communicate to family tends to be overly optimistic. Yet, the majority of patients and families prefer to discuss prognosis with physicians, even in the face of uncertainty. The consequences of failing to communicate prognosis with patients and their surrogates are great. For instance, patients are more likely to receive aggressive end-of-life care and less likely to receive symptom-directed care when they have a poor understanding of their prognosis.

The SPIKES mnemonic is one way to help remember key steps in delivering bad news such as a poor prognosis (Table 4–4), similar to having a framework for goals of care discussions, as discussed earlier. Technical language should be avoided. For example, most individuals do not understand the term *median survival* when used by their physicians. Similarly, vague language such as "good" or "poor" chance of survival may also lead to misinterpretations. Combining

Table 4–4. The SPIKES mnemonic for delivering bad news.

S	Setting up the interview
P	Patient's Perception (assessing what they understand of their illness and prognosis)
I	Obtain the patient's Invitation (ask about the readiness to discuss prognostic information)
K	Give Knowledge and information (give prognosis in the context of the patient's illness)
E	Address the patient's Emotions with empathic response
S	Strategy and Summary (establish and summarize a clear care plan)

both qualitative and numeric language may improve comprehension of prognostic statements.

Exploring patient and surrogate understanding and personal beliefs about prognosis is imperative in these discussions. Few surrogates report basing their view of their loved one's prognosis solely on the physician's prognostic estimate. Rather, most attempt to balance the physician's judgment of prognosis with other factors, including (1) their own knowledge of the patient's intrinsic qualities and will to live; (2) their observations of the patient; (3) their belief in the power of their support and presence; and (4) optimism, intuition, and faith. Furthermore, even in the face of poor prognostic information, patients and surrogates remain optimistic and overestimate survival.

SUMMARY

Accurate prognostication allows clinicians to provide patients and families with realistic options for care given current medical circumstances and aids in determining which interventions offer little chance of benefit because of competing risks of morbidity and mortality. The use of structured approaches, such as SPIKES, is one way to ensure that this information is delivered in an effective and empathic manner. Prognostic information should be used along with consideration of other health priorities, such as maintaining independence, as part of shared decision making with older adults and their family members.

Abadir PM, Finucane TE, McNabney MK. When doctors and daughters disagree: twenty-two days and two blinks of an eye. *J Am Geriatr Soc.* 2011;59(12):2337-2340.

Baile WF, Buckman R, Lenzi R, et al. SPIKES: a six-step protocol for delivering bad news: application to the patient with cancer. *Oncologist.* 2000;5(4):302-311.

DeForest A. Better words for better deaths. *N Engl J Med.* 2019;380(3):211-213.

Feudtner C. The breadth of hopes. *N Engl J Med.* 2009;361(24):2306-2307.

Glare P. A systematic review of physicians' survival predictions in terminally ill cancer patients. *BMJ.* 2003;327(7408):195-198.

Lee DS, Austin PC, Rouleau JL, Liu PP, Naimark D, Tu JV. Predicting mortality among patients hospitalized for heart failure: derivation and validation of a clinical model. *JAMA.* 2003;290(19):2581-2587.

Lee SJ, Go AS, Lindquist K, Bertenthal D, Covinsky KE. Chronic conditions and mortality among the oldest old. *Am J Public Health.* 2008;98(7):1209-1214.

Mack JW, Weeks JC, Wright AA, Block SD, Prigerson HG. End-of-life discussions, goal attainment, and distress at the end of life: predictors and outcomes of receipt of care consistent with preferences. *J Clin Oncol.* 2010;28(7):1203-1208.

Mitchell SL, Miller SC, Teno JM, Kiely DK, Davis RB, Shaffer ML. Prediction of 6-month survival of nursing home residents with advanced dementia using ADEPT vs hospice eligibility guidelines. *JAMA.* 2010;304(17):1929-1935.

Setoguchi S, Stevenson LW, Schneeweiss S. Repeated hospitalizations predict mortality in the community population with heart failure. *Am Heart J.* 2007;154(2):260-266.

Silveira MJ, Kim SY LK. Advance directives and surrogate decision making before death. *N Engl J Med.* 2010;362(13):1211-1218.

Yourman LC, Lee SJ, Schonberg MA, Widera EW, Smith AK. Prognostic indices for older adults: a systematic review. *JAMA.* 2012;307(2):182-192.

USEFUL WEBSITES

EFFECT Heart Failure Mortality Prediction tool. http://www.ccort.ca/Research/CHFRiskModel.html. Accessed March 5, 2020.

ePrognosis. www.eprognosis.org (a repository of geriatric prognostic indices). Accessed March 5, 2020.

Palliative Care Fast Facts and Concepts. https://www.mypcnow.org/fast-facts/ (accessible and clinically relevant monographs on palliative care topics). Accessed March 5, 2020.

Seattle Heart Failure Model. http://depts.washington.edu/shfm/. Accessed March 5, 2020.

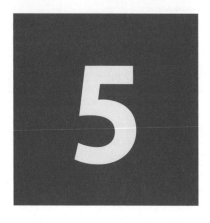

Functional Assessment & Functional Decline

Marlon J. R. Aliberti, MD, PhD

Kenneth E. Covinsky, MD, MPH

THE DISABLEMENT PROCESS

Older persons consistently indicate that maintaining independence is their top priority. The capacity to complete a series of day-to-day actions and tasks with as little difficulty as possible, irrespective of having chronic illnesses, determines good health and quality of life and is an important element of successful aging. However, for almost everyone, aging brings functional challenges that can compromise independence. Chronic and acute conditions, which are increasingly common as people age, are the trigger points for the disablement process. These conditions cause the development of impairments in specific body systems, which then result in functional limitations, eventually culminating in disability (Figure 5–1). Disability is defined as difficulty or need for help doing activities in any domain of life (from personal care to hobbies) due to a health or physical problem. For example, diabetes (chronic condition) leads to peripheral neuropathy (impairment), which then leads to poor balance and mobility (functional limitation), which finally leads to an inability to bathe in the tub/shower (disability).

For chronic diseases such as diabetes and hypertension, the linkage to disability is indirect and often distant, spanning years to decades. For other chronic diseases, such as knee osteoarthritis and dementia, the linkage is more direct and less distant, spanning months to years. For acute diseases and injuries, such as infections and fall-related injuries, the linkage is often direct and happens suddenly.

This process leading to disability is always influenced by an individual's intrinsic factors (socioeconomic status, lifestyle, behavioral and psychological aspects) and environmental factors (access to medical care, medications and other therapeutic regimens, devices and structural modifications for accessibility). Although some risk factors are nonmodifiable, such as advanced age and female gender, most of them are potentially modifiable such as current smoking, excessive alcohol consumption, sedentary lifestyle, limited access to health care and social services, polypharmacy and the use

of potentially inappropriate medications (eg, anticholinergic drugs and benzodiazepines), and challenges in home structure (eg, broken flooring and stairs without handrails).

Disability should not be considered a personal characteristic but instead a gap between personal capability and environmental demand. It is important to distinguish between intrinsic disability and actual disability. With intrinsic disability, one might be disabled without environmental modifications or adaptive equipment, but providing these modifications and assistance restores independence. With actual disability, one is disabled even with these modifications and assistance. This distinction notes the importance of detecting modifiable factors, especially those external to the individual, that influence the capacity of a person to keep their function. For example, persons with diabetes and peripheral neuropathy who have difficulty bathing could maintain their independence for a longer time if provided adequate access to health care assistance and if they receive physical rehabilitation and simple home modifications (eg, grab bars in the bathroom).

EPIDEMIOLOGY OF FUNCTIONAL DISABILITY

Among older people, disability in activities of daily living (ADLs) is common and highly morbid. Nearly one in three older adults in the United States, representing almost 17 million people, has difficulty performing or receives help with one or more basic ADLs. ADLs include tasks, such as bathing, toileting, dressing, eating, getting in/out of chairs, and walking across the room, that are essential for personal care and independence (Box 5–1). The prevalence increases to 50% or more among those 85 and older, making the problem even more significant as the oldest old people represent the fastest-growing segment of the population. The rates are also substantial for difficulty or need for help doing instrumental activities of daily living (IADLs) and walking one-quarter of a mile (Figure 5–2). IADLs comprise essential

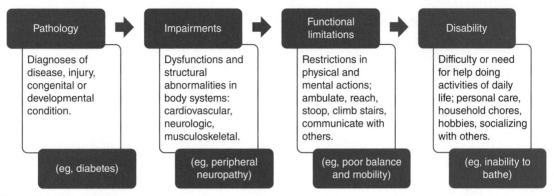

▲ **Figure 5–1.** The disablement process.

Box 5–1. Activities of Daily Living
Basic Activities of Daily Living (ADLs)

Activity	Independent	Needs Help	Example of Needing Help
Dressing			Needs help with any item of clothing
Bathing			Needs help getting in or out of the tub
Toileting			Needs help transferring or cleaning
Transferring			Needs help moving from bed to chair
Grooming			Needs help with daily hygiene
Eating			Needs help getting food to the mouth

Instrumental Activities of Daily Living (IADLs)

Activity	Independent	Needs Help	Example of Needing Help
Shopping			Needs to be accompanied
Housework			Does not perform any housekeeping
Transportation			Requires assistance for travel
Using the Telephone			Does not use the telephone
Managing Finances			Can't handle money day-to-day
Managing Medications			Requires medications are prepared

skills for an individual living independently in a community such as managing money, using the telephone, shopping, using transportation, preparing meals, and cleaning and maintaining the house (Box 5–1). Regardless of the type of activity assessed, the prevalence of disability is consistently higher among women than men (Figure 5–2).

Although disability in older adults is often thought to be progressive and permanent, more recent research has shown that many individuals who experience one episode of disability regain their independence, at least temporarily. Disability is a dynamic process, and episodes are often transient. Approximately one in three community-dwelling older adults who are independent in their ADLs will report at least one episode of needing help in any ADL during a 1-year follow-up. Among those who develop new ADL disability, 81% regain independence within 12 months of their initial disability episode. Even among those who experience 3 consecutive months of disability, 60% recover independence. While most older individuals experiencing new disability can be reassured that they will restore independence, those who recover from one episode are at high risk for recurrent disability.

Functional disability is often seen as a problem affecting people 65 years or older and especially the oldest old (≥85 years). However, it is also common in middle-aged adults. Nearly 15% of adults 55 to 64 years have difficulty performing at least one ADL, a group that includes people with longstanding impairments that are congenital or developed in young adulthood, as well as people with impairments that are newly acquired in middle age.

It is noteworthy that functional disability, even for brief episodes lasting 1 or 2 months, is strongly linked to multiple adverse health outcomes, such as depression, social isolation, hospitalization, poor quality of life, nursing home placement, further disability progression, and death. Compared to older adults with no ADL disability, those with ADL disability are five times more likely to be institutionalized and three times more likely to be deceased 2 years later. In addition, the yearly

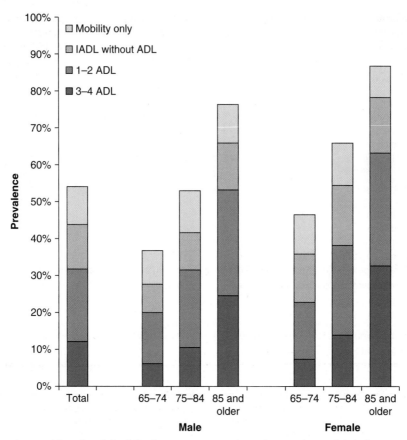

▲ **Figure 5–2.** Prevalence of functional disability by age group and gender. Activities of daily living (ADL) disability refers to difficulty or need for help doing one or more of the following tasks: bathing, dressing, eating, getting in/out of chairs, walking, or using the toilet. Instrumental activities of daily living (IADL) disability refers to difficulty or need for help doing one or more of the following tasks: using the telephone, light housework, heavy housework, meal preparation, shopping, or managing money. Mobility-related disability refers to difficulty or need for help walking one-quarter of a mile.

cost in the United States of caring for older people with disability in the community ranges from $5531 for the least disabled to >$46,480 for the most disabled who need a home health aide full time. An estimated $450 billion in unpaid care is provided by family or informal caregivers assisting older persons in performing everyday self-care tasks. An additional $350 billion each year is spent on nursing home care for individuals unable to function independently. As the population ages, the costs associated with ADL disability will continue to climb. Moreover, even among people between 50 and 64 years of age, difficulty performing ADLs has important clinical implications indicating increased risk for hospitalization, nursing home admission, and death. Thus, the focus of health care should shift from illnesses management to preventing disability and restoring function. The focus on function is the key to promoting successful aging and maintaining older adults' independence as long as possible.

ASSESSMENT OF FUNCTIONAL STATUS

Functional status can be assessed by a self-report or proxy report, by physical performance tests, or by direct observation of task performance. These different methods provide complementary information. A practical screen starts with a simple observation of the older adult's transfers and ambulation during the medical appointment. In addition, simple questions may be asked during the medical interview, such as (1) "Do you need help taking a bath or shower?"; (2) "Is getting dressed difficult for you?"; and (3) "Do you need help taking your medications?" Clinicians should also think of function in terms of important activities necessary for personal care (ADLs) and for living independently in the community (IADLs). In older adults with evidence of cognitive impairment, it is essential to confirm self-reported ability to perform ADLs with a caregiver or other appropriate informant. Proxy informants tend to overestimate disabilities, but their accuracy improves as their amount of contact with the patient increases.

Some validated tools for functional assessment can be particularly helpful for clinicians to detect disabilities in ADLs and IADLs and monitor function over time. These instruments are very useful in creating a common language about patient function for all health care providers involved in overall care planning and discharge planning. Table 5–1 presents some of the most commonly used functional assessment tools in older adults. In some settings, the assessment of function is part of standard protocols, such as the Minimum Data Set (MDS)–ADLs for residents in nursing homes, and the Outcome and Assessment Information Set (OASIS) Functional Assessment, composed of ADLs and IADLs, for patients assisted by home care agencies.

Simple physical performance measures have been shown to be helpful in different settings to identify older individuals at high risk of developing new disabilities. The ability to detect a latent disability is crucial since interventions may be more effective early in the disablement process. Among available measures, the physical frailty phenotype, the Short Physical Performance Battery (SPPB), and gait speed have been well-validated in different scenarios across different countries. The physical frailty phenotype comprises five components (0–5)—weight loss, exhaustion, weakness, slowness while walking, and low levels of activity—and stratifies older adults as robust (0), prefrail (1–2), and frail (3–5). Individuals classified as physically frail even if still nondisabled are vulnerable to multiple adverse outcomes (eg, ADL disability, hospital admission, institutionalization, death). The SPPB combines three tests of lower limb physical capability: (1) gait speed, (2) chair-stands test, and (3) balance test. This physical battery scores from 0 to 12, with higher scores indicating better function. It has been used as a practical tool to identify community-dwelling and hospitalized older adults at moderate (5–8 points) and high (0–4 points) risk for new disability and death. Gait speed alone, which can be easily measured with a stopwatch and 2-meter distance markings on the floor, is also highly correlated with subsequent disability

Table 5–1. Commonly used functional assessment tools.

Tool	Description	Reference
Barthel Index	This tool measures functional independence and needs for assistance in 10 items comprising basic activities of daily living (ADLs) and mobility (ie, feeding, bathing, grooming, dressing, bowel control, bladder control, toileting, chair transfer, ambulation, and stair climbing). Each performance item is rated by a self-report or proxy report. The instrument was introduced in 1965 with a score of 0–100 and modified in 1988 for a score from 0 (totally dependent) to 20 (fully independent), with each domain scored in 1-point increments. In the updated version, changes of >2 points in the total score reflect a clinically meaningful difference. This index signifies one of the first contributions to the functional status literature, and its effectiveness to detect disabilities and changes in function over time has been well documented in different settings, including hospital, home care, rehabilitation facilities, and community.	Barthel 1965 Collin 1988
Katz Index	This instrument assesses the level of independence in ADLs. The tool ranks adequacy of performance in the six functions of bathing, dressing, toileting, transferring, continence, and feeding. Patients are scored yes/no for independence in each of the six functions by a self-report or proxy report. This index has been widely used across all settings to assess the need for assistance for personal care and to measure the change in functioning over time.	Katz 1970
Lawton Index	This tool is a useful instrument to assess independent living skills (instrumental activities of daily living), which are considered more sophisticated than ADLs. There are eight items of function measured, including telephone use, shopping, meal preparation, housekeeping, laundry, transportation, medication management, and managing finances. Patients are scored according to their highest level of functioning (self or proxy) reported in each category. A summary score ranges from 0 (low function, dependent) to 8 (high function, independent). This instrument is widely used in community and hospital settings.	Lawton 1971
Functional Independence Measure (FIM)	The FIM is an 18-item scale of physical, psychological, and social function that is used to assess disability and changes in patients' status in response to medical and rehabilitation interventions. This instrument evaluates bowel and bladder control, transfers, locomotion, communication, social cognition, and ADLs (feeding, grooming, bathing, dressing, toileting). Each item is scored from 1 (total assistance) to 7 (complete independence). The total score of the instrument indicates the level of independence or burden of care and has been shown to track changes in the functional status of patients from the onset of rehab and medical care through discharge and follow-up.	Dodds 1993

and mortality. Clinical cut points for gait speed make it easily interpretable: faster than 1.0 m/s suggests intact mobility and between 0.6 and 1.0 m/s indicates high risk. Most older adults with a gait speed <0.6 m/s already have ADL difficulties.

RISK FACTORS FOR FUNCTIONAL DISABILITY

Many factors are associated with functional disability in addition to demographic characteristics such as advancing age and female gender. The socioeconomic disadvantage, linked to lower access to education, health care, and social support, is a significant risk factor for disability. Older adults with higher comorbidity, more depressive symptoms, cognitive deficits, obesity, malnutrition, and hearing and visual impairments are all more likely to experience functional decline and subsequent disability. Among comorbid conditions, arthritis, chronic cardiopulmonary disease, neurologic diseases, and chronic pain place patients at greater risk. Polypharmacy, especially in older persons using potentially inappropriate medications (eg, anticholinergic drugs and benzodiazepines), is associated with functional decline. Habits such as current smoking, excessive alcohol consumption, low physical activity, and minimal social interactions also are associated with increased risk of disability.

In particular, problems with mobility, such as walking a quarter mile or climbing stairs, and upper extremity limitations, such as difficulty lifting an object over one's head or grasping small objects, often precede difficulty in ADLs and put older adults at risk for further functional disability. Falls, even without injury, are associated with subsequent fear of falling, leading to activity restriction and disability. Early detection of mobility difficulty, upper extremity limitations, or declines in performance measures, such as gait speed and grip strength, allow physicians to identify still-independent individuals who are at high risk for incident ADL disability.

The development of disability is conceptualized on the knowledge that environmental factors such as characteristics of the home, social support, and availability of services, in concert with an older person's capabilities, influence the likelihood of developing disabilities. Environmental demands in the home (eg, steps, slippery floors, bathtubs, unreachable appliances) and in the community (eg, curb cuts, uneven walking surfaces, lack of wheelchair ramp to access buses) are risk factors strongly associated with disability.

Previous transient episodes of disability are also associated with a higher risk for new ADL dependence. Compared to older adults with no recent disability, older adults who had experienced a prior episode of ADL dependence are twice as likely to experience a subsequent episode of disability.

Acute diseases, particularly those requiring hospitalization, are the most common events that precipitate the onset of functional disability. More than one-third of older adults admitted to hospitals for an acute medical condition experience decline in their ability to perform ADLs during and after hospitalization. The immobility, poor nutrition and hydration, and delirium that frequently accompany hospital care put older adults at high risk for deconditioning and functional decline. Restricted activity, such as staying in bed or cutting back on usual activities, is the most important risk factor for the development of disability in acute care settings.

PREVENTION OF FUNCTIONAL DECLINE

▶ Community-Dwelling Older Adults

Increased physical activity is the most effective intervention to prevent functional disability or improve functional status in older adults. Progressive resistance training, aerobic exercise, and balance training have all been shown to prevent functional decline in older adults. The National Institute on Aging has produced a handbook for older adults that provides information about the health benefits of exercise, as well as information to help start and maintain a safe program of physical activity. Older adults without acute cardiac symptoms generally do not need additional testing before beginning an exercise program. Although standard group exercise can be beneficial in higher-functioning older adults, most successful interventions in frail older adults involved individualized exercise programs developed by a physical therapist or other trained professional.

Comprehensive geriatric assessment that includes a multidimensional evaluation of risk factors and follow-up visits has been shown to prevent functional decline. First, the management of cardiovascular risk factors may prevent functional decline among relatively healthy older adults. Treating diseases (eg, diabetes, hypertension, osteoarthritis, osteopenia) associated with disability can also have a positive impact on function. In addition, older people should receive routine screening for hearing and visual impairments and timely provision of adequate interventions (eg, hearing aids, comprehensive eye care). Cognition should be screened in those with memory complaints, and cognitive stimulation (eg, reading newspapers, training orientation using sticky notes and alarm devices, exercising memory with computer games, and enabling the individual to share their experiences and values) can be offered to help older people cope with cognitive challenges. Although there is an ongoing debate in the literature, no good evidence supports that nutritional supplements prevent functional decline in community-dwelling older adults. Finally, home safety assessment and modification interventions (eg, ramp, grab bars, antislip flooring) are effective in reducing environmental demands and thereby improving function. Environmental interventions also include those in the community, such as providing safe spaces for walking, ensuring easy access to local facilities and services, seeing people of a similar age exercising in the same neighborhood, and regular participation in exercise with family and friends.

▶ Hospitalized Older Adults

Many interventions have been developed to prevent functional disability in hospitalized older adults (discussed in Chapter 28, "Hospital Care"). Key features of successful interventions include assessment of risk factors; nursing protocols to improve self-care, continence, nutrition, mobility, sleep, skin care, and cognition; daily interprofessional team rounds; careful attention to hydration and nutritional status; minimization of catheterization, potentially inappropriate medications, and mobility restrictors (lines, tubes, and restraints); environmental enhancements (handrails, uncluttered hallways, large clocks and calendars, elevated toilet seats); and encouraging getting out of bed and walking. Acute care for the elderly units and geriatric evaluation and management programs, which incorporate many of these features, have reduced hospitalization-associated functional decline in some studies. The Hospital Elder Life Program, designed to prevent delirium, has also been effective at avoiding functional disability.

REHABILITATION: THE TREATMENT OF FUNCTIONAL DISABILITY

Like other geriatric syndromes, functional disability is usually multifactorial, and rehabilitative care must address multiple medical, psychological, and social factors. A comprehensive assessment must identify potential diseases, symptoms, and impairments, as well as the personal and environmental factors contributing to an individual's functional disability. The treatment plan is then tailored to the patient's specific needs. For example, a patient whose improvement in function is limited by symptomatic heart failure may benefit from more intensive medical management, which should also include cardiac rehabilitation physical therapy. However, a patient having difficulty bathing and using the toilet could benefit from home improvements such as prioritizing the shower instead of a bathtub, installing tailored bathroom safety equipment, and raising toilet seats.

Settings for rehabilitative care vary depending on the circumstances and the patient's needs. Older adults with functional difficulties in the outpatient setting can receive an office-based comprehensive geriatric evaluation and can be referred to home-based or outpatient physical and occupational therapy. Upon discharge, hospitalized older adults can receive rehabilitative services in an inpatient rehabilitation facility, in a skilled nursing facility, through home health agencies, or as outpatients. Regardless of the setting, the interprofessional nature and the key components of rehabilitation are similar.

Each member of the interprofessional team has an important role in rehabilitation. In addition to the treatment of uncontrolled acute or chronic medical conditions, medical and nursing assessment of the rehabilitation patient should include factors that may impede functional recovery, such as orthostatic hypotension, poor pain control, delirium, and depressive symptoms. A pharmacist can provide valuable assistance in review of the medication regimen to identify potentially inappropriate medications or medications contributing to delirium, fatigue, or mobility difficulty. Physical and occupational therapists evaluate and treat deficits in balance, strength, range of motion, and endurance. They also use modalities such as heat, cold, electrical stimulation, and ultrasound to treat pain and as adjuncts to therapeutic exercise. Therapists also determine the most appropriate assistive device for an individual and provide training in the proper use of these devices. Occupational therapists focus on functional tasks and can provide adaptive equipment and recommend environmental improvements (eg, installing grab bars, lowering household tools to reachable heights) to promote safety and independence. Nutritionists can assist in the assessment of nutritional status and provide dietary recommendations. Speech therapists also help ensure adequate nutrition by assessing the mechanics of eating; in addition, they can provide cognitive therapy for patients with cognitive deficits.

The interprofessional team must also include family members and other informal caregivers of care-dependent older people. Psychological support, intervention, and training should be offered for caregivers responsible for the care of older persons with disabilities, particularly but not exclusively when the need for care is complex and extensive or there is significant caregiver strain.

Chatterji S, Byles J, Cutler D, Seeman T, Verdes E. Health, functioning, and disability in older adults—present status and future implications. *Lancet.* 2015;385(9967):563-575.

Collin C, Wade DT, Davies S, Horne V. The Barthel ADL Index: a reliability study. *Int Disabil Stud.* 1988;10(2):61-63.

Dodds TA, Martin DP, Stolov WC, Deyo RA. A validation of the functional independence measurement and its performance among rehabilitation inpatients. *Arch Phys Med Rehabil.* 1993;74:531-536.

Gill TM. Disentangling the disabling process: insights from the precipitating events project. *Gerontologist.* 2014;54(4):533-549.

Katz S, Downs TD, Cash HR, Grotz RC. Progress in development of the index of ADL. *Gerontologist.* 1970;10(1):20-30.

Kogan AC, Wilber K, Mosqueda L. Person-centered care for older adults with chronic conditions and functional impairment: a systematic literature review. *J Am Geriatr Soc.* 2016;64(1):e1-e7.

Lawton MP. The functional assessment of elderly people. *J Am Geriatr Soc.* 1971;19(6):465-481.

Schulz R, Eden J, eds. *Families Caring for an Aging America.* Washington, DC: National Academies Press; 2016.

Szanton SL, Xue QL, Leff B, et al. Effect of a biobehavioral environmental approach on disability among low-income older adults: a randomized clinical trial. *JAMA Intern Med.* 2019;179(2):204-211.

Verbrugge LM, Jette AM. The disablement process. *Soc Sci Med.* 1994;38(1):1-14.

USEFUL WEBSITES

Go4Life. An exercise and physical activity campaign from the National Institute on Aging that offers exercises, motivational tips, and free resources to help older adults get ready, start exercising, and keep going. The Go4Life campaign includes an evidence-based exercise guide in both English and Spanish, an exercise video, and many other resources. http://go4life.nia.nih.gov/. Accessed March 5, 2020.

Hartford Institute for Geriatric Nursing. ConsultGeri. Assessment Tools: Try This. A series of articles describing assessment tools for use in older adults, many with videos demonstrating their use. https://consultgeri.org/tools/try-this-series. Accessed March 5, 2020.

The Hospital Elder Life Program (HELP). http://www.hospitalelderlifeprogram.org/public/public-main.php. Accessed March 5, 2020.

World Health Organization (WHO). WHO provides recommendations that consider different starting points and levels of capacity for physical activity to maintain health. https://www.who.int/dietphysicalactivity/factsheet_adults/en/. Accessed March 5, 2020.

World Health Organization (WHO). WHO Guidelines on Integrated Care for Older People (ICOPE): Ageing and life-course. https://www.who.int/ageing/publications/guidelines-icope/en/. Accessed March 5, 2020.

Falls & Mobility Impairment

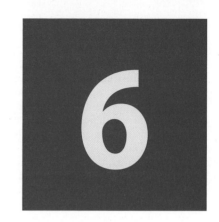

6

Deborah M. Kado, MD, MS

Daniel Slater, MD, FAAFP

Jean Y. Guan, MD

ESSENTIALS OF DIAGNOSIS

▶ Older adults who report more than one fall in the past year or a single fall with injury or gait and balance problems are at increased risk for future falls and injuries.

▶ Acute factors (infectious, toxic, metabolic, ischemic, or iatrogenic) may contribute to falls and mobility disorders. Falling can be a sign of medical illness and is commonly the presenting symptom in older adults.

▶ Medications, particularly psychotropic drugs, increase the risk for falls.

▶ Common modifiable fall risk factors important to consider include visual acuity, home environmental hazards, and footwear.

▶ General Principles

As people age, their risk of falling increases. Approximately 30% of people older than the age of 65 years and 50% of people older than age 80 years fall each year. Almost 60% of those with a history of falls in the previous year will suffer from a subsequent fall. Up to 50% of falls result in some type of injury, the most serious of which includes hip fractures, head trauma, and cervical spine fractures. Injuries that occur as a result of falls rank seventh as a cause of accident-related deaths in the United States. This is continuing to rise, with a 30% increase in fall death rates in older adults from 2007 to 2016. If this trend continues, we can anticipate several fall deaths every hour by 2030. Multiple risk factors account for the increased rate of falls observed in older persons, and as such, falls are considered a geriatric syndrome.

One major risk factor for falls includes problems with mobility. The risk for developing a mobility disorder increases with age. Mobility disorders range from subclinical to obvious, and within this range, fall risk is elevated. Because the risk for mobility disorders and falls is increased in older persons, clinicians should be particularly aware of how to prevent and treat both. This chapter discusses falls and associated mobility disorders with regard to the background, epidemiology, risk factors, clinical evaluation, prevention, treatment, and prognosis of older persons who may be at risk or who have already developed mobility problems and recurrent falls.

An international fall outcomes consensus group, the Prevention of Falls Network Europe (ProFaNE), defines a fall as "an unexpected event in which the participant comes to rest on the ground, floor, or lower level." Most falls do not result in serious physical injury, but those who fall are twice as likely to have a recurrent fall. In addition, many who experience an initial fall develop a fear of falling that itself can lead to an increased fall risk. Thus, it is particularly important to query about a history of falls when evaluating an older patient so that an appropriate evaluation and recommendations for prevention and treatment can be made before a significant injury occurs.

Mobility disorders refer to any deviation from normal walking. To walk normally, control of balance and posture both at rest and with movement is necessary. Thus, normal gait requires a complex integration of adequate strength, sensation, and coordination. For a normal healthy adult, walking is almost automatic. However, the control of gait and posture is both complex and multifactorial, and a defect at any level can result in mobility problems.

The incidence and health impact of falls vary depending on age, sex, and living status. As stated earlier, the incidence increases with age, with about a third of the population older than age 65 years and half of the population older than age 80 years reporting a fall in the previous year. Men and women tend to fall in equal proportions, but women are more likely to suffer from an injury. Similarly to those older than age 80 years, approximately 50% of residents in long-term care settings fall each year. Of the 10% to 20% of falls that result in serious injury, the most common complications include major lacerations, head trauma, and fractures.

Fall-related injuries are the major reason that clinicians need to be acutely aware of this widespread problem that affects older patients. Although the majority of falls do not result in serious physical injury, in those 65 years and older, falls account for 62% of nonfatal injuries leading to US emergency department visits, and approximately 5% lead to hospitalization. Patients who suffer from fall-related injuries are more likely to experience a decline in functional status and an increase in medical service utilization. In addition, they have an increased likelihood of long-term nursing home placement.

Special mention of hip fractures is deserved because they are among the most common and costly of fall-related injuries in older adults. More than 90% of all hip fractures occur as a result of a fall, often from falling sideways. Falls resulting in hip fractures are known to roughly double the 1-year mortality rate compared to matched older people without hip fractures. The 1-year mortality rate ranges from 12% to 37%, and approximately half of those who fall and fracture a hip are unable to regain the ability to live independently.

Mobility disorders affect approximately 15% of those 60 years and older and 80% of those 85 years and older. One simple measure of mobility is to assess walking speed; in one observational study of about 900 older men and women (average age: 75 years; range: 71–82 years), gait speed averaged 1.2 m/s and declined approximately 5% over 3 years. In general, slower gait speed is a risk factor for falls among older adults, but there is a U-shaped relationship in that those with faster walking speeds (≥ 1.3 m/s) also experience an increased rate of falls. Approximately 17% of falls in older persons can be attributed to balance, leg weakness, or gait problems. Of those with mobility problems, the causes are multifactorial in nature, with sensory deficits, myelopathy, and multiple infarcts being among the top three categories reported in the literature.

▷ Prevention

Fall prevention strategies appear to work in both institutional and community settings according to recent comprehensive systematic reviews published by the Cochrane Collaboration. Single and multifactorial intervention randomized controlled trials have been conducted, and while not uniformly in agreement, the preponderance of evidence demonstrates positive benefit with fall rate declines. However, the effect of these interventions on fall-related outcomes is unclear. Multifactorial interventions, usually including exercise (ie, gait training, balance and strengthening exercises) and targeted physical therapy, appear to have the greatest benefit. In addition, if these fall prevention strategies can be implemented in populations at risk for injurious falls, society on the whole will enjoy cost savings.

Thus, many organizations have taken on falls as a preventable health condition, and resources have been put toward implementing fall prevention programs. Since 2004, the National Council on Aging (NCOA) has been leading the Falls Free Initiative in the United States to address the growing public health problem of falls and fall-related injuries among older adults by collaborative leadership. Initially, representatives from 58 national organizations, professional associations, and federal agencies collaborated to develop a blueprint for reducing falls and fall-related injuries that included 36 strategies. Since its inception, NCOA has developed coalition workgroups, one of which was responsible for having the US Senate delegate the first day of fall as National Fall Prevention Awareness Day, initially established in 2009. That same year, the American Geriatrics Society (AGS) and British Geriatrics Society (BGS) expert panel on fall prevention provided updated recommendations that health care providers follow a step-by-step process of decision making and intervention to manage falls among older persons assessed to be at high fall risk (see algorithm, Figure 6–1).

For preventive strategies to be most cost-effective, they should target those who are at highest risk for developing the outcome. Multiple studies have shown that the strongest risk factors for falling include: (1) previous falls; (2) decreased muscle strength; (3) gait and balance impairment; and (4) specific medication use. With the exception of previous falls, muscle strength, gait and balance, and medication use are all potentially modifiable risk factors. Other potentially modifiable risk factors include visual impairment, depression, pain, and dizziness. Difficult to modify or nonmodifiable fall risk factors are age, female sex, activities of daily living disabilities, low body mass index, urinary incontinence, cognitive impairment, arthritis, and diabetes.

Although advanced age is a risk factor for developing mobility disorders in general, there are no particular risk factors to highlight as the root cause of disabling gait disorders. Gait disorders are most often unknown and/or multifactorial in etiology. As an example, weakness leading to mobility problems could stem from upper motor neurons (dysfunction of the cord and/or higher central motor pathways), lower motor neurons (problems with spinal motor neurons or peripheral nervous system), or primary myopathic problems. Some of the most disabling gait disorders result from serious neurologic disease and are beyond the scope of this chapter. However, because each of these diseases is also associated with an increased fall risk, they are listed for completeness: (1) extrapyramidal disorders (eg, Parkinson disease); (2) cerebellar ataxia (eg, cerebrovascular disease); (3) vestibular dysfunction (eg, acoustic neuroma); and (4) frontal lobe dysfunction (eg, normal pressure hydrocephalus).

Besides aging and/or deconditioning leading to muscle weakness and mobility problems, there are other nonneurologic medical problems that can lead to mobility disorders. Examples of these include visual loss, morbid obesity, orthopedic problems, rheumatologic disorders, pain, medications, and

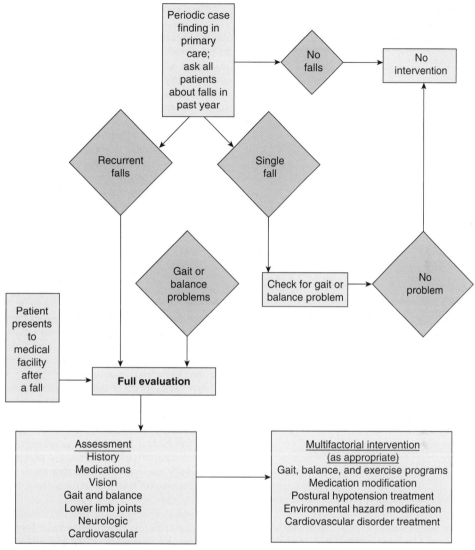

▲ **Figure 6–1.** Fall prevention algorithm. (Reproduced with permission from Guideline for the prevention of falls in older persons. American Geriatrics Society, British Geriatrics Society, and American Academy of Orthopaedic Surgeons Panel on Falls Prevention, *J Am Geriatr Soc* 2001 May;49(5):664-72.)

cardiorespiratory problems. Thus, in performing a clinical evaluation of an older patient, it is important to take into account these underlying systemic medical conditions that can adversely affect mobility and, hence, lead to an unwanted fall.

Clinical Findings

A. Symptoms & Signs

In the clinical evaluation of a geriatric patient, it is important to keep in mind identified independent risk factors for

falling (Table 6–1). In addition, falls in older adults typically are not due to a single cause, but occur when there is an additional stress, such as an acute illness, new medication, or an environmental hazard, that makes an older person unable to compensate as well as a younger person, and thus more likely to fall. The activity profile of the older person also will affect their risk for falling. Sedentary individuals may have multiple risk factors for falling but not be at danger because they modify their behavior to avoid the opportunity for falls. More active older adults may be less cautious and therefore be at increased risk for falling because they may not be able

Table 6–1. Independent risk factors for falling among community-dwelling older adults.

Risk Factor	Modifiable
Previous falls	No
Balance impairment	Yes
Decreased muscle strength	Yes
Visual impairment	Maybe
More than four medications or psychoactive medication use	Yes
Gait impairment or walking difficulty	Maybe
Depression	Maybe
Dizziness or orthostasis	Maybe
Functional limitations (ADL disabilities)	Unlikely
Age >80 years	No
Female	No
Low body mass index	Unlikely
Urinary incontinence	Maybe
Cognitive impairment	Unlikely
Arthritis	Maybe
Diabetes	Unlikely
Pain	Maybe

Risk factors listed in order of the strength of prediction, with the strongest at the top and weakest at the bottom.

ADL, activities of daily living.

Data from Tinetti ME, Kumar C: The patient who falls: "It's always a trade-off", *JAMA* 2010 Jan 20;303(3):258-266.

to compensate as well as a younger person for threats against postural stability.

To help prevent falls in older persons, multifactorial risk assessments have been advocated by the AGS/BGS and other organizations. These assessments begin with a basic falls history that inquires whether the patient experienced any fall in the past year. The ProFaNE consensus group recommends asking individuals about falling using the following wording, "Have you had any fall, including a slip or trip, in which you lost your balance and landed on the floor or ground or lower level?" If a fall is reported, important details with regard to the activity that led to the fall, any prodromal symptoms (eg, lightheadedness, imbalance), and where and when the fall occurred should be obtained. Patients should be asked about the number of falls in the past year, whether any injuries were sustained from any of the falls, and if they suffer from a fear of falling. Finally, patients should be asked if they suffer from any difficulties with walking or balance. All of the above questions are important because a "yes" answer to any would indicate a high likelihood of sustaining a future fall.

When inquiring about a specific fall, if there was an associated loss of consciousness, then orthostatic hypotension or underlying cardiac or neurologic causes should be considered as precipitating factors. Other chronic medical conditions associated with an increased fall risk should be considered and include cognitive impairment, dementia, chronic musculoskeletal pain, knee osteoarthritis, urinary incontinence, stroke, Parkinson disease, and diabetes. Another crucial part of the medical history for an older person who might be at increased risk for falling includes a functional assessment of the activity of daily living skills, including use of adaptive equipment and mobility aids. In a patient who reports multiple falls, an inquiry into alcohol use is warranted as most patients would not volunteer this information freely, and frequent alcohol consumption could increase fall risk. Finally, physicians should perform an up-to-date and careful review of the patient's medication list that should include current prescriptions and over-the-counter medications. One large observational study of 4260 older community-dwelling men demonstrated that 82.3% of participants reported inappropriate medication use (eg, polypharmacy, inappropriate medicine consumption, underutilization). In addition, both polypharmacy (five or more medications) and taking one or more potentially inappropriate medications were associated with having had a fall in the past year, highlighting the importance of addressing inappropriate use of medications as a modifiable fall risk factor.

Once the history is obtained, clinicians should make sure that orthostatic vital signs, visual acuity, cognitive status, and cardiac system be included in a basic physical exam. Of vital importance is the evaluation of gait and balance. There are quite a few balance and mobility assessments that are effective at assessing fall risk but are not practical in a busy clinical setting. Such tests include the Performance-Oriented Mobility Assessment (POMA; Table 6–2), Short Physical Performance Battery (SPPB), Berg Balance Scale (BBS), and Safety Functional Motion Test. The POMA (sometimes referred to as the Tinetti Test or Tinetti Assessment Tool) is a validated, comprehensive evaluation of gait and balance that takes 10 to 15 minutes to complete. Each task is scored on a scale of 0 (most impairment) to 2 (independence). A score of <19 suggests high fall risk, 19 to 24 indicates medium fall risk, and 25 to 28 indicates low fall risk. However, there are two other tests, the Get Up and Go and the Functional Reach tests, that are more frequently used because they each take less than a minute to administer. For the Get Up and Go test, the physician should ask the patient to rise from a standard armchair (without the use of arms if possible), walk a fixed distance across the room (3 meters), turn, walk back to the chair, and sit down. Besides observing the patient for unsteadiness, if it takes >13.5 seconds to complete this task, the patient is considered at increased risk for future falls. The Functional Reach test (Figure 6–2) requires using a yardstick mounted on a wall at shoulder height. The patient is asked to stand close to the wall at a comfortable stance with an outstretched

Table 6–2. Performance-Oriented Mobility Assessment (POMA) of balance.[a]

Maneuver	Response		
	Normal	Adaptive	Abnormal
Sitting balance	Steady, stable	Holds onto chair to keep upright	Leans, slides down in chair
Arising from chair	Able to arise in a single movement without using arms	Uses arms (on chair or walking aid) to pull or push up; and/or moves forward in chair before attempting to arise	Multiple attempts required or unable without human assistance
Immediate standing balance (first 3–5 s)	Steady without holding onto walking aid or other objects for support	Steady, but uses walking aid or other object for support	Any sign of unsteadiness[b]
Standing balance	Steady, able to stand with feet together without holding object for support	Steady, but cannot put feet together	Any sign of unsteadiness regardless of stance or holds onto object
Balance with eyes closed (with feet as close together as possible)	Steady without holding onto any object with feet together	Steady with feet apart	Any sign of unsteadiness or needs to hold onto an object
Turning balance (360 degrees)	No grabbing or staggering; no need to hold onto any objects; steps are continuous (turn is a flowing movement)	Steps are discontinuous (patient puts one foot completely on floor before raising other foot)	Any sign of unsteadiness or holds onto an object
Nudge on sternum (patient standing with feet as close together as possible, examiner pushes with light even pressure over sternum 3 times; reflects ability to withstand displacement)	Steady, able to withstand pressure	Needs to move feet, but able to maintain balance	Begins to fall, or examiner has to help maintain balance
Neck turning (patient asked to turn head side to side and look up while standing with feet as close together as possible)	Able to turn head at least halfway side to side and be able to bend head back to look at ceiling; no staggering, grabbing, or symptoms of lightheadedness, unsteadiness, or pain	Decreased ability to turn side to side to extend neck, but no staggering, grabbing, or symptoms of lightheadedness, unsteadiness, or pain	Any sign of unsteadiness or symptoms when turning head or extending neck
One-leg standing balance	Able to stand on one leg for 5 s without holding object for support		Unable
Back extension (ask patient to lean back as far as possible, without holding onto object if possible)	Good extension without holding object or staggering	Tries to extend, but decreased range of motion (compared with other patients of same age) or needs to hold object to attempt extension	Will not attempt or no extension seen or staggers
Reaching up (have patient attempt to remove an object from a shelf high enough to require stretching or standing on toes)	Able to take down object without needing to hold onto other object for support and without becoming unsteady	Able to get object but needs to steady self by holding on to something for support	Unable or unsteady
Bending down (patient is asked to pick up small objects, such as pen, from the floor)	Able to bend down and pick up the object and is able to get up easily in single attempt without needing to pull self up with arms	Able to get object and get upright in single attempt but needs to pull self up with arms or hold onto something for support	Unable to bend down or unable to get upright after bending down or takes multiple attempts to upright
Sitting down	Able to sit down in one smooth movement	Needs to use arms to guide self into chair or not a smooth movement	Falls into chair, misjudges distances (lands off center)

[a]The patient begins this assessment seated in a hard, straight-backed, armless chair.
[b]Unsteadiness defined as grabbing at objects for support, staggering, moving feet, or more than minimal trunk sway.

Reproduced with permission from Tinetti ME: Performance-oriented Assessment of Mobility Problems in Elderly Patients, *J Am Geriatr Soc* 1986 Feb;34(2):119-126.

A   B

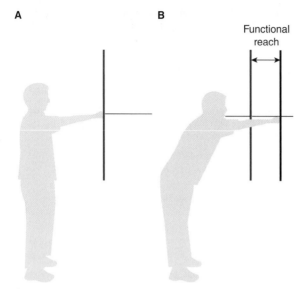

Functional
reach

▲ **Figure 6–2.** Functional Reach test. (**A**) The patient is asked to stand close to the wall at comfortable stance with the shoulders perpendicular to the yardstick and an outstretched arm. (**B**) The patient is then instructed to extend the arm forward as far as possible without taking a step or losing balance; the functional reach is the distance between the light blue line and the dark blue line and is measured along the yardstick in inches.

arm with the shoulders perpendicular to the yardstick. The patient is then instructed to extend the arm forward as far as possible without taking a step or losing balance; the functional reach is measured along the yardstick in inches, and if <10 inches in men, there has been reported a two times greater risk for falling. If there is sufficient time to perform multiple assessments, a recent meta-analysis shows that two assessment tools used in combination, preferably one with good sensitivity (eg, POMA or Get Up and Go test) and another with good specificity (eg, BBS), will maximize the predictability of each test.

Finally, also important to the physical exam is the examination of the feet and footwear. High heels, floppy slippers, and shoes with slick soles can predispose people to trip and fall. Ill-fitting footwear that is too big, without sufficient grip or too much friction, and/or without proper fixation (untied or loosely tied shoes) will also contribute to increasing someone's fall risk. When selecting shoes, the upper shoe should be soft and flexible with smooth lining. The toe box should be deep enough to allow for toe wiggle room. The sole should be strong and flexible for a good grip. The heel should provide a broad base for stability and be no higher than 4 cm. Finally, the fastening should provide a stable fit with some flexibility to allow for unusually shaped feet or swelling.

B. Diagnostic Tests

In completing a workup for an older patient with falls or determined to be at increased risk for falling, other than a general medical workup, there is no standard diagnostic evaluation. However, laboratory tests for hemoglobin to rule out clinically significant anemia, a chemistry panel to rule out electrolyte disorders and/or hyper- or hypo-osmolar states, thyroid-stimulating hormone (TSH) to rule out hypothyroidism, and vitamin B_{12} level to rule out B_{12} deficiency (linked to proprioceptive problems) could be considered appropriate. In addition, falling can be a sign of medical illness, and it is not uncommon for older patients to present with a fall to the emergency department and later be diagnosed with an underlying urinary tract infection or pneumonia. Basic laboratory testing (ie, complete blood count and basic metabolic panel as a starting point), a standard urinalysis, or chest radiograph might be appropriate depending on the clinical scenario, especially if the patient suffers from significant cognitive impairment or dementia.

Fewer than 10% of falls are caused by a loss of consciousness, but when there is a history of such, a different approach to evaluation and prevention might be indicated. An electrocardiogram to evaluate for significant cardiac pathology should be included; routine Holter monitoring has not been shown to be effective. However, if a crescendo-decrescendo systolic murmur is appreciated at the right upper sternal border, then echocardiogram would be indicated to rule out clinically significant aortic stenosis that, when critical, can present with syncope. Carotid sinus sensitivity has also been linked to falls, and pacemaker placement might be considered in patients who experience carotid sinus massage–induced heart rate pauses of >3 seconds. Contraindications to carotid sinus massage include presence of carotid bruits, recent myocardial or cerebral ischemia, and previous ventricular tachyarrhythmias.

In patients who present with falls who have new or unexplained neurologic findings on examination, imaging with head computed tomography (CT) or magnetic resonance imaging (MRI) may be indicated to rule out stroke, mass, normal pressure hydrocephalus, or other structural abnormality. If the patient has significant gait abnormalities, then spine radiographs or even MRI may help exclude cervical spondylosis or lumbar stenosis as a cause of falls. Clinical signs consistent with cervical spinal spondylosis include neck stiffness, deep aching neck, arm and shoulder pain, and possibly stiffness or clumsiness while walking. If the condition is chronically progressive, there may be significant associated muscle atrophy. The hallmark symptom of cervical spondylotic myelopathy is weakness or stiffness in the legs, and patients may present with gait instability; characteristically, there should be evidence of hyperreflexia, and a stiff or spastic gait would be expected in advanced cases. Lumbar spinal stenosis usually presents with pain, muscle weakness, and tingling of the legs in the L4-S1 distribution with classic symptoms of pseudoclaudication, more recently referred to as neurogenic claudication (pain improves with sitting, worsens with standing or walking).

Treatment

There are multiple interventions that can be implemented to decrease a patient's fall risk, and each needs to be tailored to the particular patient's needs. Overall, a multifactorial approach should be taken as modifiable factors, both intrinsic and extrinsic to the patient, have been shown to decrease fall rates. Of the interventions, medication reduction, physical therapy, and home safety modifications have demonstrated the best efficacy in fall prevention.

Starting with intrinsic modifiable fall risk factors (Table 6–3), visual impairment should be corrected if possible. The evidence supporting treatment of visual problems is not conclusive as a single intervention, but cataracts commonly affect older patients, and correction of vision may not only help to decrease the risk of falls, but also improve quality of life. In patients with cardioinhibitory carotid sinus hypersensitivity who experience recurrent falls, dual-chamber pacemaker placement is probably indicated. In all patients, but particularly in patients with postural hypotension, a careful review of medications should be done. A goal should be to reduce the total number of medications and/or dose of individual medications. Psychoactive medications, including sedative-hypnotics, anxiolytics, antidepressants, and antipsychotic medications, should be minimized and appropriately tapered and withdrawn if possible. If after discontinuation of predisposing medications a patient still has postural hypotension, then recommendations for adequate hydration, advice to slowly change positions, and the addition of a medication such as fludrocortisone may be considered. Vitamin D supplementation is no longer routinely recommended for fall prevention in patients older than 65 years without osteoporosis or vitamin D deficiency.

Extrinsic modifiable factors include checking the home environment to remove obvious fall hazards and ensuring that proper footwear is worn. In evaluating the home environment, removal of clutter (eg, loose floor rugs) to minimize tripping hazards, making sure there is adequate lighting, and installation of safety measures like shower bars and/or raised toilet seats are helpful to decrease fall risk. In assessing the footwear, foot problems can also be screened for and patients referred for treatment if necessary. Patients should be advised that they should wear well-fitting shoes of low heel height and high surface area.

Table 6–3. Recommended management of modifiable risk factors.

Risk Factors	Management
Intrinsic	
Vision	Check acuity and for cataracts, refer to ophthalmology if indicated; advise to avoid multifocal lenses while walking
Postural hypotension	Reduce medications, rule out dehydration, advise to change positions slowly, consider fludrocortisone if previous three interventions do not work
Cardiovascular	Medical management, consider dual-chamber cardiac pacing if carotid-induced hypersensitivity >3-s pauses
Neurologic	Consider neuroimaging with MRI/CT, medical management as indicated
Arthritis	Medical management, consider physical therapy/occupational therapy referral, assistive devices as appropriate
Balance or gait impairment	Referral to physical and/or occupational therapy for progressive strength, balance, and gait training
Other medical conditions (eg, cognitive impairment, depression)	Medical management as indicated
Psychoactive medications	Eliminate or reduce dose of as many sedatives, antidepressants, anxiolytics, and antipsychotics as possible as these are associated with an increased fall risk
Other medications	Eliminate or reduce dose of as many medications as possible, paying close attention to: (1) antihypertensives, which can lead to orthostasis/lightheadedness; and (2) antihistamines, anticonvulsants, and opioids, which can lead to confusion or impaired alertness
Extrinsic	
Home environmental hazards	Ideally, physical therapy/occupational therapy referral can assess home safety and make recommendations for safety improvements (eg, grab bars in shower, reaching devices, adequate lighting)
Footwear	Advise to wear well-fitting shoes with low heel height and high surface contact area

CT, computed tomography; MRI, magnetic resonance imaging.

In addition to reviewing and treating intrinsic and extrinsic modifiable fall risk factors, patient education and information programs are helpful in falls prevention. For example, simple advice, such as a removal of multifocal lenses while walking or on stairs, can reduce the risk of falls. Perhaps most important is education and recommendations regarding physical activity. Although there is a lot of information available to the general public with regard to proper diet and exercise and good health, many probably do not link this beneficial information directly to fall risk reduction. Therefore, clinicians should make a specified recommendation regarding exercise and fall risk reduction as it has the best evidence for reducing fall rates. The National Institute on Aging recommends at least 150 minutes of exercise weekly.

If during the clinical evaluation the patient demonstrates balance or gait instability, referral to physical therapy is warranted. Physical therapy should consist of progressive standing balance and strength exercise, transfer practice, and gait interventions, including use of appropriate assistive devices. Patients should also be trained on how to get up from the floor after a fall. Once mastering of these skills is accomplished, focusing on maintenance and building endurance should be encouraged. For all community-dwelling older patients, clinicians should recommend an individually tailored exercise program to maintain function, possibly increase endurance, and decrease their risk for falls. In the most recent systematic review on the topic, 43 trials tested the effect of exercise on falls. In trials of exercise classes that employed gait training, balance, and strengthening, there was a 17% risk reduction in falling (n = 14 trials; 2364 participants; 95% confidence interval, 0.72–0.97). A recent meta-analysis of 10 trials that examined the effects of Tai Chi on the risk and rate of falls showed a 43% risk reduction with practicing Tai Chi. However, the impact of Tai Chi on time to first fall is yet to be well established.

Separate mention of treatment in acute and long-term care settings is warranted because this patient population clearly would be expected to be at an increased fall risk, and yet studied interventions in these patients have not demonstrated clear benefit. In particular, the use of bedrails, restraints, fall-alert bracelets, and bed alarms has not been shown to decrease fall rates and may potentially increase fall risk. Even so, the AGS/BGS still provides the recommendation that multifactorial/multicomponent interventions should be considered in the long-term care setting; within this recommendation, exercise programs are also suggested but should be implemented with caution due to risk of injury in frail persons.

▶ Prognosis

There is significant morbidity and mortality associated with falls in older persons. The prognosis for a single fall is less severe than with repeated falls. Those who had fallen one or more times at home in the preceding 3 months were more than three times as likely as nonfallers to require institutional care within the subsequent year. Fallers had an overall three-fold increase in subsequent fracture, with recurrent fallers age 60 to 74 years having an eightfold increased risk of subsequent fracture. Additionally, recurrent fallers older than age 60 years had an overall risk of death about twice that of nonfallers. This was not simply a function of subsequent risk of fracture. In fact, recurrent fallers age 60 to 74 years have a fivefold increased mortality independent of fracture.

Besides recurrent falls, inability to get up from a fall also portends a poor prognosis. Among 1103 community-dwelling residents in New Haven, Connecticut, there were 313 uninjured fallers, of whom 47% were unable to get up on their own. Even when they were not injured as a result of a fall, those unable to get up without help were more likely to suffer a lasting decline in activities of daily living (35% vs 26%). Not surprisingly, over an average follow-up of 16 months, compared with nonfallers, these individuals were also more likely to be hospitalized.

Older adults who fall also suffer from a worse quality of life. Confusion and sadness are four times more common in recurrent fallers than nonfallers, and it appears that decisions to enter institutional care are often driven by fear of future falls and being unable to get up, rather than actual demonstrated disability. The negative impact of fear of falling should not be underestimated. Another study reported that compared with falls and fractures, fear of falling had the largest negative effect on health-related quality of life.

Although recurrent falls, inability to get up after a fall, and psychological implications following falls all are associated with poor prognosis, each is potentially modifiable. Careful attention should be made to underlying medical disorders that may contribute to an individual's fall risk. In one randomized controlled trial, a focused history and physical assessment by nurse practitioners following a fall led to identification of modifiable medical conditions and decreased hospitalization rates over 2 years of follow-up.

In this chapter, we discussed the underlying predisposing risk factors, clinical evaluation, prevention, and treatment of falls in older persons. Although chronologic aging is inevitable, the ability to prevent falls in aging patients is not. The astute practitioner who is aware of fall risk factors takes the time to do a proper assessment, and is knowledgeable about treatment can help our older population avoid falling and its associated ill-health consequences.

Bringole M, Moya A, de Lange FJ, et al. 2018 ESC Guidelines for the diagnosis and management of syncope. *Eur Heart J.* 2018;39(21):1883.

Centers for Disease Control and Prevention. Important facts about falls. https://www.cdc.gov/homeandrecreationalsafety/falls/adultfalls.html. Accessed February 1, 2018.

Davis JC, Robertson MC, Ashe MC, Liu-Ambrose T, Khan KM, Marra CA. Does a home-based strength and balance programme in people aged > 80 years provide the best value for money to prevent falls? A systematic review of economic evaluations of falls prevention interventions. *Br J Sports Med.* 2010;44(2):80-89.

Delbaere K, Crombez G, Vanderstraeten G, Willems T, Cambier D. Fear-related avoidance of activities, falls and physical frailty. A prospective community-based cohort study. *Age Ageing.* 2004;33(4):368-373.

Hopewell S, Adedire O, Copsey BJ, et al. Multifactorial and multiple component interventions for preventing falls in older people living in the community. *Cochrane Database Syst Rev.* 2018;7:CD012221.

National Institute on Aging. Prevent falls and fractures. https://www.nia.nih.gov/health/prevent-falls-and-fractures. Accessed February 1, 2018.

Panel on Prevention of Falls in Older Persons, American Geriatrics Society, British Geriatrics Society. Summary of the updated American Geriatrics Society/British Geriatrics Society clinical practice guideline for prevention of falls in older persons. *J Am Geriatr Soc.* 2011;59(1):148-157.

Park SH. Tools for assessing fall risk in the elderly: as systematic review and meta-analysis. *Aging Clin Exp Res.* 2018;30(1):1-16.

Quach L, Galica AM, Jones RN, et al. The nonlinear relationship between gait speed and falls: the maintenance of balance, independent living, intellect, and zest in the Elderly of Boston Study. *J Am Geriatr Soc.* 2011;59(6):1069-1073.

Tolea MI, Costa PT Jr, Terracciano A, et al. Associations of openness and conscientiousness with walking speed decline: findings from the Health, Aging, and Body Composition Study. *J Gerontol B Psychol Sci Soc Sci.* 2012;67(6):705-711.

US Preventative Services Task Force. Interventions to prevent falls in community-dwelling older adults: US Preventative Services Task Force recommendation statement. *JAMA.* 2018;319(16):1696-1704.

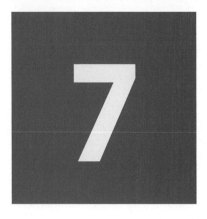

Managing Vision Impairment

Meredith M. Whiteside, OD

Tonse A. Kini, MD

Andrew G. Lee, MD

General Principles

Vision impairment is relatively rare in people younger than 65 years of age, but its incidence steadily increases to almost 24% of those 80 years and older. Not surprisingly, vision impairment can have a significant impact on a patient's quality of life. It is associated with social isolation, anxiety, depression, and a loss of independence. It can affect balance, leading to more frequent falls, and has been shown to negatively affect physical activity.

The following three levels are used to categorize the severity of vision loss[*]:

1. Normal vision: Visual acuity ≥20/40
2. Visual impairment: Visual acuity <20/40 but <20/200
3. Legal blindness: Acuity ≤20/200 in the better eye, or total visual field <20 degrees

NORMAL CHANGES IN THE AGING EYE

Clinical Findings

Although not meeting the definition of vision impairment, there are still a number of changes in the aging eye leading to diminished vision. Changes in refractive error in older adults may cause reduced vision. In all adults, the crystalline lens gradually becomes less flexible and less able to change its curvature (accommodate) with age. This results in the condition known as presbyopia, in which patients lose the ability to focus their eyes on near objects. Contrast sensitivity is the ability to distinguish objects from the background when they are similar in brightness, and this ability decreases slightly with age. A real-life example of contrast sensitivity

is the ability to see a curb when the sidewalk is similar in color and brightness. In eyes with no significant pathology, the loss of contrast sensitivity with aging exists but is not significant enough to cause problems seeing curbs in well-lit conditions. Notably, the ability to see well in dim light also becomes diminished in older adults. When combined with reduced contrast sensitivity, this reduced sensitivity in dim illumination may explain why older drivers may have difficulty seeing pedestrians at night. Both the change in contrast sensitivity and the reduced ability to see in dim illumination result from a combination of decreases in pupil size and progressive increases in the light absorption of the lens. This age-related reduction in retinal illumination is substantial. A typical 60-year-old's retina receives only about one-third of the light that a typical 20-year-old receives. As a result of the tendency for opacities to form in the aging lens and cornea, older adults are increasingly sensitive to glare caused by scattered light in the eye. In addition, largely due to neural changes in the retina, there is an age-related reduction in the ability to adapt to sudden changes in illumination. Finally, dry eye, especially in older women, is also common. Symptoms include a mild foreign-body sensation, burning, small fluctuations in vision, and even (reflexive) tearing because of mild corneal irritation. Table 7–1 includes suggested vision screening tests for older adults.

Treatment and Prognosis

Although a number of normal, age-related changes have a negative impact on vision, there are simple ways to compensate for many of them. Starting in the mid-40s, reading glasses may be required to manage presbyopia. In epidemiologic studies, 40% to 60% of older adults have vision worse than 20/40 simply because of problems with their eyeglasses, a problem easily remedied through ensuring regular eye examinations.

---

[*]It is assumed the patient is wearing the best glasses (or contact lens) correction.

Table 7–1. Suggested vision screening tests for older adults.

Procedure	Description	Causes of Abnormal Findings
Visual acuity	Test left eye (OD), right eye (OS) separately Use habitual glasses to test distance Use bright ambient light	Cataract, uncorrected refractive error, retinal or optic nerve disease, other neurologic disease
Visual field by confrontation	Test OD, OS separately Patient fixates on examiner's eye opposite of the patient Examiner shows fingers in four quadrants of patient's visual field Patient counts fingers	Monocular defect = disorder of retina, optic nerve Binocular defect = chiasm, cortex or bilateral eye disease
Pupils	Check direct and consensual response to light Swinging flashlight test	Asymmetric responses = optic nerve or autonomic nervous system disorder
Extraocular motility	Observe patient with both eyes open for strabismus Test motility of OD, OS separately: patient looks up/down, right/left with head fixed	Deviations or restricted movement = binocular vision disorder, nerve palsy, trauma, or previous ocular surgery
External observation	Observe lids, lashes, conjunctiva, cornea Instill fluorescein, illuminate eye with cobalt blue filter on direct ophthalmoscope	Discharge, crusting of lids or conjunctival injection = infection or allergy Significant corneal staining = abrasion or foreign body
Direct ophthalmoscopy	Darken room illumination Observe red reflex in pupils Examine optic disc, macula, and vasculature	Darkened red reflex often caused by cataract Large cupping = possible glaucoma Disc pallor = optic atrophy or end-stage glaucoma Hemorrhages = possible diabetic or hypertensive retinopathy White spots = macular degeneration or exudate due to diabetes or hypertension

Careful selection of glasses to correct refractive error is important. Epidemiologic studies show that multifocal progressive glasses or bifocal wearers are twice as likely to fall compared to single-vision wearers—especially so when navigating outdoor activities. Thus, single-vision distance glasses are recommended when negotiating an unfamiliar area or when an older adult predominantly spends time in outdoor activities. For those who spend more time indoors, the use of a multifocal prescription that is set toward correcting distance and intermediate vision can help maintain safety indoors. Other ways to compensate for normal age-related losses of vision include providing bright, indirect (ie, nonglare) lighting, use of larger text with both books and electronic devices, and making objects as high contrast as possible from their background. These strategies can significantly improve visual function in most older adults. Finally, since dry eye tends to be chronic and associated with many medications used by older adults, nonprescription artificial tears, liquigels, or ointment at bedtime can help relieve symptoms. If the eye drop contains a preservative, which is true of most eye drops in bottles, the general recommendation is to use it no more than four times daily since chronic exposure to preservatives can cause a toxic keratitis. In contrast, preservative-free eye drops, which typically come in single-use vials, can be used as needed (eg, one to two times hourly).

Elliott DB. The Glenn A. Fry award lecture 2013: blurred vision, spectacle correction, and falls in older adults. *Optom Vis Sci.* 2014;91(6):593-601.

Owsley C. Vision and aging. *Annu Rev Vis Sci.* 2016;2:255-271.

CONDITIONS REQUIRING URGENT REFERRAL TO AN EYE CARE SPECIALIST

Red flags indicating the need for urgent referral include significant changes in vision and moderate or worse eye pain. Changes in vision may include a sudden onset of decreased visual acuity (even with correction), a report of distorted vision (eg, in metamorphopsia, straight lines appear curved or irregular), or the sudden appearance of a scotoma or a visual field defect. Careful review of the ocular history is important. The patient should be questioned about which eye is affected and the timing and onset of symptoms such as pain, decrease in vision, or photophobia. If the primary symptom is pain, ask about a history of recent eye surgery, trauma, chemical injury, photophobia, or recent use of contact lenses. If there is a reduction in vision, ask about the location of the loss. A reduction in central vision suggests macular involvement and may be a result of macular degeneration, diabetic retinopathy, vascular occlusive disease, or optic neuropathy.

Table 7-2. Visual symptoms indicating the need for referral.

Symptom	Possible Etiology	Need for Referral

Decreased central vision
Marked loss
Rapid onset
Monocular (usually)
	Wet age-related macular degeneration
	Macular edema or hemorrhage caused by diabetes
	Vascular occlusion
	Ischemic optic neuropathy
	   Arteritic = patients with temporal arteritis
	   Nonarteritic = patient often has diabetes or hypertension
		ASAP[a]

Decreased central vision Mild loss Slow onset Bilateral (usually)	Dry age-related macular degeneration Cataracts Diabetic retinopathy Refractive error change	Less Urgent (4–6 weeks)
Ocular pain Monocular Moderate-to-severe photophobia (possibly)	Infection (eg, herpetic keratitis) Corneal abrasion Uveitis Endophthalmitis (usually also reduces vision) Chemical or mechanical trauma Angle-closure glaucoma	ASAP[a]
Loss of peripheral vision Monocular	Retinal detachment[a] Glaucoma (usually bilateral, but asymmetric)	ASAP[a] or urgent
Loss of peripheral vision Binocular	Lesion in central visual pathway (from chiasm to cortex)	Urgent

[a]ASAP: telephone consult or referral for in-person evaluation by an eye specialist within the hour.

If the vision loss is peripheral, establish whether it is monocular or binocular. If it is monocular, suspect either a retinal or optic neuropathy. In cases of bilateral loss of vision, consider a neurologic cause or, less likely, concomitant bilateral eye disease (Table 7–2).

▼ ABNORMAL CHANGES IN THE AGING EYE

The leading abnormal ocular changes that cause vision impairment in older adults are cataracts, AMD diabetic retinopathy, and glaucoma.

CATARACTS

▶ General Principles

A cataract is a clouding of the lens and is a leading cause of vision impairment in the United States and globally. Cataracts progress gradually and may require removal. By age 80 years, more than half of all people in the United States either have a cataract or have had cataract surgery. Risk factors for cataracts include advanced age, diabetes, cumulative exposure to ultraviolet (UV) B radiation, smoking, current or previous long-term use of corticosteroids, previous eye surgery, or a history of eye injury.

▶ Prevention

Decreasing UV exposure by wearing sunglasses and hats, encouraging smoking cessation, and good glycemic control may delay the onset and progression of cataracts. Currently, there is no evidence that medication or nutritional supplementation prevents, delays the progression of, or cures cataracts.

▶ Clinical Findings

Typical symptoms of cataracts include a gradual onset of blurred vision and increased sensitivity to glare (especially when driving at dusk or night). A common sign of a sight-limiting cataract is an insensitivity to subtle color differences such as those caused by food stains on clothing in an otherwise neatly dressed patient. Observing a white haze in the pupil during pupil testing suggests a moderate or worse cataract. With the pupil dilated, the red eye reflex may exhibit focal or diffuse areas of darkness when viewed with the direct ophthalmoscope or a slit lamp.

▶ Differential Diagnosis

Patients with significant cataracts often present with a history of painless, gradual, and progressive deterioration of vision and a normal-appearing external eye. Other possibilities include uncorrected refractive error, diseases of the macula or optic nerve, or diabetic eye disease. If vision loss is sudden, unilateral, and painless, the most common differential includes vascular/ischemic disorders such as nonarteritic ischemic optic neuropathy or a central retinal artery or vein occlusion. When sudden vision loss is associated with physical symptoms such as scalp tenderness, a headache, jaw claudication, weight loss, and/or malaise, giant cell arteritis should be considered and constitutes an ophthalmic emergency requiring prompt evaluation and treatment.

▶ Management and Treatment

Cataracts usually develop slowly, and in the early stages, an updated spectacle correction often will improve vision. Environmental modifications, such as avoiding high-glare situations (eg, night driving), use of antiglare sunglasses, and providing adequate ambient light, can help patients cope. The only treatment for cataracts is removal. Surgery is usually indicated when a patient's daily activities are compromised by reduced vision (often ~20/40), despite best correction. The decision for surgery should take into account other pathologies, such as macular degeneration or diabetic retinopathy, which may limit postsurgical vision.

A. Pre- & Postoperative Care

Most older adults can tolerate cataract surgery. Patients should be medically stable and ideally be able to lie supine for 30 minutes. Postoperative care typically requires the administration of antibiotic and anti-inflammatory eye drops, as well as follow-up office visits. For patients with comorbidities such as chronic obstructive pulmonary disease, poorly controlled blood pressure, coronary artery disease, or diabetes, the ophthalmologist will typically request a medical evaluation by the patient's primary care physician. Although preoperative laboratory testing for any medical problems indicated by the history and physical examination is appropriate, studies show that routine medical testing before cataract surgery does not improve outcomes.

Cataract surgery is an outpatient procedure. In patients deemed to have a reasonably healthy cornea, the incision is made through the cornea, which results in minimal or no blood loss and usually requires only topical anesthesia and minimal systemic medications. Because of this, anticoagulant or antiplatelet therapy may be continued, based on the preferences of the eye surgeon and primary care physician.

B. Complications

Serious postoperative complications from cataract surgery are rare (<1.5%). Symptoms of pain or a decrease in vision in the days following surgery suggest intraocular infection (endophthalmitis), and an increase in floaters or flashes of light could signal retinal detachment. Both of these conditions require immediate ophthalmologic consultation. While less vision threatening, two common complications, cystoid macular edema and the development of opacities on the posterior capsule of the lens, also require consultation because they can reduce visual acuity. Cystoid macular edema may occur 4 to 6 weeks after surgery at a rate of 1.2% to 11% in the weeks following cataract removal. Whereas patients initially appreciate an improvement in vision after cataract surgery, as cystoid macular edema develops, they will note a gradual decrease in vision over 1 or more weeks. Once detected, the typical treatment is topical anti-inflammatory medications. Posterior capsular opacities (sometimes called secondary cataracts) can develop several months to years following lens removal surgery and occur at a rate of 12% to 28%. As the opacity grows, vision slowly degrades over months. Once vision loss is significant, a laser is used to ablate the area of membrane that blocks vision.

▶ Prognosis

Age-related cataracts typically progress slowly over time. Through regular evaluations, an optometrist or ophthalmologist can monitor their progress and recommend when the risks of cataract surgery are justified by its potential benefits in terms of ensuring the patient's visual capacities continue to meet the demands of daily living. If there are no comorbid ocular conditions present, surgical outcomes from cataract surgery are very good and vision will return to normal. Studies show that cataract surgery leads to an improvement in vision-related quality of life, which may translate to ability to perform real-life daily activities such as reading and driving.

Liu YC, Wilkins M, Kim T, Malyugin B, Mehta JS. Cataracts. *Lancet.* 2017;390(10094):600-612.

AGE-RELATED MACULAR DEGENERATION

▶ General Principles

Age-related macular degeneration (AMD) is a disease that progressively destroys the macula, impairing central vision. It accounts for 54% of all legal blindness and is the leading cause of irreversible vision loss in people over 65. Although the etiology of AMD is unknown, it is likely an inherited disease with contributing environmental factors. Risk factors include advancing age, white race, a family history of AMD, and smoking. There are two forms of AMD: nonneovascular (also known as nonexudative or dry) and neovascular (also known as exudative or wet). Ninety percent of patients have the dry form of AMD, which causes a gradual loss of vision. Even though wet AMD is less common, leakage from the newly growing vessels results in rapid vision loss and is responsible for the majority of cases of legal blindness.

Prevention

Although there are no definitive preventive treatments for either dry or wet AMD, studies suggest that people who eat a diet rich in green, leafy vegetables and fish may have a lower risk of developing AMD. Smoking doubles the risk of AMD. Because severe vision loss is typically associated with the wet form of AMD, the best prevention of blindness is prompt diagnosis and treatment of neovascularization.

Clinical Findings

In its early stages, AMD has no symptoms. As dry AMD progresses, patients note a gradual blurring of central vision and increased difficulty reading fine print, recognizing faces, or seeing street signs. In contrast, wet AMD often presents as a rapid loss of central vision, with metamorphopsia (images that appear distorted) or central scotomas. Even with advanced wet or dry AMD, patients maintain navigational mobility. In dry AMD, drusen—cream-colored lesions that represent a buildup of metabolic waste products within the retina—are seen in the macula. Other signs include pigmentary changes or chorioretinal atrophy of the macula. In wet AMD, abnormal blood vessels grow and hemorrhage, causing macular swelling, loss of retinal function, and scarring.

Differential Diagnoses

Other conditions causing a reduction in visual acuity with changes in the appearance of the macula include diabetes and hypertension, each of which might cause retinal hemorrhages and/or the deposition of exudates, which may or may not be in the macula.

Complications, Treatment, and Prognosis

Loss of central vision is the main complication of AMD. In wet AMD, vision loss rapidly deteriorates, requiring urgent consultation. Evaluation and treatment for wet AMD frequently involve visualizing the retinal vasculature with fluorescein angiography and then laser photocoagulation of abnormal blood vessels. Unfortunately, while the laser stops leakage and destroys new blood vessels, it also destroys the underlying retina. The development of anti–vascular endothelial growth factor (anti-VEGF) medications such as bevacizumab that inhibit neovascularization has markedly changed the management of wet AMD. These drugs are injected intravitreally and may be used alone or in conjunction with laser treatment. With prompt recognition and referral to a retinal ophthalmologist, many patients treated with anti-VEGF intravitreal injections will maintain or even have mildly improved vision. Patients who develop unilateral wet AMD have a 30% 6-year risk of neovascularization in the contralateral eye, so frequent follow-up evaluations are recommended.

For patients with dry AMD, vision loss progresses slowly. In mild cases, there is no treatment. For patients who have been diagnosed with intermediate or advanced dry AMD, the 10-year clinical trial Age-Related Eye Disease Study (AREDS) showed that a specific formulation of antioxidants (commonly referred to as AREDS2 vitamins, which include vitamins C and E, lutein, and zeaxanthin, among others) lowered the risk of progressing to advanced AMD and the development of severe vision loss. The AREDS formulation is not a cure, nor does it restore vision loss caused by AMD; it simply may delay the onset of advanced AMD and help maintain stable vision.

Mitchell P, Liew G, Gopinath B, Wong TY. Age-related macular degeneration. *Lancet.* 2018;392(10153):1147-1159.

Wu J, Cho E, Willett WC, Sastry SM, Schaumberg DA. Intakes of lutein, zeaxanthin, and other carotenoids and age-related macular degeneration during 2 decades of prospective follow-up. *JAMA Ophthalmol.* 2015;133(12):1415-1424.

DIABETIC RETINOPATHY

General Principles

Diabetic retinopathy is characterized by a progressive series of abnormal changes in the retinal microvasculature. The early phase of the disease is called nonproliferative (or background) retinopathy. Changes in the microvasculature causing damage to small vessel pericytes and endothelium lead to increased vasopermeability, which causes the appearance of microaneurysms and hemorrhages. If the disease progresses, retinal hypoxia can cause upregulation of vasoproliferative growth factors and leads to proliferative diabetic retinopathy. At this stage, there is a pathologic propagation of fragile retinal vessels that can break and bleed extensively. Overall, ~35% of persons with diabetes have some stage of diabetic retinopathy. The longer one has diabetes, the more likely it is that retinopathy will develop.

In areas where there is inadequate access to eye care specialists, fundus photographs reviewed via telemedicine can be a sensitive and effective screening tool for identifying patients with diabetic retinopathy who need to be prioritized for referral to specialty eye care. Specialty diabetic eye examinations typically include retinal examination for subtle signs of macular edema, assessing the location and amount of hemorrhages, and assessing the vascular abnormalities that help stage the severity of either nonproliferative or proliferative retinopathy.

Prevention

Good glycemic and blood pressure control are associated with decreased development and progression of diabetic retinopathy. Although diabetic retinopathy may not be completely avoidable, studies show that severe vision loss can be prevented 90% of the time with timely detection and intervention. Therefore, leading eye care organizations (the American Academy of Ophthalmology and American Optometric Association) recommend that patients with diabetes should have an annual dilated, funduscopic examination.

Clinical Findings

Diabetic retinopathy may be asymptomatic in its early, more treatable stages. Blurred vision may occur if there is macular edema, but if the contralateral eye is unaffected or the vision loss is subtle, patients may not notice changes. In cases of proliferative retinopathy, new blood vessels can bleed extensively, causing blurred vision, visual field scotomas, or loss of vision. Patients who have had extensive laser photocoagulation for treatment of proliferative disease may have an overall constriction of the visual field. Signs of diabetic retinopathy are best evaluated through dilated funduscopy and can include hemorrhages, exudates, vascular changes like beading of vessels, or neovascularization.

Vision loss caused by diabetic retinopathy is caused mainly by macular edema and proliferative retinopathy and, to a lesser extent, by macular capillary nonperfusion. Macular edema occurs when fluid leaks into the central retina and may occur with either nonproliferative or proliferative retinopathy.

Differential Diagnosis

Hypertensive retinopathy, vein occlusions, ischemic disorders, inflammatory or infectious disorders, or any other disorder that can cause retinal hemorrhages can be considered in the differential diagnosis of diabetic retinopathy.

Complications and Treatment

Management of nonproliferative diabetic retinopathy (with no macular edema) typically consists of observation by an optometrist or ophthalmologist via a dilated stereoscopic examination of the fundus. In the early stages of nonproliferative retinopathy with no macular edema, management consists of emphasizing the importance of glycemic control and timely follow-up evaluations. In more advanced cases of retinopathy, intravitreal injections of medication, laser treatment, or other medications may be indicated. In cases where macular edema or proliferative disease is present or likely to occur (such as in severe nonproliferative retinopathy), referral to an ophthalmologist (preferably one specializing in retina) is indicated. Clinical studies show that treatment of a specific subset of macular edema, clinically significant macular edema (CSME), significantly reduces the risk of moderate vision loss. In proliferative retinopathy, blood vessels can bleed extensively into the vitreous and/or undergo fibrous proliferation, causing vitreoretinal traction and tears in the retina. Treatment for both CSME and proliferative retinopathy may include laser and intravitreal injections of anti-VEGF agents.

Prognosis

Traditional treatments for most types of diabetic eye disease typically cannot restore lost vision and hence are aimed at preventing further vision loss. A few recent studies have shown that patients with CSME treated with intravitreal anti-VEGF gained a mild improvement in vision. It remains critical, however, that CSME be detected and treated in a timely manner. Regardless of the ability to improve vision, laser treatment and/or intravitreal injections for CSME reduce the future risk of moderate vision loss by 50% or more. In terms of proliferative or severe nonproliferative diabetic retinopathy, panretinal laser photocoagulation yields a 50% reduction in the risk for severe vision loss.

Hendrick AM, Gibson MV, Kulshreshtha A. Diabetic retinopathy. *Prim Care.* 2015;42(3):451-464.

Weingessel B, Miháltz K, Gleiss A, et al. Treatment of diabetic macular edema with intravitreal antivascular endothelial growth factor and prompt versus deferred focal laser during long-term follow-up and identification of prognostic retinal markers. *J Ophthalmol.* 2018;2018:3082560.

GLAUCOMA

General Principles

Glaucoma is a progressive, chronic optic neuropathy in which intraocular pressure (IOP) and other currently unknown factors contribute to a characteristic acquired atrophy of the optic nerve that, if left to progress, leads to visual field loss. There are two major forms of glaucoma: open angle, in which the intraocular drainage system is open, and closed angle, in which the system is blocked. Primary open-angle glaucoma (POAG) accounts for the vast majority of glaucoma cases. Vision loss caused by glaucoma typically occurs first in peripheral vision, and as the disease advances, central vision is lost. Glaucoma is the second leading cause of blindness worldwide, and approximately 50% of those with glaucoma are unaware they have the condition.

Besides elevated IOP, ethnicity and age are two risk important factors for glaucoma. In the United States, glaucoma is the leading cause of irreversible blindness in African Americans. Starting in early middle age (~age 45), African Americans have a prevalence of POAG that is three times higher compared to white and Hispanic/Latino persons of the same age. Older age is another risk factor for glaucoma.

Although the prevalence of glaucoma increases with age in all ethnicities, by age 80 and older, Hispanic/Latino patients have the highest prevalence rate of 12.7%.

Clinical Findings

Prevention of vision loss from glaucoma is dependent upon early diagnosis and treatment. Unfortunately, because glaucoma is often asymptomatic, most patients fail to notice changes in vision until end-stage disease. Because of this, annual eye examinations are recommended for older adults at higher risk (Table 7–3). For others, an eye examination every 1 to 2 years is recommended. Clinical examination for glaucoma includes measurement of IOP (tonometry), optic disc assessment, visual field assessment, and gonioscopy to assess whether the intraocular drainage system is "open" or "closed." In gonioscopy, a specialized lens is placed on the patient's cornea that allows the examiner to visualize the iridocorneal angle between the cornea and the iris where aqueous humor drains. IOP normally ranges from 10 to 21 mm Hg; however, IOP outside of this range is not pathognomonic for glaucoma—it is simply a risk factor associated with the development and/or progression of the disease. In angle-closure glaucoma, narrowing of the intraocular drainage system raises IOP and induces retinal nerve fiber loss, which initially leads to increased vertical optic nerve cupping and corresponding visual field defects that respect the horizontal meridian. If the rise in IOP occurs quickly, patients may complain of pain. Gradual rises in IOP may be asymptomatic. In normal-tension glaucoma, glaucomatous optic atrophy occurs in the absence of documented elevated IOP.

Optic disc examination is one of the most important ways to evaluate for glaucoma. Glaucomatous atrophy causes increased optic nerve cupping. Although most cases of glaucoma are bilateral, the presentation can vary between the two eyes. Hence, markedly asymmetric cupping between the two eyes can indicate glaucoma. In the earliest stage of glaucoma, optic disc findings are usually observed before visual field losses appear. Nonetheless, periodic visual field assessment using standardized perimetry is important for diagnosing, staging, and monitoring disease progression.

Differential Diagnosis

The differential diagnosis of glaucoma encompasses a variety of conditions that affect the optic nerve. Possibilities include optic atrophy caused by retinal vascular disease, ischemic optic neuropathies, compressive lesions including tumors, inflammatory or demyelinating conditions, and toxic, metabolic, or nutritional optic neuropathies. These conditions can be differentiated from glaucomatous atrophy in that they usually cause optic nerve pallor with less optic nerve cupping. A central scotoma, nerve fiber loss causing horizontal cupping, a visual field defect respecting the vertical midline, and a temporal field defect are more likely nonglaucomatous and require further workup to identify the underlying cause.

Complications and Treatment

Vision loss in glaucoma typically starts in the periphery and extends inward, ultimately destroying central vision until complete blindness. Treatment of primary open-angle and normal-tension glaucoma consists of lowering IOP, with the goal of preventing progressive visual field loss by slowing retinal nerve fiber loss and associated glaucomatous atrophy. Therapies to lower IOP may include topical or oral medications; laser surgery, such as iridotomy, iridoplasty, or trabeculoplasty; or incisional surgical procedures, such as a trabeculectomy with or without an iridectomy as well as tube shunts or valves. Topical medications are often the first line of treatment and work by either decreasing aqueous production or increasing aqueous outflow. As a result of their effectiveness in lowering IOP, simplicity of once-a-day dosing, and few systemic side effects, prostaglandin analogs such as latanoprost are among the most frequently prescribed first-line therapies for glaucoma. All medications used for the treatment of glaucoma may have significant local and systemic effects and should be included in the older patient's chronic medication list. (See Table 7–4 for a summary of local and systemic side effects.)

Surgery is considered when two or more topical therapies do not adequately control IOP or if the topical medications are not well tolerated. Other indications for surgical care of glaucoma include poor compliance with medications because of memory impairment or if poor manual dexterity prevents eye drop application. Finally, when compared to the cost of surgery, the annual cost of medications may be prohibitive for some.

Table 7–3. Indications for referral to an optometrist or ophthalmologist for glaucoma screening.

Patients at higher risk for glaucoma	African ancestry, especially older than age 40 years Everyone older than age 60 years, especially Mexican Americans Family history of glaucoma Prolonged corticosteroid use Elevated intraocular pressure History of eye trauma
Possible indications of glaucoma	Suspicious optic disc cupping with a cup-to-disc ratio >0.5 Asymmetric optic cup, marked interocular asymmetry in disc cupping

Table 7–4. Topical medications to lower intraocular pressure (IOP).

Class of Medication	Mechanism of Action	Example	IOP Reduction	Local Adverse Events	Systemic Adverse Events
Prostaglandin analogs	Increase outflow	Latanoprost, travoprost, bimatoprost, tafluprost, latanoprostene bunod	25%–33%	Conjunctival hyperemia Increased eyelash length Darkening lashes and iris Superior eyelid sulcus deepening Uveitis Macular edema	Minimal systemic effects
β-Adrenergic blockers	Decrease production	Timolol, betaxolol, levobunolol	20%–25%	Ocular irritation and dry eyes	Contraindicated in those with asthma, chronic obstructive pulmonary disease, and bradycardia Depression Impotence
α-Adrenergic agents	Decrease production Increase outflow	Brimonidine, apraclonidine	14%–19%	Ocular irritation, dryness Allergy	Caution with patients with cerebral or coronary insufficiency, postural hypotension, and renal or hepatic failure Central nervous system effects and respiratory arrest in young children
Carbonic anhydrase inhibitors	Decrease production	Brinzolamide, dorzolamide	15%–20%	Corneal endothelial compromise Ocular irritation, dryness Burning sensation	Topical systemic effects are rare and may include: Stevens-Johnson syndrome Toxic epidermal necrosis
Cholinergic agonists	Increase outflow	Pilocarpine, carbachol	20%–25%	Ocular irritation Reduced vision or poor vision at night due to miosis and/or ciliary spasm in younger patients	Headaches due to ciliary spasm in young patients
Rho kinase inhibitors	Increase outflow	Netarsudil	20%–25%	Conjunctival hyperemia Corneal deposits (visually insignificant) Subconjunctival hemorrhage, mild	Minimal systemic effects
Combination medications	(See individual medications)	Brimonidine and timolol, dorzolamide and timolol, brinzolamide and brimonidine	Varies	(See individual medications)	(See individual medications)

Data from Weinreb RN, Aung T, Medeiros FA. The pathophysiology and treatment of glaucoma: a review. *JAMA*. 2014;311(18):1901-1911; Mantravadi AV, Vadhar N. Glaucoma. *Prim Care*. 2015;42(3):437-449; and Konstas AGP, Katsanos A, Quarantet L, et al. Twenty-four hour efficacy of glaucoma medications. In: Bagetta G, Nucci C, eds. *Progress in Brain Research: New Trends in Basic and Clinical Research of Glaucoma: A Neurodegenerative Disease of the Visual System, Part B*. New York, NY: Elsevier; 2015;221:297-318.

Prognosis

Without treatment, glaucoma causes a progressive loss of vision that will eventually lead to complete blindness. Patients who are diagnosed before extensive glaucoma optic nerve atrophy and who are able to achieve good IOP control have a good prognosis for vision.

Biousse V, Newman NJ. Diagnosis and clinical features of common optic neuropathies. *Lancet Neurol.* 2016;15(13):1355-1367.

Weinreb RN, Aung T, Medeiros FA. The pathophysiology and treatment of glaucoma: a review. *JAMA.* 2014;311(18):1901-1911.

NEURO-OPHTHALMIC MANIFESTATIONS IN OLDER ADULTS

The most common cause of unilateral painless loss of vision in older individuals with cardiovascular disease associated with a disc edema in the involved eye is nonarteritic anterior ischemic optic neuropathy (NA-AION). Currently, there is no proven treatment for NA-AION; however, ongoing clinical trials have shown some promising results. Because patients with NA-AION have a 15% risk of involvement of the other eye over the next 5 years, it is important to control cardiovascular risk factors including hypertension and diabetes (if applicable) as well as diet control, exercise, low-dose aspirin (if there are no contraindications), and management of obstructive sleep apnea.

Berry S, Lin WV, Sadaka A, Lee AG. Nonarteritic anterior ischemic optic neuropathy: cause, effect, and management. *Eye Brain.* 2017;9:23-28.

Anterior Ischemic Optic Neuropathy

A less common but more vision-threatening cause of acute painful loss of vision in older adults is giant cell arteritis, which causes arteritic anterior ischemic optic neuropathy (A-AION). Common symptoms may include headache, jaw claudication, fever, weight loss, temporal tenderness, and a previous history of polymyalgia rheumatica. Less common symptoms include diplopia or transient vision loss. Unlike NA-AION, A-AION is an ophthalmic emergency requiring hospital admission and prompt administration of high-dose intravenous steroids since the risk of contralateral eye involvement is high if left untreated. Examination of these patients may reveal poor vision in the involved eye with a relative afferent pupillary defect. Funduscopy reveals a pale and swollen optic nerve. Laboratory investigations reveal an elevated erythrocyte sedimentation rate and C-reactive protein. A definitive diagnosis is made by characteristic pathologic findings on temporal artery biopsy. Patients with a positive biopsy are treated with long-term steroids or may be considered for alternate steroid-sparing regimens.

Central Retinal Artery Occlusion

Central retinal artery occlusion can cause sudden painless loss of vision due to emboli arising either from a cardiogenic source or from vessels. Symptoms preceding artery occlusion may include a transient loss of vision or amaurosis fugax lasting seconds at a time followed by complete resolution of vision. It is important to recognize these symptoms as these individuals are at high risk of developing a cerebrovascular attack (CVA) and require emergent admission for an evaluation for a CVA.

NEURODEGENERATIVE DISEASE AND THE EYE

Patients with age-related neurodegenerative diseases can have associated ocular findings. Visual variant Alzheimer disease, also known as posterior cortical atrophy (PCA), is a condition where there is predominantly atrophy of posterior cortical areas of the brain that result in visual cognitive disorders such as simultanagnosia (inability to understand the complete scene but can see individual parts of the scene), prosopagnosia (inability to recognize faces), and visual disorientation. The presentation is often confusing to the clinician as the patient might be able to see 20/20 size letters but is unable to read them and/or is unable to drive. These patients may have homonymous visual field defects but without a structural correlate to the field changes. These symptoms can disrupt daily activities and are very distressing to patients. Poor awareness of the condition by clinicians can lead to underdiagnosis. Drugs used in Alzheimer disease management such as donepezil, rivastigmine, galantamine, and memantine have been tried with some success in PCA, and when suspected, patients should be referred to a neurologist for further evaluation.

Parkinson disease is an age-related neurodegenerative condition in which patients can present with visual disabilities including difficulty reading, writing, and driving despite normal vision. These patients have a higher incidence of convergence insufficiency, which can manifest as eye strain, headache, double vision when trying to read, and difficulty concentrating on objects that are closer to the patient. In addition, these patients may have dry eyes, blepharitis, and a reduced blink rate. Treating the dry eye and blepharitis and providing specialized glasses for convergence insufficiency can help with symptomatic relief. Patients with visual-cognitive dysfunction with either PCA or Parkinson disease can be referred to low-vision services in addition to visual rehabilitation to help with activities of daily living and to potentially regain some driving ability.

Ekker MS, Janssen S, Seppi K, et al. Ocular and visual disorders in Parkinson's disease: Common but frequently overlooked. *Parkinsonism Relat Disord.* 2017;40:1-10.

Maia da Silva MN, Millington RS, Bridge H, James-Galton M, Plant GT. Visual dysfunction in posterior cortical atrophy. *Front Neurol.* 2017;8:389.

INTERACTIONS BETWEEN SYSTEMIC AND OCULAR DISEASE

SYSTEMIC MEDICATIONS AND GLAUCOMA

The use of corticosteroids, such as cortisone and prednisolone, can increase IOP. Although the majority of patients taking corticosteroids do so without a subsequent elevation in IOP, risk factors for developing increased IOP include a personal or family history of glaucoma, current status as a glaucoma suspect, and route of administration and duration of the corticosteroid treatment. Topically or intravitreally applied corticosteroids pose the highest risk. Other routes of administration in order of descending risk are intravenous, parenteral, and inhaled routes. Corticosteroid use for <2 weeks generally does not require special monitoring of IOP. However, patients taking corticosteroids chronically or at risk for glaucoma should have at least an annual eye evaluation.

Most medications that list glaucoma as a contraindication or adverse effect are concerned with the relatively uncommon, narrow-angle form of glaucoma in which the anterior chamber angle drainage system is narrow. These medications can narrow the drainage system even further, sometimes to the point of closure, which causes a rise in IOP. Classes of medications that have the potential to induce angle closure are antihistamines, antiparkinsonian drugs, antipsychotic medications, antispasmolytic agents (eg, hyoscyamine), tricyclic antidepressants, monoamine oxidase inhibitors, and topical mydriatics (eg, phenylephrine). Consultation with an eye specialist may reveal that the above medications can be used safely. These medication warnings do not apply to most glaucoma patients who have the primary open-angle form of the disease.

SYSTEMIC EFFECTS OF EYE MEDICATIONS

Medications used in ocular disease management can have significant systemic effects because drug elimination through the kidney and the liver is slower in older adults. Thus, although some medications may be safe in a younger patient, they should be avoided or administered at reduced dose in older adults. One of the most underrecognized risks of topical eye medications in older adults accompanies the use of the antiglaucoma medication timolol. Timolol is a nonselective β-blocker used in both open-angle and angle-closure glaucoma due to its efficacy in reducing aqueous production and thus lowering IOP. Timolol is known to increase the risk of falls in older adults due to bradycardia, orthostatic hypotension, cardiac failure, and possible syncope. This effect is likely due to the drug entering the nasolacrimal duct and reaching the nasal mucosa, where it is absorbed immediately into circulation by bypassing the first-pass metabolism, thus increasing the risk of acute changes in heart rate and blood pressure. As a result, a careful risk-benefit decision should be made, and if possible, an alternative antiglaucoma agent with less systemic cardiovascular effects should be considered for older adults with a history of falls, bradycardia, cardiac conduction block, or orthostatic hypotension. In cases where the indications of use outweigh the risk, systemic absorption may be decreased by instructing patients to close their eyes and block their lacrimal punctum for about 3 to 5 minutes after instillation of eye drops, which will substantially decrease systemic absorption.

Mäenpää J, Pelkonen O. Cardiac safety of ophthalmic timolol. *Expert Opin Drug Saf.* 2016;15(11):1549-1561.

SYSTEMIC MEDICATIONS AFFECTING THE EYE

A variety of medications prescribed for the treatment of systemic disease may affect the eye. One example is diphenhydramine (Benadryl), a first-generation sedating antihistaminic drug that may be taken for allergies. This medication should be avoided due to its sedative effects as well as the tendency to cause dry eyes. Hydroxychloroquine prescribed for the management of rheumatoid arthritis is associated with maculopathy. Ethambutol used to treat tuberculosis is associated with optic neuropathy. Patients using these medications should be closely monitored for signs of ocular toxicity, and if there are signs or symptoms indicating ocular involvement, consideration should be made about discontinuing the treatment. Amiodarone is a systemic agent used in the treatment of ventricular arrhythmias and is associated with ocular toxicity. One effect may be benign corneal deposits called cornea verticillata, which does not require discontinuation. Another effect is amiodarone-associated optic neuropathy (AAON), a potentially reversible cause of optic neuropathy that presents with gradual progressive unilateral or, more commonly, bilateral vision loss. In patients with AAON, a prompt referral to an ophthalmologist for additional evaluation is recommended. Cessation of amiodarone in consultation with the patient's cardiologist should be considered because over half of patients with AAON have some restoration of vision following cessation. Finally, medications to treat erectile dysfunction, such as phosphodiesterase inhibitors, used alone or in conjunction with other blood pressure–lowering agents, are known to increase the risk of development of NA-AION, which can lead to permanent vision loss. Although the evidence is not conclusive, these medications should be used with caution in patients with chronic conditions such as diabetes and hypertension, and patients should be informed of the risks.

Liu B, Zhu L, Zhong J, Zeng G, Deng T. The association between phosphodiesterase type 5 inhibitor use and risk of non-arteritic anterior ischemic optic neuropathy: a systematic review and meta-analysis. *Sex Med.* 2018;6(3):185-192.

Passman RS, Bennett CL, Purpura JM, et al. Amiodarone-associated optic neuropathy: a critical review. *Am J Med.* 2012;125(5):447-453.

Wasinska-Borowiec W, Aghdam KA, Saari JM, Grzybowski A. An updated review on the most common agents causing toxic optic neuropathies. *Curr Pharm Des.* 2017;23(4):586-595.

CONSIDERATIONS FOR VISUALLY IMPAIRED OLDER ADULTS

When working with older patients with or without vision impairment, there are two simple ways to maximize their vision: increase contrast and provide adequate lighting. As mentioned earlier, contrast sensitivity refers to the ability to distinguish an object from its background. Low-contrast objects are harder for older persons to detect, but these objects are markedly more difficult in those with vision impairment. Patients may demonstrate adequate acuity when tested with a high-contrast, black-on-white eye chart, and yet perform poorly when reading a low-contrast chart with light gray letters on a white background. This latter test more closely resembles the everyday situation an older adult faces when trying to step off the curb at the edge of a sidewalk. Providing adequate lighting for these patients means using a light source that brightly illuminates the object of regard without shining directly into the eyes or producing excessive reflections. This typically involves use of an indirect, high-wattage light source.

In addition to receiving medical eye care, patients with vision impairment will often benefit from referral to a low-vision specialist. These eye doctors specialize in maximizing the patient's remaining functional vision through customized optical devices, such as strong reading glasses, telescopes, magnifiers, and electronic devices that enlarge and project reading material onto a video screen. Their efforts often include collaboration with rehabilitation specialists who, in addition to working directly with visually impaired patients, can recommend the use of nonoptical aids, such as large-print books and newspapers, free library audiobooks, and special telephones, clocks, or dials (eg, oven or cooktop) equipped with large, high-contrast numerals.

USEFUL WEBSITE

Lighthouse (provides more information on visual rehabilitation services, education, research, prevention, and advocacy). http://www.lighthouseguild.org. Accessed March 8, 2020.

Managing Hearing Impairment

8

Lindsey Merrihew Haddock, MD
Margaret I. Wallhagen, PhD, GNP-BC

ESSENTIALS OF DIAGNOSIS

▶ Hearing loss is a common but underrecognized medical problem in older adults.

▶ Screening can and should be done during routine office visits and takes just a few minutes.

▶ Patients with a positive screen should be referred to an audiologist and counseled on the impact hearing loss has on overall health.

▶ Providers can take simple steps to improve communication with individuals with hearing loss, including making their setting hearing friendly through minor modifications.

▶ General Principles

Hearing loss is highly prevalent in older individuals but is often overlooked as a potential contributor to morbidity in this population. In the United States, an estimated 26.7 million adults 50 years of age or older suffer from bilateral hearing loss of 25 decibels (dB) or greater. The prevalence of hearing loss increases dramatically with age, affecting approximately 45% of adults in their 70s and up to 80% of adults over age 85. Interestingly, the percentage of older adults who self-identify as hearing impaired is much lower; only about one-third of older adults in their last 2 years of life report fair or poor hearing. Although the hearing of many of these individuals could be helped with current technology, evidence suggests that this population is vastly undertreated. For example, approximately 67% to 86% of adults in the United States who might benefit from hearing aids do not use them. The stigma associated with hearing loss and hearing aid use impacts access to care and use of hearing aids and reinforces the importance of the health care

provider's role in helping individuals realize that hearing loss is a health concern.

Hearing loss affects an individual's ability to communicate effectively but is often erroneously perceived as a normal part of aging, both by patients and health care providers. However, current evidence points out its negative health effects. Studies show that hearing loss can lead to social isolation, depression, and increased cognitive effort. It has also been associated with poorer cognitive function and increased falls. Older individuals in their last 2 years of life who self-report hearing loss also report lower life satisfaction when compared to peers. Such significant negative outcomes warrant routine screening for and treatment of hearing loss in patients.

▶ Prevention

Age-related hearing loss (ARHL) in older adults represents the sequelae of multiple insults that can progressively damage the cochlea over time superimposed on age-related changes. Although many of these factors cannot be modified (eg, intrinsic aging of the cochlea, sex, genetic predisposition), several factors (eg, noise exposure, ototoxic medication use, cardiovascular health) can be controlled and are discussed in the following sections.

▶ Clinical Findings

A. Symptoms & Signs

1. Patient interview—Patients are often unaware of their hearing loss, especially when it progresses gradually over many years. It is useful to ask a patient if they have difficulty hearing in large groups or in loud, crowded venues; if they have trouble on the phone; if they often ask people to repeat what they have said; or if others have suggested they may have trouble hearing. The interviewee may note that they can hear but that people mumble or just speak too softly. Answers to these questions can provide clues about the presence of hearing loss. If the patient is aware of the hearing loss, the time course and nature of the progression can provide insights into the etiology. To obtain information that helps differentiate ARHL from other conditions that have hearing loss as a concurrent symptom (discussed later under differential diagnoses), it is important to ask about ringing or buzzing (tinnitus), ear pain (otalgia), ear drainage (otorrhea), dizziness (vertigo, disequilibrium), other neurologic deficits, and cranial neuropathies. Asking about a history of intense and/or prolonged noise exposure, chemotherapy exposure, ear trauma, head trauma, ear surgery, or ear infections (even remotely as a child or young adult) is an important component of any interview and can help identify possible risk factors for hearing loss.

2. Family member/friend interview—The impetus for the hearing loss–related office visit may be an insightful family member or friend. They are often the first to notice that the patient is asking others to repeat themselves or misunderstanding words or entire conversations. They may note that they have to speak louder to interact with the patient, that the patient may not hear them when speaking from a different room, or that the patient turns the radio or television volume to a level that sounds too loud to other listeners. Interviewing people who spend time with the patient can be helpful in detecting more subtle hearing impairments.

3. Physical exam findings—The ear should be inspected with an otoscope and the external auditory canal (EAC) and tympanic membrane (TM) fully visualized. Cerumen can accumulate in the EAC and cause some hearing loss if it fully occludes the EAC. Of note, cerumen can vary depending on a person's background. Cerumen in persons identifying as white or black tends to be yellow and sticky, while those identifying as Asian or Native American tend to have cerumen that tends to be dry and white. However, in general, the ear canal can become more constricted with age, and cerumen tends to become drier and less mobile; these changes can increase the likelihood of cerumen impaction in older adults. The EAC can also be occluded by other masses, such as tumors, granulation tissue, cysts, polyps, or even a foreign body. The TM should be translucent and grayish in color. Any perforation of the TM, drainage from the TM or middle ear, masses behind the TM (in the middle ear), middle ear effusion, or significant thickening of the TM is abnormal and may cause hearing loss. A tuning fork exam should also be performed, ideally with a 512-Hz tuning fork, using two techniques. A Weber test is performed by placing the tuning fork on a bony prominence in the midline, most often on the upper forehead, to identify any lateralization of sound. A normal test is heard equally in both ears. A Rinne test compares bone conduction to air conduction of each ear by, first, placing the tuning fork on the bony prominence at the tip of the mastoid behind the ear (bone conduction) and, then,

Table 8–1. Interpretation of tuning fork tests.

Results of Weber Test	Results of Rinne Test	Interpretation
Sound does not lateralize	Air conduction greater than bone conduction bilaterally	No hearing loss or equal sensorineural hearing loss bilaterally
Sound does not lateralize	Bone conduction greater than air conduction bilaterally	Equal conductive hearing loss bilaterally
Sound lateralizes to one side	Air conduction greater than bone conduction bilaterally	Sensorineural hearing loss on the side opposite of the lateralization
Sound lateralizes to one side	Bone conduction greater than air conduction on the side of lateralization	Conductive hearing loss on the side of lateralization
Sound lateralizes to one side	Bone conduction greater than air conduction bilaterally	Bilateral conductive hearing loss, greater on the side of lateralization

comparing its sound when held lateral to the patient's ear (air conduction). A normal (positive) Rinne test demonstrates air conduction greater than bone conduction. Table 8–1 demonstrates how to interpret the findings of tuning fork tests.

B. Special Tests

1. Screening tests—Screening can be accomplished by asking a simple question, "Do you have difficulty with your hearing?" Because individuals are often unaware of the extent of their hearing loss, it is helpful to combine the single-item question with a standardized whispered voice test or a finger rub test (Box 8–1). The Hearing Handicap Inventory for the Elderly–Screening Version (HHIE-S) (Box 8–2) is a well-validated, more detailed questionnaire that assesses the social and emotional impact of hearing loss, although notably some patients may find the questions to be dated. Data suggest that persons who screen high on the HHIE-S are more likely to be receptive to treatment and the use of hearing aids than those who score lower on the scale. Screening can also be done with a handheld instrument such as an otoscope with a built-in audiometer, and hearing screening apps are becoming available on cellular phones. In August 2012, the US Preventive Services Task Force reported that current evidence was insufficient to assess the balance of benefits and harms of screening for hearing loss in asymptomatic adults aged 50 and older; however, the topic is currently being updated. Although there is little published evidence showing a benefit to screening asymptomatic individuals, screening may help patients recognize hearing problems and offer an opportunity to provide counseling and education on the value of

Box 8–1. Standardized Whispered Voice and Finger Rub Test

Have patient seated in a quiet exam room with space behind the patient for the examiner to stand.

Whispered Voice Test	Finger Rub Test
• Tell the patient you will be saying a three-item combination of letters and numbers in a very soft, whispered voice, which they will be asked to repeat.	• To make the sound, rub the thumb across the middle fingers of the same hand.
• Demonstrate by saying "four K two" in a normal voice (making sure the patient knows you will be actually be whispering the sequences for this assessment).	• Demonstrate the sound, and have the patient raise the hand on the side of the perceived signal when they hear the sound.
• Have patient close eyes and press on the tragus to occlude the ear canal of the nontested side.	• Have patient close their eyes, and stand behind the patient. Hold both arms extended laterally, equidistant from examiner and patient's ears (about 27 inches from ears).
• Stand at arm's length behind the patient.	• Perform a strong finger rub by rubbing fingers as strongly as possible without snapping for approximately 5 seconds on one side.
• Quietly exhale, and then whisper "eight M three" and ask the participant to repeat what was said.	• If the patient reports hearing the sound, the test is complete for that ear. If not, perform a second time. If the patient hears it the second time, perform a third time.
• If response is correct, test is complete. If incorrect, whisper "K five R."	• Perform on both ears.
• Perform on second ear, using "two J seven" for the first test and "S four G" for the second test if needed.	• Patients who do not hear the first finger rub are considered at risk for possible hearing loss for that ear unless they hear the rub on both the second and third attempts.
• If two or fewer items are correctly identified for one ear, the patient is at risk for loss in that ear.	

Data from Pirozzo S, Papinczak T, Glasziou P. Whispered voice test for screening for hearing impairment in adults and children: systematic review. *BMJ* 2003 Oct 25;327(7421):967 and Torres-Russotto D, Landau WM, Harding GW, et al. Calibrated finger rub auditory screening test (CALFRAST), 2009 May 5;72(18):1595-1600.

Box 8–2. Hearing Handicap Inventory for the Elderly–Screening Version

Instructions: Do not skip questions if you avoid a situation due to a hearing problem. If you use a hearing aid, answer based on how you hear without the hearing aid.

Possible responses are "yes," "sometimes," and "no," scored as 4, 2, and 0 points, respectively.

Does a hearing problem cause you to feel embarrassed when meeting new people?

Does a hearing problem cause you to feel frustrated when talking to members of your family?

Do you have difficulty hearing when someone speaks in a whisper?

Do you feel handicapped by a hearing problem?

Does a hearing problem cause you difficulty when visiting friends, relatives, or neighbors?

Does a hearing problem cause you to attend religious services less often than you would like?

Does a hearing problem cause you to have arguments with family members?

Does a hearing problem cause you difficulty when listening to TV or radio?

Do you feel that any difficulty with hearing limits or hampers your personal or social life?

Does a hearing problem cause you difficulty when in a restaurant with relatives or friends?

Scoring: 0–8, no handicap; 10–24, mild/moderate handicap; 36–40, severe handicap.

Reproduced with permission from Ventry IM, Weinstein BE. Identification of elderly people with hearing problems, *ASHA* 1983 Jul;25(7):37-42.

assistive technology and communication techniques. Screening may also be valuable in populations at high risk for hearing loss such as individuals on ototoxic medications or with a history of noise exposure. In addition, with data increasingly documenting the negative health effects of hearing loss, the value of screening is becoming clearer.

2. Referral to audiology and otolaryngology—Patients who acknowledge they have hearing loss or are identified as at risk for hearing loss should be referred to an audiologist with master- or doctoral-level training for formal audiometric testing. Referral to a hearing aid dispenser (or hearing aid specialist) can also be considered. The training for these

Table 8–2. Indications for otolaryngologic referral.

Impacted cerumen that cannot be removed
Mass in the external auditory canal
Significant otorrhea
Persistent otalgia
Persistent perforation of the tympanic membrane
Persistent middle ear effusion
Mass in the middle ear
Severe infection of the external auditory canal or middle ear
Associated vertigo or disequilibrium
Associated cranial neuropathies
Asymmetric hearing loss
Fluctuating hearing loss
Hearing loss for which an audiogram does not provide adequate explanation

individuals varies from state to state, with some having only a high school degree. Referral to an otolaryngology physician is warranted when a medical concern exists (Table 8–2).

▶ Differential Diagnosis

Sensorineural hearing loss (SNHL) constitutes 92% of hearing loss in older adults, with the remainder being conductive or mixed (both sensorineural and conductive components). In the vast majority of cases, hearing loss in older adults is multifactorial, and many etiologies concurrently lead to hearing loss over time. Of note, subjective tinnitus, a perception of sound or noise in the absence of an external source, can accompany any type of hearing loss. The sound is often perceived as some form of buzzing, ringing, or hissing, but can be perceived as similar to other noises and varies greatly in how bothersome it is to the individual. Because tinnitus can have a significant impact on an individual's quality of life and functional ability, it is important to assess how bothersome it is and how much it interferes with the individual's life and refer for further assessment and treatment as needed.

A. Sensorineural Hearing Loss (Inner Ear Disease)

1. Presbycusis—An audiogram typical of presbycusis (ARHL) shows a down-sloping SNHL, in which the higher frequencies (toward 8 kHz) are more severely affected than lower frequencies (toward 250 Hz) (Figure 8–1). This has important implications for speech understanding because consonants tend to be higher frequency and give language meaning while vowels tend to be lower frequency and give language audibility, as depicted in the figure. Thus, patients often are unaware of their degree of hearing impairment because of its gradual progression over many years but also because they "hear" parts of words but they can be muffled or misinterpreted, thus leading to misunderstandings. In some patients, hearing loss may be accelerated due to hereditary factors.

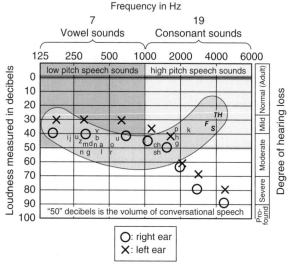

▲ **Figure 8–1.** Audiogram of presbycusis (age-related hearing loss) with an overlying diagram showing the frequency at which different speech sounds are heard. Higher frequencies tend to be more affected by age-related hearing loss than the lower frequencies. Because consonants tend to be higher frequency and are especially important to speech understanding, age-related hearing loss can significantly impair a patient's ability to understand the meaning of what is said.

2. Noise damage—Noise-induced hearing loss can result either from prolonged exposure to noise, in which case the hearing loss would be permanent and develop gradually over months to years, or from brief, sudden exposure to intense noise, in which case the hearing loss may be immediate but be temporary or permanent. However, even if hearing returns to baseline after brief exposure to a very loud sound, such as at a concert or sports event, data suggest there may be ongoing damage occurring in the inner ear that can have long-term effects on hearing capacity. Noise-induced hearing loss may be prevented or minimized with avoidance and use of earplugs and other hearing protective devices.

3. Other medical causes—There are numerous medical problems that can cause or contribute to hearing loss, including infection, autoimmune inner ear disease, systemic and vascular disease, chronic conditions such as diabetes and HIV, trauma, and acoustic neuroma. Acoustic neuroma should be excluded in patients with unilateral hearing loss.

4. Ototoxic medications—Signs and symptoms that a patient may be experiencing ototoxic effects include the development of new tinnitus, vertigo or disequilibrium, and difficulty hearing. If these symptoms develop, the patient should be evaluated and the drug should be stopped

Table 8–3. Common ototoxic medications.

Aminoglycoside antibiotics
Gentamicin
Amikacin
Neomycin
Streptomycin
Vancomycin
Erythromycin
Antimalarials
Chloroquine
Quinine
Platinum-based chemotherapy agents
Cisplatin
Carboplatin
Loop diuretics
Furosemide
Torsemide
Nonsteroidal anti-inflammatory drugs
Aspirin
Ketorolac

immediately if possible. Additionally, if a patient is on ototoxic medications or has had recent exposure to an ototoxic medication, such as chemotherapy, screening for hearing loss periodically is recommended. Table 8–3 lists some of the most common ototoxic medications.

5. Ménière disease—This condition is characterized by episodic rotational vertigo that is typically debilitating and lasts from 20 minutes to 24 hours, but usually 1 to 2 hours. It is associated with fluctuating low-frequency hearing loss, aural fullness, and tinnitus. The symptoms almost always begin unilaterally, but the contralateral ear may become involved in up to 50% of patients over time. The natural history is a relapsing and remitting course with the disease often "burning out" over time. Recurrent attacks can lead to a permanent SNHL.

6. Sudden sensorineural hearing loss—Sudden SNHL is a sudden decrease in hearing thresholds of 30 dB or greater at three contiguous audiometric frequencies occurring over 72 hours or less. It is an otologic emergency that occurs in an estimated 5 to 20 per 100,000 people per year. The primary goal in managing these patients is the prevention of permanent SNHL through prompt referral to an otolaryngologist for confirmation and treatment with steroids within 24 to 48 hours. Distinguishing between sudden SNHL (requiring immediate referral) and an acute conductive loss from an ear infection or middle ear effusion (treated with simple antibiotics or a nasal steroid spray and not requiring urgent referral) can often be done using the tuning fork tests described earlier and a careful ear exam.

7. Radiation—A history of radiation to the head or neck, either for a neoplastic process or as a result of environmental exposure, can lead to SNHL by direct damage to the inner ear and auditory nerve.

B. Conductive Hearing Loss (Middle or External Ear Disease)

Conductive hearing losses are far less common than SNHLs in older adults and can often be diagnosed in the clinic by otoscopic examination or through tuning fork testing. Common causes include EAC obstruction (eg, cerumen), TM perforations, middle ear effusions, and ossicular chain pathology. Middle ear effusions caused by eustachian tube dysfunction can often be treated with intranasal steroids and oral antibiotics (if there is a concern for acute otitis media) and followed conservatively for 2 months. Failure of resolution or concern for any other etiology for a conductive hearing loss warrants referral to an otolaryngologist.

► **Complications**

Hearing loss impairs verbal communication, can lead to poorer social functioning and isolation, and strains relationships between partners and family members. Partners may initially feel ignored before they realize that the person has a hearing loss. They frequently get frustrated from having to repeat all the time and are not aware of, or forget to use, effective communication strategies. Both partners can experience fatigue because of the effort it takes to listen and understand.

In addition to impairing verbal communication, epidemiologic evidence demonstrating that ARHL is independently associated with cognitive and physical functioning in older adults is beginning to surface. ARHL has now been found to be independently associated with poorer neurocognitive functioning on both verbal and nonverbal tests of executive function and memory, accelerated cognitive decline, and incident dementia. Cognitive resources are also critical for gait, balance, and other tasks, such as driving. Recent studies demonstrate that ARHL is associated with poorer balance, falls, and impaired driving ability. These relationships may be mediated through the effects of hearing on cognitive load or from reduced awareness of the auditory environment. In addition, ARHL impairs one's ability to hear high-frequency sounds used to communicate danger such as sirens and smoke alarms, and thus impacts the safety of older adults with hearing loss.

Hearing loss not only affects the safety and physical, cognitive, and social functioning of older adults, but also their health care costs. Recent studies have shown that adults with untreated hearing loss experience significantly higher health care costs and higher health care utilization rates than those without hearing loss and have higher rates of 30-day readmissions.

► Treatment

Most often, the difficulty in treating or attempting to address hearing loss in older adults is convincing them, first, that they have a hearing loss and that it has potentially significant implications for healthy aging and, second, that current treatment can help them to hear better and improve many aspects of their lives.

A. Adaptive Techniques

There are numerous adaptive techniques that can be employed to improve communication with individuals with hearing loss; strategies that providers can use when communicating with individuals with hearing loss are outlined in Table 8-4.

Table 8-4. Improving communication with individuals with hearing loss.

Positioning
- Face the patient directly.
- Keep your mouth visible; do not to cover your mouth with your hand, look down, or turn away when speaking (especially when you are typing on a computer).

Lighting
- Use adequate lighting; the light should shine on your (the speaker's) face and not be behind you.

Correct visual impairment
- Make sure that glasses are worn when needed.

Attention
- Make sure you have the patient's attention.
- Introduce the topic or subject matter and indicate if the subject shifts focus.

Speech
- Speak at a normal volume; don't shout.
- Enunciate clearly without using exaggerated lip movements.
- If possible, lower the pitch of your voice if it tends to be high.

Repetition
- Rephrase sentences instead of repeating them. If the individual says "what" or indicates they did not understand, use different words that may be heard more clearly.

Assistive listening devices
- Use a pocket talker (personal amplifier).
- If hearing aids are used, make sure they are in place and that the batteries are charged; batteries have a relatively short life span of a few days, especially if the hearing aid is heavily used or streaming and blue tooth are actively used.

Assessing understanding
- Beware of misunderstandings that may be perceived as cognitive impairment.
- Provide written information.
- Have the individual repeat what they heard and understood.

Home safety
- Elicit input on best ways to communicate about an emergency.
- Consider recommending low-frequency home alarms and captioned phones.

Individuals with hearing loss should directly face the person with whom they are speaking and stand so the light is behind them and shines on the person's face to whom they are speaking. Family members and friends can be encouraged to speak at a normal volume, enunciate clearly, keep hands and other items away from in front of their mouths, and rephrase sentences instead of repeating them when asked. Also, training in speech reading, word recognition, and active listening has shown some benefit in these patients. Individuals can also benefit from aural rehabilitation classes and local support groups, such as local chapters of the Hearing Loss Association of America.

B. Environmental Modifications

People with hearing loss should place themselves at the center of the conversation, away from background noise. A setting with minimal background noise should be chosen for gatherings or conversations if possible. Selecting a table and sitting with one's back to the wall can also minimize background noise. Lighting should be adequate to see the faces of those speaking.

Clinicians who care for patients with hearing loss should consider making their practice "hearing friendly" by arranging exam rooms such that providers can continuously face patients and do not have to turn away from the patient to use the computer or access the medical record. Most patients with hearing loss note difficulty hearing their name called in a waiting room, so staff should be trained to seat patients with hearing loss closest to where their name will be called. Other strategies include "looping" the check-in counter for use with persons with T-coils (discussed later) and using devices that can be given to the person that will flash a light or vibrate when their name is called. Arrangements should be made for persons who have difficulty on the phone if calls are made to discuss treatments or to confirm or make appointments. Information related to important test results, treatment, and follow-up should be provided in writing.

C. Assistive Listening Devices

Multiple devices exist that allow for improved communication through personal amplification without hearing aids. These can be useful in a patient who would like hearing aids but cannot afford or manage them. Assistive listening devices (ALDs) typically use a microphone placed close to the desired sound and transmit this sound to the patient. One device is a personal amplifier or "pocket talker," which amplifies nearby sound and sends it to the user through earphones. All providers who work with patients with hearing loss should have access to a pocket talker and be familiar with its use. Many public venues also have listening systems that send sound from the speaker or area of interest to the user through infrared or frequency modulation (FM) signals. Other devices include amplified telephones, telecommunication devices for the deaf (also known as text telephones), closed captioning for television, vibrating alarm clocks, and visual alarm systems (eg, doorbells and smoke alarms). Persons with hearing loss may also be eligible for home captioned phones. These are phones with screens that allow the person with hearing loss to read as well as listen to what is said. It is possible to now use other screens such as computers. This is a free service that is paid for by a charge included in all phone bills. Further, captioning is increasingly available on cellular phones through a variety of apps.

D. Audiologic Evaluation

The goal of the audiologist or hearing aid specialist is not to simply fit a hearing aid, but to ensure that a patient can effectively communicate in all settings. The hearing rehabilitative process, therefore, entails counseling, proper fitting of hearing aids and amplification devices, rehabilitation, and training in the use of other systems such as ALDs, amplified telephones, and hearing loop induction systems. To identify an audiologist or hearing aid specialist who shares these goals, ask the following: Do they offer regular audiologic rehabilitation sessions for their patients? Do they have an induction loop system installed in their office? Are they a member of the Academy of Rehabilitative Audiology, an organization focused on the comprehensive management of hearing loss? Given the fee-for-service model of most audiologic services that are rarely covered by insurance, it is vital to distinguish between audiologists committed to comprehensive rehabilitative care from those who are focused only on hearing aids.

E. Hearing Aids

Up to 67% to 86% of adults in the United States who might benefit from hearing aids use do not use them, despite the evidence for improved speech perception, understanding, and hearing-related quality of life, including social, emotional, and mental well-being. This may be a result of hearing aids' cost, appearance, comfort, and performance in different environments. Many patients also do not realize that it will require a period of adjustment and that they need to work closely with their audiologist to maximize the benefit from using a hearing aid. It can be helpful to reinforce to the individual that their brain has to relearn how to listen, especially if they have had untreated hearing loss for some time, and that hearing aids are *aids*—they do not cure or fix the underlying damage that has occurred to the inner ear. However, another barrier is that, in the United States, most insurance carriers do not cover the cost of hearing aids, which on average cost approximately $1500 each, with premium models costing $3000 to $5000 each. It is important for the individual to check prices because they can vary significantly between practices and settings. Increasingly, large pharmacies and other businesses, such as CVS or Costco, are offering hearing services at lower prices. In 2017, Congress passed the Over-the-Counter Hearing Aid Act, which will allow adults with mild to moderate hearing loss to purchase hearing aids over the counter. These will come on the market once the

standards, guidelines, and labeling are finalized. Not everyone will be eligible for these devices, so guidance will be needed when they begin to be sold.

1. Types of hearing aids—Digital hearing aids have become standard over the past decade and offer size and performance advantages over the bulky analog hearing aids commonly used a decade ago. There are four main types: behind the ear, in the ear, in the ear canal, and completely in the ear canal.

2. Selection and fitting of hearing aids—When patients are referred to audiology, they should be counseled on the expected course of adjustment and the need for multiple visits to optimize the performance of their hearing aids. Generally, after a comprehensive audiometric assessment, the audiologist will adjust the hearing aid to the patient's specific type of hearing loss. Efforts are made to maximize the patient's hearing capacity in settings that they feel are most essential for their functioning with consideration of their preferences for appearance, functionality, and cost. However, what is most important is that the individual select the hearing aid that best addresses their hearing loss and not choose a hearing aid based on its visibility. Once the hearing aid is chosen and fitted, the patient should take part in aural rehabilitative training, which audiologists should offer to all their patients. During aural rehabilitation, patients are educated in the proper use of the hearing aid and its management in different environments, effective strategies to enhance speech perception and communication, and strategies to cope and deal with difficulties that may arise during use. Successful amplification requires an ongoing effort by the audiologist and the patient over multiple visits. Patients also need to understand that batteries have a limited life and need to be changed frequently, depending on use and the types of assistive devices used with the hearing aid.

3. Assistive listening devices for use with hearing aids—Although hearing aids perform well when the sound source is within a 6-foot radius, at farther distances, they perform less well. Some public venues are equipped with technology that can transmit sound directly to hearing aids through FM, infrared, or induction loop systems. These improve sound quality by increasing the signal-to-noise ratio. That is, the "signal," or what one wants to hear, is significantly louder or more prominent than the background or interfering sounds (noise). Of particular interest, induction loops or "hearing loops" directly transmit sound to the two-thirds of hearing aids currently equipped with a telecoil, dramatically improving sound quality. The system involves a thin wire that is placed around the periphery of a room or area, allowing sound to be transmitted to the telecoil through induction. Such systems are installed in concert halls, ticket booths at train stations, houses of worship, and anywhere background noise or proximity to the sound of interest may interfere with communication. Persons purchasing a hearing aid should discuss the types of assistive devices that might be more appropriate and that are also compatible with the hearing aid. They should also be told about assuring that any cellular phone they purchase is compatible with their hearing aid and that they have a right to test compatibility.

4. Cochlear implants—Cochlear implants are surgically implanted neuroprosthetic devices that are used to treat profound SNHL in patients who do not gain appreciable benefit from optimized hearing aid use. The surgery is typically a 2-hour outpatient operation performed by an otolaryngologist who implants an electrode array into the cochlea by way of a mastoidectomy. The electrode array is a form of technology that sends electric signals from an implant device directly to the cochlea. Unlike hearing aids, cochlear implants directly stimulate the auditory nerve, functionally replacing the role of the impaired cochlea. Cochlear implantation can substantially improve the ability of older adults to communicate. Many older adults improve from no word comprehension preoperatively (without the aid of visual cues) to 100% comprehension several months after surgery. There are no age contraindications to cochlear implant surgery, with many implant centers routinely performing cochlear implantation in adults in their 80s and 90s. Candidates for cochlear implantation are those who have severe-to-profound SNHL even while using optimized bilateral hearing aids. Typically, even while maximally aided, these patients score <40% to 50% on word or sentence recognition testing. Patients should be counseled on the need for aural rehabilitation after cochlear implantation to adjust to a different sound quality; patients who benefit most from this procedure have the cognitive ability and motivation to engage in aural rehabilitation.

▶ **Prognosis**

ARHL generally progresses over time and, if left untreated, can contribute to social isolation, cognitive load, and morbidity in older adults. Although there is currently no definitive evidence on whether treating hearing loss can mitigate these negative outcomes, data suggest that use of hearing aids can improve quality of life, social engagement, and relationships. Furthermore, data increasingly suggest that treating hearing loss may decrease health care costs and improve patient experiences in the health care settings. Practitioners can play an important role in promoting hearing health care by being aware of the prevalence and importance of hearing loss to health, using simple screening measures, and referring patients who screen positive or acknowledge hearing loss to qualified hearing care specialists for treatment.

SUMMARY

Hearing loss is a common but underrecognized condition in older adults that is often incorrectly dismissed as a part of normal aging. However, hearing loss has important consequences for older adults' cognitive and physical functioning, in addition to their quality of life. Providers can help recognize hearing loss by screening patients and then referring those who screen positive to audiologists for further treatment. The provider also plays a critical role in reducing stigma around hearing loss and educating patients on the importance of treating hearing loss to improve function and quality of life. Communication with persons with hearing loss can be improved with simple adaptive techniques, environmental modifications, and ALDs. All patients with hearing loss should be evaluated by an audiologist to determine if hearing aids are appropriate, and patients should be referred to audiologists who offer comprehensive aural rehabilitation to help patient adapt to their hearing aids to receive the maximum benefit from their use.

Bainbridge KE, Ramachandran V. Hearing aid use among older U.S. adults; the national health and nutrition examination survey, 2005-2006 and 2009-2010. *Ear Hear.* 2014;35(3):289-294.

Chang J, Weinstein B, Chodosh J, Blustein J. Hospital readmission risk for patients with self-reported hearing loss and communication trouble. *J Am Geriatr Soc.* 2018;66(11):2227-2228.

Loughrey DG, Kelly ME, Kelley GA, Brennan S, Lawlor BA. Association of age-related hearing loss with cognitive function, cognitive impairment, and dementia: a systematic review and meta-analysis. *JAMA Otolaryngol Head Neck Surg.* 2018;144(2):115-126.

National Academies of Sciences, Engineering, and Medicine, Blazer D, Liverman C, Domnitz S, eds. *Hearing Health Care: Priorities for Improving Access and Affordability.* Washington, DC: National Academies Press; June 2, 2016.

Reed NS, Altan A, Deal JA, Yeh C, Kravetz AD, Wallhagen M, Lin FR. Trends in health care costs and utilization associated with untreated hearing loss over 10 years. *JAMA Otolaryngol Head Neck Surg.* 2019;145(1):27-34.

Smith AK, Ritchie CS, Miao Y, Boscardin WJ, Wallhagen ML. Self-reported hearing in the last 2 years of life in older adults. *J Am Geriatr Soc.* 2016;64(7):1486-1491.

Strawbridge WJ, Wallhagen MI. Simple tests compare well with a hand-held audiometer for hearing loss screening in primary care. *J Am Geriatr Soc.* 2017;65(10):2282-2284.

US Preventive Services Task Force. Final update summary: hearing loss in older adults: screening. September 2016. https://www.uspreventiveservicestaskforce.org/Page/Document/UpdateSummaryFinal/hearing-loss-in-older-adults-screening. Accessed March 8, 2020.

Wallhagen MS. Stigma: what does the literature say? *Hear J.* 2018;71(9):14-16.

Cognitive Impairment & Dementia

9

Kaycee M. Sink, MD, MAS

Kristine Yaffe, MD

ESSENTIALS OF DIAGNOSIS

- ▶ Impairment in at least two of the following cognitive domains: memory, executive function, language, visuo-spatial function, and personality/behavior.
- ▶ Significant impairment in social or occupational functioning.
- ▶ Significant decline from previous level of function.
- ▶ Deficits not occurring solely in the presence of delirium or accounted for by major psychiatric disorder.

▶ General Considerations

The prevalence of dementia approximately doubles every 5 years after 60 years. Among community-dwelling elders older than 85 years, the prevalence is estimated to be 25% to 45%. Prevalence is even higher in nursing homes (>50%). Approximately 60% to 70% of dementia cases are attributable to Alzheimer disease (AD), either alone or mixed with Lewy body dementia (DLB) or vascular dementia (VaD), the next two most common forms of dementia in older adults. Fronto-temporal dementia (FTD) is typically thought of as a common cause of early-onset dementia (age of onset <65 years old) and is less common in older adults, although likely underdiagnosed.

Cognitive function in older adults is considered a spectrum and ranges from cognitive changes seen in normal aging to mild cognitive impairment (MCI) to dementia. Compared with younger adults, older adults often perform more slowly on timed tasks and have slower reaction times. Mild memory changes may be present with subjective problems such as difficulty recalling names or where an object was placed. In the case of normal aging, however, the person usually remembers the information later and has intact learning, and any deficits in memory function are subtle, relatively stable over time, and do not cause functional impairment.

MCI is a disorder in which cognitive function is below normal limits for that patient's age and education but is not severe enough to qualify as dementia. MCI is characterized by subjective cognitive complaints, preferably corroborated by someone else; evidence of objective cognitive impairment in one or more cognitive domains (eg, memory, language, executive function); and intact functional status. When MCI involves memory (amnestic MCI), it is associated with an increased risk of AD and often represents a very early AD process. Among patients with amnestic MCI, 10% to 15% per year convert to AD compared with 1% to 2% of age-matched controls. Although many patients with MCI will progress to AD with time, it is a clinically heterogeneous group, with some patients progressing to other types of dementias and others remaining cognitively stable. The most severe type of cognitive impairment is dementia. This diagnosis requires deficits in multiple domains of cognitive functioning (at least two) that represent a significant change from baseline and that are severe enough to cause impairment in daily functioning (see "Essentials of Diagnosis," earlier).

Dementia often goes undiagnosed or undocumented in primary care settings, especially early in the course of the disease. Cognitive impairment and dementia should be detected as early as possible in older patients so that secondary causes of cognitive impairment can be identified and addressed. Drug therapy for AD remains symptomatic (not disease modifying) and may improve a patient's quality of life, extend the period of relatively good function, and delay nursing home placement. In addition, early diagnosis allows patients and caregivers to plan future needs and for primary practitioners to adjust medication regimens and assess treatment goals.

McKhann GM, Knopman DS, Chertkow H, et al. The diagnosis of dementia due to Alzheimer's disease: recommendations from the National Institute on Aging-Alzheimer's Association workgroups on diagnostic guidelines for Alzheimer's disease. *Alzheimers Dement.* 2011;7(3):263-269.

Prevention

At this time, there are no proven strategies to prevent MCI or dementia. However, control of vascular risk factors such as hypertension, hyperlipidemia, and diabetes may reduce the risk of both AD and VaD. Recent results from a large hypertension treatment trial (SPRINT) showed that treating systolic blood pressure to a goal of <120 mm Hg resulted in statistically significant reduction in risk of MCI (hazard ratio [HR], 0.81) and in the combined outcome of MCI or all-cause dementia (HR, 0.85) after a median of 3.3 years of treatment. In addition, evidence is accumulating that regular physical activity (including walking) may be an important behavioral strategy for reducing the risk of cognitive impairment and dementia. Cognitive activity such as mental exercises, moderate alcohol intake, and nutritional strategies may also reduce risk, but more data are needed. Both depression and smoking are linked to increased risk of dementia, and they should be screened for in older adults. Gingko biloba, nonsteroidal anti-inflammatory drugs (NSAIDs), statins, estrogens, and vitamin E are *not* recommended for prevention because they have failed to delay or prevent dementia in large clinical trials and, in some cases, may cause harm.

Livingston G, Summerland A, Ortega V, et al. Dementia prevention, intervention, and care. *Lancet.* 2017;390:2673-2734.

The SPRINT-MIND Investigators for the SPRINT Research Group. Effect of intensive vs standard blood pressure control on probable dementia: a randomized clinical trial. *JAMA.* 2019;321(6):553-561.

Yaffe K. Modifiable risk factors and prevention of dementia: what is the latest evidence? *JAMA Intern Med.* 2018;178(2):281-282.

Clinical Findings

A. Patient History

The history is the most important part of the evaluation of a patient with possible cognitive impairment or dementia. Although it may be unreliable, eliciting the history first from the patient can be very informative and useful. Allowing patients to give their version of the history also enables assessment of recent and remote memory. Questions about their medical and surgical history as well as current medications may help to assess both recent and remote memory. For example, if a patient has denied any medical or surgical history, the discovery of a large abdominal surgical scar on examination is very informative.

Because the history from a patient with cognitive impairment can be incomplete and incorrect, it is crucial to also obtain history from a family member, caregiver, or other source. The history should focus on how long the symptoms have been present, whether they began gradually or abruptly, and the rate and nature (stepwise vs continual decline) of their progression. Specific areas on which to focus include the patient's ability to learn new things (eg, use of a microwave or

a remote control), language problems (eg, word-finding difficulties or absence of content), trouble with complex tasks (eg, balancing the checkbook, preparing a meal), spatial ability (eg, getting lost in familiar places), and personality changes, behavioral problems, or psychiatric symptoms (eg, delusions, hallucinations, paranoia). Obtaining a good functional assessment (see Chapter 2, "Overview of Geriatric Assessment") will help to determine the severity of impairment and the need for caregiver support or, in patients without caregivers, the need for more supervised living setting. This should include an assessment of the activities of daily living (ADLs) and instrumental activities of daily living (IADLs; eg, cooking, cleaning, shopping, managing finances, using the telephone, managing medications, and driving or arranging transportation). In addition, the clinician should assess the patient's family and social situation because information obtained may be important in developing a treatment plan.

It is crucial to obtain a detailed medication history and history of comorbid conditions, including symptoms of depression and alcohol and other substance use. Although potentially reversible causes of dementia account for <1% of cases, a large part of the workup is directed toward identifying and treating these causes. Table 9–1 summarizes the key elements of the history and physical examination.

B. Symptoms & Signs

Early signs and symptoms of dementia are often missed by both physicians and families, especially in AD, in which social graces are often retained until moderate stages of the disease. Subtle hints of early dementia or MCI may include frequent repetition of the same questions or stories, reduced participation in former hobbies, increased accidents, financial mistakes or unpaid bills, and missed appointments. Poorly controlled chronic conditions may suggest lack of adherence to medication prescriptions because of memory problems, especially if these conditions were previously well controlled. Self-neglect, difficulty handling money, and getting lost are more obvious signs.

1. Alzheimer disease—The classic triad of findings in AD is memory impairment manifested by difficulty learning and recalling information (especially new information), visuospatial problems, and language impairment, which, in combination, are severe enough to interfere with social, occupational, or daily functioning. Classically, AD patients have little or no insight into their deficits, which may be a result of their compromised executive functioning (planning, insight, and judgment). Early in the course of disease, patients with AD typically retain their social functioning and ability to accomplish overlearned, familiar tasks, but often have difficulty with more complicated tasks, such as balancing a checkbook or making complex decisions. Because symptoms are insidious and family members often dismiss the short-term memory loss as normal aging, several years may pass before the patient receives medical attention. Disorientation is common

Table 9–1. Key elements of the history and physical examination.

History

Duration of symptoms and nature of progression of symptoms

Presence of specific symptoms related to:
- Memory (recent and remote) and learning
- Language (word-finding problems, difficulty expressing self)
- Visuospatial skills (getting lost)
- Executive functioning (calculations, planning, carrying out multistep tasks)
- Apraxia (not able to do previously learned motor tasks, eg, slicing a loaf of bread)
- Behavior or personality changes
- Psychiatric symptoms (apathy, hallucinations, delusions, paranoia)

Functional assessment (activities of daily living and instrumental activities of daily living)

Social support assessment

Medical history, comorbidities

Thorough medication review, including over-the-counter medications, herbal products

Family history

Review of systems, including screening for depression and alcohol/substance abuse

Physical Examination

Cognitive examination

General physical examination with special attention to:
- Neurologic examination, looking for focal findings, extrapyramidal signs, gait and balance assessment
- Cardiovascular examination
- Signs of abuse or neglect

Screen for impairments in hearing and vision

---

among patients with AD and typically begins with disorientation to time, then place, and ultimately to person. Patients develop a progressive language disorder that begins with subtle anomic aphasia and ultimately progresses to fluent aphasia and may become nonverbal at the end stages of the disease. They have difficulty with visuospatial tasks and may be prone to getting lost, even in familiar surroundings. The disease is slowly progressive, and patients show continual decline in their ability to remain independent.

Behavioral changes are common in AD, as in most dementia subtypes, and no neuropsychiatric symptom or behavioral disturbance is pathognomonic. Early changes may be manifested by apathy and irritability (up to 70% of patients) and depression (30%–50% of patients). Agitation becomes more common as the disease progresses and may be especially notable regarding issues of grooming and dressing. Psychotic symptoms, such as delusions, hallucinations, and paranoia, are also common, affecting up to 50% of patients in moderate to advanced stages.

2. Dementia with Lewy bodies—DLB is another common form of dementia, affecting up to ~20% of patients with dementia. The core features of DLB are parkinsonism, fluctuation in cognitive impairment, recurrent visual hallucinations, and rapid eye movement (REM) sleep disorder along with dementia. These symptoms should occur in the absence of other factors that could explain them. The presence of one of these features suggests possible DLB, and the presence of two to three suggests probable DLB. Severe sensitivity to antipsychotics, severe autonomic dysfunction, syncope, and repeated falls are some of the supportive features. Biomarker evidence is not required for a diagnosis of DLB, but indicative biomarkers include polysomnographic confirmation of REM sleep disorder without atonia and reduced dopamine transporter uptake in basal ganglia demonstrated by single-photon emission computed tomography (CT) or positron emission tomography (PET) imaging (DaTscan).

The parkinsonism in patients with DLB generally presents after, or concurrent with, the onset of the dementia. This is in contrast to the Parkinson disease (PD)–related dementia, which generally occurs later in the disease. Parkinsonism in DLB is manifested primarily by rigidity and bradykinesia; tremor is less common (<10%–25% of patients in a large series). The development of parkinsonism late in the stages of a dementia is not specific for DLB because many patients with advanced AD also develop increased tone, bradykinesia, and tremor.

Like AD, DLB is insidious in onset and progressive, although it classically has a fluctuating quality on a day-to-day basis. The fluctuation is seen in the level of alertness, cognitive functioning, and functional status. Early in the course, memory and language deficits are less prominent than in AD. In contrast, visuospatial abilities, problem solving, and processing speed are more significantly impaired than in AD at the same stage. Visual hallucinations occur in 60% to 85% of autopsy-confirmed DLB patients compared with 11% to 28% of autopsy-confirmed AD patients. They are classically very vivid and often are of animals, people, or mystical things. Unlike typical psychosis, early in the course of illness, many patients with DLB can distinguish hallucinations from reality and tend not to be disturbed by them. Caution is advised in the use of antipsychotic medications to treat hallucinations or delusions because patients with DLB are exquisitely sensitive to neuroleptics (even atypical antipsychotics), and a dramatic worsening of extrapyramidal symptoms may occur. Neuroleptics should not be given as a diagnostic test because deaths have been reported among those with DLB.

3. Vascular dementia—In general, the diagnosis of VaD is based on the presence of clinical or radiographic evidence of cerebrovascular disease in a patient with dementia. Sudden onset of dementia after a stroke or stepwise, rather than continuous, decline is supportive of the diagnosis in the context of cortical strokes and focal neurologic findings on examination. However, because a considerable percentage of patients have subcortical vascular disease, the course may appear to be more gradual. In addition, many patients have mixed AD and VaD, and mild, progressive, non-VaD may suddenly be unmasked by the occurrence of a stroke.

Memory impairments in VaD are often less severe than in AD. Patients with VaD have impaired recall but tend to have better recognition and benefit from cueing in contrast to AD patients. On formal neuropsychiatric testing, "patchy" deficits may be found, often with predominant difficulty on speeded tasks and tests of executive function. As in AD, behavioral and psychological symptoms are common. Depression may be more severe in patients with VaD.

4. Frontotemporal dementia—FTD (formerly known as Pick disease) develops at a relatively young age (mean age of onset is in the late 50s). It is estimated that FTD accounts for approximately 25% of early-onset dementias. FTD is clinically (and neuropathologically) heterogeneous with three main subtypes: behavioral variant, a language variant that includes progressive nonfluent aphasia, and semantic dementia.

Behavioral variant FTD (bvFTD) is characterized by early changes in personality and behavior with relative sparing of memory and is often misdiagnosed as a psychiatric disorder. However, some symptoms are highly specific for bvFTD (eg, hyperorality, early changes in personality and behavior, early loss of social awareness [disinhibition], compulsive or repetitive behaviors, progressive reduction in speech [early], and sparing of visuospatial abilities) and reliably distinguish it from AD. The hyperorality may be manifested by marked changes in food preference (often toward junk food and carbohydrates) or simply excessive eating.

Cognitive testing in patients with FTD may reveal normal Mini-Mental Status Examination (MMSE) scores early in the disease. More formal neuropsychiatric testing reveals deficits in frontal systems tasks such as verbal fluency and other language abilities, abstraction, and executive functioning, and these deficits are seen earlier than in a typical patient with AD. In contrast to patients with AD, FTD patients tend to show preserved visuospatial abilities and relatively preserved memory, especially recognition or cued memory.

5. Other dementias—Many other diseases are associated with cognitive impairment and dementia, such as PD and its related disorders, Huntington disease (HD), HIV, and alcoholism. Approximately 30% of patients with PD develop dementia. This generally occurs late in the course of PD and is characterized by slowing of mental processing, impaired recall (but usually preserved recognition memory), executive dysfunction, and visuospatial problems. HD is a rare autosomal dominant disorder characterized by motor (chorea, dystonia), behavioral, and cognitive impairments. With the advances in HIV care and the increasing numbers of long-term survivors, HIV-associated neurocognitive disorder should be considered in the differential diagnosis of cognitive impairment. With the use of combination antiretroviral therapy, the prevalence of HIV-associated dementia has declined, but up to 60% of HIV-infected persons may suffer from some degree of cognitive impairment. Although chronic alcohol abuse impairs cognitive functioning, there is controversy as to whether a true dementia syndrome related to alcohol exists (separate from thiamine deficiency and head trauma), partly because there have been no large-scale studies.

6. Advanced & end-stage disease—The advanced symptoms of most dementias appear similar, and in late stages, it is often nearly impossible to distinguish between different types of dementia. In advanced dementia (typically with a score <10 on the MMSE), language skills are significantly impaired. There may be very little meaningful speech, and comprehension is very impaired. Some patients will progress to the point of mutism. Patients with advanced dementia have progressive difficulty with even the most basic ADLs, such as feeding themselves, and may progress to the point at which they are incontinent of bowel and bladder and are completely dependent in all ADLs. Symptoms of parkinsonism such as rigidity are common. Gait is impaired, and ultimately, patients may stop walking, leading to a bed-bound state. The risk of seizures increases with disease severity but is generally higher in AD patients throughout the course of illness than older adults without AD. Patients who do not die of other comorbidities tend to develop concomitant complications (eg, malnutrition, pressure ulcers, recurrent infections). The most common cause of death in advanced dementia is pneumonia.

Bang J, Spina S, Miller BL. Frontotemporal dementia. *Lancet.* 2015;386(10004):1672-1682.

McKeith IG, Boeve BF, Dickson DW, et al. Diagnosis and management of dementia with Lewy bodies: fourth consensus report of the DLB Consortium. *Neurology.* 2017;89(1):88-100.

McKhann GM, Knopman DS, Chertkow H, et al. The diagnosis of dementia due to Alzheimer's disease: recommendations from the National Institute on Aging-Alzheimer's Association workgroups on diagnostic guidelines for Alzheimer's disease. *Alzheimers Dement.* 2011;7(3):263-269.

C. Physical & Mental Status Examination

The physical examination of a patient with cognitive impairment or dementia focuses on identifying clues to the cause of the dementia, comorbid conditions, conditions that may exacerbate the cognitive impairment (eg, sensory impairment or alcoholism), and signs of abuse or neglect. The neurologic examination should be directed at identifying evidence of prior strokes, such as focal signs; eye movements; and evidence of parkinsonism, such as rigidity, bradykinesia, or tremor, keeping in mind that, late in the course of dementia, increased tone and brisk reflexes are nonspecific. Gait and balance are an important part of the examination and should be assessed routinely. A careful cardiovascular evaluation, including measurement of blood pressure and examination for carotid disease and peripheral vascular disease, may help in supporting the diagnosis of VaD. Some patients without dementia who have significant hearing or visual impairments may demonstrate behavior that suggests dementia and have a low score on mental status testing. Therefore, it is important to identify and correct, if possible, sensory impairments before making a diagnosis of dementia.

D. Screening Tests

The public health benefit of screening asymptomatic patients for dementia is controversial. However, for patients with a high risk of dementia (eg, patients 80 years and older) or for those who report memory impairment, screening with a standardized and validated tool is recommended.

1. Mini-Mental Status Examination—The MMSE, a 30-point tool that tests orientation, immediate recall, delayed recall, concentration/calculation, language, and visuospatial domains, has been the most widely used screening test of cognition. However, the MMSE is copyright protected, and forms should be purchased from Psychological Assessment Resources. The MMSE, like many screening tests, is a culturally and language-biased test, and adjustments should be made for age and level of education. When scores are adjusted for age and education, the MMSE has a high sensitivity and specificity for detecting dementia (82% and 99%, respectively). Because it is administered verbally and patients are asked to write and draw, hearing, visual, or other physical impairments may make the scoring less valid. A patient with early cognitive impairment may score within normal limits for age and education; however, if the test is repeated every 6 to 12 months, the MMSE can detect cognitive decline and suggest a diagnosis of MCI or dementia. Among patients with AD, MMSE scores decline an average of 3 points per year, whereas for those with MCI, 1 point per year is more typical. In patients who are aging normally, MMSE scores should not decline much from year to year. As a general guideline, scores above 26 are normal, scores of 24 to 26 may indicate MCI, and a score <24 is consistent with dementia. However, it is best to compare each patient's score with age- and education-adjusted median scores and to monitor for change in addition to assessing for functional decline.

2. Montreal Cognitive Assessment—The Montreal Cognitive Assessment (MoCA) is another commonly used screening test for cognitive impairment. Similar to the MMSE, it is a 30-point screening test that assesses a variety of cognitive domains including memory (with a five-word recall task), orientation, visuospatial function, concentration, calculation, attention, abstraction, language, and executive function (which is not well represented on the MMSE). It is more sensitive than the MMSE, particularly for detecting MCI. The test and directions can be downloaded for free at www.mocatest.org in multiple languages, as well as for the blind. The form shows a cutoff score of 26 (≤25 indicates impairment), but this value is likely too high for most US populations. For example, in a large, ethnically diverse sample of adults in the Dallas Heart Study, the mean score for a 70-year-old with high school education is about 21. MoCA test scores are highly influenced by education level. Normative data are accumulating, and providers should consult the literature for tables that provide age- and education-stratified means and standard deviations for populations similar to the patient being tested.

3. Mini-Cog—Attempts have been made to create brief, focused screening tools that are less time consuming than the MMSE or MoCA (which typically take 10 minutes or so) and are freely available. Two commonly used tests are the Clock Draw Test (CDT) and the Three-Item Recall; when used together, this is called the "Mini-Cog." In the Mini-Cog, the patient is asked to draw a clock face with the hands set at a designated time. Several CDTs are available, each with a different scoring system. However, evidence suggests that a simple dichotomy between normal and abnormal clocks has a relatively good sensitivity (~80%) for detecting dementia, even for inexperienced raters. Normal clocks have all the numbers in the correct position and the hands correctly placed to display the requested time. Using the Mini-Cog is quick and easy, and if both parts are normal, it essentially rules out dementia. The Mini-Cog may be particularly useful in poorly educated or non–English-speaking patients for whom the MMSE and MoCA are not so helpful

E. "Bedside" Cognitive Assessment

The cognitive assessment of a patient with cognitive impairment or dementia should be paired with the medical and physical examination. Patients are less likely to be threatened or offended by questions about cognitive abilities if the questions are framed as part of the physical examination. In addition to administering a standardized assessment tool such as the MMSE or MoCA, providers should also assess domains of cognitive functioning that are not well represented in the MMSE or MoCA, such as judgment and insight. The diagnosis of dementia requires that there be impairment in two or more cognitive functions such as memory, language, visuospatial function, and executive functioning. Language can be assessed by simply listening for a lack of content in the patient's dialogue or the use of vague terms to replace nouns, such as "thing" or "it." Asking the patient to name common things in the room may be helpful if the language seems normal. Evidence of impaired executive functioning is often discovered in the history and can be assessed during the examination as well. For example, if the patient is not able to describe a complex function that the patient may normally do (or used to do) in fine detail, there may be a problem with executive functioning.

When to refer patients for formal neuropsychological testing is discussed later in this chapter.

Borson S, Scanlan J, Brush M, Vitaliano P, Dokmak A. The mini-cog: a cognitive "vital signs" measure for dementia screening the multilingual elderly. *Int J Geriatr Psychiatry.* 2000;15(11):1021-1027.

Nasreddine ZS, Phillips NA, Bédirian V, et al. The Montreal Cognitive Assessment, MoCA: a brief tool for mild cognitive impairment. *J Am Geriatr Soc.* 2005;53(4):695-699.

Rossetti HC, Lacritz LH, Cullum CM, Weiner MF. Normative data for the Montreal Cognitive Assessment (MoCA) in a population-based sample. *Neurology.* 2011;77(13):1272-1275.

F. Laboratory Findings

In the evaluation of a patient with cognitive impairment or newly diagnosed dementia, laboratory studies are generally used to rule out potentially treatable causes of dementia (Table 9–2). Vitamin B_{12} deficiency and hypothyroidism are common in older adults and can affect cognitive functioning. Treatment of these conditions is warranted, although few cases of dementia are actually caused by (or improved with treatment of) vitamin B_{12} deficiency or hypothyroidism. Most clinicians will also perform complete blood count, electrolytes, creatinine, glucose, calcium, and liver function tests. One should screen for latent syphilis and HIV if there is a high index of suspicion of these conditions.

G. Imaging

Structural brain imaging with noncontrast magnetic resonance imaging (MRI; or noncontrast CT if MRI is contraindicated or unavailable) is recommended by most guidelines in the evaluation of cognitive impairment to rule out treatable causes of dementias, such as subdural hematoma, normal pressure hydrocephalus, and tumor. In addition to looking for structural lesions, imaging may be helpful in the diagnosis of the particular type of dementia, with MRI being more sensitive for vascular changes and measures of hippocampal volume. Neuroimaging is likely to be of low yield in patients with a typical clinical appearance of AD and symptoms that have been present for >1 to 2 years. Advantages and disadvantages of neuroimaging can be discussed with patients and families.

Imaging studies for VaD are also nonspecific. This is because many older patients will have some degree of small-vessel ischemic disease on CT or MRI. In fact, by 85 years, nearly 100% of patients will have white matter hyperintensities on imaging studies. Therefore, simply seeing evidence of vascular disease does not warrant diagnosis of VaD. If, however, there is extensive disease, multiple infarcts, or infarcts in

Table 9–2. Potentially treatable causes of cognitive impairment.

B_{12} deficiency	Subdural hematoma
Thyroid disease	Normal pressure hydrocephalus
Hypercalcemia	Central nervous system neoplasms
Depression	Drug effects
Alcoholism	Heavy metals

key anatomic locations (eg, thalamus) in a patient with a history or neuropsychological findings consistent with VaD, it is probable that the imaging findings are clinically relevant. In FTD, there is classically asymmetric volume loss of the frontal or anterior temporal lobes in comparison to the overall atrophy seen in AD.

Fluorodeoxyglucose PET (FDG-PET) scans measure glucose metabolism in specific areas of the brain and may be helpful in distinguishing early AD from FTD or DLB. Although FDG-PET has been shown to improve diagnostic accuracy of pathologically confirmed AD, it is not considered standard in the workup of AD and is generally not needed to make a diagnosis. In addition, Medicare currently only pays for FDG-PET when used to distinguish AD from FTD. Several amyloid-binding PET tracers are now clinically available, and amyloid PET scans can be used to detect intracerebral amyloid. While routinely used in Alzheimer clinical trials, amyloid PET imaging is not covered by Medicare, and thus, the role of its use in the clinical diagnosis of AD is yet to be determined. It is important to note that although it may be useful in the differential diagnosis of cognitive impairment, it is not recommended as a screening test for asymptomatic individuals in part because up to 30% of cognitively "normal" older adults test positive for brain amyloid and because there is currently no treatment that will delay or prevent the onset of symptoms. New ligands targeting the tau protein and other processes are under investigation but have not been established for clinical practice.

Rabinovici GD, Gatsonis C, Apgar C, et al. Association of amyloid positron emission tomography with subsequent change in clinical management among Medicare beneficiaries with mild cognitive impairment or dementia. *JAMA.* 2019;321(13):1286-1294.

H. Special Tests & Examinations

1. Neuropsychological testing—Neuropsychological testing is generally performed by neuropsychologists and consists of an in-depth battery of standardized examinations that test general intelligence and multiple cognitive domains, including memory, language, visuospatial abilities, attention, reasoning, and problem solving, as well as other measures of executive function. The diagnosis of dementia can generally be made by obtaining a detailed history and physical examination (including a brief cognitive evaluation) and does not require neuropsychological testing. However, there are instances in which referral for formal neuropsychological testing can be particularly helpful (eg, when patients have early or mild symptoms, especially if they have high premorbid intelligence and are performing "normally" on tools such as the MMSE). Neuropsychological testing can also be helpful in patients with low intelligence or education and in those with depression, schizophrenia, or other psychiatric illness in which it may be hard to determine how much the condition is contributing to the apparent cognitive deficits. Likewise, in patients with atypical features, such as early language impairment, neuropsychological testing may be helpful in the differential diagnosis of an unusual type of dementia. In addition, a more thorough cognitive battery can identify relative strengths that may be important to patients and their caregivers and may be useful for establishing a baseline from which to reassess.

2. Kohlman Evaluation of Living Skills— A Kohlman Evaluation of Living Skills (KELS), generally performed by occupational therapists, assesses a patient's ability to perform tasks required for safe independent living. For example, a patient is asked to write a check for a mock bill, use the telephone, or identify dangerous situations in pictures and state what he or she would do. This evaluation may be helpful when a patient with known or suspected dementia is living alone and there is concern about whether the patient needs to move to a more supervised setting such as assisted living.

3. Genetic testing— Tremendous advances have been made in elucidating the genetics of AD. Two categories of genetic defects have been defined: those that cause classic autosomal dominant familial AD and those involved in late-onset or sporadic AD. Familial AD is rare and accounts for <5% of all AD cases. Patients with familial AD usually develop dementia in their 40s to 50s and almost always before 65 years. Because early-onset AD is often familial, it is important to obtain a detailed family history of dementia. Familial AD is inherited in an autosomal dominant fashion. Mutations that cause early-onset AD have been identified in three genes thus far: presenilin 1 (*PSEN1*), presenilin 2 (*PSEN2*), and amyloid precursor protein (*APP*) on chromosomes 14, 1, and 21, respectively. A mutation in *PSEN1* is the most common. Testing for genetic mutations in a patient with early-onset AD is not clinically useful for that patient because it will not alter the management of the disease. However, if the patient has children who wish to know whether they have inherited a gene that causes AD, the family should be referred for genetic counseling. In addition, genetic testing of patients with early-onset AD may be valuable for research.

In contrast to early-onset AD, late-onset/sporadic AD (>60–65 years) is associated with genes that increase the risk of AD, but not in an autosomal dominant fashion. Physicians may be asked by patients or family members for the "Alzheimer blood test," most likely referring to apolipoprotein E (*APOE*) genotyping, although many other genes have recently been implicated in increased risk of AD and polygenic risk scores are being developed. The association between *APOE* and risk of AD is well established and is the strongest genetic risk factor discovered to date (not including the mutations causing familial AD noted earlier). The presence of one ε4 allele increases the risk of AD by about two to three times, whereas the ε2 allele may be protective. It is important to keep in mind that *APOE*-ε4 is only a genetic risk factor for AD; therefore, the absence of an ε4 allele does not rule out the diagnosis nor does the presence of homozygous ε4/ε4 rule it in. In fact, most patients with AD do not carry the ε4 allele. There is broad consensus that *APOE* testing be reserved for research purposes only, although the test is now commercially available direct to consumers via in-home genetic testing kits.

Brothers KB, Knapp EE. How should primary care physicians respond to direct-to-consumer genetic test results? *AMA J Ethics*. 2018;20(9):E812-E818.

Marshe VS, Gorbovskaya I, Kanji S, et al. Clinical implications of APOE genotyping for late-onset Alzheimer's disease (LOAD) risk estimation: a review of the literature. *J Neural Transm (Vienna)*. 2019;126(1):65-85.

▶ Differential Diagnosis

The differential diagnosis of dementia includes the potentially treatable causes of dementia listed in Table 9–2, among them metabolic abnormalities, structural brain lesions, medications, alcoholism, and depression. The differential diagnosis also includes delirium, uncorrected sensory deficits, amnestic disorders, and other psychiatric conditions.

A. Depression

Depression commonly coexists with dementia (up to 30%–50% of patients), but it may also be the only cause for cognitive deficits and, therefore, must be ruled out or treated before a diagnosis of dementia can be made. A patient's memory complaints that are disproportional to objective deficits should alert a provider to the possibility of depression. This is in contrast to dementia, in which patients tend to minimize (or be unaware of) their deficits. It is important to keep in mind that older patients who develop reversible cognitive impairments while depressed are at high risk for dementia over the next few years.

B. Delirium

Delirium is a common cause of confusion in older adults, particularly in those who are hospitalized, and may be incorrectly labeled as dementia. In contrast to dementia, delirium is characterized by abrupt onset of altered cognition and consciousness, decreased attention, perceptual disturbances (commonly visual hallucinations), and impressive fluctuations in symptoms. Table 60–4 in Chapter 60, "Confusion," contrasts delirium, depression, and dementia. If delirium is suspected, underlying causes should be sought and treated. Dementia is one of the key risk factors for delirium. If cognitive deficits persist after the resolution of delirium, further workup for dementia should be pursued.

C. Medications & Sensory Deficits

Medications are commonly associated with confusion in older adults. Many classes of drugs have been implicated, including opiates, benzodiazepines, neuroleptics, anticholinergic drugs (many unsuspected medications have significant anticholinergic properties), H$_2$ blockers, and corticosteroids. Clinicians should ask patients or caregivers to bring in all medications, including nonprescription medicines, for review. Drug-drug interactions and appropriateness of doses should be assessed. In addition, any nonessential medications should be discontinued. Reassessment of the patient may reveal marked improvement in cognition and function. Similarly, correction of sensory deficits (visual or hearing impairments) in patients who have been misidentified as having dementia can be equally rewarding.

D. Alcohol Abuse

Patients with cognitive impairment, disorganization, frequent accidents, or failure at home or work should be screened for alcohol abuse. Years of heavy alcohol use may contribute to permanent cognitive impairment, possibly through direct toxic effects on the brain or thiamine deficiency or from complications of alcohol abuse such as head trauma related to falls or violence. However, alcohol abuse may also be responsible for more acute declines in a patient's level of function; improvement in cognition and function may be seen on cessation of drinking.

E. Other Psychiatric Conditions

Chronic psychiatric conditions such as schizophrenia or bipolar affective disorder may also be included in the differential diagnosis of dementia, especially when behavioral changes and psychiatric symptoms such as delusions and hallucinations predominate. In addition, older patients with chronic schizophrenia are more likely to develop dementia than unaffected adults. The pattern of cognitive deficits seen in geriatric schizophrenia patients is distinct from AD, and autopsy series confirm that AD does not account for the cognitive impairments.

▶ Complications

A. Delirium

Delirium, as well as being considered in the differential diagnosis of dementia, is also a major complication of dementia. Risk factors for delirium include cognitive impairment, severe medical illness, polypharmacy, elevated blood urea nitrogen (BUN)-to-creatinine ratio, and visual or hearing impairment, among others. When patients with dementia are hospitalized, it is critical to be aware of their high risk for delirium and to take measures to avoid precipitating factors, such as the use of physical restraints and bladder catheters, malnutrition, and use of multiple new medications.

B. Behavioral and Psychological Symptoms of Dementia

Behavioral and psychological symptoms of dementia (BPSDs) are very common, eventually affecting nearly all patients with dementia, usually as the disease progresses (although they may be early manifestations of FTD and LBD). These symptoms, which are associated with worse prognosis, earlier nursing home referral, greater costs, and increased caregiver burden, include the following:

- Agitation and aggression
- Disruptive vocalizations
- Psychotic features (delusions, hallucinations, paranoia)
- Depressive symptoms
- Apathy
- Sleep disturbances
- Wandering or pacing
- Resistance to personal care (bathing and grooming)

Although agitation and psychosis are common in dementia, especially as the disease progresses, any new behavioral symptoms should be evaluated before being attributed solely to the dementia. Precipitating causes of new agitation may include delirium, untreated pain, fecal impaction, urinary retention, new medications, sensory impairment, and environmental causes (eg, new environment, excessive stimulation).

The delusions seen in patients with AD are usually not as complex or bizarre as those of schizophrenia. Table 9–3 lists some common delusions of dementia. More than 50% of patients with AD will have psychosis at some point, occasionally requiring drug therapy. However, in many patients, the psychosis is self-limited. Thus, it is important to attempt periodically to withdraw any drug therapies being used to manage agitation or psychosis. In fact, there are federal regulations governing the duration of as-needed (PRN) and daily use of such medications in patients residing in nursing homes so they are not inadvertently prescribed indefinitely.

C. Complications Related to Caregiver Stress

Informal caregivers provide the majority of care to patients with dementia at considerable financial and personal costs. The risk of caregiver stress rises with the patient's advancing severity of dementia, increased dependence in ADLs, and presence of problem behaviors. Clinicians should assess caregivers for stress because stress is associated with poor outcomes

Table 9–3. Common delusions in patients with dementia.

Paranoid Delusions	Misidentifications
People are stealing things	Misidentifies familiar people (eg, believes daughter is wife)
Accusations of infidelity	Current home is not their home
Belief that someone is trying to harm them	Impersonation (eg, spouse is an impersonator)

for both patients and caregivers, including increased risk of placement in a nursing home, increased risk of patient neglect or abuse, and increased risk of depression among caregivers (reported to affect 30%–50%). Stress can be reduced with therapeutic interventions such as respite care and caregiver support. Please see Chapter 17 for more on caregiving.

▶ Treatment

In the management of patients with cognitive impairment or dementia, the goals are to preserve function and autonomy for as long as possible and to maintain quality of life for both the patient and the caregivers. The medications currently available offer modest symptomatic benefit. There are currently no disease-modifying drugs on the market despite tremendous effort over the past two decades.

A. Cognitive Impairment

1. Cholinesterase inhibitors—Cholinesterase inhibitors (ChEIs) are currently the mainstay of treatment for AD of any severity (mild to severe): donepezil, rivastigmine, and galantamine. All have been shown to modestly improve cognitive function and delay functional decline in mild to moderate AD and are likely of benefit even in moderate to severe dementia. Off-label use of ChEIs in MCI is common, especially for the amnestic type, but not approved by the US Food and Drug Administration (FDA). Clinical trials indicate that there may be some symptomatic benefit in MCI, although they do not prevent progression to AD. In addition, although the ChEIs are FDA approved only for AD and PD dementia, benefit has also been shown in patients with DLB and mixed AD plus VaD. All of the ChEIs have the same relative efficacy in AD and generally differ only in their half-lives (and, therefore, dosing regimen) and specificity for receptors (rivastigmine also inhibits butyrylcholinesterase). Gastrointestinal side effects, including nausea, vomiting, and diarrhea, are a class effect and are the most common reason for discontinuation. These side effects can usually be ameliorated by slow titration of the drug over 8 to 12 weeks. Sleep disturbance and nightmares are also reported. In addition, ChEIs appear to increase the risk of syncope. Caution should be used when prescribing to patients with bradycardia. Table 9–4 lists the recommended initial doses and target doses for each of the ChEIs. Donepezil 23 mg is not recommended over 10-mg dosing because there are increased side effects and lack of added clinical benefit.

Assessing effectiveness of therapy with ChEIs in individual patients has not been formally standardized for clinical practice. Effect sizes are modest in clinical trials, with only 40% to 50% of patients showing evidence of improvement on measures of cognitive functioning, ADL scores, or subjective clinician ratings. Stable or improved MMSE or MoCA scores over 6 to 12 months suggest the drug may be effective. Although switching ChEIs because of lack of efficacy or

Table 9–4. Cholinesterase inhibitors.

Drug	Starting Dosage	Target Dose
Donepezil[a]	2.5–5.0 mg daily	10 mg daily (increase every 4 weeks)[b]
Rivastigmine[c]	1.5 mg twice a day	6 mg twice a day (increase by 1.5 mg twice a day every 2 weeks)[d]
Galantamine[e]	4 mg twice a day	8–12 mg twice a day (increase every 4 weeks)

[a]Also available in orally dissolving tablets and in combination with memantine.
[b]Donepezil 23 mg has not been shown to be more effective than 10 mg and risk of side effects is greater.
[c]Also available in a patch. Starting dose is 4.6 mg/24 hours. Increase to 9.5 mg after 4 weeks.
[d]Retitrate from 1.5 mg twice a day (oral) or 4.6 mg (patch) if treatment is interrupted for more than several days.
[e]Also available in extended release form for once-daily dosing. Start at 8 mg daily, increase by 8 mg every 4 weeks to max of 16–24 mg daily. Oral solution (twice daily) also available.

intolerable side effects may be beneficial for some patients, there is little evidence to support doing so.

The appropriate length of treatment with ChEIs is still unknown, but many experts recommend that therapy be continued indefinitely (or until there is no function left to lose) if improvement or stabilization is noted. Clinicians and caregivers may notice a decline in function if ChEIs are discontinued. If the patient reaches a stage of illness where they can no longer safely swallow a tablet or capsule, it is reasonable to have a conversation about discontinuing the therapy. However, if continued therapy is desired, tablets and capsules should not be crushed; nonpill formulations are available (Table 9–4).

2. Memantine—Memantine, an *N*-methyl-D-aspartate (NMDA) antagonist, is FDA approved for the treatment of moderate to severe AD. It is often added to ChEI therapy when the dementia reaches moderate severity. Memantine is generally well tolerated. Headache is the only side effect reported in controlled clinical trials that occurred in at least 5% of patients and at twice the placebo rate (6% with memantine compared to 3% in placebo group). Dizziness, confusion, and constipation may also be reported infrequently.

3. Other treatments—There has been interest in antioxidants, such as ginkgo biloba and vitamin E (α-tocopherol), for the treatment of dementia because they have a plausible mechanism of action. Studies of ginkgo suggest it may be of mild benefit in dementia, but the evidence is inconsistent. Large-scale, high-quality, randomized controlled trials have found that neither ginkgo biloba nor vitamin E is effective for prevention of dementia in older adults with normal cognition or MCI.

Although NSAIDs, statins, and estrogen looked promising as treatments for AD in observational studies, randomized controlled trials have failed to show benefit of these agents for the treatment of AD.

Dietary supplements such as B vitamins, coconut oil, and fish oils have not been shown in randomized clinical trials to be of benefit in the treatment of dementia. In addition, in general, it is better to eat your antioxidants (fresh fruits and vegetables), vitamins, and healthy fats (omega-3 fatty acids; high in foods such as salmon, flaxseed, walnuts) than to take them as supplements. The Mediterranean diet, which is high in fruits, vegetables, whole grains, and nuts and seeds, along with fish and healthy oils, is currently the most promising diet for brain health.

B. Vascular Dementia

No drug therapies have been specifically approved for the treatment of VaD. The principles of treatment of VaD rely on the treatment of stroke risk factors such as smoking, diabetes, hyperlipidemia, and hypertension. However, there is no consensus on the appropriate target blood pressure for patients with existing VaD due to lack of robust clinical trial data and some observational data suggesting that, once dementia is present, permissive mild hypertension (up to systolic blood pressures in the 150s) may be better for cognitive function than lower blood pressures. ChEIs and memantine may be of modest benefit in VaD.

Kaviragan H, Schneider LS. Efficacy and adverse effects of cholinesterase inhibitors and memantine in vascular dementia: a meta-analysis of randomized controlled trials. *Lancet Neurol.* 2007;6(9):782-792.

C. Problem Behaviors

1. Nonpharmacologic approaches— Because BPSDs are common and may adversely affect both patient and caregiver quality of life, it is important to manage them as dutifully as the cognitive symptoms. Once precipitating causes (eg, delirium, pain, fecal impaction, broken hearing aids) of new behavioral problems have been treated or ruled out, it is critical to try to identify what the behavior may represent. When patients are agitated or displaying other problem behaviors, it is often because they do not have the language skills to express their needs. Providers and caregivers should try to learn what the behaviors for a patient with dementia may represent and then attempt to address underlying needs. Keeping a behavior log may be useful. Federal regulation requires that the least-restrictive methods for behavior problems be tried first for nursing home residents. For all patients, nonpharmacologic treatments should be attempted before initiating drug therapies.

A few strategies that may be helpful in reducing agitation in patients with dementia include music, reminiscence therapy, exposure to pets, outdoor walks, and bright light exposure. One of the unifying themes in many of these strategies is that the therapy works best if it is tailored to the patient. For example, with music therapy, playing music that is consistent with patients' prior preferences seems to be superior to playing a standard selection for everyone. One study confirmed an intuitive assumption that providing intensive education and training on understanding and treating BPSD for nursing assistants or care providers also significantly decreases agitation among patients with dementia in nursing home settings.

Table 9–5 presents less evidence-based but more practical tips for both caregivers and medical providers of patients with dementia-related difficult behaviors.

2. Pharmacologic approaches— If nonpharmacologic approaches fail, it may become necessary to add drug therapy. However, there are no approved pharmacologic therapies for BPSD, and modest benefits must be weighed against potential harms. Several classes of drugs are used for BPSD, including antipsychotics, antidepressants, mood stabilizers, and ChEIs. Table 9–6 lists drugs and doses commonly used to treat BPSD.

Antipsychotics: The atypical antipsychotics olanzapine and risperidone have the best evidence for effectiveness (which is modest), but side effects and risks should be considered and weighed against potential benefits. There is a boxed warning on all atypical antipsychotics for increased risk of death when used in patients with dementia, and thus these drugs should be used with caution and only in refractory cases or where there is a serious risk of the patient harming self or others, using the lowest possible dose for the shortest possible time. A discussion with the patient's decision maker about the risks and benefits of using antipsychotics should be documented. In addition to stroke and mortality, side effects to consider are extrapyramidal symptoms and tardive dyskinesia (at higher doses), sedation, weight gain, diabetes mellitus, and hyperprolactinemia. Low-dose typical antipsychotics (eg, haloperidol) may be used in the acute care setting but should be avoided as a chronic medication due to the risk of irreversible tardive dyskinesia. In one study, even low-dose oral haloperidol (1.5 mg/day) resulted in tardive dyskinesia in 30% of older patients at 1 year and >60% of patients at 3 years.

Selective serotonin reuptake inhibitors (SSRIs): The SSRI citalopram has been shown to significantly improve agitation as measured by several different outcomes in patients with AD when compared to placebo. However, the trial was conducted using 30 mg/day, and the FDA has since advised against using >20 mg/day in older adults due to dose-dependent risk of QT prolongation. A large phase III trial of escitalopram (up to 15 mg/day) for agitation in AD is currently underway with results expected in 2022.

Mood stabilizers: Mood stabilizers such as carbamazepine and valproic acid have shown benefit for some secondary outcomes in small trials. However, because of side effects, drug-drug interactions, and necessary blood test monitoring, these agents are not recommended as first-line treatments.

Table 9–5. Dementia-related difficult behaviors: practical tips for caregivers and medical providers.

Maintain familiarity and routines as much as possible.
Any change in the routine can produce anxiety and distress for patients with dementia. Changes in living arrangement, going on vacation, or being hospitalized may provoke agitation and other undesirable behaviors.

Decrease number of choices.
Patients with dementia may become overwhelmed with too many choices and become frustrated by their inability to sort things out. Limiting choices may be helpful. A good example is the case of a patient who resists changing clothes or insists on wearing the same clothes every day. In this case, it might be helpful for the caregiver to lay out only one outfit or to give the patient two choices: eg, "Would you like to wear the blue blouse or the red blouse?" Similarly, simplifying conversation and environment is also important. Too much input is often overwhelming or misinterpreted.

Tell; don't ask.
At first glance, this recommendation may seem uncomfortable to some. However, with the apathy that is commonly associated with dementia, it may be a struggle to get patients with dementia to agree to do anything. Instead of asking, "Do you want to go to dinner now?" which may often result in a "no" answer followed by an argument, it may be more effective to say, "It is time to go to dinner now." Similarly, patients may be more agreeable if things are framed in positive rather than negative terms. For example, use "come with me" rather than "don't go there."

Understand that they *can't*, rather than they *won't*.
Family members and caregivers often believe that the patient with dementia is being stubborn and willfully making things difficult. Caregivers can waste much time and energy trying to "teach" something to patients who have difficulty learning. Helping caregivers understand the limitations of their loved one may improve quality of life for both.

Don't try logic or reason.
Because of the executive dysfunction that accompanies dementia, there is a relatively early loss of the ability to reason and use logic, which becomes more profound as the illness progresses. Trying to rationalize with someone with dementia often leads to frustration on the part of both parties. This is particularly true for delusions. If the patient has a nonthreatening delusion, arguing with the patient and trying to get the patient to see that it does not make sense is often fruitless and frustrating for both parties.

Always keep the goals in mind.
Is it really important if grandma thinks it is 1954 or that her daughter is her sorority sister? Why can't she wear that raincoat in the house if she wants to? By keeping the goals and "big picture" in mind, some conflict may be avoided. It is also important for caregivers and physicians to remember that most behaviors do not last indefinitely but are rather temporary stages.

Table 9–6. Off-label pharmacotherapy for behavioral and psychological symptoms of dementia.

Drug	Starting Dosage	Maximum Recommended Dosage[a]
Haloperidol[b,c]	0.25–0.5 mg daily	2–3 mg/day
Risperidone[c,d]	0.25 mg twice a day	1–1.5 mg/day
Olanzapine[c,e]	2.5 mg daily	5–10 mg/day
Trazodone	25 mg every night at bedtime	50–100 mg every night at bedtime
Citalopram	10 mg daily	20 mg/day
Divalproex sodium[f]	125 mg twice a day	~1000 mg/day

[a]Use the lowest dose that achieves benefit.
[b]Also available in intravenous formulations.
[c]CAUTION: Antipsychotics have a boxed warning from the US Food and Drug Administration for increased risk of death. Use should be limited to refractory cases or imminent risk of harm to self or others.
[d]Also available in liquid form (do not mix with cola or tea) and orally dissolving tablets.
[e]Also available intramuscularly and in orally dissolving tablets.
[f]Also available in sprinkles.

If attempts at nonpharmacologic approaches and use of more common drug classes have failed, referral to a geriatrician or geropsychiatrist should be considered.

Benzodiazepines are not recommended for the chronic management of BPSD. They have not been found to be more efficacious than other classes of drugs. In addition, adverse effects associated with benzodiazepine use, such as increased risk of falls, sedation, withdrawal, and occasionally paradoxical excitation, make them a particularly poor choice.

Lanctôt KL, Amatniek J, Ancoli-Israel S, et al. Neuropsychiatric signs and symptoms of Alzheimer's disease: new treatment paradigms. *Alzheimers Dement.* 2017;3(3):440-449.

Porsteinsson AP, Drye LT, Pollock BG, et al. Effect of citalopram on agitation in Alzheimer disease: the CitAD randomized clinical trial. *JAMA.* 2014;311(7):682-691.

▶ **Management**

A. Advance Directives

Establishing advance directives and having the patient appoint a durable power of attorney (DPOA) for health care should be a part of the management plan of patients with dementia. It is particularly important to have this discussion as early as possible so that patients can participate in decisions to direct their end-of-life care. Even patients with moderate dementia may be able to consistently state preferences and choices, including the appointment of a DPOA. In addition to preferences regarding resuscitation, specific interventions such as the use of artificial hydration and nutrition should be addressed and included. Patients may also want to appoint a DPOA for finances. Consultation with an elder law attorney or estate planner may be helpful.

B. Safety Issues

1. Driving—Cognitive impairment has been shown to adversely affect driving ability, even among patients with mild dementia. Some states require reporting of AD and "related conditions" to the department of public health or the state's department of motor vehicles. Primary care providers should familiarize themselves with their state's law on reporting. If a patient with dementia is involved in a motor vehicle accident, the practitioner may be held liable if required reporting has not been done.

2. Home safety—Home safety should be assessed by interviewing a reliable informant or, preferably, by a home visit from a visiting nurse or occupational therapist. Specific safety measures to consider implementing include grab bars in the bathrooms, good lighting, clear pathways through the house, reducing clutter, and disabling stoves if there is concern for potential kitchen fires. If there is any indication that a patient may not be safe in the home or there is evidence of self-neglect or concern about elder abuse by others, the provider should contact adult protective services, which has a variety of resources and can quickly develop a plan for ensuring patient safety.

3. Wandering—Patients with dementia may wander and become lost. Some form of identification (eg, sewn-in clothing, identification bracelet) is recommended. The Alzheimer's Association has a program called Medic Alert + Safe Return. When registered, patients receive identification products including a wallet card and jewelry. The Medic Alert + Safe Return program maintains a 24-hour toll-free emergency line for help in locating and reuniting missing patients with loved ones. Registration can be done through the Alzheimer's Association for a nominal cost.

4. Caregiver assistance—Caring for a patient with dementia can be exhausting and stressful and can lead to physical and mental health problems in the caregiver and the risk of abuse to the patient. After making a diagnosis of dementia, the primary care provider should make a referral to a knowledgeable social worker or office on aging for a list of resources to assist the caregiver. In addition, an assessment of caregivers at each follow-up appointment is warranted. If caregiver stress is detected, caregivers should be asked about their use of resources and provided additional referrals as needed. If caregiver stress is severe, referral to a 24-hour respite program (either nursing home or assisted-living facility) may be helpful. Please refer to Chapter 17 for more on caregiving and caregiver well-being.

Lee L, Molnar F. Driving and dementia: efficient approach to driving safety concerns in family practice. *Can Fam Physician.* 2017;63(1):27-31.

Moye J, Sabatino CP, Weintraub Brendel R. Evaluation of the capacity to appoint a healthcare proxy. *Am J Geriatr Psychiatry.* 2013;21(4):326-336.

▶ Prognosis

The prognosis of dementia is variable depending on the cause and presence of comorbid conditions. Estimates of survival from time of onset or diagnosis of AD have been broad. Median life expectancy is 3 to 15 years. Patients with earlier ages of onset tend to have longer survival, and patients with VaD may have slightly shorter survival. Death is commonly a result of terminal pneumonia in the degenerative dementias and of cardiovascular events in VaD. It may be useful to use a staging scale such as the Functional Assessment Staging (FAST staging) for AD to help families understand the progression of the disease. There are seven stages in the FAST staging system, with stage 7 being end-stage dementia. This scale is widely available online, and the Alzheimer's Association website features it for patients and families. When patients reach stage 7, referral for hospice may be indicated.

As many as 90% of patients with dementia are eventually institutionalized and this has great variability depending on sociocultural factors, financial resources, and other factors. The median time to nursing home placement is 3–6 years from diagnosis. Dementia severity, dependence in ADLs, difficult behaviors, and caregiver age and burden are significant risk factors for placement. Interventions that include caregiver support and education in managing difficult behaviors may extend time to nursing home placement.

USEFUL WEBSITES

Alzheimer's Association (extensive informational materials for patients and caregivers as well as a link to clinical trials in your area). www.alz.org. Accessed March 8, 2020.

Alzheimer's Disease Education and Referral Center (of the National Institutes of Health and National Institute on Aging). www.nia.nih.gov/health/alzheimers. Accessed March 8, 2020.

Family Caregiver Alliance (provides information, support, and guidance for family and professional caregivers; includes topic-specific newsletters, information on care facilities and legal issues, and online discussion lists). www.caregiver.org. Accessed March 8, 2020.

Montreal Cognitive Assessment (download the MoCA test form and directions in many languages for free). www.mocatest.org. Accessed March 8, 2020.

Urinary Incontinence

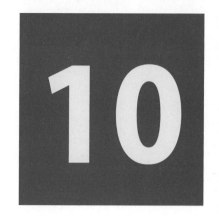

Anne Suskind, MD
G. Michael Harper, MD

ESSENTIALS OF DIAGNOSIS

► Urinary incontinence is the involuntary loss of any amount of urine.

► Urinary incontinence is a syndrome caused by medical conditions, medications, lower urinary tract disease and dysfunction, or functional and cognitive impairment, often in combination.

General Principles

Older women and men are more likely to experience urinary incontinence (UI) than younger adults; however, it is not an inevitable product of aging. Approximately 15% to 30% of community-dwelling older adults experience some urinary leakage. The prevalence is nearly 50% in frail community dwellers and between 50% and 75% in nursing home residents. UI occurs more frequently in women than in men in most age groups, but the prevalence of UI increases with age in both men and women. Leading risk factors for UI in older adults include increasing age, female sex, cognitive impairment, genitourinary surgery, obesity, and impaired mobility.

Patients often do not report UI because of embarrassment, the misconception that it is a normal part of aging, or a lack of knowledge of potential treatment options, and clinicians rarely ask about it. Less than 20% of incontinent adults are assessed for this condition by primary care providers. The reasons cited for lack of inquiry are time constraints, underappreciation of the prevalence, and uncertainty about the management.

The financial impact of incontinence is substantial. Contemporary direct cost estimates of UI are hard to find. The best available cost data are over 20 years old, and in 1995 dollars, the annual direct cost was estimated to be over $16 billion in the United States. These costs include continence supplies, diagnostic evaluation, medical and surgical treatment, and complications. Based on the growth of the geriatric population and the prevalence of UI, the cost in current dollars is likely to be substantially greater.

UI has long been classified as a geriatric syndrome: a symptom complex found more frequently in older adults that is often multifactorial in etiology and that requires a multidimensional approach to risk factor modification and treatment. To understand how to prevent, diagnose, and treat the condition accurately, it is important to understand the normal physiology of voiding and how normal voiding can be disrupted.

Normal Voiding

To maintain continence, a person must have intact cognitive, neurologic, muscular, and urologic systems. Consciousness, motivation, comprehension, and attention are needed to properly recognize the need to void and sequence the necessary steps to pass urine in an appropriate time and location. Diseases such as dementia, depression, stroke, and delirium can disrupt the cognitive function needed to exert control over voiding. Muscular dexterity is needed to manipulate clothing and toileting supplies and to physically reach a toilet or urinal. Arthritis and muscular conditions, which impair ambulation and joint functioning, can result in incontinence episodes.

Neurologically, micturition is a coordinated balance between the spinal cord sympathetic and parasympathetic systems (Figure 10–1) and cerebral signaling. The pontine micturition center coordinates the cognitive inhibition/disinhibition to void and the spinal cord response to urinary tract stimulation. Innervation to the detrusor muscle and distal urethra/pelvic floor comes from the sacral 2–4 nerve roots, and the innervations to the proximal urethra come from the thoracic 11–lumbar 2 nerve roots. The sympathetic system allows urinary storage by contracting the urethral sphincter and relaxing the detrusor muscle.

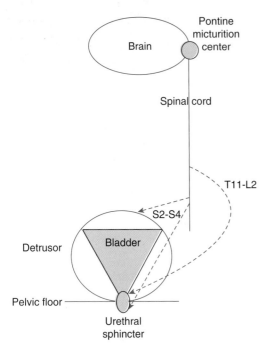

▲ **Figure 10–1.** Neurologic mechanism for continence control.

The parasympathetic system allows voiding by contracting the detrusor and relaxing the urethral sphincter. Diseases, such as spinal cord injury and multiple sclerosis, can impede the neurologic balance between the bladder wall and sphincter. The genitourinary organs and tissues can be diseased or damaged to a degree that impairs controlled urination. Prostatic enlargement, bladder prolapse, urethral strictures, bladder stones, and estrogen-deficient tissue atrophy can cause anatomic abnormalities that lead to incontinence.

Prevention

Because UI has many different etiologies, triggers, and risk factors, the timing, frequency, and severity of symptoms can be quite variable. Prevention thus focuses on reducing the impact of chronic disease on incontinence-related risk, as well as preventing the development of UI itself. It may not be possible to completely prevent UI, but measures to reduce the impact and frequency of the condition may be reasonable goals. Prevention of symptoms or events often requires a multifactorial approach designed to eliminate the factors that lead to incontinent episodes.

There are few studies that target primary prevention of UI. Most treatment trials target secondary prevention by attempting to reduce the number of episodes in those who already have some degree of UI. In one primary prevention study of poststroke patients, a multidimensional approach that included dedicated rehabilitation and a continence care team was found to reduce the development of UI. Another study of continent older women who were taught pelvic floor exercises showed a reduction in the later development of UI. A small trial of weight loss reduced the development of UI in some obese patients, but increased exercise led to increased UI in others. Diabetes is associated with higher rates of UI. In one trial of obese women with prediabetes (average age 50 years old), intensive lifestyle therapy that included a healthy diet, reduced weight, increased activity levels, and smoking cessation was associated with a lower subsequent prevalence of weekly stress, but not urge, incontinence symptoms. In a subgroup of women 60 years of age and older, there was no benefit in the intensive lifestyle group, but this group was small, limiting the ability to draw any firm conclusions.

▶ Clinical Findings

A. Symptoms & Causes

UI is the involuntary loss of any amount of urine and is considered to be a geriatric syndrome. The most common types of UI are urge UI, stress UI, and mixed UI. Additional less common forms of UI in older adults include functional incontinence, in which the individual has difficulty getting to the bathroom due to physical or cognitive impairment, and overflow incontinence, which can be caused by either an underactive bladder or bladder outlet obstruction (or a combination of the two).

1. Urgency UI (UUI)

- *Symptoms*: The report of involuntary loss of urine associated with a sense of urgency.
- *Potential causes*: Idiopathic or associated with neurologic disorders (eg, stroke, multiple sclerosis, Parkinson disease), bladder irritants, stones, infection or tumors.

2. Stress UI (SUI)

- *Symptoms*: The description of involuntary loss of urine associated with effort or physical exertion such as coughing or sneezing.
- *Potential causes*: Failure of the urethral sphincter mechanisms, insufficient pelvic support in women, or prostate surgery in men.

3. Mixed UI (MUI)

- *Symptoms*: The experience of involuntary loss of urine associated with urgency and also with effort or physical exertion such as coughing or sneezing.
- *Potential causes*: A combination of causes discussed earlier for SUI and UUI.

B. History

All adults with UI should undergo a thorough and focused incontinence-related history. Questions should assess both bladder storage symptoms (eg, urgency, urgency incontinence, frequency, nocturia) and bladder emptying symptoms (eg, hesitancy, straining to urinate, prior history of urinary retention, force of stream, intermittency of stream). The type of UI should be assessed with questions such as, "Do you ever leak urine with coughing, laughing, or sneezing?" (indicating SUI) or "Do you ever have a strong need to urinate and can't get to the bathroom in time, and if so, does this result in leakage?" (indicating UUI). Understanding the frequency, duration, and severity of UI is also important because treatment plans should be guided by the degree of bother experienced by that patient. Bladder questionnaires may be helpful in subjective symptom assessment both at baseline and to follow patients over time and track response to therapy. Fluid intake should also be assessed. This includes understanding both the amount and type of fluid consumed during the day and night, with particular attention to ingestion of known bladder irritants such as caffeine and alcohol. Additionally, it is important to understand an individual's access to the toilet and whether or not the individual has any physical or cognitive limitations that may impair their ability to reach the toilet in a timely fashion.

It is also important to perform a thorough urologic, medical, surgical, and obstetric/gynecologic (in females) history in all older adults with UI. As part of the urologic history, it is important to rule out hematuria and nephrolithiasis and to obtain any pertinent oncologic history and history of radiation treatment. Certain medical and neurologic conditions such as diabetes, stroke, Parkinson disease, and lumbar disk disease may contribute to UUI, whereas other conditions such as strong coughing from chronic pulmonary disease may exacerbate SUI. A bowel history is also important to obtain, because addressing bowel issues such as constipation or diarrhea may also improve bladder symptoms.

A thorough review of medications is also essential, particularly in older adults who take multiple medications, some of which may contribute to UI or may interact with potential incontinence treatments (Table 10–1).

C. Physical Examination

Physical examination should include general, neurologic, and genital/gynecologic exams. A cardiovascular exam should evaluate for evidence of congestive heart failure or peripheral edema, which may lend themselves to symptoms of nocturia. The abdominal exam should assess for a palpable bladder suggestive of urinary retention or incomplete bladder emptying. A brief neurologic exam should address mental status and evaluate motor and sensory deficits that may correlate with bladder dysfunction. In men, a rectal exam may be helpful to assess the prostate for enlargement, nodules, or tenderness, in addition to rectal tone. Assessment of the penis for possible phimosis, paraphimosis, balanitis, or meatal stenosis (ie, scarring) is also warranted. In women, a pelvic exam may be helpful to assess for vaginal atrophy, pelvic organ prolapse, pelvic floor strength, urethral hypermobility, and SUI. To assess for SUI, a supine empty stress test should be performed, whereby

Table 10–1. Medications that can contribute to urinary incontinence.

Medication/Class	Mechanism
Antihistamines Antimuscarinics Antispasmodics Antipsychotics Antiparkinson Muscle relaxants Tricyclic antidepressants	Anticholinergic effects on bladder wall/sphincter
Diuretics	Increased urinary volume and diuresis
Sedative-hypnotics Benzodiazepines	Sedation; impaired cognition
Opioids	Opioid receptor–induced bladder dysfunction
α-Adrenergic agonists	Urethral sphincter constriction
α-Adrenergic antagonists	Urethral sphincter relaxation
Calcium channel blockers	Decrease bladder smooth muscle contractility

a patient is laying in the lithotomy position with a full bladder and is asked to cough or bear down. Visualization of leakage on this test is indicative of SUI. Inspection of the perineal skin should be performed in both men and women to assess for rash or any skin breakdown.

D. Urinalysis

Urinalysis is part of the American Urological Association (AUA) guidelines on the diagnosis and treatment of overactive bladder and should be performed. If hematuria is found on dipstick, urine should then be sent to the lab for formal microscopic urinalysis. The presence of at least three red blood cells on microscopic urinalysis warrants referral to a urologist for further workup and evaluation for any genitourinary pathology such as cancer or nephrolithiasis, typically by performing upper tract imaging and cystoscopy. If urinary tract infection is suspected, urine should be sent for culture and sensitivity and treated accordingly. Asymptomatic bacteriuria is not associated with UI and should not be treated with antibiotics.

E. Postvoid Residual

Assessment of a postvoid residual (PVR) is important in the evaluation of UI in order to rule out incomplete bladder emptying. This can be assessed immediately after the patient voids either via a catheter or an ultrasound bladder scanner, which is less invasive for the patient. While the threshold for what constitutes an elevated PVR is not clearly defined, incomplete bladder emptying may raise red flags and warrant further workup and evaluation by a specialist.

F. Bladder Diaries

Bladder diaries can be helpful to document fluid intake and voiding behavior in some patients, particularly in those who have difficulty describing their voiding habits. It is typically recommended that a patient complete a diary for a minimum of 3 days (consisting of three full 24-hour periods) wherein they document the time and volume of each void and incontinence episode. This can also be a useful tool to evaluate the effect of certain treatments over time and to assess for nocturnal polyuria. A sample bladder diary from the National Institutes of Health can be found at **www.niddk.nih.gov/-/media/Files/Urologic-Diseases/diary_508.pdf**.

G. Further Evaluation

Further evaluation with urodynamics should be used at the discretion of the specialist and is not recommended for all patients with UI. Urodynamics is the dynamic evaluation of bladder storage and emptying. It is an interactive test between the clinician and the patient and can be helpful to obtain more objective functional information in certain individuals in whom history and physical exam are not sufficient. This test is minimally invasive and involves the placement of two catheters, one in the bladder and one in the rectum, and electromyogram patches on the perineum to assess pelvic floor activity. The bladder is filled via the urethral catheter, and bladder pressures are measured during both storage and voiding phases.

For the assessment of UUI, urodynamics may be indicated (1) for patients who have failed multiple treatments; (2) when it is important to determine if altered bladder compliance, detrusor overactivity, or other abnormalities are present (or not); (3) for individuals in whom potentially irreversible treatments are being considered; (4) to rule out bladder outlet obstruction; or (5) to help counsel patients with UUI or MUI. For the assessment of SUI, urodynamics may be indicated (1) to assess urethral function, (2) to evaluate individuals who have an elevated PVR, or (3) to evaluate patients in whom invasive therapy is being considered.

▶ DIFFERENTIAL DIAGNOSIS

UI is often the result of a primary genitourinary organ or tissue dysfunction; however, certain diseases or conditions may secondarily cause UI (Table 10-2). In most cases, secondary causes affect the neurologic innervation, structural integrity of the genitourinary tissues, or volume of urine, and thus overwhelm normal bladder functioning. The DIAPPERS mnemonic is a handy way to think of categorizing the transient causes (Box 10-1). Delirium inhibits the ability to know when and where to void and is common in hospitalized older adults. Urinary tract infection, although not commonly a cause of UI, should be considered in patients with dysuria and sudden-onset UI. Atrophic vaginitis or urethritis can cause a variety of genitourinary symptoms including dryness, burning, and itching, along with urinary frequency and

Table 10-2. Conditions that can exacerbate urinary incontinence.

Condition	Mechanism
Constipation Fecal impaction Cystocele Rectocele Uterine prolapse	Mass effect impeding bladder neck and urethra
Dehydration Recurrent urinary tract infection Nephrolithiasis	Mucosal and bladder wall irritation
Pulmonary edema Peripheral edema Hypercalcemia Hyperglycemia	Increased urinary volume
COPD/asthma Chronic bronchitis	Cough-induced weakening of pelvic musculature
Delirium Dementia Depression	Impaired cognition, consciousness, or motivation to remain dry
Spinal cord injury Multiple sclerosis Parkinson disease Spinal stenosis Cerebrovascular accident	Disrupted neurologic coordination to bladder/sphincter
Tremor Osteoarthritis/rheumatoid arthritis Cerebrovascular accident Frailty	Impaired mobility and dexterity
Urogenital atrophy	Loss of estrogen to tissues

COPD, chronic obstructive pulmonary disease.

Box 10-1. DIAPPERS Mnemonic for Transient Causes of Urinary Incontinence	
D	Delirium
I	Infection
A	Atrophic vaginitis/urethritis
P	Pharmaceuticals
P	Psychological disorders (particularly depression)
E	Excess urine output
R	Restricted mobility
S	Stool impaction

Data from Resnick NM, Yalla SV. Management of urinary incontinence in the elderly, *N Engl J Med* 1985 Sep 26;313(13):800-805.

incontinence. Many medications, as listed in Table 10–1, can cause UI. Psychological disorders, particularly depression, have been linked to UI, although the mechanism is not well understood. Excess urine output can occur for a variety of reasons including heart failure, hyperglycemia, and excess fluid intake. Restrictions in mobility impede the ability to get to the toilet in a timely manner, and stool impaction can lead to both UI and fecal incontinence.

▶ Complications

UI can have significant physical and psychological effects on older adults. Older adults with UI are more likely to self-report an overall poor health status. Studies demonstrated that depressive symptoms are more prevalent in incontinent older adults and the severity of depressive symptoms correlates positively with the severity of UI. Men with lower urinary tract symptoms have higher rates of anxiety, depression, and sexual dysfunction. Women with UI may also report a negative impact on sexual function, especially with mixed-type incontinence. UI can cause embarrassment and social withdrawal. Older adults may avoid leaving home or curtail social activities because of fear of incontinence. If medications, such as diuretics, exacerbate UI, adherence to medications and control of comorbid diseases may be reduced. Chronic skin wetness from UI may compromise skin integrity. Dermatitis, candidiasis, cellulitis, and skin breakdown may occur when the skin is repeatedly moist.

Depending on the type of incontinence, certain complications may be more common. A systematic review demonstrated that UI is associated with an increase in falls for adults with an urge but not stress incontinence. Sleep disruption can occur as a result of nocturia with overflow and UUI, especially in the setting of excessive nocturnal diuresis. Overflow incontinence, if caused by severe urinary retention, may result in hydronephrosis and renal dysfunction. Urinary retention is also a risk factor for the development of delirium in older adults.

▶ Treatment

Treatment for UI should begin with lifestyle modification and proceed to behavioral interventions, followed by pharmacologic and device or surgical treatment. With all types of UI, it is also important to maximize treatment for comorbid conditions that can exacerbate urinary symptoms. Medications that contribute to bladder dysfunction and polyuria should be modified if possible (Table 10–1).

A. Lifestyle Modifications

Reducing dietary diuretics, such as caffeine and alcohol, and bladder irritants, such as spicy foods or acidic fruits, can reduce urinary symptoms. Cautious avoidance of excess liquid intake at certain times of the day may be useful. In obese women with SUI, evidence strongly supports weight reduction.

B. Behavioral Therapy

Bladder training and pelvic floor muscle exercises are two approaches with an established evidence base for the treatment of UUI, SUI, and MUI.

1. Bladder training—With this training, scheduled voiding is combined with relaxation techniques to reduce the sense of urgency. The goal is to gradually lengthen the time between scheduled voiding and to reduce the number of UI episodes. The initial schedule should be based on the shortest voiding interval recorded on a bladder diary to maintain dryness, often about 2 hours. With this approach, patients are taught that when the urge to void occurs to relax and allow the urgency to wane before walking to the bathroom. Techniques include slow deep breathing and focusing on calming thoughts. The voiding interval can usually be increased by 15 to 30 minutes per week. To be successful, patients must be cognitively intact and motivated because this approach takes time, patience, and encouragement.

2. Pelvic floor muscle exercises—Pelvic floor muscle exercises have been demonstrated to reduce UI episodes and improve the quality of life in women with UI. The key is to correctly identify and train the muscles of the pelvic floor as one would any skeletal muscle under voluntary control. The pelvic muscles are contracted for 8 to 10 repetitions of 6 to 8 seconds each. One method to ensure the proper muscles are being exercised is to instruct patients to "hold back" the urine flow while voiding on the toilet. These muscles can be contracted for progressively longer times, up to 10 seconds if possible. Three sets of these contractions should be performed three to four times daily to augment the closing pressure of the pelvic floor–urethral sphincter mechanism. Some women have difficulty localizing the pelvic floor muscles that are used for continence control. Specially trained gynecologic physical therapists can assist women in isolating and appropriately exercising these muscles. Techniques, such as biofeedback, electrical stimulation, and the insertion of weighted vaginal cones, can be used to improve pelvic floor strength.

C. Pharmacotherapy

Pharmacotherapy is most effective for the treatment of UUI and in the management of obstructive uropathy that can lead to overflow incontinence (Table 10–3). No medications are currently approved by the US Food and Drug Administration for the treatment of SUI. In many cases, medications modulate the bladder wall and sphincter function through antimuscarinic or anticholinergic effects on sympathetic or parasympathetic pathways. Because many older adults have mixed type of incontinence, medications must be used cautiously, as improvement in one type of UI (eg, urge type) may worsen another form (eg, overflow type).

Topical estrogen may improve UI in women with vaginal atrophy; however, the evidence to support a strong

Table 10–3. Medications used to treat urinary incontinence.

Medication	Dosing	Type of Incontinence
Estrogen		Stress; urge
Estradiol ring	2-mg ring; every 90 days	
Estrogen vaginal cream	0.5–2 g daily to twice weekly	
Antimuscarinics		Urge
Darifenacin (IR/ER)	7.5–15 mg daily	
Fesoterodine (IR/ER)	4–8 mg daily	
Oxybutynin 　IR oral 　ER oral 　Patch 　Topical gel	 2.5–5 mg twice/three times daily 5–30 mg daily 3.9 mg daily 1 g daily	
Solifenacin	5–10 mg daily	
Tolterodine 　IR oral 　ER oral	 1–2 mg twice daily 2–4 mg daily	
Trospium 　IR oral 　ER oral	 20 mg twice daily 60 mg daily	
β$_3$-Adrenergic Agonists		Urge
Mirabegron	25–50 mg daily	
α$_1$-Adrenergic Antagonists		Overflow
Doxazosin	1–8 mg daily	
Terazosin	1–20 mg daily	
Alfuzosin	10 mg daily	
Silodosin	8 mg daily	
Tamsulosin	0.4–0.8 mg daily	

ER, Extended release; IR, immediate release.

recommendation is lacking. Nevertheless, many experts will recommend a trial. Topical estrogen is usually supplied through vaginal suppositories and creams. For some women, however, ring devices impregnated with estrogen that are placed in the vagina for up to 3 months can be more practical than daily estrogen administration. Systemic (oral) estrogen is not beneficial for control of UI and, in fact, may worsen urinary symptoms.

1. Antimuscarinic agents—The mainstay of pharmacotherapy for urge incontinence is the use of medications with anticholinergic effects through inhibition of muscarinic postganglionic cholinergic sites on the bladder wall. This reduces bladder wall contraction and thus increases bladder capacity. Numerous medications are now available in this category. These medications may be available in sustained-release oral and transdermal formulations, which are generally better tolerated; however, efficacy is not superior to the immediate-release formulations. Given the heterogeneity in studies and a variety of clinical outcomes measured, it is difficult to say with certainty, even with meta-analysis data, that any one medication is truly superior to another. The anticholinergic side effects of these medications can be troublesome to older adults and include dry eyes and mouth, constipation, headache, dizziness, orthostatic blood pressure changes, and confusion.

2. β$_3$-Adrenergic agonists—Mirabegron is approved for the treatment of UUI and acts by relaxing the detrusor muscle and increasing bladder capacity. Its efficacy and safety are similar to the antimuscarinic agents. Because it can increase blood pressure, it should be used with caution in hypertensive patients and avoided in patients with uncontrolled hypertension.

3. α-Adrenergic antagonists—The prostate, bladder neck, and urethral tissue contract under the stimulation of α-adrenergic receptors. Alpha blockade allows relaxation of these tissues to improve urine flow and is used most frequently in men with bladder outlet obstruction caused by benign prostatic hyperplasia (BPH). The literature clearly demonstrates the benefit of α-blockers in reducing urinary retention in this population. A number of α-blockers are available. Most of these medications are "nonselective" for urinary tract tissue and also block the α-receptors on the vascular system, causing vasodilation and hypotension. Tamsulosin and silodosin are "selective" α$_{1A}$-blockers, with minimal binding to nonurinary tissues and thus less potential to cause hypotension. These medications are considered preferential for older men because of their more favorable side effect profile.

Because α blockade allows for urethral relaxation, these medications have potential for use in non-BPH overflow incontinence from neurogenic bladder, urethral obstruction, or urethral noncompliance. Studies show benefit in urinary symptoms and flow rates with use of α-blockers in these conditions.

4. Other agents—The serotonin-norepinephrine reuptake inhibitor duloxetine was studied in the treatment of SUI, and high-quality evidence did not show improvement when compared to placebo. Vasopressin for the treatment of nocturia should be avoided in older adults because of the risk of hyponatremia.

D. Devices

Incontinence pads and disposable absorbent undergarments are regularly used to manage UI in both men and women. It is estimated that $4.4 billion are spent annually in US nursing homes alone for these products in addition to laundry service and other continence care expenses. Urethral catheter placement is not a recommended treatment for UI in either gender, due to high risks of urinary tract infection and urethral erosion. However, a condom (external) catheter may be appropriate for men with UI but has been shown to be associated with higher rates of urinary tract infection compared to the use of disposable absorbent undergarments alone. Another option in males with UI is penile clamps, the most common of which is a Cunningham clamp. These clamps have been shown to be comfortable and effective; however, they can result in penile skin breakdown in some cases and should be monitored closely, particularly in older men with cognitive impairment. Of note, some level of both cognition and manual hand dexterity is required by the patient in order for this to be a viable treatment option.

For women with SUI, a pessary with a continence knob may be helpful. These devices are fitted by an experienced clinician to optimize comfort and success. The device works by compressing the bladder neck and urethra, hence decreasing the loss of urine. They require regular cleaning and inspection by a clinician over time, often necessitating frequent visits to the clinic for proper hygiene and maintenance.

E. Minimally Invasive Procedures & Surgery

1. UUI in males & females—Invasive treatments for UUI exist for individuals who have failed more conservative behavioral treatments and pharmacotherapy and in whom other disease processes have been ruled out. Peripheral tibial nerve stimulation (PTNS) is a minimally invasive form of neuromodulation that can be performed in the office setting. A fine-needle electrode is inserted in the inner aspect of the lower leg, just medial to the medial malleolus, into the tibial nerve. A grounding pad is placed and the needle is connected to a pulse generator. A treatment typically lasts 30 minutes and is performed weekly for 12 weeks. Studies have shown subjective and objective success rates of approximately 60%, which is comparable to pharmacotherapy but without the side effects. Unfortunately, this therapy has not been extensively studied in older adults; however, the favorable side effect profile may make this treatment attractive to many older individuals. The main limitation of this therapy is the need for weekly treatments over the course of 12 weeks, potentially followed by maintenance sessions.

Sacral neuromodulation is another form of neuromodulation that is used for the treatment of UUI. This typically involves two outpatient procedures that can be performed under monitored anesthesia care and/or local anesthesia. This procedure involves placement of a tined electrode through the S3 foramen that directly and continuously stimulates the sacral nerve roots innervating the bladder. Control and setting of the device require a cognitively intact individual or help from a family member or caregiver. Limited studies report symptom improvement in older adults, albeit slightly decreased compared to younger (<65 years of age) individuals.

Intradetrusor onabotulinumtoxinA injections act directly on the detrusor (bladder) muscle by blocking the release of acetylcholine from vesicles in the presynaptic nerve, causing temporary chemodenervation and subsequent detrusor muscle relaxation. Dosing varies from 100 to 300 units, and treatment lasts 3 to 12 months. Injections can be performed either in the office setting or in the operating room. The main downsides of onabotulinumtoxinA injections are risks for urinary tract infection and urinary retention, or incomplete bladder emptying, due to detrusor muscle denervation. While retention occurs in only 6% to 10% of individuals receiving the 100-unit dose, patients who are not good candidates for or who are unwilling to perform intermittent catheterization should not undergo this treatment. Limited studies have been performed in older adults undergoing onabotulinumtoxinA injections. Compared to younger adults undergoing this therapy, older adults demonstrated beneficial reductions in UUI, albeit with slightly higher rates of urinary tract infections and elevated PVRs. While these study findings are indeed promising, more studies on outcomes related to PTNS, sacral neuromodulation, and onabotulinumtoxinA in older adults are needed in order to be able to make any generalizable conclusions on the use of these therapies in this patient population.

2. SUI in females—Surgical treatments for SUI in females include urethral bulking agents and sling procedures. Urethral bulking agents are a minimally invasive treatment that can be performed endoscopically either in the office or in the operating room. The aim of the bulking agent is to restore the normal mucosal coaptation of the urethra. The ideal bulking agent is easily injectable, cost effective, biocompatible, and nonmigratory and would cause little to no tissue inflammation. The most common agents currently available are polydimethylsiloxane (Macroplastique), polyacrylamide hydrogel (Bulkmaid), and calcium hydroxylapatite (Coaptite). Objective success rates range from 25% to 73%. The most common adverse event with urethral bulking agents is urinary tract infections. Another limitation is that injections are not permanent and often lose efficacy over time. Due to their minimally invasive nature, however, they may be a good option for older adults who suffer from SUI and do not wish to undergo a more involved surgical procedure.

While urethral bulking agents are less invasive, the gold standard treatment for SUI in females remains the midurethral sling. Midurethral sling procedures are typically performed in an outpatient setting and address urethral hypermobility as a cause of SUI. The aim of the sling is to use a small piece of polypropylene mesh to reinforce the functional pubourethral ligaments and proper fixation of the midurethra to the pelvic bone. Mesh slings are considered to be less invasive compared to nonmesh slings and have shorter operative times, reduced surgical pain, shorter hospitalization, and reduced rates of voiding dysfunction. Mesh-related complications are considered to be acceptably low (<3%). Midurethral slings typically have one vaginal incision and either two lower abdominal incisions (retropubic) or two groin/thigh incisions (transobturator). There is also a "mini-sling" procedure that is performed via one vaginal incision; however, evidence regarding efficacy and safety is immature. While subjective success rates following midurethral sling placement are overwhelmingly high across all ages, older women have been shown to have slightly lower satisfaction, increased UUI symptoms (both persistent and de novo), higher rates of intermittent catheterization, and higher rates of complications. Despite this finding, overall complication rates are low, and midurethral slings remain a good option among older women with SUI.

3. SUI in males—The two main types of surgery for SUI in men are the male sling and the artificial urinary sphincter (AUS). The male sling is a synthetic mesh sling based on the concept of external urethral compression. This surgery is best suited for men with mild to moderate SUI and for men who wish to avoid an AUS.

The AUS remains the most effective treatment for male SUI. The AUS is a surgically implanted device used to treat more moderate to severe SUI. It is designed to supplement the function of the urinary sphincter to restrict the flow of urine. The device consists of a urethral cuff, a pump, and a balloon arranged in a closed system. The urethral cuff wraps around the urethra and is "closed" when it is filled with fluid. The pump, which sits in the scrotum, moves fluid away from the urethral cuff when activated, allowing for the urethra to open and urine to flow. The balloon typically sits in the retropubic space and serves as a reservoir to hold the fluid while the cuff is deactivated (fluid shifts from the cuff to the reservoir to allow the cuff to open). When a patient wishes to urinate, he squeezes the pump in the scrotum, which moves fluid from the urethral cuff to the reservoir, allowing the cuff and urethra to open. The urethra stays open for 3 minutes and then closes automatically.

Compared to the male sling, the AUS requires a more active role of the patient to operate, necessitating intact cognition and good manual dexterity. The main downside of the AUS is the need for periodic revisions over time due to mechanical failure, urethral atrophy, infection, and erosion. These are important considerations among older adults considering both options. Men with cognitive and/or physical limitations may not be good candidates for an AUS and may receive more benefit from a male sling, although it is a less effective procedure.

▶ Prognosis

The outcome of treatment for UI is affected by many factors, including the type of UI, severity of symptoms, and underlying comorbidities. In general, significant reduction in symptom burden can be achieved with the appropriate treatment. If an inciting trigger for incontinence can be identified and alleviated, clinical cure may be possible. Surgical interventions for UI is very favorable but is generally indicated for stress-type incontinence alone. Behavioral interventions can be helpful and require a motivated and sustained effort on the part of the patient or caregiver. Pharmacologic treatments also can substantially reduce symptom burden but are generally not expected to provide a complete clinical cure for all urinary symptoms. Complete dryness may not be possible, but reducing the number and severity of episodes can have a substantial benefit on quality of life and caregiver burden.

American Urological Association (AUA). AUA Position statement on the use of vaginal mesh for the surgical treatment of stress urinary incontinence (SUI). AUA Website. October 2018 (revised). https://www.auanet.org/guidelines/use-of-vaginal-mesh-for-the-surgical-treatment-of-stress-urinary-incontinence. Accessed March 15, 2019.

Cody JD, Jacobs ML, Richardson K, et al. Oestrogen therapy for urinary incontinence in post-menopausal women. *Cochrane Database Syst Rev.* 2012;10:CD001405.

Culbertson S, Davis AM. Nonsurgical management of urinary incontinence in women. *JAMA.* 2017;317(1):79-80.

Engen M, Svenningsen R, Schiotz HA, Kulseng-Hanssen S. Midurethral slings in young, middle-aged, and older women. *Neurourol Urodyn.* 2018;37:2578-2585.

Gormley EA, Lightner DJ, Faraday M, Vasavada SP. Diagnosis and treatment of overactive bladder (non-neurogenic) in adults: AUA/SUFU guideline amendment. *J Urol.* 2015;193(5):1572-1580.

Kobashi KC, Albo ME, Dmochowski RR, et al. Surgical treatment of female stress urinary incontinence: AUA/SUFU guideline. *J Urol.* 2017;198(4):875-883.

Lukacz ES, Santiago-Lastra Y, Albo ME, Brubaker L. Urinary incontinence in women: a review. *JAMA.* 2017;318(16):1592-1604.

Madhuvrata P, Cody JD, Ellis G, Herbison GP, Hay-Smith EJ. Which anticholinergic drug for overactive bladder symptoms in adults. *Cochrane Database Syst Rev.* 2012;1:CD005429.

Natalin R, Lorenzetti F, Dambros M. Management of OAB in those over age 65. *Curr Urol Rep.* 2013;14:379-385.

Pratt TS, Suskind AM. Management of overactive bladder in older women. *Curr Urol Rep.* 2018;19:92.

Qaseem A, Dallas P, Forciea MA, et al. Nonsurgical management of urinary incontinence in women: a clinical practice guideline from the American College of Physicians. *Ann Intern Med.* 2014;161(6):429-440.

Siddiqui ZA, Abboudi H, Crawford R, Shah S. Intraurethral bulking agents for the management of female stress urinary incontinence: a systematic review. *Int Urogynecol J.* 2017;28:1275-1284.

Sung VW, Borello-France D, Newman DK, et al. Effect of behavioral and pelvic floor muscle therapy combined with surgery vs surgery alone on incontinence symptoms among women with mixed urinary incontinence: the ESTEEM randomized clinical trial. *JAMA.* 2019;322(11):1066-1076.

Vaughan CP, Goode PS, Burgio KL, Markland AD. Urinary incontinence in older adults. *Mt Sinai J Med.* 2011;78:558-570.

Winters JC, Dmochowski RR, Goldman HB, et al. Urodynamic studies in adults: AUA/SUFU guideline. *J Urol.* 2012;188(6 suppl):2464-2472.

Sexual Health & Dysfunction

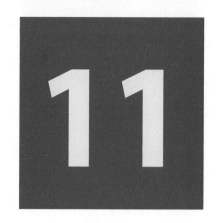

11

Elizabeth Waring, MD

Angela Gentili, MD

Michael Godschalk, MD

ESSENTIALS OF DIAGNOSIS

▶ Sexual dysfunction is common among older persons and is caused by a combination of physiologic changes, lifestyle choices, psychological factors, and aging-related diseases.

▶ In older men, the most common type of sexual dysfunction is erectile dysfunction, and the most common etiology is vascular disease.

▶ In older women, sexual dysfunction is often multifactorial, including lack of estrogen causing vaginal dryness and lack of testosterone decreasing libido.

▶ Evaluation of sexual dysfunction consists of a complete sexual history, review of medications, a targeted physical exam, and selected laboratory tests.

▶ General Principles

Older men and women are still interested in sex, yet sexual activity can decline with age. In the National Social Life, Health, and Aging Project (NSHAP), Lindau and colleagues found that self-reported sexual activity decreased with age; 73% of respondents aged 57 to 64 years described themselves as being "sexually active," as compared to 26% of those aged 75 to 85. It is of interest, however, that of those who identified as being sexually active, the frequency of sexual activity was similar to that of younger counterparts; 54% reported sexual activity at least two to three times month, with 25% stating frequency of at least weekly. These findings run counter to the stereotypes of older adults who are often mislabeled as sexless and uninterested in intimacy.

In men, age-related physiologic changes impact sexual function. Alterations in the pituitary–hypothalamic–gonadal axis may result in hypogonadism and decreased libido.

Changes in penile innervation reduce penile sensitivity to touch, make it more difficult to achieve a rigid erection, increase the time it takes to reach orgasm, diminish forcefulness and volume of ejaculation, and prolong the refractory period (the time it takes to have an erection after ejaculation). The prolonged time to orgasm may be beneficial in men with a history of premature ejaculation.

Masters and Johnson in 1966 first described the sexual response in four distinct stages: excitement, plateau, orgasm, and resolution. The female physiologic response may change with aging in the setting of hypoestrogenism following menopause. During the excitement phase, there is decreased genital engorgement. Vaginal lubrication may decrease, necessitating longer foreplay and use of supplemental lubrication for penetrative intercourse. During the plateau phase, there is less expansion and vasocongestion of the vagina. During orgasm, the strength and frequency of the perineal muscle contractions may diminish, although the ability to achieve multiple orgasms is retained. During the resolution phase, vasocongestion is lost more rapidly.

In women, for whom the stages may overlap or even be absent, the characterization of "normal" sexual response as one that culminates in orgasm is a limiting lens through which to view satisfactory sexual intimacy. Some older persons may engage in sexual activity not out of desire for sex but out of desire for closeness with their partners. A positive experience may increase motivation for future encounters, whereas a negative one (eg, from dyspareunia) may decrease one's interest in sex. When sexuality is redefined such that the goal is not necessarily orgasm but rather sexual touch and intimacy, the overall satisfaction with sexual health improves greatly.

In addition to the physiologic changes that occur with aging, lifestyle choices, psychological factors, availability and health of a partner, and aging-related diseases and their treatment may affect sexual function and activity in both men and women. In a survey of men and women aged 75 to 85 years, 78% of men identified as having an available partner, but this number decreased to 40% for women, likely reflecting the differences seen in life expectancy.

Prevention

A. Men

The most common cause of sexual dysfunction in older men is erectile dysfunction (ED). The National Institutes of Health (NIH) defines ED as the consistent inability to achieve and/or maintain an erection sufficient for satisfactory sexual activity. More than 60% of men age 70 years are unable to achieve a rigid erection. ED is the most common chronic disease in older men, and vascular disease is the most common cause of ED.

Risk factors for vascular disease include lack of exercise, diabetes mellitus (DM), hyperlipidemia, hypertension, and smoking. In many cases, these diseases are preventable by dietary and lifestyle changes. Because of the correlation between ED and vascular disease, ED is a marker for future vascular events, such as myocardial infarction and stroke. ED is a powerful predictor of cardiovascular disease in men younger than 60 years of age and in patients with DM.

The second most common causes of ED are neurogenic. The autonomic dysfunction seen in DM and Parkinson disease prevents penile vasodilatation and erection. Neurogenic ED is frequently seen after prostatectomy or radiation therapy for prostate cancer. In treating prostate cancer, nerve-sparing surgery reduces this risk.

DM has the greatest impact on sexual function in men since it may cause both vascular and neurogenic ED. Approximately two-thirds of diabetic men age >60 years report ED. The risk of ED is directly related to the duration of diabetes, the hemoglobin A1c level, and increasing age. Early aggressive control of DM may prevent ED or delay its onset.

Another common cause of ED is medications. Anticholinergics, such as antipsychotics and oxybutynin, block parasympathetic-mediated vasodilatation. Antihypertensives, including β-blockers and thiazides, also increase the risk of ED. Angiotensin-converting enzyme inhibitors and calcium channel blockers do not have an adverse impact on erections. In addition to ED, medications such as α-blockers, used as antihypertensives and/or to treat lower urinary tract symptoms (LUTS), may cause ejaculatory disorders. Antidepressants such as the selective serotonin reuptake inhibitors (SSRIs) are associated with ED, decreased libido, delayed ejaculation, and anorgasmia. Bupropion and mirtazapine are the antidepressants least likely to cause sexual dysfunction.

Psychogenic ED is the least common etiology in older men. Patients with psychogenic ED usually describe the sudden onset of ED related to an event in their lives (eg, argument with their partner, losing a job). Of note, men with ED caused by a nonpsychogenic etiology may have performance anxiety and/or depression because of the ED.

Testosterone's role in ED is controversial. Low testosterone is associated with decreased libido, but hypogonadal men can still achieve an erection, and most men with ED have normal testosterone levels. Studies in animals suggest that testosterone is needed for a rigid erection. Studies also show that testosterone replacement in hypogonadal men improves their response to phosphodiesterase type 5 inhibitors.

Premature ejaculation (PE) occurs in approximately 30% of men, also referred to as "rapid ejaculators." PE is defined as orgasm with minimal stimulation. The most common cause is neurophysiologic. PE may also be psychogenic. Most PE is chronic. Patients with acute onset of PE may have a prostate infection (prostatitis). PE is often associated with psychological distress and can result in decreased intimacy. As men age, PE becomes less of a problem because of changes in penile innervation resulting in decreased penile sensation.

Retrograde ejaculation is a common complaint in men who have DM or have undergone transurethral prostatic resection. In both cases, the proximal sphincter does not close during ejaculation and semen goes into the bladder.

Orgasmic failure is uncommon in men. When it does occur, it may be a result of nerve damage (prostate cancer, radical prostatectomy, or DM) or may be medication induced (gabapentin). Apart from stopping gabapentin, treatment is usually unsuccessful.

B. Women

The physiologic changes in sexual function with age constitute a "dysfunction" only if they cause significant distress to the woman. Given that the average Western woman will spend almost 30 years in a postmenopausal state, it is important to address the physiologic changes associated with hypoestrogenism as a normal part of the sexual lifespan, rather than as a dysfunction. As such, the term *genitourinary syndrome of menopause* (GSM) was adopted in 2014 by the International Society for the Study of Women's Sexual Health and the North American Menopause Society. GSM replaces the previous terms of *vulvovaginal atrophy* or *atrophic vaginitis* when describing the genitourinary symptoms associated with prolonged states of hypoestrogenism.

Due to a common embryologic origin, the female genitalia and lower urinary tract (including the urethra and bladder) share common estrogen receptor function. The vaginal and urethral epithelium is comprised of nonkeratinized stratified squamous epithelium that stores glycogen in the presence of estrogen, increasing compliance and elasticity. The vaginal wall releases stored glycogen, which is then hydrolyzed to glucose. It is this glucose that maintains the natural vaginal flora, being metabolized by *Lactobacillus* into lactic acid and acetic acid, maintaining the acidic pH of the vagina. The acidity of the vagina, in turn, provides natural protection against urinary tract infections and vaginitis. Although glucose plays a role in maintenance of vaginal health, it is beneficial only when moderated by physiologic levels of estrogen;

in older women with poorly controlled diabetes, chronic glucosuria may precipitate recurrent and recalcitrant vulvovaginal candidiasis and/or cystitis.

In the absence of sufficient estrogen, the vaginal pH becomes more alkalotic and the vaginal flora composition can change significantly, leading to malodorous discharge (vaginitis); there is decreased blood flow within the vulvovaginal microvasculature and thus decreased lubrication; and the epithelium thins and becomes pale, friable, and prone to fissures and tears that may cause dyspareunia.

The prevalence and burden associated with GSM are significant. In the recent Vaginal Health: Insights, Views, and Attitudes (VIVA) international survey, 63% of postmenopausal women reported vaginal symptoms related to menopause. Of these women, 48% identified vaginal discomfort or pain as their predominant symptom, with dryness (83%) and dyspareunia (42%) identified as the most common etiology of their discomfort. In women who reported vaginal discomfort, 80% considered vaginal discomfort to negatively impact their lives, with a negative effect on sexual intimacy (75%), ability to have a loving relationship (33%), self-esteem (26%), and an overall decrease in quality of life (25%). Despite the high symptom burden, however, 40% of women affected by GSM reported waiting >1 year before seeking advice from their provider.

Once GSM and female sexual dysfunction have been identified, it is important to counsel patients on options regarding further treatment. GSM is a progressive and chronic disease; early identification and intervention with topical hormonal or nonhormonal treatments can have a significant impact on the sexual health of a patient for the remainder of her life.

Another change in sexual function observed in the aging female not associated with GSM is a decrease in libido. As in men, androgens are thought to have a role in women's libido. The ovaries and adrenals are the main sources of androgens; a decrease in the production of androgens and dehydroepiandrosterone with aging can lead to a decrease in libido, arousal, and genital sensation. The association between sexual function and androgen levels in women has been weak at most and of limited clinical significance. Because there are no normative data on plasma total and free testosterone in women and there is no well-defined clinical syndrome of androgen deficiency, the Endocrine Society does not recommend making a diagnosis of androgen deficiency in women.

Painful intercourse, or dyspareunia, can be caused by psychological and/or organic factors. The most common cause of dyspareunia is GSM. Other causes of dyspareunia include vaginismus (involuntary muscle spasm), vaginal infections, cystitis, or history of prior sexual trauma. Once experienced, the fear and anticipation of recurrent pain may perpetuate the symptoms, thus creating a positive feedback loop that needs to be specifically addressed by the provider, patient, and partner.

▶ Clinical Findings

A. Symptoms & Signs

1. Men—The evaluation of sexual dysfunction in men includes taking a good sexual history, a physical exam, and a few lab tests. Patients may be reluctant to talk about their sexual function, and the International Index of Erectile Function (IIEF-5) can be used to start this discussion. The IIEF-5 is self-administered and consists of five questions about sexual function during the past month. The IIEF-5 can be given to male patients to complete before the visit.

Obtaining a thorough history is the most important part of the evaluation of sexual dysfunction. The first step is to determine the specific nature of the problem. Does the patient have decreased libido, difficulty obtaining and/or maintaining an erection, PE, retrograde ejaculation, or anorgasmia?

The patient should be then asked about the onset (gradual vs sudden) of the problem, the presence or absence of sleep-associated erections, and about any treatments that he has tried (both prescription and nonprescription). In men with ED, the onset and presence or absence of sleep-associated erections (SAEs) can help distinguish among psychogenic, medication-induced, and organic (vascular, neurogenic, and endocrine) ED. Patients with psychogenic ED will describe a sudden onset but will still have SAEs. Men with medication-induced ED will also report a sudden onset but will deny having SAEs. Finally, patients with organic ED will have a gradual onset and absent SAEs.

The physical exam targets signs of hypogonadism and vascular and neurologic disease. Signs of hypogonadism include gynecomastia, decreased body hair, scant pubic hair, or a female escutcheon. The vascular exam involves listening for bruits and palpating pedal pulses. The neurologic exam includes rectal sphincter tone, bulbocavernosus reflex (performed by squeezing the glans penis, which should result in anal sphincter contraction), and deep tendon reflexes. During the rectal exam, the prostate should be palpated for nodules. Finally, the penis should be examined for plaques (Peyronie disease).

2. Women—As for men, a detailed sexual health history is of paramount importance in women. Asking specific questions related to sexual health and function alleviates the patient from the burden of having to initiate discussion of symptoms that may be difficult or embarrassing. Normalization of changes in vaginal lubrication, increased incidence of urinary and fecal incontinence, and changes in arousal, orgasm, and libido by the medical provider is the first step in obtaining a detailed and accurate review of systems. An example of such a directed interview is provided in Table 11–1.

Each of these questions creates a branching pathway of follow-up queries that can further delineate the needs of the patient while encouraging patients to disclose their symptoms without having to initiate the conversation.

Table 11–1. Example of a sexual history in older women.

Question	Rationale
1. Are you currently sexually active?	• Identification of current degree of sexual activity and partner availability
2. Are you sexually active with men, women, or both?	• Address partner sexual dysfunction specific to gender • Education about transmission of sexually transmitted diseases from opposite- and same-sex behaviors (contact with bodily fluids, shared sex toys, oral-genital contact, penetrative intercourse)
3. Have you noticed any difficulties with lubrication or achieving orgasm?	• Assessment of symptoms related to hypoestrogenism (genitourinary syndrome of menopause [GSM])
4. Do you ever lose control of your bowel or bladder? Has this ever happened during intercourse?	• Identification of urinary and/or fecal incontinence as well as impact on sexual activity and health
5. Have you experienced pain or bleeding with penetrative intercourse?	• Assessment of dyspareunia versus vestibulodynia or vaginismus, screen for possible malignancy with postcoital bleeding versus symptoms related to GSM
6. Have you ever been forced to have sex? 7. Have you ever been touched in a sexual way without your consent?	• Screen for prior sexual trauma or abuse

A thorough medical history is also important as several chronic illnesses can result in sexual dysfunction: diabetes and rheumatologic disease can cause debility and decreased physical function, and a history of breast cancer with mastectomy may result in a change in a woman's self-image, as may pelvic organ prolapse or urinary and/or fecal incontinence. Estimates of coital urinary incontinence, defined as involuntary loss of urine that occurs with arousal, penetration, and/or orgasm, occurs in 24% to 66% of women with underlying stress or urge urinary incontinence. Fecal incontinence, which affects 15% of older women but is reported to providers <30% of the time, has an even more severe negative effect on sexual health and function.

The clinician should elicit a complete drug history because several medications can contribute to sexual dysfunction, including SSRIs, antipsychotics, antihypertensives, antiestrogens, antiandrogens, alcohol, and several illicit/recreational drugs. Chronic use of opioids can affect sexual function by causing opioid-induced androgen deficiency. Anticholinergic drugs, often used for overactive bladder/urge urinary incontinence, decrease normal vaginal lubrication and may precipitate or worsen dyspareunia.

The physical exam is directed by symptoms elicited during the history and is particularly important in older women who may not have received regular medical care. An external vulvar exam should be considered in every patient, whereas an internal vaginal exam is only indicated with complaints of vaginal dryness or dyspareunia in which GSM is suspected. The exam should also include blood pressure and peripheral pulses as vascular disease affects arousal, a musculoskeletal exam as rheumatologic disorders can cause pain and difficulty with sexual activity, thyroid exam as hypothyroidism can cause decreased desire or arousal, and screening

for neuropathy as neurologic disorders can cause decreased desire and arousal, or anorgasmia.

B. Laboratory Findings

1. Men—The laboratory evaluation of men with sexual dysfunction should include a hemoglobin A1c, a lipid panel, and total testosterone (if there are signs and/or symptoms of hypogonadism). Because of its diurnal secretory pattern, testosterone should be obtained between 8 AM and 10 AM. If the testosterone is low, it should be repeated and luteinizing hormone (LH) level obtained. If the testosterone is low and the LH is high, the problem is at the level of the testes. If testosterone is low and LH is low or normal, the patient has a hypothalamic or pituitary disorder and will need further testing.

2. Women—Routine laboratory testing is not necessary or indicated in the evaluation of female sexual function. Testosterone levels do not correlate with sexual function. Prolactin and thyroid-stimulating hormone levels should be only be obtained if the history or physical exam is suggestive of underlying abnormalities.

▶ Treatment

1. Men—The choice of treatment in men depends on the etiology of the sexual dysfunction. In men with psychogenic ED, discussion and reassurance are frequently effective. If the patient continues to have ED, referral to a sex therapist may be necessary.

In men with decreased libido who are hypogonadal, testosterone replacement therapy (TRT) may improve their sex drive. Contraindications to testosterone treatment include a history of prostate or breast cancer, polycythemia, severe LUTS, or obstructive sleep apnea. There is controversy about whether TRT increases cardiovascular risk in hypogonadal men. Of note, in 2015 the US Food and Drug Administration (FDA) required that manufacturers of testosterone products add information to the labeling about a possible increased risk of heart attacks and strokes.

Neurophysiologic PE is treated with behavioral therapy ("stop-start" and "squeeze") and medications that delay ejaculation. These include SSRIs, α-blockers, and topical anesthetics. If a patient has prostatitis, an antibiotic usually cures the PE. In men with psychogenic PE, psychotherapy may help.

Retrograde ejaculation is a benign condition. Reassurance is the main treatment. The patient should be reminded that even without visible ejaculate, impregnation is still possible with a fertile partner.

The most common cause of sexual dysfunction in men is ED. However, before treating ED, clinicians need to determine if it is safe for the patient to engage in sexual intercourse. The person on top during intercourse expends the equivalent of the energy needed to climb two flights of stairs. If a patient is sedentary and has cardiac risk factors (hypertension, DM, hyperlipidemia, or tobacco use) and/or known cardiovascular disease, a cardiac evaluation including a stress test may be needed before starting treatment for ED.

In men with drug-induced ED, if possible, the offending drug should be discontinued or changed to another agent/different drug class. For example, replace a β-blocker with an erection-sparing agent, such as a calcium channel blocker. Of note, patients with drug-induced ED frequently have underlying vascular disease, now unmasked by the drug. If the ED is longstanding, patients may not see improvement in their erectile function with the change in agents.

However, in most cases, ED is caused by vascular and/or neurologic disease. The only FDA-approved treatments for ED are vacuum devices, phosphodiesterase type 5 inhibitors, and alprostadil (prostaglandin E$_1$) given as an intraurethral suppository or an intracavernosal injection (ICI) (Table 11–2).

a. Vacuum constrictive device—The vacuum constrictive device (VCD) was patented in 1917. It works by having the patient insert his penis in a plastic tube that is connected to a pump. He then pumps the air out of the tube and the resultant vacuum pulls blood into the penis and makes it erect. A rubber ring is slipped off the tube onto the base of the penis. The ring traps the blood in the penis and thereby maintains the erection. Patients or their partners may be reluctant to try VCDs because they are mechanical and take the spontaneity out of sex. However, VCDs are successful in 70% to 80% of patients who try them. Men should be warned not to leave the ring on for more than 30 minutes because the rings act

Table 11–2. Nonsurgical treatment for ED.

Treatment	Route	Dosage	Cost/Dose	Common Adverse Effects	Serious Adverse Effects
Vacuum devices	EXT	–	$95–$350	Penis cool to touch Ring may cause vaginal irritation	Ring left on for <30 minutes may cause penile ischemia Do not use in patients with sickle cell anemia
Sildenafil	PO	25–100 mg	$85	Erythema, flushing, indigestion, headache, insomnia, visual disturbance, epistaxis, nasal congestion, rhinitis	MI, sickle cell anemia with vaso-occlusive crisis, NAION, sudden hearing loss, priapism
Vardenafil	PO	5–20 mg	$62	Flushing, dizziness, headache, rhinitis	Chest pain, MI, prolonged QT interval, seizure, NAION, sudden hearing loss, priapism
Tadalafil	PO	2.5–20 mg	$12–$76	Flushing, indigestion, nausea, backache, myalgia, headache, nasopharyngitis	Angina, Stevens-Johnson syndrome, CVA, seizure, NAION, sudden hearing loss
Avanafil	PO	50–200 mg	$75	Flushing, backache, headache, nasal congestion, nasopharyngitis	Priapism, NAION, sudden hearing loss
Alprostadil	TU	125–1000 mcg	$71–$86	Urethral discomfort, pain in penis, pain in testicle	Priapism
Alprostadil	ICI	10–40 mcg	$92–$156	Pain in penis, pain in testicle, fibrosis of penis	Priapism

CVA, cerebrovascular accident; EXT, external; ICI, intracavernosal; MI, myocardial infarction; NAION, nonarteritic ischemic optic neuropathy; PO, oral; TU, transurethral.

Cost data for medications from UpToDate; cost data for vacuum devices from the Internet; drug adverse events from MicroMedex.

like a tourniquet. VCDs with a battery-powered pump are available for patients who have arthritis or another condition that limits their ability to use a manual pump.

b. Phosphodiesterase type 5 inhibitors—When a man becomes aroused, there is stimulation of the penile nerve that results in the activation of nitric oxide synthase. Nitric oxide synthase catalyzes the production of nitric oxide from L-arginine. Nitric oxide diffuses into penile smooth muscle cells and activates guanyl cyclase, which produces cyclic guanosine monophosphate (cGMP). cGMP relaxes smooth muscle, resulting in vasodilatation and erection. cGMP is metabolized by phosphodiesterase type 5 (PDE5). PDE5 inhibitors prevent the breakdown of cGMP, thereby increasing vasodilation and erection.

There are four FDA-approved PDE5 inhibitors in the United States: avanafil (Stendra), sildenafil (Viagra), tadalafil (Cialis), and vardenafil (Levitra). Avanafil, sildenafil, and vardenafil are taken "on demand." Tadalafil has both "on demand" and daily dosing. Except for daily tadalafil, these medications are taken 30 to 60 minutes before initiation of sexual activity. The starting doses are 100 mg for avanafil, 25 mg for sildenafil, 10 mg for tadalafil, and 5 mg for vardenafil. The starting daily dose of tadalafil is 2.5 mg.

Side effects are usually mild and related to smooth muscle relaxation. They include headache, flushing, esophageal reflux, and rhinitis. Sildenafil may cause "blue haze," a transient disturbance in color vision, because of its effect on retinal PDE6. Tadalafil may cause muscle aches and back pain from its effect on PDE11. Vision loss, from nonarteritic anterior ischemic optic neuropathy, and sudden hearing loss have been reported in a small number of men taking PDE5 inhibitors. The relationship between these events and PDE5 inhibitors is unclear. However, patients should be warned to stop taking PDE5 inhibitors and seek immediate medical attention for a sudden decrease or loss of vision or hearing.

Because of their mechanism of action, PDE5 inhibitors potentiate the effects of nitrates and may cause profound hypotension and death. Use of PDE5 inhibitors with any form of nitrates is contraindicated. In addition, because PDE5 inhibitors are vasodilators, they may augment the hypotensive effects of antihypertensives. Patients should be warned about possible orthostatic symptoms. Doses of PDE5 inhibitors should be decreased in patients with significant liver or kidney disease or in men taking P450 inhibitors.

There are many oral, nonprescription, non–FDA-approved treatments for ED. Yohimbine is one of the most commonly used nonprescription treatments for ED. It blocks presynaptic α_2-receptors and may improve libido and increase blood flow into the penis. Based on reports from the authors' patients, yohimbine is not an effective treatment of ED.

If patients fail VCDs and PDE5 inhibitors, the next step may be transurethral alprostadil (Medicated Urethral System for Erection or MUSE). Alprostadil (prostaglandin E_1) increases cyclic adenosine monophosphate, resulting in vasodilatation and erection. Alprostadil can be given as an intraurethral pellet or by penile injection. The pellet is inserted into the urethra using a plastic applicator. It dissolves and is absorbed into the surrounding tissue producing an erection. It works in approximately 50% of older patients. Side effects include urethral burning, prolonged erections (priapism), and hypotension.

Alprostadil (Caverject or Edex) given as an ICI is a very effective treatment for ED. Unfortunately, it is the least popular treatment because it requires an injection into the penis each time the patient wants to have intercourse. Penile pain, priapism, and penile fibrosis (Peyronie disease) are some of the side effects seen with ICI.

2. Women—As previously mentioned, GSM is a chronic and progressive disease that occurs in the setting of hypoestrogenism following menopause. Early identification is crucial to prevent further sequelae, and prompt initiation of treatment is encouraged when physical signs are present, even in the absence of distressing symptoms. Current recommendations for treatment of GSM start with nonhormonal therapy, followed by escalation to hormonal interventions for patients with refractory symptoms thereafter following assessment of risk/benefit.

a. Nonhormonal therapies—Vaginal moisturizers are readily available and may be purchased without a prescription. They are recommended for regular, daily to thrice weekly use, with the goal of maintaining a lipophilic barrier along the vaginal epithelium. Women using a vaginal moisturizer should use an additional lubricant during penetrative intercourse. Although water-based lubricants are most common, silicone lubricants are becoming more readily available and may be preferred by many patients. Oil-based lubricants, including baby oil and food-grade coconut oil, may also be used safely; however, patients using latex barriers for prevention of disease transmission should be counseled that oil will compromise the efficacy of the barrier. Vaginal patency is best maintained with regular sexual activity, either with penetrative intercourse, digital insertion, or use of a dilator. Allowing increased time for foreplay may also be useful to achieve greater arousal and lubrication in the setting of delayed vasocongestion and engorgement.

b. Hormonal therapies—Refractory symptoms of GSM generally respond well to low-dose topical estrogen therapy (Table 11–3); systemic hormonal replacement therapy is not indicated in the postmenopausal female. The absorption of vaginal estrogen creams depends on the dose. In 2008, the FDA approved a low-dose conjugated estrogen cream regimen (0.3 mg twice weekly) because it does not cause significant proliferation of the endometrial lining (unopposed estrogen is contraindicated in women who have a uterus due to risk of endometrial hyperplasia). Vaginal estradiol rings or tablets deliver low-dose estrogen locally with low systemic absorption. In a Cochrane review, women favored

Table 11–3. Low-dose topical hormone therapies with minimal systemic absorption.

Vaginal Hormone Therapy	Dose	Comment
Conjugated estrogen cream (Premarin)	Continuous regimen: 0.5 g (0.3 mg conjugated estrogen) twice weekly	Correct doing with applicator may be cumbersome. doses >0.5 g twice a week are considered high dose and more likely to have systemic effects.
Estradiol softgel capsule 4 µg or 10 µg (Imvexxy) or tablet 10 µg (Vagifem or generic Yuvafem)	4 or 10 µg softgel capsule or 10 µg tablet daily × 2 weeks then twice weekly	Softgel capsule does not need use of an applicator.
Ring: Estradiol ring 2 g (Estring)	7.5 µg/24 h over 90 days; provider or patient replace the ring every 90 days	Not to be confused with the higher dose estradiol ring (50–100 µg/day, Femring), which provides systemic estrogen therapy. Well tolerated and does not interfere with intercourse.
Prasterone (synthetic DHEA, Intrarosa) 6.5 mg vaginal suppository	6.5 mg daily	FDA approved in 2016 for dyspareunia in the setting of GSM.

DHEA, dehydroepiandrosterone; FDA, US Food and Drug Administration; GSM, genitourinary syndrome of menopause.

the vaginal ring because of ease of use and comfort. According to the 2019 American Geriatrics Society Beers Criteria, low-dose vaginal estrogens (estradiol <25 µg twice weekly) are likely safe in women with a history of breast cancer who do not respond to nonhormonal therapies (moderate quality of evidence). The American College of Obstetricians and Gynecologists (ACOG) recommends short-term use of topical estrogen therapy in this patient population for moderate to severe symptoms that have failed first-line nonhormonal treatment options, and only following appropriate counseling with the patient's oncologist regarding potential risks and benefits.

Dyspareunia has recently been targeted by two new medications. Ospemifene (Osphena), a selective estrogen receptor modular, is the only oral medication approved by the FDA for the treatment of moderate to severe dyspareunia resulting from vulvovaginal atrophy. A once-daily 60-mg dose has been shown to improve dyspareunia in clinical trials; however, no appreciable effect on libido, arousal, or quality of orgasm was found. It is contraindicated in women with a history of breast cancer or severe hepatic impairment and is associated with many of the same risks as seen in systemic estrogen therapy (eg, increased risk of thromboembolic events, although to a significantly lower degree). The only non–estrogen-based treatment for any symptom of GSM is prasterone (Intrarosa), a 6.5-mg synthetic dehydroepiandrosterone vaginal insert FDA approved for treatment of moderate to severe dyspareunia in postmenopausal women. The vaginal insert is placed via applicator once daily and may take up to 12 weeks of use prior to appreciable effect. Although a study of systemic sex steroid and metabolite levels following 12 weeks of use (including estradiol/E2) remained at or below average normal postmenopausal values, vaginal prasterone is currently contraindicated in women with a history of or current breast malignancy.

Several studies have looked at the effect of testosterone on libido in postmenopausal women with mixed results (Table 11–4). Randomized trials have demonstrated that low-dose testosterone patch improves sexual desire in women with decreased libido, with or without concurrent use of estrogens/progestins, and either surgically induced or natural menopause. Androgenic side effects such as acne and hirsutism were uncommon, and there was no decrease in high-density lipoprotein cholesterol as seen in studies using oral methyltestosterone. In two large randomized trials, testosterone gel for 6 months did not improve sexual function compared to placebo. Because of lack of data on long-term safety, the FDA did not approve the testosterone patch for women, and no formulations are available in the United States.

Because the cause of sexual dysfunction is often multifactorial, a team approach may be the most helpful. The primary care provider addresses medical issues and medication review. Physical/occupational therapists can improve function in older women with limited mobility, especially those trained in pelvic physical therapy. A gynecologic referral is indicated if symptoms persist despite treatment with the current standard of care or if physical findings warrant expert evaluation (eg, suspicious lesions or postcoital bleeding). A referral to urogynecology as available for evaluation of persistent urinary and/or fecal incontinence as well as pelvic organ prolapse may also be indicated. A sex therapist can educate the older couple about sexuality and changes with aging, while a couples therapist can address conflicts or poor communication between the couple. If there is underlying depression, anxiety, or substance abuse, other mental health referrals may be appropriate.

3. Sexually transmitted infections (STIs)—Sexually active older men and women should be warned about the risk for STIs. Older persons may be at increased risk of STIs due to

Table 11–4. Treatment options for sexual dysfunction in older women.

Symptom	Common Causes	Therapy
Decreased desire	Low testosterone from menopause Chronic illness Depression Relationship problems Medications	Testosterone patch is not FDA approved in women Treatment of underlying illness Antidepressant medication Marital therapy Review of drugs ingested
Decreased lubrication	Vaginal dryness or atrophy from postmenopausal status Antiestrogen and anticholinergic medications	Longer foreplay, regular intercourse, lubricants, topical estrogens Review of medications, including OTC drugs
Delayed or absent orgasm	Neurologic disorders, diabetes Psychologic problems	Treatment of underlying illness Cognitive-behavioral therapy, masturbation, Kegel exercises
Pain with intercourse	Organic cause Vaginal dryness, atrophy Vaginismus (involuntary vaginal contractions)	Treatment of underlying physical condition Longer foreplay, regular intercourse, lubricants, topical estrogens or topical DHEA, oral estrogen receptor modulator (ospemifene) Psychotherapy, cognitive-behavioral therapy

DHEA, dehydroepiandrosterone; FDA, US Food and Drug Administration; OL, Off Label; OTC, over-the-counter.

Gentili A, Godschalk M. Sexuality. In: Harper GM, Lyons WL, Potter JF, eds. Geriatrics Review Syllabus: *A Core Curriculum in Geriatric Medicine*, 10th ed. New York, NY: American Geriatrics Society; 2019. http://geriatricscareonline.org. Reprinted with permission.

multiple or new partners (sometimes after divorce or death of partner), lack of knowledge about STI risk factors, and physiologic changes such as vaginal atrophy. Before starting treatment for sexual dysfunction, warn patients about STIs, including HIV, and offer testing if they are at risk.

Davis SR, Robinson PJ, Jane F, White S, White M, Bell RJ. Intravaginal testosterone improves sexual satisfaction and vaginal symptoms associated with aromatase inhibitors. *J Clin Endocrinol Metab.* 2018;103(11):4146-4154.

Duralde ER, Rowen TS. Urinary incontinence and associated female sexual dysfunction. *Sex Med Rev.* 2017;5(4):470-485.

Erectile dysfunction. *Nat Rev Dis Primers.* 2016;2:16004.

Faubion SS, Sood R, Kapoor E. Genitourinary syndrome of menopause: management strategies for the clinician. *Mayo Clin Proc.* 2017;92(12):1842-1849.

Food and Drug Administration. FDA Drug Safety Communication. FDA cautions about using testosterone products for low testosterone due to aging. www.fda.gov/Drugs/DrugSafety/ucm436259.htm. Accessed March 11, 2020.

Jannini EA, Nappi RE. Couplepause: a new paradigm in treating sexual dysfunction during menopause and andropause. *Sex Med Rev.* 2018;6(3):384-395.

Kouidrat Y, Pizzol D, Cosco T, et al. High prevalence of erectile dysfunction in diabetes: a systematic review and meta-analysis of 145 studies. *Diabet Med.* 2017;34:1185-1192.

La Torre A, Giupponi G, Duffy D, Conca A. Sexual dysfunction related to psychotropic drugs: a critical review—Part I: antidepressants. *Pharmacopsychiatry.* 2013;46:191-199.

Lindau ST, Schumm LP, Laumann EO, Levinson W, O'Muircheartaigh CA, Waite LJ. A study of sexuality and health among older adults in the United States. *N Engl J Med.* 2007;357:762-774.

Martin C, Nolen H, Podolnick J, et al. Current and emerging therapies in premature ejaculation: where we are coming from, where we are going. *Int J Urol.* 2017;24(1):40-50.

Masters WH, Johnson VE. Sex and the aging process. *J Am Geriatr Soc.* 1981;29(9):385-390.

Morton L. Sexuality in the older adult. *Prim Care Clin Off Pract.* 2017;44(3):429-438.

Rahn DD, Carberry C, Sanses TV, et al. Vaginal estrogen for genitourinary syndrome of menopause: a systematic review HHS public access author manuscript. *Obs Gynecol.* 2014;124(6):1147-1156.

Shifren JL, Davis SR Androgens in postmenopausal women: a review. *Menopause.* 2017;24(8):970.

Thompson IM, Tangen CM, Goodman PJ, Probstfield JL, Moinpour CM, Coltman CA. Erectile dysfunction and subsequent cardiovascular disease. *JAMA.* 2005;294(23):2996-3002.

Thompson JC, Rogers RG. Surgical management for pelvic organ prolapse and its impact on sexual function. *Sex Med Rev.* 2016;4(3):213-220.

Trompeter SE, Bettencourt R, Barrett-Connor E. Sexual activity and satisfaction in healthy community-dwelling older women. *Am J Med.* 2012;125(1):37-43.e1.

Depression & Other Mental Health Issues

12

Mary A. Norman, MD

Bobby Singh, MD

DEPRESSION

ESSENTIALS OF DIAGNOSIS

▶ Depressed mood.

▶ Loss of interest or pleasure in almost all activities.

▶ Unintentional weight change, lack of energy, change in sleep pattern, psychomotor retardation or agitation, excessive guilt, or poor concentration.

▶ Suicidal ideation or recurrent thoughts of death.

▶ Somatic rather than mood complaints in the elderly.

▶ General Principles

According to the World Health Organization, approximately 15% of adults aged 60 and over suffer from a mental disorder, with depression affecting 7% of the world's older population. The prevalence of major depression is estimated at 1% to 2% for elders in the community and 10% to 12% for those in primary care settings. However, even in the absence of major depression as defined by *Diagnostic and Statistical Manual of Mental Disorders* (fifth edition; *DSM-5*) criteria, up to 27% of elders experience substantial depressive symptoms that may be relieved with intervention. For institutionalized elders, the rates of major depression are much higher: 12% for hospitalized elders and 50% for permanently institutionalized elders.

The World Health Organization Primary Care Study reported that 60% of primary care clinic patients treated with antidepressant medication still met criteria for depression 1 year later, with similar efficacy rates for antidepressants reported in older adults and those younger than the age of 60 years. However, depression is often missed or inadequately managed in older adults, sometimes because of the belief that depression is an inevitable process of aging or because

treatment may be risky or ineffective. Indeed, there are several reasons why optimal treatment of depression in the geriatric population may differ from that for younger populations. Higher rates of physical and cognitive comorbidity in older adults, different social circumstances, greater potential for polypharmacy, and age-related pharmacodynamic and pharmacokinetic susceptibility all suggest that this population should be considered separately.

Women are twice as likely to experience major depression as men. Other risk factors include prior episodes or a personal family history of depression, lack of social support, use of alcohol or other substances, and a recent loss of a loved one. Several medical conditions are also associated with an increased risk of depression, including Parkinson disease, recent myocardial infarction, and stroke. These conditions share common threads of loss of control of body or mind, increasing dependence on others, and increased social isolation.

Depression is associated with poorer self-care and slower recovery after acute medical illnesses. It can accelerate cognitive and physical decline and leads to an increased use and cost of health care services. Among depressed older adults who have had a stroke, rehabilitation efforts are less effective and mortality rates are significantly higher.

▶ Clinical Findings

A. Symptoms & Signs

Major depression is defined as depressed mood or loss of interest in nearly all activities (anhedonia) or both for at least 2 weeks, accompanied by a minimum of three or four of the following symptoms (for a total of at least five symptoms): insomnia or hypersomnia, feelings of worthlessness or excessive guilt, fatigue or loss of energy, diminished ability to think or concentrate, substantial change in appetite or weight, psychomotor agitation or retardation, and recurrent thoughts of death or suicide. Severity of depression varies and is important in determining optimal treatment and prognosis. Mild depression is marked by few, if any, symptoms in excess of the minimum number required to meet the diagnostic criteria defined above, and it is accompanied by minimal impairment in functioning. Moderate depression includes a greater number and intensity of depressive symptoms and moderate impairment in functioning. Patients with severe depression experience marked intensity and pervasiveness of depressive symptoms with substantial impairment in functioning. Patients with less severe depressive symptoms who do not meet criteria for major depression may also benefit from psychotherapy and pharmacotherapy.

B. Screening Tools

Older patients can have fewer mood and more somatic complaints, which are often difficult to differentiate from underlying medical conditions. Special screening tools that consider this difference have been developed for the older population. The Geriatric Depression Scale is widely used and validated in many different languages. Its shortened 15-item scale (Table 12–1) is often used for ease of administration. A separate two-item scale consisting of two questions about depressed mood and anhedonia has also been shown to be effective in detecting depression in older adults (Table 12–1). The Patient Health Questionnaire-9 (PHQ-9) may be used to both screen for depression and monitor response to treatment with sensitivity and specificity of 88%. Screening alone has not been found to benefit patients with unrecognized depression, but in combination with patient support programs, such as frequent nursing follow-up and close monitoring of adherence to medication, it improves outcomes.

▶ Differential Diagnosis

Diagnosing depression in older adults can be challenging because of the presence of multiple comorbid conditions. Many patients with mild cognitive impairment may have predominantly depressive symptoms. With effective treatment of depression, their cognitive performance frequently improves; however, their risk for developing dementia in their lifetime is roughly double the risk of nondepressed seniors. Bereavement often manifests with depressed mood, which may be appropriate given a patient's recent loss. However, if depressive symptoms persist, further evaluation may be warranted.

Older patients who experience delirium caused by an underlying medical illness may have mood changes. Other comorbid psychiatric illnesses must also be considered, such as anxiety disorder, substance abuse disorder, or personality disorders. Patients with bipolar disorder or psychotic disorders may have depressed mood; thus, it is important to ask patients about prior manic episodes, hallucinations, or delusions.

Depression can also be confused with other medical conditions. Fatigue and weight loss, for example, may be

Table 12–1. Geriatric depression scale (short form).[a]

Depression Scale	
1. Are you basically satisfied with your life?	Yes/**No**
2. Have you dropped many of your activities and interests?	**Yes**/No
3. Do you feel that your life is empty?	**Yes**/No
4. Do you often get bored?	**Yes**/No
5. Are you in good spirits most of the time?	Yes/**No**
6. Are you afraid that something bad is going to happen to you?	**Yes**/No
7. Do you feel happy most of the time?	Yes/**No**
8. Do you often feel helpless?	**Yes**/No
9. Do you prefer to stay at home rather than going out and doing new things?	**Yes**/No
10. Do you feel that you have more problems with memory than most?	**Yes**/No
11. Do you think it is wonderful to be alive now?	Yes/**No**
12. Do you feel pretty worthless the way you are now?	**Yes**/No
13. Do you feel full of energy?	Yes/**No**
14. Do you feel that your situation is hopeless?	**Yes**/No
15. Do you think that most people are better off than you are?	**Yes**/No
SCORE: _____	

Directions: Score 1 point for each bolded answer. A score of 5 or more is a positive screen for depression.

Two-Question Case-Finding Instrument[b]	
1. During the last month, have you often been bothered by feeling down, depressed, or hopeless?	**Yes**/No
2. During the last month, have you often been bothered by having little interest or pleasure in doing things?	**Yes**/No

Directions: Yes to either question is a positive screen for depression.

[a]Adapted with permission from Yesavage JA, Brink TL, Rose TL, et al. Development and Validation of a Geriatric Depression Screening Scale: A Preliminary Report, *J Psychiatr Res* 1982-1983;17(1):37-49.
[b]Data from Whooley MA, Avins AL, Miranda J, et al. Case-finding Instruments for Depression. Two Questions Are as Good as Many, *J Gen Intern Med* 1997 Jul;12(7):439-445.

associated with diabetes mellitus, thyroid disease, underlying malignancy, or anemia. Patients who have Parkinson disease may first present with depressed mood or flat affect. Sleep disturbances as a result of pain, nocturia, or sleep apnea may also lead to daytime fatigue and depressed mood.

A complete history and physical examination, including assessment of cognitive status, is critical in the evaluation of depression in older adults. Because depression is a clinical diagnosis, no routine laboratory tests are indicated. Testing may be tailored to each patient based on their underlying comorbidities and presenting symptoms. A complete review of medications, both prescription and nonprescription, is essential. Medications, such as benzodiazepines, opioid analgesics, glucocorticoids, interferon, and reserpine, may cause depressive symptoms. Contrary to earlier beliefs, β-blockers have not been proven to cause depression. Screening for alcohol and other substance use or addiction is another important part of the medical history. Substance use can interfere with compliance and contribute to high relapse rates, although active substance abuse should not preclude treatment for depression. For patients who struggle with addiction, "dual diagnosis" programs (alcohol or other substance dependence and psychiatric disorder) may be optimal.

▶ Treatment

A. Patient & Family Education/Supportive Care

Educating patients and families about depression is the cornerstone of successful treatment. Depression continues to carry a stigma in many communities and cultures. Appropriate education can help patients understand that their condition results from a combination of inherited factors and personal and environmental stressors. Providers should also emphasize that physical symptoms and sleep disturbances are characteristic of depression; thus, relief of depression could make other physical symptoms more bearable. Encouraging physical activity with a family member or friend can be a simple, effective step toward improving social support and overall well-being.

Involving families in the care of older patients is crucial for both diagnosing depression and developing an effective treatment plan. However, caregivers of older patients, especially if impaired physically or cognitively, may experience considerable stress and depression as well. Referred to as caregiver burden, this is an all-encompassing term used to describe the physical, emotional, and financial toll of providing care. In particular, when patients with dementia have depression, their caregivers report higher levels of burden. Many programs are available that may alleviate stress and promote positive social interactions for patients. Adult day programs, senior centers, and senior support groups can be helpful resources for patients and their families, and geriatric social workers can assist with finding appropriate programs for each patient. Caregiver support groups and formal respite programs are also available in many communities.

B. Pharmacotherapy

1. Antidepressants

a. **Selection**—Overall, antidepressants, including tricyclic antidepressants (TCAs), selective serotonin reuptake inhibitors (SSRIs), and selective serotonin-norepinephrine reuptake inhibitors (SNRIs), are equally effective in the treatment of geriatric depression. However, because of side effect profiles and propensity for drug interactions, monoamine oxidase inhibitors (eg, phenelzine and tranylcypromine) and tertiary amine TCAs (eg, amitriptyline, imipramine, and doxepin) are rarely used in older adults. The SSRI class includes citalopram, escitalopram, fluoxetine, paroxetine, and sertraline; examples of SNRIs are venlafaxine, desvenlafaxine, and duloxetine. Fluoxetine is generally avoided in older adults because of its long half-life and inhibition of the P450 system. Choice of therapy among the remaining drugs is generally determined by side effect profile and the patient's comorbid symptoms such as anxiety, insomnia, pain, and weight loss, although anxiety and insomnia do not necessarily predict a better response to more sedating medications. Renal and hepatic functions are also important considerations in older adults and should be assessed before initiation of therapy.

SSRIs are relatively safe in overdose. Thus, they are a reasonable first choice in treating older patients with depression. However, the SSRI citalopram (Celexa) has been associated with increased QT interval prolongation and torsade de pointes in older patients when used in higher doses and carries a warning issued by the US Food and Drug Administration (FDA) to limit maximum daily dose to 20 mg for all patients older than age 60 years. The warnings do not apply to its racemic drug, escitalopram (Lexapro), which is the S-enantiomer of the citalopram molecule.

Other agents offer unique advantages: mirtazapine stimulates appetite and can help with insomnia, and bupropion can reduce craving in smoking cessation. Secondary amine TCAs (eg, nortriptyline, desipramine) can offer beneficial effects for patients with neuropathic pain, detrusor instability, or insomnia. SNRIs, which have serotonergic and noradrenergic activity, are other effective alternatives that may also be useful in treating anxiety and neuropathic pain.

b. **Dosage**—In general, older patients should begin an antidepressant by taking half of the manufacturer-recommended starting dose (to minimize side effects), but the medication should be titrated to the recommended target dose in weekly increments. Older patients are frequently undertreated because the provider fails to adequately titrate the dose to a therapeutic level. If minimal or no benefit occurs by 4 to 6 weeks and side effects are tolerable, the dose should be increased. The full effect may not be seen for 8 to 12 weeks in older patients. If a therapeutic dose has been reached and maintained for 6 weeks and the patient has not adequately responded, one should consider switching to a different agent or augmenting with an additional agent. Although serum drug levels are not useful for SSRIs, levels of TCAs can be measured to assess adherence.

c. **Side effects**—Side effects differ depending on the type of antidepressant. Most side effects lessen within 1 to 4 weeks from the start of therapy, but weight gain and sexual dysfunction may last longer. For the SSRIs, the most common side effects include nausea and sexual dysfunction. Sexual dysfunction may respond to treatment with sildenafil, but switching antidepressant medication or lowering the dose of SSRI and augmenting with an additional agent may be necessary. The TCAs have more anticholinergic properties and may lead to dry mouth, orthostasis, and urinary retention.

d. Cautions & interactions

1. Cardiovascular disease—TCAs can be associated with orthostatic hypotension and cardiac conduction abnormalities, leading to arrhythmias. Citalopram has been implicated in potentially dangerous arrhythmias. Therefore, electrolyte and/or electrocardiographic monitoring is recommended for patients at risk for arrhythmias if these agents are considered.

2. Hypertension—Venlafaxine and desvenlafaxine may increase systolic and diastolic blood pressure.

3. Electrolyte abnormalities—SSRIs may induce hyponatremia.

4. Hepatic disease—Most antidepressants are hepatically cleared and should be used with caution in patients with liver disease. Nefazodone, in particular, should not be used in patients with liver disease or elevated transaminases because it has been associated with an increased risk of hepatic failure and interacts with other hepatically cleared medications, including simvastatin and lovastatin.

5. Falls—SSRIs and SNRIs have been associated with an increased risk in falls, particularly in older patients with dementia. Fall risk assessment should be included as part of the overall medical evaluation.

6. Bleeding risk—SSRIs may increase bleeding risk and interact with anticoagulant medications such as warfarin. International normalized ratio levels should be closely monitored with initiation of treatment with SSRIs.

7. Cognitive impairment—TCAs and certain SSRIs, such as paroxetine, have stronger anticholinergic effects and should be avoided in patients with cognitive impairment to avoid increasing confusion.

8. Seizure disorders—Bupropion lowers seizure thresholds.

9. Suicidal ideation—TCAs are lethal in overdose and should be avoided in actively suicidal patients. SSRIs and SNRIs are relatively safe in overdose.

10. Serotonin syndrome—Use of serotonergic antidepressants may lead to serotonin syndrome, a potentially life-threatening condition associated with increased serotonergic activity in the central nervous system. Although classically described as a triad of mental status changes (headache, confusion, agitation), autonomic hyperactivity (diaphoresis, hypertension, tachycardia, nausea, diarrhea), and neuromuscular abnormalities (tremor, myoclonus, hyperreflexia), serotonin syndrome can span a spectrum of clinical findings ranging from benign to lethal. Given the increased use of serotonergic agents in medical practice and the syndrome's potential for rapid onset, with its clinical course developing over 24 hours, providers are advised to remain vigilant for this condition. The central principles to the management of suspected serotonin syndrome are (a) discontinuation of all serotonergic agents and (b) supportive care aimed at normalization of vital signs.

2. Psychostimulants—Psychostimulants, such as dextroamphetamine (5–10 mg/day) or methylphenidate (2.5–5 mg/day), are sometimes indicated as either a primary or an adjuvant treatment for depression with predominant vegetative symptoms. Modafinil (Provigil), which increases monoamines, has also been used as an adjunct to traditional antidepressants. With its additional histaminergic effects, modafinil is considered by some to be a "wakefulness-promoting agent," and unlike the classic amphetamine-like stimulants, it is considered to have limited abuse potential. At the end of life, patients may not have time to wait 4 to 6 weeks for the benefits of antidepressant medication, and psychostimulants may offer more immediate relief. In the setting of depression after an acute medical illness, psychostimulants may offer a faster means to enhance recovery and participation in rehabilitation. Typical side effects include insomnia and agitation, but these may be lessened by taking the medication early in the day in divided doses (morning and noon). Another common side effect is tachycardia.

3. Herbal remedies—Many herbal remedies claim to be effective in treating depression, but further evidence is still needed to determine whether these "dietary supplements" (eg, *Hypericum perforatum* [St. John's wort]) have a role in the treatment of depression. *H perforatum* should not be used in conjunction with SSRIs because the combination may lead to serotonergic syndrome, which is characterized by changes in mental status, tremor, gastrointestinal upset, headache, myalgia, and restlessness. It may lower the concentration of certain drugs, such as warfarin, digoxin, theophylline, cyclosporine, and HIV-1 protease inhibitors. Other common herbal remedies such as kava kava and valerian root have not been proven effective for treating depression. Herbal remedies should not be substituted for proven depression therapies.

C. Psychotherapy

Cognitive-behavioral therapy (CBT), problem-solving therapy, and interpersonal psychotherapy are effective treatments for major depression, either alone or in combination with pharmacotherapy. CBT focuses on identifying negative thoughts and behaviors that contribute to depression and replacing them with positive thoughts and rewarding activities. Problem-solving therapy teaches patients techniques to identify routine problems, generate multiple solutions, and implement the best strategy. Interpersonal psychotherapy focuses on recognizing and attempting to resolve personal stressors and relationship conflicts that lead to depressive symptoms.

Typically, these therapies should be continued once or twice weekly for 6 to 16 sessions. In patients with severe depression, combination therapy with psychotherapy and pharmacotherapy is superior to either treatment alone. Psychoanalytic and psychodynamic therapies have not proved effective for treatment of major depression.

D. Electroconvulsive Therapy

Electroconvulsive therapy (ECT) is an effective treatment for geriatric depression. Response rates for refractory depression are quite high at 73% for the young-old (age 60–74 years) and 67% for the old-old (age >75 years). Typical side effects include confusion and anterograde memory impairment, which may persist for 6 months. ECT may be first-line therapy for severely melancholic patients, for those at high risk for suicide, and for medically ill patients whose hepatic, renal, or cardiac diseases preclude the use of other antidepressants. Other brain stimulation therapies such as repetitive transcranial magnetic stimulation (rTMS), deep brain stimulation (DBS), and vagus nerve stimulation (VNS) have yet to be proven beneficial in randomized clinical trials in older adults.

E. Psychiatric Therapy

Psychiatric consultation is recommended for patients with a history of mania or psychosis, for those who have not responded to a trial of one or two medicines, and for those who require combination therapy or ECT. Many depressed older adults contemplate suicide. Primary care providers must recognize the risk factors for suicide in patients with major depression. Immediate psychiatric evaluation is required for any patients who, after probing, admit to having active plans to harm themselves. Risk factors for suicide in older patients with major depression include older age; male gender; marital status of single, divorced, or separated and without children; personal or family history of a suicide attempt; drug or alcohol abuse; severe anxiety or stress; physical illness; and a specific suicide plan with access to firearms or other lethal means (eg, stockpiled medications). If medications and weapons are present and cannot be removed from the patient's home, consider adding "weapon at home" to the patient's problem list to highlight potential suicide risk. Actively suicidal patients with intent and plan require emergent psychiatric evaluation either through emergency departments or local psychiatric crisis units.

F. Follow-Up

1. Pharmacotherapy—Older patients should be monitored closely during the initial 3 months of treatment. Many medical outpatients who receive a prescription for an antidepressant terminate treatment during the first month, when side effects may be at a maximum and before therapeutic effects are evident. Older patients should be monitored closely in the first 1 to 2 weeks of therapy to assess side effects and encourage continued therapy. They should have a minimum of three visits (in person or by telephone) during the first 12 weeks of antidepressant treatment.

Older patients must be informed that antidepressants usually take 4 to 6 weeks, but may take 8 weeks or longer, to have a full therapeutic effect and that only approximately 50% of patients respond to the first antidepressant prescribed. Patients who have not responded after an adequate trial of medication or who have had intolerable side effects may switch either to another medication within the same class (different SSRI) or to a different class of medications. When switching among SSRIs or between TCAs and SSRIs, no washout period is required (with the exception of switching from fluoxetine, because of its long half-life). However, abrupt cessation of shorter-acting antidepressants (eg, citalopram, paroxetine, sertraline, or venlafaxine) may result in a discontinuation syndrome with tinnitus, vertigo, or paresthesias. Referral for psychiatric consultation is recommended if a patient fails to respond to two different medication trials.

Once remission has been achieved, antidepressants should be continued for at least 6 months to reduce the risk of relapse. Patients who are at high risk of relapse (two or more episodes of depression in the past or major depression lasting >2 years) should be continued on therapy for 2 years or possibly indefinitely. Many recommend lifelong therapy, even if it is the patient's first episode of major depression and especially if depression is severe and related to life changes that are not expected to improve. Follow-up visits should be arranged at 3- to 6-month intervals. If symptoms return, the medications should be adjusted or changed or the patient referred for psychiatric consultation.

If the patient and physician agree to a trial discontinuation of therapy, medications should be tapered over a 2- to 3-month period, with at least monthly follow-up by telephone or in-person. If symptoms return, the patient should be restarted on medications for at least 3 to 6 months.

When patients fail to respond to adequate trials of two medications for major depression, a diagnosis of treatment-resistant depression is considered. One must review the case and consider that the original diagnosis may be inaccurate. What first appeared as depressive symptoms may be a manifestation of underlying anxiety or cognitive impairment. Apathy may be one of the first symptoms seen in dementia prior to more obvious cognitive symptoms. One must then verify that the patient actually received the medication that was prescribed. A simple investigation may reveal that the patient never filled the prescription or was never given medication by caregivers. Finally, one must ensure that the patient had adequate trials of medications (6–8 weeks) and that this trial was performed at a therapeutic dose.

Any patient who has severe depressive symptoms including active suicidal ideation, who has depression with psychotic features, or who has had an adequate trial of two different medications without acceptable response should be referred to a psychiatrist for urgent evaluation. As shown from the federally funded Sequenced Treatment Alternatives to Relieve Depression (STAR*D) trial, the largest real-world study of treatment-resistant depression, patients with persistent depression have the potential to improve after several medication treatment trials; however, the odds of remission diminish as additional treatment strategies are needed. Lithium may be used in low doses in older adults with careful monitoring of side effects. Small doses of liothyronine (T$_3$) can be used safely in euthyroid patients. In addition, combinations of two antidepressant medications may be synergistic, with low doses of one antidepressant enhancing response to an antidepressant of another class.

2. Structured psychotherapy—Patients who have been referred to psychotherapy must still be monitored closely by their primary care clinicians because patients tend to discontinue therapy even more frequently than antidepressant treatments. The benefits of psychotherapy are generally evident by 6 to 8 weeks. The addition of pharmacotherapy should be considered for patients who have not fully responded to psychotherapy alone by 12 weeks. A combination of psychotherapy and pharmacotherapy may be more effective for moderate depression than either treatment alone.

▶ Prognosis

Depression is often a chronic or relapsing and remitting disease. Greater severity of depression, persistence of symptoms, and a higher number of prior episodes are the best predictors of recurrence. The lifetime risk of suicide in patients with major depression is 7% for men and 1% for women.

BIPOLAR DISORDER

ESSENTIALS OF DIAGNOSIS

▶ History of manic episode: grandiosity, decreased need for sleep, pressured speech, racing thoughts, distractibility, increased activity, excessive spending, hypersexuality.

▶ May be associated with psychosis.

▶ Depressive episodes may alternate with mania.

▶ Mania may present for the first time in elderly patients, usually in those with a history of depressive episodes.

▶ General Principles

Bipolar disorder is a less common diagnosis in older adults, with an overall low prevalence of <1% in community-dwelling elders, but a 10% rate in some nursing home populations. Many patients with bipolar disease require special considerations as they age because of comorbid conditions and diminished ability to tolerate psychiatric medications. Late-onset mania is often secondary to underlying medical conditions and is frequently associated with neurologic abnormalities such as cerebrovascular accident and cognitive impairment. Older patients with bipolar disorder have an increased 10-year mortality rate compared with those who have depression alone (70% vs 30%).

▶ Differential Diagnosis

Bipolar disorder is diagnosed when a patient meets criteria for a manic episode. A manic episode is defined as a distinct period of abnormally and persistently elevated, expansive, or irritable mood and abnormally and persistently increased goal-directed activity or energy, lasting at least 1 week and with at least three of the following symptoms: inflated self-esteem or grandiosity, decreased need for sleep, pressured speech, racing thoughts, distractibility, increase in goal-directed activity or psychomotor agitation, and excessive involvement in pleasurable activities that have a high potential for painful consequences. Although major depressive episodes are common in bipolar disorder, they are not required for the diagnosis. The presence of mania is key to the differentiation between depressive disorder and bipolar disorder.

A variety of conditions may mimic a manic episode. Patients with dementia, particularly frontotemporal dementia, may be disinhibited and hypersexual. Brain tumors, cerebrovascular accidents, and partial-complex seizures may also lead to bizarre, disinhibited behaviors. Older patients who are prone to delirium can have waxing and waning levels of consciousness with some periods of hyperarousal. In addition, some medications may have unexpected effects in older patients. Glucocorticoids, thyroxine, and methylphenidate may lead to acute mania. Even sedative medications (eg, benzodiazepines) may have a paradoxical effect in older adults and lead to agitation. As in younger populations, substance intoxication or withdrawal from cocaine, alcohol, or amphetamines and endocrine disorders, such as hyperthyroidism or pheochromocytoma, can lead to symptoms consistent with mania.

▶ Treatment

Mood stabilizers have been the hallmark of treatment for bipolar disease. Valproic acid, carbamazepine, and lithium are typically first-line treatments with choice dependent on comorbid disorders and contraindications (eg, avoid lithium with renal impairment and avoid valproate with hepatic

Table 12–2. Mood stabilizers.

Generic Name	Trade Name	Initial Dose	Target Dose	Comments
Lithium	Lithobid, Eskalith	300 mg QD or BID	600–1200 mg/day in divided doses BID or TID	Monitor drug levels, renal function, thyroid function; diuretics and ACE inhibitors increase levels; avoid dehydration and many NSAIDs because of toxicity
Carbamazepine	Tegretol	200 mg QD or BID	400–1000 mg/day	Monitor blood count, liver function tests, drug levels
Valproic acid	Depakote	250 mg QD or BID	500–1500 mg/day	Monitor blood count, liver function tests, drug levels

ACE, angiotensin-converting enzyme; BID, twice a day; NSAIDs, nonsteroidal anti-inflammatory drugs; TID, three times a day; QD, every day.

disease) (Table 12–2). Antipsychotic medications are also first-line treatment of manic episodes associated with bipolar, maintenance treatment of bipolar, or when psychotic features are present. In general, the newer antipsychotic agents, such as olanzapine and quetiapine, are better tolerated by older adults than the older neuroleptics with their extrapyramidal side effects and high risk of tardive dyskinesia, especially in women. Among the atypical antipsychotics, olanzapine, risperidone, quetiapine, ziprasidone, and asenapine are approved for acute treatment of mania and as adjunctive treatment with lithium or valproate. Antidepressants are often used as an adjunct to mood stabilizers for patients with depression but should not be used alone because of the risk of transforming a depressive episode into a manic episode.

ANXIETY AND STRESS DISORDERS

1. Panic Disorder

▶ Sudden, recurrent, unexpected panic attacks, characterized by an abrupt surge of intense fear or intense discomfort, reaching a peak within minutes.

▶ Attacks may include palpitations, sweating, trembling, choking sensation, chest pain, nausea or abdominal distress, feeling dizzy or light-headed, chills, paresthesias, derealization or depersonalization, fear of losing control, and/or fear of dying.

▶ Persistent worry about future attacks or their consequences.

▶ Maladaptive change in behavior related to the attacks.

General Principles

The lifetime prevalence rate of panic disorder is 1.5% to 2%, increasing to 4% in the primary care setting. The rate among community-dwelling older adults is <1%. Depression is also present in 50% to 65% of patients with panic disorder; the suicide rate for these patients is 20% higher than that for depressed patients without panic disorder. Panic disorder may be associated with agoraphobia, which can be particularly disabling in older adults.

Differential Diagnosis

A panic attack is defined as an abrupt surge of intense fear or discomfort with four or more of the symptoms from the list above (second item under the "Essentials of Diagnosis." *DSM-5* criteria for panic disorder include recurrent unexpected panic attacks, with at least one of the attacks having been followed by 1 month or more of either one or both of the following: persistent concern or worry about additional attacks or their consequences, or a significant maladaptive change in behavior related to the attacks.

Because the likelihood of physical disease is much higher than in younger populations, panic disorder is more difficult to distinguish from other life-threatening events in older patients. Acute coronary syndromes, cardiac arrhythmias, acute bronchospasm, and pulmonary embolism may lead to symptoms consistent with panic attacks. Endocrine disorders, particularly hyperthyroidism and pheochromocytoma, can mimic panic disorder. In acutely hospitalized patients, alcohol, caffeine, and tobacco withdrawal may present as agitation, worry, and other physical symptoms. Abrupt discontinuation of a short-acting antidepressant, anxiolytic, or opioid analgesic medication may also trigger panic symptoms. Older patients who suffer from panic disorder often have comorbid psychiatric diagnoses such as posttraumatic stress disorder (PTSD), generalized anxiety disorder, and depression.

Treatment

CBT has been proven effective for the treatment of panic disorder. Patients often go into a complete remission after as few as 12 weekly sessions. CBT is particularly helpful in preventing relapse and treating agoraphobia. Antidepressants, particularly SSRIs and TCAs, are helpful, although the latter are more likely to cause problematic side effects.

Benzodiazepines may also be used as a brief adjunctive therapy while awaiting the clinical response to antidepressants or CBT. Whenever possible, long-term therapy with benzodiazepines should be avoided because of the potential risk of falls, cognitive impairment, and dependence.

Perhaps the most important aspect of treatment is education for the patient and family. Understanding the symptoms of panic disorder and developing ways of coping are essential for effective management of the disease.

2. Social and Specific Phobias

 ESSENTIALS OF DIAGNOSIS

▶ A phobia is an irrational fear leading either to intentional avoidance of a specific feared object, event, or situation, or enduring the object, event, or situation with intense fear or anxiety.

▶ Exposure to this phobic object may result in symptoms similar to those of a panic attack.

▶ Patient is aware that his or her fear is irrational.

▶ General Principles

The prevalence of phobias is 5% to 6% in older adults. Phobias present with features similar to panic disorder but are triggered by a specific event. Late-onset phobias are often associated with a recent life event, such as a fall or injury. Social phobias affect 3% of older adults and can lead to increasing isolation. Simple phobias are thought to be more common than social phobias, affecting 5% to 12% of the general population.

▶ Differential Diagnosis

Social phobia, also known as social anxiety disorder, is defined by *DSM-5* criteria as a marked and persistent fear or anxiety about social situations, exposure to which almost always provokes these feelings. The patient fears that the patient's response to the social situation will be negatively evaluated, and either avoids the situation or endures it with great anxiety. The avoidance, fear, or anxiety associated with the situation is disproportionate to any actual posed threat and interferes with the patient's occupation or relationships. Specific phobia is a fear or anxiety about certain objects or situations that is disproportionate to the actual danger posed by such and may lead to impairment in a patient's ability to function normally.

In older adults, new phobic symptoms may represent delusions associated with dementia or delirium. Patients with dementia or delirium are not typically aware of the irrational nature of their delusions in contrast to patients with phobia. Less common causes of phobia include brain tumors or cerebrovascular accidents. The psychiatric differential diagnosis of phobia includes depression, schizophrenia, and schizoid and avoidant personality disorders. Social phobia and alcohol dependence often coexist; therefore, probing for alcohol use is an important part of the assessment. Although both phobic disorders and panic disorder may present with panic attacks, patients with phobias do not experience recurrent unexpected attacks; rather, their anxiety symptoms are always associated with a specific object or situation.

▶ Treatment

The first-line therapy for specific phobias is behavioral therapy. Techniques may include relaxation therapy, cognitive restructuring, and systematic exposure to the feared object or situation. Use of antidepressants, particularly SSRIs, may be beneficial for generalized social phobia. β-Adrenergic antagonists such as propranolol may also be effective treatments when administered before a foreseeable feared event or situation. Benzodiazepine use may be necessary but, in general, should be used with caution because of adverse effects on balance and cognition. Most patients can adapt to or overcome their phobias and can lead relatively normal lives; if not, they should be referred for evaluation by a mental health specialist.

3. Generalized Anxiety Disorder

 ESSENTIALS OF DIAGNOSIS

▶ Excessive anxiety and worry.

▶ Worry is recurrent and difficult to control.

▶ Physiologic symptoms of restlessness, fatigue, poor concentration, irritability, muscle tension, and sleep disturbance may be present.

▶ General Principles

Anxiety symptoms are often a normal reaction to the surrounding environment. Anxiety disorders tend to begin in early adulthood and continue throughout a patient's lifetime with periods of relapses and remissions. The lifetime prevalence of generalized anxiety disorder is 5%; estimates in older patients range from 2% to 7%. Anxiety may increase in older adults as a result of isolation, loss of independence, illness, disability, and bereavement.

▶ Differential Diagnosis

The diagnosis of generalized anxiety disorder is characterized by the following according to *DSM-5* criteria:

• Excessive anxiety and worry about a number of events or activities occurring more days than not for at least 6 months.

- Worry is difficult to control.
- Anxiety and worry are associated with at least three of the following: restlessness, easy fatigability, difficulty with concentration, irritability, muscle tension, sleep disturbance.

Diagnosing generalized anxiety in elders can be complicated because many underlying illnesses may have similar symptoms. The differential diagnosis for generalized anxiety disorder includes the physical illnesses discussed previously for panic disorder. In addition, chronic medication or substance use and subsequent withdrawal may lead to anxiety symptoms. Caffeine, nicotine, and alcohol are common culprits. Older patients are much more sensitive to commonly used nonprescription medications such as pseudoephedrine, which may cause restlessness, anxiety, and confusion. Up to 54% of patients who suffer from generalized anxiety disorder have comorbid depression. Obsessive-compulsive disorder, somatoform disorder, and personality disorders may also present with symptoms of anxiety. Psychiatric consultation should be initiated if the diagnosis is in question.

▶ Treatment

CBT is one of the most effective treatments for generalized anxiety disorder. Relaxation techniques and biofeedback may also alleviate symptoms. Several antidepressants (paroxetine, extended-release venlafaxine) also have significant anxiolytic properties and may be effective for both anxiety and depression. When depression and anxiety occur together, one should treat the depression first; doing so may improve the symptoms of both disorders. Anxiolytic medications such as buspirone (5–30 mg twice daily) may be effective. Benzodiazepines should be used with caution in older adults because they can cause a paradoxical effect and may also lead to falls and cognitive impairment.

4. Posttraumatic Stress Disorder

ESSENTIALS OF DIAGNOSIS

- ▶ History of exposure to a traumatic event.
- ▶ Intrusive thoughts, nightmares, flashbacks, cue-induced physiologic and psychological distress.
- ▶ Avoidance of stimuli associated with the traumatic event.
- ▶ Negative alterations in cognitions and mood.
- ▶ Symptoms of arousal and reactivity.
- ▶ Frequently associated with depression and substance abuse.

▶ General Principles

According to the National Comorbidity Survey, the lifetime prevalence rates of PTSD are 9.7% for females and 3.6% for males. For older (60+ years) adults, the rate is noted to be 2.8%, significantly lower than the overall younger adult rate of 6.8%. Some studies have shown that increased age may protect against the development of PTSD. Other protective factors include marriage, social support, and higher socioeconomic status. However, lower rates of diagnosis in older patients may also be due to other factors. For instance, many older patients are reluctant to acknowledge or conceptualize their problematic symptoms as PTSD due to the stigma associated with the diagnosis, especially among certain age groups or cohorts. Among older patients, it is not uncommon to see the expression of PTSD symptoms in somatic or physical terms. There may also be significant provider reluctance to directly assess for PTSD due to a lack of expertise and/or limited time, especially due to other possible medical needs of older patients. It is important to remember that although the initial traumatic event may have taken place decades ago, symptoms of PTSD may persist into older age. In addition, symptoms can remain hidden until an older age when patients have new experiences (deaths, medical illness, disability) that trigger memories of former events or lose the capacity to compensate for lifelong symptoms because of cognitive impairment or other medical illness. Furthermore, many older patients are exposed to certain potentially traumatic events, such as unexpected death or serious illness among family and/or friends. The presence of PTSD may increase the risk of cardiovascular disease and diabetes, although definitive evidence is still lacking. Some recent studies also indicate an increased likelihood of chronic pain and a higher risk of developing dementia, at least among veterans, in the presence of PTSD.

▶ Differential Diagnosis

Per *DSM-5* criteria, the patient has been exposed in one or more of the following ways to a traumatic event involving actual or threatened death, serious injury, or sexual violence. Symptoms may be grouped into four categories and may persist for >1 month.

1. Intrusive symptoms with at least one of the following: recurrent and intrusive recollections, dreams, dissociative reactions (eg, flashbacks), distress at exposure to cues to the event, or marked physiologic reaction to such cues.

2. Avoidant symptoms with one or both of the following: avoiding memories, thoughts, or feelings associated with the trauma; or avoiding external reminders (eg, people, places, activities) associated with the trauma.

3. Negative alterations in cognition and mood, with more than two of the following: inability to remember aspects of the trauma; exaggerated negative beliefs or expectations about oneself, others, or the world; distorted blaming of oneself or others; persistent negative emotions (eg, fear, anger, guilt, shame); diminished interest or participation in activities; feeling of detachment or estrangement from others; or inability to experience positive emotions.

4. Arousal symptoms indicated by at least two of the following: irritability or outbursts of anger, reckless or self-destructive behavior, hypervigilance, exaggerated startle response, difficulty concentrating, or sleep disturbance.

Other anxiety disorders can present with symptoms of hyperarousal similar to those in patients with PTSD. Major depressive disorder and adjustment disorders can also present with numbing or avoidant symptoms. During a period of bereavement, patients can have visual/auditory hallucinations or dreams about the deceased. Other psychotic disorders may be confused with PTSD, but patients with PTSD may also experience transient psychotic symptoms during severe episodes. Substance use or withdrawal may contribute to symptoms. Organic brain syndrome resulting from prior head injury may be associated with symptoms similar to those of PTSD; the presence of visual hallucinations is particularly suggestive of an organic cause. Patients with delirium may also appear hyperaroused or be prone to illusions/hallucinations. There is a high comorbidity of depression and alcohol abuse among patients with PTSD.

Treatment

Antidepressants, particularly SSRIs and, to a lesser extent, SNRIs, are used as the first-line treatment of PTSD. Antiadrenergic agents such as clonidine may be helpful for symptoms of increased arousal, although one must consider related side effects such as orthostasis. Prazosin, an α_1-adrenergic receptor antagonist, has been used for years to manage nightmares associated with PTSD; however, a recent study showed no significant benefit over placebo. Nonetheless, for selective patients, it may be worth attempting. Benzodiazepines can often worsen symptoms of PTSD and generally should be avoided. Antipsychotic medications are occasionally necessary for the treatment of associated psychotic symptoms (see Table 12–2); however, these should be used with caution in light of their potential side effect profile and limited evidence of efficacy. Both individual and group CBT is also effective in the treatment of PTSD and may be used alone or in combination with pharmacologic therapy. In particular, the strongest evidence-based for PTSD-specific therapies include prolonged exposure, cognitive processing therapy, and eye movement desensitization reprocessing.

SCHIZOPHRENIA AND PSYCHOTIC DISORDERS

 ESSENTIALS OF DIAGNOSIS

► Prominent delusions or auditory or visual hallucinations.
► Diminished emotional expression and/or avolition.
► Disorganized speech, thought processes, or behavior.

General Principles

Psychotic symptoms may be attributable to a longstanding psychotic illness that has persisted into older age or may present for the first time in later life in association with underlying medical conditions, especially dementia. Estimates for schizophrenia in the older population range from 0.1% to 0.5%. The prevalence of other psychotic syndromes, such as paranoid ideation, is higher, estimated at 4% to 6% in the older population, and is frequently associated with dementia. Patients with Alzheimer disease have a particularly high incidence of psychosis; 50% manifest psychotic symptoms within 3 years of diagnosis.

Differential Diagnosis

The diagnostic criteria for schizophrenia include at least two of the following characteristic symptoms present for at least 1 month: delusions, hallucinations, disorganized speech, grossly disorganized or catatonic behavior, or negative symptoms such as flattened affect. These symptoms must also be associated with dysfunction in such areas as work, relationships, or self-care. Patients commonly will not volunteer psychotic symptoms unless specifically asked by their provider after a trusting relationship has been established. If psychosis is suspected, it is important to ask patients and family members specifically about auditory and visual hallucinations, delusions, ideas of reference, and paranoid ideation. Visual hallucinations are associated more strongly with underlying organic cause.

Especially in older adults, new psychotic symptoms carry a vast and complicated differential. New-onset psychotic symptoms can be attributed to medications; changes in environment; organic causes, including dementia; or a combination of these factors. Because psychosis may be the presenting sign of dementia, any older patient with new-onset psychosis should have a thorough cognitive screen. Prominent visual hallucinations are one of the hallmarks of Lewy body dementia. Patients with Alzheimer disease frequently have fixed delusions regarding people stealing their possessions or marital infidelity. The dementia associated with Parkinson disease may include negative symptoms of schizophrenia, such as flat affect.

Other central nervous system diseases, such as brain tumors, partial seizures, multiple sclerosis, or cerebral systemic lupus erythematosus, can also cause psychotic symptoms. Patients with major depression or bipolar disorder may experience psychotic features. Infections, endocrinopathies (thyroid, diabetes, adrenal), and nutritional deficiencies (vitamin B_{12}, thiamine) may lead to psychosis. Finally, older patients can be especially sensitive to medications that trigger psychotic symptoms such as steroids or levodopa. Because of the large differential diagnosis, collateral information regarding the patient's baseline mental status, psychiatric history, and onset of symptoms is critical in the evaluation of psychotic symptoms.

▷ Treatment

A. Pharmacotherapy

Atypical antipsychotic agents, such as risperidone, olanzapine, quetiapine, ziprasidone, and aripiprazole, are the mainstays of treatment for psychotic symptoms and are approved for use in schizophrenia and bipolar disease (Table 12–3). Newer atypical antipsychotics, such as asenapine, iloperidone, lurasidone, and paliperidone, have not been rigorously studied in older patients, and most clinicians have limited experience prescribing them in a geriatric setting. Because of their lower incidence of extrapyramidal side effects, the atypical antipsychotics agents are generally much better tolerated than the older antipsychotic agents, such as haloperidol and

trifluoperazine. Recent data from multiple studies highlight the increased all-cause mortality rates in seniors with use of antipsychotic medications, particularly when used in patients with dementia. Unlike older neuroleptics, which mainly treat positive symptoms (eg, delusions, hallucinations), many clinicians believe that the newer agents are better at managing both positive and negative psychotic symptoms (eg, flat affect, social withdrawal). The main acute side effects of newer agents are sedation and dizziness. Patients may experience akathisia and parkinsonism (eg, stiffness and rigidity) and, with longer term use, tardive dyskinesias, although the risk of such side effects is lower than with high-potency traditional antipsychotic drugs. One of the most serious long-term side effects of the atypical antipsychotics is an increased risk of metabolic syndrome. Patients may experience weight gain, dyslipidemia, and/or glucose dysregulation. Therefore, close, routine monitoring of patients is strongly recommended. These agents have also been associated with an increased incidence of strokes in patients with dementia. Unlike most other newer agents, ziprasidone does not appear to cause weight gain and may be useful in the treatment of obese patients. However, it is associated with QT prolongation and thus should be avoided in patients with underlying conduction disease and QT prolongation at baseline. Clozapine is often the treatment of choice for patients with severe resistant psychosis and those with disabling tardive dyskinesias. Clozapine, however, carries a 1% to 2% risk of agranulocytosis and, therefore, requires weekly blood monitoring for at least the first 6 months and

Table 12–3. Commonly used antipsychotics.

Generic Name	Trade Name	Initial Dose (mg)	Target Dosage[a] (mg/day)	Available Routes of Administration
Older agents				
D$_2$-Antagonists—high potency[b]				
Haloperidol	Haldol	0.5	0.5–1	PO, IV, IM, depot
Newer agents:				
Serotonin dopamine receptor antagonists[c]				
Risperidone	Risperdal	0.5	1–1.5	PO, depot
Olanzapine	Zyprexa	2.5	2.5–5	PO, IM
Quetiapine	Seroquel	25	50–200	PO
Quetiapine XR	Seroquel XR	50	50–200	PO
Ziprasidone	Geodon	20 BID	80 BID	PO (with food), IM
Aripiprazole	Abilify	2.5	15	PO

BID, twice a day; IM, intramuscular; IV, intravenous; PO, oral; XR, extended release.

[a]Target dose is the usually effective dose for organic psychosis or agitation in the elderly. Patients with formal thought disorder may require higher doses in consultation with a psychiatrist.

[b]Typical antipsychotics carry an increased risk, relative to atypical antipsychotics, of extrapyramidal side effects, including akathisia, bradykinesia, rigidity, and tardive dyskinesia.

[c]Atypical antipsychotics may increase glucose and cholesterol levels. Consider monitoring lipids and glucose after initiation of these medications.

less frequent but ongoing monitoring after that. Dosages of antipsychotics used in older patients with dementia or acute delirium tend to be lower than those required for management of other psychotic disorders and may be only necessary for short periods of time (see Table 12–3) as these medications now carry an FDA black box warning for treatment of behavioral symptoms in older patients with dementia. (See Chapter 9, "Cognitive Impairment & Dementia," for further details on dementia and antipsychotics use.)

Neuroleptic malignant syndrome (NMS) is a life-threatening emergency associated with the use of neuroleptic agents. NMS is characterized by a distinctive clinical syndrome of mental status change, rigidity, fever, and autonomic instability, and is associated with elevated plasma creatine phosphokinase. Although NMS is most often seen with the typical high-potency neuroleptic agents (eg, haloperidol, fluphenazine), every class of neuroleptic agents has been implicated, including the low-potency (eg, chlorpromazine) and the atypical antipsychotic drugs (eg, risperidone, olanzapine), as well as the antiemetic metoclopramide. NMS may even occur when dopaminergic drugs, such as levodopa, are abruptly reduced or discontinued. Developing from over a few days to the first 2 weeks of neuroleptic therapy, this syndrome should be suspected when any two of the four following cardinal clinical features occur in the setting of neuroleptic use: mental status change, rigidity, fever, or autonomic instability. When there is any suspicion of NMS, neuroleptic agents should be withheld, and patients should have close inpatient monitoring of clinical signs and laboratory values.

To decrease inappropriate use of psychotropic medications and improve the quality of care in long-term care facilities, the Health Care Finance Administration's 1987 Omnibus Reconciliation Act (OBRA) outlined indications and prescribing guidelines for psychoactive medications used in the treatment of psychotic disorders and agitated behaviors associated with organic brain disorders. OBRA requires documentation of response in terms of specific target symptoms and careful monitoring of side effects. To avoid long-term side effects such as tardive dyskinesia, OBRA also recommends trial dose reductions of neuroleptics unless clinically contraindicated because of severity of symptoms.

B. Behavioral Therapy

Behavioral therapy may be helpful for the management of psychosis and after the acute episode has resolved. Many studies suggest cognitive remediation therapy and social skills therapy can address many of the deficits seen in patients with schizophrenia. Providing a stable living environment is critical to the successful treatment of psychosis. Medical compliance is difficult without close supervision by a family or staff member. Adult day facilities provide structured programs for patients and give critical respite to caregivers, thus allowing patients to remain in the community longer than they would otherwise be able to without nursing home care.

American Geriatrics Society. 2019 Updated Beers Criteria for potentially inappropriate medication use in older adults. *J Am Geriatr Soc.* 2019;67(4):674-694.

American Psychiatric Association. *Diagnostic and Statistical Manual of Mental Disorders.* 5th ed. Washington, DC: American Psychiatric Association; 2013.

Cohen CI, Meesters PD, Zhao J. New perspectives on schizophrenia in later life: implications for treatment, policy, and research. *Lancet.* 2015;2(4):340-350.

Cook JM, McCarthy E, Thorp SR. Older adults with PTSD: brief state of research and evidence-based psychotherapy case illustration. *Am J Geriatr Psychiatry.* 2017;25:522-530.

Jeste DV, Maglione JE. Treating older adults with schizophrenia: challenges and opportunities. *Schizophr Bull.* 2013;39(5):966-968.

Kaiser AP, Wachen JS, Potter C, Moye J, Davison E, Hermann B. PTSD assessment and treatment in older adults. U.S. Department of Veteran Affairs: National Center for PTSD: https://www.ptsd .va.gov/professional/treat/specific/assess_tx_older_adults.asp. Accessed on October 18, 2019.

Khan WU, Rajji TK. Schizophrenia in later life: patient characteristics and treatment strategies. *Psychiatric Times.* 2019;36(3): Digital Edition

Moye J, Rouse SJ. Posttraumatic stress in older adults: when medical diagnoses or treatments cause traumatic stress. *Clin Geriatr Med.* 2014;30(3):577-589.

USEFUL WEBSITES

Agency for Healthcare Research and Quality. AHCPR Supported Guidelines for Diagnosis and Treatment of Depression in Primary Care. http://www.ahrq.gov/professionals/clinicians-providers/guidelines-recommendations/archive.html. Accessed March 11, 2020.

American Association for Geriatric Psychiatry. http://www .aagponline.org. Accessed March 11, 2020.

Depression and Bipolar Support Alliance. https://www.dbsalliance .org/. Accessed March 11, 2020.

Depression Awareness, Recognition, and Treatment (DART) program of the National Institute of Mental Health. http://www .nimh.nih.gov/health/topics/depression/index.shtml. Accessed March 11, 2020.

Geriatric Mental Health Foundation. http://www.gmhfonline.org/ gmhf. Accessed March 11, 2020.

International Foundation for Research and Education on Depression (iFred). http://www.ifred.org. Accessed March 11, 2020.

National Alliance on Mental Illness. http://www.nami.org/. Accessed March 11, 2020.

National Center for PTSD. http://www.ptsd.va.gov/. Accessed March 11, 2020.

National Mental Health Association (Campaign on Clinical Depression). http://www.mentalhealthamerica.net/go/depression. Accessed March 11, 2020.

Defining Adequate Nutrition

13

Meera Sheffrin, MD, MAS

Michi Yukawa, MD, MPH

▶ General Principles

Adequate nutrition is an important part of older adult health. However, nutritional needs may change with aging, and both obesity and malnutrition are prevalent in later life. Previous studies have reported that 35% to 65% of hospitalized geriatric patients and up to 60% of geriatric residents in institutions suffered from malnutrition. Although there has been an increase in the prevalence of obesity in older adults over the past 20 years, obese older adults experiencing involuntary weight loss lose lean mass and are similarly at risk for functional decline and other medical complications compared to nonobese older adults.

In general, body weight in men tends to increase from age 30 to 60 years, plateaus for the next 10 to 15 years, and then slowly declines. In women, the pattern of weight change is similar, except that changes occur approximately 10 years later in life. Lean body mass (primarily skeletal muscle) begins to decline by middle age as a result of many factors, including decreasing exercise and age-related declines in hormone levels (eg, testosterone, estrogen, and growth factors), metabolism, and muscle protein synthesis. Even during healthy aging, daily energy requirements decline with age. This is a result of decreases in muscle mass and decreases in physical activity.

▶ Caloric Needs and Recommended Dietary Allowances for Older Adults

There are many formulas to estimate resting caloric needs of older adults (Table 13–1). All of these estimations should take into account activity levels and underlying illness severity.

Recommended dietary allowances (RDAs) of vitamins and minerals for geriatric patients are similar to those for middle-age adults, although older adults are recommended to have higher calcium and vitamin D intake. (Table 13–2). For men and women older than age 70 years, recommended

calcium intake is 1200 mg/day, and recommended daily dosage of vitamin D (cholecalciferol) is 800 IU. Micronutrient deficiencies of vitamin B_{12} and vitamin D and inadequate calcium intake are common in older adults. However, unless it is clear an older adult is not meeting his or her micronutrient needs due to low overall intake, routine multivitamin supplementation is controversial. Older adults should be encouraged to increased intake of calcium and vitamin D in their diet through food, and supplementation remains warranted for older adults who do not consume adequate amounts in their diet.

The RDAs of macronutrients for older adults are similar to those for middle-age adults (Table 13–2). Protein requirements may fluctuate and are influenced by activity level, medications, nonprotein content of the diet, and health status. For example, corticosteroid use, bed rest, injury, infection, and inflammation all increase the risk of negative nitrogen balance, which can lead to rapid loss of lean body mass. The standard RDA for protein for men and women 51 years of age and older is 0.80 g/kg/day. For example, a 70-kg man should eat 3 to 4 oz of protein per meal to meet that requirement. Older hospitalized persons who are very ill or recovering from trauma or major surgery may require ≥1.5 g/kg/day of protein to maintain their nitrogen balance. For example, a 70-kg man should eat 5 to 6 oz of protein per meal. Monitoring protein intake becomes challenging in medical conditions requiring protein restriction, such as liver or renal disease. In these situations, patients and families have to work closely with dietitians to provide adequate protein intake without worsening patients' hepatic or renal failure.

Serum lipid levels remain a strong predictor of risk for coronary heart disease in older adults as in middle-age adults. Most current recommendations for a healthy diet suggest a diet in which 25% to 30% of total calories come from fat. Some fat in the diet is required for the absorption of fat-soluble vitamins (A, D, E, and K). Based on current data, in nonfrail older adults, fat intake should not exceed 30% of total calories

Table 13–1. Estimation of daily resting caloric (kcal) requirements.

Male: $661.8 - (9.53 \times$ age [y]) = PAC $\times$ (15.91 $\times$ weight [kg] + 539.6 $\times$ height [m])

Female: $354.1 - (6.91 \times$ age [y]) = PAC $\times$ (9.36 $\times$ weight [kg] = 726 $\times$ height [m])

PAC, physical activity coefficient (sedentary PAC = 1.0; low activity PAC = 1.12; active PAC = 1.27; very active PAC = 1.45); y, age in years.

Data from Institute of Medicine and National Academies Press. Dietary Reference Intakes for Energy, Carbohydrate, Fiber, Fat, Fatty Acids, Cholesterol, Protein, and Amino Acids. 2005. https://www.nal.usda.gov/sites/default/files/fnic_uploads/energy_full_report.pdf. Accessed March 10, 2019.

consumed, polyunsaturated and monounsaturated fats should predominate, and saturated fat and partially hydrogenated fat intake should be reduced. In addition, essential fatty acids must be consumed because they cannot be synthesized in the body. There are two general categories of essential fatty acids: omega-6 type and omega-3 type. Omega-6 fatty acids have proinflammatory properties and are the substrate for arachidonic acid, prostaglandins, thromboxanes, and leukotrienes. Omega-3 fatty acids, including eicosapentaenoic acid, docosahexaenoic acid, and prostacyclin, decrease platelet aggregation and vasoconstriction and have anti-inflammatory properties. However, in frail older adults who are at high risk for weight loss, fat intake of all types should be encouraged so as to increase total calorie intake.

Carbohydrate requirements are generally calculated after determining total caloric, fat, and protein requirements.

Thus, carbohydrates generally make up approximately 55% of total caloric intake. Unrefined, whole-grain products should be emphasized, with decreased intake of simple sugars.

Several specific diets can be considered for older adults. A Mediterranean diet, consisting of a high intake of plant foods such as leafy and other vegetables, nuts, whole grains, and olive oil, has been shown to decrease cardiovascular events and may help reduce frailty and positively impact mortality in older adults. The DASH diet (Dietary Approaches to Stop Hypertension), which is high in fruits, vegetables, and low-fat dairy and provides <25% of calories from fat, is recommended to reduce blood pressure (http://dashdiet.org). In general, increasing whole-grain food intake improves fiber intake. A higher intake of fiber is associated with improved bowel function and is associated epidemiologically with a decreased risk for cardiovascular disease, diverticular disease, and diabetes mellitus type 2.

► Findings of Malnutrition and Obesity and Clinical Assessment of Nutrition

A. Anthropometrics

1. Adverse effects of unintentional weight loss & malnutrition— Among community-dwelling older adults, significant weight loss is defined as 5% to 10% weight loss over 6 to 12 months or rapid weight loss of >5% in 1 month. For older adults living in skilled nursing homes, the definition of significant weight loss is either ≥10% weight loss over 6 months or ≥5% weight loss over 1 month. Adverse effects of involuntary weight loss and malnutrition include functional decline, increase in mortality rate (9%–38% within 1–2.5 years),

Table 13–2. Dietary reference intake for older adults age >70 years.

A. Recommended dietary allowances for vitamins and minerals for older adults										
	Vitamin A (µg/day)	Vitamin B₁ (Thiamine) (mg/day)	Vitamin B₂ (Riboflavin) (mg/day)	Vitamin B₆ (Pyridoxine) (mg/day)	Vitamin B₁₂ (mg/day)	Vitamin C (mg/day)	Vitamin D (IU)	Vitamin K (µg/day)	Niacin (mg/day)	Calcium (mg/day)
Males	900	1.2	1.3	1.7	2.4	90	800	120	16	1200
Females	700	1.1	1.1	1.5	2.4	75	800	90	14	1200

B. Recommended dietary allowances for macronutrients for older adults					
	Carbohydrates (g/day)	Total Fiber (g/day)	n-6 Polyunsaturated Fatty Acids (g/day)	n-3 Polyunsaturated Fatty Acids (g/day)	Protein and Amino Acids (g/day)
Males	130	30	14	1.6	56
Females	130	21	11	1.1	46

Data from Dietary References Intakes from Food and Nutrition Board, Institute of Medicine, National Academies; National Agricultural Library, Agricultural Research Service, US Department of Agriculture US Department of Health and Human Services, and US Department of Agriculture. 2015–2020 Dietary Guidelines for Americans, 8th ed. December 2015.

increased risk for hospitalization, increased risk for developing pressure ulcers, postural hypotension, poor wound healing, cognitive decline, and increased risk for infection as a result of poor immune function. Physical signs of malnutrition besides weight loss include peripheral edema caused by protein malnutrition, alopecia, glossitis, loss of subcutaneous fat and muscle bulk, skin desquamation, and dry depigmented hair.

2. Adverse effects of obesity in older adults—In the United States, approximately 27.6% of women >65 years old and 28.4% of men >65 years old are obese. Black (36.5%), American Indian/Alaska Native (35.3%), and Hispanic (32.8%) older adults in America have the highest rates of obesity. The lowest rate of obesity in older adults in the United States is found in the Asian population. Obesity is associated with an increase in the all-cause mortality rate in community-dwelling older adults. There remains controversy regarding the appropriateness of advocating for weight loss in older adults with body mass index (BMI) greater than 35 kg/m². In geriatric patients living in skilled nursing homes, increased mortality was found for those with a BMI ≥35 kg/m², but not for those with BMI between 30 and 35 kg/m². Obesity in middle age can increase the risk for developing hypertension, dyslipidemia, diabetes mellitus, coronary artery disease, stroke, osteoarthritis, and sleep apnea. Increased risk for breast, prostate, and colon cancers has also been associated with obesity. In addition, obesity has been associated with increased knee pain from osteoarthritis. Interestingly, recent studies showed that obese older adults had lower in-hospital mortality after cardiothoracic and breast cancer surgeries compared to non-obese patients. This may be due to higher mortality rate after surgery in older adults with weight loss and malnutrition.

BMI, rather than body weight, is a better measure for determining an individual's nutritional status. BMI adjusts weight in relation to height; however, it does not identify persons who have replaced muscle mass with adipose tissue, nor does it distinguish persons with central obesity. Central obesity is associated with negative health outcomes, and thus, some researchers believe that waist circumference may be a better measure than BMI for assessment of obesity in older adults.

B. Laboratory Assessment

The initial laboratory assessment of unintentional weight loss should include a complete blood count, glucose, electrolytes, renal and liver function, thyroid-stimulating hormone level, urinalysis, and chest x-ray film. These initial tests should rule out metabolic, endocrine, or infectious causes of weight loss.

Although serum albumin is commonly ordered to assess protein nutrition or status, serum albumin levels have poor sensitivity and specificity as a measure of nutritional health. The half-life of albumin is approximately 3 weeks. Levels respond slowly to adequate nutritional intervention and may never normalize if inflammation is ongoing. Increasing the serum albumin with intravenous albumin replacement does not improve prognosis. However, measurement of serum albumin does have clinical value: a low serum albumin, although not a good indicator of nutritional status, may be a powerful predictor of overall illness severity and mortality.

In the past, prealbumin (transthyretin) was used as a more sensitive marker than albumin in evaluating acute nutritional change. However, prealbumin is neither sensitive nor specific enough to screen for or diagnose malnutrition and may not be consistently responsive to nutritional interventions or correlated with health outcomes. While a progressively rising prealbumin level may help to confirm improving nutritional status, the clinical exam remains the best indicator. Serum cholesterol <160 mg/dL is a marker for increased risk of morbidity and mortality but not a good measure of nutrition.

C. Clinical Assessment

A comprehensive clinical assessment of nutritional status is the most useful way to identify malnutrition, and several assessment instruments exist. The Mini Nutritional Assessment (Figure 13–1) is well validated and has become widely used to evaluate nutritional status in geriatric patients. Other screening tools include Seniors in the Community: Risk Evaluation for Eating and Nutrition (SCREEN) (https://www.phsd.ca/resources/research-statistics/research-evaluation/reports-knowledge-products/seniors-community-risk-evaluation-eating-nutrition) and the Simplified Nutrition Assessment Questionnaire (SNAQ) (https://www.msdmanuals.com/professional/multimedia/figure/nut_simplified_nutritional_assessment).

▶ Differential Diagnosis of Impaired Nutritional Status

A. Potential Causes of Unintentional Weight Loss

As in most geriatric syndromes, unintentional weight loss in older adults is often caused by multiple factors. Possible causes can be categorized into medical, psychosocial, and pharmacologic (Table 13–3). Underlying or previously undiagnosed cancer could be the cause of involuntary weight loss in 16% to 36% of cases according to some studies. Gastrointestinal malignancy such as esophageal, pancreatic, and gastric cancer is more common than other cancers. Other malignancies that are associated with weight loss include lymphomas and lung, prostate, ovarian, and bladder cancers. Nonmalignant causes of weight loss include chronic illnesses such as dementia, congestive heart failure, chronic obstructive pulmonary disease, endocrine disorders (diabetes mellitus, hyperthyroidism), and end-stage kidney or liver failure. Depression and dementia are major causes of weight loss in older adults and may account for 10% to 20% of weight loss in community-dwelling older adults and in 58% of nursing home residents. People who have dementia lose weight and decrease food intake as a result of impaired access to food,

Mini Nutritional Assessment
MNA®

Nestlé
NutritionInstitute

Last name:			First name:		
Sex:	Age:	Weight, kg:	Height, cm:	Date:	

Complete the screen by filling in the boxes with the appropriate numbers. Total the numbers for the final screening score.

Screening

A Has food intake declined over the past 3 months due to loss of appetite, digestive problems, chewing or swallowing difficulties?

0 = severe decrease in food intake
1 = moderate decrease in food intake
2 = no decrease in food intake ☐

B Weight loss during the last 3 months

0 = weight loss greater than 3 kg (6.6 lbs)
1 = does not know
2 = weight loss between 1 and 3 kg (2.2 and 6.6 lbs)
3 = no weight loss ☐

C Mobility

0 = bed or chair bound
1 = able to get out of bed/chair but does not go out
2 = goes out ☐

D Has suffered psychological stress or acute disease in the last 3 months?

0 = yes   2 = no ☐

E Neuropsychological problems

0 = severe dementia or depression
1 = mild dementia
2 = no psychological problems ☐

F1 Body Mass Index (BMI) (weight in kg) / (height in m²)

0 = BMI less than 19
1 = BMI 19 to less than 21
2 = BMI 21 to less than 23
3 = BMI 23 or greater ☐

IF BMI IS NOT AVAILABLE, REPLACE QUESTION F1 WITH QUESTION F2.
DO NOT ANSWER QUESTION F2 IF QUESTION F1 IS ALREADY COMPLETED.

F2 Calf circumference (CC) in cm

0 = CC less than 31
3 = CC 31 or greater ☐

Screening score (max. 14 points)

12 - 14 points: Normal nutritional status
8 - 11 points: At risk of malnutrition
0 - 7 points: Malnourished ☐☐

References
1. Vellas B, Villars H, Abellan G, et al. Overview of the MNA® - Its History and Challenges. *J Nutr Health Aging.* 2006;**10**:456-465.
2. Rubenstein LZ, Harker JO, Salva A, Guigoz Y, Vellas B. Screening for Undernutrition in Geriatric Practice: Developing the Short-Form Mini Nutritional Assessment (MNA-SF). *J. Geront.* 2001;**56A**:M366-377.
3. Guigoz Y. The Mini-Nutritional Assessment (MNA®) Review of the Literature - What does it tell us? *J Nutr Health Aging.* 2006; **10**:466-487.
4. Kaiser MJ, Bauer JM, Ramsch C, et al. Validation of the Mini Nutritional Assessment Short-Form (MNA®-SF): A practical tool for identification of nutritional status. *J Nutr Health Aging.* 2009;**13**:782-788.
® Société des Produits Nestlé, S.A., Vevey, Switzerland, Trademark Owners © Nestlé, 1994, Revision 2009. N67200 12/99 10M
For more information: www.mna-elderly.com

▲ **Figure 13–1.** The Mini Nutritional Assessment (MNA) short form. (© Société des Produits Nestlé SA 1994, Revision 2009.)

Table 13–3. Potential causes of involuntary weight loss.

Medical factors	**Cancer:** GI malignancy (esophageal, pancreatic, and gastric cancer) Lung Lymphoma Prostate Ovarian Bladder	**Noncancer:** GI disorders (motility or swallow dysfunction, mesenteric ischemia, peptic ulcers, gallstones) Congestive heart failure Dementia COPD Endocrine disorder (hyperthyroidism, diabetes mellitus) Stroke End-stage renal failure End-stage liver failure Alcoholism Rheumatoid arthritis Oral or dental problems
Psychosocial factors	**Social:** Poverty Inability to shop or cook Inability to feed Social isolation Lack of ethnic food variety	**Psychological:** Depression Alcoholism Bereavement Paranoia
Medications	**Anorexic:** Antibiotic (erythromycin) Digoxin Opiates SSRIs (fluoxetine) Amantadine Metformin Benzodiazepines **Dry mouth:** Anticholinergics Loop diuretics Antihistamines	**Nausea/vomiting:** Antibiotic (erythromycin) Bisphosphonates Digoxin Dopamine agonist Levodopa Opiates Tricyclic antidepressants SSRIs **Alter taste or smell:** ACE inhibitors Calcium channel blockers Spironolactone Iron Antiparkinsonian medications (levodopa, pergolide, selegiline) Opiates Gold Allopurinol

ACE, angiotensin-converting enzyme; COPD, chronic obstructive pulmonary disease; GI, gastrointestinal; SSRIs, selective serotonin reuptake inhibitors.

Data from McMinn J, Steel C, Bowman A. Investigation and management of unintentional weight loss in older adults. *BMJ.* 2011;342:d1732; and Chapman IM. Weight loss in older persons. *Med Clin North Am.* 2011;95(3):579-593.

dysphagia, the inability to self-feed, and the excess energy expenditure caused by agitation and wandering. Oral and dental problems, such as ill-fitting dentures or poor dentition, can also lead to weight loss.

Social factors, such as financial constraints, inability to shop or cook, social isolation, and lack of ethnic foods in institutional facilities, can contribute to unintentional weight loss. Many medications can lead to weight loss from side effects of anorexia, nausea/vomiting, dry mouth, or altered taste or smell (see Table 13–3).

▶ Interventions for Impaired Nutritional Status

A. Improve Malnutrition & Weight Loss

Successfully motivating undernourished persons to eat requires a multidimensional approach, including assessing and treating for pain and depression, increasing social supports, and adapting to individual food preferences and meal times. Simple exercise, such as daily walking, may improve appetite in some patients.

Older adults often eat better, and more, when fed by family members. One reason for this is the length of time the family member dedicates to unhurriedly feeding and encouraging the patient. Older people also eat more if they are eating with others. Studies have shown that older adults receiving delivered meals (eg, Meals on Wheels) eat more if the delivery person stays with them.

1. Oral supplements—A variety of commercial liquid and powder supplements are used when patients are unable or unwilling to consume enough regular food. Although the most recent Cochrane review on oral nutritional supplements did not show improvement in survival rate, studies using dietary advice with or without oral nutritional supplements have shown some improvements in weight and body composition. Nutritional supplements are most effective when consumed at least 1 hour before meals, so patients do not substitute supplement intake for regular meals. Powder formulations allow the supplement to be masked by mixing it with other food. A major barrier to canned supplements is cost, even with generic brands. For patients with no history of lactose intolerance, instant breakfast powders mixed in milk are a satisfactory and less expensive alternative.

2. Appetite stimulants—Several medications have been promoted as helping to improve appetite and increase weight; however, none have proven satisfactory or effective in older adults.

Megestrol acetate has been shown to increase appetite and weight in AIDS and cancer patients; however, it has only been associated with a minimal increase in weight in older adults. There are significant potential harms of megestrol acetate, including the risk of deep venous thrombosis, suppression of the hypothalamic-pituitary adrenal axis, worsening of congestive heart failure, and additionally, a possible increase in mortality in nursing home patients. Megestrol acetate is listed on the 2019 American Geriatrics Society Beers Criteria for Potentially Inappropriate Medication Use in Older Adults.

Mirtazapine, an antidepressant associated with weight gain, is commonly prescribed for management of depression and weight loss in older adults. However, the impact of mirtazapine on weight among older adults has not been rigorously evaluated. Persons with persistent anorexia may benefit from a trial of antidepressant therapy such as with mirtazapine to treat possible underlying depression.

Most other medications have limited or uncertain effects on weight or have significant side effects in older adults. Dronabinol has not been well studied in older adults, and in several small trials, older adults were unable to tolerate the central nervous systems effects and dysphoria associated with dronabinol use. Cyproheptadine has not been shown to be effective in older adults. Anabolic agents such as growth hormone and insulin-like growth factor are expensive and associated with frequent side effects. Ghrelin use in clinical trials has increased body weight and lean body mass in older adults; however, it is currently only available for research purposes. Androgen therapy with testosterone or its analogues also has many side effects, and thus its use for weight gain remains experimental.

3. Artificial tube feeding—Before discussing the use of artificial tube feeding, patients and their family members should discuss overall goals of care. Some clinicians initiate artificial feeding as a therapeutic trial for a limited and predetermined duration with the understanding that if certain goals are not achieved (eg, the person will begin to voluntarily consume sufficient calories for survival), the intervention will be discontinued. In certain clinical situations, temporary use of tube feeding can be beneficial, such as during treatments for head neck cancer or recovery from an acute stroke. However, the benefits of artificial feeding by tube in many clinical situations are uncertain.

In patients with advanced dementia, initiation of artificial tube feeding does not increase survival, improve functional status, or improve wound healing. Furthermore, no method of tube feeding (G-tube or J-tube) will prevent aspiration or pneumonia in patients with dementia. Retrospective cohort studies of patients with neurologic illness have shown high rates of aspiration pneumonia in tube-fed patients. (For more on the use of feeding tubes, see Chapter 9, "Cognitive Impairment & Dementia.")

4. Treatment of obesity—Community-dwelling older adults who are obese and have poorly controlled hypertension, diabetes mellitus, functional impairment, or lower extremity arthritis may benefit from gradual weight reduction. Sustained weight loss generally requires a combination of healthy diet and exercise. Several studies of older obese adults who were placed on a weight loss diet along with exercise (aerobic exercise and resistance training) demonstrated ability of these subjects to lose weight without losing significant lean body mass. The use of weight loss medication (amphetamines, sibutramine, orlistat) in older adults has not been investigated adequately, and thus these medications should not be used or should be used with significant caution. Amphetamines and sibutramine should be avoided in patients with cardiac disease.

Although the effects of obesity have been studied extensively in older adults living in the community, little is known about the effects of obesity in the nursing home. One study showed that nursing home residents with BMI >40 kg/m² had increased mortality compared to those with normal weight (BMI of 19–28 kg/m²). Because of concerns about potential malnutrition and decrease in bone density, weight loss programs for nursing home residents should be initiated with caution. Having a low BMI (<19 kg/m²) is associated with increased mortality rates among nursing home patients, and nursing home residents with a BMI of 30–35 kg/m² have been shown to have a higher mortality rate.

5. Interaction between medications and food—Certain foods can inhibit or potentiate the effects of commonly prescribed medications for older adults (Table 13–4). Grapefruit juice can inhibit cytochrome P450 3A4 and thus lead to increased serum levels of statins, calcium channel blockers, and phosphodiesterase inhibitors (sildenafil, vardenafil, and tadalafil) (see Table 13–4). Grapefruit juice affects certain statins more than others; there is a large effect on simvastatin and atorvastatin; however, there is little to no effect on the serum levels of pravastatin and rosuvastatin, which can be taken with grapefruit juice safely. Dairy products or calcium supplements can diminish the effectiveness of some antibiotics if taken at the same time, including fluoroquinolones, cefuroxime, and tetracyclines (see Table 13–4). These antibiotics should be taken at least 2 hours before or 6 hours after calcium supplements or calcium-rich foods. For community-dwelling older adults, a local pharmacist is often a good person to consult for how many hours to wait until a food or drink can be consumed after taking a medication. Table 13–4 lists other interactions between food and medications.

SUMMARY

Adequate nutrition is an important part of older adult health. The RDAs of vitamins, minerals, and macronutrients for geriatric patients are not significantly different than those for younger adults except for increased need for calcium and vitamin D supplements. A Mediterranean diet or the DASH diet may serve as a good guideline for healthy older adults to follow. Involuntary weight loss and obesity in older adults can increase morbidity and mortality. Improving malnutrition and weight loss in geriatric patients requires a multistep approach. Assessing social issues, potential psychiatric illnesses including depression and cognitive impairment,

Table 13–4. Food and drug interactions.

Food	Medications	Interaction
Grapefruit juice	Atorvastatin Simvastatin Lovastatin	Decreased metabolism Increased risk for muscle toxicity (myalgia, myopathy, rhabdomyolysis)
	Calcium channel blockers: 　Amlodipine 　Nifedipine 　Nicardipine 　Verapamil 　Felodipine	Decreased metabolism Increased risk for orthostatic hypotension
	Phosphodiesterase inhibitors: 　Sildenafil 　Vardenafil 　Tadalafil	Increased serum concentration Priapism, hypotension, visual disturbances
	Benzodiazepines: 　Diazepam 　Temazepam 　Midazolam	Increased serum concentration Increased central nervous system depressant effect
	Amiodarone	Decreased metabolism Increased risk for bradycardia, CHF, hypotension
Caffeine	Ciprofloxacin	Ciprofloxacin can potentiate the effect of caffeine Increase risk for insomnia
	Cimetidine	Cimetidine can increase caffeine levels
	Theophylline	Caffeine inhibits the metabolism Increase risk for anxiety, insomnia, and cardiac arrhythmia
Dairy products or calcium supplements	Fluoroquinolones: 　Ciprofloxacin 　Levofloxacin Cefuroxime Tetracycline	Decreased absorption
	Bisphosphonates: 　Alendronate 　Risedronate 　Ibandronate	Low bioavailability and drug absorption when taken with dairy products or calcium supplements
Protein-rich foods	Propranolol	Increased bioavailability of propranolol Increased risk for bradycardia, hypotension, and bronchoconstriction
	Carbidopa/levodopa	Decreased serum concentration
	Theophylline	Decreased serum concentration
Fiber	Metformin	Decreased serum levels if taken with large amounts of fiber
Tyramine-containing foods (cheese and red wines)	MAOIs: 　Selegiline 　Phenelzine 　Isocarboxazid 　Tranylcypromine	Potentiate the effect of these medications. Can contribute to serotonin syndrome
	Linezolid	Some MAOI properties
	Isoniazid	MAOI effects
	Tramadol	Weak MAOI
Green, leafy vegetables	Warfarin	Rich in vitamin K and thus reduce the efficacy of warfarin

CHF, congestive heart failure; MAOI, monoamine oxidase inhibitor.

underlying medical conditions, and medications is essential. A combination of healthy diet and exercise should be recommended for obese community-dwelling older adults. For obese nursing home residents, weight loss programs should be initiated with caution.

America's Health Rankings. www.americashealthrankings.org. Accessed April 20, 2019.

Anton SD, Manini TM, Milsom VA, et al. Effects of a weight loss plus exercise program on physical function in overweight, older women: a randomized controlled trial. *Clin Interv Aging.* 2011;6:141-149.

Attar A, Malka D, Sabate JM, et al. Malnutrition is high and underestimated during chemotherapy in gastrointestinal cancer: an AGEO prospective cross-sectional multicenter study. *Nutr Cancer.* 2012;64(4):535-542.

Baldwin C, Weekes CE. Dietary advice with or without oral nutritional supplements for disease-related malnutrition in adults. *Cochrane Database Syst Rev.* 2011;9:CD002008.

Chapman IM. Weight loss in older persons. *Med Clin North Am.* 2011;95(3):579-593.

Cullen S. Gastrostomy tube feeding in adults: the risks, benefits and alternatives. *Proc Nutr Soc.* 2011;70(3):293-298.

DiFrancesco V, Fantin F, Omzzolo F, et al. The anorexia of aging. *Dig Dis.* 2007;25(2):129-137.

Flegal KM, Carroll MD, Kit BK, Ogden CL. Prevalence of obesity and trends in the distribution of body mass index among US adults, 1999-2010. *JAMA.* 2012;307(5):491-497.

Gioulbasanis I, Georgoulias P, Vlachostergios PJ, et al. Mini Nutritional Assessment (MNS) and biochemical markers of cachexia in metastatic lung cancer patients: Interrelations and associations with prognosis. *Lung Cancer.* 2011;74(3):516-520.

Li A, Heber D. Sarcopenic obesity in the elderly and strategies for weight management. *Nutr Rev.* 2011;70(1):57-64.

McMinn J, Steel C, Bowman A. Investigation and management of unintentional weight loss in older adults. *BMJ.* 2011;342:d1732.

Moore AH, Trentham-Dietz A, Burns M, et al. Obesity and mortality after locoregional breast cancer diagnosis. *Breast Cancer Res Treat.* 2018;172:647-657.

Rutter CE, Yovino S, Taylor R, et al. Impact of early percutaneous endoscopic gastrostomy tube placement on nutritional status and hospitalization in patients with head and neck cancer receiving definitive chemoradiation therapy. *Head Neck.* 2011;33(10):1441-1447.

Saragat B, Buffa R, Mereu E, et al. Nutritional and psycho-functional status in elderly patients with Alzheimer's disease. *J Nutr Health Aging.* 2012;16(3):231-236.

Vargo PR, Steffen RJ, Bakaeen FG, et al. The impact of obesity on cardiac surgery outcomes. *J Cardiol Surg.* 2018;33:588-594.

Villareal DT, Chode S, Parimi N, et al. Weight loss, exercise, or both and physical function in obese older adults. *N Engl J Med.* 2011;364(13):1218-1229.

Yaxley A, Miller MD, Fraser RJ, Cobiac L. Pharmacological interventions for geriatric cachexia: a narrative review of the literature. *J Nutr Health Aging.* 2012;16(2):148-154.

Principles of Prescribing & Adherence

Michael A. Steinman, MD

Holly M. Holmes, MD, MS, AGSF

WHAT IS "GERIATRIC" ABOUT PRESCRIBING FOR OLDER ADULTS?

On the surface, prescribing for older adults is similar to prescribing for younger adults, requiring understanding of drug indications, dosing, potential adverse reactions, and drug-drug interactions. However, prescribing for older adults is complicated by a variety of factors. Physiologic changes as patients get older result in alterations in drug metabolism and susceptibility to adverse events. The presence of multiple chronic conditions and multiple medications leads to potentially complex drug-drug and drug-disease interactions, as well as the need to balance multiple competing recommendations. Changes in cognitive function, manual dexterity, and social supports complicate adherence to medications, and heterogeneous goals of care require special attention. Because clinical trials that inform many practice guidelines are often conducted in younger patients, there can be ambiguity about the extent to which these evidence-based recommendations apply to older adults. Thus, mastering prescribing for older patients requires expertise not only in technical elements of drug use, but also in synthesizing evidence and biomedical and psychosocial factors into a coordinated plan of care that meets each individual's unique needs. More details about extrapolating the evidence from clinical research to older patients can be found in Chapter 24, "Applying Evidence-Based Care to Older Persons."

DRUG METABOLISM AND PHYSIOLOGIC EFFECTS IN OLDER ADULTS

▶ Pharmacokinetics

Pharmacokinetics refers to how the body handles a drug from the time it is ingested to the time it is excreted. This includes the processes of absorption, distribution, metabolism, and elimination. While each of these processes can vary with age, they are typically more influenced by genetic factors and by an individual's diseases, environment, and other medications. For most older patients, changes in renal function have the greatest impact on pharmacokinetics.

A. Absorption

Absorption of drugs is impacted by the size of the absorptive surface, gastric pH, splanchnic blood flow, and gastrointestinal (GI) tract motility. Most of these are relatively unaffected by age but can be substantially affected by certain diseases and medications. Some medications, including vitamin B_{12}, calcium, and iron, have decreased absorption in older adults as a result of reduced activity of active transport mechanisms.

B. Distribution

Older patients have an increased fat-to-lean body mass ratio, decreased total-body water, and sometimes decreased serum albumin. Drugs that distribute in fat (eg, diazepam) may thus have a larger volume of distribution. Hydrophilic medications (eg, digoxin) will have a decreased volume of distribution, resulting in higher serum levels. Drugs that bind to serum proteins reach an equilibrium between bound (inactive) and free (active) drug. Use of two or more drugs that compete for protein binding (eg, thyroid hormone, digoxin, warfarin, phenytoin) can result in higher levels of free drug, requiring careful monitoring of drug levels and effects. In the case of testosterone, age-associated increases in sex hormone–binding globulin can result in normal serum levels of total testosterone, even while levels of serum-free testosterone (the bioactive form) are reduced.

C. Metabolism

The cytochrome P450 system assists with drug metabolism through oxidation and reduction (known as phase I metabolism). There typically are not major changes in the function of this system with advancing age. Instead, the cytochrome

P450 system is typically far more impacted by genetic polymorphisms that result in some individuals being "fast" or "slow" metabolizers and by the use of other drugs and foods that can inhibit or induce specific P450 enzymes, resulting in slowed or accelerated drug metabolism. (See the section "Adverse Drug Reactions" later in this chapter for information on cytochrome P450–mediated drug-drug interactions.) Phase II hepatic metabolism, otherwise known as conjugation, follows phase I metabolism. It typically makes drugs biologically inactive and facilitates their excretion. It is not affected by age. Pharmacogenetic testing can identify an individual's cytochrome P450 system genotype to determine whether certain drugs are likely to be metabolized quickly or slowly and thus aid in drug dosing, although in most settings, such testing is not widely used.

D. Excretion

Renal function often decreases with age, involving loss of both glomerular filtration rate and tubular function. Because muscle mass declines in older age, renal function can often be substantially impaired even in the presence of a normal serum creatinine. Thus, estimation of creatinine clearance (or the closely related estimated glomerular filtration rate [eGFR]) is essential. Mathematically complex formulas such as the Chronic Kidney Disease Epidemiology Collaboration (CKD-EPI) and Modification of Diet in Renal Disease (MDRD) formulas tend to more accurately reflect renal function compared to the Cockcroft-Gault equation (shown below). However, each is imperfect and should be interpreted as providing only a rough estimate of renal function. In situations of rapidly changing renal function, neither formula performs well. In general, it is far better to have (and use) an easy-to-obtain rough estimate of renal function than none at all. Where there is substantial uncertainty about the true eGFR or need for precise quantification, cystatin C–based lab assays can provide accurate estimates.

$$\text{Creatinine clearance} = \frac{(140 - \text{age}) \times \text{weight (kg)}}{\text{Serum creatinine} \times 72}$$

(multiply by 0.85 for women to allow for 15% less muscle mass).

Pharmacodynamics

Pharmacodynamics refers to how a drug affects the body; that is, the physiologic effects exerted by a drug's action on end-organ receptors. Older adults are more sensitive to medications that depress the central nervous system, which can result in delirium, confusion, and agitation. The frequent use of multiple medications in older adults often leads to the simultaneous use of two or more drugs that have mutually reinforcing physiologic effects, which can result in harm. Examples include bleeding with simultaneous use of anticoagulant drugs and aspirin and orthostatic hypotension with various blood pressure medications and first-generation α-blockers.

GERIATRIC THERAPEUTICS

Adverse Drug Reactions

A. Epidemiology & Risk Factors

Adverse drug reactions (ADRs) are substantially more common in older than in younger adults. Up to 35% of ambulatory older adults experience one or more ADRs annually, 9% of hospital admissions in older adults are ascribable to ADRs, and roughly one in five hospitalized adults experience an ADR during their inpatient stay. Simply being old does not meaningfully increase ADR risk. Rather, it is the number of medications taken and the burden of disease (which often, but not always, increases as patients get older) that are the strongest risk factors for ADRs in the outpatient setting. The risk of ADRs may also increase with specific drugs that can interact with specific impairments. For example, central nervous system–acting drugs may have a particularly high risk of causing ADRs in patients with underlying cognitive impairment.

A note on terminology: "Adverse drug reactions" refers to the unwanted effects of drugs at normal dosage and use. "Adverse drug events" refers to a broader range of potential harms associated with the drug, including overdose, withdrawal reactions from abrupt discontinuation of a drug, and more.

B. Causes of Adverse Drug Reactions

ADRs are commonly classified into two predominant types. Type A ADRs result from expected yet unwanted or exaggerated physiologic effects of the drug. For example, β-blockers may cause bradycardia that results in syncope. Type B ADRs, which are less common, result from idiosyncratic effects unrelated to the drug's usual physiologic targets; for example, anaphylaxis to penicillin.

In older adults, type A ADRs often arise from the interaction of a drug and underlying characteristics of the patient. Medications with a narrow therapeutic index and prolonged half-life cause the most trouble for the older patient. Older adults with multiple medications, disease states, and/or subclinical physiologic changes associated with aging can be more susceptible to unwanted effects of a drug.

Drug-drug interactions can lead to ADRs by pharmacokinetic and pharmacodynamic mechanisms. In the former, an interaction can affect absorption, distribution, metabolism, or excretion. For example, diltiazem inhibits cytochrome P450 isoenzyme 3A4 (CYP3A4). Atorvastatin and several other (but not all) statin medications are metabolized by CYP3A4. Thus, if a patient is taking both diltiazem and atorvastatin, atorvastatin will accumulate because the enzyme that metabolizes it has been rendered less active. Tissue levels of atorvastatin will rise, potentially to the level where they cause substantial toxicity (ie, increased risk of rhabdomyolysis and liver injury). Other common culprits that inhibit P450 activity include antimicrobials such as ciprofloxacin, fluconazole, and clarithromycin; some selective serotonin reuptake inhibitors (SSRIs); amiodarone; and verapamil.

Cytochrome P450 isoenzymes can also be induced ("sped up"). This results in rapid clearance and thus decreased effectiveness of drugs metabolized by the affected isozyme. Medications that are potent inducers of P450 enzymes include rifampin, barbiturates, carbamazepine, and phenytoin. In general, cytochrome P450–mediated interactions are most important when induction or inhibition is potent (eg, greater than five-fold change in enzyme activity) and the substrate drug has a narrow therapeutic index (eg, warfarin, sulfonylureas). Drug interactions that involve weak induction or inhibition and a substrate drug with a wide safety margin are less likely to be clinically relevant.

Use of two or more drugs with mutually reinforcing physiologic effects can also result in harms (ie, a pharmacodynamic interaction). For example, third-degree heart block may occur in a patient prescribed digoxin and an α-blocker, as both suppress conduction of atrial impulses through the atrioventricular node.

Drug-disease interactions occur when an underlying disease state makes a patient more susceptible to the unwanted physiologic effects of a drug. Not every potential interaction results in harm. For example, many patients with mild or moderate chronic obstructive pulmonary disease can tolerate β-blockers without adverse effects, although some will develop worse pulmonary symptoms in this setting.

In addition to ADRs, an expanded range of adverse events can occur from misuse of drugs. This can include complications of excessive doses of a drug, failure to prevent or treat disease because of nonadherence to or insufficient dosing of a drug, or withdrawal reactions caused by abrupt discontinuation of a drug to which the body has physiologically adapted (ie, chronic opioids or corticosteroids).

C. Preventing Adverse Drug Reactions & the Role of Monitoring

Only a fraction of ADRs in ambulatory older adults are a result of clinicians making clearly inappropriate prescribing decisions. Rather, most ADRs result from drugs that were reasonable to prescribe and represent the known but unwelcome potential adverse reactions of a given drug. Anticoagulants, antiplatelets, and oral and injectable antihyperglycemics are among the most common causes of ADRs severe enough to precipitate an emergency department visit. Nonetheless, these drugs have an important place in the therapeutic armamentarium for older adults. In fact, anticoagulants are often underprescribed because for many patients the benefits of preventing a stroke or pulmonary embolism outweigh the risk of hemorrhage.

True prevention is difficult in this setting because it can be difficult to precisely predict which patients will be helped or harmed by a drug. Yet, many ADRs can be detected and managed early, sparing the patient prolonged symptoms or

a cascade of ever-worsening adverse effects (eg, untreated orthostasis resulting in a fall with fracture). Monitoring older adults for emerging ADRs thus plays a critical role in reducing the burden of ADRs yet is often not done well. One important impediment to monitoring is that both patients and physicians may falsely attribute a new symptom to an underlying disease state or "getting old," rather than recognizing it as an ADR. This leads patients to underreport potential ADRs and to physicians not properly diagnosing a symptom as an ADR even when the patient reports it. The mantra "any symptom in an older adult is a medication side effect until proven otherwise" provides a useful reminder to always keep ADRs on the differential diagnosis when evaluating a new or worsened complaint.

> *Any symptom in an older adult is a medication side effect until proven otherwise.*

Dedicated nurse-led and pharmacist-led programs are effective strategies for ADR monitoring, best exemplified by anticoagulation clinics. Although few data are available to support simple in-office or bedside tools for ADR monitoring, expert opinion suggests that several strategies may be helpful. These include: (1) at the time a drug is prescribed, warning the patient of which adverse reactions to watch for; (2) at the next patient encounter, use a combination of open-ended questions and specific prompts to query for adverse reactions (eg, "Are you having any side effects or problems from Drug X?" followed by specific questions about dangerous and common adverse reactions); and (3) using a similar strategy to query for adverse reactions during annual medication review.

▶ Multiple Medication Use (Polypharmacy)

A. Epidemiology & Potential Harms & Benefits of Using Multiple Medicines

In the United States, 39% of adults age 65 years and older use five or more medications. This use of multiple medications is commonly referred to as *polypharmacy*. This term lacks a universally accepted definition but is often used to refer to the concurrent use of five or more medications, although in clinical practice, it is typically better to think of polypharmacy as a continuum. The concept of polypharmacy carries a pejorative connotation, in part for good reason. Use of multiple medications substantially increases the risk of drug-drug interactions and of adverse drug events, potentially imposes substantial cost burdens on patients, complicates adherence, and contributes to increased risk of using inappropriate medications. However, older patients often have multiple chronic conditions that can be substantially helped by medications. In many such patients, the use of multiple drugs is an appropriate therapeutic choice. Thus, although use of multiple medications is a risk factor for medication problems—and should prompt close attention to reducing unnecessary medications—the focus on reducing medications needs to be balanced with the potential benefits that medications can provide to longevity and quality of life. This is often a highly individualized calculus based on a patient's conditions, ability to tolerate and adhere to multiple medications, likelihood of drug benefits and harms, and goals and preferences.

B. The Prescribing Cascade

One important contributor to multiple medication use is the "prescribing cascade," in which the adverse effects of one drug are treated with another drug, which itself causes adverse effects that are treated with a third drug, and so forth. This can result from misinterpreting a sign or symptom as the manifestation of an underlying disease process, rather than as an adverse drug effect. As noted earlier, remembering the mantra "any symptom in an older adult is a medication side effect until proven otherwise" can help guard against potential prescribing cascades. Except in unusual circumstances, it is typically better to withdraw or substitute the offending drug rather than treating its adverse effects with another drug.

▶ Overuse, Misuse, and Underuse of Medications

For many older adults, the question is not whether a patient is taking too many or too few medications, but whether the patient is taking the right medications given her or his diseases, preferences, and ability to adhere. Deviations from an optimal regimen can be viewed as problems of overuse (use of a drug where no medication therapy is needed), misuse (use of a drug where a better alternative is available), and underuse (nonuse of a drug that would be beneficial).

A. Overuse & Misuse

Overuse and misuse of drugs are common. Approximately 20% to 35% of older ambulatory adults in the United States and other developed countries use at least one drug that consensus criteria recommend avoiding in older patients. Expert review of medication regimens in outpatient, inpatient, and nursing home settings has also identified large proportions of patients taking drugs that are not indicated, ineffective for the condition being treated, or otherwise problematic. It is common for drugs to be continued long after they are no longer necessary. For example, roughly half of US patients who are started on a proton pump inhibitor for stress ulcer prophylaxis during a hospital stay are continued on these medications after discharge, for no discernible reason.

Several explicit criteria, commonly called "drugs-to-avoid lists," have been developed to identify medications that are potentially inappropriate for older adults. These tools have proved useful for quality improvement, including flagging instances of such prescribing for special scrutiny and review. Nonetheless, clinical judgment needs to be applied for individual patients, as there are situations in which use of many of these drugs is reasonable.

The American Geriatrics Society *Beers criteria* of potentially inappropriate medications are shown in Table 14–1. The most frequently cited part of these criteria concern drugs that are potentially inappropriate in any setting. Commonly used medications on this "drugs-to-avoid" list include first-generation antihistamines (eg, diphenhydramine and hydroxyzine), benzodiazepines and the sedative-hypnotic "Z drugs" (eg, zolpidem), tertiary-amine tricyclic antidepressants, long-acting sulfonylureas (eg, glyburide), and chronic use of nonsteroidal anti-inflammatory drugs (NSAIDs).

The *STOPP* (Screening Tool of Older Person's Prescriptions) *criteria* define an extensive list of specific clinical situations in which drug use is potentially inappropriate (Table 14–2). Examples include use of loop diuretics for ankle edema in the absence of heart failure; SSRIs in patients with a history of hyponatremia; and use of NSAIDs in patients with heart failure or moderate-to-severe hypertension. There is substantial overlap between the American Geriatrics Society Beers criteria and the STOPP criteria.

B. Underuse

Older adults are less likely to receive indicated medications than their younger counterparts, even after accounting for contraindications to these therapies. Excessive fear of causing adverse events, distraction by other clinical issues, a sense of futility, and unrecognized ageism likely contribute to this pattern. In addition, treatable conditions are often underdiagnosed in older patients, and symptoms such as pain, fatigue, depressed mood, or orthostasis may be incorrectly attributed to "getting old."

The *START* (Screening Tool to Alert to Right Treatment) *criteria* are consensus criteria that identify potential underuse of beneficial medications in older adults (Table 14–3). As with other explicit criteria, these are intended as a guide but not as a substitute for clinical judgment for individual patients. Examples of drugs that the START criteria recommend should routinely be used include anticoagulation for chronic atrial fibrillation (in the absence of contraindications); regular inhaled β-agonist or antimuscarinic bronchodilator for patients with mild to moderate asthma or chronic obstructive pulmonary disease; and bisphosphonates, vitamin D, and calcium in patients on chronic corticosteroid therapy.

▶ High-Risk Medications

The following medications are often associated with adverse reactions and merit special caution in prescribing.

Table 14–1. Potentially inappropriate medications in older adults—Beers criteria (selected examples).[a]

Criterion	Rationale
First-generation antihistamines (eg, diphenhydramine, hydroxyzine)	Highly anticholinergic; risk of confusion, dry mouth, constipation, and other anticholinergic effects
Digoxin >0.125 mg/day	In heart failure, higher dosages associated with no additional benefit and may increase risk of toxicity; slow renal clearance may increase risk of toxic effects
Tertiary tricyclic antidepressants (eg, amitriptyline)	Highly anticholinergic, sedating, and cause orthostatic hypotension
Antipsychotics for behavioral problems of dementia unless nonpharmacologic options have failed and patient is a threat to self or others	Increased risk of cerebrovascular accident (stroke) and mortality in persons with dementia
Benzodiazepines	Older adults have increased sensitivity to benzodiazepines and slower metabolism of long-acting agents. In general, all benzodiazepines increase risk of cognitive impairment, delirium, falls, fractures, and motor vehicle accidents in older adults
Nonbenzodiazepine, benzodiazepine receptor sedative-hypnotics (eg, the "Z drugs" such as zolpidem, eszopiclone)	Adverse events similar to those of benzodiazepines in older adults (eg, delirium, falls, fractures); minimal improvement in sleep latency and duration
Male androgens unless indicated for moderate to severe hypogonadism	Potential for cardiac problems and contraindicated in men with prostate cancer
Long-acting sulfonylureas (eg, glyburide, chlorpropamide)	Risk of severe prolonged hypoglycemia
Meperidine	Not an effective oral analgesic in dosages commonly used; can cause neurotoxicity
Non–cyclooxygenase-selective NSAIDs; avoid chronic use unless other alternatives are not effective and patient can take gastroprotective therapy (eg, proton pump inhibitor)	Increases risk of gastrointestinal bleeding and peptic ulcer disease; use of proton pump inhibitor or misoprostol reduces, but does not eliminate, risk
Skeletal muscle relaxants	Poorly tolerated by older adults because of anticholinergic adverse effects; sedation, risk of fracture

[a]For the full list of Beers criteria, see the American Geriatrics Society 2019 Updated AGS Beers Criteria® for Potentially Inappropriate Medication Use in Older Adults. https://onlinelibrary.wiley.com/doi/abs/10.1111/jgs.15767. Accessed March 15, 2020.

Table 14-2. Potentially inappropriate medications in older adults—STOPP criteria (selected examples).[a]

Criterion	Rationale
Loop diuretic for dependent ankle edema only (ie, no clinical signs of heart failure, liver failure, renal failure, or nephrotic syndrome)	Leg elevation and compression stockings usually more appropriate
Use of diltiazem or verapamil with NYHA class III or IV heart failure	May worsen heart failure
Aspirin in combination with anticoagulant in patients with atrial fibrillation	No added benefit from aspirin
Acetylcholinesterase inhibitors with history of persistent bradycardia, heart block, recurrent unexplained syncope, or concurrent treatment with drugs that reduce heart rate	Risk of cardiac conduction failure, syncope, injury
SSRIs with current or recent significant hyponatremia	Risk of exacerbating or precipitating hyponatremia
Drugs likely to cause constipation (eg, antimuscarinic/anticholinergic drugs, oral iron, opioids, verapamil, aluminum antacids) in patients with chronic constipation where nonconstipating alternatives are available	Risk of exacerbation of constipation
Bladder antimuscarinic drugs with dementia or cognitive impairment	Risk of increased confusion, agitation
Use of oral or transdermal strong opioids (eg, morphine or fentanyl) as first-line therapy for mild pain	World Health Organization analgesic ladder not observed
Use of regular opioids without concomitant laxative	Risk of severe constipation

COPD, chronic obstructive pulmonary disease; NYHA, New York Heart Association; SSRI, selective serotonin reuptake inhibitor.

[a]For the full list of STOPP criteria, see the STOPP/START Criteria for Potentially Inappropriate Prescribing in Older People: Version 2. https://psnet.ahrq.gov/issue/stoppstart-criteria-potentially-inappropriate-prescribing-older-people-version-2. Accessed March 15, 2020.

Table 14–3. Medications that should be used in older adults, barring extenuating circumstances—START criteria (selected examples)

- Anticoagulants in the presence of chronic atrial fibrillation[a]
- Antiplatelet therapy with a documented history of coronary, cerebral, or peripheral vascular disease
- Angiotensin-converting enzyme (ACE) inhibitor in heart failure with reduced ejection fraction and/or documented coronary artery disease[a]
- Regular inhaled β_2-agonist or antimuscarinic bronchodilator for mild to moderate asthma or chronic obstructive pulmonary disease
- L-DOPA (levodopa) or dopamine agonist in idiopathic Parkinson disease with functional impairment and resultant disability
- Antidepressant (other than tricyclic antidepressant) in the presence of persistent major depressive symptoms
- Proton pump inhibitor with severe gastroesophageal reflux disease or peptic stricture requiring dilatation
- Bisphosphonates, vitamin D, and calcium in patients taking long-term systemic corticosteroid therapy

[a]For the full list of the START criteria, see the STOPP/START Criteria for Potentially Inappropriate Prescribing in Older People: Version 2. https://psnet.ahrq.gov/issue/stoppstart-criteria-potentially-inappropriate-prescribing-older-people-version-2. Accessed March 15, 2020.

A. Oral Anticoagulants

The benefits of anticoagulation for stroke prevention in atrial fibrillation and for the treatment of venous thromboembolism (VTE) outweigh the risk of hemorrhage for most patients, even for patients older than age 80 years and patients with a history of falls. Yet, anticoagulants are among the most common medications implicated in emergency department visits and hospitalizations for ADRs. Safe use requires close monitoring to help patients avoid drug-drug and drug-diet interactions that can affect bleeding risk, ongoing evaluation of renal function to ensure that doses are still appropriate, and in the case of warfarin, frequent blood tests to ensure that the level of anticoagulation remains in the desired range. The vast number of drug-drug and drug-diet interactions involving warfarin and need for frequent blood checks and dose adjustments pose special challenges, although the medication remains a reasonable choice for many older adults. The direct oral anticoagulants (DOACs) such as apixaban, rivaroxaban, dabigatran, and edoxaban pose fewer challenges in these domains but still confer risk of bleeding and, depending on the specific DOAC, are either contraindicated or require dose adjustment for people with impaired renal function and, in certain cases, additional adjustments based on indication, age, and weight. Although definitive data are lacking, concerns over increased bleeding risk associated with dabigatran and rivaroxaban compared to alternatives have resulted in inclusion of these two drugs in the 2019 version of the American Geriatrics Society Beers criteria as "drugs to use with caution"; specifically, caution is advised for use in the treatment of VTE or atrial fibrillation in adults age 75 years and older (see Chapter 44, "Anticoagulation").

B. Insulin

Older age is associated with increased risk of drug-induced hypoglycemia, and insulin is a common cause of ADRs that lead to emergency department visits in older adults. Although insulin has a useful place in the treatment of diabetes, caution in prescribing is merited. Special attention should be paid to factors that may increase the risk and consequences of severe hypoglycemia. These risk factors include diminished renal function, use of medications that may interact with insulin's effects, and impaired cognitive function (which may interfere both with proper use and with the patient's ability to obtain help if hypoglycemia begins to occur). Long-acting basal insulins (eg, insulin glargine and insulin detemir) are less likely to cause hypoglycemia than neutral protamine Hagedorn (NPH) and regular insulin. Sliding-scale insulin (ie, use of short-acting insulin to "chase" current blood sugar levels, without concurrent use of a long-acting basal insulin) should be avoided, as it increases the risk of hypoglycemia without yielding improved glycemic control. (See also Chapter 51, "Diabetes.")

C. Long-Acting Sulfonylureas

All sulfonylureas have the potential to cause hypoglycemia. In older adults, the risk of adverse events is particularly high with the long-acting sulfonylureas, including glyburide (also known as glibenclamide), glimepiride, and chlorpropamide. If a sulfonylurea is used, a shorter-acting version, such as glipizide, is preferred.

D. Digoxin

Digoxin toxicity is common, often manifesting as neurologic abnormalities (including fatigue, confusion, or changes in color perception) and/or GI disturbances. Toxic effects including arrhythmias are accentuated in the presence of hypokalemia, which commonly occurs in patients who are also receiving loop diuretics. Impaired renal function and drug-drug interactions often result in elevated serum digoxin levels in older adults, although toxicity can occur even at serum digoxin levels within the normal range. Other agents are typically preferred for management of heart failure and atrial fibrillation with rapid ventricular response, although digoxin may be appropriate in select patients. If used, digoxin should be prescribed at doses ≤0.125 mg/day and patients carefully monitored for serum digoxin levels (aiming for the low-normal range), electrolytes (particularly hypokalemia), and clinical signs of toxicity. New or worsening neurologic, GI, or cardiac signs or symptoms in a patient taking digoxin should be considered an ADR until proven otherwise.

E. NSAIDs

NSAID-induced peptic ulcer disease and renal impairment occur more commonly in older adults than in younger adults. In addition, these drugs exacerbate hypertension, promote fluid retention in patients with heart failure, and antagonize the cardioprotective effects of aspirin through competitive inhibition of the cyclooxygenase (COX)-1 enzyme. The American Geriatrics Society Beers criteria and pain guidelines from the American Geriatrics Society discourage regular, chronic use of systemic NSAIDs in older adults. NSAIDs are contraindicated in patients with heart failure or renal dysfunction and in those at high risk of peptic ulcer–induced GI bleeding. Risk of this latter complication increases substantially in patients also taking anticoagulants, SSRIs, or systemic corticosteroids. If NSAIDs are used for longer than brief episodic use, the following considerations are advised: (1) use at the lowest dose and for the shortest duration possible; (2) coadminister proton pump inhibitors or misoprostol for gastroprotection; (3) maximize the time between taking cardioprotective aspirin and taking an NSAID (ie, take aspirin upon awakening, delay taking NSAIDs until at least 2 hours later); and (4) consider follow-up in 2 to 4 weeks after starting an NSAID to evaluate for renal dysfunction, fluid retention, and blood pressure elevation. NSAIDs with a balanced inhibition of COX-1 and COX-2 are preferred in patients who are at risk of cardiovascular disease. Consistent with this, some data suggest that naproxen has one of the most favorable cardiovascular risk profiles. The degree of systemic absorption, and thus potential for toxicity, remains uncertain for topical NSAIDs such as topical diclofenac gel, and likely has substantial person-to-person variability. However, overall, the risk from topical administration is likely lower than from oral administration.

F. Anticholinergics

Drugs that block the action of acetylcholine include first-generation antihistamines, tricyclic and certain other antidepressants, antipsychotics, bladder and GI antispasmodics, muscle relaxants, and certain antiemetics (see examples in Table 14–4). Several lists of anticholinergic medications have been developed, with some differences between lists; see references later in this chapter and the useful websites at the end of this chapter. The cumulative burden of multiple anticholinergic drugs has been associated with an increased risk of falls, functional decline, and impaired cognition in older persons. If a medication with anticholinergic properties is considered necessary, substitution with a less anticholinergic medication in the same therapeutic category should be attempted when possible.

G. Opioids

Opioids can be useful to treat moderate to severe pain in older persons, yet raise important safety concerns, including those seen in younger adults (eg, risk of addiction, respiratory suppression) as well as adverse effects of special relevance to older adults including impaired cognition, delirium, falls, and constipation. Risk of addiction and death from overdose in older adults remains incompletely characterized, although overall risks of these outcomes appear to

Table 14–4. Medications with strong anticholinergic properties (partial list).

Drug Type	Strong Anticholinergic Properties
Antiemetics	Promethazine (Phenergan) Prochlorperazine (Compazine)
Antidepressants	Amitriptyline (Elavil) Desipramine (Norpramin) Doxepin (at doses >6 mg/day) Nortriptyline (Pamelor)
Antihistamines, including antivertigo medications	Chlorpheniramine (Chlor-Trimeton) Dimenhydrinate (Dramamine) Diphenhydramine (Benadryl) Hydroxyzine (Atarax) Meclizine (Antivert) Scopolamine (TransDerm Scop)
Antipsychotics	Clozapine (Clozaril) Olanzapine (Zyprexa)
Gastrointestinal antispasmodics	Dicyclomine (Bentyl)
Muscle relaxants	Cyclobenzaprine (Flexeril) Orphenadrine (Norflex)
Parkinson disease	Benztropine (Cogentin) Trihexyphenidyl (Artane)
Urinary antispasmodics	Oxybutynin (Ditropan) Tolterodine (Detrol)

This is a partial list. Data from the Anticholinergic Cognitive Burden Scale (2012) and 2019 American Geriatrics Society Beers Criteria; see the original scales for a complete list of medications with anticholinergic properties.

be less common than in younger adults. Opioid prescribing can be particularly challenging for older adults, since chronic use of NSAIDs is typically not recommended (see previous section on NSAIDs), thus leaving fewer alternatives. As with younger adults, subacute and chronic pain can often be best controlled with the fewest adverse effects through use of nonpharmacologic therapies or with local therapies for localized pain (see Chapter 63, "Persistent Pain"). If opioids are needed to achieve adequate pain control, for most patients starting at a low dose and avoiding escalation to large doses is prudent, as risk of serious adverse effects increases with higher doses. It is almost always helpful to prescribe concurrent anticonstipation therapy in a patient on opioids, since this adverse effect is so common. Poorly controlled pain despite escalating doses of opioids for conditions such as joint or back pain should often prompt de-escalation of opioid treatment and pursuit of another, more effective and safer modality for pain control, although high doses may be needed for treatment of cancer pain and other selected conditions. Opioids should not be prescribed for a patient taking benzodiazepines, since the combination of these medications can lead to serious adverse effects. Similarly, concurrent use of gabapentinoids (eg, gabapentin or pregabalin) in patients using opioids (or vice versa) is contraindicated due to risk of serious adverse events including sedation and mortality and should be avoided except when these medications are being cross-titrated. Finally, drug-drug interactions need to be kept in mind, as many opioids are substrates for P450 enzymes. For those with substantial renal impairment, morphine should be avoided, and hydromorphone, fentanyl, and methadone may be preferred alternatives.

H. Antipsychotics in Dementia

The use of antipsychotics to treat behavioral and psychological symptoms of dementia is associated with increased likelihood of myocardial infarction, stroke, falls, fractures, VTE, and mortality. As a result, US Food and Drug Administration warnings, practice guidelines, and initiatives from the Centers for Medicare and Medicaid Services have decreased their use. Older antipsychotics also have significant anticholinergic and extrapyramidal side effects. When possible, behavioral and psychological symptoms of dementia should be treated by nonpharmacologic means. When antipsychotics are deemed necessary for refractory symptoms causing severe distress or harm, benefits and risks should be discussed with a patient's family or caregiver, the discussion should be clearly documented, and the antipsychotics should be used for a minimum duration of therapy with attempts to taper and discontinue the medication when possible.

Boustani M, Campbell N, Munger S, Maidment I, Fox C. Impact of anticholinergics on the aging brain: a review and practical application. *Aging Health*. 2008;4(3):311-320

Gray SL, Hart LA, Perera S, Semla TP, Schmader KE, Hanlon JT. Meta-analysis of interventions to reduce adverse drug reactions in older adults. *J Am Geriatr Soc*. 2018;66(2):282-288.

Gurwitz JH. Polypharmacy: a new paradigm for quality drug therapy in the elderly? *Arch Intern Med*. 2004;164(18):1957-1959.

Hilmer SN, Mager DE, Simonsick EM, et al. A drug burden index to define the functional burden of medications in older people. *Arch Intern Med*. 2007;167:781-787.

Kantor ED, Rehm CD, Haas JS, Chan AT, Giovannucci EL. Trends in prescription drug use among adults in the United States From 1999-2012. *JAMA*. 2015;314(17):1818-1831.

Mallet L, Spinewine A, Huang A. The challenge of managing drug interactions in elderly people. *Lancet*. 2007;370(9582):185-191.

Merel SE, Paauw DS. Common drug side effects and drug-drug interactions in elderly adults in primary care. *J Am Geriatr Soc*. 2017;65(7):1578-1585. Erratum in: *J Am Geriatr Soc*. 2017;65(9):2118.

O'Mahony D, O'Sullivan D, Byrne S, O'Connor MN, Ryan C, Gallagher P. STOPP/START criteria for potentially inappropriate prescribing in older people: version 2. *Age Ageing*. 2015;44(2):213-218.

Rudolph JL, Salow MJ, Angelini MC, McGlinchey RE. The anticholinergic risk scale and anticholinergic adverse effects in older persons. *Arch Intern Med*. 2008;168(5):508-513.

The 2019 American Geriatrics Society Beers Criteria® Update Expert Panel. American Geriatrics Society 2019 Updated AGS Beers Criteria® for Potentially Inappropriate Medication Use in Older Adults. *J Am Geriatr Soc*. 2019;67(4):674-694

PRESCRIBING FOR OLDER ADULTS

Explicit drugs-to-avoid criteria, attention to specific high-risk medications, and an understanding of technical elements of prescribing are important. Yet, these discrete skills address only a small proportion of potentially inappropriate prescribing in older adults. Several principles can be extremely useful for guiding optimal prescribing decisions for older adults.

▶ Goals of Care

In younger and physically robust adults, there are typically standardized guidelines about the use of common drugs. These guidelines (both formal and informal) are based not only on the risks and benefits of drug therapy for an average patient, but also on the expectation that most people share similar values about what benefits and potential harms are most important to them. In contrast, older patients may have a different profile of benefits and risks than the "average" adult. Moreover, older adults hold widely varying views about what benefits they want their drugs to achieve and what harms are most important for them to avoid. For example, some older adults place great value on extending longevity and preventing future disease, whereas others are more interested in minimizing current symptoms and place a lower priority on life extension. Careful elicitation of a patient's goals of care—and keeping these goals of care in mind when prescribing—can help target therapy to achieve the goals most important to the patient and minimize the unwanted consequences most concerning to them.

▶ Time to Benefit

Medications used to prevent future health events (eg, fracture, myocardial infarction, or renal failure) typically have a delayed time to benefit, with a meaningful reduction in risk not achieved until 1 to 2, or more, years after the patient starts taking the drug. In contrast, adverse drug effects typically begin soon after a drug is started. Patients with limited life expectancy may thus spend the final period of their lives exposed to the harms of a drug, without living long enough to reap the benefits. (See tools for estimating life expectancy in Chapter 4, "Goals of Care & Consideration of Prognosis.") General estimates of time to benefit include:

- Glycemic control for patients with diabetes—at least 3 years for macrovascular complications (eg, myocardial infarction, stroke) and up to 9 years for microvascular complications (eg, nephropathy, neuropathy)

- Bisphosphonates for osteoporosis—1 year to prevent fracture
- HMG-CoA reductase inhibitors ("statins") for patients with chronic cardiovascular disease—benefits can take 1 to 2 years for composite cardiovascular events and >3 years for stroke.

Attention to Dose

Because older adults are more susceptible to adverse drug effects, it is often helpful to "start low and go slow," meaning to use a low starting dose and to advance the dose slowly. For many drugs, it is useful to start at half the regular adult starting dose. This can often be accomplished by splitting tablets using an inexpensive pill splitter. Some patients with limited manual dexterity have difficulty splitting pills, and most pills with sustained-release delivery mechanisms should not be split.

Careful attention should be placed on renal dysfunction and other characteristics that may result in increased serum levels, and dose escalation should stop at the lowest effective dose. Nevertheless, some older adults require the full dose of a drug, and many older patients are undertreated as a result of clinician reluctance to escalate dose. Thus, continued dose escalation to the maximum dose is usually advisable if lower doses do not yield the desired effect and the patient is tolerating the drug.

Monitoring

At the time a clinician prescribes a medication, she or he makes an educated guess that the probability of benefit exceeds the probability of harm, without definitively knowing which beneficial and harmful outcome(s) will occur. Monitoring for benefit and harm can help determine to what extent a drug is actually helping or harming a patient, and thus plays a key role in individualizing care. Unfortunately, monitoring is often not consistently performed.

Few guidelines are available to guide the frequency of monitoring, either for laboratory values or for signs and symptoms. In the absence of evidence-based recommendations, a general approach can be helpful. Patients often underreport ADRs, and clinicians often misinterpret these symptoms as markers of aging or an underlying disease. Thus, once the decision is made to prescribe a drug, patients should be educated and activated to understand and report medication-related problems (Figure 14–1). Then, at regular intervals, the drug should be monitored for potential adverse effects and effectiveness, for adherence, and to assess whether the drug is still needed. Although ongoing monitoring is important, in many cases, adverse effects and effectiveness become apparent within the first several weeks of use, so particular attention should be paid to monitoring during this time. It is almost always useful to inquire about drug effectiveness, harms, and adherence in the first follow-up visit after a drug is started or changed.

Adherence

Medications are not useful if patients don't take them. See "Adherence" section later in this chapter.

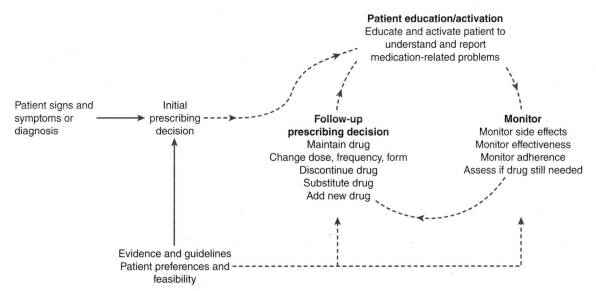

▲ **Figure 14–1.** Approach to monitoring for drug effectiveness, adverse events, and adherence. (Reproduced with permission from Steinman MA, Handler SM, Gurwitz JH, Schiff GD, Covinsky KE. Beyond the prescription: medication monitoring and adverse drug events in older adults, *J Am Geriatr Soc* 2011 Aug;59(8):1513-1520.)

Applying Clinical Trial Evidence and Evidence-Based Guidelines

Clinical trials that have established the efficacy of commonly used therapies have largely been conducted in relatively young and otherwise healthy populations. As a result, many have questioned the applicability of these findings to the care of clinically complex older adults. In addition, many clinical practice guidelines provide limited guidance about how their recommendations apply to adults who are frail or in the upper reaches of life span.

Despite this uncertainty, many therapies are likely beneficial for the majority of older adults. In some cases, older adults may achieve greater benefits from drugs than younger populations, particularly for preventive medications, because older patients typically have a greater risk of developing the outcomes the drug is used to prevent and thus the same relative reduction in risk translates to a greater absolute reduction in risk. Thus, although older adults can be more likely to suffer harms from drug therapy, in many cases, they can have the most to gain. (See also Chapter 24, "Applying Evidence-Based Care to Older Persons.")

Prescribing at the End of Life

Prescribing for patients with limited life expectancy typically requires a rebalancing of the benefits and harms of drug therapy. For many patients near the end of life, prevention of long-term outcomes through drugs used to prevent myocardial infarction, fracture, and other such outcomes is less relevant because of delayed time to benefit. Goals of care may shift to prioritizing quality of life and the minimization of medical interventions, and drugs to alleviate symptoms may continue to be highly valued. Difficulty swallowing can also complicate the delivery of oral therapies.

Several consensus recommendations have been published recommending drugs to be avoided in patients with limited life expectancy (typically <6 months to 1 year) and/or advanced dementia. Although there is no universal consensus, several groups recommend against routinely using bisphosphonates, cholesterol-lowering therapy, and warfarin. In contrast, bothersome symptoms are often underrecognized and undertreated in the patient in the terminal phase of life, and careful attention should be paid to pain control, constipation, and other symptoms. (See also Chapter 22, "Geriatric Palliative Care.")

Boyd CM, Darer J, Boult C, Fried LP, Boult L, Wu AW. Clinical practice guidelines and quality of care for older patients with multiple comorbid diseases: implications for pay for performance. *JAMA*. 2005;294(6):716-724.

Holmes HM, Hayley DC, Alexander GC, Sachs GA. Reconsidering medication appropriateness for patients late in life. *Arch Intern Med*. 2006;166(6):605-609.

Schiff GD, Galanter WL. Promoting more conservative prescribing. *JAMA*. 2009;301(8):865-867.

Steinman MA, Handler SM, Gurwitz JH, Schiff GD, Covinsky KE. Beyond the prescription: medication monitoring and adverse drug events in older adults. *J Am Geriatr Soc*. 2011;59:1513-1520.

ADHERENCE

Medication adherence refers to the extent to which a patient takes medication that is part of a therapeutic plan agreed upon by a health care provider and the patient. Persistence refers to a patient taking a therapy for a necessary duration of time. Nonadherence and nonpersistence are common problems, especially in the treatment of chronic, asymptomatic conditions such as hypertension or hyperlipidemia. Nonadherence is associated with failure to achieve disease control, misdiagnoses, increased emergency department visits and hospitalizations, increased health care costs, and in some cases, higher mortality. Up to half or more of older adults do not take their medications as prescribed, and failure to appreciate this could result in overprescription of additional medication. It is thus important to assess adherence regularly during clinical visits.

Assessing adherence may be a difficult task during a clinical encounter. Patients may be reluctant to admit that they are not taking medications adequately or correctly. Assessing adherence in a nonjudgmental fashion, such as asking how many doses are missed in a week, is a quick way to gauge adherence. Other methods to assess adherence include doing pill counts during a brown bag medication review (see later in this chapter), asking patients to keep a diary (which can be unreliable and most likely will overestimate adherence), and subjective approaches using surveys or questionnaires. Commonly used tools include the Brief Medication Questionnaire, the Medication Adherence Questionnaire, and the Morisky Medication Adherence Scale, although the latter requires a license to use in most settings. These are brief tools that can quantify the degree of adherence and elicit barriers to adherence.

Major risk factors for nonadherence in chronic disease therapy include patients' beliefs that medications are not necessary or are harmful, side effects, cost and copays, and increased number of medications. Cognitive impairment and other reasons for not understanding how to use a drug and/or not remembering to take it are also common contributors to nonadherence, but far from the sole explanation for many older adults. Understanding the reason for nonadherence is essential for designing strategies to improve adherence. For example, if a patient is nonadherent because of high out-of-pocket costs for obtaining the drug, less-expensive drug alternatives or pharmaceutical assistance programs may be useful to consider. If a patient is nonadherent because the patient does not know what the drug is for or believes that the drug is not providing benefit, educating the patient can be helpful. (Alternatively, if a patient taking a drug used to control symptoms believes the drug is not helping, this may be a sign to try another drug.) If a patient has difficulty keeping track of which drugs to use when, a pill organizer can often be helpful, and depending on the situation, family, caregiver, or nurse or pharmacist assistance may be needed to fill the organizer correctly at the beginning of each week. Drugs that require dosing three or four times per day can be difficult to take, and switching patients to a drug regimen that requires only once- or twice-daily dosing has proven to be one of the most successful strategies for improving adherence.

Marcum ZA, Gellad WF. Medication adherence to multidrug regimens. *Clin Geriatr Med.* 2012;28(2):287-300.

Osterberg L, Blaschke T. Adherence to medication. *N Engl J Med.* 2005;353(5):487-497.

MANAGING COMPLEXITY

Optimizing prescribing for older adults is a complex process that requires balancing multiple considerations. Several strategies can be helpful to unpack this complexity and approach these issues in a systematic manner.

▶ Regular Medication Review

Experts recommend that regular medication review occur at least annually. Patients with multiple medication changes may benefit from more frequent reviews.

A. Brown Bag Review

A highly effective technique for medication review is the "brown bag review," in which the patient is instructed to put all of his or her medications (including over-the-counter, herbal, and other products) into a bag and bring it to clinic for inspection. In addition to reconciling the medications taken by a patient, this review provides a valuable opportunity to assess patient understanding and adherence. Multiple bottles of the same medicine, prescriptions whose label indicates that they were dispensed many months (or years) ago, and other clues can help identify potential problems. For each drug, asking "What is this medication for?"; "How do you take this?"; and "How often do you not take it or miss a dose?" (and if yes, inquiring why) can provide valuable clues to improve adherence. Asking the patient "Are you having any problems with this drug?" and probing for common and dangerous adverse effects can help elicit previously underreported adverse drug effects.

B. Critically Reviewing the Medication List

Another important goal of medication review is to provide the clinician an opportunity to think critically and holistically about the medication regimen, rather than the piecemeal

Table 14–5. Questions to consider during a medication review.

1. Is there an indication for the drug?
2. Is the medication effective for the condition?
3. Is the dosage correct?
4. Are the directions correct?
5. Are the directions practical?
6. Are there clinically significant drug-drug interactions?
7. Are there clinically significant drug-disease/condition interactions?
8. Is there unnecessary duplication with other drugs?
9. Is the duration of therapy acceptable?
10. Is this drug the least-expensive alternative compared with others of equal utility?

Adapted with permission from Hanlon JT, Schmader KE, Samsa GP, et al: A Method for Assessing Drug Therapy Appropriateness, *J Clin Epidemiol* 1992 Oct;45(10):1045-1051.

approach that often accompanies a typical visit in which the focus is on one or two specific diseases. This holistic review can include identifying drugs that are no longer needed (ie, overuse), drugs with inadequate or excessive doses or instances where an alternative drug is likely to be safer or more effective (ie, misuse), and omissions of potentially beneficial drugs (ie, underuse). The Medication Appropriateness Index provides a useful list of 10 questions to consider for each drug a patient is taking (Table 14–5).

A helpful strategy for reviewing the medication list is to group medicines by the patient's diseases or syndromes they are used to treat. This way of organizing medication information can highlight potential problems. If the patient is taking a drug with no corresponding disease on the patient's problem list, it may be unnecessary. For example, if a patient is taking a proton pump inhibitor and does not have a diagnosis of gastroesophageal reflux disease or is not a chronic user of NSAIDs, the drug may be unnecessary. If a patient has a disease with no corresponding medication, this may represent underuse. For example, if an older man has bothersome lower urinary tract symptoms that persist despite lifestyle modifications, a trial of an α-blocker may be warranted. If a patient has poorly controlled disease for which the patient is taking multiple medications, this might indicate suboptimal doses, poor adherence, or a complicating factor. For instance, if an older patient has poorly controlled hypertension and is taking four antihypertensive medications, further investigation for nonadherence and potential secondary causes of hypertension may be useful. Finally, careful review of medications can identify other potential problems. For example, if a patient is taking a medication with strong anticholinergic properties, it is worth inquiring about anticholinergic side effects and considering if there is another medicine that can provide the same benefit with less potential for harm.

▶ Interprofessional Care

Careful attention to pharmaceutical care for older adults is time consuming and is best done using a team approach where feasible. Pharmacists can play an essential role, bringing both content expertise and dedicated time to assessing potential medication problems, reconciling medications, and evaluating and improving patient adherence. Multiple models of care are increasingly integrating pharmacists into primary care clinics, providing opportunities to share workload and expertise. Under Medicare Part D (the prescription drug benefit), health plans in the United States are required to offer medication therapy management services to high-risk older adults, including comprehensive medication review conducted in person or by phone at least annually. Eligibility criteria and services provided vary from plan to plan and can typically be found on the plan's website. Community pharmacists can work with prescribers and patients, and consultant pharmacists (expert consultants in geriatric pharmacotherapy) can be engaged to provide comprehensive medication review and reconciliation, monitor medications, improve adherence, identify appropriate Medicare Part D plans and prescription assistance programs to help lower drug costs, and more. In the inpatient setting, hospital pharmacists rounding with teams reduce ADRs, and pharmacists have been widely engaged to support medication reconciliation at admission and discharge.

In addition to pharmacists, other members of the health care team can be engaged to support optimal pharmaceutical care. Nurses can assess adherence, reconcile medications, screen for adverse events, and monitor drug effectiveness (eg, through structured protocols for hypertension management, keeping track of overdue laboratory tests for drug monitoring). Visiting home nurses can also assess how medicines are actually being used in the home environment and provide medication counseling and support (eg, helping to fill and teaching patients how to fill medication organizers, ordering pharmacy refills). Occupational therapists can help troubleshoot problems with opening medication bottles, and speech therapists can clarify questions about the safety of swallowing pills. Informal and paid caregivers can serve as "eyes and ears" for the clinician to identify medication challenges at home and help implement solutions.

Scott IA, Gray LC, Martin JH, Mitchell CA. Minimizing inappropriate medications in older populations: a 10-step conceptual framework. *Am J Med.* 2012;125(6):529-537.

Steinman MA, Hanlon JT. Managing medications in clinically complex elders: "there's got to be a happy medium." *JAMA.* 2010;304:1592-1601.

DEPRESCRIBING

Deprescribing refers to a systematic process of reviewing and withdrawing harmful or unnecessary medications, under the supervision of a health care professional, with a goal of improving patient outcomes. This term has been used both for efforts to comprehensively review a patient's medication list and for efforts that focus on a single class of medications. The focus of this section is on the former, although similar principles are involved in both. Although seemingly simple, effective deprescribing requires specific skills and approaches.

A framework by Scott and colleagues (Figure 14–2) provides useful guidance for how to approach the deprescribing process. First is assessing what medications a person is taking and the reasons for each one (see previous section on brown bag review). Understanding reasons for use is essential as it provides valuable clues about which medicines may no longer be needed, and which medicines may initially seem ill-advised but are in fact serving a valuable purpose. The second step is calibrating the intensity of intervention. This reflects the fact that deprescribing can be time intensive, and the greater the opportunity to benefit, the more time is worthwhile to invest. Patients currently exposed to significant harm from multiple medications may need a more rapid, more intense deprescribing plan. Other factors that often indicate substantial opportunity to benefit include characteristics of the drug regimen, including the presence of polypharmacy and use of high-risk drugs (including Beers criteria medications and drugs with high risk of serious adverse events such as insulins or anticoagulants). Patient characteristics are also important to consider, including advanced age, multimorbidity, cognitive or functional impairment, multiple prescribers, and a history of nonadherence or medication misuse.

The third step is assessing each medication and whether it merits a trial of discontinuation. Several situations are useful to consider (see Figure 14–2).

- A drug that lacks a current indication—the clinician does not know why the patient is taking it and neither does the patient—is a good candidate to consider stopping. This can be difficult to assess when a patient is seen by multiple specialists, but the presumption should not automatically be that the drug is necessary because someone else prescribed it. In such situations, communicating with the relevant specialist(s) to clarify the drug's purpose and necessity is essential.

- Drugs that may be part of a prescribing cascade (see the earlier section "The Prescribing Cascade") or that are causing adverse effects disproportionate to their benefits are also good candidates for a discontinuation trial.

- Drugs whose actual or potential harms outweigh their benefits should be strongly considered for deprescribing.

- Drugs that are intended to control symptoms or markers of disease activity (eg, blood pressure) and that did not achieve their intended effect are natural candidates to consider stopping. The success of symptom control may be assessed by asking the patient, "Did you feel better

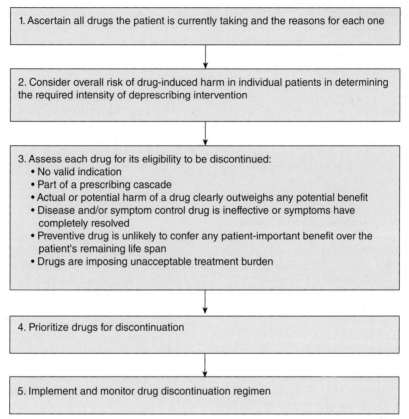

1. Ascertain all drugs the patient is currently taking and the reasons for each one

2. Consider overall risk of drug-induced harm in individual patients in determining the required intensity of deprescribing intervention

3. Assess each drug for its eligibility to be discontinued:
   - No valid indication
   - Part of a prescribing cascade
   - Actual or potential harm of a drug clearly outweighs any potential benefit
   - Disease and/or symptom control drug is ineffective or symptoms have completely resolved
   - Preventive drug is unlikely to confer any patient-important benefit over the patient's remaining life span
   - Drugs are imposing unacceptable treatment burden

4. Prioritize drugs for discontinuation

5. Implement and monitor drug discontinuation regimen

▲ **Figure 14–2.** **The process of deprescribing.** (Data from Scott IA, Hilmer SN, Reeve E, et al. Reducing Inappropriate Polypharmacy: The Process of Deprescribing, *JAMA Intern Med* 2015 May;175(5):827-834.)

after you started taking this drug?" or "Do you feel this is helping your [symptom]?" If the patient is not sure, it is often reasonable to try stopping the medication and monitor closely to see if symptoms worsen. The same principles apply to disease-control medications, such as blood pressure response after initiating an antihypertensive. Conversely, if symptoms or signs of a disease have completely resolved, it may mean the drug is no longer needed.

- Medicines intended to prevent long-term future adverse events (eg, blood pressure medications, antiplatelets, antihyperglycemic medications, medications for osteoporosis) should be evaluated in the context of remaining life expectancy and the balance of benefits and harms (see Chapter 4, "Goals of Care & Consideration of Prognosis").
- Patients should be asked which of their drugs are particularly burdensome (eg, due to high out-of-pocket costs,

frequency of administration, difficulty of use, or requirements for monitoring), and the clinician should explore whether these burdens outweigh the drug's presumed benefits.

The fourth step is prioritizing which drugs to discontinue first. Priority can be determined by considering which drugs have the most adverse balance of harms to benefits, which are easiest to discontinue, and which are not aligned with patient preferences. It often is useful to discontinue one drug at a time, so that if adverse withdrawal reactions occur, they can be ascribed to a specific drug. However, this has to be balanced against the dangers of clinical inertia that can arise from going too slow, the simplicity of discontinuing multiple medications at once that are unlikely to lead to withdrawal reactions, and more urgent situations such as delirium or rapid weight loss where medications are a potential culprit but it is unclear which one to blame.

The final step is implementing and monitoring the deprescribing plan. Several considerations are key for success. First and foremost is engaged patient communication and understanding of patients' preferences, fears, and priorities. Many patients are reluctant to stop dangerous or unnecessary medications out of fear that symptoms will return, cognitive dissonance from being told to stop a medication after years of clinicians telling them they need to take it, and fear that their clinicians are giving up on them. To counter this, clinicians should elicit patient perceptions and concerns, correct misconceptions, and frame deprescribing as a positive step to optimizing the patient's health care (ie, as an improvement, not a "taking away"). Similarly, it can be important to offer alternative pharmacologic or nonpharmacologic strategies for controlling bothersome symptoms. For example, discussion of deprescribing benzodiazepines used for insomnia should focus as much on what can be done to help this troublesome symptom (eg, cognitive-behavioral therapy) as one stops the medicine. Patients' buy-in, shared decision making, and maintaining a therapeutic alliance are essential in deprescribing, and except in unusual cases, patients should not be forced off medications against their will.

Once buy-in has been achieved, patients should be provided with a clear action plan. This can include instructions for tapering, which are required for a number of drugs including many central nervous system–active medications (eg, sedative-hypnotics, antipsychotics, antidepressants), glucocorticoids, proton pump inhibitors (to prevent rebound hyperacidemia), and others. The action plan should also include instructions on what to do if concerns arise or symptoms recur and expectations for how the clinician will follow up to monitor the patient's progress. Other key elements of deprescribing are clear communication with other health care providers and with caregivers and family members and clear documentation. Although the evidence base for how to optimally deprescribe is sparse for many medications, evidence-based guidelines on how to deprescribe medications, such as benzodiazepines, antipsychotics, proton pump inhibitors, and more, have been developed by Canadian and other groups focused on this topic (see www.deprescribing.org and https://www.primaryhealthtas.com.au/resources/deprescribing-guides/).

Reeve E, Farrell B, Thompson W, et al. Deprescribing cholinesterase inhibitors and memantine in dementia: guideline summary. *Med J Aust.* 2019;210(4):174-179.

Scott IA, Hilmer SN, Reeve E, Potter K, et al. Reducing inappropriate polypharmacy: the process of deprescribing. *JAMA Intern Med.* 2015;175(5):827-834.

MEDICARE PART D

Most older adults in the United States receive medications at a reduced cost through the Medicare Part D prescription drug program, a voluntary benefit for people with Medicare. Other common sources of prescription drug insurance for older adults in the United States include employer-sponsored plans and the VA health care system. Drug coverage can be very confusing for both patients and clinicians, and because of this, patients often do not choose plans that best suit their needs and budget. Information on the Medicare website can help patients compare the costs and coverage of Part D plans in their area (https://www.medicare.gov/find-a-plan/questions/home.aspx). State health insurance assistance programs (which can be located at www.shiptacenter.org) provide help from trained counselors free of charge. Clinicians can also help their patients by having a basic familiarity with how Part D coverage works.

For people enrolled in fee-for-service Medicare, Part D is provided through a stand-alone prescription drug plan selected by the patient. The choice of plan can be changed annually. For those enrolled in Medicare Advantage (ie, Medicare Managed Care), Part D services are linked with their Medicare Advantage services as a Medicare Advantage prescription drug plan (MA-PD). All Part D plans have to offer a standard benefit and can provide enhanced benefits. The standard benefit is a set deductible, coinsurance rate, and initial coverage limit beyond which beneficiaries enter a coverage gap (the so-called "donut hole")—all of which change annually and are available at Medicare.gov. At the beginning of each coverage year, patients first pay their deductible and then fixed copayments and/or a proportion of drug costs. Once spending hits a certain threshold, the patient enters the coverage gap, in which beneficiaries bear a greater proportion of their drug costs. With ongoing spending, another limit is reached—the catastrophic threshold—after which the enrollee pays a maximum of 5% of total drug costs. Enrollees with low incomes and low assets are eligible for low-income subsidies, which provide additional help with premiums, deductibles, and copays. Part D plans cover the vast majority of prescription drugs, although each plan may have a formulary or a preferred tier system with financial incentives for beneficiaries to choose one medication over another. Most plans use some form of utilization management, including quantity limits, step therapy requirements, and prior authorizations.

PRESCRIBING ACROSS THE CARE CONTINUUM

Although general principles of prescribing apply to different care settings, certain considerations merit special mention in the hospital and nursing home.

▶ Prescribing in the Hospital

Hospitalized older adults are particularly prone to medication misadventures for a number of reasons. Errors in medication reconciliation and communication between providers commonly occur during transitions, including admission, transfer between hospital units, and discharge. Ensuring that patients continue to receive the right medications as they move between providers and locations is critical. Hospital-based pharmacists have been shown to be helpful in improving outcomes related to medication reconciliation during these transitions and should be involved when possible. Medications started for transient reasons during hospital stays are often mistakenly continued at discharge and may become a permanent fixture on the patient's medication regimen. Careful attention should be paid to discontinuing proton pump inhibitors that may have been started for stress ulcer prophylaxis (itself a questionable indication), analgesic medications for pain that is no longer present, and so forth. Discharge from hospital to skilled nursing or rehabilitation facilities is commonly associated with miscommunication about medications and a frequent source of medication errors, so it is incumbent on the hospital-based health care team to ensure that complete information on medications, including those intended only for short-term use, is communicated to the post-acute care facility.

Clinicians may be tempted to change medication regimens for chronic diseases during hospital stays. In many cases, this temptation should be resisted. Data indicating inadequate chronic disease control measured during a hospital stay (eg, elevated blood pressure or serum glucose) may not be representative of the patient's usual status, and contextual factors, such as contraindications for a drug, may not be known by the inpatient team. Changing multiple medications also increases the risk of adverse drug events. Yet, if important quality gaps are identified, hospital stays can provide an opportune time to rectify these problems if done in consultation with the patient's primary care clinician.

Sedative-hypnotic drugs or anticholinergic agents such as diphenhydramine have been prescribed "as needed" to hospitalized older adults to aid sleep. These drugs increase the risk of falls and delirium and should be avoided if possible. Instead, environmental interventions such as limiting night-time vital signs and reducing noise and light stimulation are preferable.

▶ Prescribing in Nursing Homes

Patients in long-term care often have multiple medical conditions, physical frailty, and/or cognitive impairment and frequently use multiple medications. Prescribing for such patients is complex, and they are at high risk of adverse drug events. In addition, features of the health system require special attention. For example, consultants to patients in nursing homes may not be able to prescribe medications directly but rather need to communicate treatment recommendations to a nursing home provider to order. More broadly, the full range of supportive living environments for older adults

can vary widely in policies and procedures around medication ordering and administration, and understanding local circumstances is essential to providing high-quality care. For example, many assisted living facilities that assist with medication management require that prescriptions be sent to partnered pharmacies and require a separate written order to nursing staff to administer each medication.

Antipsychotic medications are prescribed to roughly one in six nursing home residents in the United States, often to manage behavioral problems of dementia. These drugs confer a substantially increased risk of death in older adults with dementia. Use should be avoided for behavioral management unless nondrug interventions have failed and the patients are threats to themselves or others. Because psychotropic medications have long been prescribed at inappropriately high rates to nursing home patients, federal regulations require that each patient receiving these medicines has ongoing documentation of the reason for treatment, how medication effectiveness and adverse effects will be monitored, and plans for dose reduction or treatment continuation.

Federal regulations also require a pharmacist to conduct monthly medication review of patients in long-term care facilities. Unfortunately, such reviews have at times been found to be deficient and should not be relied on to catch prescribing problems.

USEFUL WEBSITES

American Delirium Society. Anticholinergic cognitive burden scale. https://americandeliriumsociety.org/files/ACB_Handout_Version_03-09-10.pdf. Accessed March 15, 2020.

American Geriatrics Society. AGS Beers Criteria 2019 (explicit criteria to identify potentially inappropriate medication use). https://www.ncbi.nlm.nih.gov/pubmed/30693946 or https://geriatricscareonline.org/ProductAbstract/american-geriatrics-society-updated-beers-criteria-for-potentially-inappropriate-medication-use-in-older-adults/CL001. Accessed March 15, 2020.

American Society of Consultant Pharmacists. Medication management. http://www.ascp.com. Accessed March 15, 2020.

Anticholinergic drug scale. http://www.ncbi.nlm.nih.gov/pubmed/18332297. Accessed March 15, 2020.

DailyMed (information from package inserts). http://dailymed.nlm.nih.gov. Accessed March 15, 2020.

Evidence-based guidelines and other resources for deprescribing. https://deprescribing.org and https://www.primaryhealthtas.com.au/resources/deprescribing-guides/. Accessed March 15, 2020.

GlobalRPh. Calculators including renal function online calculator. http://www.globalrph.com/multiple_crcl.htm. Accessed March 15, 2020.

Health in Aging Foundation. Medications and older adults (patient-facing resources about medication use for older adults). https://www.healthinaging.org/medications-older-adults. Accessed March 15, 2020.

Indiana University Department of Medicine. Cytochrome P450 Drug Interaction Table (drug-drug interactions). http://medicine.iupui.edu/clinpharm/DDIs/. Accessed March 15, 2020.

Medline Plus. Drugs, Supplements, and Herbal Information (drug information for patients). http://www.nlm.nih.gov/medlineplus/druginformation.html. Accessed March 15, 2020.

National Council on Patient Information and Education (NCPIE) and BeMedWise.org. Medication Use Safety Training (MUST) for Seniors. http://www.bemedwise.org/health-education-resources/older-adults. Accessed March 15, 2020.

Proprietary drug–drug interaction programs, including www.epocrates.com (free), and www.lexicomp.com (subscription only) and www.micromedex.com (subscription only). Accessed March 15, 2020.

STOPP and START Criteria (explicit criteria to identify potentially inappropriate medication use [STOPP] and potentially underused medications [START]). https://www.ncbi.nlm.nih.gov/pubmed/25324330. Accessed March 15, 2020.

Addressing Multimorbidity

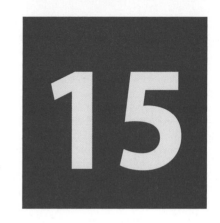

Cynthia M. Boyd, MD, MPH
Christine Seel Ritchie, MD, MSPH

BACKGROUND AND DEFINITIONS

Multimorbidity is often defined as the presence of two or more chronic co-occurring conditions. Although this is the formal definition, most clinicians consider multimorbidity to be particularly vexing when it involves a broad array of conditions and is also accompanied by functional limitations, cognitive impairment, or mental health concerns, as well as interactions between the conditions themselves and their treatments.

Among older adults, multimorbidity is the rule rather than the exception: almost half of those 65 to 69 years old have two or more chronic conditions; this proportion increases to 75% among those age 85 years or older. Thanks to public health interventions, technology, and overall population aging, the proportion of older adults with multimorbidity has grown significantly in the past decade. Among those age 65 years or older, the number of those with two or more conditions (from among nine measured conditions: hypertension, heart disease, diabetes, cancer, stroke, chronic bronchitis, emphysema, current asthma, and kidney disease) grew 22%. Clearly, multimorbidity will play a growing role in routine medical practice.

MULTIMORBIDITY AND HEALTH OUTCOMES

Multimorbidity is associated with a number of negative health outcomes, including accelerated declines in functional status, increased symptom burden, reduced quality of life, and mortality. Increasing numbers of chronic conditions place older adults at higher risk of hospitalization and nursing home placement. Accordingly, increased costs of care follow increased numbers of chronic conditions. In a study of more than one million Medicare beneficiaries, when seven conditions were considered, average per-person cost of care increased from $211 per year with no chronic conditions to $1870 with two or more conditions to $8159 for those with five conditions. Those with seven or more conditions averaged >$23,000 in costs per year. As health care systems become increasingly accountable for care across care settings, development of effective approaches to support older adults with multimorbidity will likely become a growing priority.

CLINICAL CHALLENGES

Clinicians caring for older adults with multimorbidity face a number of challenges in their management. This is true for both specialists and primary care clinicians. First, there is a disturbing lack of evidence for specific treatments among those with multiple chronic conditions as these individuals are commonly excluded from clinical trials. In a study examining a sample of randomized controlled trials (RCTs) published from 1995 to 2010 in the five highest-impact-factor general medical journals, individuals with multimorbidity were excluded in 63% of the 284 RCTs identified. In a separate examination of 11 Cochrane reviews evaluating clinical trials of treatments for four chronic diseases (diabetes mellitus [DM], heart failure, chronic obstructive pulmonary disease [COPD], and stroke), less than half described the prevalence among trial participants of any comorbidity co-occurring with the index condition. In addition to being excluded from many RCTs, multimorbidity is often not accounted for in clinical guidelines. If clinical practice guidelines for a particular condition acknowledge the presence of comorbid conditions, they often do not offer recommendations that take into account these other co-occurring conditions. This is particularly true if the condition is discordant (ie, the condition is pathophysiologically distinct from the condition of interest and therefore does not share treatments), in contrast to treatment-concordant conditions that share treatments, such as DM and hypertension (HTN). For suggestions about how to apply clinical evidence from research to the older patient, see Chapter 24.

Second, older adults with multimorbidity frequently present special management challenges. Their medical and social complexity often leads to complicated treatment regimens that are difficult for patients and/or caregivers to understand and challenging for clinicians to explain. Communication requirements are often intensified as a result of the need to coordinate with other clinicians and interact with patients, their family members, and caregivers. Goal setting and discussion of benefits and burdens of treatment also become more demanding when benefits of one treatment potentially contribute to burdens of another condition. Cognitive impairment amplifies all of these challenges. Time demands leave many clinicians feeling like they cannot go in depth with these patients and contribute to frustration and a sense of incompetence.

Finally, financial compensation for patients with multimorbidity rarely corresponds to the time and effort required to appropriately care for these patients. Even with extended visit codes, the effort required to review long medication lists and medical records, communicate with other clinicians, and interact with family members generally exceeds reimbursement, particularly as many of these tasks fall outside of the in-person visit itself.

GENERAL CONSIDERATIONS

Despite the challenges intrinsic to caring for someone with multimorbidity, provision of higher quality, more gratifying care can occur when a few guiding principles are taken into account. These guiding principles were initially developed by a national expert panel on multimorbidity of the American Geriatrics Society (AGS). The panel performed an extensive review of the literature and synthesized these findings into practical perspectives for clinicians. We discuss three steps that can support clinicians in their care of older adults with multimorbidity: ascertainment of prognosis, elicitation of patient preferences, and assessment and management of treatment complexity.

Because in older adults with multimorbidity, tension exists between benefit from a particular intervention and possible harm from complications or interactions with other conditions, it is very important to ascertain as best as possible the older person's prognosis. Prognosis ideally should be considered not just for survival but also for function and quality of life (see Chapter 4, "Goals of Care & Consideration of Prognosis," for more details). Determination of prognosis can provide the appropriate context for elicitation of preferences for particular treatments. It offers the backdrop for decisions related to (1) disease prevention or treatment (eg, whether or not to start or stop a medication or insert or replace a device); (2) disease screening (eg, whether or not to start, stop, or continue screening for cancer); and (3) use of specific services (eg, whether or not to admit a patient to the hospital or enroll them into hospice).

Elicitation of patient preferences can help guide the management of older adults with multimorbidity. Patient preferences take many forms: preferences regarding the importance of any one condition over another, preferences regarding states of being and how much burden is acceptable in order to achieve a particular state of being (also called an outcome; eg, survival, higher functional status, or better quality of life), and preferences regarding particular treatments in light of potential benefits and burdens associated with that treatment.

Involving patients and their caregivers (who may sometimes be a surrogate, and when appropriate) is particularly important when treatment decisions are preference sensitive. Preference-sensitive decisions are those that relate to (1) therapies that might help one condition but lead to worse outcomes in another (eg, anti-inflammatory agents that might reduce pain but increase the risk for gastrointestinal bleeding); (2) therapies that may be beneficial over the long term but are at risk for causing short-term harm (eg, anticoagulants for stroke prevention but that increase risk of bleeding); or (3) therapies that may include multiple medications with potential harmful interactions (eg, medications for heart failure and COPD). Table 15–1 offers some language for elicitation of preferences.

It is also important that patients and their caregivers understand as well as is possible the potential benefits and harms of a particular treatment. Unfortunately, the evidence

Table 15–1. Language for eliciting patient preferences.[a]

Question Purpose	Question
To understand patient's view of their quality of life	How would you consider your current quality of life?
To understand patient's view of their future	What sort of things have you been thinking about, especially as you think about the future?
To learn patient's values	What kinds of things are important to you now? (*Or if surrogate [meaning a person acting in lieu of a patient who does not have capacity]:* If your loved one were able to tell us what she or he is thinking, what things would she or he think are important now?)
To learn patient's preferences	Some people want to live as long as possible no matter the risks, including being willing to accept hospitalizations and less independence. Other people are less willing to compromise their quality of life or independence and would defer treatment knowing this may limit their survival. Do you have an idea of what kind of person you might be? (*Or alternatively:* Would you share your preferences?)

[a]Older adults may wish to involve family or friends (who may or may not be a caregiver or surrogate) in decisions even when they retain capacity.

Table 15–2. Strategies to communicate risks and benefits of treatments or diagnostic tests.

Do	Don't
Use numerical likelihoods	Use words like "rarely" and "frequently"
Provide the likelihood of an event both occurring and not occurring	Provide the likelihood in only one direction either in favor of benefit or harm
Provide absolute risks	Provide relative risks
Offer visual aids and assess understanding	Assume the patient understands

base for risks and benefits for many treatments is not evaluated in the context of multimorbidity and must be extrapolated from single-condition studies and observational studies. Regardless, it is incumbent on clinicians to communicate what is known in language that makes sense to patients. Table 15–2 provides some general suggestions for ways to communicate benefits and harms.

Treatment complexity is common in patients with multimorbidity. The Medication Regimen Complexity Index (MRCI) captures some of the elements of complexity by capturing (1) the steps in the task, (2) the number of choices, (3) the duration of execution, (4) the process of administration, and (5) the patterns of intervening and potentially distracting tasks. It highlights the multiple dimensions of treatment patients have to contend with when managing their conditions. For clinicians who strictly follow individual clinical practice guidelines, regimens for patients can be both complex and also onerous and costly. Boyd and colleagues described the implications of following individual practice guidelines for an older woman with the following conditions of *moderate severity*: COPD, HTN, DM, osteoporosis, and osteoarthritis. If clinical practice guidelines were followed, the patient would be taking 19 doses per day at four different time points. In 2010, assuming no prescription drug coverage, this regimen would have cost US$407 per month and US$4877 per year. Complex treatment regimens increase the risk for nonadherence, adverse reactions, reduced quality of life, financial burden, and caregiver stress.

Given the problems associated with complex treatment regimens, it is worthwhile to consider ways to reduce or mitigate treatment burden or complexity. A number of tools have been developed that can assist the provider in both identifying complex medication regimens that pose potential difficulties for patient self-management along with strategies to reduce treatment complexity and optimize outcomes. Table 15–3 lists tools that can be used to assess treatment complexity and ability to manage it. Table 15–4 identifies a few approaches that can be used by a patient's clinical team to address candidate medications to discontinue to decrease treatment complexity.

Table 15–3. Tools to identify medication regimen complexity and challenges with medication management.

Tool	Description
Medication Management Ability Assessment	Role-play task that simulates a prescribed medication regimen, similar in complexity to one to which an older person is likely to be exposed
Drug Regimen Unassisted Grading Scale	Drugs: (1) *identification:* showing the appropriate medications, (2) *access:* opening the appropriate containers, (3) *dosage:* dispensing the correct number per dose, and (4) *timing:* demonstrating the appropriate timing of dose
Hopkins Medication Schedule	Role play that includes the following: "Read the medication instructions below. Assume that you eat breakfast, lunch, and dinner at the following listed times. Please indicate at what times you should take each medication and how many you need to take. Also, indicate when you should drink water and eat any snacks."
Medication Management Instrument for Deficiencies in the Elderly	20-item assessment that covers three domains relevant to medication adherence (knowledge of medications, how to take medications, and procurement) and yields a total score of 13 or less

Table 15–4. Strategies to reduce treatment complexity and burden.

Tool	Description
Screening Tool to Alert to Right Treatment and Screening Tool of Older Persons' Potentially Inappropriate Prescriptions (START/STOPP)	Algorithm of medications that should be considered in certain conditions and medications that may be inappropriate to use in certain conditions
Good-Palliative Geriatric Practice (GP-GP) algorithm	Series of questions that can provide guidance of the ongoing utility or value of continuing a medication based on the patient's prognosis or the underlying evidence base

SPECIFIC OPPORTUNITIES

▶ Deprescribing

Deprescribing, the process of withdrawal of an inappropriate medication, supervised by a health care professional with the goal of managing polypharmacy and improving outcomes, is an essential component of safe and effective health care for older adults. Even with the most intensive efforts, it is difficult to prevent older adults from being started on medications that are likely to cause more harm than benefit. In addition, medications that were once helpful for older adults may no longer be advisable to continue, either because the person has developed adverse effects or because their clinical conditions, overall health, and/or goals of care may have changed since the medication was first prescribed. One framework by Scott and colleagues for approaching deprescribing describes five steps (see Chapter 14): "(1) ascertain all drugs the patient is currently taking and the reasons for each one; (2) consider overall risk of drug-induced harm in individual patients in determining the required intensity of deprescribing intervention; (3) assess each drug in regard to its current or future benefit potential compared with current or future harm or burden potential; (4) prioritize drugs for discontinuation that have the lowest benefit-harm ratio and lowest likelihood of adverse withdrawal reactions or disease rebound syndromes; and (5) implement a discontinuation regimen and monitor patients closely for improvement in outcomes or onset of adverse effects." Deprescribing may be particularly helpful in the setting of multimorbidity to improve adherence and safety and to decrease complexity of medication regimens.

▶ Patient Priorities Care

The Patient Priorities Care approach interprets treatment options through the lens of what matters most to each patient. Free online training is available through the American College of Physicians. This approach is further informed by a recent translation of the AGS Guiding Principles for the Care of Older Adults with Multimorbidity into a framework of Actions and accompanying Action Steps for decision making for clinicians who provide both primary and specialty care to older people with multimorbidity, or multiple chronic conditions. A work group of geriatricians, cardiologists, and generalists (1) described the core Actions and the Action Steps needed to carry out the Actions; (2) provided decisional tips and communication scripts for implementing the Actions and Action Steps, using common situations; (3) performed a scoping review to identify evidence-based, validated tools for carrying out the Actions and Action Steps; and (4) identified potential barriers to, and mitigating factors for, implementing the Actions. The recommended Actions included: (1) identifying and engaging in communication regarding patients' health priorities and health trajectory; (2) stopping, starting, or continuing treatment based on health priorities, potential benefit versus harm and burden, and health trajectory; and (3) aligning decisions and care among patients, caregivers, and other clinicians with patients' health priorities and health trajectory (Figure 15–1).

SUMMARY

Addressing multimorbidity in clinical practice is essential to good-quality care. Cumulatively adding treatments and interventions for individual conditions in persons with multimorbidity may be harmful for patients by increasing the

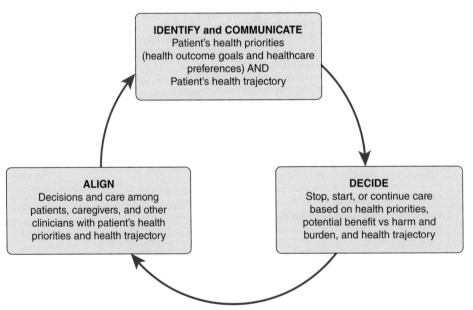

▲ **Figure 15–1.** Patient priorities–aligned decision making for older adults with multiple chronic conditions. (Reproduced with permission from Boyd C, Smith CD, Masoudi FA, et al: Decision Making for Older Adults With Multiple Chronic Conditions: Executive Summary for the American Geriatrics Society Guiding Principles on the Care of Older Adults With Multimorbidity, *J Am Geriatr Soc* 2019 Apr;67(4):665-673.)

risk for interactions between treatments and between treatments and other conditions, as well as by affecting adherence and quality of life. Thus, an individualized approach to care is necessary to make the complex decisions about which treatments and interventions are most likely to help an individual patient and is based on the elicitation of patient preferences, assessment of prognosis for all outcomes, and minimization of treatment complexity and burden.

American Geriatrics Society. 2019 Updated AGS Beers Criteria® for Potentially Inappropriate Medication Use in Older Adults. *J Am Geriatr Soc.* 2019;67(4):674-694.

American Geriatrics Society Expert Panel on the Care of Older Adults with Multimorbidity. Guiding principles for the care of older adults with multimorbidity: an approach for clinicians. *J Am Geriatr Soc.* 2012;60(10):E1-E25.

Boult C, Wieland GD. Comprehensive primary care for older patients with multiple chronic conditions: "nobody rushes you through." *JAMA.* 2010;304(17):1936-1943.

Boyd CM, Darer J, Boult C, et al. Clinical practice guidelines and quality of care for older patients with multiple comorbid diseases: implications for pay for performance. *JAMA.* 2005;294(6):716-724.

Boyd C, Smith CD, Masoudi FA, et al. Decision making for older adults with multiple chronic conditions: executive summary for the American Geriatrics Society Guiding Principles on the Care of Older Adults With Multimorbidity. *J Am Geriatr Soc.* 2019;67(4):665-673.

Jadad AR, To MJ, Emara M, Jones J. Consideration of multiple chronic diseases in randomized controlled trials. *JAMA.* 2011; 306(24):2670-2672.

O'Mahony D, O'Sullivan D, Byrne S, O'Connor MN, Ryan C, Gallagher P. STOPP/START criteria for potentially inappropriate prescribing in older people: version 2. *Age Ageing.* 2015;44(2):213-218.

Orwig D, Brandt N, Gruber-Baldini AL Medication management assessment for older adults in the community. *Gerontologist.* 2006;46(5):661-668.

Reeve E, Gnjidic D, Long J, Hilmer S. A systematic review of the emerging definition of "deprescribing" with network analysis: implications for future research and clinical practice. *Br J Clin Pharmacol.* 2015;80(6):1254-1268.

Scott IA, Hilmer SN, Reeve E, et al. Reducing inappropriate polypharmacy: the process of deprescribing. *JAMA Intern Med.* 2015;175(5):827-834.

Wolff JL, Starfield B, Anderson G. Prevalence, expenditures, and complications of multiple chronic conditions in the elderly. *Arch Intern Med.* 2002;162(20):2269-2276.

USEFUL WEBSITES

American College of Physicians. Patient priorities care: aligning care with what matters to patients. https://ethosce.acponline.org/patient-priorities-care. Accessed March 15, 2020.

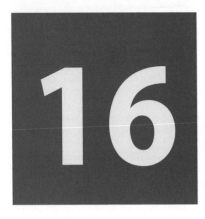

Atypical Presentations of Illness

Michael Goldrich, MD

Amit Shah, MD

▶ General Principles

Traditional education of clinicians hinges on typical presentations of common illnesses. The teaching of these classic presentations influences clinicians' "illness scripts," or preformed outlines on how a patient should present with a particular disease. Yet, what is often left out from medical training is the frequent occurrence of atypical presentations of illness in older adults. These presentations are termed atypical because they lack the usual signs and symptoms characterizing a particular condition or diagnosis. In older adults, so-called "atypical" presentations are actually quite common and can range from one-fifth to one-half of all presentations. For example, a change in behavior or functional ability is often the only sign of a new, potentially serious illness. Failure to recognize atypical presentations may lead to worse outcomes, missed diagnoses, and missed opportunities for treatment of common conditions in older patients. As in other illnesses, some of the reasons for delayed recognition may also be caused by social factors, such as lack of caregiver, lack of transportation, the fear of being hospitalized, and the risk of losing independence.

The lack of specificity of some atypical presentations, however, can also lead to unnecessary workups, treatments, and hospitalizations. For example, always treating the feared possibility of a bacterial infection in the setting of nonspecific symptoms can prompt improper use of antibiotics that can cause harm to the patient and create drug resistance in the long run. Awareness of atypical presentations of common diseases is fundamental to high-quality care of older adults and also offers a unique opportunity to introduce key geriatric principles to trainees at all levels. Furthermore, identifying atypical presentations of common diseases in the older adult is a recommended minimum geriatrics competency for medical students, internal medicine residents, family medicine residents, surgery residents, and geriatric medicine fellows.

DEFINING ATYPICAL PRESENTATIONS

One definition of an atypical presentation of illness in an older person is: *when an older adult presents with a disease state that is missing some of the traditional core features of the illness usually seen in younger patients.* Atypical presentations usually include one of three features: (1) vague presentation of illness, (2) altered presentation of illness, or (3) nonpresentation of illness (ie, underreporting).

IDENTIFYING PATIENTS AT RISK

The prevalence of atypical presentation of illness in older adults increases with age. With the aging of the world's population, atypical presentations of illness will represent an increasingly large proportion of illness presentations. The most common risk factors include:

- Increasing age (especially age 85 years or older)
- Multiple medical conditions ("multimorbidity")
- Multiple medications (or "polypharmacy")
- Cognitive impairment
- Residing in a care institution or functional dependence

Understanding which patients may be more at risk of atypical disease presentation will guide clinicians to more astutely pick up subtle signs of illness. Rather than approaching a patient visit in the traditional way of a system-focused review, the clinician needs to expand beyond the typical evaluation and begin to assess nonspecific but serious symptoms and incorporate questions about changes from baseline that correlate with an atypical presentation (Table 16–1). For example, recognition of an atypical presentation of illness requires a clinician to pay more attention to small changes in cognition compared to baseline. In the case of a patient with dementia, this can be difficult to determine as some older

Table 16–1. Symptoms characteristic of an atypical presentation and potential questions to uncover atypical presentations

Nonspecific Symptoms	Questions to Ask
• Acute confusion (ie, delirium) • Anorexia • Generalized weakness/fatigue/dizziness • Change in mobility • New urinary incontinence • New functional decline • Falls	• Is the patient usually quiet and nonconversant or is this a change? • Have you noticed the patient to be less or more active? • Has there been in any change in what the patient is able to do in their daily routine? • Has there been change in weight? Change in appetite? • Are there any new medications that were started when the symptoms started? • In the past, when the patient has had an infection, what signs has the patient had?

adults with dementia still experience minor daily variations in cognition. Gathering this baseline level of information requires patience, time, and having reliable caregivers and family member informants. Often, in order to arrive at an accurate history of present illness, the clinician will have to undertake a systematic investigative approach, of which one example is detailed later in this chapter.

► Examples of Common Atypical Presentations

The first step to assessing an older person for atypical presentation of disease is to recognize the common warning signs and symptoms frequently present across a wide spectrum of illness in the older adult. In an older adult, a common warning sign of a looming infection or critical illness may be a new decline in function (eg, new incontinence, new difficulty walking). Similarly, a change in behavior (eg, agitation or increased confusion) in either cognitively impaired or intact people may be the only indication to caregivers or family members (who are most in tune with the individual's normal cognition and behavior) that "something is going on." Other indicators of a new, potentially serious illness include, but are not limited to, falls, anorexia, and generalized weakness. One retrospective observational study of emergency department patients showed that more than half of elderly patients presented with an atypical presentation of illness, most of which were falls.

► Atypical Presentations of Common Conditions

Examples of atypical presentations exist across a variety of disease states, including infectious, pulmonary, cardiovascular,

and psychiatric diseases. In the care of an older adult, atypical presentations of illness are often more common than a classic textbook presentation, such that a clinician must maintain a wide differential diagnosis and be prepared to find coexisting new diagnoses before too rapidly arriving at a single explanation for the clinical findings. The principle of "Occam's razor," in which there exists one unifying diagnosis to explain all of the patient's symptoms and findings, is a rarity in geriatric care. "Hickam's dictum" provides the often true counterargument that a patient can have any number of diseases rather than a unified diagnosis. For example, a patient with a new productive cough and kidney failure may have community-acquired pneumonia with acute urinary retention rather than the pneumonia alone causing kidney dysfunction.

Ultimately, atypical presentations occur because of a combination of factors that coexist in older adults, including physiologic changes of aging, loss of physiologic reserve, multiple comorbidities, and geriatric syndromes, which all converge to confound the diagnosis and make the presentation of an illness uncharacteristic. Common examples of typical and atypical presentations of common illnesses are included in Table 16–2, and others are described in more detail in the following sections because of either their overall prevalence or greater risk with missed diagnosis.

A. Dehydration

Dehydration is the most common fluid and electrolyte problem in older adults and is a major risk factor for delirium, which may obscure the underlying diagnosis. This risk for dehydration is a result of normal age-related physiologic changes, which include decreases in total-body water, alterations in thirst perception, and reduced renal function leading to decreased urine-concentrating ability. Older adults will be more prone to dehydration with infection, tube feedings, and medication-related side effects. Additional risk factors for dehydration include delirium and mobility disorders, both of which can lead to decreased fluid intake. As in other atypical presentations, the signs and symptoms of dehydration in the older adult may be vague or even absent. Vital signs may not be revealing; cardiac conduction disturbances or medications such as β-blockers may mask the usual tachycardic response seen in volume depletion. Skin turgor in the older adult is unreliable, and intake–output charts may be inaccurate in the setting of incontinence. Lastly, oral dryness may be misleading given the prevalence of mouth breathing or mouth dryness as a result of medications with anticholinergic properties. Consequently, the clinician must be aware of the vulnerability posed by older adult physiology and the possibility that dehydration may manifest itself only as constipation or slight orthostasis. In most cases, the clinician will need to rely on a combination of symptoms, signs, and possible laboratory abnormalities in order to accurately detect severe dehydration.

Table 16–2. Examples of altered presentations of illness in older adults

Illness	Typical Presentation	Atypical Presentation
Urinary tract infection	Dysuria Increased urinary frequency Urinary urgency	Absence of fever Sepsis without leukocytosis (often bandemia or leukopenia) Urinary retention Abdominal pain
Pneumonia	Cough Fever Shortness of breath	Absence of fever Sepsis without leukocytosis (often bandemia or leukopenia) Abdominal pain if lower lobe (pleurisy)
Acute abdomen	Abdominal pain Rebound/guarding	Absence of symptoms (silent presentation) Constipation Tachypnea and vague respiratory symptoms
Myocardial infarction	Chest pain Nausea Radiating arm/neck pain	Absence of chest pain and radiation Dyspnea Dizziness Fall
Heart failure	Orthopnea Dyspnea on exertion Lower extremity swelling	Abdominal fullness Weight loss
Hyperthyroidism	Anxiety Tachycardia Diarrhea Tremor	"Apathetic thyrotoxicosis" (ie, fatigue and slowing down) Confusion Agitation
Depression	Depressed mood Anhedonia Psychomotor retardation	Somatic complaints: appetite changes, vague gastrointestinal symptoms, constipation, and sleep disturbances Hyperactivity Sadness misinterpreted as normal consequence of aging or medical problems that mask depression
Gout	Monoarticular Acute	Polyarticular Fever Subacute course

B. The Acute Abdomen

Acute abdominal pain in older adults is often underrecognized, with some studies indicating that as many as 40% of older patients are misdiagnosed. Some of the most common causes of abdominal pain in the older adult include cholecystitis, bowel obstruction, diverticular disease, complications of cancer, and medication side effects. In these medical conditions, rather than having localizing signs to specific abdominal quadrants, pain may be more diffuse, mild, or absent altogether. Patients may also lack a fever or even present with hypothermia. They may lack an elevated white blood cell count and have reduced rebound secondary to decreased abdominal wall musculature. For example, in one study of older patients with appendicitis, patients with a ruptured appendix had the classic presentation only 17% of the time (with fever, white blood cell count elevation, and abdominal pain) and 35% of the time completely lacked abdominal pain. In cholecystitis, only 25% of adults actually present

with biliary colic; consequently, a wide differential should be considered when older adults present with vague abdominal complaints. In addition to different and vague symptom presentation, the diagnosis of acute abdomen in the older adult may be difficult as a result of challenges in obtaining an accurate history, and confounding signs and symptoms because of presentation later in the illness course; multiple comorbid conditions; and illness-related complications. Because of delayed presentations and difficult diagnoses, the mortality rate and complications of the acute abdomen are much greater in older adults.

C. Infection

Although a new infection can present in the usual way with fever and leukocytosis in older adults, it is just as common for an older adult to present with vague symptoms, no fever, no elevation in white blood cell count, and no localizing signs. Older adults generally have a lower basal body temperature due to reduced muscle and diminished meal-induced thermogenesis. A temperature cutoff as low as 37.3°C has been associated with underlying infection in older adults. Although leukocytosis is less common in older adults, a left shift is usually observed even in the absence of an elevated white blood cell count and indicative of infection.

Often a change in functional status and mental status is the only sign of underlying infection. However, to complicate the picture, a nonspecific symptom such as fatigue or a change in mental status alone does not necessarily increase the chance of infection being the etiology for the symptom. The urinary tract infection (UTI) is one of the most common clinical dilemmas and best exemplifies this phenomenon. Rather than presenting with dysuria and urinary frequency, both older men and older women may instead present with confusion, incontinence, and anorexia. Frighteningly, half of the patients with bacteremia from a urinary source did not have urinary symptoms at all. However, the rate of asymptomatic bacteriuria is similarly high in older adults. When a patient presents with altered mental status, the positive urinalysis may lead to premature closure and the assumption that UTI is the cause when a more serious condition may be the cause of delirium. Since the presentations of UTI are protean in older adults, the diagnosis of UTI is also often used as a scapegoat for nonspecific symptoms and makes clinical decision making difficult.

Similarly, pneumonia can present with the absence of cough, incomplete radiographic findings, or shortness of breath and often presents with general malaise and confusion. Attending to these subtle cues is important as the consequences of missing atypical infectious presentations could lead to sepsis, prolonged hospitalization, and even death.

D. Cardiovascular Disease

Classic symptoms of substernal chest pain associated with myocardial infarction are hard to miss. But in the older adult, myocardial infarction can present with the complete absence of pain and can even occur in the absence of other associated symptoms such as nausea or dyspnea. Myocardial infarction in older adults can present as new-onset fatigue, dizziness, or even confusion. This can lead to delay in the treatment for acute myocardial infarction. In contrast to younger adults in whom female sex or diabetes is classically associated with an atypical presentation, older patients are most at risk of atypical presentations of acute myocardial infarction when they have multimorbidity, cognitive impairment, and reduced functional status.

Similarly, although heart failure is increasingly prevalent in older age groups, clinicians must be attuned to both the typical and atypical presentations of heart failure. Common symptoms in older patients can include fatigue and loss of appetite rather than dyspnea. In vascular illnesses, such as peripheral artery disease, comorbidities may obscure typical symptoms, such as claudication. For example, preexisting neuropathy can lead to a baseline alteration in pain perception, and a relative lack of physical activity can make it easy for clinicians to miss this common and potentially dangerous diagnosis.

E. Depression

The prevalence of depression among older adults in medical outpatient clinics ranges from 7% to 36% and increases to 40% in those who are hospitalized. Because early treatment of depression may improve quality of life and functional status, the recognition of depression is important. The typical symptoms of depression such as malaise and depressed mood are well-captured in the Patient Health Questionnaire-9. In older adults, more common, atypical symptoms may include anxiety, diminished self-care, irritability, weight loss, new cognitive impairment, and higher rates of somatic symptoms. Depression in older adults is often overlooked or misdiagnosed because some of these symptoms are erroneously labeled as a normal part of aging. Additionally, atypical causes of secondary depression such as apathetic thyrotoxicosis are more common in elderly patients.

▶ An Approach to the Older Adult with Nonspecific Symptoms

We propose a framework to the approach of an older adult presenting with nonspecific symptoms that may indicate atypical illness presentations (Figure 16–1). Nonspecific symptoms present a very difficult management situation. The same nonspecific symptom that can herald a serious illness can also be an atypical presentation of a self-resolving, benign cause. Regardless of the etiology, nonspecific symptoms should *always* prompt a thoughtful differential and assessment from the clinician.

The first step in any clinical management decision is determining acuity. The old adage of determining if a patient is "sick or not sick" is as important in geriatrics as any other field. In the face of physiologic aging and comorbidities, determining severe illness is more difficult, but distinctions in severity of nonspecific symptoms can be made. For example, a patient complaining of feeling "a bit off" is a very different clinical scenario than a patient who is difficult to arouse in the office. Additionally, any signs of vital sign instability, taking into account baseline values and coexisting mediations such as β-blockers, should prompt a swift workup.

In the face of uncertainty, trials of diagnostics and treatment are often warranted. These segmental workups in order of priority require deliberate action and can avoid the expensive "shotgun" approach to evaluation where multiple, expensive diagnostic tests are ordered all at once. For example, treating all older adults with an episode of emesis with a full cardiac and infection workup with electrocardiogram, troponins, urinalysis, and blood cultures may trigger

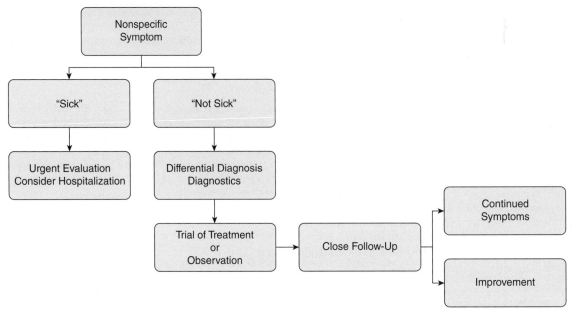

▲ **Figure 16–1.** An example approach to the older adult with an atypical presentation.

an unnecessary stress testing or treatment of asymptomatic bacteriuria or a blood culture contaminant. In the right clinical scenario, treating with hydration and supportive care with careful follow-up to reassess need for further testing may provide the least invasive route to diagnosis and avoid unnecessary treatment.

Equally important to the diagnostic and treatment plan is close follow-up. Patient and caregiver education about next steps and return precautions allows room for diagnostic delay and avoids the possibility of premature closure.

SUMMARY

Recognizing atypical presentations of illness in older adults is an underappreciated but essential component of high-quality geriatric care. Delay in the recognition of acute illness can lead to adverse health outcomes such as prolonged hospitalization, iatrogenesis, and increased risk of death. As the population ages, increasing numbers of adults with geriatric syndromes and multiple medical conditions will present to hospitals and primary care offices with serious illnesses in the absence of typical clinical features. Recognition of common serious illnesses in the setting of atypical presentations in older patients is becoming an increasingly essential skill in clinical diagnosis and treatment. Optimal treatment of older adults with an atypical presentation of disease fundamentally requires knowledge of the manners in which illness

may present atypically in the older adult; recognition of the common signs and symptoms of acute disease presentation in the older adult; and familiarization with the common conditions presenting atypically in older adults. By becoming more familiar with these common, yet underrecognized, presentations, health care clinicians can optimize the care of older adults and more effectively train future health care clinicians to do the same.

Brening A, Negers A, Mora L, et al. Determinants of clinical presentation on outcomes in older patients with myocardial infarction. *Geriatr Gerontol Int.* 2018;18:1591-1596.

Caterino JM, Kline DM, Leininger R, et al. Nonspecific symptoms lack diagnostic accuracy for infection in older patients in the emergency department. *J Am Geriatr Soc.* 2019;67(3):484-492.

Chang CC, Wang SS. Acute abdominal pain in the elderly. *Int J Gerontol.* 2007;1(2):77-82.

Emmett KR. Nonspecific and atypical presentation of disease in the older patient. *Geriatrics.* 1998;53(2):50-52, 58-60.

Hofman MR, van den Hanenberg F, Sierevelt IN, Tulner CR. Elderly patients with an atypical presentation of illness in the emergency department. *Neth J Med.* 2017;75(6):241-246.

Khouzam HR. Depression in the elderly: when to suspect. *Consultant.* 2012;March:225-240.

Leuthauser A, McVane B. abdominal pain in the geriatric patient. *Emerg Med Clin N Am.* 2016;34:363-375.

Lyon C, Park D. Diagnosis of acute abdominal pain in older patients. *Am Fam Physician.* 2006;74(9):1537-1544.

Oudejans I, Mosterd A, Bloemen JA, et al. Clinical evaluation of geriatric outpatients with suspected heart failure: value of symptoms, signs and additional tests. *Eur J Heart Fail.* 2011;13(5):518-527.

Ouellet GM, Geda M, Murphy TE, et al. Pre-hospital delay in older adults with acute myocardial infarction: the SILVER-AMI study. *J Am Geriatr Soc.* 2017;65(11):2391-2396.

Tseng Y, Hwang L, Chang W. Delayed diagnosis in an elderly patient with atypical presentation of peripheral artery occlusion disease. *Int J Gerontol.* 2011;5:59-61.

van Duin D. Diagnostic challenges and opportunities in older adults with infectious diseases. *Clin Infect Dis.* 2012;54(7):973-978.

Waterer GW, Kessler LA, Wunderink RG. Delayed administration of antibiotics and atypical presentation in community-acquired pneumonia. *Chest.* 2006;130(1):11-15.

Weinberg AD, Minaker KL. Dehydration. Evaluation and management in older adults. Council on Scientific Affairs, American Medical Association. *JAMA.* 1995;274(19):1552-1556.

Woodford HJ, Graham C, Meda M, Miciuleviciene J. Bacteremic urinary tract infection in hospitalized older patients-are any currently available diagnostic criteria sensitive enough? Letter to the editor. *J Am Geriatr Soc.* 2011;59(3):567-568.

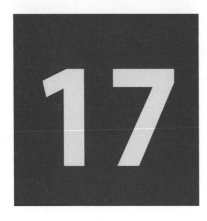

17

Caregiving & Caregiving Support

Dawn Butler, JD, MSW
Todd C. James, MD

Caregiving is receiving increased attention as the world experiences demographic shifts that favor older adults. For many seniors, caregivers are vital to maintaining independence. Assessing and supporting caregivers is becoming essential for efforts to improve the quality of health care and patient experiences.

Unfortunately, important and vital contributions of caregivers often go unrecognized and unsupported by health care teams and providers. Indeed, health care systems often do not have mechanisms for recognizing, addressing, and supporting caregiver needs. These gaps are most apparent in the situations that require intensive support over extended periods of time, such as for patients with dementia, heart failure, frailty, and chronic conditions.

This chapter describes the sometimes surprising demographics about caregivers and the unexpected roles that they undertake. We provide an update on methods for assessing them and explore some of the supports available in health systems and communities. We suggest activities that will be useful in clinical environments and review the topic of patient privacy and the Health Insurance Portability and Accountability Act (HIPAA).

First, it is important to consider terminology. When we think of caregiving, we often delineate between formal caregivers (ie, those who are usually trained and compensated for care, such as certified nurse assistants, physiotherapists, nurses, social workers) and informal caregivers (ie, those who are usually unpaid and untrained, such as family members, friends, or neighbors). This chapter is focused on informal caregivers.

▶ Importance of Caregivers

Caregivers assist with a vast array of tasks, including medication management, health system coordination, complex medical tasks such as wound care, and more. They often feel invisible and are frequently a shadow workforce, operating outside of usual professional practice and regulatory frameworks. Indeed, they frequently report inadequate support, strain, and low confidence in managing tasks. Caregivers have been shown to face risks to their health and well-being, such as increased rates of emotional distress, financial strain, depression, anxiety, and social isolation. It is hard work. Nonetheless, caregivers are partners in high-value care and are often involved in crucial decisions such as when to seek emergency care.

Caregivers are increasingly important to health systems. As health systems prioritize value-based reimbursements, quality reporting, and a focus on what matters to patients, the engagement of caregivers will be vital. In the United States, the new Quality Payment programs of Medicare will measure quality in ways for which continuity of care will be important (eg, posthospitalization visits). Continuity of care may be directly related to the coordination of care that caregivers provide, such as transportation to a posthospitalization appointment.

Despite high burdens, research has shown that 80% of caregivers report positive experiences and exhibit satisfaction with their efforts. Some sources of fulfillment come from providing regular care, supporting the wishes of the recipient, giving back to someone who cared for them, and continuing a family tradition. In reality, a majority of caregivers will have mixed experiences. Thus, it is often appropriate to help identify approaches to minimize strains of caregiving and to maximize gains.

▶ Invisibility of Caregivers

Health care teams frequently encounter caregivers. However, historical conceptions of medical care have stressed the patient as the sole focus of attention. In a narrow understanding of the clinical relationship between the medical provider and the patient, caregivers are considered by some as bystanders.

Patients, especially vulnerable seniors with chronic medical conditions, are often embedded in family and community networks and are not entirely autonomous. In daily life, most are enmeshed in partnerships and relationships, such as in marriage, family, communities of faith, clubs and social organizations, among others. Current institutional frameworks and practices often do not reflect an understanding of who caregivers are, what they do, or how they help. Primary care medical home models have stressed the importance of a focus on both patients and their families, but the medical record often has limited options for recording names, activities, and contact information for various caregivers, and many systems have no mechanisms for including caregivers on the health care team.

Improving the effectiveness of medical-caregiver interactions can improve patient care, improve quality, decrease suffering, and lower costs. Caregivers and patients can be viewed as dyads working together through the medical, physical, and emotional aspects of the patient's health condition. As burdens of clinical complexity and chronic disease care increase, the importance of engaging caregivers as members of the team increases in importance as well. This engagement will include assessment of a caregiver's readiness, preparedness, knowledge, and skills to take on and to carry on caregiving roles and to meet their own needs.

DEMOGRAPHICS OF CAREGIVING

With over 44 million Americans as caregivers and 34 million caring for someone over the age of 50, caregiving is a role that many will experience. According to recent comprehensive surveys in the United States, caregivers are about 60% women and 40% men. One-half are employed at jobs outside of their caregiving role. About 22% of caregivers felt their health had declined; only about 33% had ever been asked by a health care professional about what was needed for them to succeed.

Most caregivers spend about 24 hours per week providing care, and 23% provide 41 or more hours per week. For activities of daily living (ADLs), 59% of caregivers helped with at least one task; frequently, the task was getting in or out of beds and chairs and getting dressed. For independent activities of daily living (IADLs), 99% of caregivers helped with at least one task, for instance, shopping or managing medications. Fully 57% of caregivers are doing medical or nursing tasks, often with little training.

Most caregivers are married or living with a partner. The average age of caregivers of older adults is 63, with one in seven over the age of 75. Most individuals serve in this capacity for 4 years, with 30% serving <1 year. Changing family structures have led to predictions of an impending dearth of caregivers. People are marrying less, and 20% of adults >25 years old have never married, compared to 9% in 1960. Almost 20% of women are childless today, compared to 10% in 1970. Overall, the number of vulnerable seniors without a surviving child is expected to increase to >20%. In addition,

Table 17–1. Risk factors for caregiver burden.

1. Long hours caring for someone with dementia
2. Lack of choice about caregiving role
3. Caregiver poor health
4. Caregiver lack of social support
5. Physical home environment making care tasks difficult
6. Low socioeconomic status
7. High levels of perceived suffering of care recipient
8. Living with the care recipient
9. Depression in the caregiver
10. Poor coping strategies
11. Perceived patient distress
12. Social isolation
13. Financial stress
14. Long duration of caregiver hours

Data from National Academies of Sciences, Engineering, and Medicine. *Families Caring for an Aging America.* Washington, DC: The National Academies Press; 2016.

the divorce rate of those over age of 50 has been increasing, and this may further diminish the pool of available caregivers.

Eighty-five percent of the care recipients are a parent, relative, or loved one, with parents being the most common care recipients. Most caregivers live close to the care recipient, with distance being closest as the caregiver age increases. Alternatively, about 15% of caregivers provide care long distance, with 7% being >450 miles away from the care recipient. Long distances can increase the challenges of coordinating and managing care. See Table 17–1 for risk factors for caregiver burden.

When working with caregivers, we must recognize that they often do not identify as a "caregiver." When asked, they will frequently share their relationship status to the care recipient such as wife, partner, son, granddaughter, or friend. Yet, as a practical matter, the relationship may bear little relation to the tasks. Clinicians add value when they both inquire about and identify the functional roles of caregivers. This clarifies communication, identifies the teaching needed, and increases the likelihood of successful care plans. The following section describes caregiver roles in depth.

CAREGIVER ROLES

When someone becomes a caregiver, this new identity is in addition to continuing to fulfill other life roles and responsibilities in the context of their personal and work lives. Becoming a caregiver can be either a gradual process with care needs slowly increasing over time or a sudden new role due to unexpected illness, diagnosis, or accident.

Factors such as one's abilities, strengths, and available resources impact the roles that caregivers assume. Responsibilities are often shared by more than one person, leading to a network of support accessed by the older adult. Additionally, when one assumes the role of the caregiver, relationships between the caregiver and the older adult change, which can cause emotional and psychological stress to both parties.

In the following sections, we describe five primary caregiver roles. Within each domain, there are many tasks routinely undertaken, often without training and support from the health care teams.

Assistance with Household and Self-Care Tasks

Assistance with household and self-care tasks includes the realm of ADLs and IADLs. The majority of time is spent on activities including bathing, dressing, grooming, and toileting. Providing ADL assistance can be stressful for both the caregiver and care recipient, with many reporting having difficulty providing personal care. Another common task is serving as an attendant to provide support or be close by in case of an emergency. Caregivers often assume the role of helping to manage the household, including cooking, cleaning, shopping, and errand running. Providing transportation can be important for access to medical appointments or social gatherings. On average, caregivers are handling four out of seven household tasks. Although support through formal services and community agencies is available, many caregivers are not accessing these resources. Health care teams should help identify community resources where available. Both the caregiver and older adult should be asked if they are comfortable with the tasks the caregiver is being asked to complete.

Assistance with Medical or Nursing Tasks

Recent surveys have revealed the increasingly complex medical and nursing tasks that caregivers undertake, frequently serving as another member of the health care provider team (see Table 17–2 for examples of medical and nursing tasks assigned to caregivers). Caregivers report feeling pressured to perform these complex tasks, including self-imposed pressure due to lack of other resources. They report concern over making mistakes or causing harm to their loved ones. As a result, health care teams need to provide education and support on the medical and nursing tasks being asked

Table 17–2. Examples of medical and nursing tasks assigned to caregivers.

Managing and administering medications	Flushing intravenous lines
Conducting wound dressing changes	Operating medical equipment such as hydraulic lifts, hospital beds, braces
Overseeing home dialysis	Managing telehealth equipment

of caregivers. Caregivers should be provided with an opportunity to demonstrate knowledge of the requested task and have resources available to answer questions.

Emotional or Social Supports

In addition to the physical tasks that caregivers undertake, they are often called upon to provide companionship and help facilitate leisure activities for the older adult. The burden of physical and emotional demands can lead to depression, anxiety, irritability, and anger. Health care teams can help caregivers by ensuring they have an outlet for having their own emotional and social needs met. This can be achieved through referrals to support groups, providing education on the need for self-care, and encouraging respite time away.

Care Coordination and Advocacy

Care coordination involves arranging, scheduling, and managing services, appointments, and supplies. Many of these responsibilities fall on caregivers. Even in the most well-intentioned health systems, fragmented service delivery and communication lapses can leave the caregiver having to navigate and coordinate multiple systems and providers. Caregivers often provide valuable background information and advocacy not only with health care teams, but also with service providers, insurance companies, and legal services. In surveys of caregivers, about 50% report conducting advocacy work on behalf of the care recipient. Caregivers are often doing their own research on illnesses, treatment, and available services. Bureaucratic language, insurance options, institutional arrangements, and disjointed care programs may result in complex trade-offs rather than simple answers. As a result, caregivers often serve as health care interpreters helping to communicate the older adult's needs and wishes and translating medical terminology for the patient.

Surrogacy

Probably the most recognizable role for family caregivers is the role of a surrogate. Health care teams often are more aware of the surrogate caregivers than the other members of the informal care team. Surrogates have a tremendous amount of decision-making responsibility that may include health care and financial decisions and location and type of living arrangements.

To help with this surrogate role, health care teams are encouraged to help facilitate discussions early between the older adult and their surrogates on care preferences and health goals (see Chapter 4, "Goals of Care & Consideration of Prognosis"). This will help ensure decisions made later by the surrogate are consistent with the wishes and preferences of the older adult.

Caregivers are in the unique position to help older adults understand and work through the identification of health priorities as part of guided facilitation such as the Patient Priorities Care Project. Patient values and preferences are the pathways for guiding care toward realistic health and life goals, which is the essence of person-centered care for older adults with complex care needs.

ASSESSMENT OF CAREGIVERS

Caregivers are frequently among the patient's most consistent supports across care settings and in the home. Welcoming caregivers as members of the care team is a best practice in all settings, including outpatient care, specialty clinics, hospitals, social service agencies, managed care health insurance plans, and sites of long-term services and supports (LTSS). Culturally sensitive assessment of caregivers must cover multiple domains and address language barriers and health care disparities, as appropriate.

An assessment plan can improve efficiency as well as gauge the willingness, stresses, confidence, abilities, and supports needed by caregivers. The assessment can also be therapeutic, as it helps the caregiver to begin to define their role more formally. The patient remains at the center of care. At the same time, the caregiver's capacities are recognized and considered in the care plan.

Depending on the situation, availability, and structures in individual health systems, assessments may be done by social workers, case managers, nurses, physicians, and others. Effective assessments may work best when they can be recorded and referenced; however, few electronic health records have been designed with this capability, and adaptations are needed.

The Family Caregiver Alliance National Consensus Report (2006), "Caregiver Assessment: Principles, Guidelines and Strategies for Change," advised that a family caregiver assessment should contain seven domains:

1. Context, including relationship, employment, living arrangements, and intensity

2. Caregiver's perception of health and functional status of care recipient, including ADLs/IADLs, psychosocial needs, and cognitive impairments

3. Caregiver values and preferences, including willingness, motivation, and limitations

4. Well-being of the caregiver, including health conditions, symptoms of depression, and quality of life

5. Consequences of caregiving, including perceived challenges, such as social, work, and emotional strains, and perceived benefits, such as satisfaction, meaningfulness, improved relationships, and new skills

6. Skills, abilities, and knowledge to provide care recipient with needed care, such as personal confidence and training for household, medical, and nursing tasks

Table 17–3. Suggested responses for addressing caregiver burden.

1. Acknowledge caregiver efforts
2. Express appreciation
3. Encourage caregiver self-care and respite
4. Direct caregiver toward local, regional, and national resources

7. Potential resources that caregiver could choose to use, such as helping networks, social supports, financial supports, and community services

A tool to capture the degree of stress and strain that caregivers experience is useful, especially one that has a numeric scoring. Such tools include the Short Form Zarit Burden Interview (ZBI-12), the Kingston Caregiver Stress Scale (KCSS), and the Modified Caregiver Strain Index (MCSI). These are available in a number of languages.

Formal assessment tools can reframe understanding and language regarding caregiving tasks. As mentioned earlier, many caregivers may not perceive themselves in this role but may identify by their relationship status such as spouse, daughter, or brother. The work of caregiving should be understood as independent of the relationship. Broadening understanding in this way may increase their awareness of belonging to a larger group with potential resources from health systems and society. Caregiving can be normalized to recognize that caregivers are not alone. See Table 17–3 for suggested responses for addressing caregiver burden.

While providing a structure for evaluation of caregiver stress and burden, current tools do not fully capture the positive and negative impacts of this role. Spiritual needs, financial strain, perception of locus of control, and meaningfulness are largely absent from caregiver assessments.

EXAMPLES OF INSTITUTIONAL SUPPORT FOR CAREGIVERS

Formal education for caregivers has been scarce. A study published in 2019 found that only 7.3% of caregivers of community-dwelling US Medicare beneficiaries received any training. Caregiver training was most likely if the care recipient had been hospitalized in the prior year or if the caregiver received some compensation. Home health agencies can provide excellent education and training to caregivers during an episode of care at home.

The Veterans Administration (VA) has among the most sophisticated supports for caregivers. Their programs provide training, education, and tools. A telephone support line, monthly telephone conferences, online workshops, and peer supports create a community to help caregiving be sustainable for families of veterans. The VA program may offer compensation for caregivers in certain circumstances. The VA system is a model for future improvements in other systems.

Some health systems are expanding evidence-based caregiver support protocols into disease management programs (eg, for dementia and cancer care). Examples of caregiver support programs, especially for dementia, include the New York University Caregiver Intervention (NYUCI), Indiana University's Aging Brain Care Medical Home, the University of California San Francisco Care Ecosystem, Jefferson University's Care of Persons with Dementia and Their Environments (COPE) program, and many others. These programs, as well as other geriatric care management models that include a special focus on caregivers, share similar themes of caregiver support responses. These themes include direct communication with the caregiver; encouragement of self-care and respite services; provision of educational information including connection to support groups; and assistance in the development of caregiving and emergency plans.

As a result of the inclusion and care of the caregivers, multiple programs have shown improved well-being, improved knowledge and skills, and reduced burden. Indeed, bolstering patients and caregivers with the knowledge, skills, and attitudes to empower their activities can lead to overall improvements to align the care delivered with the care that is desired by patients.

PUBLIC MANDATES TO SUPPORT CAREGIVERS

To improve caregiver visibility and effectiveness, the American Association of Retired Persons (AARP) developed model legislation to give new supports to caregivers and those for whom they are caring. This legislation is called the Caregiver Advise, Record, and Enable (CARE) Act. Since 2014, 40 states in the United States have passed CARE Act legislation. In general, the CARE Act asks hospitals to provide patients the opportunity to identify a caregiver in the record, to advise the caregiver about discharge plans, and to offer the caregiver instructions on medical or nursing tasks that may need to be undertaken. Since hospitalization is often a time of acute changes in responsibilities, caregivers benefit from the assessment to address their needs and equip them with the skills they need.

The Recognize, Assist, Include, Support, and Engage (RAISE) Family Caregivers Act of 2018 requires the US Secretary of Health and Human Services to develop, maintain, and update an integrated national strategy to support caregivers. It will take some time for this to be fully implemented.

Caregivers are the primary source of LTSS in America, providing an estimated 80% of LTSS. In many states, Medicaid LTSS are delivered by managed care companies under contract to states. Increasingly, LTSS contract conditions include stipulations regarding supportive caregiver services such as information and education regarding chronic conditions, education and training for direct care skills, respite care, counseling, and assistive technologies. Caregivers, as identified by the plan members, are natural allies for improving coordination and increasing advocacy with LTSS managed care. This may lead to better care for the member.

CAREGIVERS AND PATIENT PRIVACY

Health care providers have an obligation to honor patient privacy, which is codified in HIPAA legislation. HIPAA gives guidance for sharing private health information and has an impact on working with caregivers.

Many patients will have provisions that grant formal access to health care information. These may include advance directives, including powers of attorney, CARE Act designations, HIPAA authorizations, and others. Yet, no set of formal documents is likely to encompass the entire team of caregivers. Given the varied roles that caregivers undertake, especially regarding complex medical or nursing tasks, every health professional will need to develop an approach for appropriately sharing information.

The most important guidance for sharing information is that when patients give explicit permission, sharing is straightforward. This assent might be as simple as a nod of the head. If there is doubt about what is to be shared, ask the patient in private what they would like to have shared. When the patient cannot be present, use professional judgment about what information you believe the patient will want you to share.

Without question, health professionals must continue to address patient autonomy and privacy as the American College of Physicians and others have outlined in ethical guidelines. Yet, frequently HIPPA and other concerns have been used as obstacles to limit communication, perhaps, at times, with the idea that this will limit workload in already stressed health care settings. Yet, impeding or eliminating caregiver engagement and communication for the convenience of the health care system is inappropriate, counterproductive, and unethical. Frequently, caregivers are seeking to convey information and coordinate care. See Table 17–4 for recommended solutions to perceived barriers of working with caregivers.

CAREGIVER RESOURCES

Caregiver resources and supports are widely available, and access often begins with the local social worker or case manager. Several national organizations have created empowering educational and supportive resources, which are generally freely accessible. See Table 17–5 for a list of caregiver resources and useful websites.

In addition to national organizations, caregivers can often find resources within their local communities. The Elder Care Locator can assist with connecting family caregivers with organizations in their city. Additionally, the Area Agency on Aging (AAA) network serves as a portal for home- and community-based services. Through the local AAA, patients

Table 17–4. Recommended solutions to perceived barriers of working with caregivers.

Topic	Perceived Barrier	Recommended Solution	Explanation
Relationship	The caregiver is not the patient or client.	Caregivers are members of the care team.	The success of care plans and interventions for those with chronic conditions and functional impairments depends on the support they are getting from one or more caregivers.
Workflow	Caregiver interactions will be burdensome.	Acknowledging the caregiver is an opportunity to focus attention on the patient.	Caregiver information and insight may rapidly improve the success of clinical care plans.
Authority	HIPAA precludes involvement of third parties such as caregivers.	Patients can give verbal assent or even a nod of agreement.	Patients often readily give verbal permission to share information and usually want optimal outcomes. Whenever in doubt, bring the patient into the conversation.
Caregiver program	Our office/health care system does not offer programs for caregivers.	The office can offer community resources for caregivers.	Multiple regional and national organizations have significant resources for caregivers (eg, Family Caregiver Alliance, Managed Care Organizations, AARP).
Too many caregivers	Families have multiple caregivers, and our office cannot keep providing similar information to multiple individuals.	Assist families to create plans to streamline communication.	Caregivers are usually open to getting education and skills training for coordinating care and interacting with the health care system.
Office visit schedule	More people in the exam room will mean longer visits.	Encourage caregivers and patients to set a visit agenda.	Attempt to engage patients and caregivers to prepare for the visit with an agenda-setting tool, such as one developed by Wolff and colleagues ("Patient–Family Agenda Setting for Primary Care Patients with Cognitive Impairment: The SAME Page Trial").
Caregiver stress assessment	Our clinic has not adopted caregiver assessment tools.	Caregiver assessment tools are readily available online.	Consider starting with the Short Form Zarit Burden Interview (ZBI-12) or Kingston Caregiver Stress Scale (KCSS).

AARP, American Association of Retired Persons; HIPAA, Health Insurance Portability and Accountability Act.

Table 17–5. Useful websites and caregiver resources.

- American Geriatrics Society. Caregiver health: basic facts. HealthinAging.org website. https://www.healthinaging.org/a-z-topic/caregiver-health/basic-facts
- Elder Care Locator is a public service of the US Administration on Aging connecting to services for older adults and their families: https://eldercare.acl.gov/Public/Index.aspx
- Family Caregiver Alliance (FCA). Caregivers count too! A toolkit to help practitioners assess the needs of family caregivers. Family Caregiver Alliance website. https://caregiver.org/caregivers-count-too-toolkit
- Home Alone Alliance has created an educational video series and other resources for caregivers: https://www.aarp.org/ppi/initiatives/home-alone-alliance.html
- National Alliance for Caregiving is a coalition of organizations with extensive resources and links to organizations for research, innovation, and advocacy: https://www.caregiving.org
- Schwartz S, Darlak L. *Selected Caregiver Assessment Measures: A Resource Inventory for Practitioners*. 2nd ed. Family Caregiver Alliance and Benjamin Rose Institute. https://caregiver.org/sites/caregiver.org/files/pdfs/SelCGAssmtMeas_ResInv_FINAL_12.10.12.pdf
- United Hospital Fund has created a resource for patients and providers, which includes educational documents, videos, and links: https://www.nextstepincare.org

All websites accessed March 16, 2020.

Table 17–6. Recommendations for health care teams regarding caregivers.

1. Ask patients who is helping them at home.
2. Record caregivers in the medical record.
3. Include caregivers as members of the health care team.
4. Use a formal assessment tool to gauge caregiver stress and burden.
5. Educate caregivers on specific roles and tasks.
6. Refer to caregiver community services.

and caregivers can receive information on homemaker services, home modification programs, home-delivered meals, transportation, respite services, and more.

SUMMARY

Caregivers play a significant role in the lives of patients, taking responsibility for everything from assisting with bathing to coordinating care across health systems. The roles of caregivers are varied, and although associated with stress, caregivers also frequently report satisfaction in their work.

Assessment of caregivers can be done with numerous tools by varied health professionals, depending on the setting. A growing evidence base of successful caregiver support programs provides a pathway to help caregivers obtain the skills, tools, and supports that enable them to succeed. See Table 17–6 for recommendations for health care teams regarding caregivers.

Since caregiving arrangements may persist for many years, sustainability for family caregivers is crucial. Health care systems are increasingly focused on value, and new public mandates and health systems programs are moving to support and sustain caregivers. Engagement of caregivers, with the patient's permission and with the patient as the center of attention, will lead to better outcomes.

Adelman RD, Tmanova LL, Delgado D, Dion S, Lachs MS. Caregiver burden: a clinical review. *JAMA.* 2014;311(10):1052-1060.

Bell JF, Whitney RL, Young HM. Family caregiving in serious illness in the United States: recommendations to support an invisible workforce. *J Am Geriatr Soc.* 2019;67(S2):S451-S456.

Borson S, Mobley P, Fernstrom K, Bingham P, Sadak T, Britt HR. Measuring caregiver activation to identify coaching and support needs: extending MYLOH to advanced chronic illness. *PLoS One.* 2018;13(10):e0205153.

Feinberg L. Caregiver assessment. *J Social Work Educ.* 2008; 44(Suppl 3):39-41.

Huang L, Smith AK, Wong ML. Who will care for the caregivers? increased needs when caring for frail older adults with cancer. *J Am Geriatr Soc.* 2019;67(5):873-876.

National Academies of Sciences, Engineering, and Medicine. *Families Caring for an Aging America.* Washington, DC: The National Academies Press; 2016. doi:10.17226/23606

National Alliance for Caregiving, AARP Public Policy Institute. Caregiving in the U.S. 2015. https://www.aarp.org/content/dam/aarp/ppi/2015/caregiving-in-the-united-states-2015-report-revised.pdf. Accessed April 8, 2019.

Reinhard SC, Levine C, Samis S. Home alone: family caregivers providing complex chronic care. AARP Public Policy Institute and United Hospital Fund. https://www.aarp.org/content/dam/aarp/research/public_policy_institute/health/home-alone-family-caregivers-providing-complex-chronic-care-rev-AARP-ppi-health.pdf. Accessed April 8, 2019.

The Social Context of Older Adults

18

Evie Kalmar, MD, MS

Helen Chen, MD

Care of older adults occurs within the context of their community and social environment, of which health care generally plays only a small role. Geriatric care is most effectively provided within the framework of an integrated care team who understands the social factors that influence the health and quality of life of older adults and have expertise and knowledge regarding community resources available to assist them and their caregivers. This is particularly important for older adults facing functional decline, cognitive decline, or frailty. This chapter discusses the significance of the social context as it affects the health and care of older adults, focusing on the following areas:

- Loneliness and social isolation
- Food insecurity
- Housing and long-term services and support
- Finances
- Legal issues

LONELINESS AND SOCIAL ISOLATION

▶ Definitions and Epidemiology

Loneliness and social isolation are increasingly recognized to adversely affect health and quality of life. Loneliness is a subjective feeling of isolation with a discrepancy between actual and desired social relationships, whereas social isolation is an objective measure of social relationships and connection. People can be both lonely and socially isolated, but these conditions do not always coexist. Both conditions are prevalent, with the prevalence of loneliness estimated at nearly half of community-dwelling older adults and up to 15% for social isolation. Together and independently, loneliness and social isolation have been shown to have a negative association with function, independence with activities of daily living (ADLs), specific health outcomes such as cardiovascular disease and dementia, and mortality. Social isolation has also been shown

to be associated with increased Medicare spending compared to nonisolated individuals.

▶ Screening and Intervention

As health care providers, screening for loneliness and social isolation can help identify these risk factors and prompt referrals to connect patients with appropriate resources. The 20-item University of California Los Angeles (UCLA) Loneliness Scale, the Revised UCLA Loneliness Scale, the UCLA Loneliness Scale (version 3) (Table 18-1), and the three-item loneliness scale in the Health and Retirement Study Psychosocial and Lifestyle Questionnaire (https://depts.washington.edu/uwcssc/sites/default/files//hw00/d40/uwcssc/sites/default/files/UCLA%20Loneliness%20Scale.pdf) are all validated screening tools. Although we do not yet have evidence for the most effective interventions for loneliness and social isolation, there are many options. Some focus on the individual such as improving social support, increasing opportunities for social interactions, and addressing maladaptive social skills. Communities may have senior centers, adult day programs, or friendly visitors. Other options work to minimize barriers such as screening for impaired hearing and recommending hearing aids if present, or using technology to increase connection and communication opportunities for older adults with limited mobility or community resources. Some older adults may be receptive to the use of simplified video devices or digital assistants to improve communication access with friends or family members (Table 18–2).

FOOD INSECURITY

▶ Definitions and Epidemiology

Even though most older adults do not live in poverty, they may still have difficulty meeting their basic needs. The US Department of Agriculture (USDA) describes four levels of

Table 18–1. UCLA Loneliness Scale (version 3).

Instructions: The following statements describe how people sometimes feel.

For each statement, please indicate how often you feel the way described by writing a number in the space provided.

Here is an example: How often do you feel happy? If you never felt happy, you would respond "never"; if you always feel happy, you would respond "always."

Never	Rarely	Sometimes	Always
1	2	3	4

Question	Answer
*1. How often do you feel that you are "in tune" with the people around you?	
2. How often do you feel that you lack companionship?	
3. How often do you feel that there is no one you can turn to?	
4. How often do you feel alone?	
*5. How often do you feel part of a group of friends?	
*6. How often do you feel that you have a lot in common with the people around you?	
7. How often do you feel that you are no longer close to anyone?	
8. How often do you feel that your interests and ideas are not shared by those around you?	
*9. How often do you feel outgoing and friendly?	
*10. How often do you feel close to people?	
11. How often do you feel left out?	
12. How often do you feel that your relationships with others are not meaningful?	
13. How often do you feel that no one really knows you well?	
14. How often do you feel isolated from others?	
*15. How often do you feel you can find companionship when you want it?	
*16. How often do you feel that there are people who really understand you?	
17. How often do you feel shy?	
18. How often do you feel that people are around you but not with you?	
*19. How often do you feel that there are people you can talk to?	
*20. How often do you feel that there are people you can turn to?	

Scoring: Items that are asterisked should be reversed (ie, 1 = 4, 2 = 3, 3 = 2, 4 = 1), and the scores for each item then summed together. Higher scores indicate greater degrees of loneliness.

Used with permission from Daniel W. Russell, 1996.

food security: (1) high food security—no indication of problem with access to food; (2) marginal food security—anxiety about food supply but minimal impact on diet or food intake; (3) low food security—decreased variety, quality, or desirability of food, with minimal reduction of food intake; and (4) very low food security—significant change in eating patterns and decreased food intake. By these definitions, 13.6% of older adults in the United States were considered marginally food insecure, 7.7% were considered food insecure, and 2.9% were considered to have very low food security in 2016. The risk of being food insecure is higher for Hispanic or African American older adults, those who live alone or in rural areas, and those in households with children, as well as those in southern US states. Population studies demonstrate that older adults who are food insecure are at higher risk for chronic disease, functional impairment, and cognitive impairment.

▶ Screening and Intervention

Given the linkages between adequate nutrition and positive outcomes for chronic conditions such as diabetes and cardiovascular disease, health care professionals who care for older adults should routinely assess for issues related to food access or food preparation (see Chapter 2, "Overview of Geriatric Assessment").

Table 18–2. Selected resources to promote social connection.

Resource	Sample Services Available	Cost/Coverage
Senior centers	Activities, classes, meals	Free or small donation for meals
Adult day health centers	Skilled nursing, physical therapy/ occupational therapy, activities, meals	Medicaid, self-pay, some have sliding scale
Support groups (eg, Alzheimer's Association caregiver support groups)	Peer support	Free
Friendly visitors programs (eg, Little Brothers, Friends of the Elderly)	Volunteer social visits	Free
Friendship line (eg, Institute on Aging Friendship Line)	24/7 phone line	Free
Local meal delivery service (eg, Meals on Wheels)	Delivered meals	Donation-based, "pay what you can afford"
Transportation programs	Subsidized public transportation, van or taxi services	Self-pay, may be locally subsidized

There are federal and local resources that can provide access to food and nutrition to older adults. The Supplemental Nutrition Assessment Program (SNAP) is the largest federal program in the food safety net. It provides cash allowances for food purchases and serves people with low income and assets. The gross monthly income limit in most states in 2019 for a household size of one is $1307, or $1760 for a household size of two. Specific eligibility criteria vary from state to state, and "elderly" (defined as older than age 60 years by the USDA) adults may qualify even if they exceed the income limits based on disability, receive Supplemental Security Income (SSI), or reside in federally subsidized housing for older adults. Yet, even with expanded eligibility, older adults are less likely to participate in SNAP than the general population. According to the USDA, only 9% of SNAP participants were older than age 60 years, and only 42% of eligible older adults participate, compared with 83% of all eligible individuals. Some hypotheses of why older adults have lower participation in SNAP include being unaware of eligibility, logistical challenges related to the application process (eg, requiring in-person applications or applications being written at a high level of literacy), and social stigma.

Other options to address food insecurity in older adults include congregate meal programs such as senior center lunches, home-delivered meals services such as Meals on Wheels, food banks, or medically tailored meal programs (see Table 18–1). Although these programs are generally low cost or operate on a sliding scale, many require some payment.

HOUSING AND LONG-TERM SERVICES AND SUPPORTS

As people get older, many will need help with ADLs and instrumental activities of daily living (IADLs). Support may involve hiring caregivers (either privately paid or through programs

funded publicly, by the Veterans Affairs, or by Medicaid, if eligible), coordinating with community programs for supervision and activities during the day, or exploring alternate and more supportive housing options. These types of options fall under the umbrella of long-term services and supports (LTSS), which encompass a range of services that help people remain at home (Figure 18–1). Although nearly 97% of older adults live in the community, the percentage of people receiving LTSS increases dramatically with age, from about 1% of the population aged 65 to 74 years, to 13% of the population over the age of 85. LTSS are expensive, and the amount covered by insurance varies by service, insurance type, and location. It is estimated that between $200 and $300 billion is spent on LTSS annually in the United States, including out-of-pocket spending by older adults and their caregivers.

▶ Programs That Support Older Adults in the Community

There are many programs that focus on supporting individuals in the community, with the goal of avoiding institutional long-term care for as long as possible. These range from home health services to social adult day programs and adult day health centers (ADHCs) or comprehensive health plans such as Programs for All-Inclusive Care of the Elderly (PACE) (see Chapter 30, "Home-Based Care"). The availability, funding, and services offered by ADHCs and social adult day centers vary across states. Depending on the program and its focus, these services may include meals, socialization, transportation, activities, exercise, nursing/medical care, physical and occupational therapy, and supervision. Many of these programs are designed to allow families to manage older adults with cognitive impairments in a safe environment with social stimulation during the day when caregivers need to work outside the home.

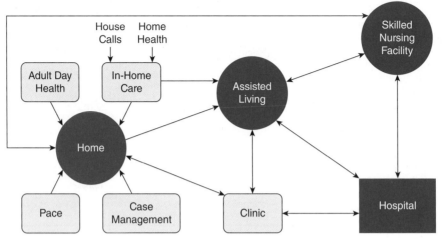

▲ **Figure 18–1.** Overview of sites and components of care of long-term supports and services. PACE, Programs for All-Inclusive Care of the Elderly. (Used with permission from Theresa Allison, MD, PhD.)

▶ Alternate Housing

Alternate housing programs include independent senior living communities (which often require significant financial resources), federally funded supportive senior housing (generally with additional services coordinated by the patient or family), and naturally occurring retirement communities (where people live in their own homes but contribute services or funds to obtain services such as housekeeping or transportation that enable them to remain safely in the community). A related housing model, co-housing, while not specifically targeted toward older adults, is designed to create communities that share resources and decision making, often with the goal of supporting affordability. Over time, progression of physical or cognitive functional impairments may preclude the ability of community-based programs to adequately meet the needs of some older adults.

▶ Assisted Living and Long-Term Care

When older adults are no longer able to live at home with the support available, assisted living or long-term care in a skilled nursing facility (SNF) becomes an option. Please see Chapters 31 and 32 for further discussion. According to the National Center for Assisted Living, >800,000 adults in the United States today reside in assisted living facilities (ALFs). According to the Administration on Aging, 1.5 million older adults (3.1% of this population) lived in an institution in 2016, meaning the vast majority of older adults who live in an institutional setting live in an SNF. *Assisted living* is not a regulated term, and its definition may vary regionally. Assisted-living services may be provided in a variety of venues—from a private home with several bedrooms to large facilities that may appear similar in concept and layout to

nursing homes. However, all ALFs differ from SNFs in that they are not licensed to provide skilled nursing care such as wound care, rehabilitation, or medication titration. ALFs may also have state-mandated regulatory restrictions limiting or prohibiting the admission of medically acute or functionally impaired residents. Long-term care in an SNF may be necessary if someone is deemed too medically complex for assisted living.

Unfortunately, the cost associated with ALFs or institutional long-term care (LTC) is significant and generally not covered by insurance. In 2018, the average national median cost for an ALF was $4000 per month or $48,000 per year, compared to nearly $100,000 per year for LTC in an SNF. Although Medicare covers a limited number of days of SNF care in association with a qualifying hospitalization, the majority of nursing home days are deemed "custodial" and are not covered. Custodial care is defined as unskilled personal care provided for patients who need assistance with ADLs, such as bathing or eating. If long-term custodial care is needed and someone does not have Medicaid, the costs are usually initially paid by individuals and families, and later by Medicaid if financial assets can be "spent down" to meet Medicaid eligibility levels. Although LTC insurance is available for purchase, many older adults may find the premiums cost-prohibitive relative to the potential benefit. Most reputable plans pay a per-diem rate for care provided either in the home or a facility. The per-diem rate may not cover the entire cost of the service but may enable some individuals to remain at home or choose a higher-quality nursing facility. There have also been highly publicized cases of insurers refusing or being slow to pay LTC insurance benefits. Patients or their families seeking to purchase LTC insurance should research the financial health and benefit payment record of insurance providers under consideration.

A physician order or recent evaluation may be needed to obtain certain services. Patients and families may be surprised to learn that Medicare does not cover all desired or needed services and may approach their health care providers for advice. While some health systems have robust social work or care management infrastructure, the primary care provider may be asked to give an opinion about appropriate LTSS services or options for LTC and housing.

FINANCIAL ISSUES

The lack of adequate financial resources is arguably one of the strongest social determinants of ill health. In 2019, in the contiguous United States, the poverty guideline is set at an annual income of $12,490 for a household of one and $16,910 for a household of two. Although adults older than age 65 years are currently the least likely age group to be officially defined as "poor," many may not have sufficient resources to pay for needed food, caregiving, health insurance coverage, medications, and housing. If older adults develop functional impairments, finances often dictate what options they have for care. In 2018, the English Longitudinal Study of Aging documented that household wealth is inversely associated with overall mortality, with the highest mortality seen in the lowest wealth group.

According to the 2017 US Census data, >7 million people aged 65 and older (14.2%) lived in poverty. This statistic has geographic variance and rises above 15% in states such as California and Florida. Older women and minorities are also more likely to live in poverty. However, even older adults who are not "poor" may struggle financially. The Elder Economic Security Index, developed at the Gerontology Institute at the University of Massachusetts Boston, is a tool that can help to assess baseline cost of living by state and county. The estimated cost of living in some metropolitan areas in California is over twice the average Social Security benefit. For example, in San Francisco, the Elder Index in 2018 was $32,568 per year. In 2018, the average monthly Social Security payment was $1413, equivalent to $16,965 yearly. This significant difference between Social Security income and the cost of living increases the likelihood that an older adult whose sole income in retirement is Social Security would have difficulty paying for basic needs.

▶ Insurance and Health-Related Costs

Medicare plays a large role in the finances of older adults. The Social Security Act was signed into law in 1935. The first monthly benefits began to be paid in 1940. Despite this benefit, more than a third of older Americans lived below the poverty line well into the 1960s. It was not until the 1970s, some 10 years after the enactment of Medicare, that this began to significantly improve, suggesting that medical issues and the lack of medical coverage were important factors in the impoverishment of older adults throughout most of the 20th century (see Chapter 79, "Age-Friendly Health Systems") Although there have been several important additions such as hospice services in 1989 and prescription drugs in 2006, Medicare continues to have notable coverage gaps. Beneficiaries are required to pay significant amounts in the form of deductibles and copayments. For lower-income beneficiaries, these out-of-pocket costs may represent a significant proportion of their monthly incomes (Figure 18–2). Some older adults, the "dual eligible," may also qualify for Medicaid, a state and federally funded health insurance program that is limited to those with very low incomes. The coverage provisions and eligibility criteria for Medicaid vary from state to state.

In 2019, even those older adults whose incomes qualify them for Medicaid face copayments for their medications. It is important for prescribers to inquire about drug coverage as some patients may practice "economic nonadherence" and self-ration, dose adjust, or fail to obtain medications because of unaffordable copayments for medications or other financial considerations such as deductibles or insurance premiums (see Chapter 14, "Principles of Prescribing & Adherence").

▶ Maintaining Financial Independence

Older adults are particularly vulnerable to financial exploitation, especially if cognitive impairment is present (see Chapter 19, "Detecting, Assessing, & Responding to Elder Mistreatment"). Health care providers can help patients maintain their financial independence by (1) screening for financial issues by openly discussing finances and related concerns; (2) including financial discussions in advance care planning at the time of diagnosis of cognitive impairment, with a focus on identification of a financial power of attorney; (3) referring to elder law practitioners or Medical-Legal Partnerships for Seniors; and (4) recommending safeguards to help streamline financial affairs such as direct deposits, automatic withdrawal for bill payment, third-party notification for late bill payments, and overdraft protection.

LEGAL ISSUES

Older adults may face medical-legal issues, including decision-making capacity, immigration status, insurance eligibility, disability rights, driving, and repercussions of elder abuse. Some of these issues are discussed in separate chapters (see Chapter 19, "Detecting, Assessing, & Responding to Elder Mistreatment"; Chapter 21, "Ethics & Informed Decision Making"; and Chapter 69, "Driving & Older Adults").

If older adults develop cognitive impairment or serious medical illness, their ability to make independent decisions

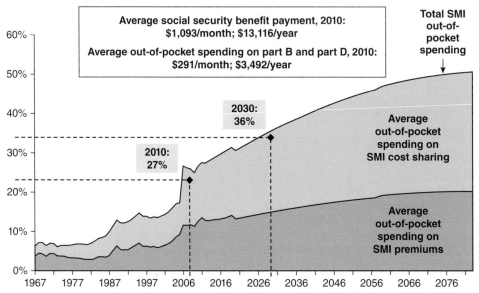

▲ **Figure 18–2.** Total Part B and Part D (supplementary medical insurance [SMI]) out-of-pocket spending as a share of the average social security benefit, 1967–2084. (Reproduced with permission from The Henry J. Kaiser Family Foundation. A primer on Medicare financing. January 2011. https://kaiserfamilyfoundation.files.wordpress.com/2013/01/7731-02.pdf.)

and manage their financial affairs may become impaired. It is important to discuss advance care planning to both elicit and document older adults' values and preferences and also to designate a surrogate decision maker to help enact these preferences (see Chapter 21, "Ethics & Informed Decision Making"). A surrogate can be designated for either or both medical and financial decisions. Situations may occur when an older adult is determined to lack capacity and there are no friends or family who are able or willing to take on these responsibilities. Then the older adult may be directed into the court system, which may require the appointment of a conservator or guardian for the incapacitated person. Although the legal requirements, paperwork, and processes vary by state, the underlying principles are the same. More detail can be found through the National Center for State Courts, listed in the references at the end of this chapter.

RECOMMENDATIONS FOR CLINICIANS

The social context and environment of their patients may be unknown to many health care professionals who do not inquire about these issues. Problems such as financial stress or lack of adequate caregiving may have a negative impact on health and functional status as much as or more than do chronic diseases. Older adults who live in the community spend <1% of their lives in contact with health care

professionals and >99% of their time self-managing their chronic conditions and functional issues in their social environment. Physicians, primary care providers, and members of the interdisciplinary team, including nurses, social workers, and pharmacists, are important sources of health-related information for older adults and may be asked to advise patients and families about their options or to refer to other services available in their own communities. Clinicians who wish to expand their effectiveness in caring for older adults should collaborate with their team and do the following:

- Ask about loneliness and social isolation and connect people to community resources.

- Assess for food insecurity and refer to SNAP, meal delivery programs, food pantries, or other sources of food.

- Become familiar with housing and LTSS options.

- Screen for financial issues and understand the health impact of limitations in Medicare coverage.

- Remain vigilant for evidence of elder abuse or mistreatment in caregiving situations.

- Learn about available community resources, for example, via the Area Agency on Aging (AAA), direct service providers, or clearinghouses for information and referrals. The national roster of AAAs can be accessed at http://www.n4a.org/.

Bishop NJ, Wang K. Food insecurity, comorbidity, and mobility limitations among older U.S. adults: findings from the Health and Retirement Study and Health Care and Nutrition Study. *Prev Med.* 2018;114:180-187.

Kollia N, Caballero FF, Sánchez-Niubó A, et al. Social determinants, health status and 10-year mortality among 10,906 older adults from the English longitudinal study of aging: the ATHLOS project. *BMC Public Health.* 2018;18(1):1357.

Masi C, Chen H, Hawkley L, Cacioppo JT. A meta-analysis of interventions to reduce loneliness. *Pers Soc Psychol Rev.* 2011;15(3):219-266.

Meals on Wheels. Fact sheet and sources 2018: the escalating problem of senior hunger and isolation. https://www.mealsonwheelsamerica.org/docs/default-source/fact-sheets/2018/2018-national/the-issue_2018-sources-and-methods_forpublication.pdf?sfvrsn=1010bc3b_2. Accessed April 2019.

National Center for Medical Legal Partnership. Homepage. https://medical-legalpartnership.org/. Accessed April 2019.

National Center for State Courts. Guardianship/conservatorship resource guide. https://www.ncsc.org/Topics/Children-Families-and-Elders/Guardianship-Conservatorship/Resource-Guide.aspx. Accessed April 2019.

National Council on Aging. Elder Index. https://www.ncoa.org/economic-security/money-management/elder-index/. Accessed April 2019.

Perissinotto C, Holt-Lunstad J, Periyakoil VS, Covinsky K. A practical approach to assessing and mitigating loneliness and isolation in older adults. *J Am Geriatr Soc.* 2019;67(4):657-662.

Perissinotto CM, Stijacic Cenzer I, Covinsky KE. Loneliness in older persons: a predictor of functional decline and death. *Arch Intern Med.* 2012;172:1078-1083.

Pooler JA, Hartline-Grafton H, DeBor M, Sudore RL, Seligman HK. Food insecurity: a key social determinant of health for older adults. *J Am Geriatr Soc.* 2019;67(3):421-424.

Russell DW. UCLA Loneliness Scale (Version 3): reliability, validity, and factor structure. *J Pers Assess.* 1996;66(1):20-40.

Shaw JG, Farid M, Noel-Miller C, et al. Social isolation and medicare spending: among older adults, objective isolation increases expenditures while loneliness does not. *J Aging Health.* 2017;29(7):1119-1143.

US Department of Agriculture Economic Research Service. Food security in the US. https://www.ers.usda.gov/topics/food-nutrition-assistance/food-security-in-the-us/definitions-of-food-security.aspx#ranges. Accessed April 2019.

US Department of Agriculture Food and Nutrition Services. Fact sheet: USDA support for older Americans. https://www.fns.usda.gov/pressrelease/2015/020215. Accessed April 2019.

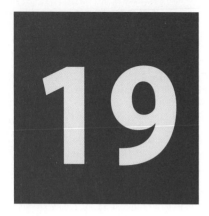

Detecting, Assessing, & Responding to Elder Mistreatment

Abigail Holley Houts, MD

Kerry Sheets, MD

Nzube Okonkwo, MD

Lawrence J. Kerzner, MD, FACP, AGSF

General Principles

Elder mistreatment is a common, yet underappreciated and underrecognized health issue affecting older adults. Mistreatment can occur at home, in nursing homes, or in other long-term care facilities. Perpetrators may be family, friends, caregivers, or other residents in a long-term care facility. In the 2008 National Elder Mistreatment Study, a random-digit dialing telephone survey, 1 in 10 community-dwelling older adults in the United States reported mistreatment in the past year; 4.6% reported emotional abuse, 1.6% physical abuse, 0.6% sexual abuse, 5.1% potential neglect, and 5.2% current financial abuse by a family member, with some respondents reporting more than one type of mistreatment. A 2017 systematic review and meta-analysis estimated the worldwide prevalence of elder mistreatment to be 15.7%. Rates of mistreatment for persons with dementia are thought to be much higher, with many estimates ranging from 40% to 60%. Rates of elder mistreatment may vary by race, ethnicity, and cultural background, although more data are needed. There are limited data estimating mistreatment rates in settings such as acute care and long-term care facilities. Recognizing the marked worldwide growth in the number of older persons and the abuse and suffering inflicted on some, the United Nations designated June 15 every year as World Elder Abuse Awareness Day.

Elder mistreatment can have a variety of impacts on the physical, emotional, and financial health of older adults. Victims of elder mistreatment have higher rates of depression and anxiety, hospitalizations, nursing home placement, and death. In the Chicago Health and Aging Project, a prospective cohort of community-dwelling older adults, those with confirmed mistreatment were two to three times more likely to be hospitalized and to die than those without a report of mistreatment. Elder mistreatment also causes emotional trauma for nonabusing loved ones, friends, and caregivers, with over two-thirds reporting personal distress related to knowing about the mistreatment.

Despite the high prevalence and health impacts of elder mistreatment, it remains underidentified and underreported. A comprehensive survey of elder mistreatment in New York State found that only 1 of every 24 cases of self-reported elder mistreatment had been reported to authorities. The information that follows will help clinicians identify, document, manage, and report suspected cases of elder mistreatment.

Acierno R, Hernandez MA, Amstadter AB, et al. Prevalence and correlates of emotional, physical, sexual, and financial abuse and potential neglect in the United States: the National Elder Mistreatment Study. *Am J Public Health.* 2010;100(2):292-297.

Breckman R, Burnes D, Ross S, et al. When helping hurts: nonabusing family, friends, and neighbors in the lives of elder mistreatment victims. *Gerontologist.* 2018;58(4):719-723.

Dong X, Simon MA. Elder abuse as a risk factor for hospitalization in older persons. *JAMA Intern Med.* 2013;173(10):911-917.

Yon Y, Mikton CR, Gassoumis ZD, et al. Elder abuse prevalence in community settings: a systematic review and meta-analysis. *Lancet Glob Health.* 2017;5(2):e147-e156.

Defining Elder Mistreatment

Elder mistreatment, also known as elder abuse, is generally defined as an act, or failure to act, by a person in a relationship of trust with an older adult that results in harm to the older adult. The World Health Organization (WHO) definition of elder abuse notes that the action or inaction need occur only once and cause harm or "distress" to an older adult. The Centers for Disease Control and Prevention (CDC) and US Administration for Community Living (ACL) expand their definitions to include actions or inactions that put older adults at serious risk for harm. The ACL also notes that the perpetrator can be a caregiver or "any other person" that has contact with a "vulnerable" adult. Each state or legal jurisdiction defines the term *vulnerable adult* differently.

Elder mistreatment comes in different forms. A recent review lists the following five "consensus" types of elder abuse: physical abuse, psychological or verbal abuse, sexual abuse, financial exploitation, and neglect. Unless otherwise noted, the following terms are derived from US National Center for Elder Abuse (NCEA), a US Administration on Aging Resource Center. Statutory definitions of elder mistreatment vary by state and jurisdiction.

A. Physical

Physical abuse is physical contact that may result in any type of pain or injury. Physical abuse may also include unwarranted administration of drugs, failure to administer needed medications, physical restraints, force-feeding, or physical punishment.

B. Sexual

Sexual abuse is sexual contact or behavior of any kind that occurs either without an older adult's consent or with an older adult who lacks capacity to give consent.

C. Psychological or Emotional

Psychological or emotional abuse involves words or actions that spur emotional stress, such as treating older adults like children or isolating them from their friends and family. Reporting psychological abuse is not required in all states (eg, California), and health professionals may wish to seek consultation with a mental health provider or social worker when psychological abuse is suspected.

D. Financial

Financial abuse is the misuse of finances or possessions of an older adult for another's gain. Financial abuse is one of the most common forms of elder abuse and may occur in any context, including among family, caregivers, or friends, and in nursing homes or long-term care facilities. Financial abuse is often accompanied by social isolation or loneliness. For example, an older adult may enter into a friendship traded for money or other material gain, or a perpetrator may isolate the older adult to exert undue influence over their finances. Older adult victims of financial exploitation may have diminished mental capacity to understand their decisions. Recent data have shown an association between decreased ability to recognize potential financial scams and incident dementia.

E. Neglect

Neglect is the failure of an informal or formal caregiver to meet the basic needs of an older adult. Neglect can be active or passive and either intentional or unintentional.

There is debate as to whether self-neglect is a form of elder abuse. Self-neglect is broadly defined as behavior by an older adult that directly endangers their safety and welfare. It is generally seen in older adults with cognitive or functional impairment and involves failure to provide oneself with basic necessities such as food, clothing, or shelter. In some cases,

failure to take medications or access medical care may be considered a form of self-neglect. Self-neglect may coincide with neglect by family or other caregivers or may occur when an older adult refuses help and/or takes efforts to conceal their inability to meet basic needs.

Boyle PA, Yu L, Schneider JA, et al. Scam awareness related to incident Alzheimer dementia and mild cognitive impairment: a prospective cohort study. *Ann Intern Med.* 2019;170(10):702-709.

Lachs MS, Pillemer KA. Elder abuse. *N Engl J Med.* 2015; 373(20):1947-1956.

▶ Prevention

Elder mistreatment is considered by some to be the largest preventable ailment affecting older adults. Despite this, there are very few data about effective prevention. A recent scoping review concluded that there is preliminary evidence for five strategies: (1) caregiver support interventions, (2) money management programs that provide financial management assistance for vulnerable older adults, (3) helplines where caregivers and patients can seek information about and assistance with elder mistreatment, (4) emergency shelters for victims of mistreatment to prevent additional mistreatment and allow time to plan for safe housing, and (5) multidisciplinary teams to facilitate coordination of available resources. Eight-year follow-up data from the National Elder Mistreatment Study suggested that social support was protective against many of the complications of elder mistreatment. Some data also suggest that social support, both in terms of companionship and built-in assistance with daily activities, may be associated with lower rates of elder mistreatment. Given the relative paucity of data regarding effective prevention of elder mistreatment, we recommend that health care providers maintain a high level of suspicion for elder mistreatment in all older adults, particularly older adults with the risk factors discussed in the next section.

Acierno R, Hernandez-Tejada MA, Anetzberger GJ, et al. The National Elder Mistreatment Study: an 8-year longitudinal study of outcomes. *J Elder Abuse Negl.* 2017;29(4):254-269.

Pillemer K, Burnes D, Riffin C, et al. Elder abuse: global situation, risk factors, and prevention strategies. *Gerontologist.* 2016;56(Suppl 2):S194-S205.

▶ Risk Factors

Elder mistreatment affects people of all genders, ethnic backgrounds, and socioeconomic status. A variety of victim, perpetrator, and environmental characteristics are associated with an increased likelihood of mistreatment. A review of international studies of elder mistreatment and the WHO European Report on Preventing Elder Maltreatment identified three levels of evidence (strong, potential, or contested) that supported these factors' contribution to risk. Strong evidence is defined as that which is validated by unanimous or nearly unanimous support from several studies. Potential evidence is supported by mixed or limited data. Contested evidence is supported by hypothesis or without a clear evidence base.

At the level of the individual (victim), mistreatment risk factors supported by strong evidence include functional dependence or physical disability, cognitive impairment, poor mental health, and low income. Gender is a potential risk factor. Women may be at greater risk of physical abuse and men at greater risk of emotional or financial abuse. In some studies in the United States, younger age is potentially a risk factor, whereas in Mexico and Europe, older age is reported to be potentially associated with increased risk. Low income is a predictor of mistreatment across many countries. US and Canadian data suggest African Americans may be at greater risk for financial and psychological abuse than Caucasians. Hispanics have lower risk of emotional abuse, financial abuse, and neglect.

Perpetrator mental illness, poor psychological health, substance abuse, and dependence on the victim for emotional support, financial help, or housing are factors supported by strong evidence for increased risk.

Aspects of the victim-perpetrator relationship that are considered risk factors vary by mistreatment type, country, and geographic location. In some countries, a spouse or partner may be the most common perpetrator of emotional and physical abuse. In other countries, children and children-in-law are more commonly the abusers. Information about marital status is mixed. Some studies suggest being married is associated with mistreatment, while others suggest increased risk in being single, separated, divorced, or widowed. Negative views about aging and normalization of violence within families are contested risk factors.

Social isolation, a commonality among all forms of mistreatment, is a strong risk factor at the environmental level. For every 1-point increase in a nine-item vulnerability risk index constructed from sociodemographic, health-related, and psychosocial factors, there was twice the risk of reported and confirmed elder abuse in the Chicago Health and Aging Project.

▶ Screening and Identification

Elder abuse is frequently unrecognized by physicians and other health care professionals. The frequency of diagnosis of elder mistreatment in emergency departments is at least two orders of magnitude lower than its prevalence in the general population. It is difficult to recognize even by home care nurses performing monthly visits. Thus, screening for elder abuse without the presence of signs or symptoms, as well as use of specifically targeted questionnaires to identify those experiencing mistreatment are areas of special interest and ongoing development.

As part of its Code of Medical Ethics, the American Medical Association recommends consideration of abuse as a possible factor in the presentation of medical complaints and for physicians to routinely inquire about abuse as part of a medical history. The specialty organizations American Academy of Neurology and American College of Obstetricians and Gynecologists support screening older patients for abuse or violence as practitioners in these areas may serve particularly vulnerable populations. The 2018 US Preventive Services Task Force (USPSTF) analysis of randomized controlled trials and systematic reviews found that current evidence is insufficient to assess the balance of benefits and harms of screening in all older or vulnerable adults. Specifically, no studies meeting the USPSTF review criteria evaluated the effectiveness of early detection and treatment or the harms of screening those without recognized signs or symptoms of abuse. Patient-related factors such as insufficient mental, physical, or financial abilities to engage in screening and dependence on perpetrators for caregiving and access to medical care are barriers to developing high-quality information about the efficacy of broad-based screening.

The most direct way to identify possible elder mistreatment during routine health care visits is to ask high-risk patients about mistreatment. Health care professionals should interview the patient and caregiver separately. In health care settings where comprehensive assessment for mistreatment is not readily available, one question, or a set of three questions, may be asked:

- Single-question screen: "Does anyone hurt you?"

- Three-question screen: "Do you feel safe where you live? Has someone not helped you when you needed their help? Who takes care of your finances or pays your bills?"

Despite limitations in current knowledge about the value of screening in primary care, numerous tools have been developed to assist with case finding. Three are highlighted by the National Elder Abuse Center and the Centers for Medicare and Medicaid Services (CMS):

- Hwalek-Sengstock Elder Abuse Screening Test (H-S/EAST): Suitable for use in the emergency department or outpatient setting, this easy-to-administer, six-item screening questionnaire can be completed by the patient or the health care professional. Because its specificity of 73% (95% confidence interval, 62%–82%) is much higher than its sensitivity, it is best used where the suspicion for mistreatment is high such as in follow up to the one- or three-question screen.

- Vulnerability to Abuse Screening Scale (VASS): With moderate reliability and construct validity, this easy-to-administer, 12-item screening questionnaire can be completed by the patient or the health care professional.

- Elder Abuse Suspicion Index (EASI): Validated in family practice and ambulatory settings, it has a sensitivity of 0.77 and specificity of 0.44. The EASI is completed by health care professionals to assess risk for and actual neglect and verbal, psychological, financial, or emotional mistreatment over a preceding 12-month period. Comprised of six items, it is also easy to administer, taking approximately 2 minutes to complete.

Another barrier to identifying elder mistreatment is provider's lack of knowledge about abuse. Enhancing medical and preprofessional (nursing, social work, criminal justice, health professions, and other) student awareness by including mistreatment in formal curricula may increase their ability to recognize and intervene when they enter clinical practice. Postgraduate medical training experiences in collaborating with Adult Protective Service (APS) workers on home visits also improve physician awareness.

Basic principles of primary care include understanding patients' home living situations and social environments. By providing continuity of care over the course of years, practitioners can monitor the trajectory of their patient's health and debilities as they age and their vulnerability to mistreatment, and mobilize resources as risk of mistreatment increases.

Burnett J, Achenbaum WA, Murphy KP. Prevention and early identification of elder abuse. *Clin Geriatr Med.* 2014;30(4): 743-759.

Committee Opinion No. 568: elder abuse and women's health. *Obstet Gynecol.* 2013;122(1):187-191.

Dong XQ. Elder abuse: systematic review and implications for practice. *J Am Geriatr Soc.* 2015;63(6):1214-1238.

Evans C, Hunold K, Rosen T, et al. Diagnosis of elder abuse in U.S. emergency departments. *J Am Geriatr Soc.* 2017;65(1):91-97.

Feltner C, Wallace I, Berkman N, et al. Screening for intimate partner violence, elder abuse, and abuse of vulnerable adults: evidence report and systematic review for the US Preventive Services Task Force. *JAMA.* 2018;320(16):1688-1701.

Fisher JM, Rudd MP, Walker RW, et al. Training tomorrow's doctors to safeguard the patients of today: using medical student simulation training to explore barriers to recognition of elder abuse. *J Am Geriatr Soc.* 2016;64(1):168-173.

Friedman B, Santos E, Liebel D, et al. Longitudinal prevalence and correlates of elder mistreatment among older adults receiving home visiting nursing. *J Elder Abuse Negl.* 2015;27(1):34-64.

Policastro C, Payne BK. Assessing the level of elder abuse knowledge pre-professionals possess: implications for the further development of university curriculum. *J Elder Abuse Negl.* 2014; 26(1):12-30.

Schulman EA, Hohler AD. The American Academy of Neurology position statement on abuse and violence. *Neurology.* 2012; 78(6):433-435.

▶ Assessment

A. History Taking

If a patient presents with a caregiver, it is useful to observe the interactions of the caregiver with both the patient and the clinic staff during the initial interview. Observations may be made of their speech, tone, and touch of the patient. Encounters with overly protective caregivers who refuse to leave the room or those seemingly lacking concern or who are hostile toward clinic staff may raise concern for abuse.

When taking a medical history from an older adult, it is preferable to conduct interviews in a private space and with the patient alone. If a patient has cognitive impairment or another limitation that may prevent them from providing a complete history, a practitioner may consider interviewing both patient and caregiver together and then requesting that a caregiver step out during some later portion of the encounter (eg, during the physical exam) to allow for private conversation with the patient. The patient and examiner should be at eye level. Assistive devices needed for communication should be provided (eg, hearing devices, amplifiers, glasses, dentures). The health care professional should be cognizant of cultural differences during the history and examination as they may contribute to varying perceptions of what constitutes elder mistreatment.

Clinicians must determine the patient's cognitive status (see Chapter 9, "Cognitive Impairment & Dementia"). Assessing the patient's level of cognitive functioning may require further evaluation.

Health care professionals need to differentiate possible signs and symptoms of abuse from medical conditions. If injuries are noted, mistreatment may be suspected when the mechanism of injury or the history provided by the patient or caregiver does not adequately explain the findings.

It is important to determine the patient's functional status and ability to perform activities of daily living. If the patient needs assistance, then it is essential to find out if the patient has access to help and who is providing the help. Collateral history from a patient's health care provider or community pharmacy regarding missed medical or home care appointments or filling of prescription medications may be helpful in ensuring that caregivers are fulfilling their obligations.

It is important to explore the patient's living arrangement as patients and potential abusers may live in the same household. Determining how long the patient has been living with the person(s), who pays the bills, and who owns or rents the living space can provide critical information regarding the potential for mistreatment. Inquiring about the financial status of the patient can help alert a physician about the potential for financial abuse. The physician should identify the person who manages a patient's finances, whether the patient is dependent on others for living and personal expenses, and whether anyone is dependent on the patient for financial assistance. Social support and engagement in community activities should be determined as victims of elder mistreatment are often socially isolated. Table 19–1 summarizes potential indicators of elder mistreatment.

B. Physical Examination

A working knowledge of the physiology of aging is useful in differentiating physical signs of abuse from expected sequelae of aging, medications, or diseases. The physical exam should

Table 19–1. Potential indicators of elder mistreatment indicated by history taking.

Items from patient history that may signal elder mistreatment
Repeated emergency department visits and hospital admissions; use of multiple different emergency departments
Explanation of injuries is inconsistent with medical findings
Prior history of similar injuries, prior mistreatment
Delays in seeking treatment
Multiple missed medical appointments and/or going to multiple medical providers
Medication nonadherence
Social isolation
Substance abuse

Patient or abuser behavior that may signal elder mistreatment
Patient seems hesitant/afraid to answer questions
Patient provides evasive or nonspecific answers
Patient seems fearful of potential abuser
Potential abuser answers all questions for the patient
Potential abuser prevents examiner from interviewing or examining patient alone
Potential abuser acts angry, demeaning, or indifferent toward the patient
Potential abuser refuses to provide necessary assistance for patient's care
Potential abuser seems overly concerned at the cost of care for the patient
Potential abuser appears to be experiencing caregiver burden

include a full examination of the patient. It should begin with general observation, including evaluation for appropriate clothing, hygiene, and signs of dehydration or weight loss. A disparity between a patient's known financial assets as obtained by history and his or her physical appearance may raise concerns about neglect or self-neglect.

A complete skin examination should include visual inspection for any evidence of physical abuse (bruising, abrasions, lacerations), evaluation of hygiene, and careful inspection for any skin breakdown or pressure sores. The pattern, number, size, location, and color of bruising and other skin lesions should be noted. When compared with accidental bruising, those on the right lateral arm and head and neck are more likely associated with abuse. Physicians should be aware that the color of a bruise may not be an indicator of its age. Tramline bruising, a unique forensic marker of elder mistreatment, should be recognized when present. It is seen when a person is struck with a linear or cylindrical object (eg, ruler, bat, iron bar) leaving a distinctive bruise with a pale central area lined on either side by linear ecchymosis or petechiae. Restraint belts also may cause tramline bruising. Basilar skull fractures are frequently overlooked and may be indicated by the finding of bruising around the eyes and ears (sometimes called Battle's sign). Clinical notes should include an opinion about whether injuries are adequately or inadequately explained by the history.

The musculoskeletal examination should focus on signs of fractures or previous fractures, including bone deformities or limitations in movement. A description of location, shape, number, stage of healing, and any delays in seeking care should be noted for injuries identified. Genitourinary and rectal exams should be completed to evaluate for evidence of sexual abuse. Neurologic examination should include screening for delirium and cognitive impairment. Psychological evaluation may include observations of affect (flat, apathetic, evasive, fearful), fear of touch, or signs of depression or anxiety.

Laboratory and radiologic evaluations should be obtained based on history and examination findings and may include diagnostic imaging for fractures, evaluation of hemoglobin, electrolytes, and renal and hepatic function for signs of dehydration or malnutrition, or testing for sexually transmitted infections. Postmortem examination physical and laboratory findings such as elevated vitreous sodium level may be indicative of dehydration and could support a finding of neglect.

Differential Diagnosis

Diagnosing elder abuse is complicated by the physiologic changes of aging, chronic illnesses, and accidental injuries that may mimic mistreatment. Consequently, it can be challenging for clinicians to make a definitive diagnosis of elder mistreatment or self-neglect. Dramatic injuries such as fractures, burns, contusions, and lacerations accompanied by a credible patient history pose no diagnostic quandary; however, subtle presentations of medical problems over long periods of time can be difficult to distinguish from elder mistreatment. Therefore, self-neglect or elder mistreatment should be included in the differential diagnosis when evaluating older adults. Table 19–2 lists possible physical findings of elder mistreatment and examples of underlying medical problems that may mimic elder mistreatment.

Baniak N, Campos-Baniak G, Mulla A, et al. Vitreous humor: a short review on post-mortem applications. *J Clin Exp Pathol.* 2015;5:1.

Gibbs LM. Understanding the medical markers of elder abuse and neglect: physical examination findings. *Clin Geriatr Med.* 2014;30(4):687-712.

Gironda MW, Nguyen AL, Mosqueda LM. Is this broken bone because of abuse? Characteristics and comorbid diagnoses in older adults with fractures. *J Am Geriatr Soc.* 2016;64(8):1651-1655.

LoFaso VM, Rosen T. Medical and laboratory indicators of elder abuse and neglect. *Clin Geriatr Med.* 2014;30(4):712-728.

Mosqueda L, Burnight K, Liao S. The life cycles of bruises in older adults. *J Am Geriatr Soc.* 2005;53(8):1339-1343.

Intervention and Treatment

Elder mistreatment is a complex medical biopsychosocial syndrome best evaluated by interprofessional assessment

Table 19–2. Types of elder abuse and associated signs.

Type of Abuse	Signs and Symptoms	Possible Physical Findings	Differential Diagnosis
Physical	Patient's report of abuse	Pattern of bruising or burns Burns in the shape of an object Bruising including bruises that encircle elder person's arms, legs, or torso; tramline bruise Bruises on head, neck, or face Broken bones, spiral long bone fractures, sprains, dislocations, internal injuries Open wounds, cuts Untreated injuries	Osteoporosis Pathologic fractures Metabolic disorders Frequent falls Coagulopathy Anticoagulant use Corticosteroid use Spontaneous bruising associated with age and thin skin
Sexual	Patient's report of sexual abuse Unusual sexual behavior Unusual or inappropriate relationship between the patient and possible abuser Patient's report of sexual assault or rape	Bruises on or around the genital area/breasts Unexplained sexually transmitted diseases or genital infections Unexplained vaginal or anal bleeding Torn, stained, or bloody underwear Pain on walking or sitting	Vaginosis, non–sexually transmitted infections like *Candida* Dementia-related behavior Hemorrhoids/lower gastrointestinal; bleeding/colon cancer Dysfunctional uterine bleeding/uterine cancer
Psychological/ emotional	Depression Anxiety Agitation Excessive fears Sleep changes Change in appetite	Passive Evasive Fear—possibly in presence of abuser Confusion Agitation Significant weight loss or gain Sudden worsening of medical conditions	Psychiatric disorders—depression, anxiety, psychosis Cognitive impairment Worsening dementia Medication side effects
Financial	Ambiguity of financial status Inability to pay bills, buy food or medications Sudden changes in legal documents (eg, will, power of attorney, or health care agent) Excessive concern regarding expenses necessary for patient's care by the possible abuser	Living well below the patient's means Discomfort/evasiveness when discussing finances	Psychiatric disorders Cognitive impairment/dementia Neurologic disorders Diminished recognition of financial scams
Neglect	Absence of assisted hearing devices, eyeglasses, dentures, or assisted walking devices Sudden changes or decline in health	Malnutrition—low BMI, muscle wasting Dehydration—skin tenting, orthostasis, tachycardia Poor hygiene Inadequate or inappropriate clothing Pressure ulcers/bedsores Moisture-associated skin damage (incontinence, intertriginous dermatitis, periwound maceration) Hypothermia/hyperthermia Burns in patient with dementia	Chronic diseases that can affect nutrition including end-stage dementia, dysphagia, Parkinson disease, amyotrophic lateral sclerosis, malabsorption syndromes, malignancy Peripheral neuropathy leading to wounds/burns Patient not allowing care or combative due to agitation from dementia or neurologic disease

BMI, body mass index.

directed towards developing an individualized intervention and treatment plan. The Abuse Intervention Model (AIM) has been recently proposed as a framework for providing guidance in understanding and intervening on three risk factor domains: (1) characteristics of the vulnerable adult, (2) characteristics of the trusted other or perpetrator, and (3) the living and care environments (Figure 19–1).

A. Medical Intervention

1. Documentation—Documentation of suspected or confirmed elder mistreatment, including abuse or neglect, should be entered in the medical record in all care settings. Since multiple types of mistreatment may coexist, documentation should address each component. The patient's chief

Abuse Intervention Model (AIM)

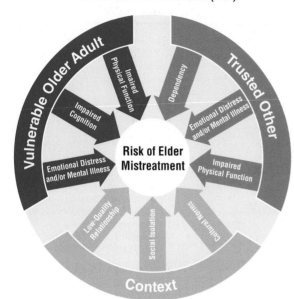

▲ **Figure 19–1.** Abuse Intervention Model (AIM).

complaints and concerns using the patient's own words, if possible, should be recorded, as should a complete medical and social history. Because repeated cancellation of scheduled clinic appointments may be a sign of mistreatment, the name of the person canceling the appointments should be noted.

If injuries are present, a detailed description of the type of injuries and possible causes should be documented. Color photographs should be obtained in compliance with local health information rules and regulations. In the United States, these regulations include those of the Health Information Portability and Accountability Act of 1996 (HIPAA), among others. Results of all laboratory and imaging studies should be recorded. Medical records frequently provide insufficient information to assist with the investigation of alleged mistreatment. Providers may use the geriatric injury documentation tool (Geri-IDT) to help guide appropriate evaluation and electronic record documentation.

The AIM provides a structure for documenting the dependency of the elder on the caregiver or trusted other, as well as any emotional distress, mental illness, physical impairment, and/or burden experienced by the caregiver. The quality of the relationship, extent of social isolation, and the cultural context should be noted. Patient behavior and family dynamics should be documented. Interviewing the patient separately from the caregiver will likely uncover additional valuable insights.

If law enforcement officers are contacted, the name of the officer, actions taken, and police incident number should be documented. The date and time the report was made to

Adult Protective Service or similar service available in countries outside the United States, and the name of the person taking the report should be recorded.

The diagnosis of elder mistreatment should be included in the medical problem list and in International Classification of Disease 10th edition coding. Documentation of resident-to-resident elder mistreatment or violent incidents occurring in nursing and assisted living facilities should also follow this outline.

2. Reporting—In the United States, public policy encourages reporting elder mistreatment to APS agencies. These are social service programs provided by state or local governments that serve vulnerable adults, including older adults and those with disabilities needing protective services. Most states designate individual physicians, health care workers, social workers, and institutions and organizations serving vulnerable adults as mandated reporters of mistreatment. Physician reports account for only 1.4% of those received by APS, the smallest percentage of any reporting group, indicating likely under-reporting of maltreatment.

The 2014 WHO global status report on a violence prevention survey of 133 countries provides an international perspective on elder mistreatment. Approximately 40% of countries report national action plans to address this problem, and one-third have APS services to investigate potential cases and assist vulnerable older adults. Less than 40% report caregiver support programs and residential care policies to lessen elder mistreatment with a wide range of differences between countries and geographic areas. Professional education and public information campaigns are even less prevalent. Laws against elder mistreatment are the least prevalent among those relating to interpersonal violence and the least fully enforced.

Potential barriers to physician reporting include limited recognition of mistreatment as historical features and signs may be subtle, patient denial of the existence of maltreatment, lack of knowledge of reporting responsibilities and processes, concern about potential adverse effects on the clinician-patient relationship, doubts about the efficacy of reporting on mitigating maltreatment or worries that it may escalate the maltreatment, and concerns about maintaining confidentiality. Many physicians are reticent to become involved with the legal system.

Providers' ambivalence toward reporting may be lessened by recognizing that APS focuses on arranging needed social and medical services using a least-restrictive-interventions framework. APS strives to balance autonomy in patient decision making with beneficence. Depending on the complexity of the situation, APS evaluations may be simple or complicated, may be brief in duration, or may extend over weeks to months. Immediate goals are to ensure safety of the vulnerable adult and to protect from emergency or urgent harmful situations.

While reporting requirements differ from state to state, some states impose legal liability for not reporting. Keeping up to date with individual state reporting requirements is crucial as these are frequently revised. The Veterans Health Administration has specific rules about reporting to APS. Practitioners should be familiar with procedures in their facilities.

3. Ongoing care planning—Elders experiencing mistreatment may be encountered in any clinical care setting, and practitioners must ensure that medical and safety needs can be met. For those seen in the office, clinic, emergency department, or home care settings, hospitalization may be needed if the situation is sufficiently urgent. If the patient does not meet hospital admission criteria, the clinician must be sure the home environment is sufficiently safe and that assistance is available for functionally and/or cognitively impaired patients. A social work or APS specialist consultation may be necessary before discharge in order to develop a safety plan. Home care services such as home nursing, therapies, and other home and community care supports, such as day programs, appropriate to patient needs should be initiated. In some geographic areas, community paramedics may be available to provide in-home evaluative services.

Elder mistreatment is often a chronic problem involving limitations in functional ability, decision-making capacity, and health and social supports. It is often best evaluated and managed by an interprofessional team from medicine, nursing, social services, legal, law enforcement, and finance areas, among others. Patients with a history of elder mistreatment should be referred to a clinician or medical team skilled in recognizing geriatric syndromes and familiar with local agencies that provide services to mistreated older patients. The referral should be to someone with whom the older adult can have an ongoing relationship. Geriatric medicine specialty consultation or comprehensive geriatric assessment and intervention may be useful in providing additional perspective and care (see Chapter 2, "Overview of Geriatric Assessment"). It may be helpful to involve an array of community resources including drug and alcohol rehabilitation services, legal assistance, and advocacy groups.

A home visit is frequently helpful as it provides the opportunity to directly observe and evaluate all aspects of the AIM including mobility, functional and cognitive abilities, medication use, food availability, home safety, pets, potential substance abuse, and interactions with others living in the home or providing assistance. Clinicians may better serve as advocates for their patients when they have first-hand knowledge of the home setting and what is most important to the patient. What may have been initially perceived as an unsafe home environment may become clarified as appropriate, at least for the moment. Indeed, specific individual patients may not consider safety their highest priority. In these circumstances, clinicians should consider avoiding setting too high a bar for safety, counsel patients to accept interventions that facilitate their goal of remaining at home, and work collaboratively with the patient and others to develop plans to identify and manage future deterioration and emergencies.

4. Assessment of decision-making capacity—The mistreated older person may be vulnerable because of chronic illnesses impairing the capacity to participate fully in medical, self-care, financial, testamentary, or other types of decision making. Any intercurrent illness affecting thinking or physical functioning may further reduce the ability to make informed decisions.

A competent individual has the right to be a fully informed participant in all aspects of decision making and has the right to refuse recommended assistance, care, or interventions. Those who lack decision-making capacity and whose expressed choices may lead to harm or death may need protection and assistance. A determination of self-neglect versus informed personal choice will hinge on the extent of the person's capacity to participate in his or her own care relative to the urgency and severity of the circumstances. It is essential to determine the patient's decision-making capacity whenever mistreatment is in question (for more discussion on informed decision making, see Chapter 21, "Ethics & Informed Decision Making").

B. Social Services & Interprofessional Intervention

APS or similar entities can provide social interventions in almost every jurisdiction in the United States. APS specialists receive reports, conduct investigations, evaluate living environments, and participate in coordinating interventions. APS obtains information from multiple sources, such as family and friends of the patient, and consults with other social workers, physicians, nurses, living facilities, home care staff, law enforcement and regulatory agencies, and legal and banking organizations. Tribal and Native American agencies may provide similar, culturally appropriate services including expanding the maltreatment framework to encompass spiritual abuse.

Working in conjunction with victims, families, ombudsmen, and other involved parties, plans are developed to ensure that services provided or interventions introduced are the least-restrictive alternatives, are reflective of the patient's preferences, and maximize independence. Those referred to APS become their "clients." When a client has the capacity to make informed decisions, APS specialists advocate for the right to refuse services if the person does not want intervention. APS specialists are bound by statutory limitations within their legal jurisdiction and may not impose services or involuntary relocation from the home if the client has the capacity to make these decisions. While in extreme circumstances petitioning the court for guardianship or conservatorship may be needed, models of providing less restrictive supported decision making are becoming more available. Obtaining a representative payee to assist in managing finances may mitigate urgencies when there are unpaid bills.

Elder mistreatment multidisciplinary teams (EM-MDT) as an evaluative and intervention framework are becoming more widespread. One hundred fifteen US and international

Table 19–3. Online accessible resources.

1. Centers for Disease Control and Prevention. Elder abuse: risk and protective factors.
   https://www.cdc.gov/violenceprevention/elderabuse/riskprotectivefactors.html
2. National Center for Elder Abuse website. https://ncea.acl.gov/
3. European report on preventing elder-maltreatment. Geneva, Switzerland: World Health Organization Regional Office for Europe; 2011. http://www.euro.who.int/__data/assets/pdf_file/0010/144676/e95110.pdf
4. World Health Organization Global Status Report on Violence Prevention, 2014.
   https://www.who.int/violence_injury_prevention/violence/status_report/2014/report/report/en/
5. American Medical Association. Code of Medical Ethics. Chapter 8, Opinions on Physicians and Health of Communities. Preventing, Identifying & Treating Violence and Abuse. https://www.ama-assn.org/delivering-care/ethics/preventing-identifying-treating-violence-abuse.
6. US Department of Justice, Elder Justice Initiative to "support and coordinate the Department's enforcement and programmatic efforts to combat elder abuse, neglect and financial fraud and scams." Multiple information areas include: Rural and Tribal Justice Resource Guide and Elder Abuse Guide for Law Enforcement
   https://www.justice.gov/elderjustice
   https://www.justice.gov/elderjustice/rural-and-tribal-resources
   https://www.justice.gov/elderjustice/eagle-elder-abuse-guide-law-enforcement
7. National Indigenous Elder Justice Initiative. https://www.nieji.org/
8. The Elder Justice Roadmap: A stakeholder initiative to respond to an emerging health, justice, financial, and social crisis. https://www.justice.gov/file/852856/download
9. American Bar Association. Legal Issues Related to Elder Abuse.
   https://www.americanbar.org/groups/law_aging/resources/elder_abuse/
10. American Bankers Association. Protecting Seniors: A Bank Resource Guide for Partnering with Law Enforcement and Adult Protective Services. https://www.aba.com/advocacy/community-programs/consumer-resources/protect-your-money/elderly-financial-abuse
11. Financial Exploitation of Seniors. Securities and Exchange Commission regulatory notice 17-11. March 2017 and Safe Seniors Act of 2018.
    http://www.finra.org/sites/default/files/Regulatory-Notice-17-11.pdf
    https://www.finra.org/sites/default/files/2019-05/senior_safe_act_factsheet.pdf
12. Department of Veterans Affairs. Reporting cases of abuse and neglect. VHA DIRECTIVE 1199. Transmittal Sheet November 28, 2017. https://www.va.gov/search/?query=Reporting+Cases+of+abuse+and+neglect+VHA+Directive+1199

All websites accessed March 15, 2020.

programs were recently cataloged describing team structure, case management, legal services, home visitation, emergency shelter, therapy/counseling, and educational characteristics. Information technology has permitted the availability of virtual statewide EM-MDT assessments and interventions. Elder mistreatment death review teams and forensic centers, hospital-based vulnerable elder protection teams, vulnerable adult–law enforcement teams, and financial abuse teams are additional developing models for resource organization, research, clinical evaluation, and service.

C. Legal Interventions

Although laws differ from state to state, law enforcement organizations are generally involved in cases in which crimes are committed against older adults, including physical abuse, neglect with malicious intent or severe adverse outcomes, financial exploitation, and other forms of elder mistreatment. Police officers investigate cases for evidence to help prosecutors pursue perpetrators. Officers of the court and judges participate in guardianship hearings when appropriate. Members of law enforcement and the legal profession help link older persons with agencies and other resources available to victims of crime. Forensic pathologists work closely with law enforcement officers to determine the cause of death in cases of suspected homicide resulting from abuse or neglect. Advocates, working through elder justice centers and other venues, participate in developing legislation to strengthen existing laws and provide additional tools to protect vulnerable adults from maltreatment. Banking and bar associations provide education for their members and advocacy. Federal Securities and Exchange Commission (SEC) rules encompass procedures mitigating potential financial exploitation of older persons.

APS participates in determining if maltreatment complaints are substantiated or not substantiated, or if the results of investigations are inconclusive. Depending on state law, institutions and individual care providers may face sanctions including exclusion from employment and participation as care providers if maltreatment allegations are confirmed.

For online accessible resources see Table 19–3.

Burnett J, Dyer CB, Clark LE, et al. A statewide elder mistreatment virtual assessment program: preliminary data. *J Am Geriatr Soc.* 2019;67(1):151-155.

Kogan AC, Rosen T, Navarro A, et al. Developing the Geriatric Injury Documentation Tool (Geri-IDT) to improve documentation of physical findings in injured older adults. *J Gen Intern Med.* 2019;34(4):567-574.

Lachs MS, Teresi JA, Ramirez M, et al. The prevalence of resident-to-resident elder mistreatment in nursing homes. *Ann Intern Med.* 2016;165(4):229-236.

Mosqueda L, Burnight K, Gironda MW, et al. The abuse intervention model: a pragmatic approach to intervention for elder mistreatment. *J Am Geriatr Soc.* 2016;64(9):1879-1883.

Rosen T, Elman A, Dion S, et al. Review of programs to combat elder mistreatment: focus on hospitals and level of resources needed. *J Am Geriatr Soc.* 2019;67(6):1286-1294.

Rosen T, Lachs MS, Teresi J, et al. Staff-reported strategies for prevention and management of resident-to-resident elder mistreatment in long-term care facilities. *J Elder Abuse Negl.* 2016;28(1):1-13.

Rosen T, Mehta-Naik N, Elman A, et al. Improving quality of care in hospitals for victims of elder mistreatment: development of the vulnerable elder protection team. *Jt Comm J Qual Patient Saf.* 2018;44(3):164-171.

Smith AK, Lo B, Aronson L. Elder self-neglect: how can a physician help? *N Engl J Med.* 2013;369(26):2476-2479.

▶ Summary

Elder mistreatment is unfortunately too common a worldwide occurrence. Medical practitioners should protect their patients from mistreatment by recognizing and reducing risk factors, being especially alert to and documenting subtle signs, engaging multidisciplinary team members, and reporting appropriately when mistreatment is suspected. Models for improving evaluation and intervention within medical care facilities and expanding team development and outreach to wide geographic areas through computer-based video technology are promising developments.

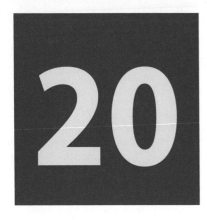

20

Prevention & Health Promotion

Dandan Liu, MD

Louise C. Walter, MD

PREVENTION FOR OLDER ADULTS

Even in older adults, preventive interventions can limit disease and disability. The heterogeneity of medical conditions, life expectancy, and goals of treatment, however, requires a thoughtful and individualized application of prevention guidelines. This approach tailors preventive interventions to an individual, balancing benefits and harms in the context of a patient's life expectancy and values rather than using a one-size-fits-all approach based solely on age.

There are many guidelines that include recommendations about preventive interventions in older adults. Since the 1980s, the US Preventive Services Task Force (USPSTF) has provided evidence-based scientific reviews of preventive interventions to guide primary care decision making. The fundamental standard applied by the task force is whether the intervention leads to improved health outcomes (eg, reduced disease-specific morbidity and mortality). Services graded A and B are recommended, whereas those with a C grade require consideration of "individual circumstances." In 1998, the Assessing Care of Vulnerable Elders (ACOVE) project began developing quality indicators specific for vulnerable older persons (defined as age >65 years and life expectancy <2 years). This project concluded that high-quality evidence about benefits and harms is often limited for interventions in older adults. The American Geriatric Society (AGS) also has published several guidelines on health promotion with a geriatric focus. Table 20–1 provides a summary of conditions for which screening or other preventive interventions have been shown to result in net benefit for some older people based on USPSTF and geriatrics-focused guidelines. The table also provides general guidance for translating national guidelines into individualized decisions with each patient.

The framework for making individualized decisions is anchored by weighing the immediate potential harms with the expected time horizon for potential benefits (benefits may not occur for 10 or more years after an intervention in the example of cancer screening; this time horizon is known

as the lag time to benefit)—all while incorporating estimated life expectancy and an older person's own values and goals (Figure 20–1). Preventive interventions should be targeted to patients whose estimated life expectancy is greater than the lag time to benefit of a preventive intervention. Also, rather than simply using average life expectancy based on age, a more accurate estimated life expectancy considers a person's health status. For example, persons with several comorbid medical conditions or functional impairments likely have a life expectancy that is lower than average for their age, whereas those without any significant medical

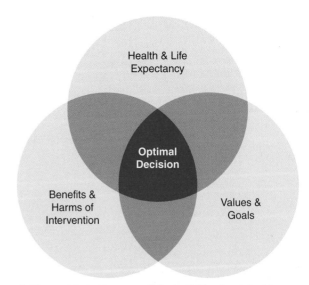

▲ **Figure 20–1.** Framework for individualized decision making. The optimal decision is a balanced amalgam of multiple variables including the potential benefits and harms of intervention, a person's health and life expectancy, and a person's own values and goals.

Table 20–1. Summary of preventive interventions incorporating framework for individualized decision making.

Topics by System	Recommendations		Individualized Decision Making (Function, Health, Prognosis, Goals)		
	Please Refer to Text for Expanded Description of Recommendations		High Independence Healthy Life Expectancy >10 Years Longevity	Limited function Multiple Chronic Conditions Life Expectancy 2–10 Years Preserving Function	Dependent End-Stage Disease Life Expectancy <2 Years Comfort Palliation
Geriatric syndromes[a]	Falls	Annually	Yes	Yes	Yes
	Depression	Annually	Yes	Yes	Yes
	Nutrition	Weigh at each visit	Maybe	Yes	Yes
	Vision	Initially, then every 2 years	Maybe	Maybe	Maybe
	Hearing	Initially, then unclear frequency	Maybe	Maybe	Maybe
	Cognition	Patient preference specific	Maybe	Maybe	Maybe
	Elder abuse	No formal screening, but be vigilant for signs of mistreatment	Maybe	Maybe	Maybe
Health-related behaviors	Exercise	Annually	Yes	Yes	Yes
	Substance use	Annually	Yes	Yes	Yes
	Sexual health	Annually	Yes	Yes	Yes
	Sleep	Unclear	Maybe	Maybe	Maybe
Immunizations	Influenza	Annually	Yes	Yes	Yes
	Pneumococcal (PPSV23 + PCV 13)	Once after age 65[b]	Yes	Yes	Yes
	Tetanus	Booster every 10 years	Yes	Yes	Maybe
	Herpes zoster	Series of two shots after age 50	Yes	Yes	Maybe
Endocrine	Diabetes	Initially if hypertension, hyperlipidemia, or obese, and then every 3 years	Yes	Maybe	No
	Osteoporosis	Initially women >65 years, men >70 years	Yes	Yes	Maybe
Cardiovascular	Hyperlipidemia	Initially, then every 5 years	Yes	Yes	No
	Hypertension	Initially, then based on blood pressure	Yes	Yes	No
	Aortic aneurysm	Once in men age 65–75 years who ever smoked	Yes	Maybe	No
	Aspirin use (81 mg)	Initially (age 50–69 for primary cardiovascular disease prevention) if outweighs risk of gastrointestinal bleeding	Yes	Maybe	No
Cancer screening	Breast	Mammogram every 2 years	Yes	Maybe	No
	Colorectal	Fecal immunochemical test (FIT) annually or colonoscopy every 10 years	Yes	Maybe	No
	Cervical	Stop at age 65	No[c]	No	No
	Prostate	Patient preference specific	Maybe	No	No
	Lung	Annually (age 55–80 with 30-pack-year smoking history or quit in past 15 years)	Yes	Maybe	No

[a]Although evidence is limited, these conditions are underdiagnosed and may reveal etiology of impaired function and quality of life.
[b]If vaccinated before age 65 years, should receive one revaccination 5 years from last dose for PPSV23. If no prior vaccination, start with PCV13 and then PPSV23 a year or more after.
[c]If no previous screening or at high risk for cervical cancer (ie, immunosuppressed), discuss with patients about their preference.

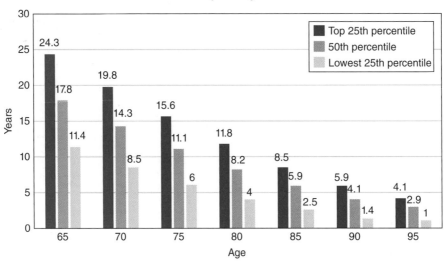

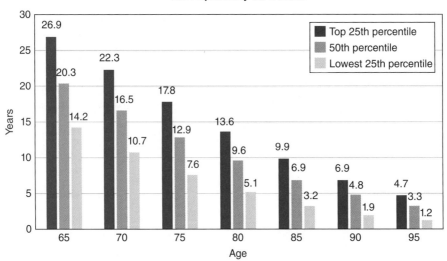

▲ **Figure 20–2.** Life expectancy quartiles by age. (Data from Walter LC, Covinsky KE. Cancer screening in elderly patients: a framework for individualized decision making, *JAMA* 2001 Jun 6;285(21):2750-2756.)

conditions or functional impairment likely will live longer than average (see Chapter 4, "Goals of Care & Consideration of Prognosis") (Figure 20–2). The risk of experiencing the adverse effects of a condition or intervention and the potential benefit from early detection and treatment should be considered in the context of a person's estimated life expectancy. The last component of the framework is to assess how individuals view the importance of these potential harms and benefits and integrate their values and goals into screening decisions.

American Geriatric Society. AGS guidelines & recommendations. www.americangeriatrics.org. Accessed March 15, 2020.

RAND Health Care. Assessing Care of Vulnerable Elders (ACOVE). https://www.rand.org/health-care/projects/acove.html. Accessed March 15, 2020.

US Preventive Services Task Force. http://www.uspreventiveservices taskforce.org/. Accessed March 15, 2020.

Walter LC, Covinsky KE, Cancer screening in elderly patients: a framework for individualized decision making. *JAMA.* 2001;285(21):2750-2756.

GERIATRIC SYNDROMES

Common geriatric conditions (called syndromes to reflect the multifactorial etiologies) include falls, depression, poor nutrition, vision and hearing loss, and cognitive impairment. These conditions are often underrecognized despite causing significant reductions in quality of life and function. Therefore, screening and treatment of these syndromes are recommended in older adults with functional limitations that may be caused by these syndromes. The benefit of screening for many of these syndromes in healthy asymptomatic older adults remains controversial, and screening decisions in this population are driven by patient preferences and values. USPSTF, ACOVE-3, and AGS guidelines are discussed here; see Chapter 2, "Overview of Geriatric Assessment," for a more detailed discussion of geriatric syndromes.

▶ Falls

The USPSTF concludes that there is strong evidence that exercise interventions (eg, gait training, resistance, flexibility, endurance training, and tai chi) and multifactorial interventions (including a comprehensive geriatric assessment of components such as postural blood pressure, gait, vision, medications, and psychological issues) reduce falls among older adults at increased risk for falls. The 2018 USPSTF guideline concluded that there is no net benefit of vitamin D supplementation in preventing falls in older adults, but later clarified that this statement does not include patients with known osteoporosis or vitamin D deficiency. The potential harms of exercise and multifactorial interventions are minimal. There are possible harms of vitamin D supplementation including hypercalcemia, toxicity, and kidney stone formation (due to increased urinary calcium excretion). The most recent AGS consensus statement on fall prevention from 2013 does recommend maintaining serum 25-hydroxyvitamin D concentration to a minimum of 30 ng/mL, but routine laboratory checks are not necessary except in persons at risk of hypercalcemia (eg, advanced renal disease, sarcoidosis, malignancy).

American Geriatrics Society Workgroup on Vitamin D Supplementation for Older Adults. Recommendations abstracted from the American Geriatrics Society consensus statement on vitamin d for prevention of falls and their consequences. *J Am Geriatr Soc.* 2014;62(1):147-152.

US Preventive Services Task Force. Interventions to prevent falls in community-dwelling older adults: US Preventive Services Task Force recommendation statement. *JAMA.* 2018;319(16):1696-1704.

▶ Depression

Depression is not a normal part of aging. It is associated with decreased quality of life, decreased function, and higher mortality. The USPSTF recommendation is to screen and implement treatment if depression screening is positive. The ACOVE-3 guideline also recommends screening at initial primary care evaluation and annually. There are several screening instruments for depression, including the Patient Health Questionnaire (PHQ) and the Geriatric Depression Scale (GDS).

The PHQ-2 is a screening tool that has been validated in adults age 65 years and older (sensitivity 100% and specificity 77%); it asks how many days over the past 2 weeks the patient (1) has been bothered by feeling down, depressed, or hopeless and (2) has had little interest or pleasure in doing things. A similar survey, called the Whooley Questions, asks these questions as yes or no questions based on the past month. If the person answers yes to either of these questions, then a more detailed assessment (eg, PHQ-9 or GDS) along with consideration of other medical explanations (eg, hypothyroidism, medication side effect, substance use, or cognitive impairment) is recommended.

Depression causes high morbidity, especially at the end of life, and a range of effective therapies exist. Treatments, including antidepressants and psychotherapy, are effective in older adults, and in contrast to young adults, antidepressants reduce suicidal behaviors. Supportive counseling and psychotherapy, when available, should be offered. When adding antidepressants, providers should consider pharmacokinetics in older adults and start with a lower dose, choose agents to minimize anticholinergic side effects, and weigh the time to benefit (usually 4–6 weeks) against a person's goals and prognosis.

Bosanquet K, Bailey D, Gilbody S, et al. Diagnostic accuracy of the Whooley Questions for the identification of depression: a diagnostic meta-analysis. *BMJ.* 2015;5(12):e008913.

Kok RM, Reynolds CF. Management of depression in older adults: a review. *JAMA.* 2017;317(20):2114-2122.

Li C, Friedman B, Conwell Y, Fiscella K. Validity of the Patient Health Questionnaire 2 (PHQ-2) in identifying major depression in older people. *J Am Geriatric Soc.* 2007;55(4):596-602.

Siu AL, US Preventive Services Task Force (USPSTF). Screening for depression in adults: US Preventive Services Task Force recommendation statement. *JAMA.* 2016;315(4):380-387.

▶ Nutrition

For the general population, the USPSTF recommends dietary counseling to reduce fats, red meat, and salt, and to increase fruits, vegetables, and grain products containing fiber because these diets are associated with better health outcomes. Counseling can improve dietary behaviors. None of the studies, however, were designed to assess the adverse effects of dietary counseling, especially in chronically ill older adults for whom protein-calorie malnutrition becomes an important concern. For older adults at risk for malnutrition or weight loss, restrictive diets should be avoided. ACOVE-3 recommends assessing weight at each visit for frail older persons to identify undernourishment.

Suboptimal levels of vitamins may be risk factors for chronic disease such as cardiovascular disease, cancer, and osteoporosis. Recent research has focused on vitamin D and calcium supplementation. While guidelines do recommend consuming at least 1000 mg of calcium per day and adequate vitamin D intake (800 IU/day), there is controversy on the role of supplement intake of calcium and the potential risk with cardiovascular events from supplementary calcium intake. Calcium supplements also carry risk of constipation, which can affect an older person's quality of life and add medication burden. It is worth noting that dietary intake of calcium can be achieved through a variety of foods (eg, yogurt, broccoli, kale, tofu, sardines, and almonds).

There is a growing recognition of different trajectories of aging. For the "healthy old," the recommendation is to focus on eating a well-balanced diet (eg, Mediterranean diet). The frail older population, however, may have comorbid conditions that increase their risk of malnutrition, such as history of gastric bypass, celiac disease, small intestinal bacterial overgrowth, and polypharmacy that can affect nutrient absorption. Studies have found associations between frailty and low micronutrient levels (including carotenoids and vitamins C and E), whereas a higher intake of protein was associated with lower frailty risk. For individuals at risk, a single multivitamin should provide adequate levels. For individuals with documented deficiencies, it is reasonable to recommend multivitamin supplements with additional vitamins D_3 and B_{12}.

Dharmarajan TS. Is vitamin supplementation appropriate in the healthy old? *Curr Opin Gastroenterol.* 2015;31(2):143-152.

Fairfield KM, Fletcher RH. Vitamins for chronic disease prevention in adults: scientific review. *JAMA.* 2002;287(23):3116-3126.

Johnson KA, Bernard MA, Funderburg K. Vitamin nutrition in older adults. *Clin Geriatr Med.* 2002;18:773-799.

Lewis JR, Sim M, Daly RM. The vitamin D and calcium controversy: an update. *Curr Opin Rheumatol.* 2019;31(2):91-97.

Lorenzo-López L, Maseda A, de Labra C, Regueiro-Folgueira L, Rodríguez-Villamil JL, Millán-Calenti JC. Nutritional determinants of frailty in older adults: a systematic review. *BMC Geriatr.* 2017;17(1):108.

US Preventive Services Task Force. Behavioral counseling to promote a healthful diet and physical activity for cardiovascular disease prevention in adults without cardiovascular risk factors: US Preventive Services Task Force recommendation statement. *JAMA.* 2017;318(2):167-174.

Vision

Up to 50% of older adults have undetected vision impairment. ACOVE-3 recommends a comprehensive eye exam (including visual acuity, pupillary dilation, intraocular pressure, and retina examination) every 2 years. There is little evidence, however, that screening for vision loss improves functional outcomes or quality of life, and some treatments carry a small risk for serious complications, including acute vision loss.

In most primary care clinics, routine screening is completed with the Snellen eye chart, which can identify impaired visual acuity (defined as best corrected vision worse than 20/50), but does not screen for macular degeneration, cataracts, or glaucoma. There is insufficient evidence for or against screening for these problems in older adults without functional limitations, given little evidence that early treatment improves vision-related function. Therefore, in clinical settings, screening for visual problems is a preference-sensitive decision.

Rowe S, MacLean CH. Quality indicators for the care of vision impairment in vulnerable elders. *J Am Geriatr Soc.* 2007;55(Suppl 2):S450-S456.

US Preventive Services Task Force (USPSTF). Screening for impaired visual acuity in older adults: US Preventive Services Task Force recommendation statement. *JAMA.* 2016;315(9):908-914.

Hearing

ACOVE-3 recommends screening for hearing loss in vulnerable adults during initial evaluation with no specific recommendation on repeat screening. The USPSTF concludes that evidence is lacking for the benefits of screening for hearing loss in asymptomatic individuals. One good-quality randomized trial showed benefit of improved quality of life with immediate hearing aids, but these individuals were symptomatic already. Screening for hearing loss carries little risk, and hearing impairment is a prevalent problem in older persons. Examples of screening include a brief question ("Would you say you have any difficulty hearing?"), finger rub (failure to identify rub in two or more of six trials), or audiometric testing. If a patient wants to pursue amplification, there are effective treatments (hearing aids); therefore, screening for hearing loss is a preference-sensitive decision.

Moyer VA. Screening for hearing loss in older adults: US Preventive Services Task Force recommendation statement. *Ann Intern Med.* 2012;157(9):655-661.

Pacala JT, Yueh B. Hearing deficits in the older patients. *JAMA.* 2012;307:1185-1194.

Cognitive Impairment

The 2014 USPSTF guidelines continue to conclude the current evidence is insufficient to assess the benefits and harms of screening for cognitive impairment. An updated guideline is in progress.

Although some screening tests have good sensitivity to detect cognitive impairment (eg, Mini-Cog, Mini-Mental Status Examination [MMSE], and Montreal Cognitive Assessment [MoCA]), the limited efficacy of therapies (both pharmacologic and behavioral) and the potential distress of being labeled with dementia in face of limited treatment options must be considered. ACOVE-3 recommends an initial cognitive assessment to allow for early implementation of nonpharmacologic interventions and earlier advanced planning, while also recognizing the lack of evidence. Given the risk of harm, the decision to screen an asymptomatic person for cognitive impairment should be preference specific and may include discussion with a caregiver to determine if this is desired by the person. If memory has been raised as a concern by the person or caregiver, then the above tests can be performed as part of an initial diagnostic workup.

Feil DG, MacLean C, Sultzer D. Quality indicators for the care of dementia in vulnerable elders. *J Am Geriatr Soc.* 2007;55(Suppl 2):S293-S301.

Moyer VA. Screening for cognitive impairment in older adults: US Preventive Services Task Force recommendation statement. *Ann Intern Med.* 2014;160(11):791-797.

▶ Elder Abuse

Although the USPSTF guidelines recommend screening for intimate partner violence in women of reproductive age, the evidence for screening for elder abuse or neglect was found insufficient.

The prevalence of elder abuse is estimated to be up to 10%. Definition of abuse includes both intentional actions that cause or increase risk of harm and failure to satisfy an older adult's needs or protect the older adult from harm. Although there is no formal recommendation for screening, there is a need for health care providers to be vigilant to the signs and symptoms of abuse.

National Center on Elder Abuse. https://ncea.acl.gov/. Accessed March 15, 2020.

US Preventive Services Task Force. Screening for intimate partner violence, elder abuse, and abuse of vulnerable adults: US Preventive Services Task Force final recommendation statement. *JAMA.* 2018;320(16):1678-1687.

HEALTH-RELATED BEHAVIORS

The health-related behaviors described in the following sections apply across the age spectrum for adults, tailored to functional and health status. This section recognizes that some tenets of healthy living are universal for persons of all ages.

▶ Exercise

Exercise recommendations are coupled with nutrition recommendations in the 2018 USPSTF guidelines. The national guidelines recommend at least 150 minutes of moderate-intensity or at least 75 minutes of vigorous-intensity physical activity per week. The benefits of as little as 30 minutes per day of walking on most days of the week to prevent coronary

artery disease (CAD), hypertension, diabetes, obesity, and osteoporosis are well established. Although a Cochrane Review of aerobic exercise did not show cognitive benefit (among those without known cognitive impairment), aerobic exercise is recognized as part of the management strategy for those with mild cognitive impairment. A different Cochrane Review of progressive resistance strength training in older adults, including persons who were healthy, frail, or institutionalized, found it improved strength and performance (gait speed and transfer from chair). Resistance training and exercises such as tai chi, dance, and yoga also have been shown to improve balance.

Howe TE, Rochester L, Neil F, Skelton DA, Ballinger C. Exercise for improving balance in older people. *Cochrane Database Syst Rev.* 2011;11:CD004963.

Langa KM, Levine DA. The diagnosis and management of mild cognitive impairment: a clinical review. *JAMA.* 2014;312(23):2551-2561.

Liu CJ, Latham NK. Progressive resistance strength training for improving physical function in older adults. *Cochrane Database Syst Rev.* 2009;3:CD002759.

Young J, Angevaren M, Rusted J, Tabet N. Aerobic exercise to improve cognitive function in older people without known cognitive impairment. *Cochrane Database Syst Rev.* 2015;4:CD005381.

▶ Substance Abuse

Tobacco, alcohol, and drug use have adverse impacts on health and are prevalent in older persons, as well as in younger persons. There is good evidence that even older smokers with low-intensity use (1–10 cigarettes per day) derive benefit from quitting tobacco, including decreased cardiovascular events. The USPSTF recommends asking all adults about tobacco use and providing tobacco cessation interventions if they screen positive. Issues specific to older adults include different pharmacokinetics with aging that may require gentle initiation of pharmacotherapy and inclusion of caregivers in counseling as they may be the source of tobacco. There are limited data to assess the potential use of e-cigarettes as a tobacco cessation tool.

Screening for alcohol use is also recommended by USPSTF, with a similar recommendation for behavioral counseling if the person screens positive for alcohol overuse. Although the prevalence of alcohol use decreases with age, an estimated 38% of people older than age 65 years drink alcohol, of whom 7.6% drink five or more servings a day. Unlike tobacco, there are safe amounts of alcohol consumption. Low-risk consumption is no more than one standard drink per day in people age 65 years and older, although in an individual with cognitive impairment, history of falls, liver disease, or a pattern of substance abuse, there may not be a safe amount. There is also controversy around the potential health benefits (reduction in heart disease, stroke, and possibly dementia) from moderate alcohol intake. Screening tests (eg, CAGE [cutting, annoyance, guilt, eye-opener], Michigan Alcoholism Screening Test–Geriatric Version, and Alcohol Use Disorders Identification Test) have been validated in primary care settings but primarily in younger populations. There also is growing interest in using a new single screening question: "In the past year, have you had any times when you had four or more drinks in one sitting?" (sensitivity 74.3% and specificity 95.6% among people age 65 years and older). The recommended follow-up to a positive screen is counseling and referral to therapy. Treatment resources in the United States can be found at www.samhsa.gov.

The updated 2014 USPSTF statement on illicit drug use screening found insufficient evidence to balance the benefits and harms of screening. Illicit substance use is a growing problem in the United States, although its prevalence remains lower in older adults than in younger adults (12.9% among age 30–34 years vs 1.1% among age 65 years and older). The question, "How many times in the past year have you used an illegal drug or used a prescription medication for nonmedical reasons?" was highly sensitive and specific for detection of a drug use disorder in one study that included participants up to age 82 years.

Inoue-Choi M, Liao LM, Reyes-Guzman C, Hartge P, Caporaso N, Freedman ND. Association of long-term, low-intensity smoking with all-cause and cause-specific mortality in the National Institutes of Health–AARP Diet and Health Study. *JAMA Intern Med.* 2017;177(1):87-95.

McCance-Katz EF, Satterfield J. SBIRT: a key to integrate prevention and treatment of substance abuse in primary care. *Am J Addict.* 2012;21(2):176-177.

Moyer VA. Primary care behavioral interventions to reduce illicit drug and nonmedical pharmaceutical use in children and adolescents: US Preventive Services Task Force recommendation statement. *Ann Intern Med.* 2014;160(9):634-639.

Siu AL, US Preventive Services Task Force. Behavioral and pharmacotherapy interventions for tobacco smoking cessation in adults, including pregnant women: U.S. Preventive Services Task Force recommendation statement. *Ann Intern Med.* 2015;163:622-634.

Smith PC, Schmidt SM, Allensworth-Davies D, Saitz R. A single question screening test for drug use in primary care. *Arch Intern Med.* 2010;170(13):1155-1160.

US Preventive Services Task Force. Screening and behavioral counseling interventions to reduce unhealthy alcohol use in adolescents and adults: US Preventive Services Task Force recommendation statement. *JAMA.* 2018;320(18):1899-1909.

▶ Sexual Health

The USPSTF recommends counseling to reduce sexually transmitted infections (STIs) in adults at increased sexual risk, meaning history of any STI in the past year or multiple sexual partners. STIs among older people are on the rise, including HIV, and assessing a person's sexual behaviors and attitudes is a way to better direct counseling. Assessing sexual health also may reveal psychosocial issues and medication side effects that may have otherwise been missed.

LeFevre ML. Behavioral counseling interventions to prevent sexually transmitted infections: US Preventive Services Task Force recommendation statement. *Ann Intern Med.* 2014;161(12):894-901.

Morton L. Sexuality in the older adult. *Prim Care.* 2017;44(3):429-438.

▶ Sleep

There is growing recognition of the association between sleep disturbances and cognitive impairment. There may be a U-shaped association where short sleep duration (<5 hours) and long sleep duration (>8 or 9 hours) are associated with increased cognitive impairment. The mainstay of treatment is modifying sleep habits, including adding daytime exercise. Evening bright light (between 7 and 9 PM) may negatively affect circadian rhythm. Melatonin maybe helpful, but in general, more studies are needed. Other pharmacologic therapies need to be weighed carefully due to potential harmful side effects in the elderly (including confusion and fall risk). The USPSTF does not recommend screening for sleep apnea among asymptomatic adults, but among those with sleep disorders or symptoms, treatment of sleep apnea can be associated with improved cognitive outcomes.

Feinsilver SH, Hernandez AB. Sleep in the elderly: unanswered questions. *Clin Geriatr Med.* 2017;33(4):579-596.

Yaffe K, Falvey CM, Hoang T. Connections between sleep and cognition in older adults. *Lancet Neurol.* 2014;13(10):1017-1028.

IMMUNIZATIONS

Several vaccinations are widely recommended because they result in net benefit for the majority of older adults. Although vaccination of older adults with moderate or severe acute illness should generally be deferred until the acute illness has improved or resolved, vaccination should not be delayed because of mild respiratory illnesses (with or without fever).

▶ Influenza Vaccines

Vaccination to prevent influenza is particularly important for adults age 65 and older, who are at increased risk for severe complications from influenza, including hospitalization and death. Among community-dwelling adults age 65 years and older, influenza vaccines are generally around 60% effective in preventing influenza. Among older long-term care residents, vaccine effectiveness in preventing influenza may only be 30% to 40%; however, it may be 50% to 60% effective in preventing pneumonia and hospitalization and

80% effective in preventing deaths. The seasonal, high-dose, trivalent inactivated influenza vaccine ("flu shot") is recommended annually for adults age 65 years and older starting in late summer or early fall—as soon as the vaccine is available. High-dose vaccine formulations have shown superior efficacy among older adults in preventing influenza compared with standard-dose formulations. Live, attenuated influenza vaccine ("nasal spray") is not recommended for adults older than age 49 years. Flu shot side effects are typically minor and last <3 days. Because the vaccine comes from highly purified inactivated influenza virus grown in eggs, influenza vaccination is contraindicated in persons with severe egg allergy.

Pneumococcal Vaccines

Two types of pneumococcal vaccines are licensed for use in the United States: the 23-valent pneumococcal polysaccharide vaccine (PPSV23), which represents 60% to 70% of the serotypes that cause invasive disease (eg, pneumonia, bacteremia, and meningitis) in the United States, and the 13-valent pneumococcal conjugate vaccine (PCV13), which contains additional serotypes. Among adults age 65 years and older, the Advisory Committee on Immunization Practices (ACIP) recommends the PCV13 vaccine first, followed by PPSV23 a year or more after receipt of PCV13. Older adults who have already received PPSV23 should receive a dose of PCV13 a year or more after receipt of PPSV23. A one-time PPSV23 revaccination is recommended for those age 65 years and older who received their initial vaccination before age 65, and this should be given a year after PCV13 and 5 or more years after their most recent dose of PPSV23. The two pneumococcal vaccines should not be co-administered. Recommendations are based on best available evidence from immunogenicity studies. The vaccines have rarely been associated with major side effects, although up to half of vaccine recipients will have a mild local reaction that usually persists for <48 hours.

Tetanus/Diphtheria and Tetanus/Diphtheria/Pertussis Vaccines

Cases of tetanus and diphtheria in the United States are rare and mostly occur in unvaccinated people. Pertussis is an acute infectious cough illness that remains endemic in the United States. ACIP recommends a booster dose of tetanus-diphtheria toxoid (Td) vaccine every 10 years for all adults. ACIP also recommends a single dose of the Tdap (tetanus, diphtheria, and acellular pertussis) vaccine be administered in place of one decennial Td booster in adults age 65 years and older. Tdap vaccine is safe to administer regardless of the interval since the most recent Td vaccine. If an adult has never been vaccinated against tetanus, diphtheria, or pertussis, then three doses are required (Tdap followed by Td ≥4 weeks later and another dose of Td 6–12 months later). Local reactions are common after these vaccines, and a nodule may be palpable at the injection site for several weeks.

Herpes Zoster (Shingles) Vaccine

Zoster ("shingles") is a localized painful cutaneous eruption that is caused by reactivation of latent varicella-zoster virus, often decades after initial varicella infection ("chickenpox"). ACIP recommends recombinant zoster vaccine (RZV) (Shingrix) for immunocompetent adults who are age 50 years and older, including those who previously received zoster vaccine live (ZVL) (Zostavax). Following the first dose of RZV, a second dose should be given 2 to 6 months after the first dose. RZV is preferred due to higher efficacy in preventing zoster, reducing the severity and duration of pain, and preventing postherpetic neuralgia. It is stored in the refrigerator and administered intramuscularly. Persons with a history of zoster (not an active episode) should be vaccinated with RZV since zoster can recur. RZV may be used irrespective of prior receipt of the varicella ("chickenpox") vaccine and does not require screening for a history of chickenpox. Serious adverse events are rare, although injection site reactions and myalgias are common. RZV is contraindicated in persons with serious allergies to any component of the vaccine.

Kim DK, Hunter P. Advisory Committee on Immunization Practices recommended immunization schedule for adults aged 19 years or older: United States, 2019. *MMWR Morb Mortal Wkly Rep.* 2019;68:115-118.

ENDOCRINE DISORDERS

Diabetes Mellitus

The USPSTF currently recommends screening for diabetes mellitus in adults aged 40 to 70 years who are overweight or obese. The American Diabetes Association (ADA) advocates screening everyone starting at age 45, or earlier based on risk factors (first-degree relative with diabetes, history of cardiovascular disease, hypertension, high-density lipoprotein [HDL] <35 mg/dL or triglyceride >250 mg/dL, physical inactivity, gestational diabetes, other condition associated with insulin resistance [eg, polycystic ovary syndrome, acanthosis nigricans]). Race and ethnicity can also increase risk for diabetes (eg, African American, Latino, Native American, Asian American, Pacific Islander). Screening can be through hemoglobin A1c (HbA1c) (glycosylated hemoglobin), fasting plasma glucose level, or oral glucose tolerance test. HbA1c has the added benefit of not requiring fasting, although its accuracy is lost if there is a comorbid condition affecting red blood cell turnover. HbA1c cutoff of 5.7% to 6.4% defines prediabetes, and ≥6.5% indicates diabetes. Both the USPSTF and ADA recommend that, if the test is negative for prediabetes, then screening should be repeated every 3 years.

The mainstay of prevention is lifestyle intervention with a goal of achieving and maintaining a 7% loss of initial body weight in obese adults and moderate-intensity physical activity (eg, brisk walking) for at least 150 minutes per week. These recommendations are based on studies such as the Diabetes Prevention Program, where it is worth noting that the oldest participant was age 61 years. Metformin therapy for preventing type 2 diabetes can be considered for those with a body mass index ≥35 kg/m², age <60, and history of gestational diabetes. Although the ADA guidelines do not have a cutoff to stop screening, they do encourage screening for complications including cognitive impairment and individualizing HbA1c goals to a person's overall health (eg, allowing HbA1c goal up to 8.5% for frail older persons). Clinical trials to prevent microvascular complications of diabetes have shown that the lag time to benefit for tight diabetes control is approximately 8 years. For asymptomatic individuals whose life expectancy is less than that, benefits of lowering HbA1c are uncertain. Treatment carries the risk of hypoglycemia and burden of injection. For some persons, quality of life may outweigh any potential benefit of treating asymptomatic diabetes.

Knowler WC, Barrett-Connor E, Fowler SE, et al. Reduction in the incidence of type 2 diabetes with lifestyle intervention or metformin. *N Engl J Med.* 2002;346(6):393-403.

Prevention or delay of type 2 diabetes: standards of medical care in diabetes–2019. American Diabetes Association. *Diabetes Care.* 2018;42(Suppl 1):S29-S33.

Siu AL, on behalf of the US Preventive Services Task Force. Screening for abnormal blood glucose and type 2 diabetes mellitus: U.S. Preventive Services Task Force Recommendation Statement. *Ann Intern Med.* 2015;163:861-868.

▶ Osteoporosis

The USPSTF recommends screening with a dual-energy x-ray absorptiometry (DXA) scan of hip and lumbar spine in women age 65 years and older and indicates that current evidence is insufficient to balance the benefits and harms of screening for osteoporosis in men. There is no clear guideline regarding screening intervals, but the USPSTF statement cites two studies that showed no benefit in repeating tests 4 to 8 years after initial screening. Past guidelines had recommended at least a 2-year gap between repeat DXA scans. Although USPSTF makes no recommendations on testing in men, other organizations have recommended DXA in men based on individual risk assessment or age >70 years. The FRAX score can further predict individual fracture risk. All guidelines emphasize that decisions to treat should be individualized because all current therapies, even calcium supplementation, although effective, do carry some potential risks. Prevention of osteoporotic fractures focuses on fall prevention, nutrition, and exercise (see previous sections).

American College of Physicians. ACP Clinical Practice Guidelines. http://www.acponline.org/clinical_information/guidelines/guidelines/. Accessed March 15, 2020.

Cosman F, de Beur SJ, LeBoff MS, et al. Clinician's guide to prevention and treatment of osteoporosis. *Osteoporos Int.* 2014;25(10):2359-2381.

US Preventive Services Task Force. Screening for osteoporosis to prevent fractures: US Preventive Services Task Force recommendation statement. *JAMA.* 2018;319(24):2521-2531.

CARDIOVASCULAR DISEASE

Cardiovascular disease (CVD) remains the leading cause of death in the United States over the past 75 years. The USPSTF recommends against screening for carotid artery stenosis or screening with resting or exercise electrocardiography (ECG) to prevent CVD events in asymptomatic adults. There is insufficient evidence to assess the benefits and harms for screening for atrial fibrillation or using nontraditional risk factors (eg, ankle-brachial index, high-sensitivity C-reactive protein, or the coronary artery calcium score) to prevent CVD events. Rather, prevention should focus on modifiable risk factors for CVD, including hyperlipidemia, hypertension, and lifestyle choices (see previous section).

▶ Hyperlipidemia

The USPSTF recommends initiating statins in adults aged 40 to 75 years who have one or more CVD risk factors (dyslipidemia, diabetes, hypertension, or smoking) and a calculated 10-year CVD event risk of 10% or greater, and to consider offering a statin if the 10-year CVD event risk is 7.5% to 10%. Adults with a low-density lipoprotein cholesterol level >190 mg/dL or known familial hypercholesterolemia may require statin use regardless of CVD risk. Example risk calculators include the 2013 American College of Cardiology (ACC)/American Heart Association (AHA) atherosclerotic CVD (ASCVD) risk calculator (but with the caveat this may overestimate risk) and the 2008 Framingham risk calculator. The Joint British Society has a 2014 risk calculator (QRISK lifetime cardiovascular risk calculator) that also incorporates the lifetime risk beyond just a 10-year window.

The Framingham equation only includes ages up to 79 years, and it is unclear if risk should be extrapolated to older adults (eg, add additional points for each 5-year category thereafter). There is also a question of a U-shaped curve with regard to total cholesterol (even when adjusted for HDL and CVD) and mortality. Observational studies previously showed an association between low total cholesterol levels and increased risk of mortality in older patients (age >80 years). The PROSPER trial, however, did show benefit of pravastatin in people aged 70 to 82 years for primary prevention of CAD.

In people with known CVD, the pattern of practice is to continue treatment. There is evidence of benefits for statins (even in patients up to age 80 years) to reduce risk of myocardial infarction, stroke, and mortality. For the oldest old and those who are frail, clinicians will need to carefully weigh life expectancy, goals of care, and potential side effects from therapies (eg, undernutrition from diet restrictions, myalgias from statins, and drug-drug interactions).

The USPSTF recommends repeat screening every 5 years. In general, 3 to 5 years of treatment are required to derive benefit from lipid-lowering therapies, suggesting that for individuals with a life expectancy of <3 to 5 years, screening is likely to cause more harm than benefit.

Shah K, Rogers J, Britigan D, Levy C. Clinical inquiries. Should we identify and treat hyperlipidemia in the advanced elderly. *J Fam Pract.* 2006;55(4):356-357.

Shepherd J, Blauw GJ, Murphy MB, et al. Pravastatin in elderly individuals at risk of vascular disease (PROSPER): a randomised controlled trial. *Lancet.* 2002;360:1623-1630.

US Preventive Services Task Force. Statin use for the primary prevention of cardiovascular disease in adults: US Preventive Services Task Force recommendation statement. *JAMA.* 2016;316(19):1997-2007.

Hypertension

The definition for hypertension (HTN) among older adults has received increased focus in recent years. While the original 2003 Joint National Committee on Prevention, Detection, Evaluation, and Treatment of High Blood Pressure (JNC7) had defined HTN as >140/90 mm Hg regardless of age, the 2013 updated JNC8 is more age-specific. Although the definition of HTN for the general population younger than 60 remains ≥140/90 mm Hg, for the general population age 60 and older, the recommendation is to not initiate treatment until blood pressure is ≥150/90 mm Hg. The USPSTF guideline continues to recommend screening for HTN in all adults older than age 18 years, with no special recommendations for those older than age 65 years. Most guidelines recommend at least two to three different office measures taken on at least two different office visits to define HTN. The automated office blood pressure may help reduce white coat HTN as it allows the patient to be in the room alone.

The ideal blood pressure goal remains a moving target. Data from previous observational studies had suggested a U-shaped curve for blood pressure. Sclerotic arteries can cause elevations in systolic blood pressure (SBP), causing "pseudo HTN," and at least one study among men age 85 years and older found SBP >180 mm Hg was associated with greater survival compared to those who had an SBP <130 mm Hg. The landmark Hypertension in the Very Elderly Trial (HYVET) randomized controlled trial, however,

demonstrated benefits of treating HTN to prevent stroke, death, and CAD in generally healthy asymptomatic people age 60 years and older. This study treated to targets of SBP <150 mm Hg and diastolic blood pressure (DBP) <80 mm Hg. One stroke resulting in death or disease was prevented for every 50 people treated over 4.5 years. Death or disease from coronary heart disease was also reduced (number needed to treat = 100 over 4.5 years). Among the very old (age >80 years), the numbers were similar for stroke (absolute risk reduction of 1.8%, with number needed to treat of 56 over 2.2 years), with no decrease in coronary heart disease. The SPRINT study evaluated more intensive blood pressure control (target SBP <120 mm Hg) compared to standard goal (target SBP <140 mm Hg), which further reduced heart failure, death from CVD, and overall mortality, even in the subgroup of participants age 75 and older. There was, however, increased risk of acute renal failure, syncope, hypotension, and electrolyte abnormalities among the intensive treatment group. The SPRINT study was able to show statistically significant differences in their end points at 2 years.

There is clear benefit in treating HTN regardless of age. For patients who are older, but with good health, prognosis, and goals to prolong life, a more intensive treatment goal may be beneficial but needs to be weighed against the potential risks (eg, falls, bradycardia, electrolyte abnormalities, and medication burden).

Beckett NS, Peters R, Fletcher AE, et al. HYVET Study Group. Treatment of hypertension in patients 80 years of age or older. *N Engl J Med.* 2008;358(18):1887-1898.

Satish S, Freeman DH Jr, Ray L, Goodwin JS. The relationship between blood pressure and mortality in the oldest old. *J Am Geriatr Soc.* 2001;49(4):367-374.

Siu AL, on behalf of the US Preventive Services Task Force. Screening for high blood pressure in adults: U.S. Preventive Services Task Force recommendation statement. *Ann Intern Med.* 2015;163:778-789.

The SPRINT Research Group. A randomized trial of intensive versus standard blood-pressure control. *N Engl J Med.* 2015;373:2103-2116.

Abdominal Aortic Aneurysm

In men age 65 to 75 years with a history of tobacco use, the USPSTF recommends a one-time screening for abdominal aortic aneurysm by ultrasound to allow early detection and elective repair. For men who have never smoked, the USPSTF recommends clinicians "selectively offer screening." The USPSTF recommends against screening women who have never smoked and concludes there is insufficient evidence to assess the benefits and harms of screening women age 65 to 75 who have smoked. An abdominal aortic aneurysm diameter of 5.5 cm or more is associated with increased risk of rupture, and interventional management is generally recommended. Both endovascular and open repair carry risks for mortality and may require substantial recovery time.

Therefore, in individuals with multiple chronic conditions or limited life expectancy, the risk of screening and intervention outweighs the benefits of early detection.

LeFevre ML, on behalf of the US Preventive Services Task Force. Screening for abdominal aortic aneurysm: U.S. Preventive Services Task Force recommendation statement. *Ann Intern Med.* 2014;161(4):281-290.

Aspirin

Currently the USPSTF concludes there is insufficient evidence for using aspirin in adults age 70 and older for the primary prevention of CVD and colorectal cancer. For adults age 50 to 59, the USPSTF does recommend initiating low-dose aspirin for primary CVD and colorectal cancer prevention, if they are not at increased risk for bleeding or have a life expectancy >10 years. For adults age 60 to 69, it is an individual decision based on the person's values.

The ASPREE trial was a randomized controlled trial in Australia and the United States that included patients age 70 years or older (or 65 years or older among blacks and Hispanics) who did not have a diagnosis of CVD, dementia, or disability. Participants were randomized to take aspirin 100 mg daily or a placebo. Over a period of 4.7 years, the study found the low-dose aspirin did not significantly lower risk of CVD more than placebo but did significantly increase risk of hemorrhage.

The 2019 ACC guidelines state that "low-dose aspirin should not be administered on a routine basis for primary prevention of ASCVD among adults >70 years." It is important to note that the recommendation for aspirin use for secondary prevention regardless of age has not changed. For frail older adults who may have poor intake and be at increased risk of gastrointestinal bleeding, the possibility of stopping aspirin could be considered together with a larger goals of care discussion.

Arnett DK, Blumenthal RS, Albert MA, et al. 2019 ACC/AHA guideline on the primary prevention of cardiovascular disease: a report of the American College of Cardiology/American Heart Association Task Force on Clinical Practice Guidelines. *J Am Coll Cardiol.* 2019;74(10):e177-e232.

Bibbins-Domingo K, Aspirin use for the primary prevention of cardiovascular disease and colorectal cancer: U.S. Preventive Services Task Force recommendation statement. *Ann Intern Med.* 2016;164:836-845.

McNeil JJ, Nelson MR, Woods RL, et al. Effects of aspirin on all-cause mortality in the healthy elderly. *N Engl J Med.* 2018;379:1519-1528.

CANCER

Breast Cancer

The USPSTF concludes that current evidence is insufficient to assess the balance of benefits and harms of screening mammography in women age 75 years and older because older women were not included in mammography trials. However, indirect evidence suggests that mammography every 2 years is likely to result in net benefit for some older women in good health. For example, older women have a higher absolute risk of dying of breast cancer, mammography is more accurate in older women, and there is no evidence that the benefit of screening ceases at a specific age. Therefore, decisions to stop screening should be individualized based on whether a woman has comorbidities that limit her life expectancy to <10 years and her values and preferences regarding the potential benefits and harms of screening. Women with limited life expectancy are at risk for harms that happen around the time of screening while they have no chance for potential survival benefit, which only happens several years after the actual screening test. Harms of screening include false-positive results that may lead to a cascade of medical testing and psychological distress, as well as the overdetection and overtreatment of inconsequential disease that would never have come to clinical attention had the woman not been screened. Therefore, a screening mammogram is likely to cause net harm and should not be performed in women with a life expectancy of <10 years and in those who place high importance on avoiding the harms of screening.

For all age groups, current evidence is insufficient to assess the additional benefits and harms of magnetic resonance imaging or clinical breast examination beyond mammography for breast cancer screening. In addition, teaching women to perform breast self-examination has been shown to cause net harm and is not recommended at any age. Of course, women should be encouraged to report breast changes or abnormalities they discover to their clinician.

Nelson HD, Cantor A, Humphrey L, et al. Screening for breast cancer: a systematic review to update the 2009 U.S. Preventive Services Task Force Recommendation. Rockville, MD: Agency for Healthcare Research and Quality; 2016 Jan. Report No.: 14-05201-EF-1.

Walter LC, Schonberg MA. Screening mammography in older women: a review. *JAMA.* 2014;311(13):1336-1347.

Colorectal Cancer

The USPSTF recommends colorectal cancer screening in adults age 50 through 75 years, and individualized decision making for adults age 76 through 85 years. It recommends against screening adults older than age 85 years. These cutoffs should be used as general guides rather than applied rigidly. For example, screening is not recommended for persons of any age who have a life expectancy <10 years, and screening may be appropriate for a very healthy 88-year-old person who has never been screened. Advancing age increases the absolute risk of dying of colorectal cancer.

There are multiple acceptable measures of colorectal cancer screening. These tests include high-sensitivity guaiac-based fecal occult blood testing (gFOBT) or fecal immunochemical test (FIT) annually, sigmoidoscopy every 5 years, or colonoscopy every 10 years. Older adults are more likely to have cancer in the right half of the colon, decreasing the sensitivity of sigmoidoscopy, which examines only the left half of the colon. Also, choice of screening test should consider service availability and individual preferences. gFOBT requires dietary and medication restrictions 7 days prior to screening, whereas FIT eliminates the need for these restrictions. Bowel preparations are required prior to sigmoidoscopy and colonoscopy. The standard follow-up of any positive test is a diagnostic colonoscopy, such that people who would never accept or tolerate colonoscopy should not be screened. Risks of colonoscopy increase with age and comorbidity burden. It is estimated that perforation, hemorrhage, or cardiovascular/pulmonary events occur in 26 per 1000 colonoscopies for adults age 65 years and older and in approximately 35 per 1000 colonoscopies for adults age 85 and older.

For all ages, there is insufficient evidence to weigh the potential benefits of computed tomographic colonography against the likely harms of the test. Barium enema is the least sensitive screening test for colorectal cancer and is not recommended for screening.

Day LW, Velayos F. Colorectal cancer screening and surveillance in the elderly: updates and controversies. *Gut Liver.* 2015;9(2):143-151.

Lin JS, Piper MA, Perdue LA, et al. Screening for colorectal cancer: updated evidence report and systematic review for the US Preventive Services Task Force. *JAMA.* 2016;315(23):2576-2594.

Cervical Cancer

The USPSTF recommends against screening for cervical cancer in women older than age 65 years who have had adequate prior screening and are not otherwise at high risk for cervical cancer (eg, women with a history of a high-grade precancerous lesion or cervical cancer, with in utero exposure to diethylstilbestrol, or who are immunocompromised). Older women with adequate prior screening are at extremely low risk for developing cervical cancer, even if they have substantial life expectancy or a new sexual partner. Adequate prior screening is defined as three consecutive negative cytology results (Papanicolaou smears) or two consecutive negative human papillomavirus (HPV) results within 10 years before cessation of screening, with the most recent test occurring within 5 years. Women older than age 65 years who have an inadequate screening history or those who have never been screened should receive screening with cytology every 2 to 5 years, ending at age 70 to 75. Women at any age who have had a hysterectomy with removal of the cervix for a benign condition are not at risk for cervical cancer and should not be screened. Harms of cervical cancer screening include false-positive results. Mucosal atrophy, which is common after menopause, may predispose older women to false-positive cytology and lead to additional testing and invasive diagnostic procedures, such as colposcopy and cervical biopsy, as well as psychological distress. In addition, many precancerous cervical lesions (eg, cervical intraepithelial neoplasia 2) will spontaneously regress such that screening may cause harm through the identification and treatment of inconsequential disease.

For cervical cancer screening in women age 30 to 65 years, HPV testing alone or combined with cytology every 5 years may be a reasonable alternative to cytology every 3 years in women who want to lengthen the screening interval. Women who have received the HPV vaccine should continue routine cervical cancer screening.

US Preventive Services Task Force. Screening for cervical cancer: recommendation statement. *Am Fam Phys.* 2019;99(4):252A-252E.

Prostate Cancer

There is considerable controversy surrounding prostate-specific antigen (PSA) screening for men of all ages because of the lack of conclusive evidence that screening reduces mortality from prostate cancer. All guidelines, however, agree that screening men with a life expectancy <10 years is not recommended because they have little chance for any potential survival benefit. While the USPSTF recommends against PSA screening in men age 70 and older, other organizations suggest screening is preference sensitive in older men in good health who value the small or uncertain benefits of screening over the substantial known harms. Guidelines generally agree that the decision to undergo PSA screening should always be informed. Clinicians should inform men of the potential benefits, limits/gaps in current evidence, and known harms of screening. Harms include false-positive results that may lead to additional testing and prostate biopsies, as well as overdetection and overtreatment of clinically inconsequential prostate cancers that would never have progressed to cause illness in a man's lifetime. In addition, treatment of prostate cancer often results in serious adverse effects in older men (eg, incontinence, impotence, radiation proctitis, or hip fractures).

For all age groups, digital rectal examination is not recommended for prostate cancer screening. Also, there is no evidence that the use of free PSA or PSA density, velocity, or doubling time improves health outcomes, and some of these strategies may increase harm.

US Preventive Services Task Force. Screening for prostate cancer: U.S. Preventive Services Task Force recommendation statement. *JAMA.* 2018;319(18):1901-1913.

Lung Cancer

One randomized trial has shown that low-dose computed tomography screening can reduce lung cancer mortality in current or former smokers age 55 to 74 years with around a

7-year lag time to benefit. However, the potential harms of screening can be substantial. Lung cancer screening among the veteran population resulted in 737 false-positive screening results per lung cancer death prevented. Workup of false-positive screening results may lead to complications from invasive diagnostic procedures, such as bronchoscopy or lung biopsy, which may be greater in older adults. There also is radiation exposure from repeated screenings that may increase the risk of future cancers. The USPSTF recommends annual low-dose computed tomography screening in a narrow population of patients at risk for lung cancer: adults age 55 to 80 years with a 30-pack-year smoking history who smoke or have quit smoking in the past 15 years. No guidelines recommend lung cancer screening in adults with severe lung disease or a life expectancy <10 years. In addition, all lung cancer prevention efforts should encourage smokers to quit.

Moyer VA, Screening for lung cancer: U.S. Preventive Services Task Force recommendation statement. *Ann Intern Med.* 2014;160:330-338.

▶ Other Cancers

The USPSTF recommends against routine screening for pancreatic or ovarian cancer for persons of all ages. There is no evidence that screening for pancreatic cancer (using abdominal palpation, ultrasonography, or serologic markers) or ovarian cancer (using CA-125 or transvaginal ultrasonography) is effective in reducing mortality, and there is potential for significant harm because of the limited accuracy of available screening tests, invasive nature of diagnostic tests, and the poor outcomes of treatment. In addition, although there is no evidence to support total-body skin examinations, clinicians should remain alert for skin lesions with malignant features (eg, rapidly changing lesions and those with asymmetry, border irregularity, or color variability).

US Preventive Services Task Force Guidelines. https://www.uspreventiveservicestaskforce.org/Page/Name/recommendations. Accessed March 15, 2020.

Ethics & Informed Decision Making

21

Krista L. Harrison, PhD

Alexander K. Smith, MD, MS, MPH

Case Vignette Part 1: Introduction and Ethical Tensions

You are in clinic seeing a longstanding patient, an 87-year-old woman with diabetes, congestive heart failure, hypertension, and mild cognitive impairment. She ambulates using a cane. The patient's adult daughter accompanies her on this visit. The daughter lives several towns away, and prior to today had not visited for several months. The daughter reports being shocked at the deteriorating condition of her mother's home. She describes a cluttered house, with trip hazards everywhere and stinking piles of garbage in the kitchen. The patient herself says she has some recent difficulty with her vision, but other than that believes she is doing fine. On examination, her blood pressure is 180/82 mm Hg, and her score on the Montreal Cognitive Assessment (MoCA) is 23/30. Laboratory tests show a HbA1c (glycosylated hemoglobin) of 12.5. A visit by a home nurse confirms the daughter's concerns about the living situation, also noting that the patient's medications have been removed from their bottles and placed together in a jar on the dresser. When you meet the patient next, you explain your concerns about her living situation and ability to care for herself. She responds that she's doing "just fine," and, "I won't move into a nursing home!"

ETHICAL ISSUES IN THE CARE OF OLDER ADULTS

Ethical tensions arise in the everyday care of older adults, where there is a high prevalence of dementia and functional dependence. These tensions require that clinicians be familiar with ethical concepts central to the care of older adults. These concepts are often cast as principles (central guidelines), professional codes (responsibilities of an ethical clinician), and virtues (qualities of the good clinician). Tables 21–1 and 21–2 provide descriptions of the major principles and virtues, with examples of how these might operate in the daily practice of caring for older adults.

As illustrated by this case, a central tension that commonly arises in the care of older adults is between autonomy and nonmaleficence/beneficence. We have a duty to protect those who cannot care for themselves, but also a duty to respect the decisions of those who still have capacity even if they may make choices that put them at some medical risk. Determination of decision-making capacity is the essential first step in such situations.

DECISION-MAKING CAPACITY AND INFORMED DECISION MAKING

Given the burden of cognitive impairment in older adults, determination of decision-making capacity is a critical skill for care of older adults. Capacity is assessed clinically for each decision and does not require specialized input from psychologists or psychiatrists. Such specialized opinions may be sought in particular cases where psychiatric or neuropsychiatric issues are a major concern, but in general most capacity questions should be answerable by generalist clinicians. Competency, in contrast to capacity, is generally based on the patient's ability to provide for food, clothing, and shelter and is a legal status determined by the courts.

Below is an outline of a practical approach to assessing decision-making capacity in older adults. The core features of determining decision-making capacity are as follows:

1. The patient must make a decision.

2. The patient must explain the reasons behind the decision.

3. The decision cannot result from delusions or hallucinations.

4. The patient must demonstrate understanding of the medical situation and the risks, benefits, and alternatives of the decision.

5. The decision must be consistent with the patient's values and preferences over time.

Several features of this strategy for assessing capacity are worth greater explanation. First, decision-making capacity is specific to the decision at hand. Some decisions are relatively

Table 21–1. Ethical principles.

Principle	What This Principle Means	Example Issues and Questions That Illustrate the Ethical Principle in the Context of the Case
Respect for autonomy	Autonomy is Greek for "self-rule." We should respect people's right to shape their own lives and make medical care decisions according to their values. Several ethical concepts follow from this principle, including informed consent, freedom from interference/control by others, and freedom from unwanted bodily intrusion (including surgery or life-sustaining treatment). Advance directives, and surrogate decision makers using substituted judgment are extensions of individual autonomy. Clinicians can enhance patient's autonomy by making sure that clinicians know their patient's goals, values, and preferences, and making sure that patients (or their proxies) understand care options and consequences. *Respect for persons* is a related principle, and includes treating people as worthy of respect, dignity, and compassion, even if they lack the decision-making capacity necessary to form autonomous preferences.	Goals and values discussions—"When you think about where you want to live going forward, what factors are most important to you?" Priority setting—"There are a number of health issues we could discuss today, including your blood pressure management, preventing falls, your diabetes, and home safety. Which of these is most important to discuss today?" Prognostic disclosure—"Would it be helpful to you to talk about how much time you might have left? Would you like someone else to be a part of this discussion?"
Nonmaleficence and beneficence (best interests)	*Nonmaleficence* ("do no harm") and the related concept *beneficence* (promote benefit) as applied to medicine are guidelines that forbid clinicians from providing therapy that on balance does more harm than good, is ineffective, or stems from malicious or selfish acts. Clinicians, as professionals with special training, skills, and knowledge, have a fiduciary duty ("held in trust") to patients to act in their best interests. Clinicians have an obligation to promote well-being of those who cannot look out for themselves.	Balancing harms, risks, and benefits—"It doesn't make sense to aim for really tight blood sugar control anymore—you would be at risk for the harms of low levels like fainting or falling, and you're unlikely to benefit given your health condition." Concern about living environment—"I worry about you continuing to live in your home. I know maintaining your independence is important to you, but if you fall at home or suffer a stroke you will almost certainly end up in a hospital and skilled nursing facility for a long time—things you also want to avoid."
Justice	Clinicians have an obligation to be prudent stewards of scarce health care resources. Reasonable people disagree about how to distribute resources fairly: Does it mean to each according to their needs? According to their preferences and life stage? This also includes the principle that physicians should treat similarly situated patients equally and consistently (eg, attending to implicit bias and discrimination within the overall health care system).	Organizations or insurance programs that use value-based payments or population health strategies (eg, per diem or bundled payments as practiced by accountable care organizations or the Medicare Hospice Benefit), may need to consider the needs and associated costs of one older adult against the overall average costs of the patient panel. Clinicians are increasingly asked to take leadership roles in financial stewardship.

straightforward and simple, such as timing of meals, whereas others are complex, such as the decision about safety in the home illustrated in the case. Second, even a patient with moderate dementia, suggested by a Mini-Mental Status Examination (MMSE) or Montreal Cognitive Assessment (MoCA) score in the teens, may be able to make simple decisions but lack the capacity for complex decisions making. As in the case vignette, tests of mental status such as the MMSE and MoCA may inform a decision but are not determinative. Conversely, a patient with paranoid schizophrenia may have a perfect cognitive test but completely lack capacity for complex decisions. Third, patients may be unable to speak (eg, dysarthria from stroke) yet still be able to participate in decision making by communicating using other methods.

> ## Case Vignette Part 2:
> ## Teach-Back Capacity Assessment
>
> You reiterate your concerns about the home environment. You say to the patient, "To make sure I've done a good job explaining my concerns, can you tell me what I'm worried about?" In her response, she clearly indicates understanding, acknowledging that her home environment is full of fall hazards and that she needs assistance with her medications. However, she reiterates her long-held preference for remaining in her home despite these risks. You decide that she has the capacity to make this decision. She agrees to a family meeting with her daughter and a social worker to discuss how she might receive more support at home.

Table 21–2. Virtues-based ethical concerns.

Virtue	What This Virtue Means	Example in the Context of the Case Vignette
Compassion	An active regard for another's welfare with sympathy, tenderness, and discomfort at suffering.	Caring enough to make time for this patient and her daughter, time to really understand why she so deeply wants to remain at home and fears of institutionalization. Asking if the patient wants to know about her prognosis and respecting preferences.
Discernment	Bringing insight, judgment, and understanding to a clinical situation. "Practical wisdom."	Sorting through the long list of chronic conditions and medications to focus on what is most important to the patient's health and well-being.
Trustworthiness	Essential in medical care where patients place themselves in the doctor's care. Being trustworthy means meriting confidence in one's character and conduct.	Keeping up to date with diabetes guidelines and treatments in older adults so clinical advice is sound. Keeping promises to patients and caregivers, while also acknowledging the limits of those promises.
Truth-telling	Within the bounds of what the patient and family ask to know, being truthful about the patient's diagnosis, prognosis, and expected trajectory of functional independence.	Disclosing the need to report concern about elder neglect to Adult Protective Services. Giving honest (rather than optimistic) assessments of prognosis.
Fidelity	Being faithful to the patient's interests, even if they do not align with the interests of the clinician.	Spending time talking with patients and families even if not reimbursed well. Not ordering remunerative tests that don't help the patient or pose risk.

How much knowledge of the risks and benefits of treatment and the alternatives must a patient demonstrate? The answer to this question has practical implications not only for the clinician's assessment, but also for the amount and manner in which they communicate information to the patient. While the extent of what constitutes an "informed" decision is a subject of some debate, we advocate that clinicians consider the following points when deciding how much information to provide.

1. Be aware of the risks of providing too much information (so-called information dumping). Patients do not need a mini-medical school curriculum to make an informed decision. The major concerns relative to the patient's circumstances should be discussed.

2. Prognosis is a critical component of informed decision making with older adults. Clinicians should routinely offer to discuss prognosis (see Chapter 4, "Goals of Care & Consideration of Prognosis"). It is important to ask permission before discussing prognosis; patients can choose to not learn this information. While many patients would prefer to hear prognostic information, some do not; either way, their preferences should be respected.

3. How information is presented may influence the patient's decision. In one study, for example, participants who were told the risks of a surgical intervention in terms of the likelihood of dying were less likely to choose that intervention than those who were presented the same risks as likelihood of survival. Consider the possibility that how the information is framed may introduce bias and

offer alternative presentations of the risks and benefits to minimize such bias.

4. Disclosure of information is different from informed decision making: what the patient understands or believes may differ from what is disclosed. Check in with the patient about the patient's understanding in a nonjudgmental way, using the teach-back method illustrated in the case.

ADVANCE CARE PLANNING AND ADVANCE DIRECTIVES

Advance care planning is the process of a patient understanding and sharing their goals, values, and preferences for future care, often through with the patient's surrogates, loved ones, and/or clinician. These plans may be codified in official forms called *advance directives* or *living wills*. These official documents may include designation of a surrogate decision maker (see later discussion) and preferences for future care. Physician orders for life-sustaining treatment (POLST) are also used to document patient preferences and are specific medical orders valid across settings (eg, homes, nursing homes, first responders to 911 calls, hospitals). Nearly every state now has or is developing POLST programs. Advance directives and surrogate decision making allow for a form of "extended" autonomy, in that they facilitate making decisions in alignment with what the patient might have wanted after they are no longer able to communicate.

Early excitement about advance directives was blunted by data showing directives were rarely completed and rarely followed. In addition, data showed that surrogates perform no better than chance at anticipating patient preferences. Emphasis has since shifted from completion of the advance directive documents themselves to repeated discussions in preparation for "in-the-moment" decision making by surrogates. This preparation encourages patients to think about their values and goals for future care and communicate these clearly to surrogates and clinicians. Completion of an advance directive may help stimulate these discussions or formalize conclusions, but it is the conversation, not the directive, that should take center stage.

SURROGATE DECISION MAKING

When patients lack capacity, clinicians turn to surrogate decision makers for assistance. The ideal surrogate decision maker is someone selected by the patient, in advance, who has extensive knowledge of the patient's values, preferences, and goals. The legal term for the surrogate varies by state and may be the "health care proxy" in some states and the "durable power of attorney for health care decision making" in others. In some states, the surrogate decision maker, if not designated, is determined by law in a default order (eg, spouse, then adult children, then siblings, then parents, depending on who is available and willing to serve as surrogate). Conservators are court-appointed surrogates.

A general approach to surrogate decision making for incapacitated patients is outlined in Figure 21–1. This approach is generally accepted in the ethics and clinical communities. It is not without controversy, however. The simplicity of the "hierarchical" approach—working first from known and documented patient preferences, or in absence of that information, with the surrogate making decisions in the best interest of the patient—belies some of the ethical complexities encountered in attempting to follow this algorithm in clinical practice. Sulmasy and Snyder argue that the hierarchical approach emphasizes information over empathy, emphasizes documented patient preferences (ultimately unknowable in advance) over values, and places an unfair burden on surrogate decision makers to choose from a menu of options. They argue for a "substituted interests and best judgments" approach in which the surrogate and clinician work together to determine the best course of action based on the patient's values rather than preferences.

BALANCING PROMOTION OF INDEPENDENCE AND PATIENT SAFETY

Case Vignette Part 3: Tension Between Autonomy and Nonmaleficence

After a family meeting with you, a social worker, the patient, and her daughter, the patient enrolls in a Program of All-Inclusive Care for the Elderly (PACE). This PACE program allows her to live at home at night and receive comprehensive service at a day center. A home health aide visits her weekly, and the daughter pays for a housecleaner.

In ordinary care of older adults, clinicians must balance competing demands of autonomy, respect for persons, and promotion of independence on the one hand, and patient safety and best health interests of the older adult on the other. As in the patient case, maximizing a sense of self-control or independence is central to the quality of life of many older adults, including those who reside in the community and institutional settings. In many cases, patients make choices that conflict with the clinician's sense of what is in their best interests—as, for example, in the case, choosing to reside in an unclean and possibly dangerous environment and taking poor care of one's health. This tension is evident in other

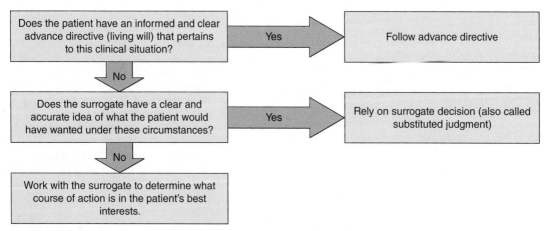

▲ **Figure 21–1.** Hierarchical approach to surrogate decision making for incapacitated patients. (*Note:* If no advance directive or surrogate is available, skip the middle step and act according to the patient's best interests.)

common issues in geriatrics; in preventing falls, for example, there is tension between patient safety and independence.

The clinician's challenge is to work with the patient to maximize independence while minimizing the risk of harms. In this case vignette, a possible solution was to recognize that the underlying value was not a refusal of assistance, but a preference to reside at home. Understanding these preferences allowed the patient, caregiver, and clinical team to come up with a plan to provide supportive services in the form of a PACE program for nursing home–eligible older adults (for more on PACE, see Chapter 25, "Ambulatory Care & Care Coordination"). The clinician in this vignette should have seriously considered reporting a case of elder self-neglect to the appropriate local agency, such as Adult Protective Services (APS), recognizing that clinicians have a duty to report when patients are at risk of being harmed. Like the clinician, these agencies ideally work with the patient to maximize independence and minimize harm. Some clinicians are reluctant to report to APS out of a fear of infringing on the autonomy of their patients. However, as one clinician told us, you do not want to wait to report until after your patient—leaving the stove on—burns down not only her own apartment, but the apartment of the family with young children next door. The risks of neglect are not only to the individual, but to society.

Even when patients have capacity for complex decision making, as in this case, family members and other caregivers often play a strong role in terms of providing and arranging services and helping the patient make decisions. In each case, the physician should look to the patient for guidance as to how involved family should be in these issues. Physicians need to be respectful of older adults who want to maintain independence in decision making, as well as those who prefer a more family-centered decision-making style. For the latter, the physician's duty to promote an informed understanding of the options and consequences of treatments and alternatives extends to the larger family unit.

This case also highlights how professional and virtue ethics work in conjunction with a principles-based approach. The time the clinician spent discussing the issue with the patient and her daughter, deliberating, setting up visiting nurses, and writing referrals to agencies has not historically been reimbursed in proportion to the effort involved. Aligning financial incentives with appropriate clinical behaviors in the best interests of both individual and society pertain to the ethical principle of distributive justice. From an individual perspective, however, the clinician in this case acted out of a sense of caring and fidelity to the patient's interests above their own. This is "good doctoring" and gratifying in its own right.

Ahalt C, Walter LC, Yourman L, Eng C, Perez-Stable EJ, Smith AK. "Knowing is better": preferences of diverse older adults for discussing prognosis. *J Gen Intern Med*. 2011;27(5):568-575.

Beauchamp TL, Childress JF. *Principles of Biomedical Ethics*. 7th ed. New York, NY: Oxford University Press; 2012.

Castillo LS, Williams BA, Hooper SM, Sabatino CP, Weithorn LA, Sudore RL. Lost in translation: the unintended consequences of advance directive law on clinical care. *Ann Intern Med*. 2011;154(2):121-128.

Farrell TW, Widera E, Rosenberg L, et al. AGS position statement: making medical treatment decisions for unbefriended older adults. *J Am Geriatr Soc*. 2017;65:14-15.

Harrison KL, Taylor HA, Merritt MW. Action guide for addressing ethical challenges of resource allocation within community-based healthcare organizations. *J Clin Ethics*. 2018;29(2):124-138.

Lo B. *Resolving Ethical Dilemmas: A Guide for Clinicians*. 4th ed. Baltimore, MD: Lippincott Williams & Wilkins; 2009.

Meier DE, Beresford L. POLST offers next stage in honoring patient preferences. *J Palliat Med*. 2009;12(4):291-295.

National POLST. National POLST Paradigm Program Designations. http://www.polst.org/programs-in-your-state/. Accessed September 30, 2013.

Siegler M. Clinical medical ethics: its history and contributions to American medicine. *J Clin Ethics*. 2019;30(1):17-26.

Smith AK, Williams BA, Lo B. Discussing overall prognosis with the very elderly. *N Engl J Med*. 2011;365(23):2149-2151.

Sudore RL, Fried TR. Redefining the "planning" in advance care planning: preparing for end-of-life decision making. *Ann Intern Med*. 2010;153(4):256-261.

Sudore RL, Lum HD, You JJ, et al. Defining advance care planning for adults: a consensus definition from a multidisciplinary Delphi panel. *J Pain Symptom Manage*. 2017;53(5):821-832.e1.

Sulmasy DP, Snyder L. Substituted interests and best judgments: an integrated model of surrogate decision making. *JAMA*. 2010;304(17):1946-1947.

Tulsky JA. Beyond advance directives: importance of communication skills at the end of life. *JAMA*. 2005;294(3):359-365.

Verma A, Smith AK, Harrison KL, Chodos AH. Ethical challenges in decision making for unrepresented adults: a qualitative study of key stakeholders. *J Am Geriatr Soc*. 2019;67(8):1724-1729.

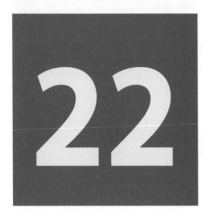

Geriatric Palliative Care

Natalie C. Young, MD
Eric W. Widera, MD

GENERAL PRINCIPLES OF GERIATRIC PALLIATIVE CARE

Most serious illness occurs in adults aged 65 years and older. These illnesses are often characterized by their chronic nature, high prevalence of untreated symptoms, progressive physical and functional decline, and extensive family caregiver needs. Geriatric palliative care integrates the core competencies of these specialized fields of medicine with a goal of improving the care and enhancing the quality of life of these older adults living with serious illness. These competencies include high-quality symptom management, coordination of care, clear communication about medical conditions, matching a patient's goals of care with the appropriate treatments, and family and caregiver support.

Specialty palliative care is provided by an interdisciplinary team including physicians, nurses, social workers, chaplains, and other individuals with expertise in palliative medicine. This model of care is patient and family centered, honoring patient and family values and preferences through a process of shared decision making. It also recognizes and attempts to address the complex multidimensional needs of patients and their families, including social, psychological/emotional, spiritual, and medical aspects (Figure 22–1).

Palliative care can be provided for any serious illness, at any stage, concurrently with life-prolonging treatments and is not prognosis dependent. Studies consistently demonstrate that palliative care can improve outcomes across diverse health care settings, including better pain management, reduced hospital utilization, and greater family satisfaction.

▶ Hospice Care

Hospice care is a form of palliative care for patients with limited life expectancy who meet certain conditions formalized under the Hospice Medicare Benefit. Hospice care provides medical, psychological, and spiritual support to the patient and family at the end of life. Under the Medicare Hospice Benefit, a patient is eligible for hospice care when a patient has an estimated prognosis of 6 months or less if the illness progresses as expected. When enrolling in hospice, the patient's treatment priorities should focus on alleviating symptoms and prioritizing comfort. Older adults with multiple chronic conditions are often not offered hospice even though it might be beneficial, because prognostication is more difficult in this population (see Chapter 4, "Goals of Care & Consideration of Prognosis"). When admitted to hospice, the hospice agency is required to provide services that are reasonable and necessary for management of terminal illness and related conditions, including physician and nursing visits, medications, medical equipment and supplies, and counseling. Hospice care is usually delivered in the patient's home or current place of residence, such as a nursing home or assisted-living community.

CHALLENGES TO PROVIDING PALLIATIVE CARE IN LONG-TERM CARE SETTINGS

Nearly 25% of deaths in the United States occur in nursing homes, and this is projected to increase to 40% by 2030. These deaths are associated with high rates of burdensome treatment and hospitalization, underuse of effective symptom management therapies, and low utilization of hospice and palliative care services. There are numerous challenges to improving end-of-life care in long-term care, including a high prevalence of comorbid conditions among residents, which complicates any diagnostic or therapeutic management plan. Alzheimer disease and other progressive neurodegenerative conditions are common, limiting the ability of residents to report symptoms and making it difficult for health care providers to evaluate for symptoms. Prognostic ambiguity and poor communication between physicians, staff, and family members can delay the transition from a restorative approach to care to one focused on comfort. A lack of physician or

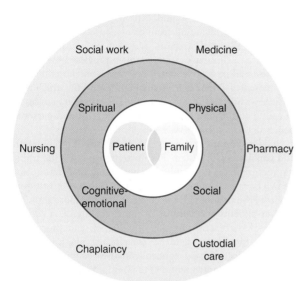

▲ **Figure 22–1.** The interdisciplinary model of care. This figure illustrates how core members of the palliative care team work together to meet the needs of the patient and family.

midlevel providers and limitations to timely diagnostic testing increase the odds that residents will be transferred to an acute care facility instead of being managed in the resident's current setting. High staff turnover decreases the effectiveness of palliative care training among nursing home staff and has been associated with lower quality of care. Additionally, current payment structures prioritize return to higher function and/or transfer of care rather than symptom relief.

While there are limited availability and underutilization of palliative care programs in US nursing homes, this trend is changing. Hospice enrollment for nursing home residents increased from 28% to 40% between 2004 and 2009. Increase in hospice use was associated with a decrease in hospital transfer, decrease in intensive care unit (ICU) utilization in the 30 days before death, decrease in feeding tube use, improved symptom management, and improved family satisfaction. (See Chapter 32, "Nursing Home Care & Rehabilitation," for more information on nursing home care of older adults.)

PSYCHOLOGICAL, SPIRITUAL, AND SOCIAL ISSUES

Patients and families express a wide variety of psychological, spiritual, and social needs during the advent of serious illness. Preserving control and independence, accessing information (eg, regarding disease progression and expectations), managing anxiety and depression, dealing with financial burdens, and spiritual support are frequently cited

concerns. Active collaboration with core members of the palliative care interdisciplinary teams, such as the social worker, chaplain, or nurse, is highly advised to help coordinate care, improve transitions between settings, and address the multidimensional needs of patients and their families. Supporting family members and informal caregivers is also a central focus of high-quality palliative care. Networks of family and friends often provide the bulk of hands-on assistance for sick and frail older adults, particularly those who are community dwelling. Thus, members of these informal care networks often require basic education about how to assist with activities of daily living (ADLs) and instrumental activities of daily living (IADLs), and knowledge of and access to community resources (see Chapter 17, "Caregiving & Caregiving Support").

COMMUNICATION, DECISION MAKING, AND ADVANCE CARE PLANNING

Good communication is critical to ensuring high-quality palliative care. Shared decision making is a process of communication between health care providers and family members that involves:

- A review of the decisions that need to be made
- Exchanging information about patient/family values, the patient's current health status, and the risks and benefits of available treatment options
- Ensuring that all parties understand the information being provided
- A discussion of preferred roles in decision making
- Reaching an agreement about treatment that is congruent with patient/family values and preferences

All pertinent health care preferences and decisions should be documented in advance directives and honored by the attending health professionals. When initiating discussions about advance care planning, it may be helpful for physicians to begin by exploring the patient's priorities in terms of comfort, longevity, and functionality. Because goals and preferences can change over time, these discussions should be considered part of an ongoing dialogue, with revision of advance directives made accordingly (see Chapter 4, "Goals of Care & Consideration of Prognosis"). In the course of caring for someone with a chronic progressive disease like Alzheimer dementia, it is imperative that these discussions occur early on with both patients and their families because a patient's capacity to make health care decisions may diminish over time.

When patients are coping with serious, complex, and life-threatening conditions, it is essential that clinicians prepare themselves to broach difficult topics, including discussion of new life-threatening illness, lack of effective treatment options, or limited prognosis. Involving members of the interdisciplinary team who have expertise in family dynamics and communication skills can facilitate an open discussion of difficult topics and decision making. When delivering bad news, the SPIKES (setup, perception, invitation, knowledge, empathize, summarize, and strategize) model provides a framework to prepare for difficult conversations.

- *Setup*: Find a private space with adequate seating, invite all members of the health team and family, and prepare the interdisciplinary team for some of the difficult questions and emotions that may arise during the meeting.
- *Perception*: Ask what the patient and family already know or what they think is going on.
- *Invitation*: Explore how much information the patient and family need and want.
- *Knowledge*: Provide medical information in clear, easy to understand language; also discuss areas of uncertainty.
- *Empathize*: Acknowledge that this is difficult news to digest and provide space to process emotion.
- *Summarize and strategize*: Review what was discussed, including any decisions that were made, and talk about next steps.

Illness, dying, and death are culturally defined phenomena, and thus, clinicians should be prepared to honor a range of diverse belief systems, which may, in some cases, conflict with conventional practice approaches. For example, discussing prognosis may be considered culturally taboo for some patients, or a shared decision-making process may be preferred over a self-directed approach to care. (See Chapter 4, "Goals of Care & Consideration of Prognosis," for more detailed approaches to communication and advance care planning.)

RESPONDING TO REQUESTS FOR PHYSICIAN-ASSISTED DYING

Physician-assisted dying (PAD) is defined as a physician providing, at the patient's request, a prescription for a lethal dose of medication that the patient can self-administer with the intention of ending life. In recent years, it has become legal in several states, including Oregon, Washington, Vermont, and California. If a patient asks about hastening death, it is helpful to have a structured approach to the conversation. Throughout this process, it is helpful to utilize open-ended questions and to respond empathetically and nonjudgmentally. Start with determining the nature of the request, including exploring if the patient is seeking immediate assistance, considering PAD as a possibility in the future, or using the request as a means to discuss challenges of living with a serious illness. Next, one should attempt to clarify the causes of suffering, which may be related to loss of autonomy, loss of control, uncontrolled symptoms, and fear of being a burden on others. Providers should explore emotional and situational factors, including feelings of depression, guilt, and social and financial stressors that may be contributing to this request. This exploration can help providers work with patients to address these underlying causes and potentially in discussing legal options to hastening their death, which may include withdrawal of certain treatments, voluntary cessation of eating and drinking, and if within the legal and personal beliefs of the clinician, PAD.

It is important to review the state's specific legislation and contact health system administration for specific training requirements if considering prescribing medications for PAD. The most common regimen for PAD that is best studied is secobarbital, although the cost has become more prohibitive for patients and families. Another regimen is a combination of diazepam, digoxin, propranolol, and morphine, although there is less evidence for efficacy. The most common side effect of these regimens is nausea, so it is important to pretreat with antiemetics 30 to 60 minutes prior to ingestion of lethal medication.

▶ Symptom Management

A. Pain

The assessment of pain in older adults begins with patient report. Patient report is the "gold standard" for assessment and should be attempted in all patients independent of cognitive status because those with moderate to severe dementia may be able to communicate the presence and severity of pain. However, self-report alone is often insufficient for individuals with cognitive impairment. It is, therefore, important to use a combination of patient report, caregiver report, and direct observation of the patient to inform a clinical assessment. Verbal descriptor scales, the pain thermometer, or Faces pain scale can be used as alternatives to verbal numeric rating scales or visual analog scales, which may be difficult to use for individuals with diminished cognitive status. Observational signs of distress may include changes in facial expressions, vocalizations, body movements, social interactions, activity patterns, and mental status. Several observational scales have been developed to assess for pain, including the Pain Assessment in Advanced Dementia (PAINAD) and the Pain Assessment Checklist for Seniors with Limited Ability to Communicate (PACSLAC).

The choice of an analgesic medication should be made based on the severity of pain, previous responses to analgesic medications, possible interactions of the analgesic with comorbid conditions or other medications, care setting, and support services. Acetaminophen should be considered the first line of therapy for mild pain, although care should be taken not to exceed a total daily dose of 3 g in most older adults. Acetaminophen should also be considered with new dementia-related behavior changes even when the presence of pain is uncertain, as there is evidence that its use may

Table 22–1. Common opioids and equivalent potency conversions.

Opioid	Oral (mg)	IV (mg)
Morphine	30	10
Hydrocodone	30	–
Oxycodone	20	–
Hydromorphone	7.5	1.5
Fentanyl[a]	–	0.1 mg (100 µg)

[a]A 25 µg/h fentanyl patch is equivalent to approximately 50 mg of oral morphine.

decrease these behaviors, as well as improve activity levels and social engagement. Nonsteroidal anti-inflammatory drugs (NSAIDs) should generally be used with caution in older adults because of the high risk of side effects, such as renal failure, gastrointestinal irritation, and worsening heart failure.

For moderate to severe pain, opioids and adjuvant pain medications such as corticosteroids, antiepileptics, antidepressants, and topical agents, such as capsaicin and lidocaine patches, should be considered. Table 22–1 lists commonly used opioids, with estimated conversions when going from one drug, or route of administration, to another. One opioid that should be avoided for all older adults is meperidine because its metabolites often lead to neuroexcitatory adverse effects such as delirium. In addition, morphine and codeine should be avoided with patients who have a history of renal insufficiency. Long-acting opioids, such as extended-release morphine or transdermal fentanyl patches, are useful when pain is persistent to ensure continuous pain relief throughout the day, with an additional short-acting immediate-release opioid to provide as-needed breakthrough pain relief. An effective and safe dose for a breakthrough opioid is approximately 10% of the total 24-hour standing dose.

Health care providers are often hesitant to use opioids in older adults because of a concern that they may exacerbate comorbid illnesses or precipitate adverse effects such as delirium. However, there is evidence that undertreatment of pain is a greater risk factor for the development of delirium than the use of opioids. In long-term care settings, in particular, the undertreatment of pain is of serious concern. This is partly because when orders are written for PRN (as-needed) pain medications, they are rarely given—not even when there is evidence of patient discomfort. Clinicians should be especially specific when drafting orders for patients in long-term care. For example, to evaluate and treat breakthrough pain, an order might state: "Observe patient every 2 hours. If patient exhibits behaviors consistent with physical discomfort (eg, grimacing, guarding, moaning), administer morphine 5 mg oral solution." or "Ask patient

to rate pain every 2 hours while awake. If patient reports a pain level of 5 or higher on a 0 to 10 scale, administer 5 mg of oral morphine." If opioids are prescribed, constipation should be aggressively managed with a stimulant laxative, such as senna. Methylnaltrexone, a multireceptor antagonist that does not effectively cross the blood–brain barrier, can be given subcutaneously as a second-line agent to reverse refractory opioid-induced constipation. (See Chapter 63, "Persistent Pain," for more detailed approaches to pain management in the older adult.)

B. Dyspnea

Dyspnea is an unpleasant or uncomfortable sensation during breathing. It is a common symptom among older palliative care patients, particularly those with chronic obstructive pulmonary disease, congestive heart failure, end-stage pulmonary disease, and lung cancer. It also is underdiagnosed and undertreated because of the patient's diminished capacity to communicate during advanced illness. Use of the Visual Numeric Scale or the Modified Borg Scale may facilitate assessment and assist with monitoring treatment efficacy.

Treatment focused on the underlying cause of dyspnea is preferred if it is consistent with the resident's goals of care. This may include antibiotics for pneumonia or furosemide for a heart failure exacerbation. There is an increase in the body of evidence supporting use of opioids to relieve the sensation of breathlessness. In opioid-naive patients, it is recommended that clinicians start at low doses of opioids (ie, 2 mg of immediate-release oral morphine) and titrate up as needed to achieve adequate symptom control. Supplemental oxygen often provides significant relief of dyspnea for individuals who are hypoxemic, although there does not seem to be similar benefit in nonhypoxic individuals with life-limiting illness.

Simple environmental changes may help patients breathe easier. For example, directing a bedside fan toward the patient's face and elevating the head of the bed can relieve feelings of breathlessness. Clinicians should note that lengthy discussions with the patient may exacerbate breathlessness. Close-ended questions, providing a nonverbal means of communication (eg, pen and paper), or relying on proxy informants can help reduce the burden of prolonged patient interviews. Shortness of breath may also be linked to anxiety or spiritual distress thus warranting judicious involvement of the interdisciplinary team. (See Chapter 66, "Dyspnea," for more detailed approaches to dyspnea management in the older adult.)

C. Nausea & Vomiting

Nausea and vomiting are prevalent symptoms near the end of life and may result from both disease processes and iatrogenic adverse effects. Identifying the likely cause of nausea is critical to developing an effective therapy. Medication- and constipation-induced nausea should always be considered

Table 22–2. Common causes of nausea and their pharmacologic treatments.

Cause	Preferred Class of Antiemetic	Examples
Gut inflammation	Serotonin receptor antagonist	Ondansetron, granisetron
Toxic/metabolic (including opioid-induced)	Dopamine antagonist	Prochlorperazine, metoclopramide, haloperidol
Chemotherapy	Serotonin receptor antagonist	Ondansetron, granisetron
Malignant bowel obstruction	Dopamine antagonist + glucocorticoids + octreotide	Metoclopramide, haloperidol; dexamethasone; octreotide
Anticipatory	Benzodiazepine	Lorazepam
Constipation	Laxatives	Stimulant (senna, bisacodyl), osmotic (lactulose)
Motion-induced/ labyrinthitis	Anticholinergic	Scopolamine, promethazine
Increased intracranial pressure	Glucocorticoids	Dexamethasone

as possible contributors to nausea. Medications commonly associated with nausea in older populations include opioids, antibiotics, antineoplastic agents, vitamins (zinc, iron), and acetylcholinesterase inhibitors. Antiemetic medications can deliver symptomatic relief for nausea. Different antiemetic medications can be used to target specific neurotransmitters to effectively treat common causes of nausea and vomiting (Table 22–2).

D. Delirium

The approach to delirium for patients with a life-limiting illness is similar to the approach for those who are not at the end of life. However, diagnostic tests and subsequent interventions need to be tailored to an individual's preferences and goals for care. The assessment of delirium at the end of life should focus on consideration of reversible causes, such as pain, adverse medication effect, urine retention, or fecal impaction. Nonpharmacologic strategies to prevent delirium remain important, including frequent reorientation, promoting daytime activity and a quiet nighttime environment, and avoiding agents that may precipitate delirium, including anticholinergic medications. Antipsychotics and benzodiazepines are frequently used to treat delirium at the end of life, but current data suggest that at best they convert a hyperactive delirium into a hypoactive delirium by sedating patients.

E. Grief & Depression

Patients receiving palliative care may exhibit signs of grief or depression; however, it can be difficult to differentiate between the two. Grief is an adaptive, universal, and highly personalized emotional response to the multiple losses that occur at the end of life. This response is often intense early on after a loss, but the impact of grief on daily life generally decreases over time without clinical intervention. Major depression, however, is neither universal nor adaptive, although it is common among persons with advanced illness. Feelings of pervasive hopelessness, helplessness, worthlessness, guilt, lack of pleasure, and suicidal ideation are key in distinguishing depression from grief. Both cognitive therapy and antidepressant medications are effective treatments in reducing distressing symptoms and improving quality of life for those with depression. Clinicians may also consider psychostimulants, such as methylphenidate, for depressed patients with a prognosis of only days to weeks.

F. Fatigue & Somnolence

Fatigue is both underrecognized and poorly treated by physicians, and yet it is considered the most distressing symptom among patients other than pain. Assessment is focused on identifying correctable causes and determining the impact of fatigue on patients and their family members. Common causes include direct effects from the advanced illness and/or its treatments, anemia, hypoxemia, deconditioning, sedating medications, and psychological issues including depression. Trials of moderate exercise have demonstrated significant benefits in patients with cancer. Improvements have been shown to include less fatigue, decreased sleep disturbance, improved functional capacity, and better quality of life. The psychostimulant methylphenidate has some evidence for its effectiveness to treat fatigue in advance illness, although trials have been small. Nondrug treatments, such as prioritizing one's activities, may also be of benefit.

G. Advanced Dementia

Hospice care for individuals with advanced dementia improves patient and caregiver outcomes, including better symptom management, fewer unmet needs, decreased hospitalizations during the last 30 days of life, and higher caregiver satisfaction with end-of-life care, compared to those receiving usual care. Unfortunately, hospice is underused in advanced dementia, in part because of the difficulty of predicting death within 6 months using current hospice eligibility criteria. Hospice should at least be considered for any nursing home patient with advanced dementia who develops a pneumonia, febrile episode, or eating problem, as these are markers of a poor 6-month prognosis (see Chapter 4, "Goals of Care & Consideration of Prognosis").

The onset and progression of eating problems are common in advanced dementia, although they can also be seen earlier in the disease trajectory. When weight loss and eating problems occur in dementia, potentially reversible conditions should be addressed according to the individual's priorities for care. Reversible conditions may include oral issues (eg, dental abscess), depression and other psychiatric comorbidities, constipation, pain, and dry mouth. Medications that commonly cause dry mouth and anorexia include anticholinergics (eg, bladder antispasmodics), antihistamines, antipsychotics, some antidepressants, and cholinesterase inhibitors used in dementia. Sometimes, family members are faced with the decision to administer food and fluids via a percutaneous endoscopic gastrostomy (PEG) tube, often during a hospitalization for pneumonia. There is no evidence that PEG tubes improve survival, prevent aspiration pneumonia, decrease the risk for pressure ulcers, improve patient comfort, or prolong life. Significant harms are associated with the use of PEG tubes in advanced dementia including the likelihood of less caregiver contact during the mealtime and high rates of physical and chemical restraint use to prevent the feeding tube displacement. Alternatives to PEG placement include careful hand feeding and proper oral care. Patients who are imminently dying may require little to no intake in the final days of life.

CARING FOR FAMILY MEMBERS: GRIEF AND BEREAVEMENT

When caring for older patients who are dying, consideration must also be given to the health and well-being of their family members, both before and after the death. Losing someone through death can be an emotionally intense, stressful, and often overwhelming experience, impacting both physical and mental health. The suffering associated with this type of loss is most intense in the first 6 months and is usually associated with feelings of disbelief, yearning, anger, and depressed mood that gradually resolve. Intense distress generally peaks by 6 months into bereavement, but occasional spikes in distress may linger for years beyond the death. Most people successfully cope with their feelings of grief without medical intervention and by relying on their own inner resources, families, friends, spiritual community, and other sources of support. It is also common for family caregivers to feel a pervasive sense of guilt after the death; however, this alone is not an indicator of a pathologic grief response.

For 10% to 20% of bereaved individuals, grief can become complicated, prolonged, and have a significant detrimental impact on their ability to function. Clinicians can recognize and treat complicated grief early on, thereby preventing psychiatric morbidity, suicidal ideation, functional disability, and poor quality of life. The symptoms of complicated or prolonged grief are distinct from normal grief, bereavement-related depression, and anxiety disorders. Key features include unusually intense separation distress with persistent yearning and longing for the deceased, as well as

dysfunctional thoughts, feelings, or behaviors related to the loss. Several psychotherapeutic treatments have been shown to be beneficial including cognitive-behavioral therapy and complicated grief treatment.

A growing body of evidence suggests that aggressive care at the end of life is associated with worse bereavement outcomes for family members. Improving physician communication with families can enhance clinical outcomes for critically ill patients, including decreasing ICU length of stay, lowering the rate of resuscitation attempts, and earlier hospice enrollment. Information about bereavement and counseling resources has been shown to improve family members' bereavement outcomes in terminally ill ICU patients.

Abernethy AP, McDonald CF, Frith PA, et al. Effect of palliative oxygen versus room air in relief of breathlessness in patients with refractory dyspnoea: a double-blind, randomised controlled trial. *Lancet.* 2010;376(9743):784-793.

American Academy of Hospice and Palliative Medicine. Position statement on physician-assisted death. *J Pain Palliat Care Pharmacother.* 2007;21(4):55-57.

Baile WF. SPIKES—A six-step protocol for delivering bad news: application to the patient with cancer. *Oncologist.* 2000;5(4):302-311.

Hall S, Kolliakou A, Petkova H, Froggatt K, Higginson IJ. Interventions for improving palliative care for older people living in nursing care homes. *Cochrane Database Syst Rev.* 2011;3:CD007132.

Hanson LC, Eckert JK, Dobbs D, et al. Symptom experience of dying long-term care residents. *J Am Geriatr Soc.* 2008;56(1):91-98.

Hui D, Frisbee-Hume S, Wilson A, et al. Effect of lorazepam with haloperidol vs haloperidol alone on agitated delirium in patients with advanced cancer receiving palliative care: a randomized clinical trial. *JAMA.* 2017;318(11):1047-1056.

Husebo BS, Ballard C, Sandvik R, Nilsen OB, Aarsland D. Efficacy of treating pain to reduce behavioural disturbances in residents of nursing homes with dementia: cluster randomised clinical trial. *BMJ.* 2011;343:d4065.

Kako J, Morita T, Yamaguchi T, et al. Fan therapy is effective in relieving dyspnea in patients with terminally ill cancer: a parallel-arm, randomized controlled trial. *J Pain Symptom Manage.* 2018;56(4):493-500.

Kehl KA. Moving toward peace: an analysis of the concept of a good death. *Am J Hosp Palliat Med.* 2006;23(4):277-286.

Meier DE, Lim B, Carlson MDA. Raising the standard: palliative care in nursing homes. *Health Aff.* 2010;29(1):136-140.

Mitchell SL, Teno JM, Miller SC, Mor V. A national study of the location of death for older persons with dementia. *J Am Geriatr Soc.* 2005;53(2):299-305.

Mitchell SL, Volicer L, Teno JM, et al. The clinical course of advanced dementia. *N Engl J Med.* 2009;361(16):1529-1538.

Parshall MB, Schwartzstein RM, Adams L, et al. An official American Thoracic Society statement: update on the mechanisms, assessment, and management of dyspnea. *Am J Respir Crit Care Med.* 2012;185(4):435-452.

Shear K, Frank E, Houck PR, Reynolds CF. Treatment of complicated grief: a randomized controlled trial. *JAMA.* 2005;293(21):2601-2608.

Steinhauser KE, Christakis NA, Clipp EC, McNeilly M, McIntyre L, Tulsky JA. Factors considered important at the end of life by patients, family, physicians, and other care providers. *JAMA*. 2000;284(19):2476-2482.

Teno JM, Plotzke M, Miller SC, Gozalo P, Mor V. Changes in Medicare costs with the growth of hospice care in nursing homes. *N Engl J Med*. 2015;372(19):1823-1831.

White DB, Braddock CH, Bereknyei S, Curtis JR. Toward shared decision making at the end of life in intensive care units: opportunities for improvement. *Arch Intern Med*. 2007;167(5):461-467.

USEFUL WEBSITES

Center to Advance Palliative Care (CAPC). www.CAPC.org. Accessed March 22, 2020.

Pain Assessment Checklist for Seniors with Limited Ability to Communicate (PACSLAC). http://www.geriatricpain.org/Content/Assessment/Impaired/Pages/PACSLAC.aspx. Accessed March 22, 2020.

Pain Assessment in Advanced Dementia (PAINAD). https://geriatrictoolkit.missouri.edu/cog/painad.pdf. Accessed March 22, 2020.

Geroscience: The Biology of Aging as a Therapeutic Target

23

John C. Newman, MD, PhD

Jamie N. Justice, PhD

GENERAL PRINCIPLES

The past 30 years have produced a revolution in the scientific understanding of the biologic processes that underlie aging. The mechanisms of aging can be elucidated, categorized, measured, manipulated in the laboratory, and, now, targeted in clinical trials to improve the health of older adults. Why consider aging itself as a therapeutic target? Simply put, aging as a risk factor for disease and disability dwarfs all others on a population level. For a litany of chronic, "age-related diseases," including heart disease, cancer, type 2 diabetes mellitus, and Alzheimer disease, age is by far the dominant risk factor, and with each decade of life over 50 years, the risk increases exponentially. Moreover, the impact of any specific disease pathophysiology is projected through the lens of aging. A broken bone is a temporary inconvenience for a young adult, but a life-changing and often fatal event for a frail older adult. Loss of independence and geriatric syndromes, such as falls, immobility, frailty, and incontinence, are rarely due to a single disease process but rather to the accumulation of physiologic dysfunctions in multiple systems for which biologic aging is the common underlying factor. Treating or preventing any one individual disease without addressing aging can often have only a limited impact, because one disease or problem will be exchanged for another. The practice of geriatric medicine targets aging at a clinical level; now the complementary field of geroscience is emerging to target aging at a biologic level.

The geroscience hypothesis posits that interventions targeting the biology of aging might prevent or delay a wide range of age-related diseases or conditions simultaneously and thus have an outsized effect on preventing disability, dependence, and death. The geroscience hypothesis is currently being tested in clinical trials. These geroscience-informed clinical trials have driven rapid advances in trial design, interventions, and biomarker development, but the underlying science has also spurred the development of unregulated and often harmful pseudomedicine. In this chapter, we will provide a concise overview of the current state of understanding of the biologic mechanisms of aging, a summary of clinical trials testing geroscience interventions, an overview of candidate biomarkers of aging, and practical suggestions for advising patients about purported aging therapies in this emerging field.

BIOLOGIC CAUSES OF HUMAN AGING

Central to the geroscience hypothesis is an emerging understanding of the biological causes of human aging. Years of exploration into how human cells and organs function led to the discovery of a set of unifying mechanisms that explain the aging process, known as hallmarks or pillars of aging (Figure 23–1). These aging mechanisms include:

- Genomic instability and buildup of DNA damage
- Epigenetic alterations, or changes in how genes are turned on or expressed
- Proteostasis and the accumulation of damaged and misfolded proteins
- Changes in pathways that regulate growth, metabolism, and nutrient sensing
- Loss of adult stem cells and ability of cells or tissues to regenerate
- Mitochondria with reduced energy production and greater damaging, oxidative by-products
- Increased maladaptive inflammation and disrupted cell-to-cell communication
- Accumulation of senescent cells that are damaged and highly proinflammatory

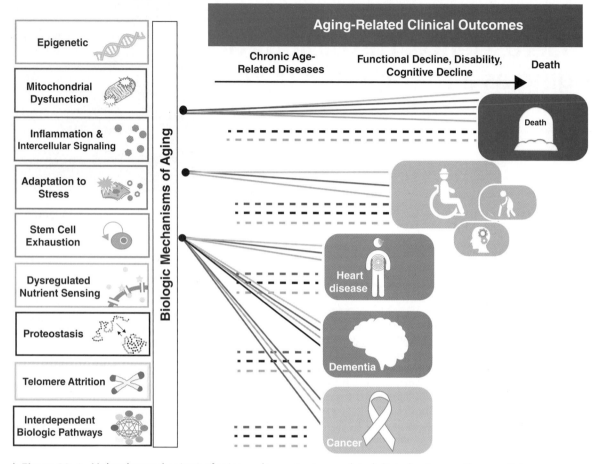

▲ **Figure 23–1.** Molecular mechanisms of aging and important age-related clinical outcomes they mediate.

The mechanisms of aging can be conceptualized in three broad themes (Figure 23–2). First is the random damage that accumulates over time, from misfolded proteins to oxidative membrane damage to DNA mutations. Second are the higher-order consequences of damage, such as mitochondrial dysfunction, loss of stem cells, and accumulation of senescent cells. Third are the endogenous pathways that attempt to repair damage and restore function, for example by recycling misfolded proteins or regenerating new mitochondria. These mechanisms and themes are not independent, but rather are highly interconnected and not easily disentangled. For example, accumulating DNA damage from the oxidative by-products of dysfunctional mitochondria or from telomere attrition can trigger a cell to activate a senescence program. Senescent cells cease cell division to prevent progenitor cells from becoming a cancer but also release proinflammatory factors that can accelerate damage in neighboring cells and contribute to age-related disease.

CLINICAL TRIALS TARGETING AGING

Biologic mechanisms of aging can be readily manipulated in the laboratory to extend lifespan and mitigate the problems of aging in diverse organisms. Some of these interventions have been advanced to humans, and the first geroscience clinical trials targeting mechanisms of aging in patients are underway or already completed.

The current candidate interventions for geroscience clinical trials fall into several categories (described in more detail later). First are drugs that manipulate nutrient signaling pathways related to repair mechanisms in aging. These include metformin, rapamycin, and other target of rapamycin (TOR) inhibitors, nicotinamide adenine dinucleotide (NAD)–related therapies, and ketone body mimetics. The second group of interventions are senolytics, drugs that selectively kill senescent cells. The third group of interventions attempts to replenish or restore the function of stem cells, either by direct administration of stem cells or through modulation of molecular

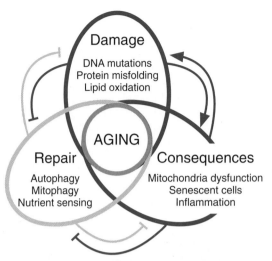

▲ **Figure 23-2.** Mechanisms that regulate aging can be organized into interconnected themes of molecular damage, higher-order consequences of damage, and endogenous repair pathways.

signals that regulate stem cells. The first generation of pharmacologic agents were found by serendipity. Metformin and rapamycin, for example, were already in clinical use for other reasons before their molecular mechanism of action was found to intersect with aging. The next generation of aging-targeting drugs is emerging from high-throughput drug screens (eg, drugs targeting senescent cells) and protein targets subjected to modern methods of drug design (eg, novel TOR inhibitors).

How should interventions that target aging be tested in clinical trials or used in patients? Proving the geroscience hypothesis by delaying or preventing several major diseases or treating a complex syndrome of aging would be transformative. There are two broad frameworks for testing aging interventions, based on the concepts of extending health span and improving resilience (Figure 23–3). Health span refers to the phase of life that is relatively free from disease and morbidity, during which the daily activities and independence of the individual are maintained. Resilience is the ability to respond to and recover from a health stress, returning quickly to the prior level of functioning and independence. Clinical trials designed to extend health span would seek to prevent the gradual or stepwise loss of health and function from accumulating chronic diseases, geriatric syndromes, or mobility and cognitive declines. For example, a nonpharmacologic analog might be a study of an exercise and nutrition program to prevent diabetes, improve cardiovascular risk factors, and enhance mobility. Clinical trials designed to improve resilience would seek to mitigate functional decline or disability after a major health stress. Common nonpharmacologic analogs are studies of periacute geriatric care systems to prevent delirium and functional decline around hospitalization. The primary outcomes of such clinical trials

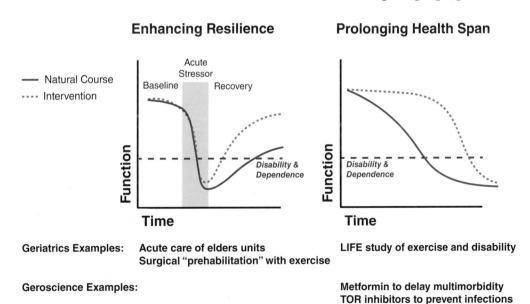

▲ **Figure 23–3.** Two major frameworks for clinical trials, targeting resilience and health span, to test geroscience interventions. TOR, target of rapamycin.

would be broadly representative of aging and might include geriatric syndromes, a composite of chronic diseases, or activities of daily living.

Although the frameworks for geroscience clinical trials would be familiar to geriatrics researchers, many barriers remain to the translation of new interventions. Chronologic "aging" as a US Food and Drug Administration (FDA) disease indication is controversial. Biologic aging processes or clinical manifestations of aging may be more appropriate. None of these have been used as indications yet, although the FDA is exploring sarcopenia and composite endpoints. Studies will also have to establish feasibility and safety specifically in older adults, a population historically excluded from drug trials. Some new drugs are being studied first for narrow disease-specific indications, although they may have broader effects on aging. Other candidate interventions already carry FDA indications and may have a long history of clinical use and a large existing body of clinical data, but require larger, prospective, randomized controlled clinical trials to assess efficacy for major indications related to aging before they can be recommended or marketed for such use.

Geroscience clinical trials have outcomes ranging from frailty and Alzheimer disease to multimorbidity and immune function (Table 23–1).

Table 23–1. Geroscience-guided clinical trials for age-related diseases, clinical conditions, or geriatric syndromes.

Disease or Indication	Intervention	Trial Name	Trial Identifier	Mechanism or Target
Nutrient Signaling Pathways				
Acute kidney injury after cardiac surgery	Calorie restriction (short-term)	Effect of a Preoperative Calorie Restriction on Renal Function After Cardiac Surgery (CR_KCH)	NCT01534364	• Cellular stress resistance • Reduce organ damage
Alzheimer disease	Resveratrol	Resveratrol for Alzheimer disease	NCT03151239	• Activate sirtuins • Lower neuroinflammation
Frailty	Metformin	Metformin for Preventing Frailty in High-Risk Older Adults	NCT02570672	• Activate AMPK • Mitochondria and energetics • Insulin/IGF-1 signaling
Metabolic syndrome	Nicotinamide mononucleotide (NMN)	Effect of NMN on Cardiometabolic Function	NCT03151239	• NAD+ precursor • Energetics
Hypertension, aging	Nicotinamide riboside (NR)	NR for Treating Elevated Systolic Blood Pressure and Arterial Stiffness	NCT03821623	• NAD+ precursor • Energetics
Immune function	Everolimus/BEZ (rapamycin)	Effects of Low-Dose Everolimus and/or BEZ235 on Vaccine Response in Elderly	ACTRN12613001351707	• Inhibit mTOR/TORC1 • Modulate immune system
Multimorbidity	Metformin	Targeting Aging with Metformin (TAME)	[proposed]	• AMPK activation • Mitochondria and energetics • Insulin/IGF-1 signaling
Aging biology	Calorie restriction	Comprehensive Assessment of Long-Term Effects of Reducing Intake of Energy (CALERIE)	NCT00427193	• Body temperature • Resting metabolic rate
Aging biology	Acarbose	Study of Acarbose in Longevity (SAIL)	NCT02953093	• Alter gene expression
Aging biology	Acarbose	Acarbose Antiaging Effects in Geriatric Subjects	NCT02865499	• Alter microbiome
Cellular Senescence & Senescence-Associated Secretory Phenotype (SASP)				
Chronic kidney disease	Fisetin	Inflammation and Stem Cells in Diabetic and Chronic Kidney Disease	NCT03325322	• Clear senescent cells • Lower inflammation
Frailty	Fisetin	Alleviation by Fisetin of Frailty, Inflammation, and Related Measures (AFFIRM-LITE)	NCT03675724	• Clear senescent cells • Lower inflammation

(continued)

Table 23–1. Geroscience-guided clinical trials for age-related diseases, clinical conditions, or geriatric syndromes. (*continued*)

Disease or Indication	Intervention	Trial Name	Trial Identifier	Mechanism or Target
Idiopathic pulmonary fibrosis	Dasatinib + quercetin	IPF Study	NCT02874989	• Lower inflammation and profibrotic factors
Knee osteoarthritis	Injection of Bcl-2/Bcl-XL inhibitor UBX0101	A Safety and Tolerability Study of UBX0101	NCT03513016	• Clear senescent cells • Lower inflammation
Stem cell transplant	Dasatinib + quercetin	Hematopoietic Stem Cell Transplant Survivors Study	NCT02652052	• Clear senescent cells • Lower inflammation
Stem Cell Exhaustion				
Frailty	Longeveron mesenchymal stem cells (LMSCs)	Phase IIb to Evaluate Longeveron Mesenchymal Stem Cells to Treat Aging Frailty	NCT03169231	• Modulate immune response • Regenerative capacity
Frailty	Allogeneic human mesenchymal stem cells (hMSC)	hMSC in Patients with Aging Frailty Via Intravenous Delivery (CRATUS)	NCT02065245	• Modulate immune response • Tissue repair
Other				
Alzheimer disease	Plasma from young donor	The Plasma for Alzheimer Symptom Amelioration (PLASMA) Study (PLASMA)	NCT02256306	• Lower circulating "geronic" factors (growth factors, inflammation)
Muscle atrophy	LY2495655 (myostatin antibody)	A Study of LY2495655 in Older Participants Undergoing Elective Total Hip Replacement	NCT01369511	• Inhibit myostatin
Muscle weakness, falls	LY2495655 (myostatin antibody)	A Study in Older Participants Who Have Fallen and Have Muscle Weakness	NCT01604408	• Inhibit myostatin
Vascular aging	High-dose trehalose	Oral Trehalose Therapy to Reverse Arterial Aging	NCT01575288	• Autophagy activator

AMPK, adenosine monophosphate-activated protein kinase (a nutrient sensor for cellular energy state); IGF, insulin-like growth factor hormone; NAD+, nicotinamide adenine dinucleotide (a key cellular energy metabolite); TOR, target of rapamycin (a nutrient sensor for proteins that controls autophagy).

Notes: Autophagy is a cellular recycling of proteins and organelles. Myostatin is a hormone that inhibits muscle cell growth. Sirtuins are enzymes activated by the cellular energy metabolite NAD+. Activating AMPK, activating sirtuins, inhibiting TOR, and inhibiting IGF all simulate a low-energy state and turn on "repair" pathways such as autophagy while turning off "growth" pathways.

▶ Calorie Restriction

Calorie restriction has been shown to extend healthy lifespan in diverse laboratory animals for almost a century. The CALERIE studies were the first large human randomized controlled trials (RCTs) of dietary restriction in healthy, nonobese, middle-aged adults. A 2-year, 25% calorie reduction intervention resulted in the expected weight loss as well as improvements in cardiometabolic risk factors, body composition, and several quality-of-life measures including mood and sleep. Ancillary analyses are studying the effects of human dietary restriction on various biomarkers of aging. A number of smaller clinical trials are investigating the effects of dietary interventions before major health stressors such as cardiac surgery or chemotherapy, but few results have yet been published.

▶ Rapamycin and TOR Inhibitors

The TOR complex is a molecular nutrient sensor that mediates many of the effects of calorie restriction. While excess dietary protein activates TOR to help build muscle bulk, reduced protein intake inhibits TOR, thereby turning on protein repair mechanisms such as autophagy. Inhibiting TOR extends healthy lifespan in species ranging from yeast to mice. Rapamycin (also known as sirolimus) and everolimus are pharmacologic TOR inhibitors approved for human clinical use at high doses as immunosuppressants in solid organ transplantation. Healthy older adults given a much lower dose of everolimus for 6 weeks showed an improved immunologic response to influenza vaccination in a RCT. A subsequent RCT found that 6 weeks of low-dose everolimus plus a second TOR inhibitor improved vaccine response and, provocatively, reduced infection rates by over one-third during the subsequent 9 months. These were two of the first examples of clinical trials targeting a syndrome of aging—immunosenescence—with a drug based on mechanisms of aging.

Metformin

The diabetes drug metformin was found to affect molecular mechanisms of aging including mitochondrial function and insulin signaling only long after its clinical introduction. Although lifespan effects are relatively modest in mouse studies, the effects on health are substantial, with improvements on tests of physical and cognitive function, cataracts, and insulin tolerance. In randomized trials, metformin prevented the onset of diabetes, improved cardiovascular risk factors, and reduced mortality. Epidemiologic studies have suggested that metformin use might reduce the incidence of cancer and neurodegenerative disease. Altogether, these molecular and clinical data suggest that metformin may have broad effects on aging aside from its effects on glycemic control. The Targeting Aging with Metformin (TAME) trial is a 6-year, double-blind, placebo-controlled, multicenter clinical trial to test if metformin slows multimorbidity. The primary outcome of TAME will be a composite of cardiovascular disease, cancer, dementia, and cognitive impairment. TAME will enroll older adults age 65 to 80 years at risk for major age-related diseases based on reduced gait speed or one prevalent major disease. The study will collect extensive secondary data on mobility, cognitive function, daily function, and potential biomarkers of aging. TAME will directly test the geroscience hypothesis. If successful, it will provide proof-of-concept for targeting aging mechanisms, as well as a template that other studies can follow for pursuing FDA indications related to aging.

NAD+ and Sirtuins

NAD+ is a normal cellular metabolite that also acts as a cofactor for the NAD-dependent sirtuin enzymes and whose abundance declines with aging. Various interventions attempt to replenish NAD+ levels, inhibit NAD-consuming enzymes, or activate sirtuins. Clinical studies of the former two strategies are at very early stages, while initial clinical studies of sirtuin activators suggest promise for managing cardiovascular risk factors.

Senolytics

Senolytics are drugs that selectively kill senescent cells. Senescence is an anticancer program in which a damaged cell shuts down its ability to divide but also releases inflammatory factors that can damage nearby cells and accelerate aging

phenotypes. A number of senolytics have been identified by high-throughput screening or by targeting unique aspects of senescent cell biology. Some are novel, and some are FDA approved for other uses. Late life intervention with senolytics in mice delays age-related functional decline and extends lifespan. Early clinical trials of senolytic drugs are targeting specific conditions to which senescent cells are thought to contribute, including idiopathic pulmonary fibrosis, knee osteoarthritis, and frailty.

Stem Cell Interventions

Several interventions seek to replenish or restore the function of stem cells, either by direct administration of stem cells or through modulation of molecular signals that regulate specific stem cell populations, such as myostatin inhibitors. Clinical trials have begun to study mesenchymal stem cell infusions as a treatment for frailty and mobility decline and myostatin inhibitors as a treatment for sarcopenia.

Barzilai N, Cuervo AM, Austad S. Aging as a biological target for prevention and therapy. *JAMA*. 2018;320(13):1321-1322.

Goldman DP, Cutler D, Rowe JW, et al. Substantial health and economic returns from delayed aging may warrant a new focus for medical research. *Health Aff (Millwood)*. 2013;32(10):1698-1705.

Justice J, Miller JD, Newman JC, et al. Frameworks for proof-of-concept clinical trials of interventions that target fundamental aging processes. *J Gerontol A Biol Sci Med Sci*. 2016;71(11):1415-1423.

Kaeberlein M, Rabinovitch PS, Martin GM. Healthy aging: The ultimate preventative medicine. *Science*. 2015;350(6265):1191-1193.

Kennedy BK, Berger SL, Brunet A, et al. Geroscience: linking aging to chronic disease. *Cell*. 2014;159(4):709-713.

López-Otín C, Blasco MA, Partridge L, Serrano M, Kroemer G. The hallmarks of aging. *Cell*. 2013;153(6):1194-1217.

Newman JC, Milman S, Hashmi SK, et al. Strategies and challenges in clinical trials targeting human aging. *J Gerontol A Biol Sci Med Sci*. 2016;71(11):1424-1434.

BIOMARKERS OF THE BIOLOGY OF AGING

Biomarkers of aging would support clinical monitoring, drug development, and clinical trials research for interventions that target the biology of aging by evaluating patient risk for aging-related outcomes and intervention efficacy. No consensus, validated set of biomarkers of biologic aging currently exist, although substantial research is underway to develop such markers. Biomarkers must do more than predict chronologic age. Clinically useful biomarkers of aging must have strong measurement reliability and feasibility, have relevance to aging mechanisms, be responsive to interventions, and have a robust and consistent ability to predict all-cause mortality and clinical and functional outcomes. Importantly, biomarkers must add power to widely used methods of assessing aging-related risk, such as frailty measures, functional assessment, and chronologic age.

Based on current evidence, the strongest candidate biomarkers for use in clinical trials include markers of inflammation (eg, interleukin-6, tumor necrosis factor-α receptor, C-reactive protein), stress response/mitochondrial health (growth differentiation factor 15), nutrient sensing (eg, insulin, insulin growth factor 1), and metabolic, cardiovascular, and kidney health (eg, hemoglobin A1c, N-terminal pro–brain natriuretic peptide, cystatin C). One investigational approach is to combine a variety of individual biomarkers into a composite marker normalized to population age-related changes. This approach demonstrated a pausing of biomarker-measured aging in a recent RCT of dietary restriction in healthy adults. Telomere length measurement is widely available but has limited evidence for clinical applicability in part due to wide individual variability. An emerging biomarker is the epigenetic clock, based on observations that patterns of DNA methylation change with age. Early studies of the epigenetic clock suggest strong predictive power for aging-related outcomes among populations. New biomarkers are being developed to assay individual aging mechanisms such as mitochondrial function or senescent cell burden.

Much like the clinical metrics now used to estimate prognosis or aging-related risk, clinically useful biomarkers of aging will likely incorporate many biologic variables, perhaps representing a number of the molecular mechanisms of aging. High-throughput "omics" technologies that measure many things at once, including genome-wide methylation patterns, transcriptomics (genes that are transcribed), proteomics (proteins that are synthesized), and metabolomics (small molecules manipulated by cellular enzymes) can comprehensively assess the interconnected pathways and molecular networks associated with aging. Investigational biomarkers of aging do not yet have validated clinical uses but are appropriate for incorporation into research studies including studies of clinical decision making based on aging-related risk.

Justice JN, Ferrucci L, Newman AB, et al. A framework for selection of blood-based biomarkers for geroscience-guided clinical trials: report from the TAME Biomarkers Workgroup. *Geroscience*. 2018;40(5-6):419-436.

DEBUNKING AGING THERAPEUTICS

Geroscience has emerged as a serious biomedical research discipline, but it exists uneasily in a sea of "antiaging" pseudomedicine and junk science. Supplement peddlers and beauty shops offer the secret ingredients to defy aging, and disreputable clinics will promise drugs and procedures available only to the select few. Some are nonsense, some have a tenuous link to promising science, none are based on rigorous clinical evidence, and many are harmful.

Dietary Supplements

There is no evidence that high doses of any vitamins or other supplements treat the problems of aging. Although oxidative damage is one of the mechanisms that drives aging, studies in animals have failed to show efficacy for antioxidants. Therapies that activate repair mechanisms have proven more promising. Large human studies have also failed to show efficacy for antioxidants, and there is evidence that some vitamins can be harmful in excessive doses or inappropriate contexts. Supplementation with vitamin E, vitamin A, or β-carotene is associated with increased mortality in meta-analyses due to cardiovascular events and lung cancer.

The link between nutrient sensing, metabolites, and aging mechanisms involves endogenous molecules like NAD+ and ketone bodies, which can lead to proposed interventions that straddle the boundary between drug and dietary supplement. In some cases, compounds are available for sale as lightly regulated dietary supplements while simultaneously being studied in clinical trials. In other cases, natural compounds have been identified in laboratory drug screens based on mechanisms of aging but are available for sale far ahead of any human scientific validation or even appropriate safety studies. There have been examples of dietary supplements that were eventually formulated as FDA-approved drugs, such as omega-3 fatty acids and niacin. Some dietary supplements that purport to affect aging may be grounded in promising science, but none yet have any demonstrated clinical utility in humans and many lack basic safety data.

Hormone Replacement

Many hormone levels decline with age, but these represent consequences rather than causes of aging, and in many cases, the decline may be adaptive. The clearest example that restoring youthful hormone levels can be harmful comes from large RCTs of estrogen/progesterone replacement in postmenopausal women. The US Preventive Services Task Force recommends against the use of estrogen/progesterone (or estrogen in women who have had a hysterectomy) for the treatment of chronic conditions, due to the risks of invasive breast cancer, coronary heart disease, and venous thromboembolism. Testosterone use in aging men is deeply controversial, with possible benefits on quality-of-life measures balanced against likely increased cardiovascular risk and risk of prostate cancer. The recent Testosterone Trials were limited to 1 year and could not sufficiently define long-term risks of chronic use. Estrogen/progesterone and testosterone therapies can be the subject of a careful and individualized risk-benefit discussion in certain contexts but are adamantly not treatments for aging.

Other anabolic hormones such as growth hormone (GH) and insulin-like growth factor (IGF) are associated with aging, but negatively. Animal studies of genetic and pharmacologic manipulation of these hormones clearly show that lower activity through the GH/IGF axis extends healthy lifespan. In fact, some of the earliest rodent models of extended longevity were the Ames and Snell dwarf mice that carry spontaneous mutations preventing GH production. Short-term clinical trials of GH therapy show small improvements in body composition but uncertain effects on strength and increased adverse events including glucose intolerance. Conversely, human mutations that reduce signaling through the GH/IGF axis appear to be more common in centenarians, and an antibody that blocks the IGF receptor is being studied as a therapy for aging-related conditions. Growth hormone supplementation has no role as a therapy for aging.

Stem Cell Procedures

Aside from bone marrow or umbilical cord blood transplants for certain cancers and hematologic diseases, there are no legitimate stem cell therapies in clinical use. In 2017, the FDA brought purported stem cell therapies under increased scrutiny following the proliferation of unregulated clinics and reports of serious harm. Stem cells and stem cell–modulating drugs remain an active and promising area of research. There is an increasing understanding of why stem cells age, the role of the systemic aging environment, methods for creating induced pluripotent stem cells (iPSCs) from human skin cells, and methods for differentiating iPSCs into many different types of tissue. Clinical trials are ongoing at reputable academic centers around the world for applications ranging from macular degeneration and Parkinson disease to frailty. These rigorous research studies using carefully regulated materials and methods are a world apart from "stem cell clinics," and much work remains to be done to see if stem cell therapies will prove clinically useful.

Young Blood Transfusions

The exposure of young animals to old blood, and vice versa, is a laboratory technique that helped show that while part of aging is intrinsic to a cell or tissue, part is also imposed by the aged systemic milieu. If factors circulating in blood can be identified that either promote or prevent aging in other tissues of the body, they could become promising drug targets. All such factors so far proposed remain controversial. In the meantime, this science has led to controversial clinical trials of blood product transfusions to treat diseases of aging and disreputable attempts to sell blood products from young adults as "antiaging" treatments. Like unregulated "stem cell" procedures, blood product transfusions carry real risk of harm. There is no evidence for using blood products outside of a research context for these purposes. The ever-tightening clinical guidelines for blood product transfusion, based on

an increasing understanding of latent harms, should strongly caution against their use outside of clinical norms.

Hellmuth J, Rabinovici GD, Miller BL. The rise of pseudomedicine for dementia and brain health. *JAMA*. 2019;321(6):543-544.

Junnila RK, List EO, Berryman DE, Murrey JW, Kopchick JJ. The GH/IGF-1 axis in ageing and longevity. *Nat Rev Endocrinol*. 2013;9(6):366-376.

Marks PW, Witten CM, Califf RM. Clarifying stem-cell therapy's benefits and risks. *N Engl J Med*. 2017;376(11):1007-1009.

Nguyen CP, Hirsch MS, Moeny D, Kaul S, Mohamoud M, Joffe HV. Testosterone and "age-related hypogonadism": FDA concerns. *N Engl J Med*. 2015;373(8):689-691.

EVIDENCE-BASED HEALTHY AGING

While many interventions that target mechanisms of aging are under study, unproven, or implausible, one intervention has abundant, rigorous, high-quality evidence: exercise. Exercise and physical activity improve mobility and quality of life, can help prevent diabetes, may slow the onset of other chronic diseases, is the most important intervention to reduce aging-related risk from surgery and chemotherapy, and is the key to maintaining mobility and independence during a hospitalization. There is no minimum effective dose for physical activity, nor any age limit. Strategies for encouraging appropriate exercise for older adults are detailed in Chapter 72.

Nutrition is closely intertwined with mechanisms of aging, but nutrition is a complex subject. There is no ideal diet for aging or panacean superfood. Healthy nutrition can strongly affect age-related syndromes such as metabolic syndrome, sarcopenia, and even dementia. Nutritional interventions such as calorie restriction that are designed to modulate aging mechanisms are being studied in clinical trials as described earlier and in Table 23–1. However, basic nutritional adequacy is often an even more pressing concern for older adults, as described in Chapter 13.

Other interventions with strong evidence for improving or preventing age-related conditions include vaccines, managing cardiovascular and metabolic risk factors, effective management of chronic diseases, strong social connections, restful sleep, and healthy nutrition (see Chapter 20). A leading-edge area of research is elucidating the biologic mechanisms that underlie lifestyle interventions, such as sleep, exercise, and social connections. Aside from guiding the care of individual patients, these interventions also have powerful public policy implications. Enabling people and communities to live active lives with strong social connections, access to healthy food, and access to medical care can all help delay or manage the problems of aging on a societal scale while we await new cutting-edge geroscience interventions.

Applying Evidence-Based Care to Older Persons

24

Lauren J. Gleason, MD, MPH
Kenneth E. Covinsky, MD, MPH

Ideally, the care of older persons should be grounded in the best available evidence about the benefits and harms of treatments. Unfortunately, high-quality evidence rarely exists. Good studies of a clinical condition often exclude older persons. Even when older persons are included, enrollment tends to be limited to healthy robust older persons who may little resemble the patient in front of you.

As a result, one can rarely practice true evidence-based medicine in older persons. Instead, one needs to examine available evidence and then critically assess the extent to which the evidence might apply to the patient being treated. To best make optimal clinical decisions, clinicians need to understand the limitations of applying the clinical research literature to their older persons and thoughtfully apply existing evidence to the individual patient they are treating.

THE CHALLENGES WITH CURRENT EVIDENCE

Clinicians are generally trained to consider outcomes from clinical trials as the gold standard for how to apply evidence-based medicine to clinical care. Ideally, clinical trials would include any patient who is a logical candidate for the therapy being examined regardless of age. Unfortunately, most clinical trials exclude patients for whom the therapy has a greater risk of side effects or patients who are at risk for not completing the trial. Study subjects excluded from clinical research represent a large proportion of patients seen in geriatric practice and often end up being the target population for the therapies being studied.

Zulman and colleagues have described a framework that outlines the reasons older persons may be excluded from clinical trials. These reasons include explicit age exclusions, implicit age exclusions, and unintentional age exclusions.

▶ Explicit Age Exclusions

Many studies have age-specific cutoffs in which all subjects above a defined age are excluded. Although these exclusions

are common, they can almost never be justified. An example of age restriction can be seen in analysis of representation of older persons in phase III clinical trials (last step required for the process of US Food and Drug Administration approval). Of the top conditions that caused hospitalizations and/or disability-adjusted life-years in older adults from 1965 to 2015, 33% had arbitrary upper age limits, and 67% reported on subjects younger than those typically afflicted by these conditions. Most studies with explicit age exclusions present absolutely no rationale to justify the exclusion.

An explicit age exclusion is only justifiable if one clearly would not offer a therapy in clinical practice to persons older than a particular age. In actual practice, most therapies tested in younger patients are eventually offered to older persons. Furthermore, explicit age exclusions ignore the vast heterogeneity in health in older persons.

▶ Implicit Age Exclusions

More often, the reasons for excluding older subjects are more subtle. Many studies without an age cutoff have exclusion criteria that differentially restrict the entry of older patients, particularly older persons who are more medically complex. Examples of implicit age exclusions include comorbidity/polypharmacy, functional impairments, cognitive impairments, and inability to give informed consent.

A. Comorbidity/Polypharmacy

Treatment studies often focus on the effect of a specific treatment on health outcomes in persons with a single condition. However, most older persons have multiple conditions (comorbidity) and are treated with multiple medications (polypharmacy). Yet many studies exclude older persons with additional health conditions other than the condition being studied. For example, a study comparing the effectiveness of bronchodilator and anticholinergic inhalers for chronic obstructive pulmonary disease (COPD) excluded persons with chronic kidney disease or hospitalizations for congestive heart failure (CHF) in the past year. This is very problematic in older persons, as many older persons with COPD have coexisting chronic kidney disease or CHF. In actual practice, comorbidity is the norm, not the exception, and most treatments are still offered to older persons despite this comorbidity. It is difficult to judge the risk and benefits of treatments studied in idealized patients when applied to real patients with complex comorbidity.

B. Functional Impairment

Many studies exclude patients with "poor performance status" or poor functional status. Although there are many simple tools available to define functional status, often studies do not include a definition of poor functional status.

Many older persons have functional limitations and, in practice, these are rarely viewed as contraindications for most therapies. Often, the goal of therapy for older persons may be to improve function or prevent further loss of function. However, functional problems, such as falls, can markedly alter the risk and benefits of therapies. The failure to account for functional impairments as a variable in analysis of most studies makes it difficult to gauge how a patient's functional impairments should affect the decision to offer a treatment. It also makes it difficult to properly weigh how different patients prioritize function, independence, and quality of life over duration of life.

C. Cognitive Impairment & Inability to Consent

Studies often exclude subjects who have cognitive impairment or are unable to provide informed consent. Often, the studies fail to describe how cognitive impairment or consent capacity was assessed.

Cognitive impairment is extremely common in older persons, and individuals with cognitive impairment are usually offered the same therapies as patients without cognitive impairment. Because most studies fail to even describe the cognitive status of their subjects, it is often impossible to know how cognitive impairment might impact the risks and benefits of a treatment. Additionally, in clinical practice, family members are often asked to consent to treatments when the patient is unable to fully understand the risks and benefits. While methods exist for enrolling these patients in studies using similar approaches for surrogate consent, surrogate consent is often not attempted.

D. Nursing Home Patients

Virtually all treatments offered in the community are offered to persons in nursing homes. It is extraordinarily rare to find a study of any therapy that even considers nursing home patients as candidates for enrollment. As a result, there is a lack of evidence to guide the most therapeutic decisions in nursing home patients.

▶ Unintentional Exclusions

Even when studies have few exclusion criteria, study processes may unintentionally exclude older persons who are potential targets for therapy. For example, many studies have complex procedures for follow-up. Follow-up procedures often require patients to report to a study center for examinations and blood draws. Many older persons no longer drive, making participation in follow-up procedures difficult. This type of subtle exclusion is important because the same factors that make study follow-up difficult may make necessary monitoring and follow-up difficult in less mobile older persons being considered for treatment. Sensory impairment may also make study enrollment and follow-up difficult for older persons. For example, older persons with hearing impairment may be excluded from studies that screen enrollees over the phone or require answers to phone-based health status questionnaires. Many studies do not budget the extra cost needed for in-person interviews for older participants who are hard of hearing.

Lastly, many researchers might not have experience in caring for older persons. Bowling and colleagues describe the **5Ts Framework** to address barriers to participation by investigators and staff with limited experience in aging research. The framework describes maximizing generalizability by enrolling participants from the **t**arget population, building **t**eams that include geriatrics and gerontology expertise, incorporating appropriate **t**ools to measure function- and patient-reported outcomes, anticipating **t**ime for longer study visits, and accommodating older participants with comorbidities by following practical **t**ips (Table 24–1).

APPLYING THE EVIDENCE TO OLDER PERSONS

Applying evidence from clinical research to an individual patient can be difficult. However, addressing a series of questions can help a clinician make the best possible inference about how existing evidence might inform the best clinical decision in their patient. In addition to addressing whether patients in existing studies are similar to your patient, one should also think about what outcomes matter to your patient and whether limited life expectancy might affect the risks and benefits of the treatment in question.

▶ New Ongoing Initiatives

National Institutes of Health (NIH) adopted the Inclusion across the Lifespan Policy on January 25, 2019. This policy was developed in response to requirements in the 21st Century Cures Act, mandating inclusion of older persons into all NIH-supported research involving human subjects. This policy requires investigators on grant applications or proposals to submit a plan for including individuals across the lifespan in clinical research and to provide rationale and justification

Table 24–1. Using the 5Ts Framework to address research challenges with older persons.

Domain	Description	Example Recommendations to Address Challenges
Target population	"At risk" or "real-world" population	• Avoid exclusions that limit study generalizability • Understand the prevalence of the studied condition in older adults
Team	Research team, family, informal caregivers	• Engage geriatrician researchers and aging experts • Connect with caregivers and community resources
Tools	Measurement tools used in aging research	• Choose appropriate measures of function, physical performance, patient-reported outcomes, and the like • Balance data collection needs and participant burden
Time	Participant and study time	• Anticipate longer study visits for some participants • May need to accommodate comorbidities during long study visit days (eg, snacks for diabetics, inform participants to bring afternoon medications) • May take longer to schedule follow-up visits if participants are dependent on others for transportation or scheduling
Tips to accommodate	Suggestions for improving recruitment and retention	• Budget for door-to-door transportation • Use pocket talkers, high-contrast print materials, large font size • Plan for higher attrition rate, which has implications for sample size/power calculations

Adapted with permission from Bowling CB, Whitson HE, Johnson TM 2nd. The 5Ts: Preliminary Development of a Framework to Support Inclusion of Older Adults in Research, *J Am Geriatr Soc* 2019 Feb;67(2):342-346.

for exclusion of a specific age range and requires the scientific review groups to assess each grantee application or proposal as being acceptable or unacceptable with regard to the age-appropriate inclusion or exclusion of individuals in the research project. Enrollment and progress reports must also include participant ages.

How Do the Characteristics of My Patient Differ from Those Patients in the Research Studies?

For a relatively healthy older person, there may be no reason to believe that a treatment that is indicated in a younger patient will not also be useful in the older person. However, this conclusion might change as one considers the comorbid burden, degree of functional impairment, and cognitive problems in a frail older person. In a patient with many comorbid conditions, it is possible that side effects of a treatment may exacerbate one of the comorbid conditions. In a patient with functional impairment, falls may be a particular concern. A medicine that causes slight problems with balance may not be a big concern in a younger patient but could precipitate a complicated fall in an older person. Thus, explicitly considering characteristics of your patient such as disease diagnoses, activities of daily living and instrumental activities of daily living function, and cognitive function, and comparing these to the characteristics of the average patient in the study can be useful in assessing whether the study is applicable to your patient

What Outcomes Matter to My Patient?

Many clinical trials focus on outcomes, such as mortality, or disease-specific outcomes, such as cardiovascular hospitalizations. Even though these outcomes are particularly relevant to older persons, other outcomes, such as preserving mobility, preventing falls, or improving quality of life, may matter more to many older persons. Because these outcomes are often not included in many studies, clinicians must often make their best inference about how a treatment impacts these outcomes.

Because quality of life is best judged by the patient, a patient's own sense of how a treatment is impacting him or her can be a crucial criterion in assessing the risks and benefits of therapy. This can be especially important for a patient taking multiple medicines. Some patients may not be bothered by taking many medicines, while for others, the addition of another medicine may be sufficiently burdensome and distressing to outweigh a small benefit seen in clinical studies.

How Does My Patient's Life Expectancy Impact the Risks and Benefits of Treatment?

Some treatments confer immediate risks to patients, whereas benefits may materialize over time. Older persons with limited life expectancy may be subject to all of the risks of treatment with few benefits. This concern becomes increasingly important with increasing age, as well as in patients with limited life expectancy as a result of major comorbidity or severe functional or cognitive impairment. These concerns are addressed in greater depth in Chapter 20, "Prevention & Health Promotion."

Overall, the exclusion of older persons in clinical research can affect the ease with which a clinician applies the evidence base to the clinician's patient. Knowing the important ways that one's patient is similar or different from participants in clinical research, as well as the quality-of-life factors that are most important to one's patient, should guide all evidence-based medical decisions in applying evidence-based medicine to older persons.

Bernard MA, Clayton JA, Lauer MS. Inclusion across the lifespan: NIH policy for clinical research. *JAMA*. 2018;320(15):1535-1536.

Bowling CB, Whitson HE, Johnson TM 2nd. The 5Ts: preliminary development of a framework to support inclusion of older adults in research. *J Am Geriatr Soc*. 2019;67(2):342-346.

Boyd CM, Darer J, Boult C, Fried LP, Boult L, Wu AW. Clinical practice guidelines and quality of care for older patients with multiple comorbid diseases: implications for pay for performance. *JAMA*. 2005;294(6):716-724.

Covinsky KE. Management of COPD: let's just pretend older patients don't exist. http://www.geripal.org/2011/03/management-of-copd-lets-just-pretend.html. Accessed March 14, 2019.

Lee SJ, Eng C. Goals of glycemic control in frail older patients with diabetes. *JAMA*. 2011;305(13):1350-1351.

Lockett J, Sauma S, Radziszewska B, Bernard MA. Adequacy of inclusion of older adults in NIH-funded phase III clinical trials. *J Am Geriatr Soc*. 2019;67(2):218-222.

Zulman DM, Sussman JB, Chen X, Cigolle CT, Blaum CS, Hayward RA. Examining the evidence: a systematic review of the inclusion and analysis of older adults in randomized controlled trials. *J Gen Intern Med*. 2011;26(7):783-790.

Ambulatory Care and Care Coordination

25

Meredith Mirrer, MD, MHS

Veronica Rivera, MD

INTRODUCTION

For many older adults, ambulatory care is a central setting of health care delivery. In response to climbing costs and health care policy changes, including the passage of the Patient Protection and Affordable Care Act in the United States in 2010, there is significant interest in improving primary care, especially for the most medically and psychosocially complex older adults, in order to achieve the Triple Aim of improving patient experience, cost, and population health. In this chapter, we will review models for ambulatory primary care for community-dwelling older adults, including the Patient-Centered Medical Home (PCMH), the Geriatric Resources for Assessment and Care of Elders (GRACE) Team Care model, the Programs of All-Inclusive Care for the Elderly (PACE) model, as well as ambulatory specialty and consultative geriatrics models. In addition, we will discuss geriatrics assessment in the ambulatory setting and the role of care coordination and quality and safety when delivering care to older adults in this setting.

AMBULATORY OFFICE-BASED PRIMARY CARE FOR OLDER ADULTS

Primary care, as defined by the Institute of Medicine in 1996, is "the provision of integrated, accessible health care services by clinicians who are accountable for addressing a large majority of personal health care needs, developing a sustained partnership with patients, and practicing in the context of family and community." Older adults require high-quality primary care to oversee chronic disease management, preventative care, and management of geriatric syndromes.

One model that aims to provide high-quality primary care is PCMH. PCMH is a care delivery model in which treatment is coordinated through a primary care physician to match the following five functions and attributes: comprehensive care, patient-centered care, coordinated care, accessible services, and commitment to quality and safety. PCMH aims to deliver team-based coordinated care, rather than fragmented care, which many patients struggle to navigate. Although this care delivery model is not specific to the older adult population, it naturally fits with the care of complex older adults. Many principles of geriatrics ambulatory care, such as strong patient-provider relationships that recognize the role of family and caregivers, interprofessional team-based care, advance care planning, and continuous care throughout life stages and health care settings, are aligned with PCMH's five functions and attributes. In the medical home, an interprofessional team of providers, discussed further in Chapter 3, is responsible for assessing and meeting each individual's health needs and providing comprehensive care. For example, team members with training in mental health, including social workers, psychologists, and psychiatrists, may screen patients for cognitive impairment, depression, loneliness, social isolation, and substance use. Physical therapists perform gait and balance testing and evaluate the need for treatments or assistive devices to prevent falls and improve function. Occupational therapists on the team assess how much assistance each patient requires for their daily activities in order to design the most appropriate care plan, including level of supervision and environment. Pharmacists and physicians work together to assess medications with a focus on reducing polypharmacy, deprescribing deliriogenic medications, and decreasing the risk of other adverse medication effects. Social workers, nurses, and physicians work together to identify what matters most for each patient and family and to develop care plans and strategies to help meet these goals. Despite the importance of each member of this interprofessional team, it is important to remember that not all PCMHs will have access to every member of this team.

Another ambulatory primary care model created for older adults is the GRACE Team Care model, which was developed at Indiana University. The GRACE Team Care model supports primary care physicians caring for low-income older adults with multiple chronic conditions to improve health and functional status, decrease overuse of health care services, and prevent avoidable long-term nursing home placement. The model includes a two-person team, called the GRACE support team, that has a nurse practitioner and a social worker, who perform a comprehensive in-home assessment on the older adult, coordinate the older adult's care, and bring the older adult's information to an expanded team. The GRACE team is led by a geriatrician and includes a pharmacist and mental health liaison, which is typically a licensed clinical social worker. This larger interprofessional team creates a care plan for the older adult based on evidence-based care protocols for 12 common geriatric conditions that include medication management, mobility issues, and depression, among others.

Another important model of care is PACE. PACE is a capitated managed care benefit under Medicare designed to provide comprehensive medical and social services to certain frail, community-dwelling adults, most of whom are dually eligible for Medicare and Medicaid and also require nursing home level of care. An interprofessional team of health professionals provides PACE participants with coordinated care. For most participants, the comprehensive PACE service package, which includes primary care, adult day health, acute care, meals, prescription drugs, diagnostic testing, rehabilitation, home care, and social work support, enables them to remain in the community, rather than receive care in a nursing home. (See Chapter 30 for additional details on PACE.)

emerging models of care include co-management models that feature geriatrics consultation by geriatricians prior to, during, and after high-risk procedures such as organ transplants and orthopedic surgeries. Furthermore, additional geriatrics training is becoming increasingly more common among clinicians from other specialties, such as cardiology, pulmonology, gastroenterology, nephrology, and oncology. These specialists have sought out extra geriatrics training because they are managing many older adults with chronic conditions in their specialties. These specialists who have additional geriatrics training can provide specialty care from the geriatrics lens.

With advancements in technology, there are now other ways for geriatrics specialists to provide consultation. Some health systems offer tools for specialists to perform electronic consultations, referred to as e-consults, that provide asynchronous, consultative, provider-to-provider communications within a shared electronic health record or web-based platform. E-consults help to improve access to specialty expertise for patients and providers without requiring a face-to-face visit. Other telemedicine models provide education and guidance to primary care providers, especially in rural settings. One such model is exemplified by the Extension for Community Healthcare Outcomes, known as Project ECHO. Unlike traditional telemedicine, in which a specialist assumes care of the patient, Project ECHO is a guided practice model that provides telemonitoring. Other uses of technology to enhance geriatric care are discussed in Chapter 33.

AMBULATORY OFFICE-BASED GERIATRICS SPECIALTY AND CONSULTATIVE CARE

Ambulatory office-based primary care is predominantly provided by general primary care providers, such as internists or family physicians. However, providers who have additional geriatrics training, such as geriatricians or geriatric nurse practitioners, also practice in the ambulatory setting as either primary care providers or as consulting specialists to meet the unique needs of older adults. Primary care geriatricians may see outpatients in a geriatrics specialty clinic, historically referred to as a senior health clinic. The senior health clinic is a specialized ambulatory service that provides primary care using an interprofessional team approach to development and implementation of a care plan. The core interprofessional clinical practice team consists of a geriatrician, nurse practitioner, and a social worker or geriatric nurse specialist. An extended team may include other professionals, such as a pharmacist, physical therapist, dietitian, and home health nurse.

Alternatively, in other ambulatory settings, geriatricians function purely as embedded consultants. Primary care providers can refer patients to geriatricians for assessment, diagnosis, and treatment of geriatric syndromes and to assist with the management of more complex patients. Other

GERIATRIC ASSESSMENT IN THE AMBULATORY SETTING

An overview of geriatrics assessment is included in Chapter 2. A comprehensive geriatrics assessment includes screening for high-risk conditions and performing functional assessments. The Geriatrics 5Ms framework for core competencies in geriatrics focuses on "mind" (mentation, dementia, delirium, and depression), "mobility" (gait and balance and falls), "medications" (polypharmacy and deprescribing), "multicomplexity" (multimorbidity), and what "matters most" (each individual's own health outcome goals and preferences) to drive many of the components of a geriatrics assessment. The outpatient clinic is an excellent setting in which to perform a comprehensive geriatrics assessment since it can be performed when an individual is at their baseline, stable health status. Also, components of the assessment can be administered over time at different visits by one core team.

In recognition of the importance of the geriatrics assessment as well as health maintenance and prevention for older adults, Medicare has supported billing codes in the outpatient setting that provide support for certain visit types, including the annual wellness visit (AWV), cognitive assessment and care planning service, and advanced care planning. In the United States, Medicare encourages the provision of preventative care for older adults through the implementation of a Medicare AWV. During this special once-a-year visit, the primary care provider completes a health risk assessment (HRA) and partners with the older adult to develop personalized wellness plans. Similar to the comprehensive geriatrics assessment described earlier, the HRA includes demographic information, a self-reported description of a patient's health status, psychosocial and behavioral health risks, and functional status. Other elements of the visit include measurement of weight and blood pressure, cognitive and depression screening, and fall and home safety risk assessments.

Another main area of focus for the management of older adults in the ambulatory setting is screening and diagnosis of major neurocognitive disorder, also known as dementia. The Health Outcomes, Planning, and Education for Alzheimer's (HOPE) Act culminated in the approval of a Medicare procedure code G0505 that took effect January 1, 2017, and was eventually replaced by the Current Procedural Terminology (CPT) code 99483 in January 2018. This code provides reimbursement to physicians and other eligible billing practitioners for a comprehensive clinical visit and includes the following: an assessment of cognition, function, and safety; an evaluation of neuropsychiatric and behavioral symptoms; a review of medications; and an assessment of the needs of the patient's caregiver. Screening for dementia, maximizing safety for patients with dementia, and supporting caregivers are essential to care for older adults in the ambulatory setting.

In addition to new Medicare procedure codes for dementia care, reimbursement is also now available for time spent discussing advance care planning, starting in 2016. Advance care planning involves a face-to-face visit with a provider to discuss advance directives and goals of care. The ambulatory setting is an excellent setting in which to review health care proxies and to discuss a patient's values and goals of care. Providers are now supported to take the time to initiate advance care planning discussions that can have a critical impact on a patient's care.

CARE COORDINATION FOR COMPLEX PATIENTS

Caring for complex older adults requires that care is coordinated and/or integrated across all elements of the complex health care system (eg, subspecialty care, hospitals, home health agencies, nursing homes) and the patient's community (eg, family, public and private community-based services). Care is facilitated by registries, information technology, health information exchange, and other means to assure that patients get the indicated care when and where they need and want it in a culturally and linguistically appropriate manner. Designated providers on the patient's care team can perform medication reconciliation and management with care coordination through telephone calls, electronic telemedicine visits, and/or traditional office visits. Telehealth services may

reduce burdens on caregivers and patients and increase efficacy in the management of chronic conditions. Successful teams work to improve communication across care settings to prevent loss of information and medication errors.

Caring for older adults requires an appreciation for the many transitions that patients and their families endure as they age, including transitions between acute care, subacute care, and home and community care, which require skillful communication among all care team members. (Transitions in care are discussed in more detail in Chapter 26.) A care transitions specialist, coach, or navigator can promote continuity of care across different care settings and health systems by assisting with timely follow-up and medication reviews upon discharge. The transitions specialists also provide direct communication with the primary care provider and outpatient team to improve continuity of care across different health systems. In recognition of the importance of this type of patient care coordination, Medicare now reimburses physicians' efforts for the time they spend on transitional care management (TCM) and chronic care management (CCM) services. TCM refers to a 30-day period following a transition back to the community, usually following discharge from a hospital or a skilled nursing facility, and involves a postdischarge phone follow-up within 2 days, care coordination services, and then face-to-face visit within 14 days. CCM provides reimbursement for coordination of care for chronic conditions that is performed by any clinician and their staff on a monthly basis that is longer than 20 minutes in duration.

QUALITY AND SAFETY

Caring for older adults requires dedicated attention to quality and safety. Tools to enhance quality in the ambulatory care setting include evidence-based resources, such as peer-reviewed research literature and databases, as well as continuous quality improvement projects of various scales and scopes and information technology to support each of these tools. Quality metrics to improve the care of older adults include the Merit-Based Incentive Payment System (MIPS). MIPS is a component of the Quality Payment Program development, part of the Medicare Access and CHIP Reauthorization Act of 2015 (MACRA), which associates payments with a wide range of quality measures, such as postdischarge medication reconciliation, assessment and plan for urinary incontinence, influenza and pneumonia immunization, fall risk assessment, and cognitive assessment.

Providing evidence-based care to older adults that aligns with their goals and preferences is a key challenge in geriatric management. Many ambulatory geriatrics providers use shared decision making as a means of improving care quality by increasing patient understanding of treatment options and making decisions that reflect patients' values. Relevant cancer screenings, for instance, are performed after careful consideration of each patient's prognosis, preferences, and unique goals. Other common ambulatory care quality metrics include rates of immunization for pneumonia and influenza; screening rates for falls, depression, and osteoporosis; and the completion and documentation of advance care planning and related conversations. A patient-centered care plan should address evidence-based quality metrics that are relevant to the older adults' health outcomes and any geriatric syndromes present, all while considering a patient's goals and values.

CONCLUSION

The application of geriatrics principles and the implementation of successful care models for older adults can contribute positively to the outcomes pursued by ambulatory care clinicians. There are many opportunities for practices to develop the care processes that may optimize outcomes for older adults, especially those burdened with multimorbidity, functional impairment, and geriatric syndromes such as falls and dementia. As we look ahead, advancements in team-based models of care and medical informatics will generate further advances in the care of older adults in the ambulatory care setting.

Bennett KA, Ong T, Verrall AM, Vitiello MV, Marcum ZA, Phelan EA. Project ECHO-Geriatrics: training future primary care providers to meet the needs of older adults. *J Grad Med Educ.* 2018;10(3):311-315.

Counsell SC, Callahan CM, Clark DO, et al. Geriatric care management for low-income seniors: randomized controlled trial. *JAMA.* 2007;298(22):2623-2633.

The John A. Hartford Foundation Change Agents Initiative. Patient-centered medical homes and the care of older adults. September 2016. https://www.johnahartford.org/images/uploads/reports/PCMH_Roadmap2016.pdf. Accessed November 18, 2019.

Rich E, Lipson D, Libersky J, Parchman M. Coordinating care for adults with complex care needs in the patient-centered medical home: challenges and solutions. White paper (prepared by Mathematica Policy Research under Contract No. HHSA290200900019I/HHSA29032005T). AHRQ Publication No. 12-0010-EF. Rockville, MD: Agency for Healthcare Research and Quality; January 2012. https://pcmh.ahrq.gov/sites/default/files/attachments/Coordinating%20Care%20for%20Adults%20with%20Complex%20Care%20Needs.pdf. Accessed November 18, 2019.

Tinneti M, Huang A, Molnar F. The geriatric 5Ms: a new way of communicating what we do. *J Am Geriatr Soc.* 2017;65(9):2115.

Wasserman M. Outpatient care systems. In: Pacala JT, Sullivan GM, eds. *Geriatrics Review Syllabus: A Core Curriculum in Geriatric Medicine.* 7th ed. New York, NY: American Geriatrics Society; 2010.

Transitions and Continuity of Care

26

Jessica A. Eng, MD, MS

Lynn A. Flint, MD

INTRODUCTION

The term *care transition* refers to the transfer of a patient's care from one setting and/or team of clinicians to another. The most-studied care transition is hospital discharge, which is often more complex than a simple return home. What follows is an example of a typical series of transitions after hospitalization: An older adult with a chronic condition, followed as an outpatient by his primary care physician and a specialist, is hospitalized for exacerbation of the chronic condition, where a hospital-based generalist and specialist physicians, nurses, and therapists care for the patient. The hospitalization is this patient's first transition. During the hospitalization, the patient may move between units within the hospital due to changing care needs, a second transition. When the patient no longer requires acute-level care, the patient may receive postacute care (PAC) from a new team, such as rehabilitation or skilled nursing care, in a facility or at home, a third transition. When the patient is discharged from the facility or home health team, a fourth transition occurs. With so many handoffs, mishaps are inevitable. *Transitional care* broadly refers to time-limited care processes aimed at avoiding such mishaps and ensuring safe and minimally disruptive transfers of care between different sites and clinicians.

BACKGROUND

Care transitions drew increasing attention in the late 20th century for a variety of reasons, including changes to the financing and structure of the US health care system and a shift in the types of illnesses prompting hospitalization, from acute episodic illnesses to exacerbations of chronic illnesses and multimorbidity. Prior to 1983, in the single disease–focused fee-for-service payment scheme, Medicare beneficiaries stayed in the hospital for longer periods of time, until near complete recovery. In 1983, to address rapidly increasing health care costs, Medicare was changed from fee-for-service payment to prospective payment. Prospective payment meant that hospitals received predetermined diagnosis-based fees for entire hospitalizations and created a financial incentive for hospitals to increase efficiency and shorten length of stay. Indeed, length of stay decreased with the reform, but patients were not only discharged "quicker," they were also discharged "sicker." Facility-based PAC use increased, as did hospital readmission rates. In one retrospective study of all Medicare beneficiaries, 22% experienced at least one care transition over the course of a year. Concurrently, fast-paced advances in hospital medicine coupled with the push to improve efficiency prompted physicians to restrict their practice to single sites (ie, clinic or hospital). Fewer primary care physicians continued to follow their patients while hospitalized. This shift in practice patterns meant that patients' care would routinely transfer care from one care team to another when moving between settings.

Finances may also subtly encourage frequent transitions between nursing home and hospital for long-term nursing home residents. Medicare-certified skilled nursing facilities (SNFs) often provide temporary skilled rehabilitation and nursing services to their residents returning from the hospital. Reimbursement for skilled services is higher than the rate paid, often by Medicaid, for room, board, and custodial care. Medicare will only pay SNFs for skilled services if patients have a preceding qualifying hospital stay. Thus, transfers to the hospital can be financially beneficial to nursing homes. In a study of Medicare claims in nursing home resident decedents, nearly one-fifth had at least one "burdensome transition" in the last 90 days of life. "Burdensome transitions" were defined as hospitalization in the last 3 days of life, multiple hospitalizations, or residing in different nursing home facilities in those last 90 days. In response to the persistent problem of high rates of health care transitions, especially hospital readmissions, the Patient Protection and Affordable Care Act (ACA) of 2010 introduced several provisions aimed at reducing hospital readmissions. These provisions include encouraging the formation of accountable care organizations in an effort to improve care coordination, and the hospital readmission reduction program, which reduces payment to hospitals with excess readmissions for six specific conditions or procedures.

Patients with life-limiting illness have unique challenges that lead to care transitions. First, serious illness comes with new and changing symptoms that can prompt multiple transitions. For example, Hunt and colleagues showed that older Medicare decedents with dementia and an unmet need for pain management had 50% more transitions to the emergency department than those without an unmet need for pain management. Second, while functional decline is expected for patients with life-limiting illness, the Medicare hospice benefit covers only limited support for assistance with activities of daily living at home, and the need for increased care can prompt transitions to the hospital and nursing home.

ADVERSE EVENTS DURING TRANSITIONS

While care transitions provide opportunities for receiving clinical teams to reevaluate ongoing problems and refine care plans, transitions are also fraught with risk. Older patients and those with multiple chronic illnesses and/or serious life-threatening illness—those who are most likely to experience multiple transitions—are particularly vulnerable to the risk of adverse events.

Older adults are vulnerable to a wide variety of adverse events related to transitions of care. A prospective observational study of hospitalized adults showed that one in five discharged patients experienced an adverse event associated with discharge. The adverse events were most frequently medication related but also included nosocomial infections, falls, and complications of procedures. Half of the adverse medication events were felt to preventable or at least "ameliorable," meaning the adverse event could have been less harmful. In a retrospective analysis of Medicare claims data, nearly one-fifth of beneficiaries who were hospitalized were readmitted within 30 days. Ninety percent of these rehospitalizations were considered "unplanned"; that is, *not* for follow-up treatments or procedures. Black patients have a higher rate of 30-day readmissions than white patients. Transitions may also drive low-value, inappropriate, costly care. For example, another study found that geographic areas with greater rates of care transitions among nursing home residents also had greater rates of feeding tube placement in patients with severe cognitive impairment, a group that is unlikely to benefit from this invasive procedure. Transfers of nursing home residents have also been associated with drug regimen changes and adverse medication effects. Another study found that avoidable readmissions, or admissions that could have been prevented, cost Medicare an estimated $17 billion over 1 year. Faced with this extremely complex problem, transitions researchers have aimed to identify the factors that contribute to transition-related adverse events, particularly readmissions, and to design interventions to decrease the rate of adverse events.

BARRIERS TO SUCCESSFUL CARE TRANSITIONS

A successful care transition is one in which receiving care teams, patients, and caregivers have timely, complete information about the hospitalization, as well as easy access to answers and support when problems arise. Coleman groups barriers to successful care transitions into three levels: systems, provider, and patient. Systems-level barriers are related to the fragmented nature of the health system and financial pressures to discharge quickly. Communication and collaboration across health care settings and between networks are challenging for many reasons—from simple lack of readily available contact information for providers at different sites to misinterpretation of laws protecting confidentiality. Information systems are often not shared between different systems, thereby slowing down the transfer of key data. Although the Health Insurance Portability and Accountability Act (HIPAA) allows transfer of information between providers for the purpose of continuing care, some clinicians and staff are not familiar with that provision. Institutional drug formularies differ based on contractual relationships with pharmaceutical companies, prompting medication substitutions with each transition, which can lead to duplications or omissions of medications upon discharge. For example, if a patient regularly takes felodipine for blood pressure, and upon admission to the hospital amlodipine is substituted for felodipine, they may inadvertently be discharged on both felodipine and amlodipine.

Provider-level barriers stem primarily from communication difficulties. The increasing prevalence of site-specific providers generates inpatient–outpatient physician discontinuity. Communication between inpatient and outpatient providers is most frequently accomplished via discharge summaries, but these often do not arrive in the receiving physician's office in a timely manner, if at all. Discharge summaries have been shown to omit key information, such as which test results are pending and which follow-up appointments have been scheduled. Hospital clinicians, who are under financial pressure to care for many patients and keep length of stay short, report that they do not have enough time to complete detailed discharge summaries. Other forms of direct communication between inpatient and outpatient providers, including between inpatient and outpatient specialists, such as telephone calls or e-mails, are infrequent.

Patient-level barriers include limitations in health literacy and self-efficacy. Discharge instructions should be written at a sixth-grade level. Patients may not know the details of their health history or the names and dosages of their medications, leading to the possibility of inaccurate medication prescription in the hospital. Additionally, with shorter inpatient stays, patients are generally still recovering and perhaps facing new diagnoses at the time of discharge. Thus, they are likely to have new self-care responsibilities, including monitoring of symptoms and signs, taking new medications, and keeping follow-up appointments either on their own or with the help of family or friends. For example, if a patient's medication for blood pressure is changed to a new medication, they may erroneously take the new one in addition to the old medication. Providers frequently overestimate patients' and families' abilities (physically, socially, and cognitively) to manage their medical conditions. All of these problems can be traced back to the limitations in provider–patient communication. Discordance between physician explanations and patient understanding has been well documented. Communication can be even less effective when patients have low functional literacy or primarily speak a language other than English.

OVERCOMING THE BARRIERS: BEST PRACTICES

Excellent transitional care is associated with reduced rates of readmission to the hospital, cost savings, and greater patient satisfaction. Readmissions can be avoided if inpatient and outpatient providers communicate effectively, medications are carefully reconciled at multiple key time points, and patients and families are educated about monitoring and care needs after discharge or transfer. The Joint Commission Guidelines for discharge summaries recommend that the following information be included: diagnoses, abnormal physical findings, important test results, discharge medications including reasons for changes, follow-up appointments, education provided to patient and family, and tasks to be completed (Table 26–1). For older adults, documentation of cognitive and functional status, skin condition including

Table 26–1. Key information to include in hospital and nursing facility discharge summaries for older adults.

Discharge diagnoses
Chronic conditions
Significant test results
Discharge condition, including cognitive and functional status, pain level, nutritional status, and notable physical exam findings, including the presence or absence of pressure ulcers
Setting of care prior to admission
Discharge disposition
Follow-up appointments
Tests still pending at discharge
Discharge medication list, with emphasis on new medications or doses, including explanation of why medications were started, changed, or discontinued
Overall goals of care and treatment preferences
Presence or absence of advance directive and/or living will
Name and phone number of surrogate decision maker
Home care services arranged

description of any pressure ulcers, nutritional status, goals of care, and surrogate decision makers are also important. Detailed medication reconciliation, with the assistance of a clinical pharmacist for patients with complex regimens, is essential to reducing adverse drug events. For patients with cognitive or functional disabilities or psychosocial challenges, a multidisciplinary team including social workers, nurse discharge planners, and physical and occupational therapists is essential. Using clear language and a trained interpreter if needed, discharging teams should counsel patients and families about medication changes, outpatient appointments, self-care, and "red flags" signaling a call to the doctor or return to the hospital. For the patient transferring to an intermediate site of care, counseling should include a description of what to expect in the next site of care. If there have been major changes in goals of care and treatment limitations, a physician order for life-sustaining treatment (POLST) form increases the likelihood that patients will have orders consistent with their wishes in the next setting. Finally, because written discharge summaries do not capture every detail, direct discussion between transferring and accepting providers can be helpful in complicated situations.

Separate from discharge summaries, which are meant for communication among health care professionals, patients and families need discharge instructions written for their level of understanding as almost half of US adults have limited health literacy skills. Health literacy may be deficient among patients and families for several reasons, including limited formal education, cultural factors, impaired short-term memory, impaired capacity for learning, and difficulty with language comprehension. In the setting of medical illness, patients' level of understanding might be impaired compared to their baseline. Health care professionals often overestimate patients' understanding of postdischarge treatment plan. Most discharge instructions are written at an eighth- to thirteenth-grade reading level, but patients on average read at a sixth-grade level. Formal health literacy screening tools are rarely employed outside of the context of a research study, and most experts advocate against routine screening of adults for limited health literacy; instead, they recommend taking a "universal precautions" approach that assumes that most adults have some degree of impairment. Experts also recommend using pictures and illustrations when possible and using the teach-back method, or asking the patient to explain their instructions for care in their own words, to screen for comprehension and also as a health literacy intervention.

The transition from one setting to another is often a good time to review overall goals of care. This type of discussion could include the patient and family's understanding of the hospitalization and what they are expecting in the next setting. Eliciting specific hopes of future therapies can help discharging providers set realistic goals with the patient and initiate discussion of alternate plans in case those goals are not met.

IMPLEMENTATION STRATEGY FOR TRANSITIONAL CARE INTERVENTIONS

Early multicomponent interventions to improve transitions focused on using additional staff to coordinate care and also encourage patient activation and self-management. A classic example is the Care Transitions Intervention, which used a "transition coach," an advance practice nurse who worked with hospitalized older adults during the admission and for 4 weeks after discharge. The aim of the intervention was to empower patients to be more involved in their own self-management. Thus, rather than act as another provider, the transition coaches helped patients and caregivers take more active roles in their care. A second component of the intervention was a personal health record, carried by patients between settings, containing key information including diagnoses, medications, allergies, and advance directives. The intervention was studied in two randomized controlled trials, one with patients enrolled in Medicare managed care plans and one with patients using traditional fee-for-service Medicare. In both studies, intervention patients had lower rates of hospital readmission at 30, 90, and 180 days.

Multiple reviews of transitional care interventions note the development of the Care Transitions Intervention and other similar models were published >15 years ago. Those early studies showed that nurse-led transitional care interventions beginning in the hospital and continuing after discharge had the potential to reduce the rate of hospital readmissions. However, since then, the health care landscape has evolved markedly with US health care systems' efforts to improve transitions to avoid nonpayment for readmissions within 30 days for the same condition for which patients were initially admitted. First, the spread of electronic medical records has improved the quantity, clarity, and timeliness of communication from inpatient to outpatient providers. Second, patient-centered medical homes have spread quickly as an effort at team-based care to provide comprehensive care, including care coordination across settings. Third, a marked increase in US postdischarge home health care agency referrals to provide home-based nursing and rehabilitation services incorporates several aspects of transitions initiatives, including early postdischarge symptoms evaluation, medication reconciliation, and nurse-led education. In this new landscape, there is no one clear transitional intervention that would work in all systems. Overall, the literature points toward successful transitional care interventions as being more comprehensive, bridging the inpatient and outpatient setting, and providing enough flexibility to respond to individual patient needs.

Transitional care interventions can be resource intensive, and systems considering implementing them should perform a needs assessment considering multiple systems-, provider-, and patient-level factors. Important considerations when implementing a transitional care intervention include the following:

1. **Patient selection:** Systems can choose to take a "universal precautions" approach by applying an intervention to their entire patient population, such as improving the health literacy levels of discharge communication, or they can apply more resources to the subset of highest-risk patients. The two most common methods of identifying subsets of patients for intervention are based either on (1) administrative data or (2) clinician judgment. These two methods often result in substantially different cohorts. Using primarily administrative data, such as calculated risk scores based on acute care utilization and chronic conditions, to identify patients for transitions interventions usually cannot take into consideration social support and health literacy, both of which are key to patients successfully following discharge instructions, including medication regimens, and attending follow-up appointments. While administrative data can predict acute care utilization, it often cannot capture whether the patient's risk can be lowered through a transitions intervention. Most clinical services rely on clinician judgment and identification. Clinical providers have knowledge of a patient's readiness to change and insight into their psychosocial context. They tend to identify patients for intervention who are older and have problems with mental health, substance use, medical decision making, and care coordination. However, provider-led identification tends to only modestly predict those at risk of rehospitalization and can miss patients who do not often access care or see the provider in order for the provider to initiate a referral. Ideally, patients are identified through use of a triangulated approach in which clinical and administrative approaches are melded to account for the inherent weaknesses in each method.

   Patients can also be divided by demographics or by clinical conditions. General medical patients, geriatric patients, and patients with heart failure are the most frequently studied groups, and there are several effective interventions in these populations. For congestive heart failure (CHF) in particular, self-management education delivered face to face, early postdischarge contact, and the ability to individually tailor the intervention are for successful interventions. Across many studies, there is little evidence that chronic obstructive pulmonary disease patients benefit from transitional care interventions. There is poor-quality evidence for transitions interventions for mental health and surgical patients.

2. **Current resources for transitions:** Since systems have a financial incentive from Medicare to decrease readmissions, systems have implemented multiple changes, and any new intervention looking to improve transitions needs to ensure it is not duplicating services. Systems should evaluate what resources are available from inpatient and outpatient services across medical, psychiatric, and surgical specialties. Having a system-wide strategy across a health care system and regular reevaluation can ensure that resources are distributed appropriately and

efficiently rather than separate programs for certain populations (eg, homeless, CHF, serious mental illness, older adults) without learning and resource sharing for those who have multiple high-risk factors.

In addition, between 2001 and 2012, home health care (HHC) referrals increased by 65%, causing Medicare spending on these services to more than double. However, HHC has become a key factor in transitions but is often not used optimally. HHC is often ordered by a hospitalist, but it is often unclear who is managing the HHC orders until primary care follow-up. This is further complicated by current regulations that allow physicians, but not physician assistants and nurse practitioners, to sign HHC orders. HHC nurses often have little access to hospital records and have difficulty accessing physicians to clarify orders. While studies show that transitions interventions are more effective if they bridge the inpatient and outpatient spheres, HHC nurses usually do not meet with patients in the hospital before discharge. In addition, HHC nurses face multiple safety issues, including addressing safety for patients with cognitive issues at home and also feeling unsafe themselves with patients with behavioral health issues; often information about cognition and behavioral health is not shared during the HHC referral process. At present, decisions about referrals for PAC, such as HHC at the time of discharge, are at the discretion of individual providers without uniform, standardized guidelines, which may promote variability in HHC referrals.

3. **Intervention intensity based on risk stratification:** Once identified, patients should be stratified by risk to allow for right sizing of intervention. While home visits can be an effective tool to address medication adherence and low health literacy issues that often play a role in poor transitions, they are time intensive and expensive to implement and maintain. Telephone-based interventions are less time intensive and less costly but might not completely assess and address the needs of complex patients. Stratifying patients based on potential needs can guide a stepped-care, population-based interventional approach that provides the optimal intervention dose for the most benefit.

An example of a well-designed, tiered intervention that uses risk stratification was published by Hoyer in 2018. The selection strategy incorporated both multidisciplinary team assessment and an evidence-based risk assessment tool. A greater percentage of patients with high-risk assessment tool scores were referred to the more intensive intervention; however, not all patients with high-risk scores were referred to the more intensive intervention, suggesting that the clinical and team assessment had an impact on risk stratification decision making. This approach recognizes the universal vulnerability experienced by all patients being discharged from the hospital. Hoyer showed that both the higher- and lower-intensity interventions reduced readmissions. Compared to those who received each intervention, those who did not receive them had greater odds of being readmitted. These results are impressive given the general difficulty in reducing overall 30-day readmissions, rather than focusing on disease-specific cohorts.

4. **Adaptation of intervention to health care system:** Intervention feasibility will be affected by many factors. Without adaptation, interventions can be a poor fit, not aligning well with the goals and interests of the health care system, individual health care personnel, patients, and families. A helpful framework when considering implementation of an evidence-based intervention is the Consolidated Framework for Implementation Research (CFIR), which has five domains. Those implementing interventions should consider the setting of the health care system, which includes payors, competition, and the regulatory environment. Implementing a transitional intervention would be very different in a government-based health care system and a private community-based hospital due to different financial incentives, possible competition from insurance-based transitional programs, and different regulations and payment models from different government-based payments and private insurances. Specific health care system factors to consider should include the culture and communication between inpatient and outpatient teams, existing inpatient discharge resources, strength of patient-centered medical home and primary care, size of catchment area, and existing geriatrics, palliative care, and home visiting programs.

An example of using this framework was published by Ritchie and colleagues, who adapted the Geriatric Resources for the Assessment and Care of Elders (GRACE) program, a home visit–based adjunct to primary care in Indiana, into a program for high-risk patients over age 18 in San Francisco. The team used CFIR to assist in making key adaptations of the original model, which included changing the target population from older adults to all adults with at least five emergency department visits or at least two hospitalizations in the last year, streamlining of standardized protocols, augmenting mental health interventions, and performing some assessments in the clinic, rather than in the home. There was a significant decline in the median number of emergency department visits and hospitalizations comparing 6 months before enrollment to 6 months after enrollment. In addition, the percentage of patients reporting better self-rated health increased from 31% at enrollment to 64% at 9 months. However, in order to maintain fidelity to the original model, they kept the six core elements of the original GRACE program with minor adaptations: comprehensive assessment performed by nurse practitioner and social work, standardized care plan developed using protocols, review of the care plan by primary care physician, implementation of care plan in collaboration with primary care physician consistent with patient goals, ongoing care management to ensure coordination of transitions, and interdisciplinary team conferences.

CONCLUSION

Older adults with complex medical conditions are at risk of adverse events as they traverse the various sites within the health care system. A number of interventions have been shown to improve postdischarge outcomes and reduce readmissions. Comprehensive changes at the patient, provider, institution, and overall system levels are needed to improve transitional care as the population ages.

Agency for Healthcare Research and Quality. Use the Teach-Back Method: Tool #5. Content last reviewed February 2015. Agency for Healthcare Research and Quality, Rockville, MD. https://www.ahrq.gov/professionals/quality-patient-safety/quality-resources/tools/literacy-toolkit/healthlittoolkit2-tool5.html. Accessed July 3, 2019.

Berkowitz RE, Jones RN, Rieder R, et al. Improving disposition outcomes or patients in a geriatric skilled nursing facility. *J Am Geriatr Soc.* 2011;59(6):1130-1136.

Coleman EA, Parry C, Chalmers S, Min SJ. The care transitions intervention: results of a randomized controlled trial. *Arch Intern Med.* 2006;166(17):1822-1828.

Gozalo P, Teno JM, Mitchell SL, et al. End-of-life transitions among nursing home residents with cognitive issues. *N Engl J Med.* 2011;365(13):1212-1221.

Hoyer EH, Brotman DJ, Apfel A, et al. Improving outcomes after hospitalization: a prospective observational multicenter evaluation of care coordination strategies for reducing 30-day readmissions to Maryland hospitals. *J Gen Intern Med.* 2018;33(5):621-627.

Hunt L, Ritchie C, Cataldo J, Patel K, Stephens C, Smith A. Pain and Emergency Department Use in the Last Month of Life among Older Adults with Dementia. *J Pain Symptom Manag.* 2018;56(6):871-877.

Jones CD, Jones J, Richard A, et al. "Connecting the dots": a qualitative study of home health nurse perspectives on coordinating care for recently discharged patients." *J Gen Intern Med.* 2017(32):1114-1121.

Ritchie C, Andersen R, Eng J, et al. Implementation of an interdisciplinary, team-based complex care support health care model at an academic medical center: impact on health care utilization and quality of life. *PLoS One.* 2016;11(2):e0148096.

USEFUL WEBSITES

Interventions to Reduce Acute Care Transfers (Interact II). http://interact2.net. Accessed March 22, 2020.

Society of Hospital Medicine. Project BOOST (Better Outcomes for Older adults through Safe Transitions). http://www.hospitalmedicine.org/ResourceRoomRedesign/RR_CareTransitions/CT_Home.cfm. Accessed March 22, 2020.

The Care Transitions Project (Coleman et al). http://www.caretransitions.org/. Accessed March 22, 2020.

Transitional Care Model (Naylor et al). http://www.transitionalcare.info. Accessed March 22, 2020.

Emergency Department Care

27

Gallane D. Abraham, MD

Corita R. Grudzen, MD, MSHS, FACEP

GENERAL PRINCIPLES

Adults age 65 years and older compose 15% of the population and are projected to grow to approximately 20% by 2030. Although older adults represent 15% of all emergency department (ED) visits, they account for almost half of all hospital admissions from the ED. Medicare data reveal that 16% to 26% of hospital admissions are considered potentially avoidable hospitalizations and account for over $5.4 billion annually. Older adults are more likely to present with urgent and emergent medical conditions confounded by multiple medical and psychosocial comorbidities. Older adults are five times more likely to be admitted as compared to younger adults. The demographic shift, increased utilization, and complex clinical presentations present a challenge for managing ED visits by older adults. Models of emergency care are evolving in response to these challenges to meet the particular needs of this growing population.

Older adults present to the ED for urgent and emergent conditions, often with atypical features or vague symptoms, multimorbidities, and polypharmacy, which require extensive rapid workups and coordinated care to determine optimal dispositions. Complex clinical presentations put older adults at risk for delays in diagnosis, adverse events, medication side effects, insufficient treatment plans, cognitive and functional decline, delirium, falls during and subsequent to their ED visit and/or hospitalization, ED revisits, and readmissions. Structural aspects of the ED and hospital environment may also increase these risks. The often complex psychosocial needs require early and intensive multidisciplinary case management to improve patient outcomes. Older adults are at risk of discharge from the ED with unrecognized illness or unmet psychosocial needs, and 20% experience a change in the ability to care for themselves after an acute illness or injury. Complications commonly ensue, with an often rapid decrease in function and quality of life; not surprisingly, 27% will experience ED revisit, hospitalization, or death within 3 months. This chapter addresses the complex needs of the older adults presenting to the ED and suggests models of care, structural enhancements, and clinical care protocols to improve quality care for older adults.

The current model of emergency care is designed to rapidly treat the acutely ill and injured. To identify and address older persons' complex medical and psychosocial needs, emergency providers must account for baseline cognitive and functional limitations, obtain the past history from and collaborate with multiple sources, and develop a broad differential. Such an intensive patient-centered approach will allow emergency providers to create appropriate care plans that place older adults' needs in context.

Ortman JM, Velkoff VA, Hogan H. An aging nation: the older population in the United States. Washington, DC: US Census Bureau; 2014:25–1140. https://www.census.gov/prod/2014pubs/p25-1140.pdf. Accessed March 22, 2020.

Shenvi CL, Platts-Mills TF. Managing the elderly emergency department patient. *Ann Emerg Med*. 2019;73(3):302-307.

Weeks WB, Weinstein JN. Medicare's per-beneficiary potentially avoidable admission measures mask true performance. *J Gen Intern Med*. 2019; doi:10.1007/s11606-019-05354-3.

MODELS OF EMERGENCY CARE

Models of geriatric emergency care are being implemented and refined as evidence-based best practices emerge. While a shared goal is to adapt the ED environment and care plans to the needs of older adults, the implementation of models differ. Elements currently include (1) geriatric-friendly structural modifications such as diurnal lighting and noise reduction, (2) universal screening and risk assessment such as the Identification of Seniors at Risk and the Timed Up and Go fall risk assessment, (3) enhanced care coordination between ED and community health care providers, and (4) linkages to community resources and postdischarge follow-up. Improved patient outcomes for such models of care illustrate the value of patient-centered coordinated emergency care;

however, no one approach has been described as superior. ED models of geriatric emergency care adapt elements from other care settings, and almost all utilize multiple strategies, including a multidisciplinary case-management approach, a collaborative comprehensive geriatric assessment (CGA), and a transitional care coordination process to improve outcomes for older adults.

In a 2011 systematic review of ED-based case management for older adults, Sinha and colleagues identified eight operational components that can inform the development of a comprehensive geriatric emergency care model. Key operational components include implementation of an evidence-based practice model; universal screening with validated risk assessment tools; nursing or midlevel clinician-directed geriatric case management; focused geriatric assessments to identify clinical and nonclinical factors that may impact care planning and future health care utilization; ED initiation of care and disposition planning; interprofessional and multidisciplinary work practices between the ED providers, hospital, primary care, and community health care providers; follow-up after discharge to maintain and facilitate care plans; and evaluation and monitoring of outcome measures for continuous quality improvement. Furthermore, capacity building through the training of existing providers in geriatric competencies can also enhance the care of older adults. In a 2019 systematic review of ED interventions for older adults, Hughes and colleagues reported positive clinical and utilization outcomes for models employing multiple components.

To operationalize evidence-based best practices for the emergency care of older adults, Carpenter and colleagues disseminated the Multidisciplinary Geriatric Emergency Department Guidelines in 2014 endorsed by the American College of Emergency Physicians (ACEP), American Geriatrics Society, Emergency Nurses Association, and Society for Academic Emergency Medicine. The guidelines identify the critical components of a geriatric ED and provide concrete structural, operational, and educational tools for implementing geriatric emergency care. In 2018, ACEP established the Geriatric Emergency Department Accreditation to standardize geriatric emergency care for accredited geriatric EDs. The requirements for accreditation include staffing, education, care protocols, quality and outcome measures, facilities, and equipment that enhance the emergency care of older adults.

American College of Emergency Physicians, et al. Geriatric emergency department guidelines. *Ann Emerg Med.* 2014;63(5):e7-25.

Carpenter C, Hwang U, Biese K, et al. ACEP Accredits Geriatric Emergency Care for Emergency Departments. ACEP Now. https://www.acepnow.com/article/acep-accredits-geriatric-emergency-care-emergency-departments/. Accessed March 22, 2020.

Carpenter CR, Bromley M, Caterino JM, et al. Optimal older adult emergency care: introducing multidisciplinary geriatric emergency department guidelines from the American College of Emergency Physicians, American Geriatrics Society, Emergency Nurses Association, and Society for Academic Emergency Medicine. *J Am Geriatr Soc.* 2014;62(7):1360-1363.

Hughes JM, Freiermuth CE, Shepherd-Banigan M, et al. Emergency department interventions for older adults: a systematic review. *J Am Geriatr Soc.* 2019;67(7):1516-1525.

STRUCTURAL ENHANCEMENTS

The environment of the ED itself places older adults at risk for iatrogenic complications. The ED is a high-risk setting that can precipitate delirium and disorientation; disrupt the sleep-wake cycle; increase anxiety, agitation, and falls; and impair communication in those with visual and hearing impairments. ED structural enhancements can improve patient outcomes, safety, and satisfaction. The ideal ED for older adults would feature nonglare nonslip flooring, pressure-reducing mattresses, sturdy bedside chairs, accommodations for visitors, and noise-reducing features of flooring and curtains. Features that reduce the risk of delirium include those that preserve orientation and the sleep-wake cycle, such as large face clocks and diurnal lighting, as well as appropriate environmental stimuli and cognitive activities. EDs can also encourage safe mobility by adding handrails, providing assistive devices, and developing clear and visible signage.

FINANCING

Comprehensive geriatric emergency care offers potential cost savings for EDs, hospitals, and health systems. Accurate assessment of the value of reducing falls, delirium, iatrogenic infections, adverse medication events on the cost of prolonged hospitalization, ED revisit, and rehospitalization, as well as the value of appropriate outpatient care utilization (eg, rapid follow-up visits, urgent care, telemedicine visits), is essential to make an evidence-based case to support financing a comprehensive geriatric ED. Collaboration with existing hospital and community health care partners to maximize available resources can result in cost savings and make financing geriatric ED interventions feasible.

CLINICAL CARE

Emergency care for the older adult involves treating both acute illnesses and injuries, as well as exacerbations of chronic disease. The most common reasons older adults present to the ED include falls, chest pain, adverse medication effects, neuropsychiatric disorders, alcohol and substance abuse, elder abuse and neglect, abdominal pain, infections, and psychosocial concerns. Older adults often present with vague symptoms, atypical presentations of common diseases, multiple acute conditions, and confounding medical comorbidities. Additionally, up to 40% of older adults have cognitive impairment that is not readily apparent to emergency providers, further complicating their medical and psychosocial evaluation as well as disposition. For this reason, innovative approaches are necessary to deliver optimal care to this population.

Universal Screening and Comprehensive Geriatric Assessments

Validated screening tools used in other care settings can rapidly identify those at high risk for poor outcomes in the ED setting. The Identification of Seniors at Risk (ISAR) (Table 27–1) is one such screening tool useful in the ED. The

Table 27–1. Adapted universal screening and risk assessment.

High risk for poor health outcomes, high utilization	**Identification of Seniors at Risk (ISAR)** *Scoring: 0–6 (positive score shown in parentheses = 1 point)* 1. Before the illness or injury that brought you to the emergency department, did you need someone to help you on a regular basis? (yes) 2. Since the illness or injury that brought you to the emergency department, have you needed more help than usual to take care of yourself? (yes) 3. Have you been hospitalized for one or more nights during the past 6 months (excluding a stay in the emergency department)? (yes) 4. In general, do you see well? (no) 5. In general, do you have serious problems with your memory? (yes) 6. Do you take more than three different medications every day? (yes) Scoring: ISAR >2 = high risk
Fall risk	**Timed Up and Go** Stand from chair Walk 10 feet Turn around Walk back 10 feet Sit in chair Scoring: <10 seconds = normal 10–29 seconds = below normal, variable mobility >30 seconds = impaired mobility
Delirium	**Confusion Assessment Method** Acute onset/fluctuating course Inattention *and either* Disorganized thinking *or* Altered consciousness

ISAR is comprised of six questions that identify older adults who are at high risk for poor health outcomes and intense health care resource utilization. Patients self-report functional capacity, need for assistance, visual acuity, memory, recent hospitalization, and their number of medications. If positive, the ISAR would then be followed by CGAs and targeted interventions to address patients' needs.

Falls

Approximately 33% of all older adults will fall annually, and 10% of such falls will result in major injuries. Falls are the leading cause of injury, resulting in significant morbidity, disability, decreased independence and quality of life, and injury-related death. ED screening with the Timed Up and Go Test (see Table 27–1) is a simple means to rapidly identify patients at risk for falls with minimal equipment, training, or professional expertise. Identifying risk factors that contribute to falls, such as gait instability and environmental hazards, is essential to create safe discharge plans for older adults.

Delirium

Delirium is a medical emergency that affects 10% of older adults in the ED and independently carries a high morbidity and mortality. Delirium can prolong hospital length of stay, can increase dependence, and is independently associated with poor health outcomes. It is underrecognized and undertreated in the ED. The Confusion Assessment Method (CAM) (see Table 27–1) is a validated tool that has been adapted for use in the ED. CAM-rated delirium is associated with falls resulting in injuries, inadequate pain control, and increased sedative or restraint use, all of which can result in prolonged hospitalization, poor functional outcomes, institutionalization, and increased mortality. This 5-minute test can differentiate delirium from dementia by the presence of mental status changes that are acute in onset and fluctuating in course, characterized by inattention, disorganized thinking, and an altered level of alertness. Older adults identified as having delirium often require admission to treat the underlying causes of delirium. If discharged without identification of the causes and treatment plans with adequate medical and psychosocial supports, they are likely unable to adhere to treatment plans on their own, placing them at risk for ED revisit and rehospitalization.

Cognitive Impairment

Between 16% and 40% of older adults presenting to the ED present with some form of cognitive impairment. In one study, 70% of those discharged home with cognitive impairment had no prior history of dementia and were less likely to have assistance with home care. Thus, older adults who present with cognitive impairments require focused ED assessment and multidisciplinary case management to minimize poor health outcomes.

▶ Multidisciplinary Care Teams

Multidisciplinary assessment and care coordination facilitate rapid ED workup, promote safe transitional care, and decrease inpatient admissions. Models of care using multidisciplinary care teams such as the Acute Care for the Elderly adapted for the ED setting include CGA performed by combinations of geriatricians, geriatric nurses, pharmacists, social workers, physical therapists, and case managers equipped to identify and address the needs of complex older adults in the ED. Sanon and colleagues describe an Acute Care for the Elderly model adapted to the ED setting that used the CGA in the ED setting to care for high-risk older adults. In addition to identifying high-risk older adults, Hwang and colleagues noted that geriatric transitional care nurses decreased inpatient admission for older adults. In a 2015 systematic review of multidisciplinary team care in the acute care settings by Hickman and colleagues, multidisciplinary team care with geriatric expertise in CGA, coordination, and communication improved ED revisits, mortality, and functional decline in older adults.

Hamilton C, Ronda L, Hwang U, et al. The evolving role of geriatric emergency department social work in the era of health care reform. *Soc Work Health Care*. 2015;54(9):849-868.

Hickman LD, Phillips JL, Newton PJ, Halcomb EJ, Al Abed N, Davidson PM. Multidisciplinary team interventions to optimise health outcomes for older people in acute care settings: a systematic review. *Arch Gerontol Geriatr*. 2015;61(3):322-329.

Hwang U, Dresden SM, Rosenberg MS, et al. Geriatric emergency department innovations: transitional care nurses and hospital use. *J Am Geriatr Soc*. 2018;66(3):459-466.

Inouye, SK, Westendorp RGJ, Saczynski JS. Delirium in elderly people. *Lancet* 2014;383(9920):911-922.

Sanon M, Hwang U, Abraham G, Goldhirsch S, Richardson LD. ACE model for older adults in ED. *Geriatrics* 2019;4(1):24.

FUTURE OF EMERGENCY CARE FOR OLDER ADULTS

Emergency care is evolving to meet the demographic changes of the 21st century by improving quality and outcomes and decreasing the cost of health care for older adults. Goals of emergency care for the older adult remain the same as for all patients: to provide appropriate, timely, and comprehensive emergency care for acute illnesses and injuries and exacerbations of chronic disease. However, multidisciplinary team care implementing universal screening and CGAs in the ED is necessary to identify older adults who are at high risk for falls, delirium, and subsequent functional or cognitive impairment. Implementing multidisciplinary team care with CGAs will continue to improve outcomes and decrease the harms associated with health care utilization. Future goals for emergency care for the older adult include implementing evidence-based best practices, improving access to ED-based palliative care services, and enhancing linkages to geriatric primary care, home care, and community resources. Implementing a multidisciplinary and multifaceted approach to emergency care for older adults not only aligns with older adults' goals of care, but also improves the quality of care by and value to health systems.

Hospital Care

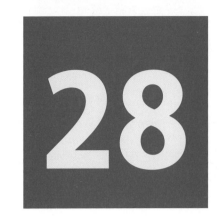

Kathryn J. Eubank, MD

Edgar Pierluissi, MD

GENERAL PRINCIPLES: HAZARDS OF HOSPITALIZATION

Almost 20% of people 65 years of age or older are hospitalized each year in the United States, a rate nearly four times that of the general population. Those 65 years of age or older account for approximately 38% of all hospital admissions, 47% of inpatient care days, and 45% of hospital expenditures. Older adults account for 74% of all in-hospital deaths and have more discharges to places other than home. Many are frail and experience disability and comorbid illnesses. Because of their medical complexity, older patients typically require services from multiple health care providers, most of whom have no formal training in geriatric medicine.

Hospitalization is a critical time for older patients, and heralds a period of high risk that extends beyond discharge, especially for the frail and the very old. Because older adults make up almost half of all inpatient care days, they are at a disproportionate risk for hospital adverse events. For example, in the landmark Harvard Medical Practice Study, patients age 65 years or older accounted for only 27% of the hospitalized population but experienced 43% of all adverse events.

Hospitalization-associated disability is a common and feared complication of hospitalization for older adults. New activities of daily living (ADL) deficits occur in as many as 30% of patients 70 years of age or older who are admitted to an acute care hospital from the community, and hospitalization accounts for approximately 50% of new disability that community-dwelling older adults experience. Hospital processes of care and environment developed without the older adult in mind contribute both to failure to recover from functional loss that occurred before admission as well as new decline during the hospitalization (Figure 28–1).

There are a number of factors that contribute to the hostile environment of hospitals. Bed rest and low mobility are major contributors to functional decline. Even short periods of bed rest can result in significant loss of muscle mass and strength in older adults. There are many reasons that bed rest occurs even when not explicitly ordered. Crowded hospital rooms, beds that are difficult to transfer in and out of either because of height or rails, hallways that are cluttered, slick polished floors, and lack of access to adaptive devices that the patient may use at home such as canes or walkers, eyeglasses, and raised toilet seats or shower chairs are all barriers to mobilization. Patients are frequently attached to peripheral devices such as intravenous line poles, oxygen tubing, urinary catheters, cardiac monitors, or other tethers that further inhibit mobility. Concerns about falls often result in inappropriate confinement to bed. Studies show that most patients will not ambulate on their own unless explicitly told to do so, yet clinicians rarely discuss exercise in the hospital with patients. In addition, older adults may experience enforced dependence when nursing staff and concerned families assist patients with ADLs regardless of the patient's underlying ability to perform them independently. Undernutrition is another factor that contributes to hospital complications. Up to a quarter of hospitalized older adults receive less than 50% of required daily protein-energy intake because of nothing by mouth (NPO) status, poor appetite, or eating an unfamiliar and unappetizing diet. Older adults are also at high risk for adverse drug events as a result of metabolism changes with age, comorbidities, and polypharmacy. Approximately 10% to 15% of older patients experience an in-hospital adverse drug event. Singly or in combination, all of these factors can result in new disability, falls, delirium, depression, pressure ulcers, and bowel and bladder dysfunction, and increase the risk for the loss of independence.

Despite the discouraging statistics, hospital care can be safer for older patients. Focused efforts have improved treatment of specific conditions such as myocardial infarction, heart failure, and pneumonia. Moreover, reengineering the microsystem of care (eg, how care is delivered on a hospital ward or how hospital care is linked to posthospital care) has been shown to improve outcomes in this vulnerable population.

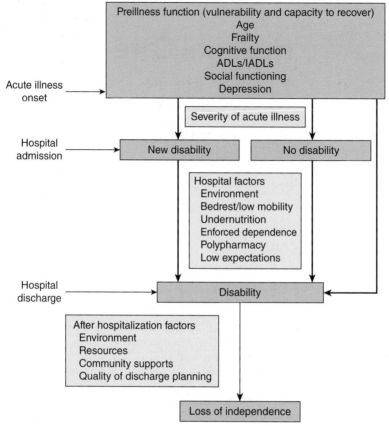

▲ **Figure 28–1.** Hospitalization, functional loss, and capacity to recover. ADLs, activities of daily living; IADLs, instrumental activities of daily living.

SUCCESSFUL MODELS OF CARE

A number of interventions that target older patients who are at high risk for hospital-associated complications have been developed to address the challenges discussed earlier. Successful care models focus on goals of care, comprehensive geriatric assessment, and interprofessional, team-based care. Attention is given to the physical environment, processes of care, and prevention of specific hospital-associated complications that are common in vulnerable older patients. These models include acute care for elders (ACE) units, Mobile Acute Care for Elders (MACE), the Hospital Elder Life Program (HELP), clinical pathways and care maps, and geriatric medicine co-management on surgical and other specialty services such as oncology or neurology.

ACE units were developed with the explicit goal to prevent functional decline and improve the quality of care for older adults during acute hospitalization. ACE units utilize comprehensive geriatric assessment and interprofessional team-based care to align care plans with patient goals and to prevent common complications of hospitalization, such as physical or cognitive decline, nutritional deficits, and polypharmacy. ACE units include a prepared environment that promotes mobility (raised toilet seats, low beds, carpeted hallways, handrails, and assistive devices) and orientation (clocks, calendars, rooms for group meals to increase socialization). Nursing protocols are deployed to promote continence, enhance sleep via nonpharmacologic means, maintain good nutrition, promote skin integrity, and provide frequent reorientation and inclusion of patients in plans of care. Emphasis is placed on discharge planning early in hospitalization with the explicit goal of returning home to community living. In addition, medical care plans are reviewed to prevent polypharmacy as well as minimize unnecessary procedures. ACE units have been shown to improve or maintain ADLs and mobility, decrease delirium, decrease discharges to long-term care, increase provider and patient satisfaction, and, in some studies, decreased length of stay, readmissions, and cost. Since the advent of ACE units and trials demonstrating their effectiveness, newer models of care have been developed that leverage the expertise of geriatrics teams to older adults throughout the hospital. MACE consists of mobile teams that implement the same geriatric assessment, nursing interventions, medication management, early focus on discharge needs, and team-based care approach as ACE but are not confined by geographic space. The e-Geriatrician model uses a linked electronic health record across hospitals to identify patients at risk for hospital-related complications. The care of these patients can be reviewed by a geriatrician who is local or geographically removed from the patient. Newer adaptations of the model are investigating "virtual" computer-based or telehealth ACE as a means to expand beyond ACE unit walls as well.

HELP is a multicomponent intervention developed specifically to prevent delirium in older hospitalized adults. Hospital volunteers implement mobility, cognitive, sleep, and nutrition protocols on general medical wards throughout the hospital. The individualized protocols are targeted to patients at medium to high risk for developing delirium based on admission risk factors. For example, sleep deprivation can lead to delirium, and measures are initiated to promote quiet environments (turning beepers to vibrate and keeping hallways quiet) and nonpharmacologic sleep protocols (warm milk and back rub for insomnia). Other risk factors addressed include immobility, visual and hearing impairment, cognitive impairment, and dehydration. Randomized trials showed a reduction in incident delirium of one-third compared to control groups, as well as improvements in delirium duration and severity. Similar results have been obtained on surgical services such as reductions in delirium following implementation of protocols in hip fracture patients on surgical wards.

Clinical pathways or care maps are problem-specific management plans that aim to standardize care across various providers and units by delineating key steps along an optimal timeline to achieve specific goals. For example, a care map for total knee replacement might include nursing-initiated pain protocols, automatic discontinuation of urinary catheters within hours postoperatively once certain predetermined criteria are met, and automatic ambulation on postoperative day 1. The Institute for Healthcare Improvement has identified standardization as a first step in developing more reliable systems independent of individual providers or unit assignment. Care maps have been shown to decrease lengths of stay for postsurgical care (knee arthroplasty, transurethral prostate resection, carotid endarterectomy), to decrease postoperative complications (cardiac surgery, femoral neck fracture), to increase physical function and ambulation at discharge (hip fracture), to decrease inpatient mortality (community-acquired pneumonia, heart failure), and to improve pain assessment and end-of-life care (inpatient hospice, acute oncology unit). Each care map or clinical pathway is problem specific and developed using evidence-based interventions shown to improve outcomes in the vulnerable older adult.

Geriatric medicine co-management is another model in which geriatricians manage the patients' medical and geriatric issues while the specialist or surgeon focuses on specialty-specific or surgical care. Geriatrician-orthopedist co-management of the patient with hip fracture repair or elective joint replacement is the most common co-management model. These services have protocols in place to optimize rapid preoperative assessment, decrease time from admission to surgery, and focus on many of the issues common to the other models discussed earlier. Most use care maps to standardize care such as thrombosis prophylaxes or time to ambulation. Trials show decreased lengths of stays, decreased postoperative complications, improved mobility, decreased inpatient mortality, and improved nursing and surgeon satisfaction.

APPROACH TO THE HOSPITALIZED OLDER ADULT

▶ Goals of Care

The goals of hospital care should be established upon admission for each patient. For older persons, these can vary widely and may include prolonging survival, relieving specific symptoms, maintaining or regaining ability to walk or care for oneself, getting help taking care of oneself, avoiding institutionalization, being reassured during a frightful experience, and providing comfort and peace while dying. Family members may share these goals but may also have additional goals, such as getting help caring for the patient, facilitating a transition in care from home to long-term care, or being protected from a frightening situation. Physicians and other professionals involved in the care of the patient may share these goals and also aim to achieve quality, efficiency, and patient satisfaction measures for inpatients, reduce hospital costs, and avoid adverse events.

Such discussions may be initiated with open-ended requests, such as: "Different patients have different goals when they are admitted to the hospital. Can you tell me about what you would like us to accomplish while you are in the hospital?" Discussions of goals of care are broader than simply cataloging do not resuscitate (DNR) decisions or reviewing options for specific therapeutic interventions. In fact, DNR and other decisions may be ill informed without first discussing the goals of care. Explicit articulation of goals of care will sometimes identify disagreements among patients, caregivers, and providers, or unattainable expectations, which can then be recognized and addressed.

▶ Comprehensive Geriatric Assessment

Hospitalized older adults require a comprehensive assessment of their physical, cognitive, psychological, and social functioning in addition to the problem-focused assessment (Table 28–1). The comprehensive assessment of key functional domains will ensure that an appropriate care plan is implemented. Because the underlying reasons for the hospitalization of an older adult may be multifactorial, the care plan must address these multiple factors.

Table 28–1. Geriatric assessment on admission.

What to Assess	How to Assess	Why It Matters	What to Do with Findings
Physical Function			
Ask about:			
Activities of daily living (ADLs)	Before you became ill, were you able to bathe, toilet, dress, eat, and transfer from bed to a chair without assistance? Currently, are you able to bathe, toilet, dress, eat, and transfer from bed to a chair without assistance?	The patient may not be getting sufficient assistance at home at baseline or may have experienced a hospitalization-associated decline in function requiring additional assistance after discharge to ensure that all ADLs are met.	Work with caregivers, social worker, and case manager to ensure patient has sufficient support that matches their functional abilities after discharge. For new-onset disability, refer to appropriate therapy service for retraining (occupational therapy). Work with nursing to implement strategies to prevent further decline while inpatient.
Mobility	Are you able to walk? Do you need to use assistive devices?	Ability to ambulate safely is important to maintain independence.	Refer to physical therapy for gait assessment and education regarding use of assistive devices. Write patient-specific activity orders to prevent decline while inpatient.
Falls	Have you fallen in the past year?	Having fallen in past year is a strong risk factor for future falls.	Assess risk factors for falls and work with primary care clinician, therapy, and home safety evaluators to ensure that appropriate interventions to reduce falls are implemented.
Cognitive Function			
Ask about:			
Cognitive symptoms	Can you tell me why you are here? The name of this place? What city and state are we in? What day is today? What is today's date, month, year? (Orientation) Serial sevens (start at 100 and subtract 7, and continue until asked to stop). Spell *world* backward. (Attention) I want you to repeat and then remember 3 words I am about to say. I will ask you to say them again in 1 minute. (3-item recall)	Delirium is present in ~15% of patients on admission and develops in another 15% during hospitalization. If delirium is present, further dementia testing is inaccurate and should be delayed until resolved. Dementia significantly increases the risk for delirium, increases the burdens and morbidity of treatment, increases risk for rehospitalization and affects planning for safe discharge, and raises concern for decision-making capacity. For patients with dementia, assess caregivers for burnout or stress.	If delirium is present, diagnose and address underlying etiologies. If dementia is present, consider further testing with the Montreal Cognitive Assessment (MoCA), neuropsychological evaluation, or an occupational therapy consultation for a Kaufmann Evaluation of Living Skills (KELS) test. Also consider referral on discharge to memory or geriatrics clinic and referral of caregivers to Alzheimer's Association and to Family Caregiver Alliance.
Psychological Function			
Ask about:			
Symptoms of depression	Over the last 2 weeks, have you felt down, depressed, or hopeless? Have you lost interest in or pleasure in doing things?	Depression and depressive symptoms are common and often underdiagnosed in the hospital, especially among patients with stroke. Depressive symptoms, especially those that persist after discharge, are associated with worse physical function and mortality after hospital discharge.	If positive, further testing can be performed using the Patient Health Questionnaire (PHQ)-9 or Geriatric Depression Scale (GDS). Evaluate for medical causes for depression such as thyroid, cardiac, neurologic, and endocrine diseases. Discuss findings with primary provider and coordinate plan for starting treatment.

(continued)

Table 28–1. Geriatric assessment on admission. (*continued*)

What to Assess	How to Assess	Why It Matters	What to Do with Findings
Social Function			
Ask about:			
Social circumstances	Where do you live? Do you live with anyone? Do you feel safe there? Do you wish to return to where you live? Is anyone coming into your home to help you with cooking, cleaning, or shopping (instrumental ADLs)? Are you satisfied with the help you are getting? Does anyone help you with your medications? How do you get to/from appointments? How are you managing your finances?	Knowledge of a patient's social situation is necessary for developing an effective home discharge plan. Any evidence of elder abuse should be reported to a local adult protective services agency.	Coordinate discharge resources with social worker, rehabilitation staff, and primary provider. Resources might include in-home caregivers, Meals on Wheels, visiting nurses, or case management services. Any evidence of elder neglect or abuse should be reported to a local adult protective services agency.

Functional assessment determines the patient's ability to walk and to perform basic ADLs (eg, bathing, dressing, transferring from a bed to a chair, using the toilet, self-feeding) both at baseline before onset of the acute illness and on admission. For some patients, an unmet need for assistance with ADLs at baseline may be a contributing factor to the hospitalization. Patients who are dependent in an ADL on admission have longer hospitalizations, higher risk for additional ADL dependence at discharge, and higher risk for death on average than otherwise similar patients who are independent in ADLs. A history of falls is also important to elicit on admission and address during the hospitalization and at discharge.

Cognitive and psychological assessment should include assessment of mental status and affect. Among hospitalized older medical patients, ≥20% have dementia, ≥15% are delirious on admission, and another 15% experience delirium during hospitalization. Symptoms of depression are common, and 33% of hospitalized older medical patients have major or minor depression.

Dementia, delirium, and depression are frequently present but infrequently recognized. If you are obtaining the history from a surrogate rather than the patient, cognitive impairment from delirium or dementia or both is likely. The presence of fluctuating mental state and impaired attention, along with altered level of consciousness and/or disorganized thinking, suggests delirium. Evidence of inattention includes difficulty focusing, being easily distracted, or failure of an attention test like subtracting serial sevens or saying the months of the year backward. The Confusion Assessment Method (CAM) is a highly sensitive and specific screening tool for delirium in hospitalized older adults. Once delirium is ruled out, serious cognitive impairment can be tested using the Mini-Cog (three-word recall plus a clock drawing). Recalling zero of three words on short-term recall is a sign of significant impairment, whereas dementia is largely ruled out by recalling all three items and accurately drawing a clock. Screening for depression consists of asking whether the patient has felt sad, depressed, or hopeless over the last 2 weeks.

It is critical for the attending physician, along with other members of the interprofessional team, to understand the patient's social context in order to develop an effective after-hospital care plan. Social isolation, loneliness, and lack of social supports are common in hospitalized older adults. This will affect the amount of in-home support services, meals, and transportation assistance a patient may require. Any hesitations or concerns should be explored further for evidence of elder neglect or abuse. The prevalence of elder abuse is higher in hospitalized settings (~14%) than in the general community (~3%–4%). Concerns about abuse should be discussed with a social worker and reported to the local adult protective services agency.

In addition to completing a functional, cognitive, psychological, and social assessment on every older adult admitted to the hospital, a geriatrics-focused review of systems may identify conditions that are commonly considered geriatric syndromes, including incontinence, falls, sensory impairment, undernutrition, and frailty. Each of these conditions should be addressed with targeted plans either during admission or at discharge.

▶ Interprofessional Care

In most cases, designing and implementing strategies to achieve the goals of care requires a team with expertise across multiple domains, including rehabilitation, pharmacology, and social and community resources. For example, consider the situation of an 83-year-old widow with chronic obstructive pulmonary disease (COPD) and mild cognitive impairment who lives alone, has declined over the past month in her ability to take care of her home and her affairs, is admitted with hypoxia and hypercarbia attributed to a COPD exacerbation, and wishes to live in her home until she dies. Although the physician may have the expertise to treat the COPD exacerbation, nursing, social work, and therapy expertise is also required to maintain and promote the patient's independent function in the hospital and at home after discharge.

THERAPY

In general, the treatment of disease should not differ according to age. Treatment should be selected on the basis of the goals of care for a particular patient and on the basis of evidence that a particular treatment regimen will achieve that specified goal.

Older patients may differ from younger patients according to their goals. For example, treatment directed primarily at amelioration of symptoms and dysfunction rather than prolongation of survival may be desired more often by patients in their 90s than by those in their 60s. Also, insofar as these choices are influenced by prognosis, which is determined in part by age, patients should be informed accurately when they desire this information. Nonetheless, the care goals may differ between patients of the same age and should be determined individually.

Evidence of the efficacy of a treatment regimen in achieving a specific patient goal should be sought. In some situations, treatment efficacy may differ by age, and older adults often have comorbidities that may affect treatment outcomes also. Medications may need to be titrated to reflect changes in body composition, volumes of distribution, and renal or hepatic function, which all change with age. The risk of side effects from many drugs and procedures also increases with age, and these risks should be considered in estimating the net benefit of a specific treatment strategy.

Unfortunately, most evidence about the efficacy of many therapies is based on studies of younger persons, and specific evidence about the efficacy of those therapies in persons age 75 years or older is sometimes inadequate. In these situations, it is reasonable to extrapolate from evidence in younger patients, taking into account age-related differences in pharmacology and increased risks of side effects when deciding on a specific treatment regimen.

PREVENTION

To prevent iatrogenic complications common in hospitalized older adults, additional assessments on admission and throughout the hospital stay are required (Table 28–2).

Functional decline is a feared, and all too common, adverse outcome of hospitalization. Many complications can be prevented through a dedicated effort to maintain mobility in the hospital. Clinicians should set walking expectations early for each patient and assess compliance daily. Although symptoms and fear of injury may limit some patients, most are motivated by avoiding functional decline and simply being asked to walk. Clinicians should also treat pain that may be inhibiting mobility; ensure assistive devices are available with appropriate training; and remove unnecessary tethers such as bladder and intravenous catheters, oxygen lines, and cardiac monitoring. Unnecessary bladder catheters, in addition to causing iatrogenic infection and limiting mobility, are associated with increased delirium risk. Delirium is preventable in many patients with simple prevention measures as outlined in Table 28–2.

TRANSITIONING FROM HOSPITAL TO HOME

It is increasingly recognized that transitions between care providers and across settings are common and fraught with hazards. This has led to a focus of care called "transitional care" (see Chapter 26) as a part of the vision for age-friendly health systems (see Chapter 79). There are numerous interventions aimed at improving the transitional care of older adults leaving the hospital. These have several key components in common, including (1) strategies to improve patient and caregiver engagement in the process starting at the time of admission; (2) early identification of postdischarge care needs and use of interprofessional teams to properly address those needs throughout the hospitalization, as well as after discharge; (3) investing time and resources into improving patient understanding about the reasons for admission, what is required to manage their health at discharge, appropriate signs and symptoms that signal a need for early intervention, and who they should contact for questions or help; (4) special attention to medication reconciliation, patient instruction, and cross-site communication of medication changes; and (5) enhanced communication between inpatient and outpatient clinicians via phone calls and improved discharge summary communication. Table 28–3 is a checklist for improving care at the time of transition from hospital to next site of care.

In addition to the topics common to the interventions discussed earlier, inpatient clinicians caring for older adults need an understanding of the multiple postdischarge sites of care available for this population. Will the patient require rehabilitation for deconditioning? If so, will the patient meet requirements for intensive rehabilitation hospitals versus skilled nursing facilities (SNFs)? Is there a skilled need that requires home services after discharge or inpatient SNF services (often this depends on the availability of a caregiver)? Has the patient declined in physical or cognitive function such that 24-hour supervision will be required at discharge? Can 24-hour supervision be done at home, or will nursing home or domiciliary placement be required? Is the patient

Table 28–2. Prevention strategies for common hazards experienced by older adults in the hospital.

Hazard	How to Assess	When to Assess	How to Prevent
Deconditioning/disability	Ask the patient or the nurse if the patient is getting out of bed for every meal and walking 3–4 times daily.	Daily	Promote mobility: Order physical therapy consultation, avoid bed rest orders, remove unnecessary catheters, write for patient to be out of bed for all meals and to ambulate at least 3–4 times daily.
Delirium	Look for signs of change in mental status, inattentiveness, disorganized thinking, or changes in level of consciousness (Confusion Assessment Method).	Daily	Promote mobility. Keep the environment bright during the day and dark and quiet at night. Provide patient with eyeglasses and/or hearing aids; provide frequent orientation with calendars and clocks. Avoid deliriogenic medications especially benzodiazepines and anticholinergics, restraints, and unnecessary catheters. Allow uninterrupted sleep at night (stop unneeded vitals, labs at night).
Falls	Have you fallen in the past 12 months?	At admission	Promote mobility. Provide patient with eyeglasses, hearing aids, assistive devices as appropriate, and frequent orientation with calendars and clocks. Avoid sedating medications, restraints, and unnecessary catheters. Address incontinence.
Urinary incontinence (UI)	Do you have trouble controlling your urine? Have you had accidents in the past 6 months?	At admission and during hospitalization for prolonged hospitalizations	Promote mobility. Use nonpharmacologic interventions such as scheduled voiding while awake. Avoid "continence aids" (diapers, catheters), which have been shown to increase the risk of ongoing UI at 6 and 12 months after discharge.
Urinary retention (UR)	Are you having any trouble emptying your bladder? Check postvoid residual.	At admission and daily	Avoid triggering medications including anticholinergics, calcium channel blockers, and opiates. Stand to void and teach maneuvers as needed to increase emptying (Valsalva, external suprapubic pressure).
Constipation	When was your last bowel movement? Review nursing documentation regarding last bowel movement.	Daily	Promote mobility. Maintain hydration. Provide fiber in diet. Provide laxatives such as sennosides for patients receiving opiates for pain or other constipating medications.
Pressure ulcers	Skin examination.	Daily	Promote mobility. Frequent position changes (every 2 hours) for patients that are bedbound. Maintain nutritional state. Keep skin dry. Consider pressure-reducing mattress.
Infection	Is bladder catheter or intravenous catheter present?	Daily	Promote mobility to stimulate deeper breathing to avoid atelectasis. Remove unnecessary bladder and intravenous catheters.
Inappropriate prescribing/polypharmacy	Review all medications for ongoing necessity, drug-drug interactions, drug-disease interactions, and age-appropriate dosing.	Daily	Review all medications for efficacy and appropriateness in older adults, considering prognosis, goals of care, side effects, and need for monitoring.
Undernutrition	See Chapter 13 for useful nutritional screening tools.	Daily	Avoid unnecessary NPO (nothing by mouth) orders; ask caregiver to bring in dentures; provide a diet that is the least restrictive possible, of the proper consistency, and that is culturally appropriate; provide nutritional supplementation for patients who are undernourished on admission.

Table 28–3. Transitional care checklist.

Patient and family education	☐	Have the patient, caregivers, and all members of the care team been included in the planning process and agree with the care plan?
	☐	Have the patient and caregiver been adequately educated about their condition, including what makes it better or worse, signs/symptoms to watch for, and when to seek medical attention?
Medications	☐	Do the patient and caregiver understand how and when to take their medications and side effects to watch for? Is proper monitoring in place for high-risk medications?
	☐	Has the medication list been properly reconciled to avoid polypharmacy and inappropriate medications?
Functional status/home environment alignment	☐	What is the patient's functional status? Does the patient need referral to therapy services, or will the patient require more supervision at discharge?
Cognitive status/home environment alignment	☐	What is the patient's cognitive status? Has there been a change? Does the patient require increased assistance or supervision after discharge?
Medical equipment	☐	Are there specific services that need to be in place prior to leaving the hospital? For example, has oxygen been delivered to the home? Durable medical equipment? Supplies?
Social circumstances	☐	Is there a plan in place to ensure adequate food and physical and financial safety and to identify and address self-neglect?
Follow-up and communication with primary provider	☐	Is follow-up arranged and occurring in a timely manner? Are the patient and caregiver aware of and in agreement with needed follow-up and referrals?
	☐	Is there a plan and direct responsibility for following up on any pending labs or studies?
	☐	Is the discharge summary completed, and has it been sent to the primary care, specialist, and receiving clinicians? If going to another facility, is the discharge summary ready and being sent with the patient and does it include who can be contacted for questions?

nearing the end of life with goals more consistent with hospice care? Most patients prefer to stay in their homes as long as possible, and good transitional care can help them achieve that goal by optimizing care at home and putting plans in place to regain and optimize functional status.

Covinsky KE, Pierluissi E, Johnston CB. Hospitalization-associated disability: "she was probably able to ambulate, but I'm not sure." *JAMA.* 2011;306(16):1782-1793.

Creditor M. Hazards of hospitalization of the elderly. *Ann Intern Med.* 1993;118(3):219-223.

Flood KL, Maclennan PA, McGrew D, et al. Effects of an Acute Care for Elders unit on costs and 30-day readmissions. *JAMA Int Med.* 2013;173(11):981-987.

Fox MT, Persaud M, Maimets I, et al. Effectiveness of acute geriatric unit care using Acute Care for Elders components: a systematic review and meta-analysis. *J Am Geriatr Soc.* 2012;60:2237-2245.

Fried TR, Bradley EH, Towle VR, Allore H. Understanding the treatment preferences of seriously ill patients. *N Engl J Med.* 2002;346(14):1061-1066.

Mendelson DA, Friedman SM. Principles of comanagement and the geriatric fracture center. *Clin Geriatr Med.* 2014;30(2):183-189.

Rochester-Eyeguokan CD, Pincus KJ, Patel RS, et al. The current landscape of transitions of care practice models: a scoping review. *Pharmacotherapy.* 2016;36(1):117-133.

Rotter T, Kinsman L, James EL, et al. Clinical pathways: effects on professional practice, patient outcomes, length of stay and hospital costs. *Cochrane Database Syst Rev.* 2010;3:CD006632.

Perioperative Care for Older Surgical Patients

29

Victoria Tang, MD, MAS

Emily Finlayson, MD, MS

GENERAL PRINCIPLES

More than half of all surgical procedures are performed in individuals older than age 65 years, and one-third of older adults undergo a procedure in the last year of life. In 2007, >4 million major operations were performed on older adults. As the aging population continues to grow, the number of older patients undergoing surgical interventions is expected to continue to increase.

SURGICAL RISK IN THE OLDER ADULT

Caring for the older surgical patient presents unique problems: older individuals present with more advanced disease, have more chronic conditions, and suffer more complications than younger patients. Careful patient selection and perioperative care are essential for optimizing surgical outcomes in this population. The benefits of the most commonly performed surgical procedures are well established. For example, colon resections increase colorectal cancer–free survival, and hip replacements significantly improve joint pain and functional ability. These benefits, however, must be weighed against the risk of mortality, morbidity, and decreased quality of life that may follow with these surgical interventions.

Nationally representative large cohort studies have highlighted the high risk of mortality in frail, older adults who undergo surgery. In a national sample of older nursing home residents undergoing breast cancer operations ranging from a lumpectomy to a mastectomy with a lymph node dissection, patients had an operative 1-year mortality of 29% to 41%, and those with the highest likelihood of mortality were those with poor preoperative function.

Major operations may also result in a diminished quality of life by causing postoperative cognitive and functional decline. The risk of postoperative cognitive dysfunction following cardiac surgery is well studied, and there is now increasing evidence that postoperative cognitive dysfunction also occurs after noncardiac procedures. Up to 10% of patients older than age 60 years suffer from memory problems 3 months out from noncardiac surgery. Recent research has shown that surgery and anesthesia exposure are not risk factors for cognitive impairment after major noncardiac surgery and critical illness, but cognitive impairment is predicted by in-hospital delirium. Functional changes following surgery can also be prolonged and irreversible. More than half of frail older patients undergoing abdominal operations experience significant functional decline that persists for up to a year after surgery. A recent study assessing functional status following breast cancer surgery in nursing home residents found that many patients suffer functional decline beyond the general expected decline seen in the nursing home population, regardless of breast surgery type. These findings emphasize the importance of addressing the risk of functional decline in all older patients, even for the most "minor" procedures. For some patients, loss of independence weighs heavier than mortality when deciding whether to undergo a high-risk operation. Awareness of these risks is essential for appropriate patient selection. It also allows clinicians to offer a realistic expectation of outcomes, which, in turn, informs decision making by the older individual and their families.

CLINICAL CARE

▶ Preoperative Assessment

The preoperative assessment may be used to optimize the possibility of a good outcome by identifying and improving upon any modifiable risk factors. Additionally, information gathered from the preoperative assessment may be used for patient and family counseling, such as surgical decision making and postoperative anticipatory guidance. The American Geriatrics Society (AGS) and American College of Surgeons (ACS) have jointly recommended preoperative evaluation specific to the geriatric surgical patient. Table 29–1 is a summary of this work. We highlight several key assessments that warrant additional discussion in the following sections.

Table 29–1. Preoperative assessment.

In addition to conducting a history and physical examination of the patient, the following assessments are strongly recommended by the American Geriatrics Society and American College of Surgeons guidelines.

- Assess the patient's cognitive ability and capacity to understand the anticipated surgery.
- Screen the patient for depression.
- Identify the patient's risk factors for developing postoperative delirium.
- Screen for alcohol and other substance abuse/dependence.
- Perform a preoperative cardiac evaluation according to the American College of Cardiology/American Heart Association algorithm for patients undergoing noncardiac surgery.
- Identify the patient's risk factors for postoperative pulmonary complications and implement appropriate strategies for prevention.
- Document the functional status and history of falls.
- Determine baseline frailty score.
- Assess patient's nutritional status and consider preoperative interventions if the patient is at severe nutritional risk.
- Take an accurate and detailed medication history and consider appropriate perioperative adjustments. Monitor for polypharmacy.
- Determine the patient's treatment goals and expectations in the context of the possible treatment outcomes.
- Determine patient's family and social support system.
- Order appropriate preoperative diagnostic tests focused on older patients.

A. Cognition

Older individuals' cognitive capacity, decision-making capacity, and risk for postoperative delirium should be assessed preoperatively. For patients without a known history of dementia, a cognitive assessment using the Mini-Cog test (see Chapter 2, "Overview of Geriatric Assessment") should be performed. This screening is the initial step in identifying patients who may lack the capacity to make medical decisions and who are at high risk for delirium. When initial evaluation identifies cognitive impairment, assessment of decision-making capacity is essential. For patients lacking capacity, advance directives or a surrogate decision maker should be used (see Chapter 21, "Ethics & Informed Decision Making"). Older adults who are at risk for delirium should be identified preoperatively. Major risk factors for delirium are dementia, hearing impairment, depression, preoperative narcotic use, preoperative delirogenic medications, medical multimorbidity, electrolyte abnormalities, malnutrition, and poor functional status. Identifying patients who are at risk for delirium is crucial as a number of preventive measures

implemented early in the patient's hospital course can reduce this risk. Co-management by a geriatrician, careful use of analgesics, and prophylactic use of atypical antipsychotics have been evaluated in clinical trials and found to significantly decrease the incidence and severity of delirium.

B. Cardiovascular

Cardiovascular complications are associated with high operative mortality rates. To identify and help reduce this risk, the American College of Cardiology and the American Heart Association (ACC/AHA) have developed recommendations for cardiac evaluation and care for noncardiac surgery. For older adults with active cardiac disease or coronary artery disease (CAD) risk factors and poor functional status who are about to undergo elective intermediate- or high-risk surgery, strong consideration should be given to noninvasive preoperative cardiac testing and evaluation by a cardiologist (Figure 29–1). Of note, routine electrocardiograms are not indicated in older patients undergoing low-risk surgical procedures in the absence of other risk factors.

C. Pulmonary

Prolonged intubation (>48 hours), pneumonia, atelectasis, and bronchospasm occur after major surgery in >15% of patients older than age 70 years. Risk factors for these complications include active pulmonary disease, current cigarette smoking, congestive heart failure, chronic renal failure, cognitive disorders, and functional dependence. To decrease the risk of pulmonary complications, smoking cessation should be initiated at least 2 months prior to elective surgery, and active pulmonary diseases should be adequately treated.

D. Functional Status

Functional dependence is an independent predictor of mortality following surgery in older adults. Robinson and colleagues reported that dependence with even one activity of daily living (ADL) significantly increased the risk of 6-month mortality (odds ratio [OR], 13.9; 95% confidence interval [CI], 2.9–65.5). The ability to perform ADLs and instrumental activities of daily living (IADLs) should be assessed preoperatively. This identifies older adults who will benefit from occupational and physical therapy in the perioperative period. In addition, the information will help inform surgical decision making and provide anticipatory guidance. Furthermore, emerging data indicate that multimodal optimization of function and mobility before surgery may improve functional recovery after surgery in older adults.

E. Nutritional Status

Older patients with functional dependence are at high risk of malnutrition. Fourteen percent of nursing home residents, 39% of inpatients, and 50.5% of individuals in rehabilitation are malnourished. All older patients should be screened for malnutrition preoperatively. Patients with unintentional weight loss of >10% to 15% over the past 6 months, body mass index (BMI) <18.5 kg/m^2, and serum albumin <3 g/dL are described as being at severe nutritional risk. Preoperative nutritional support should be provided to these patients. Enteral nutrition is the preferred route for nutritional support; when this option is not available secondary to gastrointestinal conditions, parenteral nutrition should be used.

F. Frailty

Frailty has been associated with risk of poor postoperative outcomes. Slow walking speeds have been shown to be associated with frailty, and an easy to use and practical assessment tool is the Timed Up and Go (TUG) test (see Chapter 6, "Falls & Mobility Impairment"). A TUG ≥15 seconds was associated with increased postoperative complications as compared to those whose TUG was <11 seconds (52%–77% vs 11%–13%, respectively). One-year mortality for those with a TUG ≥15 seconds was 31% as compared to 3% for those with a TUG <11 seconds. The preoperative frailty assessment helps inform surgical decision making and assess the risk of postoperative complications.

G. Patient Counseling

Given increased risk of poor postoperative outcomes in older adults, patient and family counseling about treatment goals and plans expected postoperative course, and the patient's family and social support system is imperative. Because patient preferences and expectations influence their treatment preferences, patient and family counseling on preoperative risk assessments is strongly recommended. Despite the possibility of a loss of decision-making capacity in the postoperative setting, such as from delirium, only 26% of older adults with multiple chronic conditions completed an advance directive before surgery in a health care system with a built-in provider advance directive reminder. Documenting advance directives and a designated health care proxy (or surrogate decision maker) in the medical chart prior to surgery is essential.

▶ Postoperative Care

The aim of postoperative care is to return older patients to a high level of functioning as quickly as possible. This goal is achieved with measures that promote recovery and prevent complications. The AGS and ACS have jointly issued guidelines on the basic level of postoperative care that should be provided to older patients undergoing any kind of surgery. Table 29–2 is a postoperative rounding checklist adapted from this work and highlights important aspects of routine postoperative care for older adults.

When possible, patients should be out of bed and walking by the first postoperative day. Physical therapy and occupational therapy consultation should be obtained for patients with functional impairment. Early ambulation

along with chest physiotherapy using incentive spirometers decreases the risk of pulmonary complications. Appropriate fluid resuscitation should be provided, and fluid balance should be monitored through documentation of intake, output, and daily weights. Oral or enteral nutrition should be resumed as soon as the gastrointestinal tract is functional. To prevent infectious complications, aspiration precautions should be instituted, Foley catheters should be removed within 48 hours, and the need for central lines and drains should be reviewed daily and removed once no longer needed.

A. Management of Common Postoperative Issues in Older Adults

1. Pain—Older patients are at higher risk of undertreated pain. Inadequate treatment of pain impedes recovery, prevents the patient from participating in activities, and can lead to delirium, depression, and pulmonary complications. To avoid these complications, pain levels should be assessed frequently and a pain management plan that delivers adequate analgesia while avoiding untoward effects of the analgesics should be implemented. The numeric rating scale is the preferred pain intensity rating scale for use in older adults. In those with dementia, an alternative pain assessment scale would be the facial expression scale. Postoperative pain is best managed with regional anesthesia. For patients undergoing major surgery, epidural regional analgesia with opioids and local anesthetic agents initiated intraoperatively provides the most effective pain control. Intravenous and oral analgesics such as opioids, acetaminophen, and nonsteroidal anti-inflammatory drugs (NSAIDs) also provide effective pain relief. They may be used as supplements to regional anesthesia or as the primary analgesics for less invasive operations. These medications are best delivered as patient-controlled analgesics or on a scheduled dose. This approach is preferred over as-needed doses of medication because patients spend less time in pain. Although effective pain control is important, providers need to be vigilant for side effects of analgesics. Older patients are at increased risk of hypotension, respiratory depression, oversedation, and constipation, which can occur as a side effect of analgesics. Use of regional analgesics; short-acting agents; smaller, less frequent doses; and frequent patient assessment can decrease the risk of these complications.

2. Delirium—Delirium occurs in 15% to 50% of older patients postoperatively. It is associated with increased mortality and medical complications. The physiologic conditions most commonly responsible for delirium in the postoperative setting are pain, hypoxia, hypoglycemia, electrolyte imbalance, and infection. The initial evaluation of the delirious patient should be focused on identifying these disorders. Pain should be adequately treated, serum electrolytes and glucose should be checked, an infectious workup should be performed, and other postoperative complications should

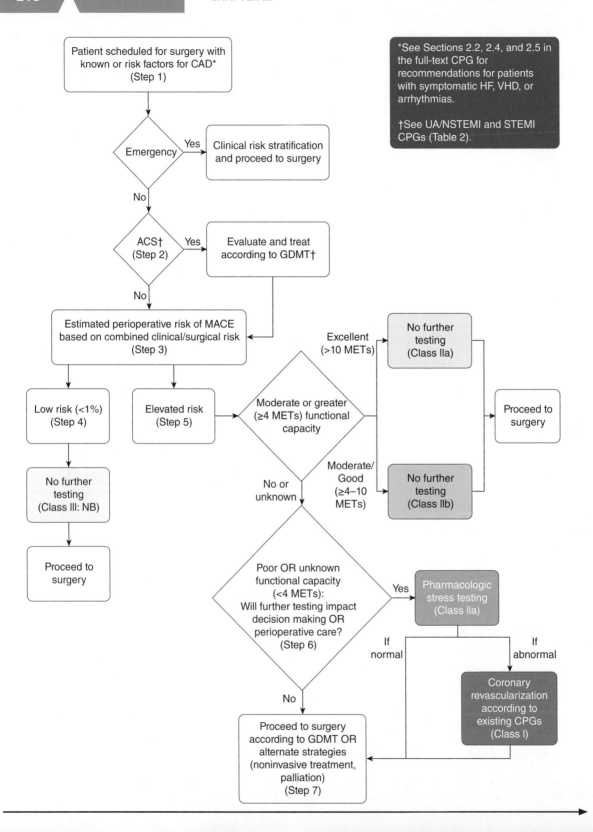

be ruled out. Further measures in the prevention and management of delirium include optimization of environmental stimuli and a review of current medications. Older patients should have their eyeglasses and hearing aids made readily available. The Beers criteria identify a number of potentially inappropriate medications for older patients. Avoiding anticholinergics, antihistamines, and benzodiazepines may help decrease the incidence of delirium in older patients. For patients with agitated delirium who are at risk of injury, frequent reorientation is required, and this may be provided by family members or a sitter; restraints should be avoided. When a multicomponent nonpharmacologic approach is unsuccessful, low doses of antipsychotics such as quetiapine or haloperidol can be prescribed. Their use, however, remains controversial, and they should be used with caution.

3. Cardiac complications—Cardiac complications occur frequently in older patients. The most common postoperative cardiac complications requiring urgent treatment are atrial fibrillation and myocardial infarction. Atrial fibrillation can occur as a result of the increased sympathetic tone associated with the stress of surgery, volume overload, hypoxia/hypercarbia, electrolyte abnormalities, or underlying heart disease. Management of new-onset atrial fibrillation begins with an assessment of hemodynamic stability and rate control. In patients with hemodynamic instability, emergent cardioversion is required. Rate control is achieved using either β-blockers or diltiazem. Intravenous amiodarone may be used when the first-line drugs are ineffective. Most cases of new-onset atrial fibrillation spontaneously revert to sinus rhythm. However, atrial fibrillation persists for more than 24 to 48 hours; anticoagulation should be considered to reduce the risk of stroke.

Perioperative myocardial infarction occurs mainly as a result of prolonged myocardial oxygen supply-demand imbalance and only rarely as a result of acute coronary syndrome. It is diagnosed based on a rise and fall of troponins in the setting of myocardial ischemia as evidenced by electrocardiogram changes, imaging findings, or cardiac symptoms. Tachycardia, tachyarrhythmias, hypertension, anemia, and hypoxia all contribute to myocardial oxygen supply-demand imbalance and can result in non–ST-segment elevation myocardial infarction (NSTEMI) in the perioperative period. When NSTEMI is suspected, management begins with heart rate and blood pressure control with β-blockers and appropriate pain control. For patients with ST-segment elevation and suspected acute coronary syndrome, immediate cardiology consultation should be obtained.

▲ **Figure 29–1.** Stepwise approach to perioperative cardiac assessment for coronary artery disease. Step 1: In patients scheduled for surgery with risk factors for or known coronary artery disease (CAD), determine the urgency of surgery. If an emergency, then determine the clinical risk factors that may influence perioperative management and proceed to surgery with appropriate monitoring and management strategies based on the clinical assessment. Step 2: If the surgery is urgent or elective, determine if the patient has an acute coronary syndrome (ACS). If yes, then refer patient for cardiology evaluation and management according to guideline-directed medical therapy (GDMT) according to the unstable angina (UA)/non–ST-segment elevation myocardial infarction (NSTEMI) and ST-segment elevation myocardial infarction (STEMI) clinical practice guidelines (CPGs). Step 3: If the patient has risk factors for stable CAD, then estimate the perioperative risk of major adverse cardiac events (MACE) on the basis of the combined clinical/surgical risk. This estimate can use the American College of Surgeons National Surgical Quality Improvement Program (NSQIP) risk calculator (http://www.riskcalculator.facs.org) or incorporate the Revised Cardiac Risk Index (RCRI) with an estimation of surgical risk. Step 4: If the patient has a low risk of MACE (<1%), then no further testing is needed, and the patient may proceed to surgery. Step 5: If the patient is at elevated risk of MACE, then determine functional capacity with an objective measure or scale, such as the Duke Activity Status Index. If the patient has moderate, good, or excellent functional capacity (≥4 metabolic equivalents [METs]), then proceed to surgery without further evaluation. Step 6: If the patient has poor (<4 METs) or unknown functional capacity, then the clinician should consult with the patient and perioperative team to determine whether further testing will impact patient decision making (eg, decision to perform original surgery or willingness to undergo coronary artery bypass graft [CABG] or percutaneous coronary intervention [PCI], depending on the results of the test) or perioperative care. If yes, then pharmacologic stress testing is appropriate. In patients with unknown functional capacity, exercise stress testing may be reasonable to perform. If the stress test is abnormal, consider coronary angiography and revascularization depending on the extent of the abnormal test. The patient can then proceed to surgery with GDMT or consider alternative strategies, such as noninvasive treatment of the indication for surgery (eg, radiation therapy for cancer) or palliation. If the test is normal, proceed to surgery according to GDMT. Step 7: If testing will not impact decision making or care, then proceed to surgery according to GDMT or consider alternative strategies, such as noninvasive treatment of the indication for surgery (eg, radiation therapy for cancer) or palliation. HF, heart failure; NB, no benefit; VHD, valvular heart disease. (Reproduced with permission from Fleisher LA, Fleischmann KE, Auerbach AD, et al. 2014 ACC/AHA guideline on perioperative cardiovascular evaluation and management of patients undergoing noncardiac surgery: a report of the American College of Cardiology/American Heart Association Task Force on practice guidelines, *J Am Coll Cardiol* 2014 Dec 9;64(22):e77-137.)

Table 29–2. Preoperative rounding checklist.

Daily Evaluation for	Prevention/Management Strategies
Delirium/cognitive impairment	• Control pain • Optimize physical environment (eg, sleep hygiene, sleep protocol, minimize tethers, encourage family at bedside) • Make sure vision and hearing aids are accessible • Remove catheters • Monitor for substance withdrawal syndromes • Minimize psychoactive medications • Avoid potentially inappropriate medications (eg, Beers criteria medications)
Perioperative acute pain	• Ongoing education regarding safe and effective use of institutional treatment options • Directed pain history • Multimodal, individualized pain control • Vigilant dose titration
Pulmonary complications	• Chest physiotherapy and incentive spirometry • Early mobilization/ambulation • Aspiration precautions
Fall risk	• Universal fall precautions • Vision and hearing aids accessible • Scheduled toileting • Appropriate treatment of delirium • Early mobilization/ambulation • Early physical/occupational therapy if indicated • Assistive walking devices
Ability to maintain adequate nutrition	• Resumption of diet as early as feasible • Dentures made available • Supplementation if indicated
Urinary tract infection prevention	• Daily documentation of Foley catheter indication • Catheter care bundles, hand hygiene, barrier precautions
Functional decline	• Care models and pathways • Structural: uncluttered hallways, large clocks, and calendars • Multidisciplinary rounds • Early mobilization and/or physical or occupational therapy • Family participation • Nutritional support • Minimize patient tethers
Pressure ulcers	• Reduce/minimize pressure, friction, humidity, shear force 　• Repositioning every 2 hours for patients who are unable to get out of bed 　• Out of bed to chair as soon as possible • Maintain adequate nutrition • Wound care

MODELS OF SURGICAL CARE

Prehabilitation, enhanced recovery programs (ERPs), and geriatric co-management are some of the innovative models being implemented to improve the outcomes of surgical care for older patients. In multimodal prehabilitation programs, older adults participate in structured programs that address frailty traits (ie, exercise, nutritional supplementation, anxiety reduction) in the weeks prior to elective surgery. These programs have been found to significantly improve older patients' preoperative functional status; decrease postoperative complications, hospitalization stay, and 30-day readmission; and enhance postoperative functional recovery. For example, Duke's Perioperative Optimization of Senior Health (POSH) program has shown a decrease in length of stay by 2 days, a lower readmission rate (2.8% vs 9.9%), greater discharge to home (62% vs 51%), and lower mean number of complications (0.9 vs 1.4). Current research on prehabilitation is focused on identifying the optimal optimization regimen and on improving compliance with the programs. ERPs are another model aimed at promoting early physiologic and physical recovery after surgery. These programs use structured evidence-based protocols to optimize preoperative patient preparation, minimize the surgical stress response, and encourage early postoperative nutrition and mobilization. ERPs decrease hospital lengths of stay and complication rates in older patients. Lastly, models in which surgeons and geriatricians work closely together to care for the older surgical patient are being developed. Collaboration should begin at the time of patient and procedure selection and continue through the recovery period. This model will certainly improve the quality of surgical care received by the older adult.

American Geriatrics Society Expert Panel on Postoperative Delirium in Older Adults AGS. American Geriatrics Society abstracted clinical practice guideline for postoperative delirium in older adults. *J Am Geriatr Soc.* 2015;63(1):142-1450.

Berger M, Nadler JW, Browndyke J, et al. Postoperative dysfunction: minding the gaps in our knowledge of a common postoperative complication in the elderly. *Anesthesiol Clin.* 2015;33(3):517-550.

Berian JR, Mohanty S, Ko CY, Rosenthal RA, Robinson TN. Association of loss of independence with readmission and death after discharge in older patients after surgical procedures. *JAMA Surg.* 2016;151(9):e161689.

Bruns ERJ, van den Heuvel B, Buskens CJ, et al. The effects of physical prehabilitation in elderly patients undergoing colorectal surgery: a systematic review. *Colorectal Dis* 2016;18(8): O267-O277.

Chow WB, Ko CY, Rosenthal RA, Esnaola NF. ACS NSQIP®/AGS Best Practice Guidelines: Optimal preoperative assessment of the geriatric surgical patient. American College of Surgeons 2016. https://www.facs.org/~/media/files/quality%20programs/nsqip/acsnsqipagsgeriatric2012guidelines.ashx. Accessed March 26, 2020.

Fleisher LA, Fleischmann KE, Auerbach AD, et al. 2014 ACC/AHA guideline on perioperative cardiovascular evaluation and management of patients undergoing noncardiac surgery: a report of the American College of Cardiology/American Heart Association Task Force on practice guidelines. *J Am Coll Cardiol.* 2014;64(22):e77-137.

Hughes CG, Patel MB, Jackson JC, et al. Surgery and anesthesia exposure is not a risk factor for cognitive impairment after major noncardiac surgery and critical illness. *Ann Surg.* 2017;265(6):1126-1133.

Launay-Savary MV, Mathonnet M, Theissen A, et al. Are enhanced recovery programs in colorectal surgery feasible and useful in the elderly? A systematic review of the literature. *J Visc Surg.* 2017;154(1):29-35.

McDonald SR, Heflin MT, Whitson HE, et al. Association of integrated care coordination with postsurgical outcomes in high-risk older adults: the Perioperative Optimization of Senior Health (POSH) Initiative. *JAMA Surg* 2018;153(5):454-462.

Tang VL, Dillon EC, Yang Y, et al. Advance care planning in older adults with multiple chronic conditions undergoing high-risk surgery. *JAMA Surg.* 2019;154(3):261-264.

Tang V, Zhao S, Boscardin J, et al. Functional status and survival after breast cancer surgery in nursing home residents. *JAMA Surg.* 2018;153(12):1090-1096.

Home-Based Care

Mattan Schuchman, MD

Jennifer Shiroky, MD, MPH

Bruce Leff, MD

INTRODUCTION

In 2011, an estimated 1 in 20 community-dwelling Medicare beneficiaries in the United States were completely or mostly homebound. This incidence will continue to rise as the number of individuals reaching older age outpaces mortality. As people age, they typically experience a higher burden of chronic diseases, symptoms, and functional limitations, all of which can contribute to homebound status.

Home-based care provides individuals who are chronically or temporarily homebound with access to a spectrum of services, including medical care. For some, home-based care may be the only way for homebound older adults to receive needed services and connect regularly with a medical provider. Home-based care can improve functional status, decrease hospitalizations, delay long-term institutionalization, and reduce mortality. It also provides unique opportunities for medical providers to assess functional capacity, social support, and safety in the home environment.

This chapter will provide an overview of the different types of home-based care available to a homebound individual. We will then describe two types of care in greater depth: home-based medical care and Medicare skilled home health care. These two complementary modes of care deliver medical provider and nursing services, respectively, to homebound individuals. We will then briefly discuss services that focus on social determinants of health or integrate medical and social services. We will conclude by reviewing new innovations and technologies advancing home-based care.

OVERVIEW OF HOME-BASED CARE

Modalities of care for older adults fall on a spectrum of increasingly specialized skills (Table 30–1). An individual may receive care through any number of these methods at a given time. Home-based care spans from informal and non-technical to highly regulated and administered by certified professionals such as physicians, nurses, and therapists.

▶ Informal Care

The dedicated labor of millions of unpaid caregivers is the cornerstone of successful care for homebound individuals. Informal caregivers, the majority of whom are women, perform essential and challenging tasks, ranging from activities of daily living (ADLs) to medication management to symptom monitoring to care coordination. The monetized value of this care in the United States alone is over half a trillion dollars annually. Please see Chapter 17, "Caregiving & Caregiving Support."

▶ Formal Care

Paid assistance can help older adults meet personal needs, such as ADLs, light housework, or errands. Over two-thirds of personal care assistants are foreign born. Often, pay is minimum wage for intensive physical work. An estimated 1.2 million Americans over 65 will have no living children, siblings, or spouses by 2020, likely increasing the demand for paid caregiving. Formal care at home is temporarily available for eligible individuals during Medicare skilled home health episodes, as detailed later, and for longer durations through Medicaid waiver programs. For most Americans, however, formal care is financed privately. Formal care is included in the cost of residence in an assisted living facility (ALF). For more information on ALFs, please see Chapter 31, "Residential Care & Assisted Living."

▶ Medicare Skilled Home Health Care

With the signed order of a physician, an older adult may receive in-home care from a home health agency for a 60-day episode. To receive this care, covered under Medicare Part A, a person must be homebound and also have a need that requires the specialized skills of a nurse or physical therapist. Once a 60-day episode has begun, other services such as

Table 30–1. Spectrum of home-based care.

Care Model	Care Providers	Annual Recipients in the United States
Informal care	Personal care provided by unpaid support networks.	15 million
Formal care	Paid personal care assistants. Often are certified medical assistants or nursing assistants.	2 million
Medicare skilled home health care	Nursing, occupational therapy, physical therapy, speech therapy, and social work.	3.4 million
Home-based medical care	Physician- or nurse practitioner–led services. Wide variety of models, some of which include additional professionals such as physician assistants, nurses, social workers, therapists, and community health workers.	0.5 million
Home hospice	Nurse-led interprofessional team including personal care assistant, social worker, chaplain, and a medical director.	1.5 million
Hospital at home and related services	Includes professionals who typically function in institutions such as hospitals, rehabilitation centers, or inpatient hospice who provide services at home.	5000

occupational therapy, speech therapy, social work, and personal care are also available. Personal care provided by Medicare skilled home health provides temporary assistance but does not replace the need for formal and informal caregiving (see later section on Medicare skilled home health).

▶ Home Hospice

Hospice care is a service, covered by Medicare, that provides additional care in order to alleviate suffering and support caregivers at the end of life. Most hospice care is provided by an interprofessional team in the home or ALF; however, inpatient hospice is available for when symptoms cannot be adequately controlled at home. Please see Chapter 22 for a more detailed discussion of hospice care.

▶ Home-Based Medical Care

Home-based medical care roughly spans four overlapping categories: (1) home-based care that takes the place of medical care provided by a physician or practitioner in a clinic setting; (2) home-based case management and transitional care that augment clinic-based care; (3) home-based care by specialists and ancillary medical services; and (4) hospital at home. We use the term *home-based medical care* to refer to care that replaces clinic-based care; this will be discussed in detail later after the other three categories are briefly reviewed.

A. Home-Based Management

Many health systems, hospitals, and insurance companies have created care and case management programs to augment clinic-based medical care. The nature of these programs varies widely, and they often target certain "high-risk" populations, such as people with certain disease states (eg, sickle cell anemia, congestive heart failure) or people who meet high-risk criteria, such as frequent admissions or frequent missed appointments. Examples of such programs include care managers to help people keep track of multiple appointments and engage in their care, deployment of community health workers to address social determinants of health and connect people to resources, pharmacist home visits, and targeted social work interventions.

B. Home-Based Specialty Services

This category of home-based medical care is composed of specialists and in-home specialty services. Examples of visiting specialists include podiatrists, optometrists, psychiatrists, and behavioral health therapists. Specialty services include in-home procedures that are typically performed in a clinical setting, such as in-home radiology and phlebotomy companies that work with clinicians to perform x-rays, ultrasound studies, electrocardiograms, Doppler ultrasound studies, and lab work. Durable medical equipment (DME) providers also offer specialized care in the home by furnishing necessary equipment, such as oxygen concentrators, mobility devices, and hospital beds, under orders of a physician. DME company representatives train homebound individuals and caregivers on appropriate device use as well. The availability of home-based specialty services varies regionally.

C. Hospital at Home & Allies

Hospital at home (HaH) models provide hospital-level services in the home setting as a substitute for a bricks-and-mortar hospital admission. In the HaH model, patients visiting the emergency department are assessed by emergency department physicians and, if deemed appropriate candidates, are admitted to HaH. Patients who are good candidates for HaH have conditions that are unlikely to decompensate or to require a high-tech oriented hospital admission. In HaH, patients receive daily care from nurses and physicians. HaH models have demonstrated benefits in mortality, length of stay, readmission rates, patient and caregiver satisfaction, and important geriatric complications, such as delirium, in comparison to in-patient hospitalization. In addition to HaH, intensive home-based care has served as a successful substitute for other facility-based services including subacute rehabilitation and emergency department observation.

HOME-BASED PRIMARY MEDICAL CARE

Home-based medical care provides access to outpatient medical care for the vulnerable and underserved population that cannot reach a clinic due to physical/mental and social/environmental barriers. Home-based practices appear in many different varieties; practitioners may work solo or in a team and may care for patients longitudinally or on an episodic basis. Recent years have shown an increase in the popularity of longitudinal, interprofessional, home-based medicine programs in the United States. These practices provide primary care, urgent care, and palliative care. In such programs, patients receive care from an interprofessional team of clinicians from multiple health professions, including, but not limited to, nurses, social workers, pharmacists, and physical and occupational therapists. Some programs also include community health workers and mental health professionals on their teams, integrating medical and social support services. In most home-based medicine practices, the team meets on a regular basis to discuss and plan patient care.

Longitudinal home-based medical care programs that use an interprofessional team approach have demonstrated reduced costs, improved satisfaction, and fewer nursing home and hospital admissions relative to clinic-based care. The Center for Medicare and Medicaid Innovation (CMMI) is studying the success of Independence at Home (IAH), a pilot program with 14 home-based medical care practices. In the first 3 years of IAH (2012–2015), participating practices saved Medicare an average of $1300 per beneficiary. Many home-based medicine practices are allied with a health system that takes on financial risk for patient care. Medicare and most insurance plans cover only cover medical providers' services but do not pay for the services of the interprofessional team members. To partially mitigate some of the financial loss from interprofessional team management, Medicare has created several billing codes that offer some level of reimbursement, such as "transitional care management," "complex care management," and "care plan oversight." CMMI is also creating new payment strategies to better compensate home-based medical care, such as Primary Care First.

In addition to increasing access to medical care for homebound patients, in-home care permits a deeper assessment of functional, social, caregiving, and environmental aspects of patient health. Inspecting the home environment—with the patient's permission—for safety concerns (eg, fall hazards, lack of adaptive equipment, lighting) and performing a medication reconciliation in situ can help the provider understand functional and medical issues that may not be apparent in a clinic setting. Observations of patient-caregiver interactions in the home are often remarkably different from those observed in the doctor's office and can provide valuable insight into caregiver engagement and patient isolation. The provider in a house call is a guest in the patient's home, which may lessen the power imbalance between patient and provider and facilitate forming a trusting therapeutic relationship that is necessary for discussion of sensitive topics, such as end-of-life preferences. Drawbacks to home-based medical care include the need to consider geography with patient scheduling and, because of travel time, the ability to see fewer patients per day than a clinic-based practice.

Home-based palliative care, which provides in-home assessment and management of symptoms resulting from serious illness, has emerged in the last decade. There is significant overlap between the skill set required to provide home-based primary care and home-based palliative care. While many functions of these programs align, they diverge in that home-based palliative care programs tend to provide mostly consultative care in the home. Home-based palliative care programs have demonstrated the ability to reduce patients' symptom burden and increase satisfaction.

MEDICARE SKILLED HOME HEALTH

Medicare Part A will pay for home health visits by nurses; physical, occupational, and speech therapists; social workers; and—during an episode of skilled care—a personal care aide. Nursing or therapy services in the home allow for expedited discharge home after a hospitalization or inpatient rehabilitation stay. Additionally, home health can serve a vital role in medical care outside of an acute care episode. For example, a homebound individual who suffered a fall may greatly benefit from physical therapy as well as a home safety evaluation by an occupational therapist. Other appropriate uses of skilled home health include management of chronic indwelling catheters, ventilators, or chronic conditions such as pressure injuries that require nursing visits to appropriately assess and treat.

To properly deploy and oversee skilled home health, physicians who care for older patients need to be familiar with Medicare's criteria for home health episodes. An overview of those criteria are as follows:

- A physician must certify that a patient is homebound and make a referral to a qualified home health agency. Nurse practitioners and physician assistants cannot independently initiate a home health episode. To meet Medicare's criteria of "homebound," a patient must have a condition resulting from illness or injury that makes it a considerable and taxing effort to leave the home without the aid of supportive devices such as crutches, canes, wheelchairs, or walkers; special transportation; or another person.
- The physician must create a care plan (reported on form CMS-485) that justifies the need for the home health episode. The care plan must make use of the specialized (or "skilled") training of a nurse or physical therapist.

An example of a "skilled" need for a nurse is to monitor a complex medical condition that requires adjustment of medications and reevaluation. An example of a skilled need for a physical therapist is to develop and implement a home exercise program to improve gait, balance, or strength. One-time services such as an infusion or drawing labs do not qualify.

- The final requirement for home health is that a provider has performed a face-to-face encounter with the patient within 90 days prior to the start of care or 30 days after the start of care. The encounter must relate to the reason for referring the patient to home health services. A detailed explanation of the Medicare home health benefit is available from the Centers for Medicare and Medicaid Services.

SOCIAL AND MEDICAL SERVICES

Older adults are often dependent on fixed incomes and on social support networks. Homebound individuals may even be more reliant on their social supports. Thus, health in the homebound population is particularly sensitive to the strength of support networks, personal finances, and available community resources. Case management and social work are both important aspects of home-based medical care and home health (described earlier). The services introduced in the following sections help address some of the resources available in the community.

▶ Area Agencies on Aging

Area Agencies on Aging (AAAs) refer to local- and state-run agencies that assist older adults in planning for and meeting their needs. AAAs act as a central point for information and access to a wide range of services, including in-home services. While specific resources vary regionally, AAAs often provide retirement planning and education, caregiver support, job placement, information on senior centers, congregate meals, adult daycare, and volunteer opportunities. Examples of in-home services include nutritional support like Meals on Wheels, assistance with personal care, shopping and housekeeping, telephone calls and personal visits for homebound adults, personal emergency response devices, financial assistance with gas and electric bills for low-income individuals, estate planning, and respite care for caregivers. Some AAAs help older adults find alternative housing if they require a supported living environment. AAAs may also provide legal assistance and investigate elder abuse charges and neglect, including self-neglect, both in the community and within long-term care facilities.

▶ Program of All-Inclusive Care for the Elderly

The Program of All-Inclusive Care for the Elderly (PACE) is a model of care focused on keeping nursing home–eligible adults in their community for as long as possible. The PACE model started at the On Lok community center in San Francisco in 1972. PACE services are organized around a day center with activities for participants, as well as a central location for participants to receive interprofessional medical care. To be eligible for participation in PACE, an individual must be older than 55, certified by the state to qualify for nursing home placement, and living within a PACE geographic service area. PACE receives capitated funding from Medicare and Medicaid for each participant. Individuals who are not eligible for Medicaid may choose to privately pay the Medicaid portion of the program expense. Once enrolled, PACE participants receive physician and nursing care, an adult day program, transportation to and from the day center, home health aides, social work, complete prescription drug coverage, respite care, and physical and occupational therapy. PACE assumes responsibility for each participant's medical costs, including inpatient expenses.

▶ Medicaid Waiver Programs

Medicaid is the largest payer of nursing home expenses. Nursing home fees compose a major portion of each state's Medicaid budget. In hopes of reducing nursing home admissions, nearly all states have launched Medicaid waiver programs to provide home-based services for nursing home–eligible patients. Within the Waiver Programs Model, the state applies funding slated for nursing home care to in-home services, with the goal of preventing or delaying nursing home admission and creating savings for Medicaid programs. States must assure the Centers for Medicare and Medicaid Services that the cost of providing these services in the home or community will not exceed that of placing individuals in an institution. Program specifics differ from state to state. Services provided include, but are not limited to, personal care, respite care, and other needed assistance in the home.

INNOVATIONS

New technology and innovative new programs are continuously improving the landscape of home-based care. Widespread high-speed internet connections and the reduced cost and miniaturization of technology have facilitated care in the home that would otherwise have to be delivered in a clinic or hospital. Additionally, the increased emphasis that Medicare and insurance companies place on value-based payments has encouraged health systems to develop cost savings programs that target the frail and homebound populations, as these have traditionally been groups with high medical expenditures.

▶ Telemedicine and Telehealth

Telemedicine refers to the practice of medicine via remote means. Telehealth is a broader construct that refers to the delivery and facilitation of health and health-related services including medical care, provider and patient education, and health information services via telecommunications and digital communication technologies. Some of the more common uses of telemedicine in home-based medical care include video conferencing with patients as a supplement to, or in lieu of, in-person provider visits and remote patient monitoring (eg, wound care). Smartphone-based apps can provide a means for virtual, on-demand medical consultation for urgent medical situations that can then lead to a house call or arranging for formal personal care services.

▶ Community Paramedicine

Community paramedicine refers to specially trained teams of prehospital emergency medicine providers, such as emergency medical technicians and paramedics, who provide emergency care in the home. Community paramedicine expands the reach of medical providers into the home by using emergency medical services as the eyes, ears, and hands of physicians. Community paramedicine teams communicate with providers through audio or video links and are able to provide in-depth assessments and administer first-line care (eg, intramuscular antibiotics, intravenous diuretics, intravenous fluid), monitoring, and transportation to the emergency department under a provider's guidance. Care from community paramedicine may reduce the need for emergency department visits or hospitalization.

▶ Community Aging in Place–Advancing Better Living for Elders

Home-based interventions that address personal and home environmental factors to lessen functional disability have demonstrated effectiveness in helping individuals achieve self-made goals while also reducing medical expenditures. The Community Aging in Place–Advancing Better Living for Elders (CAPABLE) program is a time-limited intervention of a nurse, occupational therapist, and home repair person to address patient-driven goals regarding pain control, depression, medication understanding, strength, and balance. CAPABLE has demonstrated clinically important improvements in functional status and reductions in depression symptoms and Medicaid costs.

CONCLUSION

Treating the patient as a whole person is a central tenet of geriatric medicine. Home-based care is, perhaps, emblematic of this ideal. Seeing the patient in their home environment broadens the provider's conception of the "whole person" by contextualizing the patient as part of a larger system, including caregiving, social supports, and the physical space they inhabit. This fuller picture gives the provider access to invaluable information needed to achieve goals of aging in place. Moreover, understanding the scope and benefits of home-based care is critical for everyone who works with older adults. Most people reach a time when they will no longer be able to see their provider in a clinical setting; homebound individuals are at risk of becoming invisible to the health care system when they can no longer travel to their provider. Familiarity with the concepts outlined in this chapter will enable providers to link their patients with the network of complementary resources that exist to meet the needs of homebound older adults, ensuring that they continue to receive necessary care. In doing so, providers will more effectively support a homebound individual's independence, safety, and health.

Centers for Medicare and Medicaid Services. Medicare Benefit Policy Manual Chapter 7 - Home Health Services. Updated 2019. https://www.cms.gov/Regulations-and-Guidance/Guidance/Manuals/downloads/bp102c07.pdf. Accessed May 6, 2019.

NEJM Catalyst. What is Telehealth? NEJM Catalyst Website. https://catalyst.nejm.org/what-is-telehealth/. Updated 2018. Accessed May 6, 2019.

Ornstein KA, Leff B, Covinsky KE, et al. Epidemiology of the homebound population in the United States. *JAMA Intern Med.* 2015;175(7):1180-1186.

Schuchman M, Fain M, Cornwell T. The resurgence of home-based primary care models in the United States. *Geriatrics (Basel).* 2018;3(3):10.3390/geriatrics3030041.

Stall N, Nowaczynski M, Sinha SK. Systematic review of outcomes from home-based primary care programs for homebound older adults. *J Am Geriatr Soc.* 2014;62(12):2243-2251.

Residential Care & Assisted Living

31

Katherine Wang, MD

Rebecca Conant, MD

General Principles

As adults age, they often require more assistance with physical and cognitive tasks. As mentioned in Chapter 18, "The Social Context of Older Adults," long-term services and supports encompass services that provide assistance (at home or other settings) such as caregivers, adult day services, home health nursing or therapy, or hospice. With functional decline, some older adults may decide to remain at home with this added support while others may choose to live long term in another setting with additional assistance, such as assisted living facilities or residential care homes. Residential care facilities continue to expand in popularity. As of 2014, there were 30,200 assisted living and residential care facilities in the United States housing 835,200 individuals, as compared with 15,600 nursing homes housing 1.4 million individuals (Figure 31–1). This chapter focuses on residential care and assisted living facilities. It describes their services, financing, medical care, and other considerations for individuals and families when selecting a long-term residential facility.

RESIDENTIAL CARE AND ASSISTED LIVING

Facilities

Many older adults reside in residential care facilities. While no one definition exists, typically these facilities aim to serve individuals who are largely independent but require assistance with some instrumental activities of daily living and activities of daily living. The terminology "residential care facility" differs from state to state, and facilities can choose what services they offer. Some terms that may denote the same level of care include residential care, assisted living, and adult group home (Table 31–1). Subtle differences may exist among these, but this chapter will address broad

considerations that apply to all facilities that fall under the heading of "residential care." In general, the state regulatory requirements are similar for all facilities in this category.

Some residential care facilities may exist as part of a continuing care retirement community, wherein care exists on a spectrum from independent living to assisted living to nursing home. Other residential care facilities may stand alone. Residential care facilities range in capacity from 4 to 499 beds, with an average of 15 beds. Fifty-nine percent of residential care facilities offer skilled nursing or nursing services, while only 10% reported providing social work services. A study from 2012 showed that just over half of settings with 50 or more units had a dementia care program.

Financing

In the United States, Medicare does not cover long-term care services, such as continuous home health, residential care, or nursing home care. However, depending on the state, Medicaid may provide coverage or assistance for residential care facility costs. In 2014, about 330,000 individuals in the United States, or about 15% of people in residential care facilities, received Medicaid assistance. How Medicaid is used to pay for services varies from state to state. Some states allow regular Medicaid to be used, while other states use Medicaid Home and Community-Based Services (HCBS) waivers, which allow for higher income eligibility limits and aim to keep people in the community and out of nursing homes. These programs often have enrollment caps and waiting lists.

Some residential care facilities may accept the Veterans Affairs (VA) Aid and Attendance Benefit, which is available to veterans and their surviving spouses who are eligible for a VA pension and require assistance. This benefit, which is added to the existing monthly pension, can help offset the cost of the residential care facility.

Long-Term Care Services Users

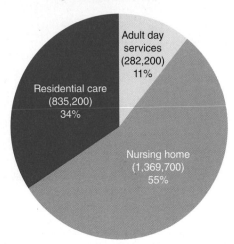

▲ **Figure 31–1.** Individuals receiving long-term care services through adult day services centers (which provide therapeutic, social, and health services to adults for some part of the day), nursing homes, and residential care settings in 2014. (Data from Harris-Kojetin L, Sengupta M, Park-Lee E, et al. Long-Term Care Providers and services users in the United States: data from the National Study of Long-Term Care Providers, 2013-2014, *Vital Health Stat 3* 2016 Feb;(38):x-xii; 1-105.)

Residential care facility costs may also be met using personal income and savings, long-term care insurance, life insurance, annuities, and reverse mortgages.

Residential care facility costs vary depending on state and facility. Typical fees may include:

- Move-in fee (one-time): $1000 to $20,000
- Room and board (monthly): typically includes meals, housekeeping and maintenance, and utilities
- Care fees: may range from $150 to $2000 per month depending on level of services (medication management, personal care), $10 to $30 per hour for home health aide

In 2018, the median cost of residential care nationally was $4000 a month for a one-bedroom unit with a single resident. Variability by state is high, with the highest median cost in Alaska, at $6300 per month, and the lowest median cost in Missouri, at $2844 per month.

▶ Oversight and Regulation

Regulatory requirements vary by state. Unlike nursing homes, which accept both Medicare and Medicaid and therefore must abide by federal and state regulatory requirements, residential care facilities are largely subject to state oversight. Thus, comparative data about services and quality may be less available. Typically, a state will issue a license to a facility after an inspection, conducted annually or semi-annually. The process is usually overseen by the state's department of health or

Table 31–1. Facility types and levels of care.

Facility Type	Other Terms	Services Provided	Payment Options
Independent living	Senior housing	Housekeeping Wellness Recreation	Out of pocket
Residential care	Assisted living Group home Adult care home Personal care home Supported living Board and care home	Room and board Assistance with ADL Housekeeping Laundry Transportation Wellness and recreation Medication management Outside services may come to facility such as podiatry, dental, home health, hospice	Out of pocket Medicaid Long-term care insurance
Nursing home		Custodial care Medical care Skilled nursing care	Out of pocket Medicaid Long-term care insurance
Continuing care retirement communities (CCRCs)	Life plan communities	Ability to transition between independent living, assisted living, and nursing home level of care	Out of pocket Medicaid Long-term care insurance

ADL, activities of daily living.

department of social services. A residential care facility website equivalent to Nursing Home Compare, the online tool providing quality data and staffing information for Medicare/Medicaid-certified nursing homes, does not exist.

Some areas that may differ between states include:

- Staff requirements for medication assistance and administration
- Staffing ratios
- Training requirements
- Depth of background checks

A 2015 governmental report comments on the variability of regulations. As one example, 40 states require direct care worker training, but the number of required training hours ranges from 1 to 80. Staffing ratios also vary widely by state and may be based on either number of staff to number of residents (eg, 1:15 during the day and 1:25 at night) or number of staff per resident per day or week. While some states mandate that a registered nurse (RN) must be available on call 24 hours a day, or that at least one RN, licensed practical nurse (LPN), or certified nursing assistant (CNA) must be on duty every shift, most states do not have a minimum requirement for nursing. In fact, only 40.1% of residential care facilities employ an RN (in contrast to 99.1% of nursing homes). Of note, not all states recommend a minimum direct care staffing ratio and may simply state "staff must be adequate to meet residents' needs."

In 2018, the US Government Accountability Office (GAO) found significant gaps in oversight and reporting; as many as 14 states could not provide information about critical incidents such as physical and sexual assault, emotional abuse, neglect, financial exploitation, medication error, or beneficiary missing/elopement. The GAO recommended that the Centers for Medicare and Medicaid Services (CMS) demand more standardized state reporting of deficiencies including annual reporting of critical incidents.

▶ Documentation

The documentation requirements for residential care facilities vary according to state regulations and the facility's policies. In general, there are standardized forms that need to be completed prior to admission, upon transitions of care, and annually. Facilities are required to show that they have notified medical providers of important changes, such as missed doses of medications, provision of as-needed medications, falls, or skin tears, by documenting and faxing the information to the medical providers. Facilities also require written orders from the medical providers for everything they do for a patient. All medication and treatment orders must be signed by the medical providers and faxed to the facilities. Simply sending a prescription to the pharmacy for delivery does not suffice as an order for the facility to administer the medication.

CLINICAL CARE

▶ Optimizing Communication

Geriatricians and primary care providers best serve individuals residing in residential care settings when communication is open and clear between the facilities, the patients, their families, and the providers. Providers and patients (particularly those who are medically complex) who transition into a residential care facility should be aware of the specific care that is available at that facility. For instance, some issues that are important for providers to recognize are as follows:

- State regulations and facility policies vary regarding medication storage and administration, as well as type of staff who may administer medications.
- Depending on staffing, it may not be possible for medications to be administered if contingent on clinical judgment (eg, sliding scale insulin, blood pressure parameters).

▶ Limitations

Due to the limited availability of licensed nursing care, individuals with particular medical needs may not be eligible for residential care settings. These individuals require a higher level of care, such as nursing homes. Some of these conditions include:

- **Advanced pressure ulcers or wounds:** In California and Arizona, for instance, individuals with a stage III or IV pressure ulcer cannot stay in a residential care setting unless they are enrolled in hospice.
- **Devices such as urinary or suprapubic catheters, feeding tubes, tracheostomies, or oxygen:** If individuals require assistance managing the devices, they may require skilled nursing and therefore be ineligible for a residential care setting.
- **Dementia:** Memory care units (available in some but not all residential care settings) may be required depending on the level of independence.
- **Functional limitations:** Some states may place admission restrictions based on independence in ambulation and ability to mobilize in emergency situations. For instance, some states, such as Rhode Island and Vermont, do not allow those who are permanently bedbound or require more than one-person assistance for ambulation to be admitted. In New York, residential care facility residents must be able to walk or use a wheelchair independently and must be able to self-transfer.

CHAPTER 31

Changes in Condition

Because licensed clinical staff may not be available, any changes in medical or cognitive status typically cannot be assessed by staff at a residential care facility. In some cases, protocols may demand that condition changes be evaluated immediately, which usually means either emergency medical services or hospice (if enrolled), which should be made clear to individuals and their families. These policies are particularly important if the patients and their families have a strong desire to avoid the emergency department and hospital.

Some individuals may have a progressive medical condition that will require additional support in the future, such as those with Parkinson disease. In such cases, the individuals and their families should be provided with anticipatory guidance about future care needs, and they should inquire about whether a particular facility is equipped to meet those needs (or if supplementary services can be added at a later time). A continuing care retirement community, which could provide for a smoother transition to a higher level of care, may be a consideration if eventual nursing home placement is likely.

Advance Care Planning and End-of-Life Considerations

Because many individuals moving into residential care facilities hope to "age in place," it is important for individuals and families to have a clear understanding of the facilities' capabilities in regard to advance care planning and end-of-life considerations.

For individuals who have completed advance health care directives and opted for a "do not hospitalize" (DNH) order, they and their families should communicate their wishes to the facilities to ensure that a system exists to honor their wishes. At that time, they should be made aware of the potential limitations of the facilities based on state regulations and facility policies. For instance, if the individual is enrolled in hospice, then a DNH order may be appropriate; if the individual is not enrolled in hospice and has uncontrolled symptoms, the individual may require transfer to a higher level of care for symptom management and stabilization until an adequate level of care can be arranged.

Depending on the state, residential care facilities may need a "hospice waiver" in order for hospice care to be provided in a facility. In the past, residential care facilities required individuals to move to nursing homes for care at the end of life. Now, most states allow hospice to provide services within residential care facilities, and about one-third of residential care residents die in place. In the event of escalating medical needs (eg, high symptom burden requiring around-the-clock administration of medications) and the desire to stay in place, individuals and their families may need to seek help from outside agencies and pay for additional attendant care out of pocket.

Geriatricians and social workers can be instrumental in realistically assessing an individual's medical, symptomatic, and custodial needs and can work with hospice providers and the facility in an interprofessional collaboration to determine if end-of-life care can be delivered in place.

GUIDING FAMILIES

Navigating the myriad of options for residential care with inconsistent state requirements can be overwhelming for patients and caregivers. To help guide patients and families, medical providers should counsel patients and families about current and future care needs and suggest some questions to ask in exploring different facilities (Table 31–2).

Social workers can be instrumental in providing support and recommendations for local resources. For families at a distance or who desire professional help organizing care, geriatric care managers can be an option. Geriatric care managers are usually nurses or social workers who can guide families with local community resources. They can help with patients living at home or in residential care. Some online resources that may be useful for providers and patients are listed in Table 31–3.

Table 31–2. Questions to ask in exploring assisted living facilities.

Questions to Ask
• How much care can the facility provide?
• Are there options to escalate services/care, and how would that affect cost?
• What are the staffing ratios? Who is available overnight?
• What outside agencies work with the facility (eg, physical therapy, hospice)?
• What happens if the resident . . . (eg, falls? require medications overnight?)
• How are advance care planning wishes (eg, POLST/MOLST) honored?
• Are residents allowed to remain at this facility at the end of life, under hospice?
• Is the comfort care kit allowed to remain in the resident's own apartment?
• Is the facility equipped for dementia care?
• What kind of dementia care training are staff required to undergo?
• Is there a designated memory care unit?

MOLST, medical orders for life-sustaining treatment; POLST, physician orders for life-sustaining treatment.

Table 31–3. Resources for information on assisted living facilities in the United States.

Online Resources
• www.ahcancal.org/ncal – National Center for Assisted Living Resource for assisted living providers as well as residents and families
• www.eldercare.acl.gov – Eldercare Locator Service of the US Administration on Aging connecting individuals with services for older adults and their families
• www.aginglifecare.org – Aging Life Care Association Professional organization for geriatric care managers
• www.n4a.org – National Association of Area Agencies on Aging Searchable database to find aging resources by geographic location
• www.seniorhomes.com/ – SeniorHomes.com Searchable database by geography. Note: This site generates income by highlighting facilities that pay a fee to the site, but does list all facilities in an area
• www.senioradvisor.com – SeniorAdvisor.com Searchable database with consumer reviews of residential care, independent living, and skilled nursing homes. Note: Operated by A Place for Mom (www.aplaceformom.com/), which receives commissions from participating facilities when clients are placed

All websites accessed March 25, 2020.

Carder P, O'Keeffe J, O'Keeffe C, RTI International. Compendium of residential care and assisted living regulations and policy: 2015 edition. US Department of Health and Human Services Office of the Assistant Secretary for Planning and Evaluation. June 15, 2015. https://aspe.hhs.gov/basic-report/compendium-residential-care-and-assisted-living-regulations-and-policy-2015-edition. Accessed July 28, 2019.

Harris-Kojetin L, Sengupta M, Park-Lee E, et al. Long-term care providers and services users in the United States: data from the National Study of Long-Term Care Providers, 2013-2014. Vital Health Stat 3. 2016;38:1-105. https://www.cdc.gov/nchs/data/series/sr_03/sr03_038.pdf. Accessed October 30, 2019.

US Government Accountability Office. Medicaid assisted living services: improved federal oversight of beneficiary health and welfare is needed. January 5, 2018. https://www.gao.gov/products/GAO-18-179. Accessed July 28, 2019.

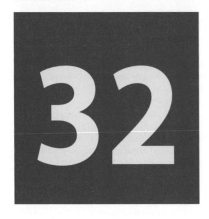

32

Nursing Home Care & Rehabilitation

Laura K. Byerly, MD

Theresa A. Allison, MD, PhD

GENERAL PRINCIPLES OF NURSING HOME CARE

Nearly half of adults in the United States over the age of 65 years will need to spend time in a nursing home, also called a care home, a long-term care home, a convalescent home, or a skilled nursing facility (SNF). Older adults often transition between levels of care, and it is easy for the older adult, families, and even clinicians to be confused by the differences in types of care available. If clinicians are going to care for the older adults who call these sites "home," even if only for a short period of time, it is important to understand the sites' teams, services, and regulations. In this chapter, we discuss the nursing home as model of care, the differences between short-term and long-term nursing home care, the composition of the interprofessional nursing home team, and some of the regulations that govern these sites.

DEFINING THE NURSING HOME

The term nursing home takes on different meaning for patients, families, and providers, depending on their experiences and perspectives. For many people, nursing home placement carries stigma. In the late 20th century, poor-quality care in nursing homes and cases of outright abuse led to the Institute on Medicine report, *Improving the Quality of Care in Nursing Homes,* and the subsequent passage of nursing home reform as part of the Omnibus Budget Reconciliation Act of 1987 (commonly known as OBRA 87). This led to the development of the minimum data set (MDS) to standardize the quality of care for nursing home residents. Soon after, a grassroots effort, the "culture change" movement, developed with the mission of improving quality of life for nursing home residents. Despite these national efforts and regular surveys and monitoring, more recent research demonstrates ongoing challenges to providing both high-quality medical care and quality of life for the people who stay in nursing homes.

Unlike residential care facilities, like assisted living facilities or group homes, the nursing home is a medical care model that is tightly regulated by state and federal guidelines. Each nursing home includes an interprofessional team of on-site licensed nurses, nursing assistants, physical therapists, occupational therapists, recreation therapists, and social workers. Other key members of the interprofessional team, including speech and language pathologists, dietitians, pharmacists, chaplains, and physicians, usually are not on site all the time. They work together to provide residents with assistance with their daily care needs, acute medical issues, and functional mobility. Despite a requirement to provide 24/7 access to medical care, the presence of physicians in nursing homes is highly variable, as is that of nurse practitioners and physician assistants. In addition to the focus on medical issues, nursing homes are also mandated to provide activities for their residents, guided by recreation therapists and sometimes with the support of volunteer services.

A nursing home is a site for people needing access to 24-hour care and assistance with activities of daily living (ADLs) that cannot be accomplished at home for social, medical, and economic reasons that differ for each individual or because they have a skilled nursing need. Differences in resident goals and payor structures create differences between short-term nursing home stays (eg, for rehabilitation, skilled nursing needs) and long-term nursing home stays (ie, when the nursing home becomes a permanent residence). Because many people live in the nursing home and truly consider it their "home" rather than a medically focused facility, they should be described as residents rather than patients.

Some nursing homes strictly cohort their long-term and short-term beds, but other nursing homes use the same beds to accommodate short-term and long-term residents, often all within the same floor or wing. In other words, it is the medical reason for the stay and the insurance coverage for the person, rather than the bed itself, that determine the payment structure. The same interprofessional care team cares for both short-term and long-term residents within the facility. Although the popularized term *SNF* relates primarily to the short-stay and rehabilitation components of nursing home, SNF more correctly refers to the enrollment of a nursing home with the Centers for Medicare and Medicaid Services.

Adding to the confusion, there are increasing numbers of continuing care retirement communities (CCRCs) in the United States. CCRCs typically include independent living, assisted living, and a nursing home unit, so that residents of the CCRC can age in place and transition to higher levels of care—sometimes temporarily in the case of rehabilitation—without having to leave the community. Some CCRCs admit outside community members to the short-stay portion of the nursing home unit; some are open only to CCRC community members.

INTERPROFESSIONAL TEAM MEMBERS OF THE NURSING HOME

Resident care at a nursing home is managed through an interprofessional team consisting of the following members:

- *Nursing:*
  - Registered nurses (RNs) have completed bachelor's level training and provide nursing assessments, pass medications, manage intravenous access, and provide skilled treatments (eg, wound care). Nursing homes are required to have at least one RN available daily for at least 8 hours per day with an RN or licensed vocational nurse on site for the remainder of the day; many states require an RN presence 24 hours a day, 7 days a week.
  - Licensed practical nurses (LPNs) or licensed vocational nurses (LVNs), with 2-year training, are licensed to pass medications and provide some treatments but do not receive the formal training in clinical assessment of RNs.
  - Certified nursing assistants (CNAs or NAs) have completed a 40-hour certification program and provide almost all of the ADL care required by older adults living in the home.
  - Certified medication aides (CMAs) pass noninjectable scheduled and PRN (as-needed) medications and provide direct basic nursing care (eg, hygiene, housekeeping, basic grooming) under the supervision of a licensed nurse. Not every state in the United States participates in CMA programs; thus, not all states have CMAs.
- *Rehabilitation:*
  - Physical therapists (PTs) assess residents and provide gait and balance training and much of the work involved in strengthening the body after a debilitating illness. Physical therapy assistants (PTAs) work with residents on already established exercise and strengthening routines.
  - Occupational therapists (OTs) assess residents and provide therapy around ADLs and instrumental activities of daily living (IADLs). Their work is highly dependent upon the functional status of the resident. OTs often work with residents experiencing cognitive, sensory, perceptual, or visual functional impairments. Occupational therapy assistants (OTAs) help residents complete already established rehabilitation activity sets.
  - Speech and language pathologists (SLPs) focus on deficits in both speech and swallowing, represent a crucial part of acute stroke rehabilitation, and work with residents with the slower neurodegenerative diseases found commonly in nursing homes.
  - Respiratory therapists (RTs) are not common in rehabilitation units unless the facility specializes in the care of ventilator-dependent residents.
- *Nutrition:* Nursing homes are required to provide at least one registered dietitian (RD) for their residents. The RD provides recommendations for nutritional supplementation, enteral and parenteral feeds, monitoring resident weight gain/loss, and individual resident education and recommendations. In some facilities, the RD partners with the kitchen staff to develop healthy menus, but this is not a federal regulatory requirement.
- *Pharmacy:* Nursing homes are required to have access to a pharmacist, but not a pharmacy. Although larger nursing homes may elect to have an on-site dispensing pharmacy, many smaller facilities contract out with local pharmacies that are willing to deliver medications, sometimes urgently or after hours. The pharmacist is required to complete drug regimen reviews, review adverse drug events, and monitor high-risk medication use, in order to prevent polypharmacy complications and to reduce the rate of medication errors.
- *Social services:* Licensed clinical social workers and social service directors assist with social, financial, and other community and systems-based issues and may provide counseling, depending on the setting. They also work with residents and families on discharge planning.
- *Recreation therapy:* Nursing home regulations mandate that the facility provide "an ongoing program to support residents in their choice of activities" to support the physical, mental, and psychosocial well-being of each resident. Activities are guided by licensed or registered recreation therapists or activities professionals.
- *MDS coordinator:* MDS coordinators are licensed nurses who have completed additional training on the MDS. MDS coordinators gather information from nursing home clinicians of different health professions and residents themselves about resident physical and emotional well-being, using the Resident Assessment Instrument (RAI). MDS coordinators monitor the care plan to ensure effectiveness for resident care and also report to

Medicare to ensure the care plan complies with Medicare's requirements.

- *Medical services:* Medical services are mandated in nursing homes, but on-site medical care is highly variable. Community physicians can provide medical care to nursing home residents, or residents can transition to a facility's in-house medical director. Physicians are required to provide the nursing home with access to an on-call provider, but they are not required to establish set hours in which to provide face-to-face care. Under Title 42, a physician must complete an initial comprehensive admission history and physical visit no later than 30 days after a resident is admitted to the facility (either for short-term or long-term care) and then every 30 days for the next 3 months. Federal regulations dictate that the physician must then see the resident every 60 days subsequently. State regulations, though, can vary wildly, with certain states requiring a physician admission exam within 48 hours of resident arrival or requiring monthly visits, only some of which may be performed by a physician assistant or nurse practitioner in a co-managed process; nurse practitioners and physician assistants cannot admit new patients.

- *Dental care:* Nursing homes must assist skilled and long-term care residents with "obtaining routine and 24-hour emergency dental care" through outside or in-house resources. This includes repairing or replacing dentures.

- *Spiritual care:* At some nursing homes, there is also chaplaincy support for the spiritual care of the residents.

- *Restorative care:* Most facilities employ restorative care programs run by nursing staff, which are designed to help residents maintain their current functional abilities, including self-care tasks, transferring, use of assistive devices, and bowel and bladder training. A restorative care nurse directs the restorative care program, and he or she is responsible for educating and training the CNAs to conduct restorative therapy at times. Depending on the size of the facility, there may be one to two restorative care staff working in a facility. Restorative care staff are different from CNAs in that they focus on helping the resident maintain function rather than assist with daily function.

The nursing home's interprofessional team, sometimes augmented by administrators, housekeepers, kitchen staff, family, and any others, are required to meet quarterly and annually with residents and their families to discuss the overall health and well-being of each person residing in the nursing home. These meetings are documented, and an individual plan of care is created. The care plan determines not only the clinical and social treatment of the resident, but also the Medicare or Medicaid reimbursement.

SHORT-TERM REHABILITATION

Nursing home care is often divided into the categories of short-term and long-term care, yet the regulatory requirements remain largely the same for both types. Table 32–1 outlines the key features between types of services provided in nursing homes. Below is an exploration of the eligibility, goals, services, and financing of short-term rehabilitation care.

▶ Eligibility and Goals for Patients

The goal of short-term care is to improve the resident's function or medical condition to where they can return to either their prior level of function, or at least to a less intensive level of care. Short-term skilled nursing and rehabilitation is a Medicare-covered benefit for residents who have had a qualifying hospital stay (3 hospital inpatient days within 30 days of the nursing home admission) and have received physician certification

Table 32–1. Comparison of key features of nursing home care models.

	Short-Stay Rehabilitation	Long-Term Institutional Care	Hospice and End-of-Life Care
Eligibility	Skilled needs (rehab or nursing) following hospitalization	24/7 assistance needs for safety or functional impairment	<6-month prognosis from terminal condition, focus on comfort
Goal for patient	Improve function or medical condition and return home	Ensure safety and necessary medical and supportive care	Symptom management, reducing care transitions at end of life
Services provided	Nursing, physical therapy, occupational therapy, recreation therapy, medicine, pharmacy, nutrition, social services	Nursing, medicine, nutrition, recreation therapy, pharmacy, social services, rehabilitation only for new functional decline and potential to improve, restorative nurse	Hospice nursing and medical care, general nursing and medical care, nutrition, pharmacy, recreation therapy, social services
Duration of stay	<100 days	Permanent	<6 months
Financing	Medicare Part A for medical care and room and board (up to 100 days)	Medicare for medical provider services; Medicaid or private pay for room and board	Medicare for hospice services; private pay for room and board

that they require daily skilled care through nursing, physical or occupational therapy, or speech and language pathology. The resident must be able to participate in at least 5 days of rehabilitation per week or require daily skilled nursing care.

Services Provided and Clinical Care

Residents in short-term care often participate in skilled nursing care (intravenous medication administration, wound care, and/or monitoring) and/or skilled rehabilitation (physical, occupational, and speech therapy). Rehabilitation services can only be provided if a resident has both a functional decline and an identifiable, achievable rehabilitation goal (eg, climbing 10 steps or transferring from bed to wheelchair with standby assistance). Occupational therapy alone will not qualify a hospitalized patient for a nursing home stay under Medicare Part A. Medical plans are overseen by a physician. Staff manages medications, equipment, and supply needs and provides transportation to appointments or services not provided within the nursing home. Labs and basic imaging are provided when needed. Social services work with residents and families to determine discharge plans or transitions to different levels of care. When a nursing home bed is used as a site for short-term rehabilitation, the institution is reimbursed only for 720 minutes of skilled rehabilitation per week (<2 hours per day). In contrast, the acute rehabilitation center (ARC) is a high-acuity, posthospital institution designed to provide a minimum of 3 hours of intensive rehabilitation each day. ARCs will be discussed more later.

Financing

The Medicare Part A benefit covers a set period for short-term nursing home care and can be invoked even if the resident is initially discharged home from the hospital. Part A benefits can also be applied if a resident is discharged from an SNF and suffers a functional decline within the first 30 days of return to home. Medicare Part A can also be invoked for a hospice patient who suffers a nonrelated illness or injury, such as a cancer patient who fractures a femur. Part A benefits cover the full cost of care for a resident's first 20 skilled days and then require that the resident pay a copayment for the remaining 100 days of coverage (days 21–100). Once this benefit has been exhausted, the resident must remain out of hospital or nursing home for 2 months before a new benefit period can be invoked.

LONG-TERM INSTITUTIONAL CARE

For every person living in a nursing home, it is estimated that two or three people with similar comorbidities are being successfully cared for in the community. Over half of long-term care nursing home residents have cognitive impairment. Some long-term care units include a memory care unit,

dementia unit or, dementia special care unit, which assists residents with cognitive impairment who need 24-hour supervision and who are at high risk of wandering or whose care plans include a stronger focus on memory loss–related deficits or dementia-related behavioral patterns. Memory care units are often egress controlled, sometimes with a coded keypad or key access, so that the residents cannot easily become lost. Following is an exploration of the eligibility, goals, services, and financing of long-term institutional care.

Eligibility and Goals for Patients

Long-term care eligibility and goals differ significantly from short-term care. In long-term care, there is little to no focus on rehabilitation and treatment to achieve prior level of function. The goal of long-term institutionalized care is to provide a safe, long-term, team-based environment for residents with cognitive and functional decline who require daily assistance. Long-term institutional care eligibility criteria are state based, but typically, eligibility is based primarily on ADL dependencies such as grooming, bathing, dressing, feeding, toileting, and transferring. Many states require residents to have dependencies in multiple ADLs. Individuals using Medicaid services to finance long-term care are required to meet the state Medicaid program's functional eligibility criteria.

Services Provided and Clinical Care

Long-term nursing home care provides 24-hour supervision and assistance with self-care for residents who cannot receive the needed level of care in the community. Long-term care residents receive nursing assistance, rehabilitative services if needed, medication management, dietary services, routine scheduled pharmacy review, personal hygiene care, scheduled activities, and medical care. Staff and the medical team provide acute care for illness, provide routine preventative services, refer for consultation both within and outside of the facility, and can set up on-site hospice services for residents at the end of their life.

Financing

The monthly national median cost of long-term care in a nursing home, as of 2019, was $8517 for a private room, with wide variability depending on facility location. Physician services are often covered by Medicare or a resident's health insurance. Costs of long-term care include room and board, nursing care, personal care, and basic services. However, residents often pay extra for private rooms, special services, or activities that are not a part of the standard resident care plan. Long-term care nursing home costs are *not reimbursed by Medicare*, so financing derives from Medicaid, personal resources, or optional long-term care insurance programs.

If people have too many assets to qualify for Medicaid, they are required to pay for long-term care privately, or "spend down," until they become indigent and meet Medicaid eligibility criteria. Each state determines the threshold for Medicaid eligibility. The Department of Veterans Affairs (VA) is the largest single-payer system to cover long-term care, but access to services is locale dependent. In addition, VA long-term care benefits are dependent on the degree of service connection, or the connection of the chronic illness or disability to the time of military service, and the financial status of the veteran.

HOSPICE AND END-OF-LIFE CARE IN THE NURSING HOME

The long-term care nursing home bed is intended to be the final resting place for the person who resides in it. Nursing homes coordinate with home hospice agencies to allow residents to spend the end of their life in the environment that they call "home." Nearly a third of deaths in the United States occur in a nursing home. Effective utilization of hospice services for nursing home residents can help with comfort and quality of life.

▶ Eligibility and Goals for Patients

A resident is eligible for hospice care if his or her prognosis from the natural course of an underlying disease process is <6 months and if the resident wishes to focus care on comfort rather than curative measures. Any resident can elect to use their hospice benefit provided a medical provider deems they meet hospice enrollment eligibility. Short-term nursing home residents may elect to transition to hospice services; however, it may affect how their nursing home costs are financed because Medicare can only pay for skilled care needs unrelated to the terminal illness.

▶ Services Provided and Clinical Care

Unlike assisted living facilities, nursing homes do not require a waiver to provide hospice care. Nursing home residents on hospice receive the same general medical and custodial care through the nursing home's interprofessional team, but additionally benefit from the in-house or contracted hospice agency's end-of-life care. Often, the hospice agency's medical director provides guidance on comfort-focused medications, such as opiates and benzodiazepines.

▶ Financing

Nursing home residents have the right to be offered hospice care, and the Medicare hospice benefit can be invoked in a nursing home. It covers, as in the outpatient setting, a visiting hospice agency and the medications, medical care, counseling,

and supplies necessary to manage the disease process's symptoms. Medicare does not cover the room, board, or 24-hour-a-day custodial care costs incurred in a nursing home. In VA or VA-contracted nursing homes, room and board costs are covered as part of the veteran's VA benefits.

ADDITIONAL MODELS OF NURSING HOME CARE

▶ Novel Models of Long-Term Care for Nursing Home–Eligible Older Adults

The nursing home is the most well-known, but not the only, form of medical institutional care. The "culture change" movement has given rise to newer, more home-like forms, the most well studied of which is the Green House Model. A green house is home to 10 or 12 nursing home–eligible older adults with caregivers who function outside of the conventional roles of nursing. Their care model is based on three values: real home, meaningful life, and empowered staff. In a green house, caregivers, called *Shahbazim*, are as likely to be found cooking or gardening with residents as to be found providing traditional bed and body care. These innovative models of care could provide a balance between necessary resident care and the independence and affordances of being at "home."

▶ Acute Rehabilitation Centers

The ARC's rehabilitation requirements are not tolerated by many older adults (requiring a minimum of 3 hours of intensive rehabilitation each day). In addition, Medicare rarely reimburses for more than a few weeks of care, making it a site of exclusively short-term care. It is important, however, to be aware of the difference between acute and subacute short-term rehabilitation in the context of stroke, because aggressive, early rehabilitation leads to earlier improvements in functional status. An older adult who would benefit from ARC, but who cannot yet tolerate the minimum rehabilitation requirements, may be admitted temporarily to a subacute short-stay rehabilitation facility for initial therapy and then transferred to an ARC once they can tolerate the higher level of participation required.

NURSING HOME AND REHABILITATION CENTER REGULATIONS

To receive reimbursement from Medicare and Medicaid, nursing homes must comply with the requirements laid out by federal regulations. To that end, nursing home teams ensure that they have staff, MDS assessments, and tailored care plans sufficient for each resident. Nursing home is expected to assist with resident care, promote quality of life, and provide the interprofessional team member services each resident is entitled to receive (eg, medical, pharmacy, dental, activities).

The Joint Commission SAFER Matrix Scoring

In January 2017, The Joint Commission launched the SAFER Matrix scoring process for health care organization accreditation (https://www.jointcommission.org/facts_about_the_safer_matrix_scoring/). The matrix is used to assess skilled and long-term care facilities in terms of the risk of harm (high, moderate, or low) and the scope of that risk (limited to a unique occurrence, a pattern with potential to impact several residents, or a widespread problem). Surveyors decide the infraction severity level based on the frequency of a finding as well as the imminent risk of harm estimate to a resident, rather than simply tallying issues they observe, thus better determining the areas on which a facility should focus corrective action.

State Surveys and Health Inspections

Nursing homes are subject to annual, unannounced surveys and health inspections by the state in which they are located. State surveyors, usually a team of health care professionals, spend days evaluating facility practice and policies related to resident care, administration, and the facility's environment. Surveys comment on both the level of severity of identified concerns, as well as the scope of the identified concern. Facilities have the opportunity to correct deficiencies identified by the survey; state surveyors conduct repeat visits to confirm correction of deficiencies. State surveys, which may take place during or after business hours, result in a report that must be posted at the nursing home and that can be accessed at http://www.medicare.gov/NursingHomeCompare.

Resident Assessment Protocols

Along with site-wide health and safety assessments, surveyors examine resident plans of care (POCs, or care plans) for residents. To prevent neglect and unnecessary restraint and to ensure that geriatric syndromes are being appropriately managed, certain conditions are identified as triggers for further treatment and documentation. These triggered conditions are addressed through a Resident Assessment Protocol (RAP), synthesized by the MDS coordinator (see Table 32–2 for the key conditions). These problems, when identified, must be addressed by the care team and incorporated into the POC. The team must explain why it is that a resident is suffering from one of these 18 conditions, as the surveyors will look closely at charts flagged with them. Reporting of every scratch and bruise on nursing home residents is mandated

Table 32–2. Illnesses/conditions that trigger a Resident Assessment Protocol (RAP).

Delirium
Cognitive loss
Change in visual function
Change in communication ability
ADL functional/rehabilitation potential
Urinary incontinence and indwelling catheter
Psychosocial well-being
Altered mood states (eg, depression)
Behavioral symptoms
Activities
Falls
Nutritional status
Feeding tubes
Dehydration/fluid maintenance
Dental care
Pressure ulcers
Psychotropic drug use
Physical restraints

ADL, activities of daily living.

and intended to prevent elder abuse and ensure that an important injury is not left unnoticed.

Minimum Data Set

The MDS is collected on each nursing home resident both to help plan care as well as to serve as a mechanism for improving quality of care. The MDS provides a comprehensive assessment of each resident's functional capabilities, which helps nursing home staff identify health-related problems to target as an interprofessional team. For example, the MDS includes sections for mood, functional status, bowel and bladder care, dentition, current medical diagnoses, and resident goal setting, all of which the team can discuss and construct plans to target any concerns or areas of decline. The MDS coordinator consolidates information based on reports from the resident and nursing home interprofessional team members.

Medicare Five-Star Quality Rating System

Based on data collected from the MDS and annual surveys and inspections, Medicare publishes, publicly, the results on a Five-Star Quality Rating System. The star rating has three components: annual Centers for Medicare and Medicaid Services (CMS) survey results including health inspections, nursing staffing to resident ratios, and CMS-driven quality metrics. The scores give an overall rating for the facility as well as ratings for health inspections, staffing ratios, and how the facility performed on Medicare-defined quality measures. (http://www.medicare.gov/NursingHomeCompare).

As of June 2018, the VA nursing homes, called Community Living Centers, are now rated on the same five-star rating to allow as close of a comparison as possible to community nursing homes in the same area. These ratings are found at www.accesstocare.va.gov. While ratings are intended to be helpful for families to make choices about where their loved ones might live, no rating system is comprehensive and all decisions should be taken in the context of the resident, his or her care needs, and the family's needs.

Penalties

The CMS has the right to penalize nursing homes, including through fines, temporary denial of payment, hold on new admissions, assigned oversight, or even the removal of nursing home certification to provide care to CMS beneficiaries (which effectively forces a nursing home to close). Facilities that did not do well on their annual survey can expect surveyors to visit their facility more frequently (within 3–6 months after their last survey).

In sum, despite its many names and associations, the nursing home is a tightly regulated medical model of care that serves multiple purposes: as a site for short-term, post-hospital rehabilitation and skilled nursing care; as a long-term residence for older adults with significant functional impairment; and as one of many places in which people with moderate to severe dementia receive 24-hour supervision. As clinicians, we should be aware that, while nursing homes cannot monitor a resident like a hospital, at their best, they are dynamic and person-centered environments that optimize function and quality of life. Our role as medical providers is to support and augment the nursing home team by providing medical guidance on acute and chronic conditions while also being mindful of the need to abide by regulatory requirements and institutional protocols.

Centers for Medicare and Medicaid Services. Title 42 CFR 483: Requirements for states and long-term care facilities. October 2017. https://www.govinfo.gov/content/pkg/CFR-2017-title42-vol5/xml/CFR-2017-title42-vol5-part483.xml. Accessed March 25, 2020.

Harris-Kojetin L, Park-Lee E. Long-term care providers and services users in the United States: data from the National Study of Long-Term Care Providers, 2013-2014. *Natl Cent Health Stat Vital Health Stat*. 2016;3:38.

Miller SC, Schwartz ML, Lima JC, et al. The prevalence of culture change practice in US nursing homes: findings from a 2016/2017 nationwide survey. *Med Care*. 2018;56(12):985-993.

Stefanacci R. Admission criteria for facility-based post-acute services. *Ann Long-Term Care Clin Care Aging*. 2015;23(11):18-20.

Teno JM, Gozalo PL, Bynum JPW, et al. Change in end-of-life care for Medicare beneficiaries: site of death, place of care, and health care transitions in 2000, 2005, and 2009. *JAMA*. 2013;309(5):470-477.

USEFUL WEB LINKS

Nursing Home Compare. http://www.medicare.gov/nursinghome-compare. The Centers for Medicare and Medicaid Services (CMS) official website for looking up information about nursing homes. Accessed March 25, 2020.

The Joint Commission. https://www.jointcommission.org/facts_about_the_safer_matrix_scoring/. Provides information about the Joint Commission scoring process and includes a downloadable file. Accessed March 25, 2020.

Genworth. http://www.genworth.com/aging-and-you/finances/cost-of-care.html. An interactive website for estimating the costs of long-term care. Accessed March 25, 2020.

Medicaid. www.medicaid.gov. Provides state-by-state requirements for determination of eligibility. Accessed March 25, 2020.

Technology in the Care of Older Adults

33

Kaitlin Willham, MD

Daphne Lo, MD, MAEd

GENERAL PRINCIPLES

- Electronic assistive technologies for activities of daily living and safety are widely available, but the evidence base is limited.

- Telemedicine includes remote patient monitoring for disease management, store-and-forward/asynchronous technology, and real-time videoconferencing.

- Age is not a major determinant of technology use; however, factors such as geography, income, and education are associated with disparate levels of access to and use of technology.

- Clinicians must participate in the ethical implementation of telemedicine technologies.

- Older adults should be included in development of technologies meant for their use.

Technology is a fundamental yet rapidly changing aspect of modern life. Technology shapes how individuals live their daily lives and receive medical care. A greater number of older adults are using technology than ever before—6 in 10 of those age 65 and older now use the internet. For older adults in particular, the potential impact of technology on health and well-being is immense. Technology may be used to support the daily needs of older adults, enabling a new wave of aging in place. Additionally, technology may overcome the challenges of accessing high-quality, geriatric-focused care. For example, telemedicine can connect older adults to the small geriatrics-trained workforce and widen the reach of geriatrics expertise across health care sites and sectors. Ultimately, it may enable older adults to receive the care they need, when and where they need it. At the same time, enthusiasm for new technologies should be tempered by careful consideration of potential downsides and ethical implications. This chapter outlines established and emerging technologies for supporting the daily life of older adults and their health care needs.

ELECTRONIC ASSISTIVE TECHNOLOGIES

Definition and Concepts

New electronic assistive technologies are continually surfacing that change the daily experience of older adults. There has been an explosion of devices, systems, and programs that rely on electronic technology to augment the performance of daily activities (Table 33–1). Automation of bill paying and direct deposit streamline the management of finances. Way-finding can be assisted by global positioning systems and mobile applications. In urban areas, ride share services may make transportation more affordable, convenient, accessible, and safe. Likewise, groceries and other goods can be directly delivered to home by most retailers. These types of services are most available to older adults who have the financial means and cognitive ability to access the internet or use a smart phone. With time, adaptations are being made to increase ease of use for all older adults. For example, ride shares can now be ordered over a push-button phone or by a remote caregiver who then receives real-time updates on the rider's status. Additionally, versions of the smart phone—a gateway to so many assistive technologies—are available that have large buttons, voice activation, and enhanced volume.

A variety of products and systems are advertised to assist with medical tasks and home safety of older adults. Electronic pillboxes organize and remind an individual when to take medications—these devices range from simple devices to complex systems that track medication adherence and update remote caregivers in real time. Fall injury prevention systems are no longer restricted to wearable devices. Instead, ambient sensors and monitors may track a person's movement within their environment. Video surveillance systems are available for remote caregivers to check the real-time

Table 33–1. Examples of electronic assistive technologies for supported living.

Instrumental activities of daily living	
Money management	Automated bill paying
Transportation	Real-time mapping/navigation systems Ride share services • Mobile device or telephone based • May provide real-time updates to a third party
Medications	Electronic pillbox • Electronic alerts/reminders • May track medication adherence and provide real-time updates to a third party
Shopping	Remote ordering and delivery of products
Cleaning	Automated vacuum
Telephone/communication	Computer or phone adapted for sensory impairment
Home safety	
Fall injury prevention	Emergency alert system • Wearable or ambient • Triggered by individual or may be automatic
Early detection of change in status	Video surveillance Wearable monitors: continuous vital signs and movement tracking
Environmental modifications	Modified appliances • Adapted with timers or other safety mechanisms • Integration and central control of all appliances Voice-activated control of home electronics and devices
Social support	Internet-based communication and social media Real-time video communication Artificial intelligence

status of older adults. The concept of the "smart home" generally refers to the integration of computer systems, sensors, and appliances to modulate the environment for safety and to enable early detection of changes in an older adult's status. With the dizzying array of available products, the clinician may be asked to provide guidance about the utility—or lack thereof—of electronic assistive technologies to older adults and their caregivers.

In addition to assisting with daily activities, technology may also be used to enhance or create social connections. Technologies that promote social connections from a distance have become more affordable and more accessible. Telephones adapted to the needs of users with vision or hearing impairment are available. Smart phones have streamlined use of videoconferencing. Videoconferencing can enable communication between older adults and remote friends, family, and support groups. Currently, 4 out of 10 adults age 65 years and older use a smart phone. Social networking sites and online social groups are also becoming more popular among adults age 65 years and older; about one in three older adults use social media sites. In addition to technologies that seek to enhance social connections, another strain of technologies seeks to replicate them. There is emerging interest—and skepticism—for products such as social companion robots. These products are generally costly and raise questions about social priorities and the value and availability of human support for older adults. Whether it is through social networking, videoconferencing, or artificial intelligence, an individual's response to any type of social technology is highly specific to their life-long social preferences.

▶ Evidence About Electronic Assistive Technologies

Electronic assistive technologies are currently vastly understudied. Most, if not all, of these types of technologies are marketed directly to the consumer. And, in many cases, the consumer is not the older adult but their caregiver. Caregivers must decide whether the product is worth the monetary cost and whether the benefits merit the infringement on privacy or autonomy. Take, for example, fall injury prevention. Fall detection systems range from wearable devices to ambient sensors that may be triggered intentionally or through infrared, video, pressure, or sound sensors. Studies have assessed reliability of various systems and rates of false-positive alerts. However, there is limited evidence that these technologies reduce injuries and no systematic evidence that they reduce falls.

While the use of electronic assistive technology is appealing to address functional limitations of cognitive impairment and dementia, there is currently no available randomized controlled trial evidence for the use of electronic assistive technology in dementia. There is also no evidence that online cognitive training prevents cognitive impairment or slows its progression. Clinicians and consumers must be aware that advertisements may overstate or misstate benefits of assistive technologies—at least one company has been penalized for falsely advertising the cognitive benefits of online games.

While technology has the potential to address aspects of social isolation, research is limited. One systematic review found that a variety of information and communication technologies had a positive effect on social connectedness and social support but not necessarily loneliness in older adults. Interestingly, heavy use of information and communication technologies such as social media may be associated with increased loneliness in older adults. It remains unclear what interventions—for example, online support groups, social networking sites, or video communication—may be helpful and to whom.

Chen YRR, Schulz PJ. The effect of information communication technology interventions on reducing social isolation in the elderly: a systematic review. *J Med Internet Res.* 2016;18(1):e18.

Van der Roest HG, Wenborn J, Pastink C, Dröes RM, Orrell M. Assistive technology for memory support in dementia. *Cochrane Database Syst Rev.* 2017;6:CD09627.

TELEMEDICINE

▶ Definition and Concepts

Telemedicine is defined as the use of telecommunications technology to deliver health care at a distance. The three main types of telemedicine are (1) remote patient monitoring, (2) store-and-forward (ie, asynchronous) technologies, and (3) real-time (ie, synchronous) videoconferencing. Remote patient monitoring often involves data collection and review coupled with an intervention to manage chronic disease or detect early clinical changes. Store-and-forward telemedicine refers to the review of patient information outside of a patient encounter. For example, store-and-forward technology may include transmission of static data such as imaging, photographs, or written communication that is later reviewed by a clinician. Store-and-forward technology also includes electronic consultations, or "e-consults," where the consulting clinician provides recommendations based on review of the patient's medical record. Real-time videoconferencing includes a two-way interaction between a patient and a clinician or between clinicians. These three types of telemedicine technologies may be employed separately or in tandem. For example, all three types of telemedicine may be integrated to provide multiple means of data collection and communication between patients and clinical teams.

While sometimes used interchangeably with the term *telemedicine*, the term *telehealth* may also refer to nonclinical services such as mobile health applications and electronic distribution of public health information.

▶ Evidence About Telemedicine

A body of evidence has emerged to outline the effects of specific telemedicine modalities on selected outcomes.

Drawing general conclusions about remote patient monitoring is challenging because of the wide variation in interventions studied. Methods of data collection, interpretation, and subsequent feedback vary and are unique to the chronic condition being monitored. One of the studies with the most robust outcomes for remote patient monitoring comes from the Veterans Health Administration's National Home Telehealth Program. The Home Telehealth Program was designed to support older veterans with diabetes, hypertension, heart failure, chronic obstructive pulmonary disease, depression, and/or posttraumatic stress disorder. Enrolled veterans, who had a mean age of 67 years, experienced a 25% reduction in number of hospital days and 19% reduction in hospital admissions in the 6 months after enrollment compared to the year prior to enrollment. The cost was $1600 per patient per year.

Store-and-forward technology is well established, and even standard, in fields that rely on visual data, such as radiology and pathology. In primary care, store-and-forward applications have also included secure messaging between patients and clinical teams and electronic collection of health histories. These types of communications may improve efficiency of data collection and interpretation and save the time of the clinician and patient. Electronic consults, or e-consults, enable a specialist to provide an assessment and recommendations based on chart review. In centers with established e-consult programs, primary care clinicians are generally satisfied with the option due to increased convenience, rapid turnaround, and improved access to specialty input. Likewise, specialists report fewer inappropriate clinic visits.

Real-time videoconferencing was originally used in circumstances when in-person visits were not available. In these cases, the benefit is indisputable; it enables access to clinical care that would otherwise not be available. Increasing access to a service, particularly when it would be difficult to receive due to limits imposed by geography, mobility, and clinician availability, remains a major strength of real-time videoconferencing. Virtual visits have been used to connect clinicians to patients in remote hospitals, clinics, subacute nursing facilities, residential care facilities, and homes. There is a long legacy of virtual visits being used in fields such as mental health, acute stroke care, and critical care medicine. However, head-to-head studies of virtual compared to in-person care are limited. In a 2015 Cochrane Review including 55 studies of interactive telemedicine as an alternative or addition to usual care, there was some evidence for improved quality of life at 3 months and lower hemoglobin A1c levels in participants with diabetes mellitus. Studies in the review evaluated the difference in mental health therapies over videoconference as compared to in person and found similar outcomes. Conclusions about cost and patient satisfaction could not be drawn. Because real-time videoconferencing is being used more and more out of convenience rather than necessity, more studies are needed to directly compare virtual to in-person visits.

Chen YRR, Schulz PJ. The effect of information communication technology interventions on reducing social isolation in the elderly: a systematic review. *J Med Internet Res.* 2016;18(1):e18.

Darkins A, Ryan P, Kobb R, et al. Care coordination/home telehealth: the systematic implementation of health informatics, home telehealth, and disease management to support the care of veteran patients with chronic conditions. *Telemed e-Health.* 2009;14(10):1118-1126.

Flodgren G, Rachas A, Farmer AJ, Inzitari M, Shepperd S. Interactive telemedicine: effects on professional practice and health care outcomes. *Cochrane Database Syst Rev.* 2015;9:CD002098.

Van der Roest HG, Wenborn J, Pastink C, Dröes RM, Orrell M. Assistive technology for memory support in dementia. *Cochrane Database Syst Rev.* 2017;6:CD009627.

Vimalananda VG, Gupta G, Seraj SM, et al. Electronic consultations (e-consults) to improve access to specialty care; a systematic review and narrative synthesis. *J Telemed Telecare.* 2015;21(6):323-330.

VIRTUAL GERIATRIC ASSESSMENT

In the use of telemedicine for geriatric clinical care, available literature sheds some light on older adults' acceptance of and satisfaction with virtual visits and provides examples of program models. There is little validation of geriatric screening tools or best practice guidelines; however, a clinician willing to adapt to the virtual setting will find that many components of the geriatric assessment are amenable to real-time videoconferencing.

What is possible during a virtual visit is dependent on the setting, the patient, additional persons present with the patient, and the technology used. When a patient is physically located in a remote clinic or facility, for example, an on-site assistant may adjust the camera, maneuver ancillary tools (eg, a virtual stethoscope), and provide printed paperwork (eg, a cognitive screener or advance directive). These options may be limited when a visit is conducted in the patient's home. However, a virtual home visit may have its own unique benefits such as providing visual information about the patient's living conditions.

In preparation for a visit, the clinician must consider how the technology will interface with the individual. A low-quality connection, small screen, or inadequate sound may decrease the value of the visit, particularly if the individual already has visual or hearing deficits. On the other hand, the right technology can be used to overcome sensory impairments—for individuals with hearing impairment, head phones can amplify sound, or, depending on the platform used, the clinician may even be able to transmit a live document for written communication. Arrangements may need to be made ahead of time for a third party to be present or for other accommodations to allow high-quality communication. Additionally, the clinician should establish a procedure in the event of technical difficulty or an emergency prior to, or at the start of, the visit.

The virtual examination of an older adult requires adaptations, and additional tools may be needed for each component of the physical examination. Vital signs, vision and hearing screenings, otoscopy, oropharyngeal, cardiac, and respiratory exams will all require specialized equipment. Patients may be able to self-perform portions of the abdominal, musculoskeletal, and neurologic exams and gait assessment. Caregivers may also be recruited to assist. Clinical judgment should always be used to determine if the necessary data can accurately be gathered through videoconferencing or if further triage is necessary.

There are several examples in the literature demonstrating feasibility of virtual cognitive assessment. One example comes from the Pittsburg Veterans Authority where an interprofessional telemedicine team conducted cognitive assessments of veterans located in rural clinics. Evaluation of the program demonstrated that most patients accepted the visit, and there were high ratings of overall satisfaction, ease of communication with providers, and willingness to use the clinic again. However, cognitive screening tools administered over videoconferencing have not been validated; one very limited study suggests variability in the standardized Mini-Mental Status Examination (MMSE) scores when administered in person versus over videoconferencing. Therefore, clinicians should interpret cognitive screening results cautiously.

Just as some tools may need to be used in yet unvalidated ways, other common geriatric assessments and screening tools may need to be modified for feasibility and safety. For example, a standardized mobility assessment may be performed when the clinician is able to confirm measurement of the appropriate distance at the patient's location such as at a remote clinic but may not be possible in the home. Whether in a clinic or a home, a third party may be needed to move the camera during gait assessment and to prevent a patient from falling.

Clinicians who practice geriatrics may particularly value close relationships between the individual, their caregiver, and the clinical team members. While telemedicine may be perceived to threaten this value, it may also facilitate contact between clinicians, patients, and caregivers. Real-time telemedicine may be used by multiple members of the geriatric clinical team—from the social worker to the occupational and speech therapists—to lessen the burden of visits on patients and their caregivers. Integration of monitoring systems, store-and-forward technology, and virtual visits may lend a greater level of support, not just to the patient but to their caregiver as well. Overall, telemedicine interventions have been shown to also have a positive impact on caregiver outcomes such as psychological health, caregiving skills, quality of life, and social support.

Chi NC, Demiris G. A systematic review of telehealth tools and interventions to support family caregivers. *J Telemed Telecare.* 2015;21(1):37-44.

Loh PK, Ramesh P, Maher S, Saligari J, Flicker L, Goldswain P. Can patients with dementia be assessed at a distance? The use of telehealth and standardised assessments. *Int Med J.* 2004;34(5):239-242.

Powers BB, Homer MC, Morone N, Edmonds N, Rossi MI. Creation of an interprofessional teledementia clinic for rural veterans: preliminary data. *J Am Geriatr Soc.* 2017;65(5):1092-1099.

BARRIERS TO IMPLEMENTATION OF TELEMEDICINE

Although older adults are using technology, disparities in technology use still exist. Adults age 80 years and older are much less likely than those age 65 to 79 years to use the internet or own a smart phone. Other factors that affect technology use include education level, household income, and rurality. About half of adults age 65 and older continue to lack high-speed internet access at home. Even when able to access the internet or a smart phone, an individual may or may not be willing to exchange health care information over these mediums. In a review of telemedicine in older adults with chronic illness, uptake was promoted by simplicity of the system, physician buy-in, and caregiver support. Barriers included lack of feedback to responses, particularly for remote monitoring.

Just as a patient's level of access and willingness to use telemedicine is critical to successful implementation, so too is the willingness of frontline clinicians. Clinical staff have varying levels of comfort with and acceptance of technology. Efforts to implement telemedicine must include strong infrastructure and technology support. Organizations must give clinicians flexibility to trial and adapt the technology to the needs of their practice and actively seek their input and feedback.

One of the major systemic barriers to implementation of telemedicine has traditionally been reimbursement. Medicare has long limited coverage of telemedicine services. Medicare fee-for-service reimburses synchronous telemedicine for patients located in nonmetropolitan or rural health professional shortage areas and only when the service is delivered at a designated clinical site such as a clinic, hospital, or skilled nursing facility. Due to this limitation, organizations that fund and administer health care, such as Veterans Affairs and Kaiser Permanente, have more robust telemedicine programs than many others. However, coverage of telemedicine services is becoming more common through private insurance and Medicaid. More than half of states have parity laws that require most private insurance plans to cover real-time videoconferencing.

State licensure regulations may also limit clinicians' ability to practice out of state. There is movement to relax these regulations—many states now offer expedited licensing to clinicians who are already licensed in a partnering state. Similarly, legislation has been proposed that would give clinicians within the Veterans Health Administration greater flexibility in providing telemedicine services across state lines. Clinicians interested in practicing out of state should acquaint themselves with local laws that regulate where they can treat patients and what kinds of treatment they can provide.

Foster MV, Sethares KA. Facilitators and barriers to the adoption of telehealth in older adults; an integrative review. *Comput Inform Nurs.* 2014;32(11):523-533.

Pew Research Center. Tech adoption climbs among older adults. 2017. http://www.pewinternet.org/2017/05/17/technology-use-among-seniors/. Accessed April 9, 2019.

Taylor J, Coates E, Brewster L, Mountain G, Wessels B, Hawley MS. Examining the use of telehealth in community nursing: identifying the factors affecting frontline staff acceptance and telehealth adoption. *J Adv Nurs.* 2015;71(2):326-337.

ETHICAL CONSIDERATIONS

Clinicians must be thoughtful about use of real-time videoconferencing and other types of telemedicine. Limitations in evidence should be balanced with willingness to critically trial new technology. The American College of Physicians (ACP) developed recommendations regarding the implementation of telemedicine in primary care in 2015. The ACP recommended that telehealth activities consider affordability, ease of use, and access to broadband infrastructure. Clinicians must use sound judgment in deciding if the necessary data can be collected through the technology and equipment at hand. The ACP recommended that telemedicine be held to the same standards of practice as in-person visits and promoted the development of evidence-based guidelines and clinical guidance for clinicians on appropriate use of telemedicine.

As advocates for older adults, clinicians should also be aware of the ethical implications of electronic assistive technologies capable of surveilling, monitoring, and reporting personal health data and activities. Many technologies propose to safeguard older adults or assist with daily activities. However, the health, safety, or functional benefits of a specific technology are often unfounded by research. Furthermore, the extent to which data will be collected, how it will be used, and the risk of security breach are often not clear to the user. These factors make the possibility of informed consent nebulous for a user of any age. In older adults, there are additional ethical considerations. Older adults are often not included in the idea generation or development of these products, and if affected by cognitive impairment or dementia, they may not be involved in the decision to use it. However, awareness of the product—such as home video surveillance—may still cause distress. We recommend careful consideration of the ethical implications of technologies with special attention paid to how the technology may impact patient autonomy and well-being prior to use.

Daniel H, Sulmasy LS. Policy recommendations to guide the use of telemedicine in primary care settings: an American College of Physicians position paper. *Ann Intern Med.* 2015;163(10):787-789.

Thilo FJS, Hürlimann B, Hahn S, Bilger S, Schols JMGA, Halfens RGJ. Involvement of older people in the development of fall detection systems: a scoping review. *BMC Geriatr.* 2016;16:42.

RECOMMENDATIONS FOR CLINICIANS

Clinicians must be involved in the implementation of telemedicine programs to ensure that they are accessible and appropriately adapted to the needs of older adults. Clinicians are well equipped to determine whether a service meets high-quality clinical standards. When virtual visits are conducted, critical consideration about the quality of the visit is of utmost importance. We recommend that clinicians advocate for use that enhances rather than degrades the therapeutic relationship and imparts satisfaction both to the patient and to the clinicians themselves. Finally, clinicians should participate in formal evaluation of health care technology and the development of guidelines.

At this time, assistive technologies are readily available, but the value added of many devices is unclear. High-quality research is required to outline benefits and drawbacks of assistive technologies. The clinician should be familiar with basic options and approach any new technology with a healthy dose of skepticism—particularly when the product comes at a high cost. Ultimately, members of the geriatric workforce must take an active role in the development and implementation of both health care technology and products for daily living. Clinicians are in the position to advocate for the equitable, ethical, and responsible use of such technologies by, and for, older adults.

Osteoarthritis

34

Ernest R. Vina, MD, MS

C. Kent Kwoh, MD

ESSENTIALS OF DIAGNOSIS

▶ History suggests noninflammatory joint pain (ie, worse with activity, better with rest).

▶ Examination suggests joint line tenderness and bony enlargement.

▶ Radiographs demonstrate joint space narrowing, osteophytes, sclerosis, and bone cysts.

▶ General Considerations

A. Prevalence & Impact

Osteoarthritis (OA) is a highly prevalent, disabling, and costly disease. More than a tenth of the adult population has symptomatic OA, and more than a quarter of those >70 years of age have self-reported arthritis. It was recently estimated that 14 million people in the United States have symptomatic knee OA. OA is also a known cause of disability, and having the diagnosis is associated with a decrease in quality-adjusted life-years. In the United States and other developed countries, the cost of OA has been estimated to account for approximately 1% to 2.5% of the gross national product. Most direct costs of OA are due to hospital stays (especially during or after joint replacement surgery) and rehabilitation care. Other direct costs are attributed to medications, provider visits, other health professional visits, and diagnostic procedures. Indirect costs are largely due to productivity losses from reduced employment rate, absenteeism, presenteeism (decrease in productivity even when at work), and early retirement. As such, OA has been designated as a serious disease by the US Food and Drug Administration (FDA) for the reasons summarized in Table 34–1.

B. Risk Factors

Several factors can increase the likelihood of developing OA, and risk factors can be divided into systemic- and joint-level risk factors (Table 34–2). Increased age is a well-known risk factor for OA, particularly among women age 50 and older. Women, compared to men, are more likely to develop hand, foot, and knee OA. African Americans, compared to whites, are more likely to develop symptomatic knee and hip OA. Certain gene variants may predispose individuals to OA development. Obesity and hyperlipidemia are risk factors for the development of knee, hip, and hand OA. High bone mineral density can increase the risk of developing lower extremity OA. Particular bone/joint shapes (eg, cam deformity) may increase the risk of developing hip and knee OA. Knee malalignment, such as varus thrust, is a known predictor of knee OA disease worsening. Particular occupations (eg, construction) and sports activities (eg, soccer) associated with joint injury can predispose people to early localized OA. Ligamental injury, meniscal tear, and cartilage damage have been associated with subsequent OA development. In research settings, joint abnormalities that are detected only by magnetic resonance imaging (MRI) as compared to plain radiography, such as synovitis, subchondral bone marrow lesions, meniscal damage, and/or extrusion, may predict OA development.

▶ Pathogenesis

Although OA was once considered "a disease of wear and tear" or a disease due mainly to cartilage damage, it is now known to be a complex condition that may affect the tissues of the entire joint. Cartilage, subchondral bone, and synovium all likely play key roles in the pathogenesis of OA:

- Cartilage architecture and biochemistry are regulated by chondrocytes in response to chemical and mechanical changes. Activated chondrocytes produce

Table 34–1. Reasons why osteoarthritis (OA) is a serious disease.

Reasons	Supportive Data
Highly prevalent globally	240 million people
Both prevalence and risk factors are increasing	Third most rapidly rising condition
No known cure	No approved treatments to stop the progression of OA
Significant impact in years of life lost due to disability (YLDs)	2.4% of all YLDs; 10% severe disability
Significant impact on and by comorbid conditions	Obesity, diabetes, depression, cardiovascular diseases
Increased risk of dying prematurely	10%–20% relative increase in mortality
Loss of productivity; early retirement; loss of retirement savings	>1% gross domestic product in the United States
High economic burden to individuals and society	TJR numbers rising globally
Natural history of disease progression with no known remission	Approximately 30% need TJR over 10 years
No proven interventions yet available to stop the progression	Weight loss and exercise as preventative measures
Current therapies have small treatment effect and are costly and associated with life-threatening adverse effects	Side effects, including NSAID-related deaths; opioid crisis

NSAID, nonsteroidal anti-inflammatory drugs; TJR, total joint replacement.

Table 34–2. Osteoarthritis (OA) risk factors.

Systemic Level	
Sociodemographic	Older age; female sex (hand, foot, knee OA); male sex (cervical spine, shoulder OA); African American race
Genetic	SNP in *ALDH1A2* gene (increased risk), *TACR1* gene (decreased risk)
Metabolic syndrome	Obesity, hyperlipidemia
Vitamins/diet	Low vitamin D, low dietary fiber
Bone density/mass	High bone mineral density
Joint Level	
Bone/joint shape	Acetabular index, cam deformity, acetabular dysplasia
Muscle strength	Low thigh muscle CSA (knee OA), high extensor CSA (patellofemoral OA)
Joint loads and alignment	Knee malalignment
Occupation and sports	Repetitive activities (eg, soccer for knee, hip OA)
Injury/surgery	Anterior cruciate ligament injury, meniscal tear, articular cartilage damage; history of joint surgery
Preradiographic lesions	Effusion, synovitis, bone marrow lesions, cartilage damage

CSA, cross-sectional area; SNP, single nucleotide polymorphism.

inflammatory response proteins, including cytokines, and matrix-degrading enzymes. The innate immune system is also activated in OA. Chondrocytes express toll-like receptors, and complement expression and activation are high in osteoarthritic joints.

- Subchondral bone is the layer of bone just below the cartilage in a joint. This structure is often abnormal in OA. Endochondral ossification is reinitiated in OA, accompanied by the formation of osteophytes and subchondral cysts. Osteoblasts, in response to mechanical stimulation, may produce inflammatory cytokines and degradative enzymes. Subchondral bone remodeling may also result from increased loading through loss of cartilage integrity. Subchondral bone is highly innervated, and structural changes in subchondral bone likely contribute to pain generation in OA.

- Synovitis is common in early OA, and synovial hypertrophy is common in late OA. Production of joint lubricants by synoviocytes is suboptimal in OA. Like chondrocytes and osteoblasts, synoviocytes also produce inflammatory mediators and degradative enzymes.

OA has been classified as either primary (idiopathic) or secondary to known causes. Certain systemic diseases are associated with the development of "secondary" OA. These include trauma, anatomic abnormalities, metabolic/endocrine disease, postinfectious arthritis, neuropathic disease, and abnormal structure and function of hyaline cartilage (Table 34–3).

A. Phenotypes

OA is a heterogeneous disease with a variety of presentations. There is growing consensus that variations of OA result from the existence of different phenotypes that may represent different mechanisms of the disease. OA may occur as the result of a number of different pathways that ultimately degenerate into joint failure. This disease process affects the total joint, including the subchondral bone, ligaments, joint capsule, synovial membrane, periarticular muscles, peripheral nerves, menisci (when present), and articular cartilage. The destruction of the joint, including loss of articular cartilage, is therefore best viewed as the final product of a variety of possible etiologic factors with one or more phenotypes being expressed in an individual (Figure 34–1). Treatment that targets the mechanism underlying one phenotype may not

Table 34–3. Systemic diseases associated with secondary osteoarthritis (OA).

Trauma

Inflammatory arthritis
- Rheumatoid arthritis
- Systemic lupus erythematosus
- Seronegative spondyloarthropathies
- Other connective tissue diseases

Metabolic/endocrine
- Hemochromatosis
- Acromegaly
- Hyperparathyroidism
- Ochronosis

Crystal deposition disease
- Gout
- Pseudogout

Neuropathic disorders
- Diabetes mellitus

Anatomical abnormalities
- Bone dysplasia

be effective for a different phenotype. Recognition of different disease phenotypes is crucial so that clinicians may tailor their disease management depending on the specific phenotype(s) present.

A cartilage-centric phenotype is manifested by loss of joint space on radiographs and cartilage damage/loss on MRI.

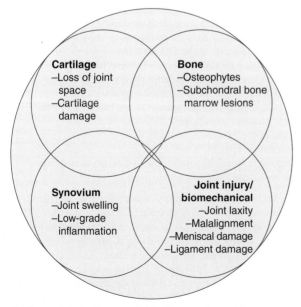

▲ **Figure 34–1.** Osteoarthritis disease phenotypes.

A bone-centric phenotype is expressed by osteophytes on radiographs and subchondral marrow lesions on MRI. A joint injury/biomechanical-centric phenotype is based on joint laxity on physical examination, malalignment on radiographs, and meniscal damage and/or ligament damage on MRI. A synovium-centric phenotype is manifested by joint swelling on physical examination and low-grade inflammation as evidenced by effusion synovitis and Hoffa synovitis (ie, inflammation of the infrapatellar fat pad) on MRI.

Prevention

Similar to other chronic diseases, prevention and early comprehensive care models are essential in treating OA. Obesity, joint injury, impaired muscle function, joint laxity, and malalignment are modifiable risk factors that are amenable to primary and secondary prevention strategies. Several strategies can be used by individuals to lose weight in the short term. The more difficult issue is maintaining weight loss over longer periods of time. Dietary restriction can successfully lead to reduced weight, but macronutrient (eg, fat, carbohydrate) manipulation seems to have only a minor effect on weight reduction. Concurrently, exercise can be helpful in maintaining weight loss. Cognitive-behavioral therapy can also be helpful with weight loss, while bariatric surgery can lead to significant weight reduction that may persist for a long time.

Prevention of joint injuries is crucial in preventing OA, especially in those who are at high risk, such as athletes. Neuromuscular and proprioceptive training programs have been successful in preventing anterior cruciate ligament injuries of the knee. Identifying target groups who may benefit from secondary prevention of knee OA (eg, those who have had knee trauma or orthopedic surgery) is also crucial. In addition to maintenance of a healthy body weight and regular physical activity, biomechanical interventions that have the ability to improve joint stability and decrease pain can be helpful. While neuromuscular exercise therapy can be helpful for this purpose, strength training is also important for minimizing muscle weakness following injury. Passive approaches to improve joint biomechanics, such as braces and foot orthotics, can also shift mechanical loads and contact stress on the knee, potentially delaying or preventing the onset of OA.

Clinical Findings

A. Symptoms & Signs

OA patients commonly present with noninflammatory joint pain. Most complain of pain that worsens with activity and is relieved by rest. The onset of symptoms is usually insidious, beginning in only one or a few joints. With more advanced disease, pain may be noted with progressively less activity, eventually occurring even at rest. The disease can also cause morning stiffness that usually resolves <30 minutes after waking up in the morning. Joint stiffness may recur following periods of inactivity, a phenomenon called "gelling." Some may report joint locking or instability. Physical examination may reveal joint line tenderness, crepitus (ie, creaking on movement), and bony enlargement. There may be joint effusion or soft-tissue swelling that tends to be intermittent and without warmth. Late in the disease, joint range of motion becomes diminished, and joint deformity and/or laxity may develop.

OA is often asymmetric and does not affect all joints equally. The most commonly affected joints are the hands, knees, hips, and spine:

- *Hand OA.* The distal interphalangeal (DIP), proximal interphalangeal (PIP), and carpometacarpal (CMC) joints are most commonly affected. Gripping, pinching, holding, or lifting objects may be particularly difficult among those with hand OA. There may be tenderness of the affected finger joints upon physical examination. Enlargement of the first CMC joint can result in a squared appearance of the hand. Prominent bony enlargements of the DIP and PIP joints are known as Heberden and Bouchard nodes, respectively.

- *Knee OA.* Patients with knee OA may have localized or, less commonly, diffuse knee pain. They may also complain of knee buckling or instability in the late stages of the disease. They may have difficulty climbing the stairs or walking for even short periods of time. Common knee joint physical exam findings include crepitus on active/passive motion, tenderness, bony enlargement, effusion without warmth, and limitation of range of motion. Increased joint effusion may lead to knee flexion and to migration into the semimembranosus bursa posteriorly, causing swelling along the posterior knee known as a popliteal or Baker cyst. Late in the disease, knee varus ("bow-legged") or valgus ("knock-kneed") deformities may be observed.

- *Hip OA.* Pain from hip OA is often manifested by pain along the anterior hip or the inguinal area. Sometimes, pain may be felt laterally or referred to the knee. Crossing legs or putting on a pair of shoes can be challenging. Upon physical examination, there is often reproducible pain with passive or active range of motion, especially with extension and internal rotation. Limited range of motion may also be observed. Some patients may develop an antalgic gait in which weight is shifted to the contralateral uninvolved hip.

- *Spine OA.* The cervical and lumbar spines are most commonly affected by OA. Cervical spine OA typically causes neck pain, but can also cause occipital headaches, upper extremity radicular pain, shoulder pain, and loss of dexterity of the hands. Rarely, large osteophytes may compromise the spinal canal, causing lower extremity spasticity and gait disturbance. Lumbar spine OA can often cause lower back pain that may radiate into the lower extremity

and worsen with bending ipsilateral to the involved joint. Lumbar facet joint osteophytes can lead to lumbar canal stenosis; symptoms of spinal stenosis are often relieved by bending slightly forward.

B. Laboratory Findings

Serum blood tests are not useful in diagnosing OA but are typically helpful in ruling out other disorders or in diagnosing an underlying disorder that has caused secondary OA (see Table 34–3). Inflammatory markers (eg, erythrocyte sedimentation rate, C-reactive protein) and immunologic tests (eg, antinuclear antibody test, rheumatoid factor) should not be routinely ordered unless there are signs or symptoms suggestive of inflammatory arthritis or autoimmune disease. Uric acid level may be ordered if gout is suspected.

Cytokines, enzymes, and extracellular matrix constituents (eg, precursors or degradation products of collagen and proteoglycan) are potential biochemical markers for OA. While many biochemical markers have been investigated, none are sufficiently well validated for use in clinical practice at present.

C. Imaging Studies

1. X-rays—History and physical examination should be sufficient to make the diagnosis of OA. Radiography is the conventional imaging modality commonly used to confirm the diagnosis of OA and assess structural severity and progression. Osteophytes, joint space narrowing (JSN), subchondral sclerosis, and cystic changes are all radiographic features of OA. Multiple radiographic views and weight-bearing views of joints of the lower extremities may increase the detection of changes consistent with OA. In hand OA, the CMC, DIP, and PIP joints may have joint space loss. Some patients with erosive hand OA will have central erosions and the classic "gull-wing" deformity in the DIP and PIP joints (Figure 34–2). Knee OA patients will typically have tibiofemoral and/or patellofemoral JSN and osteophyte formation (Figure 34–3). Osteophytes may be seen anteriorly at the distal femur and proximal tibia and posteriorly at the patella and tibia. Hip OA patients typically have JSN (superior, axial, or medial), osteophyte formation, and subchondral sclerosis. Those with lumbar or spinal OA will show intervertebral disk narrowing and osteophytes arising from the vertebral body margins. Sclerosis and cysts may also be seen.

2. MRI—Due to the limited sensitivity and specificity of radiography, many have proposed the additional use of MRI to detect and evaluate OA features. MRI can allow visualization of the articular cartilage, tendons, ligaments, epiphyseal plate, and adjacent soft-tissue envelope. There are several semi-quantitative MRI-based scoring systems that can be used to grade OA features to assess the amount of joint damage in research studies. The MRI Osteoarthritis Knee Score (MOAKS), for instance, evaluates the knee for the following

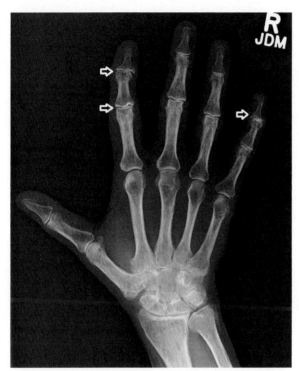

▲ **Figure 34–2.** Hand x-ray showing joint space narrowing of primarily the distal interphalangeal (DIP) and proximal interphalangeal (PIP) joints. There are also central erosions of the DIP/PIP joints of the index and small fingers (unfilled arrows).

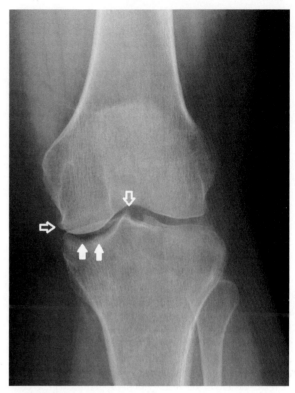

▲ **Figure 34–3.** Anteroposterior view of the right knee showing medial tibiofemoral joint space narrowing (filled arrows) and osteophytes (unfilled arrows).

components: cartilage size and depth, bone marrow lesions, osteophytes, synovitis or effusion, Hoffa synovitis, meniscal extraction, meniscal status, ligaments, periarticular cysts/bursitides, and loose bodies. Quantitative and compositional MRI measurements may also provide information on the three-dimensional shape and tissue composition of the articular cartilage. At present, MRI is more useful in research than in clinical settings.

D. Special Tests

A joint aspiration and synovial fluid analysis can be done to rule out an infectious etiology or crystalline disease in suspected cases. Synovial fluid findings in OA usually suggest a minimally inflammatory (white blood cell count <2000/mm^3) process. Under polarized microscopy, there are usually no visible crystals.

▶ Differential Diagnosis

The clinical diagnosis of OA is based on history, physical examination, and, sometimes, characteristic radiographic features.

Before making a clinical diagnosis of OA in older adults, other disorders should be excluded, as physical or radiographic finding of OA is quite common in older adults without accompanying symptoms. When an older adult presents with less typical features or has unusual joint involvement, confirming the presence of OA unequivocally can be particularly difficult. The clinician must distinguish OA from referred pain, other inflammatory joint diseases such as rheumatoid arthritis, gout or pseudogout, and soft-tissue processes such as periarticular bursitis (eg, pes anserine bursitis mimicking knee OA, greater trochanteric bursitis simulating hip OA). Such patients will benefit from imaging studies of affected joints in combination with selected laboratory tests, although most patients do not need imaging studies for the diagnosis of OA.

▶ Complications

Complications of OA in and around the joint include osteonecrosis, stress fractures, joint infection, and deterioration/rupture of ligaments and tendons around the joint. An acute onset of inflammatory arthritis may suggest a superimposed diagnosis of gout or pseudogout. Those with synovial effusion of the knee may have a dissecting or ruptured Baker cyst. The development of periarticular symptoms may be due to bursitis or inflammation of soft tissue around the joint. Moreover, there is evidence that the risk of cardiovascular disease is increased in patients with OA compared with the general population. Other chronic conditions such as depression and sleep disorders are also not uncommon in older persons with OA.

▶ Treatments

Numerous guidelines for OA management exist. The main goals of management are to minimize OA-related pain, improve physical functioning, and optimize the quality of life of patients with OA. There are nonpharmacologic, pharmacologic, and surgical treatment options. OA management should be tailored to the individual, and optimal management includes a combination of these treatment modalities.

A. Nonpharmacologic

1. Patient education and self-management—Patients should be taught about the goals of OA treatment and the different modalities of available treatment. The focus should be on initiating self-help and patient-driven treatments. There should also be an emphasis on maintaining adherence to nonpharmacologic and pharmacologic therapies. Patients may be referred to self-management programs. Regular contact to promote self-care can be particularly helpful. Other components that patients can benefit from include instructions in joint protection (especially for hand, hip, and knee OA), an evaluation of ability to perform activities of daily living, psychosocial interventions, and individualization of treatment plans.

2. Exercise and weight loss—For those with advanced OA, range of motion and isometric strengthening exercises can be initially prescribed. Beneficial isometric exercises for older adults include chair leg extensions, wall sits, and hip extensions. The exercise regimen may progress sequentially through isotonic strengthening, aerobic exercises, and, eventually, recreational exercises. Beneficial isotonic exercises include squats, wall slides, and leg presses. Regular aerobic activities for older adults include walking, bicycling, or swimming. Water-based exercise, in particular, is a low-impact activity that can be invaluable for those with severe OA and marked deconditioning. Consideration should be given to exercise in combination with manual therapy, endurance or strengthening exercises, and physical/occupational therapy referral. Weight loss should be recommended to overweight and obese individuals with knee and hip OA. A structured weight management program may be necessary for some. An effective program focuses on developing healthy eating and physical activity habits. It should include a plan to lose weight slowly and steadily and to maintain the weight loss over the long term.

3. Taping, braces, orthoses, and assistive devices—Patellar taping can be helpful in treating knee OA. A knee brace can reduce pain, improve stability, and diminish the risk of falling in knee OA patients with varus or valgus instability. Laterally wedged insoles can decrease lateral thrust in the knee of patients with medial compartment OA. Medially wedged insoles can be beneficial to patients with lateral knee OA. Walking aids (eg, canes, crutches, walkers) can benefit those with knee and hip OA. Splints may be helpful for those with trapeziometacarpal joint OA. Other devices that may also be helpful include reaching aids, elevation of chairs and beds, and grab rails for lower extremity OA, and enlarged grips and aids for opening jars for hand OA.

4. Heat and cold therapy—Thermal modalities may be effective for relieving OA symptoms, albeit the effects may be temporary. Heat can be administered by the application of heat packs or immersion in warm water or paraffin baths. Cold can be administered by application of ice packs or massage with ice. Patients should be instructed to limit the use of heat/cold therapy to 20-minute intervals.

5. Alternative and complementary modalities—Other therapies that may be helpful in treating OA include acupuncture, Tai Chi, and transcutaneous electrical nerve stimulation. Evidence supporting the efficacy of these treatments for a broad range of patients is mixed, however.

B. Pharmacologic

1. Acetaminophen—Acetaminophen/paracetamol is often the initial therapy for mild OA because it is inexpensive, relatively safe, and effective. Hepatotoxicity is a potential side effect, but, within the therapeutic range (ie, <3000 mg/day), it is seen primarily in patients with concurrent alcohol abuse or in conjunction with other hepatotoxic medications.

2. Oral nonsteroidal anti-inflammatory drugs (NSAIDs)—Among OA patients with moderate to severe levels of pain, NSAIDs can be more effective than acetaminophen. There is no convincing evidence that any particular NSAID is more effective than other NSAIDs for the treatment of hand, knee, or hip OA. Patients respond differently to different agents in terms of efficacy and toxicity. Low-cost NSAIDs with a short half-life, such as ibuprofen or naproxen, may be an appropriate initial choice, and medication dosage may be maximized after a few weeks. Switching to a different NSAID is a treatment management option after failure of any given NSAID. Potential adverse effects include peptic ulcer, gastrointestinal (GI) bleeding, renal dysfunction, edema, elevated transaminases, elevated blood pressure, cardiovascular risk, and cognitive dysfunction (especially in older adults). Presence of multiple comorbidities, including GI diseases, limits NSAID use in older patients and those on anticoagulants. The risk of GI bleeding can be lessened by use of a cyclooxygenase-2 selective agent (eg, celecoxib, meloxicam) or concomitant use of a proton pump inhibitor or misoprostol. However, gastroprotective agents are not protective below the ligament of Treitz, and lower GI bleeding risk is not uncommon with NSAID use in older adults.

3. Topical therapies—Topical capsaicin cream can be effective in treating knee OA and should only be used with caution in hand OA. Patients should be instructed to avoid inadvertent application of capsaicin in the eyes and mucous membranes. Rubefacients containing salicylates (eg, trolamine salicylate, hydroxyethyl salicylate, diethylamine salicylate) can also be used as adjunctive therapy. Skin burning and other skin reactions are potential side effects. Topical NSAIDs (eg, diclofenac sodium gel) can be an effective alternative or adjunct treatment for knee and hip OA. They may be particularly useful in patients with multiple chronic medical conditions.

4. Narcotic analgesics—Tramadol is a dual-acting weak μ-receptor inhibitor with serotonin reuptake inhibition that should be used with caution in older adults with OA and preferably only for limited duration in the lowest effective dose. It has been shown to have an additive effect with acetaminophen. Side effects include nausea, vomiting, lightheadedness, dizziness, or headache. The initial and maintenance dose should be lower in the geriatric population to minimize potential side effects. For patients with refractory OA symptoms or when other treatments are not appropriate, an opioid medication can be considered, although opioids are poorly tolerated in older patients because of increased sensitivity to adverse side effects, especially sedation, confusion, and constipation. The lowest dose of opioids should be used whenever possible. Opioid analgesics may also be considered in older adults who are either not willing to undergo or have contraindications for total joint replacement surgery after having failed all other nonpharmacologic and pharmacologic therapies.

5. Other oral agents—Use of serotonin and norepinephrine reuptake inhibitors (eg, duloxetine) appears promising for the treatment of OA. They may be used in OA patients with refractory symptoms and those with contraindications to the use of other pharmacologic therapies. There are several nutraceuticals that have been used for the treatment of OA. However, the use of glucosamine and/or chondroitin is controversial, and high-quality trials have shown little to no evidence of clinically meaningful benefit with use of these products. Other nutraceuticals that have been used in the management of OA include flavocoxid, S-adenosylmethionine (SAM-e), Boswellia, collagen hydrolysate, avocado-soybean, curcuma (turmeric), ginger, and evening primrose oil, but each of these has very limited evidence of efficacy.

6. Intra-articular therapy—Intra-articular glucocorticoid injections help to relieve pain and increase joint flexibility for variable periods of time. They may be of greater value when synovial effusions or signs of inflammation are present, and in patients with one or a few joints that are painful despite use of an oral agent. Hip joint injection requires ultrasonographic or fluoroscopic guidance, and efficacy of glucocorticoid injections at sites other than the knee or hip is less certain. Steroid injection can cause elevation in blood sugar, and septic arthritis is a rare complication. Intra-articular injection of moderate- to high-molecular-weight hyaluronan preparations, also known as viscosupplementation, is widely used to treat knee OA, but there is still some uncertainty regarding whether its use is superior to placebo, oral NSAIDs, or intra-articular glucocorticoid. Significant pain reduction may not be achieved until weeks following the initial injection. There is also a risk of postinjection reactive inflammatory synovitis and a small risk of joint infection with joint injection. Evidence concerning the use of intra-articular platelet-rich plasma is very limited.

C. Surgical Procedures

1. Joint arthroplasty—Although there are no clear criteria for surgery, surgical interventions are generally reserved for individuals with severe symptomatic OA who have marked limitations in function, such as performing activities of daily living, and who have failed nonpharmacologic and pharmacologic therapies. Potential surgical candidates should have had an adequate trial of exercise and physical therapy. Total joint arthroplasty is usually selected for OA of the hip, knee, and shoulder. Among those with severe OA at the base of the thumb, CMC joint replacement is also an option. Total knee arthroplasty, in particular, involves resection of the diseased articular knee surfaces, followed by resurfacing with metal and polyethylene prosthetic components. Contraindications include active infection, a nonfunctioning extensor mechanism, and poor lower extremity vascular flow. Preoperative evaluation includes the identification of chronic conditions that may affect the choice of anesthesia, the procedure, and potential complications. Postoperative care includes pain management, prophylaxis against infection, venous thromboembolism prophylaxis, and appropriate physical therapy. Initial improvement may be observed 6 to 12 weeks postoperatively, but full recovery typically occurs 1 to 2 years postoperatively. Complications include those common to other surgeries, as well as those specific to joint operations (eg, prosthetic joint infection, neurovascular injury, fractures). Hemiarthroplasty may be beneficial for those with unicompartmental knee OA, and excellent outcomes are often observed. There is an increased risk of mortality with hemiarthroplasty in older adults, however, and older age is related to worse function, particularly in women.

2. Other surgical procedures—In selected patients, corrective osteotomy and joint resurfacing can be considered instead of total arthroplasty. Joint lavage and arthroscopy with debridement or meniscectomy are not recommended for symptomatic knee OA because multiple randomized controlled clinical trials have shown no greater benefit than placebo for these interventions.

Prognosis

The natural course and prognosis of OA largely depend on the joints involved, underlying risk factors, presence of symptoms, and the severity of the condition. OA is generally slowly progressive but stable, responding well to medical management. A subset of patients, however, follows a progressive trajectory and eventually requires surgical therapy. There are several factors associated with relatively rapid progression of disease, but risk factors for progression vary according to the joints involved. There are no FDA-approved disease-modifying drugs for OA, and current therapeutics focus mainly on relief of pain and functional improvement. Although a multidisciplinary approach and joint replacement surgery have altered the severity of OA's impact, patients with OA still experience varying degrees of physical disability. Patient education and psychosocial support are as important as medical therapy in preventing disability, particularly in older adults.

Studies have shown moderate evidence of increased mortality among persons with OA compared with the general population. Possible explanations for this excess mortality include reduced levels of physical activity among persons with OA as a result of involvement of lower limb joints and presence of comorbid conditions (eg, cardiovascular disease), as well as adverse effects of medications used to treat symptomatic OA. Therefore, management of patients with OA and walking disability should focus on effective treatment of cardiovascular risk factors and other chronic conditions, as well as on increasing physical activity.

Demehri S, Hafezi-Nejad N, Carrino JA. Conventional and novel imaging modalities in osteoarthritis: current state of the evidence. *Curr Opin Rheumatol.* 2015;27(3):295-303.

Deveza LA, Melo L, Yamato TP, Mills K, Ravi V, Hunter DJ. Knee osteoarthritis phenotypes and their relevance for outcomes: a systematic review. *Osteoarthritis Cartilage.* 2017;25(12):1926-1941.

Global Burden of Disease Study Collaborators. Global, regional, and national incidence, prevalence, and years lived with disability for 301 acute and chronic diseases and injuries in 188 countries, 1990-2013: a systematic analysis for the Global Burden of Disease Study 2013. *Lancet.* 2015;386(9995):743-800.

Glyn-Jones S, Palmer AJ, Agricola R, et al. Osteoarthritis. *Lancet.* 2015;386(9991):376-387.

Hunter DJ, Schofield D, Callander E. The individual and socioeconomic impact of osteoarthritis. *Nat Rev Rheumatol.* 2014;10(7):437-441.

Nelson AE, Allen KD, Golightly YM, Goode AP, Jordan JM. A systematic review of recommendations and guidelines for the management of osteoarthritis: the chronic osteoarthritis management initiative of the U.S. bone and joint initiative. *Semin Arthritis Rheum.* 2014;43(6):701-712.

Osteoarthritis Research Society International. Osteoarthritis: a serious disease. Submitted to the US Food and Drug Administration. https://www.oarsi.org/sites/default/files/library/2018/pdf/oarsi_white_paper_oa_serious_disease121416_1.pdf. Accessed March 19, 2019.

Roos EM, Arden NK. Strategies for the prevention of knee osteoarthritis. *Nat Rev Rheumatol.* 2016;12(2):92-101.

Silverwood V, Blagojevic-Bucknall M, Jinks C, Jordan JL, Protheroe J, Jordan KP. Current evidence on risk factors for knee osteoarthritis in older adults: a systematic review and meta-analysis. *Osteoarthritis Cartilage.* 2015;23(4):507-515.

Vina ER, Kwoh CK. Epidemiology of osteoarthritis: literature update. *Curr Opin Rheumatol.* 2018;30(2):160-167.

Osteoporosis and Hip Fractures

35

Michele Bellantoni, MD, CMD

Meredith Gilliam, MD, MPH

ESSENTIALS OF DIAGNOSIS

▶ Osteoporosis is a systemic skeletal disease characterized by low bone mass and microarchitectural deterioration of the bone tissue, with a consequent increase in bone fragility and susceptibility to fracture.

▶ Osteoporosis is a "silent" disease, but its complications, especially hip and vertebral fractures, may result in decreased functional independence, pain, kyphosis, and diminished quality of life.

▶ The prevalence of osteoporosis and fragility fractures increases with age.

▶ Osteoporosis is more common in women than in men, but at least a fourth of fragility fractures occur in men.

General Principles

Osteoporosis is a skeletal disorder characterized by compromised bone strength, resulting in bone fragility and susceptibility to fractures. Bone strength is a function of bone mineral density (BMD) and bone quality. Bone quality refers to the architecture, bone turnover, damage accumulation, and mineralization occurring at the bony matrix. Bone mass is assessed using bone density measurements, particularly dual x-ray absorptiometry (DXA), but there is no agreed-upon way to measure bone quality in a quantitative and comparable way.

Given these limitations, the World Health Organization (WHO) has defined osteoporosis as the condition of having a BMD that is >2.5 standard deviations lower than the BMD of a sex-matched young adult. Osteoporosis may also be defined by the occurrence of its main complication, fragility fractures. Fragility fractures are bone fractures that result from poor bone strength in the setting of minor trauma or no trauma. These fractures most often result from a fall from

standing height or less and involve the thoracic and lumbar vertebrae, hip, proximal humerus, wrist, ribs, and pelvis. The skull, cervical spine, hands, feet, and ankles are less commonly affected by osteoporosis, and fractures of these bones are generally not labeled as fragility fractures.

Osteoporosis is a disease with its origin in childhood. Although genetic factors primarily account for peak bone mass, environmental factors such as nutrition and exercise can alter the genetically determined pattern of skeletal growth. Illness and medications during a person's lifetime can impact the accrual of peak mass such that individuals start at a lower peak bone mass. Modulation of peak bone mass can even occur during intrauterine life and is affected by maternal nutrition, smoking, and level of exercise. During adulthood, bone tends to have a steady state of formation and resorption with a stable bone mass. For women, menopause marks the start of increased bone resorption. For most older adults, bone resorption exceeds bone formation, and certain illnesses and medications can accelerate this process.

Older adults are particularly susceptible to complications of osteoporosis. Comorbidities, such as cognitive and gait impairments, predispose the individual to falls and the development of fragility fractures.

Epidemiology

The United States has approximately 52 million individuals with low bone mass: 10 million with osteoporosis and 43 million with osteopenia, which is a designation the WHO has given to individuals with a bone density between 1 and 2.5 standard deviations lower than a sex-matched young adult. The prevalence of osteoporosis and osteopenia increases with age for both men and women. In the United States, about 25% of women over age 65 and 5% of men over 65 have osteoporosis. Following the WHO definition, another 52% of women and 43% of men in this age group have osteopenia.

An estimated 1.5 million fragility fractures occur in the United States each year. Approximately 40% of women and

13% of men older than 50 years will have a fragility fracture or their hip, vertebra, or forearm in their remaining lifetime. The annual US health care cost of fractures is approximately $22 billion, most of it attributed to acute care hospitalization followed by subacute rehabilitation. Although the overall prevalence of fragility fractures is higher in women, men generally have a higher rate of fracture-related mortality because of associated comorbidities. Even though vertebral fractures are the most prevalent of all fragility fractures, hip fractures contribute more to significant health care expenditure and are associated with the most serious outcomes.

RISK FACTORS

Several important common clinical risk factors for osteoporosis and falls have been identified through epidemiologic studies and indicate how codependent these entities are (Table 35–1). Approximately 95% of hip fractures are caused by falls, so risk factors for falls must be considered when assessing an individual's fracture risk.

The FRAX algorithm, a fracture risk assessment tool that has been adopted by several national osteoporosis guidelines, uses some of the above clinical risk factors, BMD measurements, and country-specific fracture data to estimate a patient's 10-year probability of a fragility fracture. FRAX was developed for both postmenopausal women and men age 40 to 90 years. It is validated to be used in untreated patients only. The algorithm is accessible online for physicians to use in a primary care setting at www.sheffield.ac.uk/FRAX. The algorithm may be used with or without knowledge of an individual's BMD to estimate their risk of future fracture. The algorithm notably omits an independent estimate of fall risk in its calculation of future fracture risk.

No single physical examination finding or combination of findings is sufficient to rule in osteoporosis without further testing. Several examination findings in women, including low body weight (<51 kg), inability to place the back of the head against a wall when standing upright, self-reported humped back, having <20 teeth, and rib-pelvis distance no more than two finger breadths increase the likelihood of osteoporosis or presence of a vertebral fracture and may identify women who would benefit from screening. Height loss resulting from vertebral fractures can be measured in the clinic over time or using the patient's recalled maximal adult height, but the predictive value of height loss is unclear. Nevertheless, a loss of height >3 cm may warrant further testing such as a lateral spine film or DXA scan.

Other pertinent physical exam findings should focus on secondary causes of osteoporosis, which will depend on the clinical history and identified risk factors. In the geriatric population, a comprehensive review of medications is essential.

Table 35–1. Risk factors for osteoporosis, fractures, and falls.

Osteoporosis and Fractures	Falls
Women >65 years old	Advanced age
Men >70 years old	Dementia
White or Asian race	Personal history of falls
Low body weight (<127 lb or body mass index <20 kg/m²)	Low body weight
Family history of osteoporosis[a]	Low muscle strength
Personal history of fragility fracture[a]	Poor nutrition
Fragility fracture in first-degree relative	Polypharmacy
Long-term use of glucocorticoids	Use of long-acting benzodiazepines
Alcohol >2–3 drinks per day[a]	Poor vision
Estrogen deficiency at <45 years old	Self-rated poor health
Testosterone deficiency	Difficulty rising out of chair
Low calcium intake	Resting tachycardia
Vitamin D deficiency	Vitamin D deficiency
Sedentary lifestyle	Sedentary lifestyle
Current tobacco use[a]	

[a]Nine validated risk factors for fracture—age; sex; personal history of fracture; low body mass index; use of oral glucocorticoid therapy; osteoporosis secondary to another condition; parental history of hip fracture; current smoking; and alcohol intake of 3 or more drinks per day—are used in the FRAX algorithm.

Blume SW, Curtis JR. Medical costs of osteoporosis in the elderly Medicare population. *Osteoporos Int.* 2011;22(6):1835-1844.

Cosman F, de Beur SJ, LeBoff MS, et al. Clinician's guide to prevention and treatment of osteoporosis. *Osteoporos Int.* 2014;25(10):2359-2381.

Green AD, Colón-Emeric CS, Bastian L, Drake MT, Lyles KW. Does this woman have osteoporosis? *JAMA.* 2004;292(23):2890-2900.

Hans DB, Kanis JA, Baim S, et al. Joint official positions of the International Society for Clinical Densitometry and International Osteoporosis Foundation on FRAX. *J Clin Densitometry.* 2011;14(3):171-180.

Looker AC, Frenk SM. Percentage of adults aged 65 and over with osteoporosis or low bone mass at the femur neck of lumbar spine: United States, 2005-2010. CDC/NCHS, National Health and Nutrition Examination Survey, 2005-2010. Published August 2015. https://www.cdc.gov/nchs/data/hestat/osteoporsis/osteoporosis2005_2010.htm. Accessed April 28, 2019.

World Health Organization. *Technical Report: Assessment of Fracture Risk and Its Application to Screening for Postmenopausal Osteoporosis: A Report of a WHO Study Group.* Geneva, Switzerland: World Health Organization; 1994.

► Pathogenesis

After the attainment of peak bone mass during the third decade of life, bone mass declines at a rate of about 0.5% per year. Other genetic and environmental factors adversely affecting bone, in combination with this age-related bone loss, predispose to fractures.

Primary osteoporosis is generally classified by two distinct pathophysiologic processes. Postmenopausal osteoporosis occurs in women as a result of estrogen deprivation and affects mostly trabecular bone, which is a highly vascular form of bone found in the metaphyseal ends of long bones and in the pelvis, vertebrae, ribs, and skull. In contrast, senile osteoporosis occurs in men and women and more often affects cortical bone, which is found in long bone shafts and forms the hard exterior of bones. Both hormonal factors and age-related alteration in stem cell physiology contribute to the development of senile osteoporosis.

Bone homeostasis is maintained via the coupled actions of bone-forming cells (osteoblasts) and bone-resorbing cells (osteoclasts). The number and activity of these cells are influenced by several signaling pathways that are affected by aging. Declining estrogen levels are associated with higher levels of receptor activator of nuclear factor kappa-B ligand (RANKL) and diminished osteoclast apoptosis. Declining vitamin D levels, which is a common finding in older adults at all latitudes, is associated with secondary hyperparathyroidism and enhanced activity of osteoclasts. Sclerostin, a glycoprotein secreted by osteoclasts, is inhibited by parathyroid hormone and may have both an antianabolic and proresorptive effect on bone. With age, mesenchymal stem cells, which are the precursors of both osteoblasts and adipocytes, are more likely to differentiate into adipocytes. The rate of apoptosis among existing osteoblasts also increases. Exactly why these age-related changes result in physiologic bone loss without consequence in some individuals, and pathologic bone loss resulting in fractures in others, is not yet completely understood.

Secondary osteoporosis is bone loss caused by one or more diseases or drugs having direct or indirect effects on bone. Up to 30% of postmenopausal women and 50% to 80% of men may be found to have a secondary cause of osteoporosis. Glucocorticoid use is the most common cause of secondary osteoporosis; the risk is dose and time dependent and begins at doses as low as 2.5 mg of prednisolone daily. Other drug classes associated with secondary osteoporosis include hypogonadism-inducing agents (particularly gonadotropin-releasing hormone agonists, aromatase inhibitors, and medroxyprogesterone), antiepileptics, and calcineurin inhibitors. Proton pump inhibitors (via interference with calcium absorption), loop diuretics (via facilitation of calcium excretion), heparin, thiazolidinediones, and antiretroviral medications have also been implicated.

Disease processes associated with secondary osteoporosis are numerous. More common causes include endocrine disorders, particularly, hyperparathyroidism, hyperthyroidism, hypogonadism in men, and Cushing syndrome; alcoholism; malabsorption syndromes including Celiac disease, inflammatory bowel disease, and post–gastric bypass malabsorption; hematologic disorders including multiple myeloma; renal disorders including idiopathic hypercalciuria and renal tubular acidosis; liver cirrhosis; and autoimmune diseases including rheumatoid arthritis and systemic lupus erythematosus.

Atkins GJ, Findlay DM. Osteocyte regulation of bone mineral: a little give and take. *Osteoporos Int.* 2012;23(8):2067-2079.

Duque G, Troen BR. Understanding the mechanisms of senile osteoporosis: new facts for a major geriatric syndrome. *J Am Geriatr Soc.* 2008;56(5):935-941.

Mirza F, Canalis E. Management of endocrine disease: secondary osteoporosis: pathophysiology and management. *Eur J Endocrinol.* 2015;173(3):R131-R151.

► Clinical Findings

A. Symptoms & Signs

Osteoporosis is generally a silent disease with no clinical manifestations until there is a fracture. Osteoporosis-related vertebral fractures may also be "silent" at the time they occur but over time may contribute to certain physiologic changes, including kyphosis and height loss. Severe kyphosis may impair pulmonary function via reduced forced vital capacity and is associated with gastrointestinal problems including dysphagia, reflux esophagitis, and hiatal hernia.

B. Laboratory Evaluation

Laboratory testing in patients with presumed osteoporosis is undertaken to rule out or find common secondary causes of osteoporosis. Preliminary testing should include a complete blood count, basic chemistry panel, liver function panel, phosphate, and consideration of 24-hour urine collection of calcium. Secondary hyperparathyroidism caused by vitamin D deficiency is prevalent and all older persons should have a 25-hydroxy vitamin D and parathyroid hormone (PTH) assessment. Other testing may be considered based on clinical suspicion (Table 35–2).

1. Bone turnover markers—Additional laboratory testing includes bone turnover markers (BTMs), which are traditionally categorized as bone formation or bone resorption

Table 35–2. Laboratory tests for secondary causes of osteoporosis.

Hypogonadism	Serum testosterone, prolactin
Primary hyperparathyroidism	PTH
Secondary hyperparathyroidism	25-Hydroxy vitamin D, PTH
Multiple myeloma	Serum and urine protein electrophoresis and free light chains
Hyperthyroidism	Thyroid-stimulating hormone
Malabsorption	Tissue transglutaminase antibody
Hypercortisolism	Urinary free cortisol, others
Mastocytosis	Serum tryptase, urine N-methylhistidine, others

PTH, parathyroid hormone.

Table 35–3. Bone turnover markers.

Bone Formation Markers (Produced by Osteoblast Activity)	Bone Resorption Markers (Produced by Osteoclast Activity)
Procollagen type I N propeptide (PINP)[a]	Tartrate resistant acid phosphatase[a]
Procollagen type I C propeptide (PICP)[a]	C-terminal telopeptides (CTX)[b] N-terminal telopeptides (NTX)[b]
Osteocalcin[b] Alkaline phosphatase (bone-specific)[a]	

[a]Marker is measured in the serum.
[b]Marker is measured in the serum or urine.

Table 35–4. World Health Organization diagnostic categories.

Category	Definition by Bone Density
Normal	BMD is within 1 standard deviation (SD) of a normal young adult (T-score > −1.0)
Osteopenia	BMD is between 1 and 2.5 SDs below a normal young adult (T-score −1 to −2.5)
Osteoporosis	BMD is 2.5 SD or more below a normal young adult (T-score ≤ −2.5)
Severe osteoporosis	BMD is 2.5 SDs or more below a normal young adult *and* the person has had a fragility fracture

BMD, bone mineral density.

markers (Table 35–3). Their routine use in clinical practice remains a challenge because of their wide biologic and analytical variability; they are generally less available in the United States than in Europe due to limited access to laboratories that process the tests and higher cost. It should be noted that resorption markers must be measured in the morning on the second void urine because there is a large diurnal variation.

The established clinical use for BTMs is in monitoring treatment efficacy and adherence. BTMs change quickly and robustly in response to treatment (decrease with antiresorptive treatment and increase with anabolic treatment) and therefore provide more rapid feedback on the effects of treatment than that provided by BMD results.

C. Imaging Studies

Imaging studies are helpful in osteoporosis to both identify patients at risk and monitor the effect of pharmacotherapy.

1. DXA—In the United States, DXA measurement is the most commonly used tool to determine bone density, estimate fracture risk, identify candidates for intervention, and assess changes in bone density over time in treated and untreated patients.

DXA is most commonly used to assess BMD in the central skeleton in the lumbar spine and proximal femur. These central sites are preferred as most diagnostic criteria, therapeutic studies, and cost-effectiveness data are based on measurements at axial sites. DXA may also be used to assess the peripheral skeleton at the distal radius and heel, which may be helpful when axial measurements cannot be taken due to prior fractures or surgical hardware or central DXA is not available.

Bone density data are reported as Z-scores and T-scores. A Z-score denotes the difference, in number of standard deviations, between an individual's BMD and the mean BMD of an age-, sex-, and ethnicity-matched reference population. A T-score gives the standard deviation difference between an individual's BMD and the mean BMD of a reference population of young adults at peak bone mass. In 1994, the WHO used T-scores of the axial skeleton to classify and define BMD measurements (Table 35–4). These definitions, originally only for postmenopausal women, have been adapted by the International Society for Clinical Densiometry (ISCD) to classify BMD in premenopausal women, men, and children.

Advantages of using DXA to assess fracture risk and monitor response to therapy include its precision, noninvasiveness, and the well-defined relationship between BMD and fracture risk, with each standard deviation decrease in BMD increasing fracture risk by 1.6 to 2.6 times. DXA is a two-dimensional measurement that only measures density/area and not the volumetric density. Disadvantages of DXA include the precision error of certain instruments (approximately 1%–2%); variability between machines; need for a skilled clinician to interpret readings and identify inaccuracies due to positioning, osteoarthritic change, prior fractures, extraskeletal calcifications, and so on; and the size and cost of central DXA machines limiting their accessibility in rural locations. Due to these limitations, serial DXA measurements should be taken on the same machine and generally not more frequently than every 2 years.

2. Vertebral imaging—Vertebral fractures are frequently asymptomatic and may not present clinically, but their presence is diagnostic of osteoporosis and confers a five-fold increased risk for future fractures. Vertebral imaging may be considered when assessing a patient's initial fracture risk, when a loss of height has been noted, or other times when knowledge of incident fractures would change clinical management. Imaging may be performed using lateral thoracic and lumbar spine x-ray or lateral vertebral fracture assessment available on most DXA machines and performed at the same time as BMD assessment.

3. Other imaging—Bone x-rays in individuals with low bone mass may show bone lucency, but this finding is generally not part of the diagnosis of osteoporosis. Quantitative ultrasound of the calcaneus has also been used to screen patients at risk for osteoporosis, is inexpensive, and may be accessible in areas where central DXA is not available. However, it does not measure BMD, has not been studied in large osteoporosis trials, and generally should not be used to guide decisions about osteoporosis treatment.

Camacho PM, Petak SM, Binkley N, et al. American Association of Clinical Endocrinologists and American College of Endocrinology Clinical Practice Guidelines for the diagnosis and treatment of postmenopausal osteoporosis—2016. *Endocr Pract.* 2016;22(suppl 4):1-42.

Marshall D, Johnell O, Wedel H. Meta-analysis of how well measures of bone mineral density predict occurrence of osteoporotic fractures. *BMJ* 1996;312(7041):1254-1259.

Ross PD, Davis JW, Epstein RS, et al. Pre-existing fractures and bone mass predict vertebral fracture incidence in women. *Ann Internal Med* 1991;114(11):919-923.

▶ Differential Diagnosis

Metabolic bone diseases other than osteoporosis may also result in low BMD and fracture, and may coexist with osteoporosis. These include osteomalacia, osteitis deformans, and renal osteodystrophy.

Osteomalacia is a disorder of decreased mineralization of newly formed osteoid at sites of bone turnover and occurs as a result of hypocalcemia, hypophosphatemia, or direct inhibition of bone mineralization. Low serum calcium and phosphate and elevated alkaline phosphatase should point toward a diagnosis of osteomalacia, and osteoporosis medications should be avoided.

Osteitis deformans, also known as Paget disease of the bone, is characterized by accelerated bone remodeling at one or more foci in the skull, spine, pelvis, or long bones of the legs; diagnosis is generally made via x-rays showing cortical thickening and coarse trabecular markings, and serum alkaline phosphatase is usually elevated.

Renal osteodystrophy refers to specific changes in bone morphology associated with chronic kidney disease, having different pathophysiology than primary osteoporosis. Chronic kidney disease and osteoporosis are both common in older persons and may coexist. However, when BMD is low and glomerular filtration rate is <30 mL/min, features of chronic kidney disease–related mineral bone disorder may predominate. Hyperphosphatemia, vitamin D deficiency, and secondary hyperparathyroidism should be treated in these cases, and coordination with a nephrologist may be appropriate.

In addition, when a patient presents with a low-trauma fracture, before the diagnosis of osteoporosis is made, radiographs should be taken to exclude an underlying focal bone lesion due to a bone tumor (primary or metastatic), bone cyst, or infection.

Ketteler M, Block GA, Evenepoel P, et al. Executive summary of the 2017 KDIGO chronic kidney disease-mineral and bone disorder (CKD-MBD) guideline update: what's changed and why it matters. *Kidney Int.* 2017;92(1):26-36.

▶ Complications

Osteoporosis results in costs both to the individual and to society through associated fragility fractures. Fragility fractures are those that result from low trauma, such as a fall from standing height or less, and their presence is diagnostic of osteoporosis. Fragility fractures are distinct from pathologic fractures, which result from an underlying focal bone lesion such as a tumor, and stress fractures, which occur as the result of repetitive tensile or compressive stresses, such as running. The most common sites of fragility fractures are the hip, spine, and distal forearm. Of note, while low BMD is an important risk factor for fragility fractures, more than half of fragility fractures occur in individuals whose BMD falls in the osteopenic range (T-score between –1 and –2.5), because this condition is much more prevalent than having a T-score less than –2.5.

A. Hip Fracture

Hip fracture incidence increases with age and typically peaks after age 85. Above age 85, the annual incidence of hip fractures exceeds 2% per year, a rate that declined between 2000 and 2015 but has recently plateaued. About 70% of hip fractures occur in women. Hip fractures represent only 14% of all osteoporotic fractures but account for 72% of fracture-related medical expenses due to the severe morbidity associated with these fractures.

Hip fracture is associated with serious morbidity and mortality, often related to the consequences of hospitalization, immobilization, pain, and infection following fracture. Older adults have a five- to eight-fold increased risk for all-cause mortality during the first 3 months after a hip fracture. Mortality rates are doubled in men, with approximately 32% of men dying within a year of a hip fracture. This disparity in mortality may be attributed to a higher prevalence of comorbidities in men. Men also have poorer functional recovery in physical activities 1 year after the hip fracture. Of those who were not institutionalized before fracture, 25% remain in an institution more than a year after fracture.

Hip fractures are classified by the area of femur affected and by whether displacement is present. The types of hip fracture are intracapsular fractures, intertrochanteric fractures, and subtrochanteric fractures. The injured leg is often shortened, externally rotated, and abducted when the patient is lying flat. Plain radiographs are usually diagnostic, but if severe osteoporosis is present, magnetic resonance imaging (MRI) may be necessary to confirm the presence of a fracture.

Surgery remains the main therapeutic option and provides the best opportunity for functional recovery. Conservative therapy with avoidance of weight bearing is appropriate for patients too ill to undergo surgery. A displaced intracapsular fracture is likely to have vascular compromise to the head of the femur, resulting in nonunion and osteonecrosis, and thus often requires arthroplasty. Intertrochanteric and subtrochanteric fractures, as well as nondisplaced femoral neck fractures, can be treated with internal fixation with sliding screws or nails. If surgery is planned, completion of surgery within 48 hours of admission and early ambulation are associated with better outcomes.

B. Vertebral Fracture

Vertebral compression fractures are the most common form of osteoporotic fracture, but only one-fourth to one-third of fractures seen on imaging are diagnosed clinically. Both the prevalence and incidence of radiographic vertebral fractures increase with age. Among white women, the prevalence of vertebral fractures increases from 5% to 10% between the ages of 50 and 59 years and to >30% at 80 years of age or older.

Multiple vertebral fractures can lead to increased thoracic kyphosis with height loss and development of a humped back; protuberant abdomen as internal organs are contained in a smaller compartment; muscular neck pain because patients must extend the neck to look forward; reduction in the distance between the bottom of the rib cage and the top of the iliac crests, which may be associated with dyspnea and gastrointestinal complaints (eg, early satiety and constipation); and psychological stress.

Lateral thoracic and lumbar spine radiographs are the standard tool for diagnosing vertebral fractures. Differential diagnoses for vertebral deformities in adults include malignancy, degenerative disease, Paget disease, hemangioma, infection, and dysplastic changes.

Pain from vertebral fractures is generally managed with nonsteroidal anti-inflammatory drugs and other analgesics. Intranasal or intramuscular calcitonin has also been shown to modestly reduce pain associated with an acute vertebral fracture. Limited evidence supports the use of therapeutic exercise programs to reduce pain and improve strength, balance, functional status, and quality of life.

Vertebral augmentation procedures (vertebroplasty and kyphoplasty, procedures in which bone cement is injected into a fractured vertebra) are sometimes performed in an attempt to reduce pain and disability. Observational studies have demonstrated benefit to the procedures; however, two randomized, double-blind trials that used sham procedures as a control showed no difference in long-term pain, function, or quality of life between the treatment and control arms.

C. Other Fractures

Besides the hip and vertebrae, other common sites of fragility fractures include the distal forearm (19% of fragility fractures) and pelvis (7%), with the humerus and clavicle being other uncommon fracture sites. Wrist fractures most commonly present after a fall onto an outstretched hand, and management may involve conservative treatment or surgical treatment depending on the injury and individual's premorbid functional level.

Prior fragility fracture is a leading risk factor for future fragility fractures; in the case of hip fractures, the period of highest risk is immediately after the initial fracture has occurred. Thus, the acute management of fragility fractures should incorporate secondary fracture prevention with fall risk reduction strategies and osteoporosis management.

Brox WT, Roberts KC, Taksali S, et al. The American Academy of Orthopaedic Surgeons evidence-based guideline on management of hip fractures in the elderly. *J Bone Joint Surg Am.* 2015;97(14):1196-1199.

Burge R, Dawson-Hughes B, Solomon DH, et al. Incidence and economic burden of osteoporosis-related fractures in the United States, 2005-2025. *J Bone Miner Res.* 2007;22(3):465-475.

Ensrud KE, Schousboe JT. Clinical practice. Vertebral fractures. *N Engl J Med.* 2011;364(17):1634-1642.

Haentjens P, Magaziner J, Colon-Emeric CS, et al. Meta analysis: excess mortality after hip fracture among older women and men. *Ann Intern Med.* 2010;152(6):380.

Lewiecki EM, Wright NC, Curtis JR, et al. Hip fracture trends in the United States, 2002 to 2015. *Osteoporos Int.* 2018;29:717-722.

▶ Prevention

Effective therapies for prevention of osteoporosis and fractures are now available.

A. Peak Bone Mass

Attainment of peak bone mass is the primary strategy in preventing osteoporosis and fractures in adulthood. This includes modification of general lifestyle factors, such as a balanced diet containing calcium and vitamin D, regular exercise, smoking cessation, and avoidance of heavy alcohol use.

B. Exercise

A Cochrane analysis noted that aerobics, weight-bearing, and resistance exercises were all effective on the BMD of the spine. Walking was also found to be effective on both BMD of the spine and the hip and should be encouraged. Long-term studies to determine fracture data are required.

The positive implications of exercising in older persons extend far beyond improvements in BMD and include prevention of falls through improvements in muscle strength, balance, and posture control; increase in fitness and quality of life; and decrease in pain intensity and frequency at the spine.

C. Fall Prevention

Fall prevention is integral in fracture prevention (see Chapter 6, "Falls & Mobility Impairment").

D. Hip Protectors

Hip protectors consist of a hard or soft shell with a soft padding that covers the area over the greater trochanter of the hip. Their use should be encouraged for patients at increased risk, especially those in nursing home settings. Adherence remains an issue.

E. Calcium Supplementation

The Institute of Medicine (IOM) recommends a total daily elemental calcium intake of 1000 mg for all adults 19 to 50 years old, including pregnant and lactating women, 1000 mg for men 51 to 70 years old, and 1200 mg for women >50 years old and men >70 years old.

Cohort studies have found an association between calcium supplements and higher rates of cardiovascular events such as myocardial infarction, stroke, and cardiovascular deaths compared with when calcium is achieved through dietary sources alone. Dairy products, almond milk, and soymilk are common calcium-rich foods and beverages.

However, many adults do not tolerate dairy products. Calcium supplements are generally well tolerated, but constipation, intestinal bloating, and excess gas can occur. A slightly higher risk of kidney stones has been reported. Calcium supplements are available as salts with varying concentrations of elemental calcium. Calcium citrate does not require acid for absorption, can be taken with or without food, and is preferred in patients taking proton pump inhibitors or H_2-receptor antagonists or in those with achlorhydria. Calcium carbonate should be taken with food and in divided doses to enhance absorption.

F. Vitamin D Supplementation

Vitamin D is necessary for optimal absorption of calcium. Older adults often do not have adequate amounts from either cutaneous production or their diet. Vitamin D deficiency is associated with muscle weakness and can predispose a person to falls.

Vitamin D status can be evaluated by measuring serum 25-hydroxy vitamin D; a level of ≥30 ng/mL is considered acceptable; ≤10 ng/mL is considered severe deficiency or osteomalacia; and a range between 10 and 30 ng/mL is considered an insufficiency when accompanied by a notable rise in serum PTH. The IOM recommends a dietary allowance of vitamin D of 600 IU daily for people up to 70 years old and 800 IU daily for those ≥71 years old. Hypercalciuria and hypercalcemia can be seen with vitamin D toxicity.

The Women's Health Initiative (WHI) reported a reduction in fractures among the women who were adherent to calcium and vitamin D supplementation. The antifracture effect of vitamin D is more pronounced in institutionalized persons and involves its effect on muscle strength and fall prevention.

Screening for Osteoporosis

Screening for osteoporosis is appropriate for individuals with elevated fracture risk who do not have a prior history of fragility fracture. When a fragility fracture has been diagnosed and workup for secondary causes of the fracture has been completed, the clinical diagnosis of osteoporosis is made and focus can shift to osteoporosis treatment. The US Preventive Services Task Force (USPSTF) recommends screening for osteoporosis in women age 65 or older and in postmenopausal women under age 65 who are deemed to be at elevated risk via use of a clinical risk assessment tool such as the FRAX calculator (Grade B recommendations as of June 2018). The USPSTF concludes there is insufficient evidence to recommend for or against screening for osteoporosis in men (Grade I recommendation). The USPSTF also concludes that central DXA, peripheral DXA, or quantitative ultrasound may be considered as modalities for screening, but central DXA measurements have been most commonly studied. In the case that an initial screening test does not show osteoporosis, the USPSTF does not give any recommendations regarding rescreening interval. Some observational and modeling studies have suggested screening intervals based on baseline BMD or age, but others have shown no benefit in predicting fractures from repeat BMD testing.

Other national guideline groups have given different recommendations regarding optimal screening for osteoporosis. The American Association of Clinical Endocrinologists recommends screening the same groups recommended by the USPSTF and does not recommend screening premenopausal women or healthy young men unless there are "specific risk factors for bone loss." The National Osteoporosis Foundation recommends considering screening in women ≥65 years old, men ≥70 years old, women and men over age 50 who have clinical risk factors for fracture including any fracture over age 50, and any adults with a condition or medication associated with bone loss.

Anderson JJ, Kruszka B, Delaney JA, et al. Calcium intake from diet and supplements and the risk of coronary artery calcification and its progression among older adults: 10-year follow-up of the Multi-Ethnic Study of Atherosclerosis (MESA). *J Am Heart Assoc.* 2016;5(10):e003815.

Gourlay ML, Fine JP, Pressier JS, et al. Study of Osteoporotic Fractures Research Group. Bone-density testing interval and transition to osteoporosis in older women. *N Engl J Med.* 2012;366(3):225-233.

US Preventive Services Task Force. Screening for osteoporosis to prevent fractures: US Preventive Services Task Force recommendation statement. *JAMA* 2018;319(24):2521-2531.

Treatment

Guidelines by the National Osteoporosis Foundation recommend osteoporosis treatment in postmenopausal women or men age 50 years and older with a T-score of less than −2.5 at the femoral neck, hip, or spine; patients with low bone mass (T-score between −1.0 and −2.5) and a 10-year probability of hip fracture of ≥3% or a 10-year probability of major osteoporosis-related fracture of ≥20%, as determined by FRAX; and patients with a fragility fracture.

Current osteoporosis therapies are divided into antiresorptive and anabolic agents (Table 35-5). Antiresorptive

Table 35–5. FDA-approved agents for osteoporosis.

Agent	Efficacy	Side Effects	Dosing	Delivery
Bisphosphonates Alendronate Risedronate Ibandronate Zoledronic acid	Reduced vertebral, hip, and nonvertebral fractures (no data on ibandronate for hip fracture)	Gastrointestinal side effects Arthralgia/myalgia Renal toxicity Atypical fractures Osteonecrosis of the jaw	5–10 mg oral daily, 70 mg oral weekly 5 mg oral daily, 35 mg oral weekly, 150 mg oral monthly 2.5 mg oral daily, 150 mg oral monthly, 3 mg IV every 3 months 5 mg IV every 12 months	
Hormone replacement therapy	Reduced vertebral, hip, and nonvertebral fractures	Increased thromboembolic events, cholelithiasis, irregular uterine bleeding	Multiple oral and transdermal formulations	
Raloxifene (selective estrogen receptor modulator)	Reduced vertebral fractures	Increased thromboembolic events, hot flashes, leg cramps	60 mg oral daily	
Calcitonin	Reduced vertebral fractures	Nausea (injectable form) Rhinitis, epistaxis (nasal form)	200 IU 100 IU	Nasal spray daily (alternate each side of nostril) Subcutaneous or intramuscular every other day
Denosumab	Reduced vertebral, hip and nonvertebral fractures	Eczema, dermatitis, rash, cellulitis, atypical fractures Osteonecrosis of jaw	60 mg	Subcutaneously every 6 months
Teriparatide Abaloparatide	Reduced vertebral, hip and nonvertebral fractures	Nausea, headache, dizziness, and leg cramps; FDA warning regarding osteosarcoma	20 μg 80 μg	Daily subcutaneous injections for 24 months
Romosozumab	Reduced vertebral, hip and nonvertebral fractures	Injection site reactions, FDA warning label regarding cardiovascular events	210 mg	Two subcutaneous injections monthly for 12 months

FDA, US Food and Drug Administration; IV, intravenous.

therapies available in the United States are bisphosphonates, hormone replacement therapy (HRT), selective estrogen receptor modulators (SERMs), denosumab, and calcitonin. PTH is the only anabolic agent available in the United States.

A. Bisphosphonates

Bisphosphonates are potent antiresorptive agents that bind hydroxyapatite crystals on bone surfaces and permanently inhibit osteoclast function. US Food and Drug Administration (FDA)–approved agents are alendronate, risedronate, ibandronate, and zoledronic acid.

Bisphosphonates may be given orally on a daily (alendronate, risedronate), weekly (alendronate, risedronate), or monthly (risedronate, ibandronate) schedule or intravenously every 3 months (ibandronate) or intravenously once yearly (zoledronic acid). Oral bisphosphonates must be taken on an empty stomach because of their poor absorption and bioavailability. Patients must sit upright and fast for 30 minutes (with alendronate and risedronate) to 60 minutes (with ibandronate) after ingestion. Prior to the initiation of any bisphosphonate therapy, calcium and vitamin D must be adequately repleted because of the possibility of inducing hypocalcemia, especially in older adults.

Oral bisphosphonates are commonly associated with gastrointestinal side effects, including dyspepsia, heartburn, indigestion, and pain while swallowing. More serious gastrointestinal effects include erosive esophagitis and esophageal ulcerations; thus, patients are reminded to take a full glass of water (6–8 oz) and remain upright after the dose. Acute phase reactions (fever, myalgia, arthralgia, headache, and flulike symptoms) have been reported with both oral and intravenous bisphosphonates. Intravenous zoledronic acid has been associated with acute renal failure and should be used with caution in patients with renal impairment. Alendronate should also be used with caution in patients with severe renal insufficiency (creatinine clearance <35 mL/min). Long-term effects, including osteonecrosis of the jaw and atypical fracture, are rare, and benefits from fracture reduction outweigh the harms.

All bisphosphonates have been shown to significantly improve BMD of the spine and reduce risk of vertebral and hip fractures. There are no published data for hip fracture reductions with ibandronate in randomized clinical trials. There are no studies of comparative efficacy of the bisphosphonates with each other.

The duration of bisphosphonate therapy is not yet clear. Seven-year follow-up of patients using alendronate showed that spinal BMD continued to increase through 7 years of treatment and remained stable. After the withdrawal of treatment, there was a small increase in biochemical markers of bone turnover. It appears that skeletal benefits may be preserved for at least 1 to 2 years after cessation, but long-term follow-up studies are needed.

B. Hormone Replacement Therapy

HRT is approved for the prevention of osteoporosis in postmenopausal women, although the primary indication is for the treatment of moderate-to-severe menopausal symptoms. The exact mechanism of HRT on bone remodeling has not been elucidated; however, it is clear that the loss of estrogen during menopause results in an acceleration of bone resorption in most women.

Combined estrogen and progesterone therapy has produced a 1.4% to 3.9% increase in BMD at skeletal sites. Studies have shown that estrogen reduces the risk for vertebral and hip fracture, as well as the risk of nonvertebral fracture. In the WHI trial, treatment of postmenopausal women with combined therapy reduced the risk of hip fracture by 33%.

The timing of initiation and duration of HRT remains unclear. It is suggested that women start estrogen within 2 to 7 years of menopause. Several studies have shown that HRT begun before 60 years of age prevents nonvertebral, hip, and wrist fractures, but there is insufficient evidence that fracture risk is reduced when HRT is begun after age 60 years. Estrogen begun and continued after age 60 years appears to maintain BMD. The duration of therapy necessary to protect women against fragility fractures is indefinite. HRT can be administered as an oral or transdermal formulation. It may be given on a continuous basis, with no interruption in therapy, or as a cyclical regimen.

Compliance with HRT is typically poor because of common side effects and concern about increased incidence of breast or endometrial cancer. Women who have not undergone hysterectomy should have progestin added to the estrogen regimen to prevent endometrial hyperplasia. Low-dose HRT can reduce the amount of uterine bleeding, fluid retention, mastalgia, and headaches, making estrogen therapy much easier to tolerate.

Safety results from the WHI study showed an increased risk of coronary heart disease, pulmonary embolism, and stroke associated with the use of combined hormonal therapy in women with an intact uterus. As a result, HRT is considered second-line therapy for only prevention of osteoporosis in young perimenopausal women with menopausal symptoms.

C. Selective Estrogen Receptor Modulators

SERMs are compounds that bind to and activate estrogen receptors but have agonist/antagonist properties at different tissue sites. Raloxifene is approved for the prevention and treatment of postmenopausal osteoporosis and indicated for the reduction of invasive breast cancer.

Raloxifene at 60 mg/day has been shown to increase BMD by 2% and reduce the risk of new vertebral fracture by 40% after 2 years. However, raloxifene has not demonstrated a protective effect on nonvertebral or hip fracture risk.

D. Calcitonin

Calcitonin, an endogenous hormone secreted by the parafollicular C cells of the thyroid gland, helps to maintain calcium homeostasis. Calcitonin acts directly on osteoclasts, with inhibitory effects on bone resorption. Calcitonin is approved for the treatment of postmenopausal osteoporosis. Calcitonin nasal spray has been shown to have modest effects on spine BMD (1.5% increase) and significantly reduce the risk of new vertebral fractures by 33% in women with prevalent vertebral fractures. There was no significant effect on hip or nonvertebral fracture risk. Calcitonin is an option for women who cannot tolerate bisphosphonates or SERMs. In some patients, calcitonin has an analgesic effect, making it suitable for patients with acute vertebral fracture. Calcitonin nasal spray is generally administered once per day, alternating nostrils daily. Injectable calcitonin can be administered subcutaneously or intramuscularly.

E. Denosumab

Denosumab is a human monoclonal antibody with a high affinity and specificity for RANKL. When denosumab binds to RANKL, it prevents RANKL-RANK interaction, resulting in a decrease in osteoclastic bone resorption.

Denosumab is approved for osteoporosis treatment. Results from phase III study in women with osteoporosis showed that treatment with denosumab increased lumbar spine BMD by 6.5% and significantly reduced the risk of vertebral (68%) and hip (40%) fractures compared with placebo. Prior to starting denosumab, patients with preexisting hypocalcemia must have this condition corrected because it could worsen with treatment. Denosumab may be given to patients with renal impairment without dose adjustment.

F. PTH & PTH-Related Protein Derivatives

FDA-approved anabolic agents include teriparatide, a synthetic PTH derivative, and abaloparatide, a PTH-related protein derivative. Both stimulate bone remodeling, preferentially increasing formation over resorption, and reduce the risk of new vertebral fractures (65% reduction) and nonvertebral fractures (35%) with significant improvements in BMD of 10% to 14%.

Teriparatide and abaloparatide are administered as daily subcutaneous injections. Eleven percent of patients developed mild hypercalcemia. Osteosarcomas have been induced in rats given teriparatide or abaloparatide. However, an independent oncology advisory board concluded that the rat carcinogenicity data are very unlikely to have clinical relevance in humans being treated with these anabolic agents for a relatively short duration (FDA approval is limited to only 2 years of use).

Upon termination of anabolic treatment, sequential therapy with an oral or intravenous bisphosphonate may strengthen the beneficial effects of teriparatide. Concurrent therapy with teriparatide and oral bisphosphonates has been avoided because oral bisphosphonates have been shown to reduce the positive effects of teriparatide on bone turnover.

G. Antisclerostin Antibody

Romosozumab is a monoclonal antibody that binds to and inhibits sclerostin with a dual effect of increasing bone formation and decreasing bone resorption. In a 2-year clinical trial of postmenopausal women at high risk of fractures, women treated for 12 months with romosozumab followed by alendronate experienced 48% fewer new vertebral fractures than those treated with alendronate alone (6.2% vs 11.9%). However, serious cardiovascular adverse events were observed more often with romosozumab than with alendronate.

In summary, given a choice of pharmacotherapy, clinical risk factors for fracture and comorbidities should be taken into account when tailoring therapy for osteoporosis. Risk factors such as age and previous fracture are critical to choosing an optimal treatment strategy. Clinicians need to be aware of the safety concerns associated with each drug, and treatment should be made on an individual basis taking into account the relative benefits and risks in different patient population.

Bonaiuti D, Shea B, Iovine R, et al. Exercise for preventing and treating osteoporosis in postmenopausal women. *Cochrane Database Syst Rev.* 2002;3:CD000333.

Cauley JA, Robbins J, Chen Z, et al. Effects of estrogen plus progestin on risk of fracture and bone mineral density. *JAMA.* 2003;290(13):1729-1738.

Gillespie LD, Robertson MC, Gillespie WJ, et al. Interventions for preventing falls in older people living in the community. *Cochrane Database Syst Rev.* 2009;2:CD007146.

Gillespie WJ, Gillespie LD, Parker MJ. Hip protectors for preventing hip fractures in older people. *Cochrane Database Syst Rev.* 2010;10:CD001255.

Harvey N, Dennison E, Cooper C. Osteoporosis: impact on health and economics. *Nat Rev Rheumatol.* 2010;6(2):99-105.

Kanis JA, Johansson H, Oden A, Dawson-Hughes B, Melton LJ 3rd, McCloskey EV. The effects of a FRAX revision for the USA. *Osteoporosis Int.* 2010;21(1):35-40.

Kanis JA, Oden A, Johansson H, Borgström F, Ström O, McCloskey E. FRAX and its applications to clinical practice. *Bone.* 2009;44(5):734-743.

Link TM. Osteoporosis imaging: state of the art and advanced imaging. *Radiology.* 2012;263(1):3-17.

Liu H, Paige NM, Goldzweig CL, et al. Screening for osteoporosis in men: a systematic review for an American College of Physicians guideline. *Ann Intern Med.* 2008;148(9):685-701.

NIH Consensus Development Panel on Osteoporosis Prevention, Diagnosis, and Therapy. Osteoporosis prevention, diagnosis, and therapy. *JAMA.* 2001;285(6):785-795.

Saag KG, Petersen J, Brandi ML, et al. Romosozumab or alendronate for fracture prevention in women with osteoporosis. *N Engl J Med.* 2017;377:1417-27.

Sambrook P, Cooper C. Osteoporosis. *Lancet.* 2006;367(9527): 2010-2018.

Silverman S, Christiansen C. Individualizing osteoporosis therapy. *Osteoporosis Int.* 2012;23(3):797-809.

Siris ES, Baim S, Nattiv A. Primary care use of FRAX: absolute fracture risk assessment in postmenopausal women and older men. *Postgrad Med.* 2010;122(1):82-90.

Vasikaran S, Eastell R, Bruyère O, et al. Markers of bone turnover for the prediction of fracture risk and monitoring of osteoporosis treatment: a need for international reference standards. *Osteoporos Int.* 2011;22(2):391-420.

Wang L, Manson JE, Sesso HD. Calcium intake and risk of cardiovascular disease: a review of prospective studies and randomized clinical trials. *Am J Cardiovasc Drugs.* 2012;12(2):105-116.

Warriner AH, Patkar NM, Yun H, Delzell E. Minor, major, low-trauma, and high-trauma fractures: what are the subsequent fracture risks and how do they vary? *Curr Osteoporos Rep.* 2011;9(3):122-128.

Winsloe C, Earl S, Dennison EM, Cooper C, Harvey NC. Early life factors in pathogenesis of osteoporosis. *Curr Osteoporos Rep.* 2009;7:140-144.

Delirium

Tammy Ting Hshieh, MD, MPH
Sharon K. Inouye, MD, MPH

ESSENTIALS OF DIAGNOSIS

▶ Clinical diagnosis based on detailed history, cognitive assessment, and physical and neurologic examination.

▶ The pathognomonic feature is an acute change in baseline mental status developing over hours to days.

▶ Other key features include fluctuating course with an increase or decrease in symptoms over a 24-hour period; inattention, with difficulty focusing attention; and either disorganized thinking, such as rambling or incoherent speech, or altered level of consciousness (vigilant or lethargic).

▶ Perceptual disturbances, such as hallucinations, or paranoid delusions present in approximately 15% to 40% of cases.

▶ Search for organic or physiologic causes (eg, illness, drug related, or metabolic derangement).

▶ Delirium is often misdiagnosed as dementia, depression, or psychosis.

▶ Accepted delirium criteria provided by Confusion Assessment Method.

General Principles

Delirium is an acute disorder of attention and cognitive function that may arise at any point in the course of an illness. It is often the only sign of a serious underlying medical condition, especially in older persons who are frail or who have underlying dementia. Delirium can result in serious clinical outcomes, such as functional decline, cognitive impairment, dementia, and decreased quality of life; delirium also results in significant caregiver burden and health care expenditures.

The prevalence of delirium on admission can range from 10% to 40%. During hospitalization, it may affect an additional 25% to 50%. Delirium is the most common postoperative complication among older adults, with rates estimated at 15% to 52%. Even higher rates (70%–87%) are seen in intensive care units (ICUs). In addition, 80% of terminally ill patients become delirious before death.

Three forms of delirium have been recognized: the hyperactive, hyperalert form; the hypoactive, hypoalert, lethargic form; and the mixed form, which combines elements of both. The hypoactive form is often unrecognized but more common among older hospitalized patients; it is associated with a poorer overall prognosis. Delirium can range from mild to severe, with increased severity associated with worse outcomes.

Delirium as a geriatric syndrome is inherently multifactorial and develops as a result of interactions between predisposing risk factors and noxious insults or precipitants. Thus, it is imperative that clinicians identify and address all potential factors and observe patients closely for resolution.

Prevention

The major predisposing risk factor for delirium is preexisting cognitive impairment, specifically dementia, which increases the risk of delirium two- to five-fold. Virtually all chronic medical illnesses can predispose older persons to delirium, as can specific neurologic and metabolic disorders. A full list of risk factors is included in Table 36–1.

The foremost precipitating factor is medications, which contribute to >40% of cases of delirium. The medications most frequently associated with delirium are those with known psychoactive effects, such as sedative hypnotics, opiates, H_2 blockers, and anticholinergic drugs. A number of these medications are readily available over the counter, such as the antihistamine diphenhydramine. The American Geriatrics Society recently published their updated list, known as the *2019 Update to the AGS Beers Criteria for Potentially Inappropriate Medication Use in Older Adults*, which highlights some of these delirium-provoking medications. In

Table 36–1. Risk factors and precipitating factors for delirium.

Risk Factors	Precipitating Factors
Cognitive Status	**Drugs**
• Dementia/cognitive impairment	• All tricyclic antidepressants
• Depression	• Anticholinergic drugs
• History of delirium	• Benzodiazepines
Coexisting Medical Conditions	• Corticosteroids
• Severe/terminal illness	• H_2-receptor antagonists
• Multiple comorbidities	• Narcotics
• Neurologic disease (including	• Polypharmacy
history of stroke, intracranial	• Alcohol
bleeding, meningitis,	**Intercurrent Illnesses**
encephalitis, Parkinson disease)	• Infection
• Metabolic derangements	• Hypoxia
(including hyper-/	• Shock
hyponatremia, hyper-/	• Fever/hypothermia
hypoglycemia, hypercalcemia,	• Withdrawal
thyroid or adrenal dysfunctions,	• Low serum albumin
and acid-base disorders)	• Metabolic derangements
• Fracture or trauma	(including hyper-/
• Anemia	hyponatremia, hyper-/
• Low serum albumin	hypoglycemia, hypercalcemia,
• Infection with HIV	thyroid or adrenal
Functional Status	dysfunctions, and acid-base
• Functional dependence	disorders)
• Immobility	**Environmental**
• Low level of activity	• Admission to intensive care unit
• History of falls, gait instability	• Physical restraints
Sensory Impairment	• Bladder catheterization
• Visual	• Pain
• Hearing	• Emotional stress
Decreased Oral Intake	• Multiple procedures
• Dehydration	• Prolonged sleep deprivation
• Malnutrition	**Surgery**
Demographic	• Orthopedic
• Age 65 years or older	• Cardiac
• Male sex	• Prolonged cardiopulmonary
• Lower educational attainment	bypass

addition, delirium risk increases in direct proportion to the number of medications prescribed. Herbal therapies are being increasingly recognized as causing or contributing to delirium, especially when taken concurrently with a psychoactive medication. This is particularly true for psychoactive herbs, such as St. John's wort, kava kava, and valerian root. Table 36–1 lists other precipitating factors, including intercurrent illness, environmental, and surgery.

2019 American Geriatrics Society Beers Criteria® Update Expert Panel. American Geriatrics Society 2019 Updated AGS Beers criteria for potentially inappropriate medication use in older adults. *J Am Geriatr Soc.* 2019;67(4):674-694.

Inouye SK. Delirium in older persons. *N Engl J Med.* 2006;354(11):1157-1165.

Inouye SK, Westendorp RG, Saczynski JS. Delirium in elderly people. *Lancet.* 2014;383:911-922.

Marcantonio ER. Delirium in hospitalized older adults. *N Engl J Med.* 2017;377:1456-1466.

Oh ES, Fong TG, Hshieh TT, Inouye SK. Delirium in older persons. *J Am Med Assoc.* 2017;318:1161-1174.

Prevention of delirium using nonpharmacologic multicomponent interventions has been demonstrated to be the most effective strategy. A meta-analysis in 2015 demonstrated that nonpharmacologic multicomponent interventions significantly reduce delirium incidence (odds ratio, 0.46; 95% confidence interval [CI], 0.38–0.58), and in addition, significantly reduce in-hospital falls (odds ratio, 0.38; 95% CI, 0.25–0.60). Table 36–2 shows targeted preventive interventions, most of which can also be nonpharmacologic treatments for delirium. Prevention of delirium by targeting vulnerable patients with predisposing risk factors or precipitating factors has been shown to be effective. In addition, proactive geriatrics consultation (daily geriatrician visits and targeted recommendations based on a structured protocol) is effective in vulnerable patients with preexisting dementia or functional impairments. Geriatric-orthopedic co-management services have also been implemented in hospitals nationwide and have reduced delirium incidence when structured protocols and multidisciplinary consultations are used.

Pharmacologic prevention of delirium has been studied in a number of clinical trials with conflicting results. Spinal anesthesia during surgery has been correlated with decreased postoperative delirium in some studies. However, lighter sedation depth and electroencephalography-guided anesthesia have not been consistently associated with reduction of delirium. These results suggest the need for future study of the role of anesthesia in preventing delirium. A recent Cochrane review examined melatonin and melatonin agonists as a means of preserving sleep-wake cycle but did not find a reduced incidence of delirium. In general, the use of antipsychotics prophylactically in delirium prevention is not recommended since no study has successfully prevented delirium or demonstrated decreased morbidity. A meta-analysis of antipsychotic agents examined seven randomized trials that were highly heterogeneous and did not demonstrate a significant decrease in incidence of delirium among the intervention group; there was also no effect on length of ICU or hospital stay or mortality.

CONCLUSION

Current evidence does not support the use of antipsychotics for prevention or treatment of delirium.

Hshieh TT, Yang T, Gartaganis SL, et al. Hospital Elder Life Program: systematic review and meta-analysis of effectiveness. *Am J Geriatr Psychiatry.* 2018;26(10):1015-1033.

Table 36–2. Nonpharmacologic and pharmacologic treatments for delirium.

Nonpharmacologic (by risk/ precipitating factor)	Targeted Intervention
Sleep deprivation	Sleep protocol (back massage, relaxation techniques, soothing music, decreased light/noise, warm milk or caffeine-free herbal tea, private room, minimizing of vital sign checks/procedures/medication administration overnight) Avoid using sedatives, especially diphenhydramine Maintain sleep-wake cycle
Dehydration	Recognition of volume depletion and replenishment of fluids
Hearing loss	Proper hearing aids or amplifiers available and in use
Vision loss	Provision of proper visual aids (patient's own glasses, magnifying lenses, or adaptive equipment)
Immobility	Ambulate as soon as possible (assistance or supervision when needed) Out of bed to chair with meals Active range-of-motion exercises if confined to bed Involve in self-care (toileting, hair brushing, dressing) Minimize lines and drains (telemetry, intravenous access, bladder catheters)
Cognitive impairment	Frequent orientation to person, place, time Large updated board, calendars, clocks Family presence, private room, close to nursing station Involve patients in decisions and daily toileting Eye contact during interactions
Medications (sedating or psychoactive)	Use alternative and less harmful medications Avoid those with long half-lives Adjust for impaired kidney and liver function Use lowest dose possible Taper and discontinue unnecessary medications American Geriatrics Society 2019 Beers Criteria medications • Examples include anticholinergics, benzodiazepines, sedative hypnotics, antispasmodics, H_2-receptor antagonists, meperidine/chlorpromazine/thioridazine, etc

Pharmacologic	Targeted Intervention
Neuroleptics – Typical	
Haloperidol (Haldol)	• *Pros:* Proven/tested, intravenous/intramuscular/oral formulations, oral formulation theoretically has less QTc-prolonging effects, pharmacokinetically optimal • *Cons:* Sedation, hypotension, acute dystonia, extrapyramidal symptoms, anticholinergic side effects (dry mouth, constipation, urinary retention, confusion), worsens Parkinson disease rigidity • *Loading dose:* 0.25–0.5 mg every 20–30 minutes until patient manageable. Maximum daily dose of 3–5 mg. Peak effect in 4–6 hours (oral), 20 minutes (intramuscular/intravenous) • *Maintenance dose:* Divide loading dose by 2, give every 12 hours; taper over 2–3 days • *Caveats:* D_2 dopaminergic receptors are saturated at low doses. Thus, >5 mg/24 hours has no clinical benefit, only increases harm
Neuroleptics – Atypical	
Olanzapine (Zyprexa, Zydis)	• *Pros:* Less extrapyramidal symptoms, dissolvable tablet • *Cons:* Increased anticholinergic side effects can worsen confusion, potential QTc prolongation • *Starting dose:* 2.5–5 mg. Repeat in 20 minutes if needed
Quetiapine (Seroquel)	• *Pros:* Sedating effect helps maintain sleep-wake cycle • *Cons:* Oral formulation only, QTc prolongation • *Starting dose:* 6.25–12.5 mg
Risperidone (Risperdal)/ ziprasidone (Geodon)	• *Pros:* Sedating effect helps maintain sleep-wake cycle, oral and intramuscular formulations • *Cons:* Can be very sedating, QTc prolongation, tardive dyskinesia
Benzodiazepines	• *Pros:* Used for alcohol/sedative withdrawal; lorazepam (Ativan) is benzodiazepine of choice because of shorter half-life, no active metabolite, intravenous version • *Cons:* Generally not recommended because oversedating, worsens confusion • *Starting dose:* 0.25–0.5 mg

Hshieh TT, Yue J, Oh E, et al. Effectiveness of multicomponent nonpharmacological delirium interventions: a meta-analysis. *JAMA Intern Med.* 2015;175:512-520.

Siddiqi N, Harrison JK, Clegg A, et al. Interventions for preventing delirium in hospitalized non-ICU patients. *Cochrane Database Syst Rev.* 2016;3:CD005563.

Wildes TS, Mickle AM, Ben Abdallah A, et al. Effect of electroencephalography-guided anesthetic administration on postoperative delirium among older adults undergoing major surgery: the ENGAGES randomized clinical trial. *J Am Med Assoc.* 2019;321(5):473-483.

▶ Clinical Findings

A. Symptoms & Signs

Initial evaluation of delirium is largely based on establishing a patient's baseline cognitive functioning and the clinical course of any cognitive change. Thus, a detailed history from a reliable informant, such as a spouse, child, or caregiver, is most important. The history should seek to clarify the acuity of any mental status changes and seek clues to the underlying cause.

The cardinal historical features of delirium are acute onset and fluctuating course, in which symptoms tend to come and go or increase and decrease in severity over a 24-hour period. This is the major feature distinguishing delirium from dementia, which usually develops gradually and progressively over months to years.

1. Cognitive changes—Usually determined through cognitive testing and, most importantly, close clinical observation of the quality of the patient's response. For example, a person may score correctly on a particular cognitive task but during the task may demonstrate fluctuating attention, easy distractibility, rambling speech, or lethargy.

2. Inattention—Decreased ability to focus, maintain, and shift one's attention. For example, patients will demonstrate difficulty maintaining or following a conversation, perseverate on a previous answer, require repetition of instructions, or struggle to follow instructions on cognitive tasks (simple repetition, digit span, backward recitation of months/days).

3. Disorganized thinking—Manifested as rambling and, at its extreme, incoherent speech. Problems with memory, disorientation, or language are frequent.

4. Altered level of consciousness—Ranges from agitated, vigilant states to lethargic or stuporous states.

5. Other features—Not essential for diagnosis but commonly seen are psychomotor agitation or retardation, perceptual disturbances (eg, hallucinations, illusions), paranoid delusions, emotional lability, and sleep-wake cycle disturbances.

B. Laboratory Findings & Imaging

The algorithm in Figure 36–1 provides a systematic approach to the diagnosis and evaluation of delirium in the older person. No specific laboratory tests exist that positively identify delirium. Specific biomarkers have been gaining recognition in delirium research; understanding these potential biomarkers may reveal the underlying pathophysiologic mechanisms behind the geriatric syndrome. Current research has focused on S-100β, insulin-like growth factor-1, and neuron-specific enolase. Inflammation may play an important role in delirium, and recent studies have examined inflammatory markers, such as C-reactive protein, interleukin-6, interleukin-8, tumor necrosis factor-α, monocyte chemoattractant protein-1, procalcitonin, and cortisol.

Laboratory tests in the evaluation of delirious patients should include complete blood count, electrolytes (including calcium), kidney and liver function, glucose, and oxygen saturation. Furthermore, in searching for occult infection, blood cultures, urinalysis/urine culture, chest x-ray, and viral assays may be considered. Other laboratory tests may be pursued if specific contributing factors have not been identified in a particular patient. These include thyroid function tests, arterial blood gas, vitamin B_{12} levels, drug levels, toxicology screens, cortisol levels, and evaluation of the cerebrospinal fluid.

Brain imaging with computed tomography or magnetic resonance imaging is indicated by a history or signs of recent fall or head trauma, fever of unknown origin, new focal neurologic symptoms, anticoagulated state, or no obvious cause identified. An electroencephalogram may be indicated to evaluate for occult seizure activity. It can also be used in differentiating delirium from nonorganic psychiatric disorders.

Adamis D, Sharmab N, Whelanc PJP, Macdonald AJD. Delirium scales: a review of current evidence. *Aging Ment Health.* 2010;14:543-555.

American Psychiatric Association. *Diagnostic and Statistical Manual of Mental Disorders.* 5th ed. Washington, DC: American Psychiatric Association; 2013.

Dillon ST, Vasunilashorn SM, Dillon ST, Inouye SK, et al. High C-reactive protein predicts delirium incidence, duration and feature severity after major noncardiac surgery. *J Am Geriatr Soc.* 2017:65(8):e109-e116.

Inouye SK, van Dyck CH, Alessi CA, Balkin S, Siegal AP, Horwitz RI. Clarifying confusion: the confusion assessment method. A new method for the detection of delirium. *Ann Intern Med.* 1990;113(12):941-948.

Khan BA, Zawahiri M, Campbell NL, Boustani MA. Biomarkers for delirium—a review. *J Am Geriatr Soc.* 2011;59(suppl 2): S256-S261.

C. Physical Examination

Detailed physical examination is essential for evaluation of delirium. Delirium may often be the initial manifestation of serious underlying disease in an older person; thus, astute

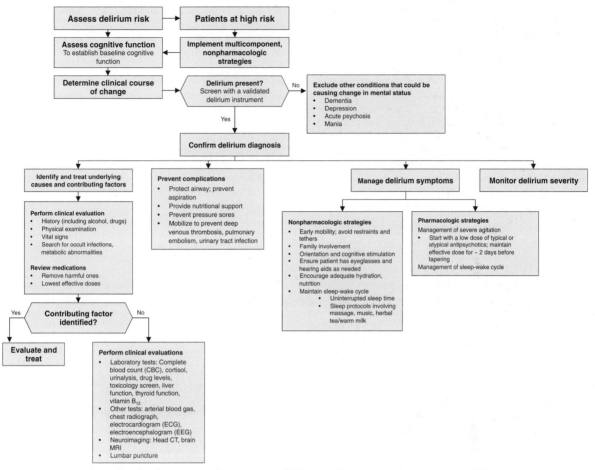

▲ **Figure 36–1.** Algorithm for diagnosis and evaluation of delirium. CT, computed tomography; MRI, magnetic resonance imaging.

attention to early localizing signs on physical examination may allow early diagnosis of a precipitating insult. A careful search for evidence of occult infections should be performed, including signs of pneumonia, urinary tract infection, acute abdominal processes, joint infections, or new cardiac murmur. A detailed neurologic examination with attention to focal or lateralizing signs is also crucial.

D. Special Tests

1. *Diagnostic and Statistical Manual of Mental Disorders*, fifth edition (DSM-5)—The American Psychiatric Association DSM-5 guidelines were developed based on expert opinion and remain the current standard for definition and diagnostic criteria for delirium.

2. Confusion Assessment Method—The Confusion Assessment Method (CAM) is a simple, validated tool currently in widespread use (Table 36–3). It has a sensitivity of

Table 36–3. Confusion Assessment Method algorithm.

(1) Acute onset and fluctuating course
and
(2) Inattention
and either
(3) Disorganized thinking
or
(4) Altered level of consciousness

Score based on cognitive testing.

See details at: www.hospitalelderlifeprogram.org.

Data from The CAM-S Score for Delirium Severity Training Manual and Coding Guide. Copyright © 1988, 2003 Hospital Elder Life Program.

94% to 100%, specificity of 90% to 100%, and negative predictive value of 90% to 100% for delirium. It has also been validated in patients with dementia. In the intensive care setting, it is feasible to perform cognitive evaluation and screen for delirium using the CAM-ICU, an adaptation of the CAM for use in mechanically ventilated, restrained, or nonverbal patients. CAM-ICU has not, however, been found to perform as well, with a sensitivity of 64% to 73% and negative predictive value of 83%; among verbal patients, the sensitivity drops to <50%. An important recent advance is the 3-Minute Diagnostic Interview for Delirium Using the Confusion Assessment Method (3D-CAM), which is a brief, user-friendly tool for detection of delirium. The Brief Confusion Assessment Method (bCAM) has been developed for emergency department patients.

3. Other instruments—Instruments developed and validated for use in identification of delirium include the Nursing Delirium Screening Scale (Nu-DESC), Delirium Symptom Interview, NEECHAM Confusion Scale, Delirium Observation Screening Scale, and Intensive Care Delirium Screening Checklist. The 4AT test was developed and validated for use in geriatric and rehabilitation settings and purportedly does not require specific training to administer. The 4AT assesses alertness, cognition (orientation and attention), and acute change in mental status; it provides a score range suggesting whether cognitive impairment may be present so that follow-up cognitive testing can be performed.

4. Delirium severity—The ability to quantitate delirium severity is critical to follow response to treatment clinically or in clinical trials, estimate prognosis, and study pathophysiologic mechanisms. Instruments developed and validated for measuring severity of delirium include the recently developed CAM-Severity (CAM-S) score, which has strong psychometric properties and direct associations with important clinical outcomes. Other delirium severity measures include the Delirium Rating Scale-98, Memorial Delirium Assessment Scale, Confusional State Examination, Delirium-O-Meter, and the Delirium Observation Scale.

Differential Diagnosis

The main diagnostic dilemma facing the clinician is differentiating delirium from dementia. This is especially difficult when knowledge of baseline cognitive function is missing or when there are known cognitive deficits and one must determine whether the current condition is caused by underlying chronic cognitive impairment or a result of delirium. Thus, it is crucial to obtain a reliable history about baseline status from an informant. Inattention and altered level of consciousness are usually not features of mild to moderate dementia, and their presence supports the diagnosis of delirium. In patients with known dementia, a history that includes

worsening confusion over and above the baseline cognitive impairment also suggests delirium.

Other important diagnoses that must be differentiated from delirium are depression, mania, and other nonorganic psychotic disorders, such as schizophrenia. These diseases do not typically arise in the context of a medical illness. Again, the history and clinical course can assist in providing important clues in differentiating these syndromes. Altered level of consciousness is not prominent in these other conditions. At times, the differential diagnosis can be quite difficult due to the presence of subtle symptoms or an uncooperative patient. Because of the potential life-threatening nature of delirium, one should err on the side of treating the patient as delirious until further information is available.

American Geriatrics Society Expert Panel on Postoperative Delirium in Older Adults. American Geriatrics Society abstracted clinical practice guideline for postoperative delirium in older adults. *J Am Geriatr Soc.* 2015;63(1):142-150.

Inouye SK, Kosar CM, Tommet D, et al. The CAM-S: development and validation of a new scoring system for delirium severity in 2 cohorts. *Ann Intern Med.* 2014;160(8):526-533.

Jones RN, Cizginer S, Pavlech L, et al. Assessment of Instruments for measurement of delirium severity: a systematic review. *JAMA Intern Med.* 2019;179(2):231-239.

Marcantonio ER, Ngo LH, O'Connor M, et al. 3D-CAM: derivation and validation of a 3-minute diagnostic interview for CAM-defined delirium: a cross-sectional diagnostic test study. *Ann Intern Med.* 2014;161:554-561.

Young J, Murthy L, Westby M, Akunne A, O'Mahony R. Diagnosis, prevention, and management of delirium: summary of NICE guidance. *BMJ.* 2010;341:c3705.

▶ Complications

Delirium is associated with adverse hospital outcomes, including increased morbidity, mortality, functional decline, and immobility and its attendant complications (aspiration pneumonia, pressure ulcers, deep venous thrombosis, pulmonary emboli, urinary tract infections). Moreover, delirium is associated with complications related to its underlying causes. All of these factors contribute to the poor long-term prognosis for delirium in older patients. Delirium is also independently associated with long-term problems, such as poor long-term functioning, mortality, increased length of stay, need for formal home health care rehabilitation services, new institutionalization, and increased costs of care.

Dharmarajan K, Swami S, Gou Y, Jones RN, Inouye SK. Pathway from delirium to death: potential in-hospital mediators of excess mortality. *J Am Geriatr Soc.* 2017;65(5):1026-1033.

Fong TG, Jones RN, Marcantonio ER, et al. Adverse outcomes after hospitalization and delirium in persons with Alzheimer Disease. *Ann Intern Med.* 2012;156:848-856.

Gleason LJ, Schmitt EM, Kosar CM, et al. Effect of delirium and other major complications on outcomes after elective surgery in older adults. *JAMA Surg.* 2015;150:1134-1140.

Witlox J, Eurelings LS, de Jonghe JF, Kalisvaart KJ, Eikelenboom P, van Gool WA. Delirium in elderly patients and the risk of postdischarge mortality, institutionalization, and dementia: a meta-analysis. *JAMA.* 2010;304(4):443-451.

▶ Treatment

Three concurrent approaches are involved in the treatment of delirium (see Figure 36–1): (1) identification and treatment of the underlying medical cause; (2) eradication or minimization of contributing factors of delirium; and (3) management of delirium symptoms.

Complete review of the medication history (including prescription, over-the-counter, as-needed, and herbal medications) is needed to identify potentially contributing medications. Drug interactions should be evaluated. Current kidney and liver function status should be assessed and medication dosage/frequency adjusted accordingly. A complete history and physical (including neurologic) examination should be performed, along with selected laboratory and radiologic screening tests to find treatable causes. Occult infection should be evaluated and treated.

If no identifiable cause or contributor is identified, further testing should be pursued, as shown in Figure 36–1. Treatment should begin with nonpharmacologic approaches in all patients.

A. Nonpharmacologic Strategies

In general, nonpharmacologic strategies should be used in all delirious patients. Table 36–2 details a number of the strategies used to prevent or treat delirium, including reorientation, therapeutic activities, fluid repletion, early mobilization, feeding assistance, sensory deficit correction, sleep hygiene, infection prevention, and pain management.

B. Pharmacologic Strategies

Pharmacologic therapy for delirium should be reserved for severely agitated individuals whose behavior threatens medically necessary care (eg, mechanical ventilation) or poses a safety hazard. All medications used in the treatment of delirium can also cause or worsen confusion; thus, a general principle is to use the lowest dose possible for the shortest period of time. The end point should be an awake and manageable patient, not a sedated patient. All too often, a medication is started for management of agitated delirium but continued indefinitely, including upon discharge. This obscures the ability to follow mental status on serial evaluation and puts the patient at significant risk for adverse drug reactions.

A comprehensive systematic review examining antipsychotic drugs did not support the use of antipsychotics in the prevention or treatment of delirium in hospitalized older adults. They may have resulted in potential harm in three of the studies where patients given antipsychotics were more likely to be institutionalized, had higher delirium symptom scores, required more breakthrough treatments, and overall had decreased survival. Table 36–2 covers the classes of medications currently recommended for the treatment and management of delirious patients.

Girard TD, Exline MC, Carson SS, et al. Haloperidol and ziprasidone for treatment of delirium in critical illness. *N Engl J Med.* 2018;379:2506-2516.

Inouye SK, Marcantonio ER, Metzger ED. Doing damage in delirium: the hazards of antipsychotic treatment in elderly persons. *Lancet Psychiatry.* 2014;1:312-315.

Neufeld KJ, Yue J, Robinson TN, et al. Antipsychotic medication for prevention and treatment of delirium in hospitalized adults: a systematic review and meta-analysis. *J Am Geriatr Soc.* 2016;64:705-714.

Page VJ, Ely EW, Gates S, et al. Efficacy and Intravenous haloperidol on the duration of delirium and coma in critically ill patients (Hope-ICU): a randomised placebo-controlled trial. *Lancet Respir Med.* 2013;1:515-523.

▶ Prognosis

Delirium has traditionally been described as a reversible syndrome, implying that patients invariably return to their baseline cognitive and functional state. Recent studies have demonstrated that delirium is not always transient and can result in long-term cognitive and functional deficits. After delirium, some patients develop persistent subjective memory complaints and demonstrate reduced performance on cognitive tests. Thus, in some patients, delirium may be associated with direct and persistent neurologic damage.

Furthermore, patients who develop delirium have been found to be more likely to be diagnosed with dementia at a later date. It appears that delirium increases the risk of developing dementia and may accelerate the rate of progression of cognitive decline in those with baseline cognitive impairment or dementia. Thus, delirium can in fact permanently alter the trajectory of cognitive decline for older persons.

Fong TG, Jones RN, Shi P, et al. Delirium accelerates cognitive decline in Alzheimer disease. *Neurology.* 2009;72(18):1570-1575.

Girard TD, Pandharipande PP, Ely EW. Delirium in the intensive care unit. *Crit Care.* 2008;12(suppl 3):S3.

Hshieh TT, Saczynski JS, Gou RY, et al. Trajectory of functional recovery after postoperative delirium in elective surgery. *Ann Surg.* 2017;265:647-653.

Inouye SK, Marcantonio ER, Kosar CM, et al. The short-term and long-term relationship between delirium and cognitive trajectory in older surgical patients. *Alzheimers Dement.* 2016;12:766-776.

Pandharipande PP, Girard TD, Jackson JC, et al. Long-term cognitive impairment after critical illness. *N Engl J Med.* 2013;369:1306-1316.

Saczynski JS, Marcantonio ER, Quach L, et al. Cognitive trajectories after postoperative delirium. *N Engl J Med.* 2012;367:30-39.

USEFUL WEBSITES

Australian Commission on Safety and Quality in Health Care. Delirium clinical care standard. 2016. https://www .safetyandquality.gov.au/our-work/clinical-care-standards/ delirium-clinical-care-standard/. Accessed March 27, 2020.

Hospital Elder Life Program. http://www.hospitalelderlifeprogram .org/public/public-main.php. Accessed March 27, 2020.

National Institute for Health and Clinical Excellence (NICE). Guidelines for delirium. http://guidance.nice.org.uk/cg103. Accessed March 27, 2020.

Network for Investigation of Delirium: Unifying Scientists (NIDUS). A collaborative, multidisciplinary network for scientific research on delirium and its mechanisms, outcomes, diagnosis, prevention and treatment. https://deliriumnetwork .org/. Accessed March 27, 2020.

Cochrane Library, Database of Abstracts of Reviews of Effectiveness. Systematic reviews of delirium studies. http:// www.cochranelibrary.com. Accessed March 27, 2020.

Parkinson Disease & Essential Tremor

37

Nicholas B. Galifianakis, MD, MPH

A. Ghazinouri, MD, CWSP

PARKINSON DISEASE

 ESSENTIALS OF DIAGNOSIS

▶ Any combination of resting tremor, bradykinesia, rigidity, and postural instability (late feature). Bradykinesia is a required feature for diagnosis.

▶ Asymmetric onset is the norm.

▶ Responds well to levodopa in most cases.

▶ Diagnostic accuracy improves with observation over time.

▶ General Principles

Parkinson disease (PD) is the second most common chronic progressive neurodegenerative disorder, after Alzheimer disease. It affects an estimated 1% of people older than age 65 years and up to 3% older than age 85 years, or approximately 1.5 million people in the United States and >5 million people worldwide. With the aging of the world's population, and with age being the strongest risk factor for PD, incidence is expected to rise dramatically in coming decades. By 2050, some researchers project >2.5 million cases in the United States.

PD is generally considered a disease of the older adult, but it can affect younger age groups. The mean age of onset is about age 60 to 65 years. Several key points should be emphasized about the care of older PD patients. The differential diagnosis of parkinsonian symptoms in patients older than the age of 75 years is mostly limited to either idiopathic PD or secondary parkinsonism, as onset of atypical etiologies is rare in this age group. Older PD patients often present with an akinetic-rigid syndrome, more nonmotor symptoms, and less tremor. Levodopa is the drug of choice in patients older than age 70 years because dopamine agonists (eg, pramipexole and

ropinirole), amantadine, and anticholinergics are poorly tolerated in this age group.

▶ Pathogenesis

The clinical presentation of PD was first described by James Parkinson in his 1817 "Essay on Shaking Palsy." It was not until the 20th century that the pathologic hallmarks of PD, α-synuclein–positive Lewy bodies and dopaminergic cell loss of the substantia nigra, were described. It is estimated that by the time the first symptoms emerge, 60% of substantia nigra neurons have already died. Neurochemically, this results in dopamine depletion in the nigrostriatal pathway. Physiologically, this leads to inhibition of the thalamus and reduced excitation of the motor cortex, manifesting as the cardinal motor features of PD (bradykinesia and rigidity).

A fundamental shift in our understanding of PD pathology has occurred in recent years. It has long been known that the pathology spreads beyond the substantia nigra as PD progresses, which explains much of the disabling nonmotor features of advanced PD, such as dementia, depression, and autonomic failure. However, we now know that even before any motor symptoms occur, pathology has spread through specific areas of the olfactory system, lower brainstem, and peripheral nervous system. This "premotor" prodrome of PD can manifest as hyposmia, sleep disorders, mood disorders, and constipation. In summary, from the earliest to the most advanced stages, PD pathology occurs in a much wider distribution of the central and peripheral nervous systems than previously thought, making PD much more than just a movement disorder.

The mechanisms of neurodegeneration in idiopathic PD are not well understood but likely include complex interactions between environmental factors and genetic predisposition. Environmental risk factors remain elusive, although exposure to pesticides is known to be a risk factor. Cigarette smoking and coffee consumption are possible protective factors.

Genetics play a role. There are now over 20 genes or loci (designated as the PARK loci) that cause or predispose people to PD. Although some of these genes account for the 5% to 10% of PD that seems to be inherited in a Mendelian pattern, some also contribute to a higher percentage of "sporadic" PD that has more complex modes of inheritance. Perhaps more importantly, discovering the function of these genes in neurons has helped elucidate several important mechanisms of pathogenesis in PD overall.

▶ Clinical Findings

PD has an insidious onset and gradually progresses, leading to increasing disability over time. The cardinal motor features include resting tremor, bradykinesia, rigidity, and gait impairment/postural instability, although the latter usually arises later in the disease. Nonmotor features are also prominent and increasingly become the main source of disability as the disease progresses.

PD is a clinical diagnosis. Bradykinesia plus one of the other cardinal manifestations must be present to diagnose idiopathic PD. Other clinical features that are supportive of the diagnosis are asymmetric presentation and a strong response to dopaminergic medications. Approximately 20% of PD cases present without tremor. Diagnostic accuracy increases to >90% in patients followed by movement disorders specialists.

A. Symptoms & Signs

Rest tremor is the most common presenting symptom of PD. It usually attenuates with use of the affected limb. However, *action tremor* is fairly common and should not steer the clinician away from a PD diagnosis if other parkinsonian features are present. In early stages, the tremor may only appear when the patient is distracted (while talking or walking), and the patient may even be able to suppress it with concentration. With progression, tremor becomes more constant, more common with actions, and higher in amplitude, impairing many activities of daily living (ADLs). On examination, tremor is a rhythmic, oscillatory, involuntary movement. Parkinsonian tremor is asymmetric, relatively slow (frequency 3–6 Hz), and tends to have a prominent pronation-supination component to it (as opposed to flexion-extension), frequently giving the tremor a "pill-rolling" quality. Examiners should observe tremor at rest, with different postures and actions, including handwriting and drawing spirals. If there is no obvious tremor, distracting tasks should be given to patients to elicit mild tremor.

Bradykinesia is defined as a slowness or lack of movement. It manifests as loss of dexterity and difficulty initiating and maintaining the amplitude and velocity of movement. ADLs, like eating and dressing, will take more time to complete. It is often described by patient as "weakness," although strength is intact. Many of the common complaints of the PD patient are direct manifestations of bradykinesia including small handwriting (micrographia), loss of facial expression (hypomimia), quiet monotone speech (hypophonia), and slower walking with shorter steps. To elicit bradykinesia, the examiner asks the patient to perform rapid repetitive movements (eg, finger taps, hand openings and closings, and heel stomps), as quickly and largely as possible. Examining handwriting and having the patient draw spirals can reveal micrographia. It is also important to take note of lack of spontaneous movements, such as blink rate, expression in speech, hand gestures while speaking, or the amount of shifting one's position.

Rigidity is subjectively experienced by the patient as "stiffness" and, when severe enough, can lead to painful aching or cramping. Patients may experience musculoskeletal complaints (eg, painful, frozen shoulder), and it is common for a patient to seek care from an orthopedic surgeon or rheumatologist before a neurologist. Rigidity is defined as the increased resistance that is felt as the examiner passively moves a body part about a joint to assess muscle tone. The increase in tone should be constant, independent of the speed or direction of the passive movement. This even increase in tone has been termed *lead pipe* rigidity, as opposed to the variable resistance felt when examining spasticity. When tremor is superimposed on rigidity, a ratcheting sensation can be sensed, giving the rigidity a "cogwheeling" component.

Postural instability and gait dysfunction are less prominent at presentation. In early PD, mild gait impairment can manifest as subtly shortened stride length, decreased arm swing, and stooped posture. In moderate PD, the gait becomes more shuffling, posture stooped, and patients turn en bloc, requiring several steps to make a turn. In advanced PD, festination (a sense that the body wants to hasten forward) or freezing of gait (the inability to take effective steps) can occur. Freezing of gait is especially sensitive to anything that requires more attention of the patient, including initiating gait, narrow spaces or doorways, turns, or even carrying something. Postural instability can be assessed with the "pull test." More than two corrective steps backward are considered abnormal. This should be done only by experienced examiners with caution, as patients can have surprising lack of postural reflexes, and may even need to be caught by the examiner. Gait dysfunction is not as responsive to treatment and can lead to falls and loss of mobility, and many patients end up wheelchair bound.

A diverse range of *nonmotor symptoms* are increasingly being recognized as characteristic of PD. Patients frequently describe hyposmia, constipation, dream enactment, and mood symptoms years before the appearance of any movement disorder. However, as the disease progresses to moderate and advanced stages, additional nonmotor problems lead to significant disability. In fact, nonmotor symptoms most strongly correlate with decreased quality of life (QOL) in PD. Cognitive and psychiatric problems are almost universal in PD, with earlier stages showing mild impairment in attention, visual-spatial, and executive function. Memory and language are relatively spared. In advanced stages, dementia and psychosis (especially visual hallucinations and delusions) are common. Most patients with PD have depression and anxiety at some point. The autonomic nervous system is greatly affected in PD, with constipation, gastroparesis, orthostatic hypotension, urinary urgency, erectile dysfunction, and sweating dysregulation. Except for constipation, autonomic complaints usually do not become prominent or disabling until later in the course, when incontinence and severe orthostatic hypotension can lead to substantial disability. Sleep can be disturbed with dream enactment, sleep maintenance insomnia, and sleep apnea, contributing to excessive daytime sleepiness and fatigue.

B. Patient Examination

On neurologic examination, extraocular eye movements, motor strength, sensory, and cerebellar examinations should be normal. The extrapyramidal examination is the central focus of the examination of a PD patient. The clinician should carefully evaluate for facial expression, speech, tremor, rapid repetitive tasks, muscle tone, gait, and balance. Details about the objective findings related to the cardinal features of PD are discussed in the previous section.

C. Laboratory Findings

At this time, there are no laboratory tests or imaging studies that can confirm the diagnosis of PD. However, PD is not a diagnosis of exclusion. To the contrary, only when certain red flags come to the attention of the clinician (especially lack of response to dopaminergic therapy) is it necessary to rule out atypical and secondary causes of parkinsonism. Genetic testing is commercially available for certain *PARK* gene mutations. Routine testing for these genes is not yet recommended, and for the most part, clinical use of genetic testing remains restricted to settings where there is a strong family history or when onset occurs before the age of 40 years.

D. Imaging Tests

The US Food and Drug Administration (FDA) has approved the use of DaTSCAN (^{123}I-ioflupane, a ligand that uses single-photon emission computed tomography [SPECT] imaging to detect presynaptic dopamine transporters) in trying to distinguish PD from essential tremor. PD patients (but also some atypical parkinsonism patients) will have a decreased DaT signal in the basal ganglia. However, DaTSCAN should not be considered a routine test, as it is no more sensitive or specific than examination by a movement disorders neurologist. Advanced functional imaging techniques remain a research tool for the vast majority of situations. Routine magnetic resonance imaging (MRI) of the brain is usually normal in early stages of PD. Only in settings when the diagnosis remains in question is an MRI ordered to investigate secondary or atypical parkinsonism.

▶ Differential Diagnosis

Idiopathic PD is the most common cause of parkinsonism. It is important to think of secondary or atypical causes when certain red flags are seen, namely symmetric presentation, lack of tremor, and the presence of atypical features that are rarely seen early in PD. The strongest alert is a lack of response to higher doses of dopaminergic medications (>1000–1500 mg/day of levodopa).

The two most common etiologies of secondary parkinsonism are vascular and drug induced. These are especially important to consider in older adults, as atypical parkinsonian syndromes rarely have onset after the age of 75 years. In fact, when exposure to dopamine-blocking drugs can be ruled out by history, idiopathic PD and vascular parkinsonism account for the vast majority of cases in older patients.

Vascular parkinsonism can result from chronic ischemic damage or multiple infarcts in the brain. Patients often present with a symmetric akinetic-rigid syndrome. Findings tend to be more severe in the legs, and gait is prominently affected. Vascular parkinsonism occasionally responds to dopaminergic medications, but not as robustly as with PD.

Drug-induced parkinsonism results from exposure to dopamine receptor–blocking agents, most commonly antiemetics and antipsychotics (both typical and atypical) or dopamine depleters (eg, reserpine or tetrabenazine). In older adults, parkinsonian features can persist for months after the offending dopamine receptor–blocking agent has been discontinued. Other secondary causes of parkinsonism are rarer (Table 37–1).

Table 37–1. Secondary causes of parkinsonism and tremor.

Parkinsonism
- Vascular parkinsonism
- Toxins (pesticides, methylphenyltetrahydropyridine [MPTP] manganese, carbon monoxide, cyanide, methanol)
- Structural brain lesions (hydrocephalus, tumor, trauma)
- Metabolic disorders (Wilson disease, hypoparathyroidism)
- Infections (AIDS, syphilis, Creutzfeldt-Jakob disease)
- Postencephalitic parkinsonism (von Economo encephalitis lethargica)

Drug-Induced Parkinsonism
- Dopamine receptor–blocking agents (antipsychotics and antiemetics)
- Dopamine depleters (reserpine and tetrabenazine)

Drug-Induced Tremor
- Amphetamines
- Antidepressants
- Antipsychotics
- β-Agonists
- Corticosteroids
- Lithium
- Amiodarone
- Methylxanthines (including coffee and tea)
- Thyroid hormone
- Valproic acid

Table 37-2. Atypical neurodegenerative causes of parkinsonism.

Condition	Clinical Features
Multiple systems atrophy (MSA)	Early autonomic failure with erectile dysfunction, urinary incontinence, syncope, cerebellar signs, spasticity, or other upper motor neuron signs
Progressive supranuclear palsy (PSP)	Prominent axial features, such as oculomotor abnormalities, especially vertical gaze impairment, early falls and dysphagia, upright posture
Corticobasal degeneration (CBD)	Persistent asymmetry, cortical sensory signs, neglect, alien limb, severe early dystonia, aphasia
Lewy body dementia (LBD)	Early dementia, visual hallucinations, delusions, fluctuating level of consciousness/cognition, extreme neuroleptic sensitivity

Atypical parkinsonism results from neurodegenerative disorders that lead to parkinsonism. They are termed *Parkinson plus* syndrome because they are associated with disabling features, such as autonomic failure, early falls, and early dementia, not usually seen in early PD. These early disabling atypical features, the lack of response to medications, and the rapid progression of these illnesses combine to give these diseases a poor prognosis. Table 37–2 lists the signs for these disorders.

A common challenge in the differential diagnosis is distinguishing between the tremor of PD and that of essential tremor (ET). The action tremor of ET tends to be more symmetric, higher frequency, and more extension-flexion as opposed to the asymmetric lower frequency, pronation-supination tremor of PD. The diagnosis can be especially difficult when one considers that a minor amount of rigidity and bradykinesia can occasionally be seen in ET. ET patients should not have the anosmia, rapid eye movement (REM) sleep behavior disorder, and more significant parkinsonism seen in PD.

▶ Complications

PD, historically viewed as a movement disorder, is now recognized as a complex condition with diverse clinical manifestations, including neuropsychiatric and other nonmotor features. As PD progresses, it can affect many parts of the central and peripheral nervous system, leading to diverse complications. Autonomic dysfunction can lead to drooling, bloating, gastroparesis, constipation, urinary dysfunction, incontinence, erectile dysfunction, temperature dysregulation, and orthostatic hypotension, which can lead to falls and syncope. Two major sources of morbidity and mortality are dysphagia and gait dysfunction. Dysphagia can lead to aspiration or choking. Postural instability and freezing of gait can lead to injurious falls or the many complications associated with immobility. Sleep dysfunction, somnolence, and fatigue are extremely common in PD. When prominent, cognitive-behavioral dysfunction is a major source of disability and results in the PD symptoms most associated with poor QOL. Furthermore, patients with advanced PD experience complications from its treatment as well.

A. Motor Fluctuations & Dyskinesia

Complications of dopaminergic therapy are significant sources of disability in moderate-stage PD patients. "Wearing off" is managed in two ways: shortening the interval between doses or adding a catechol-*O*-methyltransferase (COMT) or monoamine oxidase (MAO) inhibitor.

Dyskinesias are involuntary hyperkinetic movements that occur at "peak-dose" levodopa levels. They are most commonly choreiform (abnormal twisting, writhing, dance-like movements) but can also be dystonic (pulling into more sustained and often painful postures). Dyskinesia can be managed either by slightly reducing the amount of levodopa at each dose or by adding amantadine. If the patient is taking a long-acting (controlled-release) formulation of levodopa multiple times a day, an unpredictable "stacking effect" may contribute to dyskinesia, and conversion to a short-acting levodopa regimen should be considered. Deep brain stimulation (DBS), especially globus pallidus interna (GPi) DBS, can have a robust antidyskinetic effect. Because management of complications is complex and because DBS can alleviate both problems in some patients, prompt referral to a neurologist is strongly recommended for advanced treatment options.

B. Falls

Falls are a major source of injury, morbidity, and mortality in PD, and patients with postural instability need to be closely monitored for falls and referred promptly to physical therapy for gait and balance evaluation and management.

C. Dementia & Psychosis

Dementia occurs in a majority of patients with advanced PD. First, always distinguish delirium from dementia and rule out general medical issues, such as infections, while also looking for medications that contribute to sedation and/or confusion (eg, dopamine agonists, amantadine, muscle relaxants, pain medications, and anticholinergic medications for tremor and bladder symptoms). Cholinesterase inhibitors (eg, donepezil, galantamine, rivastigmine) are thought to be more beneficial for patients with PD than Alzheimer disease, especially for attention, bradyphrenia, and psychotic features like visual hallucinations. To treat psychosis, address medications first (eg, lowering dopaminergic medications). If needed, consider using quetiapine, clozapine, or pimavanserin (a novel, expensive serotonergic antipsychotic approved by the FDA specifically for PD psychosis). All other typical and atypical antipsychotics are contraindicated in PD, especially in older adults.

D. Depression

Selective serotonin reuptake inhibitors (SSRIs) are first-line agents for depression in PD. Although citalopram and escitalopram are widely used, in clinical practice, they are less useful for patients with PD, because they are so serotonin specific, and more importantly, dosage reductions are required for patients older than 60 years of age because of the risk of QT prolongation. Few clinical trials provide evidence for the choice among antidepressants in PD, but serotonin-norepinephrine reuptake inhibitors (SNRIs) may address a broader spectrum of neurotransmitter deficits in PD. Care should be taken to avoid drug interactions with MAO inhibitors such as selegiline.

E. Orthostatic Hypotension

Medications that contribute to orthostatic hypotension should be reduced if possible. Consider antihypertensives, which are frequently no longer needed as PD progresses. Dopaminergic drugs can also exacerbate hypotension. Salt in the diet can be liberalized and water intake encouraged. The head of the bed should be raised above 30 degrees. Eating small, frequent meals can avoid splanchnic dilatation. Hot weather, hot liquids, and hot showers should be avoided. Pharmacotherapy, such as fludrocortisone, midodrine, and droxidopa, which is FDA approved for neurogenic orthostatic hypotension, is sometimes used when the above measures fail, but causes complications in older patients and should be used with caution.

F. Gastrointestinal Complications & Constipation

Dysphagia must be monitored closely, and patients should be promptly evaluated when present. Drooling can respond to careful administration of botulinum toxin to the salivary glands. Constipation is practically universal in PD. Hydration, exercise, and a healthy, high-fiber diet should be encouraged. Laxative agents (eg, polyethylene glycol and Senokot) should be taken daily.

G. Referral Guidelines

Consider referring patients to a neurologist or movement disorders specialist when (1) the diagnosis is in question; (2) a patient is not responding to standard therapies; (3) the patient has unacceptable side effects; (4) complications occur from PD or its treatments; or (5) surgical interventions are considered.

▶ Treatment

A. Nonpharmacologic Therapy

Care of the PD patient requires a multidisciplinary team approach, including important aspects such as patient education, exercise, diet, and rehabilitation services. Patients and their families should be educated about the natural history of PD and available treatments and resources. Support groups are particularly valuable. As the disease progresses and new symptoms and complications arise, treatment regimens can become complex. Patients will need to learn to differentiate among symptoms related to PD, medication side effects, or other conditions. Exercise improves mood, strength, balance, flexibility, and mobility. A combination of aerobic, strengthening, flexibility, and balance exercises can help to maintain functional status. A well-balanced healthy diet and adequate hydration can prevent constipation and orthostatic hypotension. Furthermore, protein restriction may be necessary in some patients, as amino acids compete with levodopa for absorption, thus blocking its therapeutic effect. Involving a nutritionist may be vital, especially as weight loss and disuse atrophy can occur and are associated with poor outcomes. Physical, occupational, speech, and swallowing rehabilitation therapies aimed at improving daily function and QOL can be effective at all stages. To prevent injurious falls (a major source of PD-related morbidity and mortality), physical therapy is critical in patients with gait dysfunction. Emotional and psychological needs of the patient and family should also be addressed through counseling of a chaplain, psychiatrist, psychologist, or other mental health provider.

B. Pharmacotherapy

PD is an incurable illness, with no treatments proven to slow disease progression. However, PD is somewhat unique among neurodegenerative disorders in that it benefits from a diverse range of effective symptomatic treatments such as dopaminergic medications. The primary goal of pharmacotherapy is to reduce symptoms to maintain independence, functional status, and QOL and reduce disability. A common misconception among patients (and clinicians) is that medications will "only last for so long" once started. This now discredited belief has led to an all-too-common practice of delaying treatment as long as possible. Treatment should be initiated and tailored to adequately reduce symptoms whenever patients are bothered by their symptoms, and certainly when functional status, independence, or mobility is threatened. Many PD patients, especially young-onset and tremor/motor-predominant patients, can lead highly functional lives for many years with optimized treatment regimens. However, as the disease progresses, complications of dopaminergic medications, such as dyskinesia and motor fluctuations, occur and regimens can become complex. Especially in older adults, medications can exacerbate nonmotor symptoms, such as visual hallucinations, behavioral problems, orthostasis, and somnolence, and reductions may be necessary at the cost of decreased motor benefit.

1. Levodopa—Levodopa is the most effective and well-established drug in the treatment of PD. Converted by DOPA-decarboxylase into dopamine, it provides dopaminergic replacement. It ameliorates tremor, bradykinesia, and rigidity, thus reducing morbidity and disability. Axial features of PD such as speech and gait impairment are frequently less responsive to levodopa and other dopaminergic medications. Furthermore, in advanced PD, postural instability, speech impairment, autonomic dysfunction, dementia, and psychiatric problems are not responsive to levodopa. Although levodopa does not slow the progression of PD pathology, life expectancy in PD has improved today compared to the pre-levodopa era.

Levodopa provides a robust and consistent improvement of motor features and keeps patients highly functional for years. However, most patients will eventually experience motor complications, namely motor fluctuations and dyskinesia, manifest as inconsistent response to levodopa. In the earlier stages, patients experience "wearing off," where the duration of effect of each levodopa dose progressively shortens and requires shorter intervals between doses. Later on, more unpredictability occurs, with some doses completely failing to "kick in" and others abruptly losing effect (see earlier section on complications). Alternate formulations of levodopa—immediate-release/controlled-release capsules, duodenal gel pumps, and inhaled—have been approved and are now available. These formulations may offer benefits when administered either as an alternative to or in conjunction with oral levodopa and should be used in consultation with a neurologist. Side effects of levodopa include nausea, vomiting, lightheadedness, dizziness, somnolence, and, in more advanced patients, hallucinations and confusion. Peripheral decarboxylase inhibitors, such as carbidopa, are always included in formulations of levodopa to reduce the gastrointestinal side effects by preventing peripheral conversion of levodopa to dopamine. Isolated carbidopa can be added to prevent the nausea experienced with standard levodopa formulations. Levodopa is generally a well-tolerated medication, and most side effects can be avoided if started slowly and gradually titrated up to an effective dose. It should be taken on empty stomach at least 30 to 45 minutes before or after meals, to avoid protein blocking of absorption of levodopa. Long-acting formulations of levodopa (eg, Sinemet CR) are helpful for bedtime dosing as they can reduce nocturnal return of PD symptoms, but daytime use of these formulations can exacerbate complications.

2. Adjunct pharmacotherapies—Most other PD drugs have minimal symptomatic benefits when used alone and serve as adjunctive therapy when motor complications occur. Because most patients require these medications when they have entered the more complicated moderate to advanced stage of PD, one should consider consulting a neurologist before initiating these agents. COMT inhibitors (entacapone and tolcapone) and MAO-B inhibitors (selegiline and rasagiline) block the enzymatic breakdown of levodopa and are used to decrease motor fluctuations ("wearing off") by extending the duration of benefit of each dose of levodopa. Amantadine is the only medication with proven effectiveness for reducing dyskinesia. It reduces tremor and freezing of gait in some patients as well. Amantadine has dopamine agonist and anticholinergic properties; commonly exacerbates somnolence, cognitive impairment, and psychosis; and has limited use in older adults.

3. Dopamine agonists—Dopamine agonists directly stimulate dopamine receptors in the striatum (the postsynaptic target of nigral neurons). The older ergot derivatives such as bromocriptine and pergolide are not used in clinical practice because of serious side effects such as heart valve damage. Newer nonergot agonists, such as pramipexole, ropinirole, and transdermal rotigotine, have replaced them. Dopamine agonists are effective as monotherapy in reducing cardinal motor features of PD. However, within 2 to 5 years, most patients will require the addition of levodopa. Dopamine agonists are also used as adjunctive therapy with levodopa when motor complications occur. Because they are longer acting, they can reduce the severity of "wearing off," and because they cause less dyskinesia than levodopa, they are sometimes used in order to attempt a decreased levodopa dose.

Dopamine agonists are poorly tolerated in older adults. Although side effects are similar to levodopa (nausea, vomiting, orthostatic hypotension, somnolence, dizziness, psychiatric symptoms, hallucinations), they occur more commonly and more severely, especially in older adults. Serious consideration should be given before starting a dopamine agonist in patients older than 70 years of age because of the side effects of somnolence, cognitive impairment, and psychosis. Dopamine agonists also have additional side effects, including impulse control disorder that are rarely seen with levodopa. Patients on dopamine agonists should be educated about and frequently screened for compulsive gambling, eating, and shopping; hypersexuality; and other impulsive behaviors.

Similarly, anticholinergic medications such as trihexyphenidyl can be effective at reducing tremor, dyskinesia, and dystonia, but older patients have low tolerance for their cognitive and autonomic impairment. These drugs should not be considered options in the geriatric population.

C. Surgical Therapies

In many patients, medications become progressively less effective in relieving PD symptoms consistently, especially after the onset of motor fluctuations or dyskinesia. Some of these patients may benefit from surgical therapies. Candidacy for these interventions is complex. The ideal candidate is a patient who has a clear diagnosis of PD, continued good response to medications in the "on" state, suffers from disabling motor complications despite optimal medical management, is healthy enough to tolerate a neurosurgical intervention, has relatively intact cognition, and does not suffer from a significant or uncontrolled mood disorder. There is no firm age limit, but patients older than age 70 years are generally considered higher risk, and those older than age 80 years are rarely operated on.

1. Stereotactic lesioning—Pallidotomy (lesioning of the GPi) is effective in treating the cardinal features of PD and can drastically reduce levodopa-induced dyskinesias. Similarly, thalamotomy can reduce tremor. However, these lesioning procedures are irreversible and not adjustable, and bilateral procedures are associated with dysphagia, dysarthria, and cognitive impairment. Consequently, today these procedures are mostly used only in situations where DBS is not feasible.

2. DBS—DBS of the subthalamic nucleus (STN) or GPi has mostly replaced stereotactic lesioning procedures. Although more expensive, DBS has the advantages of being nondestructive, reversible, and programmable. Bilateral procedures are better tolerated. The DBS system is a four-contact lead implanted into each hemisphere of the brain by stereotactic technique. The leads are connected to a pulse generator in the chest wall by subcutaneous extension wires. Clinicians program the device for optimal benefit to avoid side effects by adjusting the amplitude, pulse width, frequency, and polarity of stimulation, and by changing the configuration of active contacts on each lead. Patients can also make some adjustments at home.

DBS of both targets can alleviate the cardinal features of PD, motor fluctuations, and dyskinesia. Both targets are effective at treating tremor, rigidity, and bradykinesia, especially in the limbs. However, as with medications, axial symptoms such as gait and speech are less responsive to DBS. In fact, DBS can make speech, falls, cognition, and behavioral symptoms worse, especially in high-risk patients. It is important to have extensive discussion with patients and their families before surgery to make sure that the symptoms that bother them the most (ie, their goals of treatment) match those that can be reliably alleviated by DBS. The largest randomized clinical trial found these two targets to have similar effectiveness and safety. However, STN-DBS has higher risk of falls and cognitive and mood side effects.

DBS has higher risk of infection and hardware problems than ablative procedures. Some side effects, such as speech impairment, spasticity, and mood changes, can result from stimulation of neighboring structures in the brain. Adjusting stimulation parameters often alleviates these stimulation-induced side effects.

▶ Prognosis

Caring for patients with advanced PD presents many challenges, and the prospect of having a chronic progressive debilitating disease is frightening. Patients can benefit from PD treatments for years and become disabled by nonmotor symptoms without effective treatments. Furthermore, PD drug doses frequently need to be lowered because of exacerbation of nonmotor symptoms, worsening, in turn, their motor symptoms.

A palliative care approach can be beneficial and is underused in advanced PD. PD has a variable, slow, and prolonged course, making accurate prognosis difficult.

However, some trends predict an unfavorable prognosis. Onset of PD in older age, prominent nonmotor features, and prominent akinetic-rigid syndrome with gait dysfunction are associated with more rapid progression and poor outcomes, whereas younger-onset PD, lack of nonmotor features, and tremor predominance are associated with slower progression.

Palliative care, unlike hospice, is not limited to a particular prognosis. PD causes disability, suffering, and caregiver strain. Applying palliative care principles at every stage is important.

Addressing advance directives and involving an attorney or estate planner for financial and legal issues (eg, establishing power of attorney) are important. Although it may be difficult to initiate end-of-life discussions, it is important to hear a PD patient's wishes when they are still able to share them. A palliative care approach does not preclude life-prolonging therapies but proactively focuses on relief of suffering from pain, depression, anxiety, and other psychosocial stressors for both patients and caregivers.

Ahlskog JE. Diagnosis and differential diagnosis of Parkinson's disease and parkinsonism. *Parkinsonism Relat Disord.* 2000;7(1):63-70.

Braak H, Del Tredici K, Bratzke H, Hamm-Clement J, Sandmann-Keil D, Rüb U. Staging of the intracerebral inclusion body pathology associated with idiopathic Parkinson's disease (preclinical and clinical stages). *J Neurol.* 2002;249(suppl 3): III/1-III/5.

Follett KA, Weaver FM, Stern M, et al; CSP 468 Study Group. Pallidal versus subthalamic deep-brain stimulation for Parkinson's disease. *N Engl J Med.* 2010;362(22):2077-2091.

Hallett M, Litvan I. Evaluation of surgery for Parkinson's disease: a report of the Therapeutics and Technology Assessment Subcommittee of the American Academy of Neurology. *Neurology.* 1999;53(9):1910-1921.

Hoehn MM, Yahr MD. Parkinsonism: onset, progression, mortality. *Neurology.* 1967;17(5):427-442.

Langston, JW. The Parkinson's complex: parkinsonism is just the tip of the iceberg. *Ann Neurol.* 2006;59(4):591-596.

Stern MB, Lang A, Poewe W. Toward a redefinition of Parkinson's disease. *Mov Disord.* 2012;27(1):54-60.

USEFUL WEBSITES

Family Caregiver Alliance (provides information on support groups, hiring caregivers, and issues of long-term care). http://www.caregiver.org. Accessed March 26, 2020.

National Parkinson Foundation, Inc. (provides information on educational programs, support groups, treatment options, and publications). http://www.parkinson.org. Accessed March 26, 2020.

Unified Parkinson's Disease Rating Scale (UPDRS). https://www.sciencedirect.com/topics/medicine-and-dentistry/unified-parkinsons-disease-rating-scale. Accessed March 26, 2020.

ESSENTIAL TREMOR

▶ Characterized by a bilateral action tremor of the hands and forearms and possibly the head, voice, and trunk.

▶ Other neurologic signs are absent.

▶ Positive family history in about half of cases.

General Principles

ET is the most common movement disorder, affecting 4% of adults 40 years of age and older. Age and family history are the strongest risk factors. It has been referred to as familial tremor, but a significant percentage of ET patients do not have a family history. The term *benign ET*, used to differentiate it from tremors associated with PD and other neurodegenerative diseases, has fallen out of use, as the tremor itself can be quite disabling. There is also controversy as to whether ET is a neurodegenerative disorder or a condition of normal aging of the nervous system.

Clinical Findings

ET is characterized by a postural-kinetic tremor, although rest tremor can occur. It often involves the arms, but commonly involves the head and voice as well. It is unusual for ET to be prominent in the legs, lips, or chin. Bilateral involvement is the general rule, but it can be asymmetric. An isolated head tremor can occur, but these cases are considered variants of cervical dystonia. ET progresses slowly and remains mild in a majority of cases. In fact, some estimate that <10% of people with ET seek medical attention. ET worsens with anxiety, stress, and caffeine intake and is frequently reduced by alcohol, although this can be true for all forms of tremor.

ET is a clinical diagnosis, usually made by a thorough history and examination. Other than the tremor, neurologic examination should be normal, except for possible subtle findings such as hearing loss and subtle cerebellar signs.

Differential Diagnosis

The differential diagnosis includes parkinsonism, with a resting tremor and other signs. Action tremors are also found in dystonia and Wilson disease, but these conditions are associated with other neurologic abnormalities and occur in a younger population. Secondary causes of postural and kinetic tremor should only be considered with unusual presentations of tremor. Tobacco and caffeine use, as well as certain medications (see Table 37–1), may result in an enhanced physiologic tremor that can closely mimic ET. Tremor can be

seen with alcohol or sedative withdrawal and can occur as part of a somatoform disorder or conversion disorder. Psychogenic tremors are usually interrupted on examination by distracting the patient.

Complications

ET can result in significant functional impairment and social embarrassment. ET has significant effects on functional status, especially on ADLs and IADLs, such as feeding, dressing, manual work, and household chores. Furthermore, ET can have significant psychological impact as it worsens in social situations and can result in early retirement, social isolation, and increased level of care. Tremor is not the only neurologic manifestation of ET. Recent studies show patients with additional findings, such as subtle cerebellar dysfunction (difficulty with tandem gait, slight incoordination), mild cognitive deficits, anxiety, and hearing loss. ET is also associated with a higher risk of PD and may be associated with an increased risk of dementia.

Treatment

All current treatments for ET are solely symptomatic. The goal of treatment is not to eradicate all tremor but to improve function and reduce social embarrassment. If the tremor is mild and nondisabling, treatment may not be required. Stress reduction and caffeine avoidance can ameliorate tremor and can be sufficient in mild ET. Alcohol may reduce tremor, but regular use is not recommended because of rebound tremor and long-term effects, including a higher rate of alcoholism in ET patients. Occupational therapists can provide adaptive utensils and devices that can improve QOL. All medications for tremor can cause side effects and should be started at low doses and gradually increased until satisfactory control or intolerable side effects occur. Severe, refractory, or atypical cases should be referred to a specialist for management including consideration for DBS.

A. Pharmacotherapy

1. First-line agents—Propranolol and primidone have the most evidence of efficacy in treating ET, reducing tremor by approximately 50% to 70% in patients. Propranolol is a nonselective β-blocker that crosses the blood-brain barrier and is the only agent approved by the FDA for ET. The average effective dose is 120 mg/day, up to 320 mg if tolerated. Mild ET can be treated with as-needed doses. Sustained-release preparations are equally effective. Potential side effects include bronchoconstriction, bradycardia, hypotension, lightheadedness, fatigue, erectile dysfunction, and depression. Other β-blockers are less effective than propranolol. Primidone is structurally similar to barbiturates. Most patients respond to about 250 mg daily. Adverse effects include sedation, dizziness, ataxia, confusion, and depression. Response to treatment and side effects guide dose adjustments. Combining propranolol and primidone may provide additive benefit.

2. Second-line agents—Gabapentin and topiramate are antiseizure drugs that can be added to first-line agents if tremor control is unsatisfactory. Gabapentin is well tolerated, with a typical effective dose around 1200 mg daily. Common side effects include sedation, dizziness, and unsteadiness. Topiramate is effective at doses >100 mg twice daily. Its use is limited because of cognitive side effects, reduced appetite, weight loss, and paresthesia. Zonisamide is an alternative to topiramate and is better tolerated and dosed daily. Benzodiazepines are occasionally used to control tremor, but common side effects (eg, sedation, cognitive dysfunction, hypotension, falls, respiratory inhibition, and abuse potential) limit their use, and therefore, they should be avoided. Calcium channel blockers, theophylline, carbonic anhydrase inhibitors, isoniazid, clonidine, and phenobarbital have yielded contradictory results and are not recommended as first- or second-line agents.

3. Other pharmacotherapies—The use of botulinum toxin type A to treat limb tremor has been disappointing, and its use should only be considered in rare refractory cases. However, neck injections can be quite effective in reducing head tremor. A high risk of dysphagia limits its use for voice tremor.

B. Surgical Therapies

There is extensive evidence that unilateral thalamotomy or thalamic (ventral intermediate [VIM]) DBS is effective in treating patients with disabling, medication-refractory ET. Dysarthria, disequilibrium, and cognitive impairment may occur after thalamotomy. DBS appears to be associated with fewer adverse events, and bilateral intervention is better tolerated. The decision to use either procedure depends on individual patient circumstance, perioperative risks, and access availability to ongoing stimulator monitoring and adjustments.

Koller WC, Hristova A, Brin M. Pharmacologic treatment of essential tremor. *Neurology.* 2000;54(11 Suppl 4):S30-S38.

Louis ED. Essential tremor. *N Engl J Med.* 2001;345(12):887-891.

Louis ED, Ottman R, Hauser WA. How common is the most common adult movement disorder? Estimates of the prevalence of essential tremor throughout the world. *Mov Disord.* 1998;13(1):5-10.

Zesiewicz TA, Elble RJ, Louis ED, et al. Evidence-based guideline update: treatment of essential tremor: report of the Quality Standards subcommittee of the American Academy of Neurology. *Neurology.* 2011;77(19):1752-1755.

Zesiewicz TA, Elble R, Louis ED, et al. Practice parameter: therapies for essential tremor: report of the Quality Standards Subcommittee of the American Academy of Neurology. *Neurology.* 2005;64(12):2008-2020.

38

Cerebrovascular Disease

Ivy Nguyen, MD
Anne Fabiny, MD
Bruce Ovbiagele, MD, MSc, MAS, MBA

▶ Stroke presents as a neurologic deficit or headache of abrupt onset.

▶ Hemorrhagic strokes can be intracerebral or subarachnoid.

▶ Urgent neuroimaging studies are essential for diagnosis.

General Principles

In the past decade, stroke declined from the third to the fifth leading cause of death in the United States, which is testament to a half-century of progress in cerebrovascular disease prevention and acute care. It remains, however, a leading cause of disability, with up to half of all patients who survive a stroke failing to regain independence and needing long-term health care. Stroke primarily affects older adults, and for each successive decade after the age of 55 years, the stroke rate doubles for both men and women.

Ischemic stroke, insufficient blood flow to the brain, accounts for 80% of strokes, whereas bleeding that destroys and compresses the brain parenchyma, intracerebral hemorrhage (ICH), accounts for 15%. Bleeding that occurs in the subarachnoid space, subarachnoid hemorrhage (SAH), accounts for 5% of strokes.

Clinical Findings

A. Signs & Symptoms

An ischemic stroke presents as an acute neurologic deficit. Older patients have more severe stroke deficits at presentation than do younger patients. The neurologic impairment reflects the area of the brain affected. Although the presenting focal neurologic symptoms are variable, 80% of patients present with unilateral weakness; 90% have a speech and/or motor deficit. In addition, deficits in sensation, vision, language, cognition, and balance may occur. Sudden-onset, severe headache is the classic presentation for aneurysmal SAH. In addition to focal neurologic symptoms, headache and a decreased level of consciousness may also develop in ICH if the hemorrhage becomes sufficiently large.

After the onset of symptoms, timely evaluation and diagnosis are paramount. This is because the effect of thrombolysis is time dependent. Thus, neurologic screening tools like the Cincinnati Stroke Scale (Table 38–1) can be useful in early triage. The three most predictive examination findings for the diagnosis of acute ischemic stroke are facial paresis, arm drift/weakness, and abnormal speech.

B. Special Tests

In patients suspected of stroke, diagnostics occur in two phases: (1) acute triage and (2) investigations into etiology after stroke is established as the diagnosis.

In the acute triage phase, several tests should be performed routinely in all patients with suspected stroke. This is to establish a diagnosis, identify systemic conditions that may mimic stroke, and identify conditions that influence therapeutic options. Immediate diagnostic studies in all patients should include noncontrast brain computed tomography (CT), blood glucose, serum electrolytes/renal function tests, electrocardiogram (ECG), markers of cardiac ischemia, complete blood count including platelet count, prothrombin time/international normalized ratio, activated partial thromboplastin, and oxygen saturation.

Establishing the time of ischemic stroke symptom onset is critical because it determines eligibility for acute therapies. Neurovascular imaging is important to evaluate for large-vessel occlusion in acute ischemic stroke and to detect possible aneurysm or vessel malformations in hemorrhagic stroke. Given the clinical history and examination, additional tests may be indicated. These include hepatic function tests,

Table 38–1. Cincinnati Stroke Scale.

Facial Droop
  Normal: Both sides of face move equally
  Abnormal: One side of face does not move at all

Arm Drift
  Normal: Both arms move equally or not at all
  Abnormal: One arm drifts down compared to the other

Speech
  Normal: Patient uses correct words with no slurring
  Abnormal: Slurred or inappropriate words or mute

Interpretation:
  If any 1 of these 3 signs is abnormal, the probability of a stroke
    is 72%

toxicology screen, blood alcohol level, arterial blood gas if hypoxia is suspected, and chest radiography if lung disease is suspected. For patients in whom diagnostic uncertainty remains, lumbar puncture may be performed if SAH is suspected and CT scan is negative for blood. If seizures are suspected as the cause of neurologic symptoms, an electroencephalogram (EEG) may be necessary.

Differential Diagnosis

The diagnosis of stroke can be firmly established with history, examination, and advanced imaging techniques. ICH, SAH, and subdural hematoma are visible immediately on CT (Figure 38–1). Seizures, syncope, migraine, hypoglycemia, hyperglycemia, or drug toxicity can mimic acute ischemia. Diffusion-weighted imaging (DWI) MRI sequences are approximately 90% sensitive in detecting cerebral infarction (Figure 38–2). Therefore, once the diagnosis of stroke is made, the etiology of the stroke must be determined (Table 38–2).

Whether an ischemic stroke or ICH is diagnosed, the underlying cause needs to be established to determine the most effective secondary stroke prevention measures. For ischemic stroke, the workup should aim to establish the stroke subtype: large artery atherosclerosis (ie, carotid or intracranial vessel stenosis), (cardioembolism (eg, atrial fibrillation), small-vessel occlusion (ie, lacunar stroke), stroke of other determined cause (eg, arterial dissection), or stroke of an undetermined cause (ie, cryptogenic).

For the majority of older patients with ICHs, the underlying etiology is (1) hypertension (hypertensive vasculopathy), (2) anticoagulation-related hemorrhage, or (3) cerebral amyloid angiopathy (CAA). Longstanding hypertension causes weakening of the small, deep-penetrating arteries that can rupture causing hemorrhage into the deep structures of the brain. Anticoagulation with warfarin or direct-acting oral anticoagulants (DOACs) increases the risk of ICH and

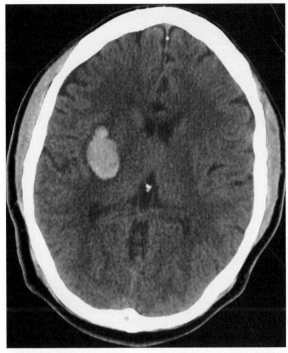

▲ **Figure 38–1.** Computed tomography scan of a patient with sudden onset left hemiplegia shows an intracerebral hemorrhage in the right basal ganglia.

worsens the severity of hemorrhage, doubling its mortality. CAA, defined as amyloid deposition in the cerebral vessel walls, may cause large and symptomatic hemorrhage or small and clinically silent hemorrhage (Figure 38–3). Severe CAA is present in 12% of patients >85 years old.

The majority of patients with nontraumatic SAH typically present with sudden-onset headache, which may be associated with nausea or vomiting, brief loss of consciousness, seizures, or meningismus. Head CT reveals the diagnosis in >90% of cases within 24 hours of bleeding onset. In patients in whom there is a strong suspicion of SAH despite a normal head CT and who present beyond 6 hours of headache onset, lumbar puncture is required to rule out SAH. Once confirmed, the etiology of SAH must be determined with vascular imaging such as CT angiography or digital subtraction angiography (DSA), which remains the gold standard for diagnosis of aneurysms or vascular malformations.

Subdural hematoma (SDH) results from tearing of bridging veins and bleeding into the dura and arachnoid membranes. Head trauma is the most common cause of SDH. The overall incidence of SDH is highest among older adults, in whom cerebral atrophy, falls, and use of antithrombotic agents are common. Acute SDH may present as focal neurologic deficits and progressive altered mental status. Chronic

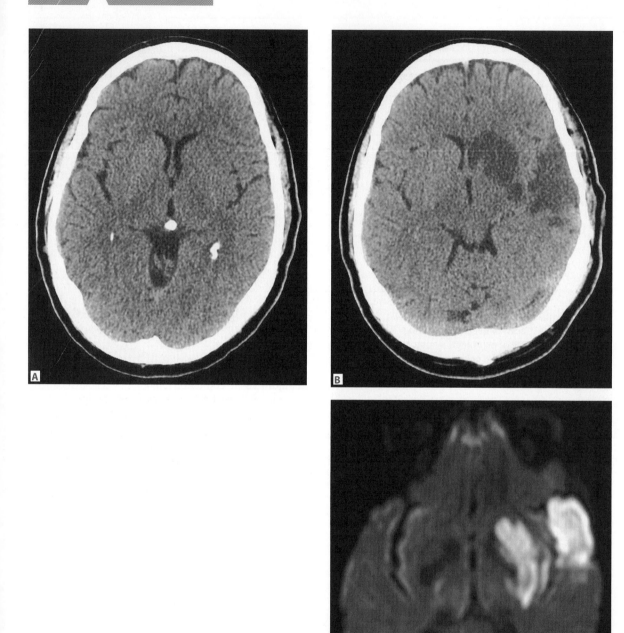

▲ **Figure 38–2.** **A.** Computed tomography (CT) scan of a patient with right hemiparesis and aphasia that started 2 hours prior; scan appears normal initially. **B.** Follow-up CT scan several days later shows an infarction in the left middle cerebral artery distribution. **C.** Diffusion-weighted magnetic resonance imaging of ischemic stroke appears bright.

Table 38–2. Common etiologies of ischemic stroke and intracerebral hemorrhage in older adults.

Ischemic Stroke
Cardioembolic (atrial fibrillation)
Large artery atherosclerosis (carotid or intracranial vessel stenosis)
Small-vessel occlusion (lacunar stroke)

Intracerebral Hemorrhage
Hypertensive vasculopathy
Cerebral amyloid angiopathy
Anticoagulation related

SDH is more likely to present as global deficits such as insidious headaches, cognitive impairment, somnolence, and occasionally seizures.

▶ Complications

Following stroke onset, some patients may deteriorate neurologically over the next few hours or days. Clinical

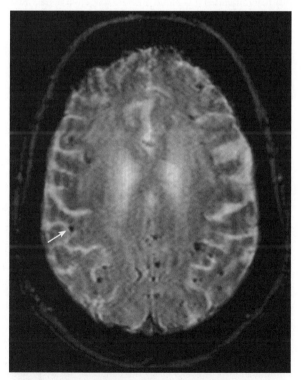

▲ **Figure 38–3.** Gradient-echo magnetic resonance imaging showing multiple chronic "clinically silent" hemorrhages (dark punctuate lesions) in cortical and cortical-subcortical regions characteristic of cerebral amyloid angiopathy.

manifestation may take the form of decreased level of consciousness, an exacerbation of the presenting neurologic deficit, or the appearance of a new deficit. Both neurologic and nonneurologic causes of deterioration are often treatable if recognized promptly.

Common neurologic causes of deterioration are progressive stroke, brain swelling, recurrent ischemic stroke, hemorrhagic transformation, and, less commonly, seizures. Large strokes of the cerebral hemisphere or cerebellum are at the highest risk for brain edema and increased intracranial pressure. Swelling in cerebellar strokes may cause obstructive hydrocephalus requiring acute neurosurgical intervention.

Medical complications are a common and important problem after acute stroke as they can be barriers to optimal recovery. During hospital admission, infection is common. Urinary tract infection or pneumonia may occur in up to one-quarter of patients, and both are associated with increasing age. The appearance of fever after stroke should prompt a search for pneumonia, as it is an important cause of death. The risk of deep venous thrombosis and pulmonary embolism is highest among immobilized and older patients with severe stroke. Pain, falls, and depression are all common during hospitalization.

▶ Treatment

A. Initial Management & Acute Ancillary Care

The acute care of patients with ischemic stroke should include (1) stabilization and initial assessment, (2) decision making regarding thrombolysis with intravenous tissue plasminogen activator (t-PA), (3) evaluation for endovascular therapies, and (4) effective communication with patients and families.

As in any emergency, the management of acute stroke starts with assessment of the "ABCs": airway, breathing, and circulation. Most stroke patients do not require intubation; however, those with a depressed level of consciousness are at the highest risk of requiring ventilator support. Acute assessment of the circulatory status includes ECG, blood pressure monitoring, and cardiac enzyme determination.

Most patients with acute ischemic stroke have an elevated blood pressure. This elevation is usually transient and helps maintain perfusion to ischemic brain tissue; therefore, rapid reduction should be avoided. No treatment is recommended unless the systolic pressure is >220 mm Hg or the diastolic pressure is >120 mm Hg. However, in patients eligible for thrombolytic therapy, blood pressure should be <185/110 mm Hg before administering intravenous (IV) t-PA.

After initial emergency department management, patients should be admitted to stroke units, because specialized care improves survival and functional outcome, regardless of age.

B. Specific Therapies

1. Acute ischemic stroke—Reperfusion of the ischemic brain is the most effective therapy for acute ischemic stroke.

By restoring blood flow to threatened tissues before they progress to infarction, reperfusion therapies salvage viable brain tissue (the ischemic penumbra) and improve clinical outcomes.

The association between thrombolysis treatment and improved outcome is maintained in all age groups, even in those over age 80. Thus, age alone should not be a barrier to treatment. Regarding the risk of ICH in older individuals, studies have varied. A meta-analysis of pooled thrombolysis data concluded that the risk of symptomatic ICH did not increase among patients older than 80 years of age despite less favorable outcomes, which were attributed to comorbidities.

The benefit of thrombolytic therapy is strongly time dependent: the more rapid the treatment, the more favorable the outcome. Patients are candidates for IV t-PA if the medicine is administered within 3 hours of symptom onset and there are no contraindications. A European study (ECASS III) showed that benefit could be extended to the 3- to 4.5-hour window, but this is only available in patients younger than 80 years of age. Patients and families should be given an explanation of the risks and benefits of t-PA.

Recently, endovascular treatment with mechanical thrombectomy has been shown to significantly improve functional outcome in patients with strokes due to anterior circulation (internal carotid artery and middle cerebral artery) large-vessel occlusion. While older patients may have worse outcomes overall, thrombectomy is just as effective in older patients as it is in younger patients. For patients who cannot be treated with thrombolytic therapy or thrombectomy, see later section, "Secondary Prevention Strategies."

2. Intracerebral hemorrhage—ICH remains the least-treatable form of stroke. Apart from management in a specialized stroke or neurologic intensive care unit, no specific therapies have been shown to improve outcome after ICH. For the majority of primary ICHs, the underlying etiology is hypertension (hypertensive vasculopathy), CAA, or anticoagulation-related hemorrhage. Acute therapy involves intensive blood pressure control (goal systolic pressure <140 mm Hg), anticoagulation reversal, and interventions for elevated intracranial pressure and mass effect as needed. Patients with symptomatic hemorrhages secondary to CAA should avoid anticoagulants and antiplatelet agents. Age is an independent predictor of outcome after ICH, with age >80 years associated with an increased 30-day mortality.

3. Subarachnoid hemorrhage—Acute management of patients with SAH involves intensive blood pressure control and aneurysm repair with surgical clipping or endovascular coiling. These patients require close monitoring for complications such as vasospasm and delayed cerebral ischemia, elevated intracranial pressure, hyponatremia, and seizures.

4. Subdural hematoma—Acute symptomatic SDH often requires surgical hematoma evacuation, especially in patients with neurologic decline attributed to brain herniation or elevated intracranial pressure. Nonoperative management of SDH may be appropriate for clinically stable patients with small hematomas (clot thickness <10 mm). Conservative management involves anticoagulation reversal, serial brain imaging, and close observation with intracranial pressure monitoring when appropriate.

C. Secondary Prevention Strategies

The successful prevention of a recurrent ischemic stroke hinges upon a comprehensive approach. This involves the identification and treatment of stroke risk factors, such as hypertension, diabetes, and hyperlipidemia. Of equal if not greater importance is the modification of lifestyles that increase the risk of a stroke, such as diet, exercise, and smoking cessation.

Antihypertensive therapy forms the cornerstone of secondary stroke prevention. A recent meta-analysis of several large trials of blood pressure reduction for secondary stroke prevention found a 20% relative risk reduction. It is generally recommended that blood pressure reduction begins after 24 hours of a stroke if the patient is neurologically and hemodynamically stable.

Long-term treatment with high-intensity statins reduces the risk of stroke and cardiovascular events.

Antiplatelet agents are the mainstay of secondary prevention in patients with a history of noncardioembolic stroke. Aspirin monotherapy is typically the first choice for initial therapy, although a combination of aspirin and dipyridamole and clopidogrel monotherapy are also reasonable options. In select patients with minor ischemic stroke or high-risk transient ischemic attack, early, short-term combination of clopidogrel and aspirin reduces risk of subsequent stroke compared to aspirin but may be associated with a possible small increase in major bleeding events.

1. Atrial fibrillation—Atrial fibrillation dramatically increases in prevalence with age and is associated with a nearly five-fold increase in stroke risk. Cardioembolic stroke related to atrial fibrillation is the most frequently encountered stroke subtype in very old patients. Warfarin reduces the stroke risk by 68%. Despite this, many clinicians assume that a combination of anticoagulation therapy and head trauma from falls leads to a substantially high risk of subdural hemorrhage and they decide not to anticoagulate their older patients whom they believe are prone to falling. Evidence contrary to this practice shows that the risk of this complication is outweighed by the benefit of stroke protection provided by oral anticoagulation.

Urgent anticoagulation (heparin infusion) with the goal of preventing early recurrent stroke is not recommended because of the risk of hemorrhage. Typically, patients are placed on aspirin during the acute phase as a "bridge" to eventual oral anticoagulation with warfarin. Anticoagulation should be initiated within 2 weeks.

DOACs, such as dabigatran, rivaroxaban, and apixaban, are at least as effective as warfarin in the prevention of stroke in patients with atrial fibrillation and are associated with lower rates of major bleeding. These agents share common properties such as high fixed oral dosing, no interaction with food, no need for anticoagulation monitoring, and rapid onset and offset of action. Because of the lower risk of intracranial hemorrhage compared with warfarin, DOACs may be preferred in older patients, but they may need to be dose adjusted based on low body weight and impaired renal function.

2. Carotid stenosis—Carotid artery stenosis is another major risk factor for ischemic stroke in the elderly. Evidence is clear that carotid endarterectomy (CEA) is more effective than medical therapy for preventing recurrent stroke in patients with symptomatic carotid stenosis (those who have had a recent stroke or transient ischemic attack), particularly in those with severe (70%–99%) stenosis. CEA is also efficacious in patients with moderate (50%–69%) symptomatic carotid stenosis, although the efficacy is less dramatic. Early surgery in symptomatic patients (within 2 weeks if possible) is recommended as the risk of a recurrent stroke is frontloaded. Recent studies show that CEA is safer than carotid artery stenting for older patients. Patients with asymptomatic carotid stenosis should receive medical management including aspirin, statin, and optimization of vascular risk factors. CEA may be considered in individuals with asymptomatic severe (>70%) stenosis of the internal carotid artery, although its effectiveness compared with contemporary best medical management alone is not well established. Results from the ongoing CREST-2 trial, a large randomized controlled trial comparing carotid revascularization versus contemporary medical management alone for preventing stroke in patients with asymptomatic high-grade carotid stenosis, will help to address this uncertainty.

3. Transient ischemic attack—In the era of advanced neuroimaging, transient ischemic attack (TIA) has been redefined from a time-based diagnosis (<24 hours) to a brain tissue–based diagnosis. A TIA is a transient episode of neurologic dysfunction caused by focal brain or retinal ischemia without acute infarction. In contrast, persistent clinical signs or characteristic imaging abnormalities define infarction—that is, stroke.

After having a TIA, the short-term risk of having a stroke is high: 10% of patients have a stroke within 90 days, with half of those occurring in the first 2 days. Thus, a TIA should trigger the same prompt evaluation and workup as a persistent neurologic deficit (ie, stroke) and requires the implementation of proven interventions to reduce this substantial short-term stroke risk.

▶ Prognosis

Advanced age increases the risk of mortality after a stroke and is also a risk factor for recurrence. Compared with younger patients, older stroke survivors recover more slowly and have more severe deficits. The severity of stroke and pre-stroke medical condition heavily influences the outcome. Of patients >80 years old who receive thrombolysis, 20% end up with no significant disability and are eventually discharged home. Of patients >70 years old who undergo mechanical thrombectomy, approximately 30% achieve functional independence at 90 days.

Chao TF, Liu CJ, Lin YJ, et al. Oral anticoagulation in very elderly patients with atrial fibrillation: a nationwide cohort study. *Circulation.* 2018;138(1):37-47.

Cordonnier C, Demchuk A, Aiai W, Anderson CS. Intracerebral hemorrhage: current approaches to acute management. *Lancet.* 2018;392(10154):1257-1268.

Emberson J, Lees KR, Lyden P, et al. Effect of treatment delay, age, and stroke severity on the effects of intravenous thrombolysis with alteplase for acute ischaemic stroke: a meta-analysis of individual patient data from randomised trials. *Lancet.* 2014;384(9958):1929-1935.

Foody JM. Reducing the risk of stroke in elderly patients with non-valvular atrial fibrillation: a practical guide for clinicians. *Clin Interv Aging.* 2017;12:127-187.

Goyal M, Menon BK, van Zwam WH, et al. Endovascular thrombectomy after large-vessel ischemic stroke: a meta-analysis of individual patient data from five randomized trials. *Lancet.* 2016;387:1723-1731.

Hao Q, Tampi M, O'Donnell M, et al. Clopidogrel plus aspirin versus aspirin alone for acute minor ischaemic stroke or high risk transient ischaemic attack: systematic review and meta-analysis. *BMJ.* 2018;18:363:k5108.

Hemphill JC 3rd, Greenberg SM, Anderson CS, et al. Guidelines for the management of spontaneous intracerebral hemorrhage: a guideline for healthcare professionals from the American Heart Association/American Stroke Association. *Stroke.* 2015;26(7):2032-2060.

Heo SH, Bushnell CD. Factors influencing decision making for carotid endarterectomy versus stenting in the very elderly. *Front Neurol.* 2017;8:220.

Jayaraman MV, McTaggart RA. Endovascular treatment of anterior circulation large vessel occlusion in the elderly. *Front Neurol.* 2018;19(8):713.

Kernan WN, Ovbiagele B, Black HR, et al. Guidelines for the prevention of stroke in patients with stroke or transient ischemic attack: a guideline for healthcare professionals from the American Heart Association/American Stroke Association. *Stroke.* 2014;45(7):2160-2236.

Nogueria RG, Jadhav AP, Haussen DC, et al. Thrombectomy 6 to 24 hours after stroke with a mismatch between deficit and infarct. *N Engl J Med.* 2018;378(1):11-21.

Powers WJ, Rabinstein AA, Ackerson T, et al. 2018 guidelines for the early management of patients with acute ischemic stroke. *Stroke.* 2018;49(3):e46-e110

Texakalidis P, Chaitidis N, Giannopoulos S, et al. Carotid revascularization in older adults: a systematic review and meta-analysis. *World Neurosurg.* 2019;S1878-8750(19):30441-30443.

Whiteley WN, Emberson J, Lees KR, et al. Risk of intracerebral haemorrhage with alteplase after acute ischaemic stroke: a secondary analysis of an individual patient data meta-analysis. *Lancet Neurol.* 2016;15(9):925-933.

Zonneveld TP, Richard E, Vergouwen MD, et al. Blood pressure-lowering treatment for preventing recurrent stroke, major vascular events, and dementia in patients with a history of stroke or transient ischaemic attack. *Cochrane Database Syst Rev.* 2018;19;7:CD007858.

Coronary Artery Disease

39

Alan H. Baik, MD

Sanket S. Dhruva, MD, MHS

ESSENTIALS OF DIAGNOSIS

▶ Presence of risk factors (hypertension, dyslipidemia, smoking, diabetes, renal disease, male, older age) accompanying symptoms.

▶ Chest discomfort or dyspnea provoked by exertion and subsiding with rest or nitroglycerin.

▶ Older adults with coronary disease often have atypical or nonspecific symptoms such as abdominal pain, dizziness, confusion, or fatigue instead of (or in addition to) more classic symptoms.

▶ Electrocardiographic changes: ST elevation, ST depression, T-wave changes, and new Q waves.

▶ Exercise or pharmacologic stress test evidence of myocardial ischemia.

▶ Angiographic evidence of coronary stenosis.

General Principles

The prevalence of cardiovascular disease (CVD), and especially coronary artery disease (CAD), is increasing and associated with both all-cause and cardiovascular mortality. In the United States, 92.1 million people have CVD. In adults aged 60 to 79 years, 69.6% of men and 68.6% of women have CVD; by age 80 years, >80% of individuals have CVD. Among people free of CVD at age 50 years, the lifetime risk for developing it is 51.7% for men and 39.2% for women.

CAD accounts for 43.8% of deaths from CVD in the United States and approximately 14% of all-cause mortality. One of the strongest risk factors for developing CAD is age, and the prevalence of CAD increases with age. Based on autopsy data, obstructive CAD (≥70% stenosis) is present in approximately 60% of people >80 years old. The good news is

that the overall rate of death attributable to CVD declined by 34.4% from 2005 to 2015, and the actual number of patients dying in the same period decreased by 17.7%. A large percentage of this decrease is related to better therapy for patients with acute coronary syndromes (ACS) and chronic stable angina. Further improvements have come from better modification of CAD risk factors, although these improvements are increasingly being offset by higher obesity and type 2 diabetes mellitus rates.

In adults aged 85 to 94 years, the average annual rate of first cardiovascular events is 24 times that of those aged 35 to 44 years. For women, first cardiovascular events occur about 10 years later in life, with the difference narrowing with advancing age. Older adults are more likely to die from CAD compared to their younger counterparts due to the higher prevalence of CAD risk factors, multivessel disease, left main CAD, and left ventricular (LV) dysfunction, along with other noncardiovascular chronic conditions. Older adults also tend to have more chronic conditions, which contribute to them having fewer surgical and interventional procedures and more adverse events from medications. They are also less frequently referred for cardiac rehabilitation. Congestive heart failure, one of the long-term complications of CAD, is the most common diagnosis on hospital discharge, and the majority of these patients are age 65 years or older.

General principles of CAD management in older patients include thoughtful and careful assessment of CAD risk factors and their management. This means that careful attention must be paid to functional status, frailty, cognitive status, and other cardiovascular and noncardiovascular chronic conditions in older adults. The risks and benefits of diagnostic tests and therapeutic interventions (both medications and surgical or percutaneous procedures) should always be considered, and older adults must be engaged in shared decision making. Although there are significant benefits to management of CAD risk factors, older adults also have higher risk of testing- and therapeutic-related adverse effects.

A. Cardiovascular Changes with Normal Aging

With normal aging, multiple changes in the heart and other organs alter function and are precursors to a variety of diseases seen in older adults (Table 39–1). These expected changes must be distinguished from changes related to diseases such as CAD and other vascular diseases. Vascular aging is associated with mitochondrial oxidative stress, alterations in endothelial homeostasis and lipid metabolism, and increased inflammation. From a molecular standpoint, cardiovascular aging is related to increased cellular apoptosis, abnormal calcium homeostasis, genomic instability, and epigenetic changes.

Table 39–1 lists the consequences of these changes. The practical effect of these aging changes on cardiac function is no change in cardiac output at rest or with moderate exercise and no change in LV ejection fraction or stroke volume. With stress (eg, trauma, disease, anemia, infection, surgery) that requires an increase in cardiac output and increase in oxygen demand, there is less ability to meet this increased demand as a result of the decrease in cardiac reserve.

B. Cardiovascular Risk Factors

Risk factors for CVD, including CAD, have been identified for decades. Because their effect on the development of CVD is directly related to the number and severity of risk factors present, the accumulation and duration of these risk factors are particularly important in the older patient. Whether a risk factor will affect the development of CVD is also partially genetically determined. For instance, everyone who smokes does not develop CAD. However, risk factor modification can reduce CAD progression in older patients.

1. Hypertension—Hypertension is highly prevalent in older patients, affecting 76.5% of patients >80 years of age. Hypertension is more common in black patients compared to non-Hispanic white, Hispanic, and Asian patients. Patients older than age 65 years with systolic blood pressure >180 mm Hg have a three- to four-fold increase in CAD compared to those with a systolic blood pressure <120 mm Hg; risk of other CVD (eg, stroke and peripheral arterial disease) also increases with blood pressure.

There is robust evidence that controlling blood pressure reduces cardiovascular events, including in older patients. The 2017 American College of Cardiology (ACC)/American Heart Association (AHA) guideline defines stage 1 hypertension as a blood pressure of 130 to 139/80 to 89 mm Hg (systolic blood pressure [SBP]/diastolic blood pressure [DBP]) and stage 2 hypertension as >140/90 mm Hg. Healthy lifestyle changes are recommended for patient with blood pressure of 120 to 129/<80 mm Hg, with reassessment in 3 to 6 months. Lifestyle changes can reduce SBP by 4 to 11 mm Hg. These lifestyle changes include weight loss, physical activity (see later in chapter), DASH (Dietary Approaches to Stop Hypertension) diet (rich in fruits, vegetables, whole grains, and

Table 39–1. Cardiovascular changes with aging and their consequences.

Change	Consequences
Decrease in arterial elasticity, increase in arterial stiffness	Increased afterload on the left ventricle (LV) and LV wall tension, systolic hypertension and the development of left ventricular hypertrophy (LVH), increased size of myocardial cells and aortic wall thickness.
Changes in the LV wall decreasing LV compliance	Prolongation of diastolic relaxation and systolic contraction.
Noncompliant LV	End-diastolic LV stiffness increases the importance of atrial systole to the filling of the LV and maintaining stroke volume. Increased LV stiffness is responsible for an S_4. With extensive LV decreased compliance, heart failure with preserved ejection fraction (HFpEF) can occur. In advanced HFpEF, patients can develop increased atrial pressure, left atrial enlargement with subsequent atrial tachyarrhythmias (which can reduce stroke volume), and secondary pulmonary hypertension (World Health Organization group II).
Increased LV wall thickness	Increased LV myocyte size and decreased number of myocytes. This can ultimately lead to increased intracardiac filling pressures and pulmonary edema.
Dropout of atrial pacemaker cells	Apoptosis of myocardial cells, including a loss of 50%–75% of atrial pacemaker cells by age 50 years, slows the intrinsic heart rate. This can result in sick sinus syndrome.
Fibrosis of the cardiac skeleton	Fibrosis of the annular valve rings and the fibrous trigones can result in various degrees of atrioventricular block. Fibrosis of the conduction system can lead to bundle branch block. Fibrosis and calcification of the aortic ring can be the first stage of aortic stenosis. Fifty percent of older patients have grades I–II systolic ejection murmurs.
Decreased responsiveness to β-adrenergic receptor stimulus and decreased reactivity of baro- and chemoreceptors	Slowing of response to position change with decreased sympathetic reflexes and postural hypotension.

low-fat dairy products), sodium restriction, reduction of alcohol intake (no more than two standard alcoholic drinks per day for men and one for women), and management of sleep apnea. In patients with an atherosclerotic CVD risk of >10% or known CVD, diabetes mellitus, or chronic kidney disease, antihypertensive medication is recommended in addition to lifestyle modifications. The blood pressure target of <130/80 mm Hg is the same for older patients, although clinical judgment, life expectancy, and patient preferences should be considered in older patients to balance benefits and risks, particularly in those with multiple chronic conditions and polypharmacy who are at increased risk for medication-related adverse events.

The Hypertension in the Very Elderly Trial (HYVET), which included almost 4000 patients older than age 80 years, showed that with blood pressure–lowering treatment, the incidence of stroke was decreased by 30% and cardiac death by 23%. The Systolic Blood Pressure Intervention Trial (SPRINT) demonstrated that in the subgroup of older adults >75 years who did not reside in a nursing home or assisted living facility, intensive blood pressure control with a SBP goal of 120 mm Hg (vs <140 mm Hg) significantly reduced the primary composite outcome of myocardial infarction (MI), non-MI ACS, stroke, acute decompensated heart failure, and cardiovascular death. There was a 34% lower relative risk in the composite outcome and 33% lower relative risk of death from any cause. The overall rates of serious adverse events were not different, although the intensive control group had higher rates of acute kidney injury, electrolyte abnormalities, syncope, and orthostatic hypotension, but not injurious falls.

2. Dyslipidemia—Dyslipidemia is another cardiac risk factor. Serum cholesterol concentration increases progressively until age 50 years in men and age 65 years in women and then begins to decline. Age-related changes in the concentration of cholesterol are mainly caused by increases in low-density lipoprotein cholesterol (LDL-C). High-density lipoprotein cholesterol (HDL-C) level remains relatively stable with age and is approximately 10 mg/dL higher in women than in men. High LDL-C and low HDL-C predict development of CAD in older adults. Clinical trial data indicate that in older patients with established CAD, LDL-C–lowering therapy, primarily with statins, is beneficial and is standard therapy for older patients who are at higher risk and otherwise in good health to be given LDL-C–lowering therapy, although benefits are smaller in those without CVD. Pharmacologic therapy to increase HDL-C has not shown clinical benefits.

3. Diabetes mellitus—As of 2015, 9.4% of the US population had diabetes mellitus, and 25.2% of patients older than 65 years had diagnosed or undiagnosed diabetes. Diabetes is the seventh leading cause of death in the United States. The prevalence of diabetes mellitus in the United States is projected to more than double from 2005 to 2050, with the largest increases in the oldest age groups, increasing by 220% in those aged 65 to 74 years and by 449% in those aged

≥75 years. Type 2 diabetes in older adults doubles the risk of CAD. Older adults are at increased cardiac risk from the constellation of signs known as the metabolic syndrome: central obesity, insulin resistance, dyslipidemia, and hypertension. More than 44% of adults >60 years old are estimated to have metabolic syndrome.

4. Smoking—Smoking is a significant public health problem and the leading cause of preventable death in the United States. Cigarette smoking is a major cause of MI, CAD, hypertension, stroke, and sudden cardiovascular death. In 2016, 8.8% of people ≥65 years of age in the United States were current smokers. Older smokers are less likely to quit smoking than younger smokers. However, when older smokers attempt to quit, they are more likely to succeed. Absolute rates of CVD incidence and mortality as a result of smoking increase steadily as age and duration of smoking increase; heavy smokers (>40 cigarettes per day) have a four-fold increased relative risk of all-cause mortality compared to non-smokers. There is no evidence that the disease consequences of smoking decrease in older adults. The proportional benefits of smoking cessation are somewhat less among older adults because of the cumulative damage of a long duration of smoking and possibly because patients susceptible to the increased risk of CAD from smoking have died at a younger age, leaving those less susceptible. However, cessation is the only way to alter smoking-related disease risk.

Electronic cigarettes, also called e-cigarettes or vapes, are being used more frequently, and it is estimated that up to 1 in every 20 Americans use e-cigarettes. These are electronic nicotine delivery systems that contain addictive nicotine and a solvent carrier, such as glycerol, which are heated to create an aerosol that is inhaled. Although long-term outcomes from e-cigarette use are not entirely known, early studies demonstrate an association with increased cardiovascular events, including MI and CAD, as well as increased oxidative stress. E-cigarette users are also at risk of nicotine dependence and tobacco use, further increasing the risk of adverse cardiovascular outcomes. Severe e-cigarette–related pulmonary disease, including deaths, has also been reported. Therefore, complete cessation of nicotine delivery systems and conventional smoking should be recommended in older patients.

5. Physical inactivity—Physical inactivity is common in patients older than age 75 years, with 38% of men and 51% of women reporting no leisure-time physical activity, and physical inactivity is a major reversible cause of death. Sedentary behavior and long periods of sitting (>8 hours/day) are associated with increased risk of type 2 diabetes, all-cause mortality, and CVD. Exercise raises HDL-C, controls obesity, lowers blood pressure, reduces insulin resistance, and improves glucose tolerance, which are all protective effects against CVD. As little as 15 minutes of daily moderate to vigorous physical activity in adults >60 years old has been shown to reduce all-cause mortality. Exercise may also prevent falls and improve muscle strength, both especially important in older patients. Adults should perform 150 to 300 minutes a week of moderate-intensity or 75 to 150 minutes of vigorous aerobic exercise per week and two sessions per week of isometric resistance exercises, although these guidelines may be modified in older adults based on their baseline level of activity and functional status. In patients with reduced exercise capacity or strength, referral to home- or facility-based cardiac rehabilitation programs can help improve physical activity levels.

6. Obesity and heart-healthy diets—Obesity is common in older patients; its prevalence was 37.7% in 2013–2014. Poor dietary habits and low activity levels contribute to obesity, diabetes, hypertension, and dyslipidemia. As of 2015, poor dietary habits contributed to all-cause mortality in 22.4% of men and 20.7% of women. In addition, obesity is associated with cardiovascular events, decreased exercise tolerance, and frailty. Therefore, older patients should be encouraged to adhere to a heart-healthy diet, defined as high intake of vegetables, whole grains, low-fat or nonfat dairy, seafood, and legumes and low intake of processed and red meats, sugar, sweetened drinks, and refined grains. Patients should be encouraged to maintain a normal body mass index to reduce the risk of CVD.

Arnett DK, Blumenthal RS, Albert MA, et al. ACA/AHA guideline on the primary prevention of cardiovascular disease. *Circulation* 2019;140:e596-e646.

Aronow WS, Fleg JL, Pepine CJ, et al. ACCF/AHA 2011 expert consensus document on hypertension in the elderly: a report of the American College of Cardiology Foundation Task Force on Clinical Expert Consensus documents developed in collaboration with the American Academy of Neurology, American Geriatrics Society, American Society for Preventive Cardiology, American Society of Hypertension, American Society of Nephrology, Association of Black Cardiologists, and European Society of Hypertension. *J Am Coll Cardiol.* 2011.;57(20):2037-2114.

Darville A, Hahn EJ. E-cigarettes and atherosclerotic cardiovascular disease: what clinicians and researchers need to know. *Current Atheroscler Rep.* 2019;21:15.

Madhavan MV, Gersh BJ, Alexander KP, Granger CB, Stone GW. Coronary artery disease in patients > 80 years of age. *J Am Coll Cardiol.* 2018;71(18):2015-2040.

Williamson JD, Supiano MA, Applegate WB, et al. Intensive vs standard blood pressure control and cardiovascular disease outcomes in adults > 75 years: a randomized clinical trial. *JAMA.* 2016;315(24):2673-2682.

ACUTE CORONARY SYNDROME

▶ General Principles

ACS has three components: ST-segment elevation MI (STEMI), non–ST-segment elevation MI (NSTEMI), and unstable angina (UA). All three share a common pathophysiologic origin related to progression of coronary plaque, instability, rupture, and thrombogenesis, resulting in reduction in or cessation of coronary blood flow and subsequent myocyte necrosis. STEMI refers to the elevation of the ST segment in at least two contiguous leads along with either biomarker evidence (cardiac troponin I or T) of myocardial necrosis or symptoms consistent with ischemia. NSTEMI has a similar definition, but without elevation of the ST segment in at least two contiguous leads. UA is chest pain or discomfort that is accelerating in frequency or severity and can occur at rest but does not result in myocardial necrosis as noted by negative cardiac biomarkers. Patients with UA are at increased risk for progression to MI due to the presence of an active coronary plaque and are generally treated similarly to patients with NSTEMI.

An estimated 720,000 people in the United States will be hospitalized with a first MI or CAD death in 2018, and 335,000 will be hospitalized with recurrent MI. Of these CAD events, 67% occur in persons older than age 65 years and 44% occur in persons older than age 75 years. The average age for first MI is 66 years in men and 72 years in women. Older patients are more likely to have NSTEMI and UA than STEMI, as well as silent (clinically unrecognized) MIs. The prevalence of silent or clinically unrecognized MI increases with age, and prevalence may be twice as high as recognized MI in older adults.

Case fatality rates after MI increase markedly with age; 80% of all MI deaths occur in persons older than age 65 years, and 30-day mortality from STEMI in older patients ranges from 13% to 30%. The incidence of MI is higher in men than in women at all ages and higher in black patients compared to white patients. However, the total number of MIs or fatal CAD events is greater in women than men older than age 75 years, reflecting the fact that the proportion of women in the surviving population increases with age.

General principles of ACS diagnosis and management in older patients include careful assessment with serial electrocardiograms and cardiac biomarkers. Older patients often have atypical symptoms, so a higher level of suspicion is required in the initial assessment, especially in those with multiple cardiac risk factors. Additional studies, including an echocardiogram and noninvasive stress testing, can help with evaluation and risk stratification. Because older patients with CAD are simultaneously at higher risk of adverse outcomes related to procedures and medications, risks and benefits of invasive procedures should be carefully weighed and initiation and up-titration of medications should be closely monitored to minimize risks associated with polypharmacy. Shared decision making about diagnostic testing and therapeutic interventions is essential.

▶ Prevention

Despite the high prevalence of CAD and ACS, these disorders are potentially preventable or can be delayed through early and aggressive management of risk factors as discussed earlier. Although some risk factors, such as age, sex, and genetics, cannot be modified, lifelong adherence to a heart-healthy lifestyle, including regular physical exercise; maintenance of desirable body weight; a diet rich in fruits, vegetables, and whole grains but low in trans and saturated fats; and avoidance of tobacco products can significantly reduce this risk.

Aspirin, adenosine diphosphatase (ADP) receptor antagonists, β-blockers, angiotensin-converting enzyme inhibitors, angiotensin receptor blockers, and statins have been shown to improve post-ACS prognosis. In addition, cardiac rehabilitation programs reduce all-cause mortality and rehospitalization after ACS. There is a dose-response association between attendance to cardiac rehabilitation and lower risk of MI and death in older adults.

▶ Clinical Findings

A. Symptoms & Signs

Typical symptoms of ACS are pressure-like, substernal chest pain at rest and provoked with exertion, lasting 5 to 30 minutes and improved with short-acting nitroglycerin. The pain can radiate to the neck, jaw, and/or bilateral arms. Associated symptoms include diaphoresis, palpitations, nausea, abdominal pain, shortness of breath, and lightheadedness. The proportion of MI patients who have chest pain declines with age; <50% of MI patients older than 80 years have chest pain. Dyspnea is often the presenting manifestation of acute MI in older adults and is the most common initial symptom in persons older than 80 years. The prevalence of atypical symptoms (eg, gastrointestinal disturbances, overwhelming fatigue, dizziness, syncope, confusion, stroke) also increases with age, as well as in patients with dementia, diabetes, and chronic kidney disease (CKD). Up to 20% of patients older than 85 years with acute MI have neurologic complaints (see Chapter 65, "Chest Pain").

Physical findings associated with ACS are nonspecific but may include signs of acute heart failure, which occur in up to 40% of older patients with MI. These signs include an S_3 or S_4 gallop, new mitral regurgitation murmur due to papillary muscle ischemia/rupture, or signs of pulmonary or systemic venous congestion, such as pulmonary rales or elevated jugular venous pressure (JVP). In patients with right ventricular infarction, the Kussmaul sign (rise in JVP with inspiration) may be present.

B. Electrocardiography

Classic electrocardiographic (ECG) features of a STEMI are ST-segment elevation of at least 1 mm in two or more contiguous leads corresponding to the anatomic distribution of a coronary artery (eg, inferior leads II, III, aVF), presence of reciprocal ST depressions (eg, anterior ST depressions with posterior ST elevation), and often subsequent evolution to pathologic Q waves. In leads V2 to V3, ST elevation must be >2 mm in men ≥40 years old, and ≥1.5 mm in women. For posterior STEMI, only 0.5-mm elevation is required in the posterior leads (V7–V9). Right-sided leads (V3R–V4R) are checked to assess for right ventricular infarction. New left bundle branch block (LBBB) alone is no longer considered to be a STEMI equivalent; however, clinical context, including hemodynamic instability, new heart failure, and elevated biomarkers, should be taken into account to determine need and urgency of reperfusion therapy. If LBBB is present, the Sgarbossa criteria should be applied to assist with the diagnosis of STEMI. Elevation in aVR often indicates left main or multivessel CAD, both of which are more common in older adults.

ST elevation is not present in NSTEMI or UA, but there can be ST-segment depression, nonspecific T-wave inversion, or hyperacute peaked T waves. ECG changes often resolve with resolution of chest pain, so a nondiagnostic or even normal ECG taken when the patient is free of symptoms does not exclude ischemia. Sensitivity for detecting ischemia is improved with serial ECG monitoring, especially with recurrence of symptoms. However, ECGs may be nondiagnostic in older adults because of preexisting conduction system disease (eg, LBBB), ventricular pacing, prior infarct, LV aneurysm, LV hypertrophy, metabolic abnormalities, drug effects (eg, hypokalemia, digoxin), or the high prevalence of NSTEMI.

Atypical symptoms and physical findings, coupled with the high prevalence of nondiagnostic ECGs, often lead to delayed presentation and recognition of ACS. This time lag increases the risk of complications and reduces the window of opportunity for timely and effective intervention. Clinicians should maintain a high index of suspicion for ACS in all older patients with a wide range of unexplained symptoms, significant physical distress, heart failure, and hemodynamic instability.

C. Cardiac Biomarkers

Definitive diagnosis of STEMI or NSTEMI requires abnormal cardiac biomarker elevation. High-sensitivity cardiac troponins I and T have become the gold standard for diagnosis because of their high sensitivity and specificity; high-sensitivity troponin assays (which are becoming widespread) have a ≥99% negative predictive value for myocardial necrosis. As such, the creatine kinase-MB isoenzyme is no longer recommended for diagnosing ACS. Serial measures of biomarkers that exceed the 99th percentile of the upper reference level and exhibit a typical rise-and-fall pattern in a patient with clinical and/or ECG features of cardiac ischemia are diagnostic of MI. MI is more likely if there is a >20% increase in serial measurements. Both the degree of rise and the absolute value of troponin measurements provide prognostic information about risk of death. Troponin levels rise within 2 to 4 hours of onset of symptoms, peak at 24 to 72 hours, and may remain elevated for up to 10 to 14 days, especially in large infarctions. Troponin levels should be drawn immediately on arrival if there is clinical concern for ACS and repeated every

3 to 6 hours to assess for a pathologic rise. It is important to consider other causes of troponin elevation in older patients, including demand ischemia (see below) and nonischemic myocardial injury (eg, myocarditis, pericarditis, trauma).

Risk Assessment

Given that older adults may present with atypical symptoms, assessment for ACS in the emergency department (ED) can be challenging. Calculators can help stratify patients into low-, moderate-, or high-risk groups to determine if the patients can be discharged from the ED or if they require additional testing or admission. These include the HEART score (https://www.mdcalc.com/heart-score-major-cardiac-events), Vancouver Chest Pain Rule (https://www.mdcalc.com/vancouver-chest-pain-rule), and GRACE score (https://www.mdcalc.com/grace-acs-risk-mortality-calculator). The HEART score estimates in-hospital and 6-week risk of major adverse cardiac events (all-cause mortality, MI, and coronary revascularization) in patients with undifferentiated chest pain and includes history, ECG changes, age, risk factors, and initial troponin. Once patients are diagnosed with NSTEMI or UA, the Thrombolysis in Myocardial Infarction (TIMI) Risk Score can be used to estimate risk of 14-day all-cause mortality, new or recurrent MI, or severe recurrent ischemia requiring urgent revascularization. Patients in the moderate- to high-risk groups should be admitted, monitored on telemetry, medically managed for ACS, and potentially revascularized. The GRACE score is a prospectively studied scoring system that estimates 6-month to 3-year mortality in patients with diagnosed STEMI or NSTEMI. It involves eight variables, including age, heart rate, SBP, creatinine, Killip class, presence or absence of cardiac arrest at admission, ST-segment deviation on ECG, and abnormal cardiac enzymes.

Differential Diagnosis

The differential diagnosis of ACS in older adults includes other cardiovascular conditions as well as pulmonary, gastrointestinal, musculoskeletal, neurologic, and psychiatric disorders (Table 39–2).

A. Type 2 Myocardial Infarction

Type 2 MI, also commonly termed *demand ischemia*, is defined as myocardial injury (ie, elevated biomarkers) due to oxygen/nutrient supply-demand imbalance to the myocardium in the absence of acute thrombotic coronary artery occlusion. It is due to insufficient blood flow to meet the metabolic demands of the heart, often reflective of underlying CAD, due to a physiologic stressor. Common stressors include sepsis, acute heart failure exacerbation, severe valvular disease, atrial fibrillation or flutter with rapid ventricular rate, bradyarrhythmia, coronary artery vasospasm, anemia, postoperative state, hypertensive emergency, respiratory failure, and pulmonary embolism. In general, the mechanisms are often complex and multifactorial. Demand ischemia is more common in older patients (>75 years old) and in patients with multiple chronic conditions, impaired baseline functional status, and CAD risk factors. Patients with CKD may have chronically elevated troponin levels due to inadequate clearance and baseline increased cardiac release from chronic myocardial injury, even without symptoms. ACS should be ruled out by monitoring ECGs and cardiac biomarkers and assessing for angina. ECG changes in demand ischemia are often nonspecific. It is expected that cardiac biomarkers will decrease with management of the underlying stressor, such as blood transfusion in anemia, respiratory support in hypoxemia, rate control in tachyarrhythmias, and diuresis in acute heart failure. In the absence of ACS, there is no clear evidence

Table 39–2. Differential diagnosis for acute coronary syndrome.

System	Differential Diagnoses
Cardiac	Aortic dissection, pericarditis, myocarditis, cardiomyopathy, acute heart failure, hypertensive emergency, severe aortic stenosis, arrhythmia (supraventricular tachycardia, VT, VF), Brugada syndrome, LV aneurysm/pseudoaneurysm, coronary artery vasospasm, blunt cardiac trauma, symptomatic aortic aneurysm, tamponade
Pulmonary	Acute pulmonary edema, pneumonia, bronchitis, pulmonary embolus, pneumothorax, pleurisy, pleural effusion, tuberculosis
Gastrointestinal	Esophagitis, esophageal spasm, esophageal rupture, GERD, peptic ulcer disease, pancreatitis, cholecystitis, cholelithiasis, biliary disease, hiatal hernia, hepatitis, splenic infarction
Neurologic	Stroke, intracranial hemorrhage, TIA, radiculopathy, altered mental status, delirium
Musculoskeletal	Muscular strain, costochondritis, injuries involving the cervical or thoracic spine, disorders of shoulder joint, chest wall trauma, herpes zoster
Psychiatric	Anxiety, panic attack, hyperventilation syndrome
Other	Cocaine, methamphetamine use

GERD, gastroesophageal reflux disease; LV, left ventricle; TIA, transient ischemic attack; VF, ventricular fibrillation; VT, ventricular tachycardia.

that patients should be treated with antiplatelet or antithrombotic agents for demand ischemia, although risk factors for CAD should be evaluated and treated. In addition, these patients are unlikely to benefit from coronary revascularization and, indeed, not all will even have obstructive CAD. After resolution of the underlying stressors and achievement of clinical stability, noninvasive stress testing may be performed to assess for obstructive CAD.

▶ Complications

Major MI complications are more common with STEMI than NSTEMI and include acute heart failure, cardiogenic shock, conduction disturbances (eg, bundle branch block, advanced atrioventricular [AV] block, ventricular arrhythmias), LV free wall or ventricular septal rupture, papillary muscle ischemia or rupture, LV aneurysm, stroke, and sudden death. Each complication is associated with worse prognosis and occurs two to four times more frequently in older patients. Ischemic mitral regurgitation affects up to 50% of patients with ACS and can lead to pulmonary edema and reduced cardiac output. LV free wall rupture, which usually occurs 3 to 6 days after MI, is a relatively rare catastrophic complication with a very high mortality rate that requires definitive emergency surgical treatment. Dressler syndrome is an immune-mediated phenomenon where patients present with signs and symptoms of pericarditis several weeks after MI.

▶ Treatment

Table 39–3 lists the major therapeutic options for all patients with ACS. In general, the following therapeutic options should be pursued in ACS: aspirin, P2Y12 inhibitor, high-intensity statin, β-blocker, and angiotensin-converting enzyme (ACE) inhibitor and mineralocorticoid receptor antagonist in patients with reduced ejection fraction. For patients with STEMI, coronary angiography with likely percutaneous coronary intervention (PCI) or thrombolysis (depending on PCI availability) is crucial.

A. STEMI

STEMI is a medical emergency that requires immediate revascularization to protect and salvage myocardium from ischemia. In general, revascularization should be attempted with a goal of door to device time of less than 90 minutes or a door to needle time for fibrinolytics of 60 minutes.

B. Non–ST-Segment Elevation ACS

Patients with non–ST-segment elevation ACS (UA or NSTEMI) should be triaged to either an early invasive or ischemia-guided strategy. Early invasive strategy (coronary angiography followed by PCI within 24 hours) should be pursued if patients have cardiogenic shock or intermediate- or high-risk features, including refractory angina, new-onset

Table 39–3. Management of acute myocardial infarction.

General measures
    Oxygen to maintain arterial saturation ≥90%
    Nitroglycerin for ischemia and heart failure
Reperfusion therapy
    Fibrinolysis (STEMI only)
    Primary percutaneous coronary intervention
    CABG
Antithrombotic therapy
    Antiplatelet
Aspirin
    P2Y12 inhibitor
    Anticoagulant
    Heparin/low-molecular-weight heparin
Glycoprotein IIb/IIIa inhibitor
β-Blockers
Angiotensin-converting enzyme inhibitors (ACEi)
Other medications
    Nitrates
    Angiotensin receptor blockers (if intolerant to ACEi)
    Calcium channel blockers
    Lipid-lowering agents (high-intensity statin preferred)
    Magnesium
    Potassium (range, 3.5–4.5 mEq/L)

CABG, coronary artery bypass graft; STEMI, ST-segment elevation myocardial infarction.

heart failure, age >75 years, transient ST-segment deviation, sustained ventricular tachycardia, GRACE score >140, or significantly elevated biomarkers. Data primarily from registries and meta-analyses indicate that older adults (>75 years) can benefit from an early invasive strategy; however, it is important to recognize contraindications to invasive procedures and to mitigate risk. Older patients are more likely to have multimorbidity, contraindications to invasive procedures, and increased risk of complications from coronary angiography (eg, contrast-induced nephropathy and bleeding). For patients with low-risk clinical features and stabilization after medical management, an ischemia-guided strategy can be appropriate; invasive procedures are deferred unless recurrent ischemic symptoms or hemodynamic instability develop. These decisions should include patient preferences and assessment of risks and benefits in older adults, taking into account frailty, overall health status, and desire for invasive procedures versus medical management.

For UA, the primary goals of therapy are symptom relief and preventing progression to NSTEMI or STEMI. Guidelines recommend that older patients receive the same treatment as younger patients with close monitoring for adverse events and with the caution that their general health, comorbidities, cognitive status, baseline functional status, and life expectancy be considered, and that increased sensitivity to hypotension-inducing drugs and possible altered pharmacokinetics be considered.

C. Critically Ill Older Adults with ACS

The highest risk, critically ill patients with recurrent or persistent ischemia despite intensive medical therapy resulting in cardiogenic shock or unstable ventricular arrhythmias may benefit from inotropes and mechanical circulatory support to improve their hemodynamics while awaiting definitive therapy. Inotropes, including dobutamine (β_1-adrenoreceptor agonist) and milrinone (phosphodiesterase-3 inhibitor), should be considered in patients with severe cardiogenic shock. Vasopressors, including norepinephrine, epinephrine, and dopamine, may be required to augment blood pressure due to the vasodilatory effects of inotropes. These agents should be used when patients have central access and continuous arterial blood pressure monitoring. Mechanical support includes intra-aortic balloon pump counterpulsation, percutaneous LV assist devices (eg, Impella), and extracorporeal membrane oxygenation. Before inotropes, vasopressors, and mechanical life support are started in older patients, their preferences and goals of care should be carefully assessed, given the high morbidity and mortality rates. Symptom management and end-of-life planning are important, and palliative care consultation is helpful.

D. General Measures

Maintenance of adequate arterial oxygenation and relief of chest discomfort are important goals. Supplemental oxygen should only be given if the patient is hypoxic (SpO_2 <92%), as studies have shown that supplemental oxygen in the absence of hypoxia is associated with higher levels of biomarkers and larger infarct sizes, likely due to increased reperfusion injury.

Angina should be initially treated with β-blockers and sublingual nitrates. Nitroglycerin should be avoided in right ventricular infarction because it may precipitate significant hypotension. Patients with persistent chest pain or signs of pulmonary congestion should receive topical nitroglycerin ointment or an intravenous nitroglycerin infusion, titrated to control symptoms while avoiding excessive blood pressure reduction. Morphine is associated with increased mortality in observational studies, and nonsteroidal anti-inflammatory drugs should be avoided because they have prothrombotic effects and are associated with worse cardiovascular outcomes.

E. Reperfusion Therapy

In STEMI, recanalization of the involved coronary artery as quickly as possible reduces mortality and morbid complications in all patients. Reperfusion can be achieved either pharmacologically with fibrinolytics or mechanically with PCI with stent implantation. In general, mechanical reperfusion is more effective than fibrinolysis if it can be achieved in a timely manner because of lower mortality, reinfarction, and stroke rates. PCI has a lower risk of intracranial hemorrhage, particularly in patients older than 75 years, in whom the risk of intracranial bleeding is 1% to 2% with fibrinolysis.

PCI benefits patients with both STEMI and NSTEMI (see later discussion), whereas fibrinolytic therapy is only effective in STEMI and is contraindicated in the treatment of NSTEMI.

Select older patients may benefit from CABG over PCI in the setting of ACS, although selection criteria are not clear in patients >80 years due to absence of randomized data in this patient population. Coronary artery bypass graft (CABG) may be preferred in low to intermediate surgical risk patients, complex multivessel CAD, unprotected left main disease, diabetes, LV dysfunction, and no prior sternotomy. In these patients, CABG has been shown to reduce future readmissions, revascularization procedures, and cardiovascular events compared to PCI, although some data suggest no significant differences in all-cause mortality, death, or MI between PCI and CABG for some clinical scenarios. The mortality rate from CABG in patients >80 years is 5% to 8%, and older patients are at increased risk of ischemic and bleeding complications and prolonged recovery time requiring postoperative rehabilitation compared to PCI. Aspirin should be continued preoperatively, whereas P2Y12 inhibitors should be held for a minimum of 5 days prior to elective CABG to reduce risk of CABG-related bleeding.

1. PCI—One of the main differences in the management of STEMI versus NSTEMI/UA is the timing of mechanical reperfusion, defined as PCI with or without stenting. In STEMI, the recommended door-to-balloon time (ie, the time from the patient's arrival in the ED to when a coronary artery guide wire crosses the culprit lesion in the catheterization laboratory) is 90 minutes. In NSTEMI/UA, the timing of PCI depends on patient risk factors and clinical features (see earlier section "Non–ST-Segment Elevation ACS"). Fibrinolysis is generally used only if a patient cannot receive PCI (including time of transfer to a PCI-capable facility) within 120 minutes. Rescue PCI should be considered for failed reperfusion (repeat ECG 90 minutes after fibrinolysis does not show improvement of ST elevation), recurrent ST elevation, and ongoing hemodynamic instability or cardiogenic shock.

In NSTEMI patients, early angiography and coronary intervention are associated with improved short- and long-term outcomes, including recurrent angina, MI, and cardiovascular death. Mechanical reperfusion, if available, is the preferred strategy in older patients with documented ACS, although it is used less often than in younger patients. Older patients have a lower rate of angiographic success and less ST-segment resolution, likely due to presence of multivessel disease. In addition, older patients also suffer from more complications, including bleeding, vascular complications, embolic and neurologic complications, and contrast nephropathy.

In both STEMI and NSTEMI, either bare metal stents (BMSs) or drug-eluting stents (DESs) can be implanted. Both provide a mechanical framework for coronary artery patency; DESs include a polymer coating with an antiproliferative drug (eg, everolimus, sirolimus). DESs are generally preferred because they have a lower long-term risk of restenosis. However, DESs require a longer duration of treatment with dual antiplatelet agents to prevent recurrent ischemic events, although at least 12 months are recommended for all patients. BMSs may be preferred in patients with poor medication compliance, elevated risk of bleeding, or semi-urgent noncardiac surgery to minimize duration of dual antiplatelet therapy.

2. Fibrinolytics—The five fibrinolytic agents approved for intravenous use for the treatment of STEMI in the United States are streptokinase, alteplase, anistreplase, reteplase, and tenecteplase. Use of fibrinolytic agents should be restricted to those who fulfill criteria for fibrinolysis and can be treated within 12 hours of symptom onset but are unable to undergo PCI within 120 minutes upon arrival to the hospital (Table 39–4). Patients who receive fibrinolytics must be treated with anticoagulation for at least 48 hours to prevent rethrombosis. Older patients have a higher likelihood of having a contraindication to thrombolytic therapy. In-hospital mortality increases with increasing age along with the risk of intracranial hemorrhage and ventricular free wall rupture in older patients receiving fibrinolytics.

F. Antithrombotic Therapy

1. Aspirin—Aspirin is indicated for all patients with ACS. It is effective in older adults and should be continued indefinitely in all patients with documented CAD to prevent further ischemic events. The recommended dosage in the acute setting of ACS is a loading dose of non–enteric-coated aspirin 325 mg, followed by 81 mg daily for long-term use.

2. Anticoagulation—Anticoagulation is indicated in patients with ACS. All patients receive anticoagulation with either unfractionated heparin or bivalirudin during PCI. Anticoagulation is indicated in patients receiving a short-acting fibrinolytic agent (eg, recombinant tissue-type plasminogen activator) for at least 48 hours to prevent rethrombosis. In medically managed ACS, anticoagulation is indicated for 48 hours. After successful PCI, anticoagulation can be discontinued unless there is another indication for ongoing anticoagulation (eg, prevention of thromboembolism in atrial fibrillation).

Anticoagulant options include weight-adjusted unfractionated heparin (UFH), bivalirudin (direct thrombin inhibitor), low-molecular-weight heparin (LMWH) agents such as enoxaparin and dalteparin, fondaparinux (selective inhibitor of activated factor X), and argatroban. LMWH provides more stable anticoagulation than UFH and offers the advantage of subcutaneous administration without the need to monitor activated partial thromboplastin time. In addition, LMWHs have been associated with improved clinical outcomes, including reduced risk of death, recurrent MI, or refractory ischemia, compared to UFH. However, LMWHs are contraindicated in renal failure and have been associated with increased bleeding in older adults, which may be due to decreased creatinine clearance. Dose adjustment for enoxaparin is recommended in patients >75 years old. Fondaparinux is contraindicated if the creatinine clearance is <30 mL/min. Argatroban, a direct thrombin inhibitor that is hepatically cleared, is generally reserved for patients with an allergy to heparin or prior heparin-induced thrombocytopenia.

Table 39–4. Criteria for fibrinolytic therapy in older adults with ST-segment elevation myocardial infarction.

Indications	Contraindications

Symptoms of acute MI within 6–12 hours of onset, particularly with very early presentation within 2 hours of symptom onset, if it is anticipated that primary PCI cannot be performed within 120 minutes of first medical contact
ST elevation ≥1 mm in 2 or more contiguous leads with exception of ≥2 mm in leads V2-V3; patients with new LBBB with symptoms consistent with ACS are also considered eligible
After fibrinolysis, all patients should be transferred to a PCI-capable center
	Absolute
	  Previous hemorrhagic stroke at any time
	  Any stroke or cerebrovascular event within 1 year
	  Known intracranial neoplasm or vascular lesion
	  Suspected aortic dissection or acute pericarditis
	  Active bleeding
	  Significant closed-head or facial trauma within 3 months
	  Severe uncontrolled hypertension
	Relative
	  Blood pressure ≥180/110 mm Hg on presentation, not readily controlled
	  History of ischemic stroke >3 months
	  Known bleeding disorder
	  Recent major trauma or internal bleeding (within 2–4 weeks)
	  Noncompressible vascular puncture (eg, subclavian intravenous catheter)
	  Active peptic ulcer disease
	  Dementia
	  Trauma or prolonged (>10 minutes) CPR

ACS, acute coronary syndrome; CPR, cardiopulmonary resuscitation; LBBB, left bundle branch block; MI, myocardial infarction; PCI, percutaneous coronary intervention.

3. Antiplatelet therapy—In addition to aspirin, most patients should receive dual antiplatelet therapy (DAPT) that includes a P2Y12 receptor inhibitor (clopidogrel, ticagrelor, or prasugrel). Dual antiplatelet therapy is indicated for all patients with ACS, including those managed medically without PCI. Antiplatelet medications reduce post-PCI stent thrombosis and recurrent ischemic events, which are higher in older adults. In addition, these agents reduce cardiovascular mortality, nonfatal MI, and nonfatal stroke by approximately 20% compared with aspirin alone during long-term therapy after NSTEMI. However, the benefits of DAPT must be weighed against increased risk of major bleeding. Clopidogrel is the most commonly used ADP receptor antagonist. The loading dose is 300 to 600 mg orally followed by 75 mg daily.

Ticagrelor and prasugrel are more potent platelet inhibitors compared to clopidogrel. Ticagrelor reduces cardiovascular events compared to clopidogrel, even in patients >75 years old, although it is associated with higher bleeding risk. The loading dose of ticagrelor is 180 mg orally once, followed by 90 mg twice daily. Prasugrel also has fewer ischemic complications compared to clopidogrel but is not recommended in patients older than 75 years, <60 kg, or with a history of intracranial hemorrhage or stroke/transient ischemic attack due to increased bleeding risk. Older adults who are at increased risk of gastrointestinal bleeding should be treated with a proton pump inhibitor while on DAPT.

Duration of DAPT is dependent on the setting in which PCI was performed (ACS vs stable ischemic heart disease) and type of stent placed (BMS vs DES). In the setting of stable ischemic heart disease, DAPT should be continued for at least 1 month after BMS placement and at least 6 months after DES placement. In the setting of ACS (with or without PCI), DAPT should be continued for at least 12 months in the absence of significant overt bleeding (ACC/AHA class I recommendation). Older patients, especially those with history of prior significant bleeding, CKD, diabetes, or low body weight, are at increased risk of severe bleeding complications. In rare cases, P2Y12 inhibitor therapy can be reduced to 3 months in stable ischemic heart disease and 6 months after ACS (ACC/AHA class IIb recommendation). Benefits of reducing ischemia, risks of stent thrombosis, and risk of bleeding with longer term DAPT should be balanced against patient preferences, including risk of polypharmacy. Interventional cardiologists performing the PCI may have more specific recommendations as well, based on coronary anatomy and PCI procedure, and should be consulted in determining antiplatelet therapy duration.

4. Glycoprotein IIb/IIIa inhibitors—These potent antiplatelet agents reversibly block the final pathway leading to platelet aggregation. Available agents include abciximab, eptifibatide, and tirofiban. Most data for these agents came prior to the routine use of P2Y12 inhibitors. Glycoprotein IIb/IIIa inhibitors were shown to reduce the risk of recurrent ischemic events and improve clinical outcomes in patients with documented MI undergoing percutaneous coronary revascularization. Risk of bleeding is higher in older adults; dosage adjustment for tirofiban and eptifibatide is necessary in patients with impaired renal function. If used, glycoprotein IIb/IIIa inhibitor therapy is given for 12 to 24 hours in addition to oral DAPT and heparin at the time of PCI. Their use is usually reserved for patients with high thrombus burden and poor arterial recanalization at time of PCI.

G. β-Blockers

Administration of β-blockers within the first 24 hours in appropriately selected ACS patients reduces mortality because of reduced sudden cardiac death and recurrent ischemic events. β-blocker therapy should be initiated as soon as possible in all patients with suspected ACS in the absence of contraindications (ie, cardiogenic shock, heart rate <50 beats/min, SBP <90–100 mm Hg, PR interval ≥240 milliseconds, heart block greater than first degree, moderate or severe pulmonary congestion, or active bronchospasm).

Cardioselective β-blockers are preferred, and metoprolol and atenolol have been approved for treatment of ACS. Patients receiving intravenous β-blockers should be carefully observed for bradyarrhythmias, hypotension, dyspnea, and bronchospasm. It is prudent to start with lower dosages and slower dose augmentation in patients older than 75 years and in those with multiple comorbidities. Dose adjustment is necessary for atenolol in renal impairment. Patients with reduced LV function should be prescribed an evidence-based β-blocker (eg, metoprolol succinate, carvedilol, or bisoprolol; see Chapter 40, "Heart Failure & Heart Rhythm Disorders").

H. ACE Inhibitors & Angiotensin Receptor Blockers

ACE inhibitors reduce mortality in patients with anterior STEMIs and MIs complicated by clinical heart failure and significant LV systolic dysfunction (LV ejection fraction <40%). They can also be considered in patients with preserved ejection fraction. Absolute contraindications to ACE inhibitors include bilateral renal artery stenosis and history of angioedema related to ACE inhibitor use. Relative contraindications include SBP <90 to 100 mm Hg, worsening renal function, and hyperkalemia; these are more common in patients >75 years old. ACE inhibitor therapy can be initiated with short-acting captopril 6.25 mg three times a day or lisinopril 2.5 mg daily. Once the maintenance dose has been achieved, changing to a once-daily agent at equivalent dosage (eg, lisinopril 20–40 mg) is appropriate. Throughout the initiation and titration phase of ACE inhibitor therapy, blood pressure, serum creatinine, and potassium should be monitored. Angiotensin receptor blockers (ARBs) are generally used for patients who do not tolerate ACE inhibitors because of cough.

I. Lipid-Lowering Agents

3-Hydroxy-3-methylglutaryl–coenzyme A (HMG-CoA) reductase inhibitors (statins) should be initiated early in the course of ACS at high doses (eg, atorvastatin 40–80 mg or rosuvastatin 20–40 mg) and continued indefinitely because they decrease mortality and recurrent ischemic events after NSTEMI and STEMI.

J. Nitrates

Nitrate preparations are effective in controlling ischemia, treating heart failure, and managing hypertension in patients with ACS due to their coronary vasodilating effects and reduction of preload and ventricular wall tension. Nitrates should be avoided in right ventricular infarction or with recent use of phosphodiesterase inhibitors (eg, sildenafil, tadalafil). As noted earlier, the options include sublingual nitroglycerin, topical nitroglycerin ointment, and intravenous nitroglycerin infusion. Nitrate tolerance generally occurs within about 24 hours.

K. Calcium Channel Blockers

Calcium channel blockers can be used for recurrent ischemia due to their coronary artery vasodilatory properties, especially if β-blockers are ineffective or not tolerated. Nondihydropyridines (eg, verapamil, diltiazem) are preferred for their antianginal effect with less likelihood of causing hypotension compared to dihydropyridines (eg, nifedipine, amlodipine). These agents should be avoided in patients with reduced LV function, impending cardiogenic shock, AV or sinus node dysfunction, and PR interval >240 milliseconds. Short-acting nifedipine should be avoided in patients with ACS as it has been associated with increased mortality in patients with CAD.

L. Mineralocorticoid Receptor Antagonists

Aldosterone antagonists (eg, spironolactone, eplerenone) should be provided to all patients after an MI who have an ejection fraction of ≤40%, diabetes, or heart failure and are already on an ACE inhibitor and β-blocker. These medications are contraindicated for men with a creatinine >2.5 mg/dL and women with a creatinine >2.0 mg/dL or potassium >5.0 mEq/L.

M. Potassium & Magnesium

Potassium should be maintained within a range of 3.5 to 4.5 mEq/L and magnesium above 2.0 mEq/L.

▶ Prognosis

Approximately 15% to 20% of patients with STEMI die before reaching the hospital, a proportion that likely increases with advancing age. Among patients with recognized ACS, both short- and long-term mortality increase progressively with age. Other factors associated with increased mortality include anterior MI, clinical heart failure, impaired LV systolic function, atrial fibrillation, complex ventricular arrhythmias, poor functional status, diabetes mellitus, and lack of guideline-based treatment. Although short-term prognosis is more favorable in NSTEMI than in STEMI, mortality rates at 2 years are similar. After ACS, patients should be referred to comprehensive cardiac rehabilitation and encouraged to slowly resume regular physical activity, as tolerated by symptoms.

Amsterdam EA, Wenger NK, Brindis RG, et al. 2014 AHA/ACC guidelines for the management of patients with non-ST elevation acute coronary syndromes: report of the American College of Cardiology/American Heart Association Task Force on Practice Guidelines. *J Am Coll Cardiol.* 2014;64(24):e139-e228.

Levine GN, Bates ER, Bittl JA, et al. 2016 ACC/AHA guideline focused update on duration of dual antiplatelet therapy in patients with coronary artery disease. *J Am Coll Cardiol.* 2016;68(10):1082-1115.

Patel MR, Calhoon JH, Dehmer GJ, et al. ACC/AATS/AHA/ASE/ASNC/SCAI/SCCT/STS 2016: appropriate use criteria for coronary revascularization in patients with acute coronary syndromes. *J Am Coll Cardiol.* 2017;69(17):2212-2241.

Thygesen K, Alpert JS, Jaffe AS, et al. Executive Group on behalf of the Joint European Society of Cardiology (ESC)/American College of Cardiology (ACC)/American Heart Association (AHA)/World Heart Federation (WHF) Task Force for the Universal Definition of Myocardial Infarction. Fourth universal definition of myocardial infarction (2018). *Circulation.* 2018;138:e618-e651.

Williams MA, Fleg JL, Ades PA, et al. American Heart Association Council on Clinical Cardiology Subcommittee on Exercise, Cardiac Rehabilitation, and Prevention. Secondary prevention of coronary heart disease in the elderly (with emphasis on patients > or =75 years of age): an American Heart Association scientific statement from the Council on Clinical Cardiology Subcommittee on Exercise, Cardiac Rehabilitation, and Prevention. *Circulation.* 2002;105(14):1735-1743.

CHRONIC CORONARY ARTERY DISEASE

▶ General Principles

Chronic CAD is defined as plaque within the coronary arteries without ACS. It is due to chronic coronary atherosclerosis that starts with intimal thickening and then progresses to a large plaque containing lipids, platelets, and apoptotic macrophages. Due to lumen narrowing and coronary artery blood flow obstruction, chronic CAD can lead to angina and exertional symptoms, such as shortness of breath and angina. Chronic stable angina is the most common form of CAD and is the initial form of presentation in 80% of patients. The overall prevalence of stable ischemic heart disease is 24.8% in patients aged 75 to 79 years old and 29.3% in patients aged 80 to 84 years old. Although the incidence and prevalence of CAD are both higher in men than in women, the rates for women increase progressively after menopause, and the greater longevity of women compared with men results in a slight predominance of women in the total number of people with CAD. Compared to younger patients, older patients are more likely to have left main CAD, multivessel CAD, and LV dysfunction.

Prevention

Primary prevention of CAD includes lifelong avoidance of tobacco products; participation in regular physical exercise; maintenance of desirable body weight; consumption of a diet rich in fruits, vegetables, and whole-grain foods; and limited consumption of foods high in trans and saturated fats and cholesterol. Early identification and aggressive treatment of risk factors, as discussed earlier, are essential.

Clinical Findings

A. Symptoms & Signs

The most common symptom of chronic CAD is central chest discomfort, often described as pressure, tightness, or heaviness, typically brought on by physical exertion or emotional stress and relieved by rest or nitroglycerin. The discomfort may radiate to or primarily be in the jaw, left or both arms, back, or epigastrium. The discomfort typically lasts longer than a few minutes and up to 20 to 30 minutes and is usually not alleviated by deep breathing, coughing, or arm movement. However, many older adults with CAD manifest atypical symptoms, including dyspnea, fatigue, weakness, dizziness, or abdominal discomfort, whereas others, particularly people with diabetes, are entirely asymptomatic. In addition, due to the high prevalence of frailty, pulmonary disease, and peripheral arterial disease in older adults, they may not experience exertional symptoms (see Chapter 65, "Chest Pain").

Myocardial ischemia occurs when the myocardial oxygen demands are not met by an increase in myocardial blood supply. The earliest events are increased myocardial stiffness of the ischemic myocardium, followed by decreased contractility, metabolic alterations resulting in increased lactic acid formation, changes in electrical repolarization, and finally the discomfort we recognize as angina. The symptoms and events created can be angina, dyspnea, or the development of malignant ventricular arrhythmias, including sudden death.

Angina is graded using the Canadian Cardiovascular Society classification system based on the level of activity required to produce symptoms (Table 39–5).

Table 39–5. Canadian Cardiovascular Society classification of angina.

Class I: No discomfort with ordinary activity (eg, walking, climbing stairs), only with strenuous exertion
Class II: Angina mildly limiting ordinary activity (eg, >2 blocks walking on level surface, >1 flight of stairs at normal pace)
Class III: Angina markedly limiting ordinary activity (eg, walking <2 blocks on level surface, <1 flight of stairs)
Class IV: Angina with any activity or at rest; inability to perform any physical activity without discomfort

The physical examination in patients with chronic CAD can be entirely normal. Some patients might have nonspecific physical findings, including an S_3 or S_4 gallop, mitral regurgitation murmur, a laterally displaced or dyskinetic apical impulse (especially in patients with prior MI), or signs of heart failure (eg, pulmonary rales, elevated JVP, peripheral edema).

B. Testing

Basic laboratory tests can reveal factors that contribute to the pathophysiology of stable angina such as complete blood count (anemia), thyroid-stimulating hormone (hyperthyroidism), B-type natriuretic peptide, and toxicology screen (eg, cocaine or amphetamine use).

1. ECG—The ECG may demonstrate pathologic Q waves in patients with prior MI. Other ECG findings, including bundle branch blocks and T-wave inversions, are nonspecific. The ECG is especially informative if performed while the patient is experiencing chest discomfort. At such times, flat or down-sloping ST depression may be seen. The ECG might be entirely normal if the patient is not experiencing angina when the ECG is performed.

2. Echocardiogram—The echocardiogram is a noninvasive ultrasound that can evaluate LV and right ventricular function, diastolic function, valvular function, and cardiac structural pathologies. Patients with CAD can have reduced LV function, myocardial wall thinning from prior infarction, and wall motion abnormalities in a coronary artery distribution. New wall motion abnormalities in a coronary artery distribution in the setting of chest pain, ECG changes, and troponin elevation indicate ACS and should prompt treatment.

3. Stress tests—Noninvasive stress testing can be used for diagnosing flow-limiting CAD in symptomatic patients (eg, including those with chest pain, negative biomarkers, and nonischemic ECG), as well as for risk stratification in patients with known CAD (eg, history of MI) and risk factors (eg, peripheral arterial disease). High-risk stress test findings are associated with a >3% cardiac mortality rate per year.

The stress modality can be exercise or pharmacologic. Exercise modalities include the treadmill (generally using the standard or modified Bruce protocol) or an upright or recumbent bicycle. If possible, an exercise test is generally preferred because the exercise duration (at least 4–6 minutes) independently predicts prognosis. In older adults, exercise duration may be limited by musculoskeletal pain, physical deconditioning, claudication, neurologic conditions, dizziness, and early fatigue. Fewer older adults can achieve 85% of maximal estimated heart rate (which is the threshold for a diagnostic study) compared to younger patients. Contraindications to exercise stress testing include high-risk UA, poorly controlled baseline hypertension (SBP >200 mm Hg), uncontrolled cardiac arrhythmias, severe aortic stenosis, recent MI or pulmonary embolus, and hypertrophic obstructive cardiomyopathy.

Pharmacologic stressors include dobutamine (positive inotrope, infusion protocol with escalating doses until 85% of maximum predicted heart rate is reached) and vasodilators, including adenosine, dipyridamole, and regadenoson. These vasoactive agents increase coronary blood flow and may provoke ischemia. Vasodilators should be avoided in patients with second- or third-degree AV block, active bronchospasm, and systemic hypotension (SBP <90 mm Hg). Competitive inhibitors of adenosine receptors, including caffeine and theophylline, should be held for 48 hours prior to vasodilator stress testing.

The detection modalities in stress testing include ECG, echocardiogram, radionuclide imaging (single-photon emission computed tomography [SPECT] myocardial perfusion imaging [MPI] or positron emission tomography), or cardiac magnetic resonance imaging (MRI). Addition of myocardial imaging increases sensitivity for detection of CAD. An ECG stress test can only be interpreted if the resting ECG is normal; baseline LBBB, paced rhythm, ventricular preexcitation, Q waves, or ST-segment changes preclude accurate diagnosis. Radionuclide imaging techniques can also assess myocardial viability, perfusion, cardiac size and global function, and transient ischemic dilation (which is a marker of multivessel CAD). Pharmacologic vasodilator stress testing is recommended in patients with LBBB, permanent pacemakers, and ventricular preexcitation. Pharmacologic SPECT MPI has a sensitivity of 88% to 91%, and a specificity of 75% to 90%. Cardiac MRI is less frequently used in the acute setting, although it can detect and localize even small areas of obstructive CAD.

4. Coronary angiography—Coronary angiography remains the gold standard for determining the presence, extent, and severity of CAD, as well as the suitability for percutaneous or surgical revascularization. Older patients are more likely to have multivessel disease and left main CAD. Complications associated with invasive coronary angiography include infection, bleeding, vascular complications (eg, aneurysm), arrhythmias, hypotension, stroke, coronary artery dissection, and death. Radial arterial access is generally preferred over femoral arterial access because it decreases risk of bleeding and vascular complications and has even been shown to have lower mortality rates.

5. Other tests—Computed tomography (CT) coronary angiography uses low-dose multidetector CT imaging to diagnose, visualize, and characterize CAD. It has 98% sensitivity and 90% specificity of detecting CAD with a very high negative predictive value.

Noncontrast low-dose CT directly measures coronary atherosclerosis and determines a coronary artery calcium (CAC) score (also called Agatston score), which improves risk prediction in older patients with multiple CAD risk factors. It is an independent predictor of CAD events, including MI and death from CAD, even in the absence of risk factors. Patients with CAC score of 0 have a very low risk of CAD

events. Higher CAC scores, particularly when combined with multiple risk factors, are associated with significantly increased risk of CAD events. In older patients with a mean age of 80 years, approximately 36% of patents have significant subclinical CAD with an Agatston score >400. CAC scores can be used to guide preventative therapies, including lifestyle modification and medications (eg, statins, aspirin).

Differential Diagnosis

Please see Table 39–2. Angina as a result of myocardial ischemia can occur whenever there is an imbalance between myocardial oxygen demand and supply. Other diseases where angina is a symptom without epicardial CAD are valvular aortic stenosis, hypertrophic cardiomyopathy, and myocarditis. With nonobstructive coronary artery plaques, an unusual increase in myocardial oxygen demand can result in myocardial ischemia and angina. Some causes include hyperthyroidism, arteriovenous fistulae, and excessive sympathetic stimulation. Patients with anemia, hypoxemia, and hyperviscosity can have decreased oxygen delivery resulting in angina.

Complications

The major complications of chronic CAD are ACS, refractory angina, development of heart failure because of the cumulative effects of myocardial injury or infarction (ischemic cardiomyopathy), and development of conduction abnormalities or arrhythmias, including ventricular tachycardia and ventricular fibrillation. Sudden cardiac death is the initial manifestation of CAD in up to 20% of cases.

Risk Stratification

The patients at highest risk are those with ACS. In patients with chronic CAD, the risk increases with higher Canadian Cardiovascular Society class; decreased LV ejection fraction; location, severity, and extent of coronary artery stenosis; high-risk noninvasive stress test; poorer general physical health; multimorbidity; poorer functional capacity; cognitive dysfunction; and uncontrolled cardiovascular risk factors.

Treatment

A. Goals of Treatment

The goals of therapy for chronic CAD are to control symptoms to allow patients to resume normal activities, prevent or slow progression, and prevent major complications. Risk factors should be aggressively managed with lifestyle and pharmacologic interventions. Given that older patients often have multiple chronic conditions and are at risk of polypharmacy, medical management can be challenging, so decision making should include patient priorities. In addition, pharmacodynamics can be altered in older patients, resulting in reduced bioavailability of medications. Because myocardial ischemia is the basis for the symptoms, the factors involved in myocardial oxygen demand must be considered. The major requirements for myocardial oxygen demand are myocardial contractility and LV wall tension, the determinants of which are the SBP, LV diastolic radius, LV wall thickness, LV end-diastolic pressure, and heart rate. The coronary blood flow to the myocardium depends on the degree of coronary artery obstruction and changes that impact patency determined by the severity of the atherosclerotic plaque, plaque rupture with platelet aggregation or thrombus, varying degrees of coronary vascular tone, and coronary spasm. The pharmacologic approach to therapy addresses the following factors:

1. *Decrease in myocardial oxygen demand:* β-blockers, ACE inhibitors, ARBs, treatment of hypertension, lowering of heart rate

2. *Increase coronary blood flow:* nitrates, Ca^{2+} channel blockers

3. *Decrease factors causing obstruction:* nitrates, antiplatelet drugs

4. *Revascularization:* coronary bypass surgery, PCI with or without stenting

Overall, optimal treatment involves lifestyle modifications, risk factor reduction, pharmacologic interventions, and in selected patients, percutaneous or surgical revascularization.

B. Lifestyle Modifications

Lifestyle modification has been shown to reduce cardiovascular risk in all age groups. Primary risk factors include cigarette smoking, elevated blood pressure, dyslipidemia (elevated LDL-C and total cholesterol, reduced HDL-C), diabetes mellitus, and calculated 10-year risk of atherosclerotic CVD. All patients with CAD should be strongly advised to discontinue all tobacco products. Gradual weight reduction through diet and regular exercise should be encouraged in overweight patients (ie, body mass index >25 kg/m²). Patients with CAD should eat a balanced diet rich in fruits, vegetables, and whole grains while limiting intake of trans and saturated fats (including partially hydrogenated oils) and cholesterol while engaging in at least 150 to 300 minutes of moderate-intensity physical activity weekly, unless limited by active cardiovascular symptoms or other medical conditions. Walking, stationary cycling, and swimming are suitable exercise modalities for older adults with mild functional impairments. When beginning an exercise program, patients should be instructed to start at a slow and comfortable pace, gradually increasing the duration and intensity over a period of weeks. Patients with a history of MI, prior PCI, or coronary artery bypass surgery should be strongly encouraged to participate in a formal cardiac rehabilitation program.

Such programs have been associated with reduced mortality, improved exercise tolerance and quality of life, and enhanced mood and sense of well-being.

C. Pharmacotherapy

1. Aspirin—Long-term use of aspirin in CAD patients reduces the risk of death, nonfatal MI, and stroke. The absolute benefit is greatest in high-risk patients, including those older than 65 years. Aspirin for primary prevention in patients >80 years old without confirmed CAD may not be beneficial due to increased risk of bleeding requiring hospitalization or transfusion. The optimal dose of aspirin is likely 75 to 100 mg once daily (in the United States, 81 mg daily is usually used), which provides benefits equivalent to higher doses with a lower risk of bleeding. In patients intolerant to low-dose aspirin, clopidogrel 75 mg daily is an acceptable alternative.

2. β-Blockers—β-Blockers reduce the risk of death and reinfarction and reduce adverse ventricular remodeling after MI. β-Blockers are also highly effective antianginal agents because they reduce myocardial oxygen demand and may reduce the incidence of coronary events in patients with chronic CAD. It is reasonable to start β-blockers in all patients with a history of ACS (for at least 3 years following ACS and indefinitely in those with LV dysfunction with or without heart failure symptoms), unless contraindicated. The therapeutic goal is to gradually increase the dose until the patient has no or minimal ischemic symptoms and the resting heart rate is <60 beats/min. Older patients may be less tolerant of β-blockers because of the effects of aging on the conduction system and the presence of comorbidities (eg, pulmonary disease); therefore, dosages should be adjusted accordingly and heart rate and blood pressure monitored for bradycardia and hypotension.

3. Nitrates—Nitrates are effective antianginal agents and can reduce pulmonary congestion, although they do not provide a mortality benefit. Sublingual nitroglycerin remains the drug of choice for treatment of an acute episode of angina. As a result of drying of the oral mucosa in older adults, nitroglycerin spray may be more effective than tablets for older patients. Older patients may also be more likely to experience orthostatic hypotension with nitroglycerin; they should be advised to take the medication in a sitting or reclining position or at bedtime. Long-term nitrates, such as isosorbide mononitrate, are effective antianginal agents. In addition, tolerance to nitrates develops rapidly, requiring a daily 6- to 8-hour nitrate-free interval. Several oral and transdermal nitrate preparations are available for chronic use. If the patient has taken a phosphodiesterase-5 (PDE-5) inhibitor within 48 hours, any organic nitrate is strictly contraindicated because of the risk of excessive hypotension.

4. Calcium channel blockers—Calcium channel blockers are effective antihypertensive and antianginal medications, but they have not been shown to improve clinical outcomes or reduce mortality in CAD patients. In addition, they may be associated with worsening heart failure and, with the exception of amlodipine and felodipine, should be avoided in patients with impaired LV systolic function. Verapamil and diltiazem slow the heart rate and conduction through the AV node, especially when used in combination with β-blocker therapy, thus increasing the risk of bradyarrhythmias and syncope in older patients with conduction system disease. Verapamil and diltiazem also impair gastrointestinal motility and can lead to constipation or ileus. Other side effects include lower extremity edema and hypotension.

5. ACE inhibitors—ACE inhibitors do not exert a direct anti-ischemic effect, but reduce mortality and major cardiovascular events, including rates of MI and death, in a broad range of patients with established vascular disease or diabetes. In addition, ACE inhibitors improve outcomes in patients with reduced LV systolic function. ACE inhibitors should be given as first-line therapy in patients with CAD who have concomitant hypertension, reduced LV function, diabetes, and/or chronic renal disease.

6. ARBs—ARBs improve outcomes in patients with diabetes and in hypertensive patients with LV hypertrophy; however, the value of these agents in patients with CAD is unproven. Currently, routine use of ARBs in patients with CAD is generally in patients who require an ACE inhibitor but are intolerant due to side effects (eg, cough).

7. Lipid-lowering agents—Statins reduce mortality and cardiovascular morbidity in patients with CAD, and the benefits extend to patients at least up to the age of 75. There are insufficient data about risks and benefits of statin use in patients who are older than 80 years. Statins have been shown to reduce adverse cardiovascular events even in CAD patients who have LDL-C <100 mg/dL. This beneficial effect has been attributed to the cholesterol-independent pleiotropic effects of statins, including improving endothelial function, enhancing the stability of atherosclerotic plaques, decreasing vascular oxidative stress and inflammation, and inhibiting the thrombogenic response.

Patients with clinical atherosclerotic CVD, including CAD, should be on a high-intensity statin (atorvastatin 40 or 80 mg or rosuvastatin 20 or 40 mg) with the goal to reduce LDL-C levels to ≤70 mg/dL if not contraindicated. As with other medications, it is advisable to start with a lower dose and titrate the drug more slowly in patients older than 75 years, while monitoring lipid levels every 3 to 12 months. Side effects of statins include earlier onset of diabetes, myalgias, severe myopathy, and myositis. Myalgias, defined as muscle aches with normal creatinine kinase levels, are a common side effect, affecting up to 15% of patients and often resulting in discontinuation of therapy. For patients with myalgias, it is recommended to reduce the statin dose or trial another statin after temporary discontinuation and

to eliminate statin interactions with cytochrome P450 inhibitors. If LDL-C remains elevated, ezetimibe can be added to maximally tolerated statin and proprotein convertase subtilisin/kexin type 9 serine protease (PCSK-9) inhibitors may also be considered.

8. Anticoagulation—Anticoagulation is often indicated in older adults for prevention of thromboembolism from atrial fibrillation, history of venous thromboembolism (pulmonary embolism/deep vein thrombosis), and/or presence of a mechanical valve.

Older patients may have an indication for anticoagulation plus antiplatelet therapy (eg, atrial fibrillation and ACS with or without PCI). Triple therapy (anticoagulant plus aspirin plus P2Y12 inhibitor) is associated with a two- to three-fold increase in bleeding complications. Therefore, triple therapy should be reduced to a minimal duration, and dual therapy with an anticoagulant plus clopidogrel should be considered based on the WOEST trial, which showed reduction in bleeding events without ischemic complications compared to triple therapy. Trials have also shown that dabigatran, rivaroxaban, or apixaban plus clopidogrel reduces bleeding complications without increasing ischemic events compared to triple therapy.

9. Ranolazine—Ranolazine, an inhibitor of the late inward sodium channel and a partial fatty acid oxidation inhibitor, is approved by the US Food and Drug Administration for management of chronic angina. Because it does not affect heart rate or blood pressure, it is useful in patients who have not responded to other maximally tolerated antianginal medications and are not good candidates for revascularization. Its use should be carefully monitored in patients with prolonged QT intervals or on other QT-prolonging medications. Its side effects include nausea and constipation.

D. Other Therapies

For select patients with refractory angina despite revascularization and antianginal medications, external counterpulsation can be considered. External counterpulsation uses cuffs wrapped around the patient's calves, pelvis, and thighs and serial inflations up to 300 mm Hg to increase arterial blood pressure and retrograde blood flow during diastole. Studies have demonstrated fewer anginal episodes and exercise-induced ischemia in patients treated with external counterpulsation. However, it is not widely available in the United States.

E. Revascularization

Patients with stable CAD who can perform ordinary activity without symptoms on optimal medical therapy and who have normal LV function can be managed medically. In the COURAGE trial, patients with stable angina, objective evidence of myocardial ischemia, and an LV ejection fraction ≥30% with coronary vessels suitable for PCI were randomized to optimal medical management or PCI with optimal medical management. With a follow-up time of 2.5 to 7 years (median, 4.6 years), there was no difference between optimal medical management with or without PCI in the composite of MI, stroke, and death. Therefore, medical therapy should be maximally uptitrated to improve symptoms as tolerated by side effects, such as dizziness, hypotension, and bradycardia.

Coronary revascularization may be warranted for coronary artery stenoses that are hemodynamically flow limiting and associated with symptoms. If the significance of a moderate coronary lesion cannot be determined by visual inspection, intracoronary physiologic testing (instantaneous wave-free ratio or fractional flow reserve) should be performed to guide decision on PCI. PCI and coronary artery bypass surgery are effective in improving symptoms and quality of life in older patients with CAD. In fact, >50% of all revascularization procedures in the United States are now performed in patients older than 65 years. On the other hand, both PCI and bypass surgery are associated with increased mortality and major complications in older adults, especially in patients older than age 80 years; thus, careful selection of candidates for revascularization procedures is of paramount importance by taking into account the patient's preferences, functional status such as renal and neurologic function, and chronic conditions. Older patients must also be able to lie flat during PCI and tolerate moderate sedation.

The decision to pursue PCI versus CABG is often not straightforward in the geriatric population given the high incidence of complex, multivessel CAD. In general, PCI is associated with lower mortality and major morbidity (including stroke and delirium) as well as much more rapid recovery compared with coronary artery bypass surgery in older patients. However, the need for repeat revascularization procedures is significantly higher after PCI compared to CABG. Thus, both procedures represent suitable options for older patients with severe symptomatic CAD, and the choice of procedure should be based on anatomic considerations (eg, multivessel CAD, left main or proximal left anterior descending artery [LAD] stenoses), prevalent comorbidities (eg, heart failure with reduced ejection fraction, diabetes mellitus), and patient preferences. Up to 50% of older patients undergoing coronary bypass surgery may experience a decline in cognitive function in the perioperative period, which may persist during long-term follow-up.

Prognosis

The prognosis of chronic CAD is highly variable. Although some patients remain minimally symptomatic or asymptomatic for decades, others experience marked disability despite multiple therapeutic interventions. Still others succumb to CAD after suffering a large MI or fatal arrhythmia. Factors that adversely influence prognosis include older age, male sex, more severe CAD, heart failure, reduced LV systolic function, more severe symptoms or functional limitations, diabetes, atrial fibrillation, and presence of significant ventricular arrhythmias. For frail patients and those with numerous comorbidities, goals of care should always be clarified.

Boden WE, O'Rourke RA, Teo KK, et al. Optimal medical therapy with or without PCI for stable coronary disease. *Circulation.* 2007;356(15):1503-1516.

Dewilde WJ, Oirbans T, Verheugt FW, et al. Use of clopidogrel with or without aspirin in patients taking oral anticoagulant therapy and undergoing percutaneous coronary intervention: an open-label, randomized, controlled trial. *Lancet.* 2013;381(9872): 1107-1115.

Lopes RD, Heizer G, Aronson R, et al; for the AUGUSTUS Investigators. Antithrombotic therapy after acute coronary syndrome or PCI in atrial fibrillation. *N Engl J Med.* 2019;380(16): 1509-1524

Patel MR, Calhoon JH, Dehmer GJ, et al. ACC/AATS/AHA/ ASE/ASNC/SCAI/SCCT/STS 2017 appropriate use criteria for coronary revascularization in patients with stable ischemic heart disease: a report of the American College of Cardiology Appropriate Use Criteria Task Force, American Association for Thoracic Surgery, American Heart Association, American Society of Echocardiography, American Society of Nuclear Cardiology, Society for Cardiovascular Angiography and Interventions, Society of Cardiovascular Computed Tomography, and Society of Thoracic Surgeons. *J Nucl Cardiol.* 2017;24(2): 439-463.

Williams MA, Fleg JL, Ades PA, et al; American Heart Association Council on Clinical Cardiology Subcommittee on Exercise, Cardiac Rehabilitation, and Prevention. Secondary prevention of coronary heart disease in the elderly (with emphasis on patients > or =75 years): an American Heart Association scientific statement from the Council on Clinical Cardiology Subcommittee on Exercise, Cardiac Rehabilitation, and Prevention. *Circulation.* 2002;105(14):1735-1743.

Heart Failure & Heart Rhythm Disorders

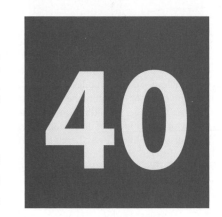

40

Sangita Sudharshan, MD

Breck Sandvall, MD

Michael W. Rich, MD

HEART FAILURE

ESSENTIALS OF DIAGNOSIS

▶ Exertional dyspnea, fatigue, orthopnea, lower extremity or abdominal swelling.

▶ Pulmonary rales, elevated jugular venous pressure, peripheral edema.

▶ Echocardiography reveals left ventricle systolic or diastolic dysfunction.

General Principles

Heart failure (HF) is a growing worldwide epidemic, affecting over 23 million individuals, and >550,000 new cases are diagnosed each year in the United States alone. The incidence and prevalence of HF increase exponentially with age, reflecting the increasing prevalence of hypertension and coronary heart disease (CHD) at older ages and the marked reduction in cardiovascular reserve that accompanies normative aging. In the United States, >60% of patients with HF are 65 years of age or older. Although the incidence of HF is higher in men than in women at all ages, women compose slightly more than half of prevalent HF cases because of the higher proportion of women among older adults and somewhat better prognosis for HF in women compared to men.

HF is currently the most common cause of hospitalization in the Medicare age group. More than 70% of the approximately one million annual hospitalizations for HF involve persons older than age 65 years, and >20% of HF patients are readmitted within 30 days. HF is also a major source of chronic disability in older adults, and it is the most costly Medicare diagnosis-related group.

Prevention

Primary prevention of HF is feasible through aggressive treatment and prevention of the major risk factors for HF (ie, hypertension and CHD). Antihypertensive therapy significantly reduces the rate of incident systolic and diastolic HF in older adults, and the greatest benefit is seen in octogenarians with systolic hypertension. Similarly, treatment of other coronary risk factors (diabetes, hyperlipidemia, tobacco use, obesity) may prevent or delay the onset of CHD, thus reducing the risk of HF.

Clinical Findings

A. Symptoms & Signs

Symptoms include exertional shortness of breath, effort intolerance, fatigue, cough, orthopnea, paroxysmal nocturnal dyspnea, abdominal bloating, and swelling of the feet and ankles. However, exertional symptoms are less prominent in older adults in part because of reduced physical activity. Conversely, altered sensorium, irritability, lethargy, anorexia, abdominal discomfort, and gastrointestinal disturbances are more common symptoms of HF in older adults (see Chapter 16, "Atypical Presentations of Illness").

Signs of HF include tachycardia, tachypnea, an S_3 or S_4 gallop, pulmonary rales, elevated jugular venous pressure, hepatojugular reflux, hepatomegaly, abdominal swelling, and dependent edema. In severe HF, the pulse pressure may be narrowed, and there may be signs of impaired tissue perfusion, such as diminished cognition or cool and clammy skin. Depending on the cause of HF, additional findings may include severe hypertension, a dyskinetic apical impulse, a murmur of aortic or mitral origin, or peripheral signs of endocarditis. As with symptoms, the signs of HF in older adults are more often nonspecific or atypical.

B. Laboratory Findings

1. Biomarkers—B-type natriuretic peptide (BNP) and N-terminal (NT)-proBNP (a precursor to BNP) are typically elevated in patients with acute HF. However, BNP and NT-proBNP levels increase modestly with age, more so in women than in men. As a result, the specificity of elevated levels declines with age. In addition, renal insufficiency is associated with higher levels of these biomarkers, whereas obesity is associated with lower levels. Levels also tend to be less elevated in patients with HF with preserved ejection fraction (HFpEF) than in those with HF with reduced ejection fraction (HFrEF).

C. Imaging Studies & Special Tests

1. Chest radiography—The chest x-ray can assess for presence of pulmonary edema or cardiomegaly and rule out other causes of dyspnea (eg, pneumonia, pneumothorax, pleural effusion). Of note, up to 40% of HF patients with elevated pulmonary capillary wedge pressure have no radiographic evidence of congestion.

2. Electrocardiography—An electrocardiogram (ECG) may reveal signs of ischemia or infarction, dysrhythmias, left ventricular (LV) hypertrophy, or left atrial enlargement. Low voltage may suggest infiltrative cardiomyopathy or pericardial effusion.

3. Echocardiography—Echocardiography is usually the preferred test for evaluating LV function. Echocardiography provides information about atrial and ventricular chamber size and wall thickness, valve function, LV diastolic function, and pericardial disorders. Less common noninvasive alternatives to echocardiography include radionuclide angiography and magnetic resonance imaging.

4. Stress test—A stress test may be considered if CHD is suspected to be the etiology of HF. Coronary computed tomographic angiography (CTA) is an alternative noninvasive method to evaluate for CHD but may be difficult to interpret in older adults with high coronary calcium burden or atrial fibrillation.

5. Cardiac catheterization—As CHD is a common cause of HF in older adults, cardiac catheterization should be considered in patients with a new diagnosis of HF, unless another etiology is more likely or there are contraindications to revascularization (including patient preference to avoid invasive procedures unless necessary). Additionally, cardiac catheterization is indicated prior to coronary revascularization or valve procedures.

6. Pulmonary artery catheterization—While not routinely recommended for evaluation of HF, right heart catheterization can help guide management in patients with cardiogenic shock and decreased perfusion when clinical markers of cardiac hemodynamics are unclear or when advanced HF therapies are being considered.

▶ Differential Diagnosis

The diagnosis of HF is straightforward in patients with severe symptoms and overt signs of congestion but may be difficult in patients with less severe HF and atypical symptoms. Other causes of dyspnea and fatigue in older individuals include acute and chronic pulmonary disease, obstructive sleep apnea, obesity, anemia, hypothyroidism, poor physical conditioning, and depression (additional details on evaluating dyspnea can be found in Chapter 66, "Dyspnea"). Lower extremity edema, in the absence of other signs of HF, may be caused by venous insufficiency, renal or hepatic disease, severe nutritional/protein deficiencies, or medications (especially calcium channel blockers). An elevated BNP or NT-proBNP level may be helpful in differentiating dyspnea of cardiac origin from that resulting from pulmonary or other causes. However, as noted earlier, BNP and NT-proBNP levels increase with age, especially in women, so the specificity of elevated levels for diagnosing HF declines with age.

In addition to establishing a diagnosis of HF and determining etiology, it is important to identify factors that may contribute to worsening HF symptoms. Common precipitants of HF exacerbations in older adults include nonadherence to dietary restrictions (ie, salt intake or fluid intake) or medications, myocardial ischemia or infarction, uncontrolled hypertension, arrhythmias (most commonly atrial fibrillation or flutter), anemia, systemic illness (pneumonia, sepsis), iatrogenesis (postoperative volume overload, blood transfusions), and adverse drug reactions (nonsteroidal anti-inflammatory drugs).

▶ Complications

Complications include progressive symptoms and functional decline, recurrent hospital admissions, supraventricular and ventricular arrhythmias (which may lead to syncope or sudden death), cognitive impairment, worsening renal function caused by hypoperfusion, deep vein thrombosis, mural thrombus with systemic embolization, and cardiac cachexia in end-stage HF.

▶ Treatment

A. Goals of Treatment

The goals of HF therapy are to alleviate symptoms, improve functional capacity and quality of life, reduce hospitalizations, and maximize functional survival. Optimal management of the older patient involves identification and treatment of the underlying cause and precipitating factors, implementation of an effective pharmacotherapeutic regimen, and coordination of care through the use of an interprofessional team. Management of HF in older adults is often complicated by comorbid conditions that may influence both the clinical course and treatment (Table 40–1). Thus, it is essential that

Table 40–1. Impact of common chronic conditions in older patients with heart failure

Condition	Impact
Renal dysfunction	Exacerbated by diuretics, ACE inhibitors; limits use of medications
Chronic lung disease	Diagnostic uncertainty, difficulty in assessing volume status
Cognitive dysfunction	Interferes with adherence and patient assessment
Depression, social isolation	Interferes with adherence, worsens prognosis
Postural hypotension, falls	Aggravated by vasodilators, β-blockers, diuretics
Urinary incontinence	Aggravated by diuretics, ACE inhibitors (cough)
Sensory deprivation	Interferes with adherence
Nutritional disorders	Exacerbated by dietary restrictions
Polypharmacy	Increased drug interactions, decreased adherence
Frailty	Exacerbated by hospitalization, increased fall risk

ACE, angiotensin-converting enzyme.

Table 40–2. Angiotensin-converting enzyme inhibitors and angiotensin receptor blockers approved for systolic heart failure.[a]

Agent	Starting Dose	Target Dose
Captopril	6.25 mg three times daily	50 mg three times daily
Enalapril	2.5 mg twice daily	10–20 mg twice daily
Lisinopril	2.5–5 mg daily	20–40 mg daily
Ramipril	1.25–2.5 mg daily	10 mg daily
Quinapril	10 mg twice daily	40 mg twice daily
Fosinopril	5–10 mg daily	40 mg daily
Trandolapril	1 mg daily	4 mg daily
Candesartan	4 mg daily	32 mg daily
Losartan	25 mg daily	100–150 mg daily
Valsartan	40 mg twice daily	160 mg twice daily

[a]Agents approved by the US Food and Drug Administration for the treatment of heart failure in the United States.

HF management be individualized, with due consideration given to concomitant illnesses, prognosis, goals of care, lifestyle, and therapeutic preferences (see Chapter 4, "Goals of Care & Consideration of Prognosis," for more on goals of care).

B. Interprofessional Care

HF is best managed with a team-based approach and interprofessional care (see Chapter 3, "The Interprofessional Team"). Common features of successful interventions include a nurse coordinator, intensive patient education and promotion of self-management skills (eg, daily weights), and close follow-up (especially after hospital discharge).

C. Systolic Heart Failure

1. Medications—Treatment of systolic HF involves multiple medications. Angiotensin-converting enzyme inhibitors (ACEIs), and subsequently angiotensin receptor blockers (ARBs), have been a cornerstone of therapy for patients with impaired LV systolic function, whether symptomatic or asymptomatic, for >25 years. Available evidence indicates that older patients treated with ACEIs or ARBs experience improved quality of life, fewer symptoms and hospitalizations, and decreased mortality. Table 40–2 lists the ACEIs and ARBs approved for treatment of HF in the United States. Potential adverse effects of ACEIs and ARBs include

worsening renal function, hyperkalemia, and hypotension. Cough occurs in up to 20% of patients receiving ACEIs and may be severe enough to require discontinuation in 5% to 10% of cases, but there is no evidence that this occurs more frequently in older adults. ARBs, on the other hand, have not been shown to induce cough. Close monitoring of renal function, electrolytes, and blood pressure is warranted during initiation and titration of these medications.

β-Blockers reduce mortality and hospitalizations in patients with HF and reduced LV systolic function. These agents are recommended for all patients with stable HFrEF in the absence of contraindications. Major contraindications include resting heart rate <45 beats/min, systolic blood pressure <90 mm Hg, markedly prolonged PR interval or heart block greater than first degree, active bronchospasm, and decompensated HF. β-Blockers approved for the treatment of HF in the United States include sustained-release metoprolol succinate, carvedilol, and bisoprolol. The starting dosage for metoprolol is 25 mg once daily; for carvedilol, it is 3.125 mg twice daily; for bisoprolol, it is 1.25 mg daily. The dose should be increased gradually to achieve daily dosages of 100 to 200 mg for metoprolol, 50 mg for carvedilol, or 10 mg for bisoprolol. With proper patient selection and dose titration, most HF patients tolerate β-blockers. However, some may experience a transient increase in symptoms, and a small minority may require discontinuation because of severe side effects. Caution should be used in titrating β-blockers in patients with severe bronchospasm as symptoms may worsen.

Spironolactone, a mineralocorticoid antagonist (MRA), reduces mortality by up to 30% in patients with advanced systolic HF with LV ejection fraction (LVEF) ≤35%. The dose of spironolactone is 12.5 to 25 mg daily. Spironolactone is contraindicated in patients with serum creatinine >2.5 mg/dL or serum potassium >5.0 mEq/L, and serum electrolytes and renal function should be assessed within 1 to 2 weeks after initiating therapy. During long-term treatment, up to 10% of patients experience painful gynecomastia requiring discontinuation. Eplerenone, a more selective MRA, has demonstrated benefit in patients with post–myocardial infarction LV dysfunction already taking an ACEI and β-blocker and in patients with New York Heart Association (NYHA) class II symptoms and LVEF ≤35%. Gynecomastia is less common with eplerenone than with spironolactone; other adverse effects are similar.

Digoxin is a mild inotropic agent that improves symptoms and reduces hospitalizations in patients with moderate HFrEF but has no effect on mortality. The benefits of digoxin in octogenarians are similar to those in younger patients. Digoxin is recommended for HFrEF patients who remain symptomatic despite other therapy. The volume of distribution and renal clearance of digoxin is reduced in older patients. As a result, a digoxin dosage of 0.125 mg daily is usually sufficient; patients with reduced renal function may require lower dosages and monitoring for symptoms of toxicity. Serum digoxin levels of 0.5 to 0.9 ng/mL are therapeutic. Higher levels provide no additional benefit but increase the risk of toxicity. Routine monitoring of serum digoxin levels is not recommended, but a level should be obtained whenever toxicity is suspected. Because of the risk of potential side effects of digoxin—including bradycardia, heart block, supraventricular and ventricular arrhythmias, gastrointestinal disturbances, and central nervous system disorders (especially visual changes)—the risks and benefits of using digoxin in the older patient should be weighed carefully. Hypokalemia, hypomagnesemia, and hypercalcemia increase the risk of digoxin toxicity, and numerous medications, including quinidine, amiodarone, dronedarone, and verapamil, are associated with an increase in serum digoxin levels.

Diuretics, with the exception of spironolactone and eplerenone, have not been shown to improve clinical outcomes in HF patients, but they are essential for relieving congestion and edema and for maintaining euvolemia. Some patients with mild HF may respond to a thiazide diuretic, but most will require a more potent loop diuretic (furosemide, torsemide, or bumetanide). Patients should be instructed to avoid excess dietary sodium intake (eg, >3 g/day), and the diuretic dosage should be adjusted to maintain euvolemia, as reflected by daily recorded weights that are within 3 pounds of the patient's predetermined dry weight. Patients with more severe HF or refractory volume overload may benefit from the addition of metolazone 2.5 to 10 mg daily. Diuretics are commonly associated with potassium and magnesium loss, and older patients are at increased risk for diuretic-induced electrolyte disturbances. Serial monitoring of electrolytes is warranted, and supplements should be prescribed as needed. Overdiuresis may result in hypotension, fatigue, muscle cramps, and worsening renal function.

Recently, two additional medications have been approved for chronic HF therapy. Sacubitril-valsartan is a neprilysin inhibitor in combination with an ARB. In a large randomized trial, sacubitril-valsartan decreased mortality and improved quality of life compared to the ACEI enalapril in patients with NYHA class II to IV HFrEF. Findings were similar in younger and older patients, including those over age 75. Based on these findings, sacubitril-valsartan is now recommended as a first-line therapy for patients with symptomatic HFrEF and as a reasonable alternative to ACEIs/ARBs in patients who have previously tolerated these classes of drugs. Due to similar side effect profiles, it is important to allow the ACEI/ARB to wash out of the patient's system for 36 hours prior to initiating sacubitril-valsartan.

Ivabradine, an inhibitor of the "funny channel" in the sinoatrial node, has been approved for management of symptomatic HFrEF in patients with sinus rhythm and resting heart rates >70 beats/min despite maximally tolerated doses of β-blockers. In these patients, ivabradine has been shown to reduce hospitalizations and HF-related deaths, with similar effects in younger and older persons.

In summary, all patients with HFrEF should receive either sacubitril-valsartan (NYHA class II–IV) or an ACEI/ARB (NYHA class I–IV) as well as a β-blocker (NYHA class I–IV) unless contraindicated. In most patients with LVEF ≤35% and at least NYHA class II symptoms, an MRA should be added unless contraindicated. Diuretics should be prescribed and the dosage adjusted to maintain euvolemia. In patients unable to tolerate a neprilysin inhibitor, ACEI, or ARB, the combination of hydralazine and nitrates provides an alternative. Although this combination has not been studied extensively in older adults, it reduces morbidity and mortality in younger patients with systolic HF, as well as in self-identified African American patients with HFrEF, for whom it has a class I recommendation. The most common side effects from hydralazine/nitrates are headache and dizziness. Low-dose digoxin can be added to the regimen of patients with persistent symptoms despite other therapeutic measures.

2. Device therapy—Patients with HFrEF are at increased risk for sudden cardiac death (SCD) from malignant ventricular arrhythmias. Implantable cardioverter-defibrillators (ICDs) are efficacious in reducing SCD in high-risk patients with systolic dysfunction. However, the benefit of ICDs in reducing all-cause mortality appears to decline with age, in part because older patients are at increased risk of death from other causes, both cardiac and noncardiac. In addition, older adults are more likely to have procedure-related complications and may be more likely to receive inappropriate shocks (eg, for atrial fibrillation), which can significantly worsen quality of life. Therefore, the decision to pursue ICD therapy in older adults must be individualized. Factors to consider in the shared decision-making process include overall prognosis, risk factors for SCD beyond LVEF (eg, CHD, left bundle branch block), prevalent comorbidities (eg, moderate to severe dementia, advanced renal insufficiency), and most importantly, individual patient's goals of care (eg, quality of life vs longevity) and personal preferences (eg, procedure avoidance). An ICD is not indicated for patients with life expectancy <1 year, and older adults with life expectancy <2 years are unlikely to derive a survival benefit from a primary prevention ICD. Similarly, older patients with substantial cognitive impairment or advanced chronic kidney disease are unlikely to derive meaningful benefits. In addition, patients should be advised that although ICDs are effective in preventing SCD, they do not improve quality of life (a common misconception). Finally, patients considering an ICD should be advised that the device can be disabled (but not removed) at any time if continued activation is no longer concordant with personal preferences and goals of care.

D. HFpEF

The prevalence of HFpEF increases with age, especially among women. HFpEF is often associated with hypertension, chronic kidney disease, diabetes, concentric LV hypertrophy, vascular stiffness, and LV diastolic dysfunction. Primary therapy entails aggressive management of hypertension and CHD. Hypertension should be treated in accordance with current guidelines, and CHD should be controlled with medications and percutaneous or surgical revascularization if appropriate. Older patients with impaired LV diastolic filling are at increased risk for atrial fibrillation (AF), and AF is a common precipitant of acute HF. In such cases, restoration and maintenance of sinus rhythm may be desirable. In patients with persistent AF, the ventricular rate should be controlled with β-blockers, calcium channel blockers (diltiazem or verapamil), or digoxin (see section on AF later in this chapter for further discussion of management).

Medical therapy for HFpEF focuses on treating hypertension, restricting sodium, and optimizing volume status. Diuretics are indicated to relieve congestion and volume overload. Overdiuresis should be avoided, as patients with HFpEF may be preload dependent, and insufficient LV preload may reduce cardiac output. Although ACE inhibitors, ARBs, and β-blockers improve outcomes in systolic HF, there is currently no evidence of survival benefit in patients with HFpEF. In a multinational, randomized, placebo-controlled trial of spironolactone in older patients with HFpEF, the drug had no effect on the composite outcome of cardiovascular death, aborted cardiac arrest, or hospitalization for HF, but significantly reduced HF admissions by 17%. In a post hoc analysis, patients enrolled in the United States, Canada, or South America derived benefit from spironolactone with respect to the composite outcome, as well as cardiovascular mortality and HF hospitalizations. Based on these findings, spironolactone now carries a Class IIB indication for treatment of HFpEF in appropriately selected patients. In September 2019, the results of the PARAGON-HF trial were reported. This study randomized patients with HF (mean age, 73 years; 52% women) and an ejection fraction ≥45% to sacubitril-valsartan or valsartan alone. The combination was associated with a 13% lower rate of the composite outcome of total HF hospitalizations or death from cardiovascular causes, but the difference was not significant ($P = .06$). More patients in the sacubitril-valsartan group experienced improved NYHA function class, and fewer patients in this group had worsening renal function. Results were similar in younger and older patients, while subgroup analysis suggested significant benefit in women but not in men.

E. Structured Exercise Programs

Structured exercise, such as a cardiac rehabilitation program, has been shown to improve exercise tolerance and quality of life when added to optimal medical treatment for patients with stable NYHA class II, III, or ambulatory class IV HF symptoms (HFpEF and HFrEF). Exercise has also been shown to modestly improve depression, although the effect attenuates after a year. Cardiac rehabilitation has not been shown to reduce hospital readmissions or mortality in patients with HF.

F. Advanced HF

Some HF patients have persistent severe symptoms and an unacceptable quality of life despite maximum medical therapy. Additional options for these patients may include palliative inotropes, cardiac resynchronization, or surgical approaches.

1. Inotropic therapy—Medications such as dobutamine and milrinone have been used to augment cardiac output in patients with advanced HF. In small studies, inotropes were found to improve quality of life measures, but overall mortality remained high. Both dobutamine and milrinone are arrhythmogenic and must be used with caution, especially in those without defibrillators. These medications are administered intravenously (IV) as a continuous infusion and can be maintained in some outpatient settings for palliation. Many nursing homes and hospice programs do not accept patients on IV inotropic therapy, which can pose challenges to the use of these agents.

2. Cardiac resynchronization therapy—In patients with moderate to severe HF symptoms, LVEF ≤35%, and prolonged QRS duration on ECG, biventricular pacing or "cardiac resynchronization" may improve symptoms and cardiac hemodynamics. Although few patients older than age 75 years were enrolled in clinical trials testing cardiac resynchronization therapy (CRT), several small observational studies have demonstrated improvements in quality of life and exercise tolerance in patients ≥75 to 80 years old. Therefore, CRT may be a reasonable therapeutic option in selected older adults with NYHA class II to IV HF symptoms.

3. Surgical management

a. Left ventricular assist devices—Left ventricular assist devices (LVADs) are surgically implanted heart pumps that provide support to the LV to increase cardiac output and reduce congestion in patients with advanced systolic HF. Implantable LVADs are approved as "bridge to transplant" (BTT) or "destination therapy" (DT; permanent use without plans for transplantation) in individuals with advanced HF who are not candidates for a cardiac transplantation; as such, these devices are increasingly being used as DT in older adults.

Randomized trials have demonstrated improved quality of life and survival in patients with refractory HF receiving LVADs as compared with medical management alone, including continuous IV inotropic therapy. However, there is considerable morbidity and mortality with LVAD therapy, especially in DT patients, who tend to be older than BTT patients. The 1- and 2-year survival rates for participants in the HeartMate II DT trial were 68% and 58%, respectively, but more recent registry data after US Food and Drug Administration (FDA) approval show 1-year survival rates exceeding 80%. Most deaths occur in the first few months after implantation, most commonly due to stroke, multiorgan failure, and HF. Older age increases the risk of complications, but age alone is not an exclusion criterion for LVAD therapy. In a retrospective analysis of the Mechanical Circulatory Support Research Network (MCSRN) registry, patients 70 years of age or older had similar rates of pump thrombosis and stroke, but had higher rates of gastrointestinal bleeding. Older age was not an independent predictor of mortality, with survival rates similar to younger individuals. Newer generation LVADs have demonstrated similarly high 1- and 2-year survival rates with decreased rates of stroke and pump thrombosis. Multidimensional preoperative assessment, including a mandatory palliative care discussion, is performed to enhance patient selection and outcomes. This assessment should be combined with individualized decision making focused on goals, risks, and benefits to determine the best approach to care for each patient. With improved patient selection and technological advances, perioperative morbidity and mortality will likely decline.

b. Heart transplantation—Heart transplantation provides definitive therapy for end-stage HF but is only available for a tiny fraction of patients because of a lack of donor availability. In 2018, there were 2940 adult heart transplants in the United States; of these, 659 (22.4%) were in patients ≥65 years of age. Although there is not a firm age cutoff for transplantation, candidacy is based on the overall clinical picture, and most centers consider advanced age a relative contraindication for transplantation. Nonetheless, the number of transplants in patients over age 65 has been increasing steadily for >15 years. Other contraindications include severe pulmonary hypertension, active infection or malignancy, severe chronic lung disease, significant renal impairment, severe peripheral vascular disease or carotid disease, severe psychiatric disease, primary

liver disease with coagulopathy, and diabetes with end-organ dysfunction.

Although older heart transplant recipients are at increased risk for posttransplantation morbidity and death, survivors report better quality of life, psychological adjustment, and adherence than younger patients. Thus, heart transplantation may be considered in highly selected patients 65 to 75 years of age with advanced HF.

c. Surgical/transcatheter valvular management

(i) Aortic stenosis (AS)—The prevalence of clinically significant AS increases with age. Traditionally, surgical aortic valve replacement (SAVR) was performed in patients with severe symptomatic AS, but older patients deemed too high risk for an open surgical procedure were limited to medical therapy alone. In the past 20 years, a less invasive, transcatheter approach to aortic valve replacement (TAVR) has been developed. In a large clinical trial of patients with severe AS deemed too high risk for open-heart surgery (mean age, 83 years; 54% women), TAVR was associated with lower mortality than medical therapy alone. More recently, TAVR has compared favorably to SAVR in high-, intermediate-, and low-risk patients with severe AS, with lower mortality and reduced hospitalizations. Accordingly, the majority of older patients with severe AS can be managed with TAVR rather than SAVR with generally shorter length of hospital stay and recovery times.

(ii) Mitral regurgitation (MR)—MR is categorized as degenerative or functional. Degenerative MR is attributable to a primary abnormality of the mitral valve or associated structures. Surgical mitral valve repair or replacement was traditionally performed in patients with severe MR and symptoms or evidence of cardiac dysfunction. In 2013, transcatheter mitral valve repair with the MitraClip was approved by the FDA for treatment of selected patients with degenerative MR, including those with prohibitive operative risk.

Functional MR is defined as MR due to ventricular dilatation and remodeling in the setting of normal valvular anatomy. In May 2019, the FDA approved the use of MitraClip for patients with severe functional MR and ventricular dysfunction who are on optimal guideline-directed HF medication and CRT (if indicated).

G. End-of-Life Care

In light of the exceptionally poor prognosis associated with established HF (worse than for most forms of cancer; see following "Prognosis" section), end-of-life issues should be addressed in all HF patients. Information should be provided about the clinical course and prognosis, and patients should be encouraged to express their preferences for end-of-life care and to assign a durable power of attorney. In patients with end-stage HF and persistent severe symptoms despite optimal medical therapy, referral for palliative care or hospice should be considered. Early contact with palliative care as part of a multidisciplinary approach has been shown to improve quality of life and relieve anxiety and depression compared to treatment that does not incorporate palliative care.

Prognosis

The prognosis for older patients with HF is poor, with 5-year survival rates of approximately 25% in patients older than age 65 years and median survival of <2 years in those older than age 85 years. The long-term prognosis is similar in patients with either HFrEF or HFpEF. Factors associated with a worse prognosis include older age, male gender, more severe symptoms, lower LVEF, ischemic etiology, AF, diabetes, hyponatremia, renal insufficiency, anemia, and ventricular arrhythmias. Progressive HF and SCD are the two major causes of death among patients with HFrEF, but rates of death have declined with the use of guideline-directed medical therapy. Mortality in patients with HFpEF is often unrelated to HF and may occur as a complication of other acute illness (eg, pneumonia, hip fracture) or associated comorbid conditions (eg, dementia).

Hess PL, Al-Khatib SM, Han JY, et al. Survival benefit of the primary prevention implantable cardioverter-defibrillator among older patients: does age matter? An analysis of pooled data from 5 clinical trials. *Circ Cardiovasc Qual Outcomes.* 2015;8(2):179-186.

Kim JH, Singh R, Pagani FD, et al. Ventricular assist device therapy in older patients with heart failure: characteristics and outcomes. *J Card Failure.* 2016;22(12):981-987.

Mack MJ, Leon MB, Thourani VH, et al. Transcatheter aortic-valve replacement with a balloon-expandable valve in low-risk patients. *N Engl J Med.* 2019;380:1695-1705.

McMurray JJ, Packer M, Desai AS, et al. Angiotensin-neprilysin inhibition versus enalapril in heart failure. *N Engl J Med.* 2014;371(11):993-1004.

O'Connor CM, Whellan DJ, Lee KL, et al. Efficacy and safety of exercise training in patients with chronic heart failure: HF-ACTION randomized controlled trial. *JAMA.* 2009;301(14):1439-1450.

Rogers JG, Patel CB, Mentz RJ, et al. Palliative care in heart failure: the PAL-HF randomized controlled clinical trial. *J Am Coll Cardiol.* 2017;70(3):331-341.

Solomon SD, McMurray JJV, Anand IS, et al. Angiotensin-neprilysin inhibition in heart failure with preserved ejection fraction. *N Engl J Med.* 2019;381(17):1609-1620.

Stone GW, Lindenfeld J, Abraham WT, et al. Transcatheter mitral-valve repair in patients with heart failure. *N Engl J Med.* 2018;379:2307-2318.

Upadhya B, Pisani B, Kitzman DW. Evolution of a geriatric syndrome: pathophysiology and treatment of heart failure with preserved ejection fraction. *J Am Geriatr Soc.* 2017;65(11):2431-2440.

Yancy CW, Jessup M, Bozkurt B, et al. 2013 ACCF/AHA guideline for the management of heart failure: a report of the American College of Cardiology Foundation/American Heart Association Task Force on Practice guidelines. *J Am Coll Cardiol.* 2013;62:e147-e239.

USEFUL WEBSITES

American Heart Association (excellent source of materials for both practitioners and patients). www.americanheart.org. Accessed April 2, 2020.

Heart Failure Society of America (source materials for physicians and patients). www.hfsa.org/. Accessed April 2, 2020.

▼ HEART RHYTHM DISORDERS

BRADYARRHYTHMIAS

ESSENTIALS OF DIAGNOSIS

▶ Exercise intolerance, shortness of breath, fatigue, palpitations, dizziness, syncope.

▶ Sinus bradycardia, sinus pauses, atrioventricular nodal conduction delay or block, paroxysmal supraventricular tachyarrhythmias accompanied by bradyarrhythmias (tachy-brady syndrome).

General Principles

Bradycardias in older adults are mainly caused by degenerative changes affecting impulse formation and conduction. Sinus node dysfunction includes sinus bradycardia, sinus pauses, chronotropic incompetence (inability to increase heart rate according to activity needs), and tachy-brady syndrome (AF or atrial flutter alternating with sinus bradycardia). Atrioventricular (AV) nodal conduction block is also a common cause of bradycardia in older adults. Pacemaker implantation is the only effective treatment for symptomatic bradycardia without reversible cause.

Prevention

Currently, there are no known measures to prevent age-related sinus node dysfunction or conduction system disease.

Clinical Findings

A. Symptoms & Signs

The most common presentation of sinus bradycardia is fatigue. Sinus pauses may result in dizziness or syncope. Patients with chronotropic incompetence may have no symptoms at rest but develop fatigue or shortness of breath with exercise. In patients with tachy-brady syndrome, the tachyarrhythmias may cause palpitations. Termination of the tachycardia may be associated with a prolonged pause and symptoms of dizziness or syncope.

Older patients often have delayed conduction in the AV node (first-degree AV block or Mobitz type I second-degree AV block), which is usually asymptomatic and benign. Mobitz type II AV block (infranodal block) may be asymptomatic but is associated with a high risk of progression to complete AV block. Complete heart block (CHB) can present with symptoms of fatigue, shortness of breath, or syncope. In older patients with CHB, stable escape rhythm, and minimal symptoms, the systolic blood pressure is usually elevated.

Carotid hypersensitivity is a common cause of unexplained falls in older patients. Gentle carotid sinus massage, after careful auscultation to rule out bruits, may elicit sinus pauses of >3 seconds in patients with carotid hypersensitivity. Pauses <3 seconds during carotid sinus massage are not considered abnormal.

B. Special Tests

1. Electrocardiography—Twelve-lead ECGs and rhythm strips may reveal sinus bradycardia, sinus pauses, AV-nodal conduction delay, or His-Purkinje system disease (left or right bundle branch block, fascicular block).

2. Ambulatory monitoring—Documentation of a rhythm abnormality temporally associated with symptoms is essential for determining therapy. Twenty-four- or 48-hour Holter monitors are useful in patients with frequent symptoms, whereas 30-day event monitors are preferable in those with less frequent symptoms. In patients with rare but potentially serious symptoms (eg, syncope), an implantable loop recorder should be considered. In a study of patients 61 to 81 years old with recurrent unexplained syncope, an implantable loop recorder established a diagnosis in 43% of cases, compared with conventional methods that were diagnostic in 6% of cases.

3. Other cardiac tests—Treadmill exercise testing can be useful in patients with suspected chronotropic incompetence. Exertional shortness of breath or fatigue associated with an inadequate increase in heart rate confirms the diagnosis. Exercise testing can also elicit Mobitz type II AV block or CHB in patients with advanced His-Purkinje system disease. Electrophysiology studies are not usually required to establish an etiology for bradyarrhythmias but can be used in select patients to determine the level of AV block (intranodal vs infranodal) and to define the need for a permanent pacemaker.

▷ Differential Diagnosis

The symptoms of bradycardia are nonspecific and may be attributable to a variety of other causes, both cardiac (HF, coronary artery disease, valvular heart disease) and noncardiac (chronic lung disease, anemia, hypothyroidism, deconditioning). Light-headedness or syncope may be caused by hypotension (especially orthostatic hypotension), autonomic dysfunction (eg, as a result of diabetes or parkinsonism),

pulmonary embolism, or neurologic events. Many medications can cause symptoms that mimic those of bradycardia. Polypharmacy, decreased renal function, and systemic absorption of topical medications (eg, β-blocker eye drops) must all be considered as potential etiologies of bradycardia.

▷ Complications

Bradyarrhythmias may result in falls or syncope with potential for serious injuries (eg, hip fracture or intracranial hemorrhage). Rarely, profound sinus arrest or CHB without an escape rhythm may be fatal.

▷ Treatment

Management of bradycardia begins with identification of potentially aggravating factors. Medications that can cause bradycardia should be discontinued, if feasible. Patients should be asked about herbal preparations that may cause bradycardia (eg, motherwort and valerian root). Evaluation and treatment for thyroid, pulmonary, or other heart disease should be undertaken if indicated.

In patients with symptomatic bradycardia from noncorrectable causes, permanent pacemaker implantation is the only effective therapy. Pacemakers are also indicated in Mobitz type II block or CHB. Asymptomatic sinus bradycardia, first-degree AV block, and Mobitz type I second-degree AV block are not indications for pacemaker implantation. Select patients with bradycardia due to a potentially reversible cause may still benefit from a pacemaker. For example, a pacemaker is indicated in patients who develop symptomatic AV block as a consequence of guideline-directed medical therapy for HF (ie, β-blockers) in the absence of an alternative treatment.

▷ Prognosis

Pacemaker implantation does not affect survival but does reduce symptoms and improve quality of life in patients with symptomatic bradyarrhythmias. Compared to patients with bradycardia alone, patients with tachy-brady syndrome have a worse prognosis as a consequence of thromboembolism and other complications from atrial tachyarrhythmias.

TACHYARRHYTHMIAS—ATRIAL FIBRILLATION AND ATRIAL FLUTTER

 ESSENTIALS OF DIAGNOSIS

▶ Palpitations, shortness of breath, chest pain, dizziness.

▶ Rapid, irregular pulse (may be regular in atrial flutter).

▶ ECG demonstrates AF or atrial flutter.

General Principles

The prevalence of AF increases with age. One study found that the prevalence of AF ranged from 0.1% among adults <55 years of age to 9% in those ≥80 years of age. In 2010, there were approximately five million people in the United States with AF, and the number is projected to double by the year 2050. In addition, it is estimated that by 2050 almost 50% of individuals with AF will be 80 years of age or older. AF is more common in men than in women at all ages, but women compose an increasing proportion of the AF population at older age. Atrial flutter (AFL) is closely related to AF, and patients frequently will have both arrhythmias at different times.

Prevention

In older adults, AF most commonly occurs in the setting of hypertension, coronary artery disease (CAD), valvular abnormalities, or HF. AF also occurs frequently in older patients with systemic illnesses, such as pneumonia, and following cardiac or noncardiac surgery. Hyperthyroidism (including subclinical hyperthyroidism), acute or chronic lung disease, sleep-disordered breathing (especially obstructive sleep apnea), pulmonary embolism, and pericardial disease are additional precipitants of AF. Prevention and appropriate treatment of these conditions can reduce incident AF.

Clinical Findings

A. Symptoms & Signs

Symptoms associated with AF are highly variable. Palpitations caused by rapid ventricular rates are common, as are shortness of breath, fatigue, and dizziness. Many patients are asymptomatic or mildly symptomatic. Acute HF caused by tachycardia and loss of atrial contraction is a common presentation of AF in older patients, especially those with impaired diastolic function. Some patients have no cardiac symptoms but present with thromboembolic events, such as a transient ischemic attack or stroke. Rarely, asymptomatic patients with AF and rapid ventricular rates present with HF symptoms as a result of tachycardia-mediated cardiomyopathy.

The cardinal physical finding of AF is an irregularly irregular rhythm. AF can be very rapid, with ventricular rates of 130 to 180 beats/min. In older patients with conduction disease, ventricular rates can be normal or even slow. AFL is often regular as a result of more organized atrial activity that conducts to the ventricles with 2:1, 3:1, or 4:1 AV block. An irregular rhythm caused by AFL with variable block is also common and may be indistinguishable from AF based on physical examination alone. Signs of volume retention and HF may be seen in patients with diastolic or systolic ventricular dysfunction in whom the loss of atrial contraction diminishes cardiac output.

B. Special Tests

1. Electrocardiography—The ECG is diagnostic in patients with ongoing AF or AFL. AF is characterized by a lack of organized atrial activity and irregular intervals between QRS complexes. AFL is more organized, and the atrial activity (ie, flutter waves) in the most common form of AFL, known as typical AFL, appears in a "sawtooth" pattern best seen in the inferior leads (II, III, and aVF). In atypical AFL, the flutter waves do not exhibit a sawtooth pattern but are still uniform, in contrast to the irregular and disorganized atrial activity of AF.

2. Echocardiography—Echocardiography is useful to assess underlying cardiac disease and chamber dimensions and to rule out LV systolic dysfunction from tachycardia-mediated cardiomyopathy. Increasing left atrial size is associated with greater risk for recurrent arrhythmias. Severe valvular disease, systolic dysfunction, and pulmonary hypertension are associated with reduced likelihood of restoring and maintaining sinus rhythm.

3. Cardiac catheterization—Cardiac catheterization is not routinely indicated in evaluation of AF but may be considered for assessment of CAD, cardiomyopathy, or valvular abnormalities.

4. Other tests—Serum electrolytes and thyroid function tests should be measured in all patients with newly diagnosed AF or AFL. In patients with a permanent pacemaker or ICD, device interrogation can provide information about rate control and overall AF burden.

Differential Diagnosis

AF and AFL must be distinguished from other types of supraventricular arrhythmias. Frequent premature atrial complexes, paroxysmal atrial tachycardia, and multifocal atrial tachycardia (MAT) may present with similar symptoms and physical findings to those seen with AF or AFL, but in most cases, the 12-lead ECG is sufficient to establish the correct diagnosis. Occasionally, vagal maneuvers or administration of adenosine may be necessary to distinguish AFL from other supraventricular arrhythmias. Some patients develop QRS widening during tachycardia (ie, aberrancy). In patients with aberrantly conducted QRS complexes and in those with baseline bundle branch block, AF or AFL may present as a wide-complex tachycardia that may be difficult to distinguish from ventricular tachycardia.

Complications

AF and AFL are not usually immediately life-threatening but can result in significant complications if not properly treated. The most devastating complication is stroke. For patients who have paroxysmal AF or AFL, stroke can occur in the presence or absence of an ongoing arrhythmia; indeed, in one major study, >60% of patients were in sinus rhythm at the time of stroke. Risk factors for stroke, as indicated by the CHA$_2$DS$_2$-VASc score, include congestive HF, hypertension, age 75 years or older, diabetes, prior stroke or transient ischemic attack (TIA), vascular disease (coronary, aortic, or peripheral arterial disease), age 65 to 74 years, and sex category (female). CHA$_2$DS$_2$-VASc assigns 2 points for stroke or TIA, 2 points for age 75 years or older, and 1 point for each of the other risk factors. Patients with no risk factors have an annual stroke risk of <1%, whereas those with 9 points have an annual stroke risk of approximately 12%. In addition to stroke and TIA, thromboembolic events attributable to AF or AFL can affect circulation to the bowel, kidney, other organs, or limbs.

In patients with chronic AF and rapid ventricular rates, tachycardia-mediated cardiomyopathy can occur. HF and SCD may result from the cardiomyopathy. In older patients with LV hypertrophy, myocardial ischemia can occur as a result of oxygen supply-demand mismatch.

▶ Treatment

A. Goals of Treatment

Management of patients with new-onset AF or AFL should begin with identification of possible precipitating causes (see earlier discussion). The primary objectives of treatment include prevention of stroke and other thromboembolic events, controlling the ventricular rate, and alleviating symptoms.

B. Antithrombotic Therapy

The risk of thromboembolic events is somewhat higher with AF than with pure AFL, but not significantly different between paroxysmal and persistent forms of AF. Stroke risk should be assessed using the CHA$_2$DS$_2$-VASc score. Of note, female sex is considered a risk modifier and is age dependent. Recent studies have shown that in the absence of other AF risk factors, women have a low risk of stroke that is similar to men. In contrast, there is an excess risk for females with two or more non–sex-related stroke risk factors. Thus, the 2019 American Heart Association/American College of Cardiology/Heart Rhythm Society guideline recommends anticoagulation for patients with AF or AFL and a CHA$_2$DS$_2$-VASc score of ≥2 in men or ≥3 in women. Based on these recommendations, anticoagulation is indicated for all men and women 75 years of age or older with AF or AFL. Furthermore, because stroke risk increases progressively with age, older patients derive the greatest absolute benefit from anticoagulation.

The greatest change in the treatment of AF and AFL over the past 10 years has been the increasing use of direct oral anticoagulants (DOACs). The four DOACs approved for the reduction of cardioembolic strokes in patients with AF or AFL can be grouped into two categories: direct thrombin inhibitors (dabigatran) and factor Xa inhibitors (apixaban, rivaroxaban, and edoxaban). Importantly, the 2019 guideline for treatment of AF and AFL recommends DOACs over warfarin in DOAC-eligible patients with nonvalvular AF or AFL (ie, in the absence of moderate to severe mitral stenosis or a mechanical heart valve, in which case warfarin remains the preferred anticoagulant). This change reflects the fact that when considered as a group, the DOACs are at least noninferior and in some trials superior to warfarin for preventing stroke and systemic embolism while being associated with lower risks of serious bleeding, including intracranial hemorrhage. In addition, a 2014 meta-analysis confirmed that the benefits of DOACs extend to patients ≥75 years of age. Additional advantages of DOACs over warfarin include fewer drug-drug interactions, fewer diet-drug interactions, and the lack of need for serial laboratory tests to ensure therapeutic anticoagulation.

The main limitation of DOACs is that the cost of all agents is substantially higher than the cost of generic warfarin, which may preclude their use in many older adults. DOACs are also contraindicated in patients with stage V chronic kidney disease (CKD), and dosage reduction is required for patients with less severe CKD. Additional studies to evaluate DOACs in patients with advanced CKD are ongoing.

Reversal of hemorrhagic complications from warfarin can be achieved with oral or IV vitamin K administration, fresh frozen plasma, or four-factor prothrombin complex concentrate (PCC). For the DOACs, idarucizumab was approved by the FDA in 2015 for reversal of dabigatran, and in 2018, andexanet alfa was approved for reversal of factor Xa inhibitors. If these agents are unavailable, PCC can be administered, with greater efficacy for factor Xa inhibitors than for dabigatran.

In older patients at high risk for stroke but with contraindications to long-term anticoagulation, percutaneous left atrial appendage (LAA) occlusion may be considered as an alternative therapy for stroke prevention. A meta-analysis comparing the FDA-approved Watchman LAA occlusion device with warfarin demonstrated that patients receiving the device had significantly fewer hemorrhagic strokes than those receiving warfarin, but there was an increase in ischemic strokes in the device group. In patients undergoing cardiac surgery for other reasons, surgical ligation of the LAA has recently been shown to reduce stroke risk.

In patients who have indications for antiplatelet therapy (ie, aspirin and/or a P2Y12 inhibitor) as well as anticoagulation, careful consideration must be given to tailor the regimen to minimize bleeding risk. The WOEST study was a large, multicenter, randomized trial that compared oral anticoagulation and clopidogrel alone (double therapy) with oral anticoagulation plus clopidogrel and aspirin (triple therapy) in patients who required anticoagulation (69% for AF) and were undergoing percutaneous coronary intervention. The primary outcome was any bleeding within 1 year of percutaneous coronary intervention; the study also evaluated a composite secondary end point of death, myocardial infarction, stroke, target-vessel revascularization, or stent thrombosis. Patients treated with double therapy had a statistically significant 64% lower risk of bleeding complications in the first year than patients receiving triple therapy (absolute risk reduction, 25%). Surprisingly, patients treated with double therapy also had a significant <44% reduction in the secondary end point. Subsequent studies have confirmed that double therapy is superior to triple therapy with respect to bleeding and is noninferior with respect to ischemic outcomes. In addition, bleeding risk is lower with DOACs than with warfarin in this setting. Taken together, these studies support avoiding triple therapy in patients who have indications for anticoagulation and antiplatelet therapy and preferring DOACs over warfarin when feasible.

Older patients with AF are at increased risk for stroke, but they are also at increased risk for major bleeding. To assess bleeding risk and to help clinicians and patients weigh the risk of major bleeding due to anticoagulation versus the benefit of reduced cardioembolic stroke, several bleeding risk scores have been developed. Among these, the HAS-BLED score created in 2010 is most widely used. In formulating this tool, major bleeding was defined as intracranial bleeding, bleeding requiring hospitalization, a hemoglobin decrease >2 g/dL, or bleeding requiring a transfusion. The score is calculated by giving 1 point for each risk factor: hypertension (uncontrolled, systolic blood pressure >160 mm Hg), abnormal renal or liver function (1 point for each), stroke, bleeding history or predisposition, labile international normalized ratios (time in therapeutic range <60%), elderly (>65 years), and drug or alcohol concomitant use (antiplatelet agents, nonsteroidal anti-inflammatory drugs; 1 point for drugs plus 1 point for alcohol excess). The annual rate of major bleeding increases from 1% in patients with a HAS-BLED score of 1 to 12.5% in patients with a score of 5. Using this information in combination with the risk of stroke as estimated by the CHA_2DS_2-VASc score can help patients and clinicians assess the net clinical benefit of anticoagulation for AF as part of a shared decision-making process.

C. Rate Control

Effective control of ventricular rate during AF and AFL is a primary goal in both acute and chronic phases of management. Optimal rate control is traditionally defined as a resting heart rate (in AF) of 60 to 80 beats/min and a heart rate of 90 to 115 beats/min with activity. However, "lenient" rate control, defined as a resting heart rate of <110 beats/min, has been shown to be noninferior to strict rate control (resting heart rate <80 beats/min) with respect to clinical outcomes, symptoms, and quality of life, and requires fewer medication adjustments. β-Blockers are the drugs of choice for rate control in patients with CAD or reduced systolic function. The calcium channel blockers diltiazem and verapamil

are effective for rate control but are not recommended in patients with depressed LV systolic function. Digoxin slows ventricular conduction through its effect on the parasympathetic nervous system but has limited efficacy in patients with high sympathetic tone, such as during physical exertion, in the immediate postoperative period, or in the setting of infection. In relatively sedentary patients, low-dose digoxin may provide adequate rate control, alone or in combination with β-blockers or calcium channel blockers. Amiodarone can be used as an adjunctive agent for rate control, but side effects are common during long-term use. In patients refractory to pharmacologic rate control, radiofrequency ablation of the AV node with permanent pacemaker implantation is an effective method of rate control and is associated with improved quality of life.

D. Rhythm Control

Restoration and maintenance of sinus rhythm is often necessary to alleviate symptoms. Rhythm control with antiarrhythmic drugs has not been shown to reduce mortality or strokes, and it does not circumvent the need for long-term anticoagulation in patients at high risk for thromboembolic events. Rhythm control is more difficult to achieve in patients with prolonged AF duration, depressed systolic function, severe diastolic dysfunction, or enlarged left atrium.

In patients who present with AF and rapid ventricular rate who are hemodynamically unstable, immediate electrical cardioversion is indicated. In stable patients, rate control with β-blockers or calcium channel blockers should be initiated. In patients who remain symptomatic, electrical cardioversion may be performed with a low risk of thromboembolic events if the duration of AF or AFL is <48 hours or if the patient has been therapeutically anticoagulated with warfarin or a DOAC for at least 3 consecutive weeks. In patients with AF or AFL for 48 hours or longer or of unknown duration in the absence of documented therapeutic anticoagulation for the preceding 3 weeks, it is recommended to perform a transesophageal echocardiogram to rule out a left atrial appendage thrombus before cardioversion. Anticoagulation must be continued for a minimum of 4 weeks after cardioversion because of continuing risk of thrombus formation from atrial stunning after cardioversion. As noted earlier, in men with a CHA_2DS_2-VASc score of ≥2 and women with a score of ≥3, anticoagulation should be continued indefinitely.

Cardioversion may be performed either pharmacologically or electrically. Direct current cardioversion is more effective and safer than pharmacologic cardioversion. The only IV agent approved by the FDA for conversion of AF is ibutilide, but there is a risk of inducing prolonged QT interval and torsades de pointes ventricular tachycardia, especially in patients with HF. Although widely used, IV amiodarone is no more effective than placebo in the acute conversion of AF to sinus rhythm (ie, within 2 hours of administration), but the conversion rate is higher with amiodarone after 6 hours.

Long-term maintenance of sinus rhythm usually requires an oral antiarrhythmic agent. Quinidine and procainamide are rarely used because of limited efficacy and multiple side effects. Disopyramide is relatively contraindicated in older adults due to prominent anticholinergic side effects. Flecainide and propafenone are relatively effective for maintaining sinus rhythm but should not be used in patients with structural heart disease. Sotalol and dofetilide are renally cleared and can prolong the QT interval; consequently, these agents must be used cautiously, especially in older women (who tend to have longer QT intervals at baseline) with decreased creatinine clearance. Amiodarone is commonly used because of its effectiveness and relative lack of short-term side effects. However, thyroid, liver, neurologic, ocular, and lung toxicity may occur during long-term use, and routine monitoring of these organ systems is essential. Dronedarone is an agent similar to amiodarone with fewer long-term organ toxicities, but rare cases of acute liver failure have been reported. Dronedarone is contraindicated in patients with active HF or persistent AF.

Radiofrequency ablation for typical "sawtooth" AFL is commonly performed with high success and low complication rates. Ablation of AF, which mainly involves electrical isolation of the pulmonary veins from the left atrium, has become a frequently performed and relatively effective procedure. The success rate, defined as freedom from recurrence of AF at 1 year, is approximately 70% for paroxysmal AF but is lower for persistent or permanent AF. Major complications, including stroke, pulmonary hemorrhage, deep venous thrombosis, pulmonary embolism, cardiac perforation or tamponade, esophageal perforation, and death, occur in 3% to 5% of cases. AF ablation has not been shown to reduce stroke risk, so it does not obviate the need for long-term anticoagulation in high-risk patients. Few studies have specifically examined the efficacy and safety of AF ablation in older patients, but limited retrospective data suggest that in selected octogenarians outcomes are similar to those in younger patients. A surgical approach for treatment of AF, the Cox-Maze procedure, has a success rate of >90% at 1 year and up to 70% at 5 years; it has also been shown to reduce strokes. In patients with a history of AF who require valvular or bypass surgery, concomitant Cox-Maze procedure should be considered.

Two recent randomized trials have investigated the benefit of catheter ablation for AF. The CASTLE-AF trial demonstrated that patients with HFrEF and AF who underwent AF catheter ablation had an improvement in a composite end point of all-cause mortality or hospitalization for worsening HF when compared to the medical therapy group, which consisted of either a rate or rhythm control treatment strategy. The absolute benefit was similar in patients older versus younger than age 65. The CABANA trial compared catheter ablation to medical therapy (rate or rhythm control) in patients with AF. By intent-to-treat analysis, there was no difference between the two arms in the primary composite end point of death, disabling stroke, serious bleeding, or cardiac arrest after 5 years, although there was a significant 17% reduction in the secondary outcome of death or cardiovascular hospitalization in the catheter ablation arm. In addition, patient-reported quality of life at 12 months was more favorable among patients randomized to catheter ablation. In subgroup analyses, there was a trend for less benefit with catheter ablation for the primary end point with increasing age ($P = .07$), especially after age 75, but effects on quality of life were similar across age groups.

Prognosis

Untreated AF is associated with increased mortality, mainly as a consequence of strokes and tachycardia-induced cardiomyopathy with resultant HF and increased risk of sudden death. In addition, hemodynamic instability and severe symptoms attributable to AF or AFL are associated with significant morbidity and high costs from recurrent hospitalizations, procedures, and antiarrhythmic medications. With appropriate treatment, the long-term prognosis of AF and AFL is excellent, and survival rates are similar in patients managed with rate control or rhythm control.

VENTRICULAR ARRHYTHMIAS

General Principles

The prevalence of ventricular arrhythmias increases with age as a result of age-related changes in the ventricular electrical system and myocardium coupled with the increasing prevalence of cardiac disease. Ventricular arrhythmias range from isolated ventricular ectopic beats or nonsustained ventricular tachycardia (NSVT), both of which are benign in patients with structurally normal hearts, to ventricular tachycardia and fibrillation, which may cause syncope or SCD.

Prevention

Because most serious ventricular arrhythmias are related to underlying cardiac disease, prevention and early treatment of myocardial infarctions and other conditions that may cause cardiomyopathy, such as hypertension and diabetes, are crucial. Early detection of cardiomyopathy is important to prevent lethal ventricular arrhythmias.

Clinical Findings

A. Symptoms & Signs

Isolated premature ventricular complexes (PVCs) are usually asymptomatic. Occasionally patients may feel "skipped" heart beats or palpitations. NSVT is defined as three or more consecutive PVCs at a rate in excess of 100 per minute and lasting <30 seconds. NSVT is often asymptomatic but can cause palpitations, transient light-headedness, or syncope. Ventricular tachycardia (VT) may cause palpitations, light-headedness, or syncope. Ventricular fibrillation (VF) is associated with hemodynamic collapse and results in syncope or SCD if not immediately treated.

Physical findings associated with PVCs include an intermittently irregular heart beat during auscultation that may be associated with lack of peripheral pulse. NSVT and VT are associated with rapid pulse and, in some cases, hypotension. VF is associated with lack of pulse or blood pressure.

B. Special Tests

1. Electrocardiography—In patients with isolated PVCs, the ECG shows wide-complex beats of ventricular origin. VT manifests as consecutive wide-complex beats, which, if sustained, are usually regular. Torsades de pointes is a polymorphic VT with waxing and waning QRS amplitude that occurs in the setting of prolonged QT interval. VF is a chaotic rhythm without discreet QRS complexes. Baseline ECGs should be examined for prior myocardial infarction or prolonged QT interval (eg, caused by medications or electrolyte abnormalities). A PVC burden of >20% of total heart beats may be associated with progression to cardiomyopathy.

2. Echocardiography, stress testing, and cardiac catheterization—These tests provide information about the presence and severity of underlying cardiac disease and the potential for serious ventricular arrhythmias. LVEF and the presence of severe ischemia are the main determinants of prognosis. Acute coronary ischemia may cause sustained VT or VF, for which emergent cardiac catheterization is indicated.

3. Electrophysiology study—The main role of an electrophysiology study (EPS) is for risk stratification of SCD in patients with structural heart disease and NSVT. In asymptomatic patients with CAD, an LVEF of 36% to 40%, and NSVT, induction of sustained VT during an EPS is associated with increased risk of SCD. In patients with syncope of unclear etiology, known CAD or a focal wall motion abnormality, and LVEF ≥40%, EPS may be considered to assess the possibility of ventricular arrhythmia as the cause of syncope. EPS is not useful for SCD risk stratification in patients with nonischemic cardiomyopathy.

Differential Diagnosis

Wide-complex ectopic beats may be ventricular or supraventricular in origin. An isolated wide-complex beat preceded by a P wave suggests supraventricular origin with aberrant conduction. Wide-complex tachycardia with AV dissociation is ventricular in origin and is diagnostic of VT. Other diagnostic criteria for VT are the presence of fusion or capture

beats (sudden narrow QRS among wide-complex beats) and left bundle branch block morphology with right axis deviation. In older patients, baseline conduction abnormalities are common. Comparison of QRS morphology during tachycardia with baseline QRS morphology during sinus rhythm may help differentiate supraventricular tachycardia with aberrancy from VT.

Complications

The most important complication of ventricular arrhythmias is SCD, which often occurs without premonitory symptoms. Ventricular arrhythmias may also be associated with syncope, falls, chest pain, dyspnea, or acute HF.

Treatment

Isolated PVCs generally do not require therapy. In highly symptomatic patients, β-blockers are the agents of choice; antiarrhythmic drugs can be used if patients are unresponsive to β-blockers. Some patients with a high burden of PVCs (eg, >20% of all beats) can develop a cardiomyopathy. In some cases, reversal of the cardiomyopathy may be achieved through adequate suppression of the PVCs, either with antiarrhythmic agents or with radiofrequency ablation of monomorphic PVCs.

The presence of NSVT is an indication for further investigation. In patients with normal LVEF, treatment is the same as for isolated PVCs. In patients with CAD, LVEF of 36% to 40%, and inducible monomorphic VT during EPS, an ICD is indicated to prevent SCD. Patients with LVEFs of 35% or less, regardless of etiology, are candidates for an ICD for primary prevention of SCD. Patients with unexplained syncope in the presence of cardiomyopathy have an indication for an ICD for secondary prevention (ie, an event likely attributable to serious ventricular arrhythmias) of SCD. Ablation of sustained VT may be performed to reduce ICD shocks in patients with recurrent arrhythmias not responsive to medical therapy. VT ablation is usually performed with the use of intravascular catheters. Recently, stereotactic radiotherapy has been used to perform VT ablations noninvasively. Additional studies of this technique are ongoing.

The role of ICDs in patients older than 75 years of age is controversial. Multiple studies and subgroup analyses have evaluated the mortality benefit of ICDs in older patients with mixed results. Although ICDs may reduce mortality in selected older patients, the absolute clinical benefit appears to be less than in younger patients due to the competing risk of death from other causes in older adults. As a result, clinicians and patients participating in shared decision making regarding ICD implantation should consider comorbidities, functional status, competing risks of mortality, and patient preferences. It should also be noted that ICD shocks are frequently painful and that effective treatment of ventricular arrhythmias may alter the mode of death from sudden to a more gradual process of living longer with reduced quality of life. Device disablement in the event of terminal illness or repetitive shocks should be discussed prior to ICD implantation and periodically thereafter, especially when there has been a major change in health status or prognosis. In addition, discussions about ICD generator changes (most commonly due to battery depletion) should include a reassessment of the risks and benefits using shared decision making.

▶ Prognosis

The prognosis of ventricular arrhythmias is governed by the nature and severity of underlying cardiac disease. In the absence of structural heart disease or depressed LVEF, the prognosis of PVCs and NSVT is excellent. The presence of NSVT in patients with decreased systolic function is a marker for increased mortality, but there is no evidence that suppression of PVCs and NSVT improves survival. In patients with LVEF ≤35%, ICDs reduce mortality in younger patients, but the mortality benefit in older patients is unclear.

Connolly SJ, Ezekowitz MD, Yusuf S, et al. Dabigatran versus warfarin in patients with atrial fibrillation. *N Engl J Med.* 2009;361:1139-1151.

Granger CB, Alexander JH, McMurray JJ, et al. Apixaban versus warfarin in patients with atrial fibrillation. *N Engl J Med.* 2011;365:981-992.

January CT, Wann LS, Calkins H, et al. 2019 AHA/ACC/HRS focused update on the 2014 AHA/ACC/HRS guideline for the management of patients with atrial fibrillation. *J Am Coll Cardiol.* 2019;74(1):104-132.

Kusumoto FM, Schoenfeld MH, Barrett C, et al. 2018 ACC/AHA/HRS guideline on the evaluation and management of patients with bradycardia and cardiac conduction delay: executive summary. *Heart Rhythm.* 2019;16(9):e128-e226.

Lampert R, Hayes DL, Annas GJ, et al. American College of Cardiology; American Geriatrics Society; American Academy of Hospice and Palliative Medicine; American Heart Association; European Heart Rhythm Association; Hospice and Palliative Nurses Association. HRS expert consensus statement on the management of cardiovascular implantable electronic devices (CIEDs) in patients nearing end of life or requesting withdrawal of therapy. *Heart Rhythm.* 2010;7(7):1008-1026.

Mark DB, Anstrom KJ, Sheng S, et al. Effect of catheter ablation vs medical therapy on quality of life among patients with atrial fibrillation: the CABANA randomized clinical trial. *JAMA.* 2019;321(13):1275-1285.

Packer DL, Mark DB, Robb RA, et al. Effect of catheter ablation vs antiarrhythmic drug therapy on mortality, stroke, bleeding, and cardiac arrest among patients with atrial fibrillation: the CABANA randomized clinical trial. *JAMA.* 2019;321(13):1261-1274.

Patel MR, Mahaffey KW, Garg J, et al. Rivaroxaban versus warfarin in nonvalvular atrial fibrillation. *N Engl J Med.* 2011;365:883-891.

Sardar P, Chatterjee S, Chaudhari S, Lip G. New oral anticoagulants in elderly adults: evidence from a meta-analysis of randomized trials. *J Am Geriatr Soc.* 2014;62:857-864.

Van Gelder IC, Groenveld HF, Crijns H, et al. Lenient versus strict rate control in patients with atrial fibrillation. *N Engl J Med.* 2010;362:1363-1373.

USEFUL WEBSITES

American Heart Association (excellent source of materials for both practitioners and patients). www.americanheart.org. Accessed April 2, 2020.

Heart Rhythm Society (source materials for physicians and patients). www.hrsonline.org. Accessed April 2, 2020.

Hypertension

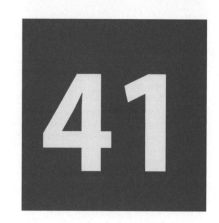

41

Saket Saxena, MD

Gina Ayers, PharmD, BCPS, BCGP

Ronan M. Factora, MD

ESSENTIALS OF DIAGNOSIS

▶ Stage 1 hypertension is defined as an average systolic blood pressure (SBP) of 130 to 139 mm Hg or an average diastolic blood pressure (DBP) of 80 to 89 mm Hg.

▶ Stage 2 hypertension is defined as an average SBP ≥140 mm Hg or DBP ≥90 mm Hg.

▶ General Principles

Per the 2017 American College of Cardiology/American Heart Association task force, blood pressure (BP) is categorized into four levels based on average SBP and DBP measurements:

- Normal (BP <120/80 mm Hg)
- Elevated (SBP 120–129 mm Hg and DBP <80 mm Hg)
- Stage 1 hypertension (SBP 130–139 mm Hg or DBP 80–89 mm Hg)
- Stage 2 hypertension (SBP ≥140 mm Hg or DBP ≥90 mm Hg)

BP measurements should be accurate, and classification should be based on at least two readings obtained on at least two occasions. Individuals with SBP and DBP in different categories should be classified based on the higher category.

Hypertension is very common among older adults and is a major risk factor for cardiovascular (CV) and cerebrovascular morbidity and mortality. In general, SBP rises with age, but DBP rises until about 55 years of age, and then gradually falls thereafter. The prevalence of hypertension is as high as 77% in those 65 to 74 years old and 85% in those ≥75 years old. In 2010, hypertension was the leading cause of death worldwide. Risk factors for hypertension include obesity, reduced physical activity, excess alcohol consumption, lower potassium intake, and excessive salt intake.

Elevated pulse pressure, which is SBP minus DBP, is increasingly being recognized as an important predictor of cerebrovascular and cardiac risk in older adults. Pulse pressure increases with age in a manner parallel to the increase in SBP.

▶ Pathogenesis

Hypertension in older adults is largely caused by increased arterial stiffness (collagen replacing elastin in the elastic lamina of the aorta) that accompanies aging, but there are other established pathophysiologic mechanisms that contribute to hypertension. Endothelial dysfunction contributes by decreasing availability of vasodilators such as prostacyclin, nitric oxide, and natriuretic peptides. In addition, age-related renal dysfunction causes alterations in the renin-angiotensin-aldosterone system, is associated with glomerulosclerosis and interstitial fibrosis, and is hastened with acute injury or chronic conditions affecting renal function. These changes are associated with increases in oxidative stress in renal and arteriolar vascular tissues. Aside from a resultant reduction in glomerular filtration rate, other homeostatic mechanisms are affected (eg, membrane sodium/potassium adenosine triphosphatase), leading to increased intracellular sodium, reduced sodium-calcium exchange, volume expansion, and resultant hypertension. Reduced renal tubular mass provides fewer transport pathways for potassium excretion, making older hypertensive patients more prone to development of hyperkalemia.

Systemic and renal vascular stiffness secondary to inflammation can be a cause and a consequence of hypertension. Elevated markers for vascular inflammation (eg, C-reactive protein, tumor necrosis factor-α, interleukin-6) have been associated with hypertension in observational

Table 41–1. Drugs potentially contributing to hypertension.

- Nonsteroidal anti-inflammatory drugs (NSAIDs)
- Glucocorticoids
- Erythropoietin analogs
- Disease-modifying antirheumatic drugs (eg, leflunomide)
- Immunosuppressants (eg, cyclosporine, tacrolimus)
- Antidepressants (eg, venlafaxine at high doses)
- Stimulants (eg, methylphenidate)
- Saw palmetto
- St. John's wort
- Licorice
- Ergotamine
- Ergot-containing herbal preparations
- Street drugs: herbal ecstasy, cocaine
- Nicotine

and prospective studies. More recent studies have identified a potential role of the innate immune system in causing inflammatory infiltrates of the blood vessels. Further understanding of these pathophysiologic mechanisms could potentially lead to improvements in personalized antihypertensive treatments. Chronic inflammatory burden from inflammatory disorders can lead to arterial stiffness and thus hypertension. In addition, a number of drugs and supplements may increase SBP; identifying these substances and discontinuing them from use may also lower BP (Table 41–1).

► Differential Diagnosis

Most older adults with hypertension have primary, or essential, hypertension. Secondary hypertension refers to hypertension with an identifiable and treatable cause such as renovascular hypertension, obstructive sleep apnea, primary aldosteronism, pheochromocytoma, and thyroid disorder. Often these secondary causes of hypertension present as resistant hypertension (discussed later in "Resistant Hypertension"). Secondary hypertension should always be considered in cases where BP remains above target despite three medications at maximally tolerated dosage and where history and physical exam suggest these disorders.

► Clinical Findings

A. Symptoms & Signs

Most older adults with hypertension are asymptomatic. A minority may present with dizziness, palpitations, or headache. A morning headache, usually occipital, may be characteristic of severe hypertension. End-organ damage, such as stroke, heart failure, or renal failure, may be the initial presentation. New-onset atrial fibrillation should require a second look at BP if diagnosis is not present.

B. Patient History

A history suggesting postprandial or orthostatic hypotension may be elicited. These syndromes may reflect longstanding hypertension or the presence of associated problems that need to be considered in treating hypertension.

Patient history should be directed toward the possibility of secondary hypertension, focusing on recent weight gain, polyuria, polydipsia, muscle weakness, history of headaches, palpitations, diaphoresis, weight loss, anxiety, and sleep history (eg, daytime somnolence, loud snoring, and early morning headaches).

Symptoms suspicious for target organ damage include headache, transient weakness or blindness, claudication, chest pain, and shortness of breath. Comorbid conditions such as diabetes mellitus, coronary artery disease (CAD), heart failure, chronic obstructive pulmonary disease, gout, and sexual dysfunction are important to elicit because they will have an impact on coronary risk factor stratification and choice of initial therapy.

Medication history should include previous BP medications, current prescription drugs, medication adherence, over-the-counter drugs (especially nonsteroidal anti-inflammatory drugs and oral decongestants), and herbal supplements (especially St. John's wort and saw palmetto). Lifestyle issues, including smoking, alcohol intake, drug use, regular exercise, and degree of physical activity, should be assessed. A dietary history targeting sodium (which can raise BP), fat intake (which can contribute to CV risk), and alcohol (which can raise BP if consumed in excessive amounts) is important as well.

C. Physical Examination

The physical examination focuses on the confirmation of hypertension and identification of possible secondary causes. Diagnosis of hypertension should be based on at least three different BP measurements on two or more separate office visits. Routine BP should be measured using an appropriate cuff size at heart level, while seated comfortably for at least 5 minutes. It is advisable to check BP at least 1 hour after any consumption of alcohol, caffeine, or tobacco.

With the availability of out-of-office monitoring devices, home BP monitoring (HBPM) and ambulatory BP monitoring (ABPM) have increasing roles in diagnosing and managing hypertension. Availability of ABPM remains a challenge in the United States in part due to issues with reimbursement. However, European studies such as TASMINH4, an unmasked randomized controlled trial, suggest that ABPM with or without telemonitoring by physicians can lead to better BP control. Teleintervention (systematic medication titration by doctors, pharmacists, or patients; education; or lifestyle counseling) leads to more meaningful long-lasting BP reduction. At home, 8 to 10 BP measurements between 1:00 PM and 5:00 PM are sufficient to give a clinically useful approximation of the daytime mean BP for an accurate diagnosis.

Secondary causes, including renal bruits (renal artery stenosis); moon face, buffalo hump, and abdominal striae (Cushing syndrome); and tremor, hyperreflexia, and tachycardia (thyrotoxicosis), should be sought out. Clinical findings suggesting a secondary cause of hypertension should be investigated.

Frail older nursing home residents may exhibit increased variability in BP readings during the day, where BP is likely elevated before breakfast and falls after breakfast. To avoid overaggressive treatments in this high-risk population, it is advisable to diagnose hypertension based on multiple readings, both before and after meals, as well as supine and standing.

D. Investigative Tests

Complete blood count, renal and metabolic panel, lipid profile, thyroid-stimulating hormone, urinalysis (to quantify proteinuria), and 12-lead electrocardiogram are included in the initial evaluation of hypertension. Evidence should be sought for end-organ target disease (ie, ophthalmologic vascular changes, carotid bruits, distended neck veins, third or fourth heart sound, pulmonary rales, and reduced peripheral pulses).

E. Complications

Older persons with hypertension have higher absolute risks of CV and cerebrovascular events. They are also more likely to have other comorbid conditions that worsen these outcomes. Thus, preventing target organ damage in older adults with hypertension is vital to reducing morbidity and mortality from hypertension. Target organ damage can occur overtly, in the form of stroke, acute myocardial infarction, heart failure, or arrhythmia, or, more subtly, in the form of a neuropsychiatric deficit such as cognitive impairment.

The pathophysiologic changes associated with hypertension predispose older adults to development of left ventricular hypertrophy and heart failure and a higher risk of developing atrial fibrillation (AF). The results from the Swedish Primary Care Cardiovascular Database (SPCCD) indicate that better BP control in hypertension is associated with a lower risk of new-onset AF. When AF is diagnosed, the first step in patient management is risk stratification of patients for stroke prevention. Because hypertension scores 1 point as a stroke risk factor on the CHA_2DS_2-VASc score, such patients should be considered for stroke prevention with anticoagulation as well as BP control. Excessive lowering of BP <110/60 mm Hg should be avoided because this is associated with higher mortality.

Other important complications include chronic renal insufficiency, end-stage renal disease, malignant hypertension, and encephalopathy. These disorders are most common with severe or poorly controlled hypertension.

Hypertension in mid-life (age 40–64 years) is a strong risk factor for cognitive impairment in late life (age >65 years). Hypertension is a known cause of vascular dementia, although the evidence behind this conclusion is more robust in women than in men.

The association between hypertension and Alzheimer disease–related dementia is not well understood. Currently, late-life hypertension does not appear to be a risk factor for incident Alzheimer disease, although multiple studies suggest that abnormally low DBP in late life may increase risk for Alzheimer disease.

Recent results of the SPRINT MIND trial suggest that ambulatory adults with hypertension (mean age, 68 years; 28% of participants were ≥75 years old) in the intensive treatment group (SBP <120 mm Hg), versus those in the standard treatment group (SBP <140 mm Hg), had similar risk of dementia but lower risk of mild cognitive impairment over the follow-up period of 5 years. Regardless of the focus, prevention of cerebrovascular disease in older adults and treating hypertension in young and middle-aged adults remain the goals of preventing cognitive decline.

► Special Situations

A. White Coat Hypertension

White coat hypertension describes elevated office BP when out-of-office BP is normal in a patient who is not receiving antihypertensive medication. White coat hypertension was associated with a higher risk for development of home hypertension during a mean follow-up of 8 years, higher risk of new CV events, and higher risk of CV-associated death. Despite these findings, current guidelines do not recommend initiating pharmacologic treatment for suspected white coat hypertension. HBPM or ABPM should confirm the diagnosis of hypertension.

B. White Coat Effect

White coat effect describes elevated office BP when out-of-office BP is normal in a patient who is receiving antihypertensive drugs. HBPM or ABPM should confirm whether intensification of the hypertensive regimen is necessary.

C. Masked Hypertension

Masked hypertension describes normal office BP and elevated out-of-office BP in a patient who is not receiving antihypertensive medication. Older patients with masked hypertension are at high risk for developing adverse CV events.

D. Masked Uncontrolled Hypertension

Masked uncontrolled hypertension describes normal office BP and elevated out-of-office BP in a patient who is receiving antihypertensive medication. Older patients with masked uncontrolled hypertension are also at high risk for developing adverse CV events.

E. Postural or Orthostatic Hypotension

Orthostatic hypotension is diagnosed by measuring a 20-mm Hg drop in SBP or a 10-mm Hg drop in DBP when checking BP 3 minutes after changing from supine to standing position. Its prevalence is approximately 20% of community-dwelling individuals >65 years of age, and it is present in 30% of those >75 years of age. It is associated with risk of falls (particularly first fall) and has also been associated with cognitive impairment. Orthostatic hypotension is associated with diabetes, hypertension, low body mass index, Parkinson disease, multiple system atrophy, Lewy body dementia, and some medications. Among antihypertensives, α-blockers, combined α- and β-blockers, nitrates, and diuretics can cause or aggravate orthostatic hypotension. In addition, antidepressants (particularly tricyclic antidepressants), some antipsychotic medications (eg, quetiapine), and monoamine oxidase inhibitors can cause orthostatic hypotension. Older adults should be screened for orthostatic hypotension on routine encounters (Table 41–2).

Identification of orthostatic hypotension should lead to a comprehensive medication evaluation, identifying potential culprit medications that should be tapered or discontinued. Knee-high compression stockings may be helpful in mild cases. Waist-high compression stockings with abdominal binders are more effective and may be needed in more severe cases. In patients with autonomic dysfunction and severe orthostasis, medications such as fludrocortisone, midodrine, or droxidopa can be considered. In older adults with orthostatic hypotension caused by deconditioning, an exercise regimen comprising swimming, recumbent biking, or rowing can help with symptoms. In elderly patient with symptomatic orthostatic hypotension, intense antihypertensive therapy should be avoided, and emphasis should be to minimize orthostasis using the above measures. Table 41–3 lists potential interventions for orthostatic hypotension.

F. Resistant Hypertension

Resistant hypertension is diagnosed when BP target is not achieved despite treatment with at least three antihypertensive

Table 41–2. Screening questions for orthostatic hypotension.

- Have you fainted or blacked out recently?
- Do you feel lightheaded on standing?
- Do you have visual disturbance on standing?
- Do your legs feel week on standing?
- Do the above symptoms improve if you sit or lie down?
- Are the above symptoms worse in morning?
- Have any of the above symptoms preceded a fall?
- Are there any other symptoms you commonly experience on standing or after 3 to 5 minutes of standing that improve on sitting or lying down?

Table 41–3. Nonpharmacologic and pharmacologic interventions for orthostatic hypotension (HTN).

Intervention	Quality of Evidence	Safety
Abdominal binder	Moderate	No concerns
Compression stockings	Low	No concerns
Midodrine	High	Supine HTN, urinary retention, headache
Droxidopa	Moderate	Supine HTN, headache, fatigue, dizziness, syncope
Fludrocortisone	Low	Supine HTN, headache, dizziness, edema, hypokalemia

agents (including a diuretic) from different classes in correct combination at the highest tolerated doses.

Resistant hypertension also includes patients whose hypertension is controlled on greater than four BP medications. It is important to exclude other causes of elevated BP, including white coat effect, patient nonadherence to medications and diet, suboptimally maximized medications, improper technique of BP measurement, and medications that increase BP. Individuals exhibiting white coat effect are excluded from resistant hypertension because their risk of CV disease complications is similar to individuals with controlled BP. Medication nonadherence should also be excluded prior to diagnosing resistant hypertension by using a combination of factors, such as patient self-report, pharmacy refill records, and pill counts. Medication adherence is generally defined as taking at least 80% of the prescribed doses. Adherence can be improved by dosing medications daily when possible, using combination medications, using generic medications to help with cost, and consolidating refills.

It is also recommended to screen for primary aldosteronism and obstructive sleep apnea (OSA). OSA is a strong and independent risk factor for development and progression of hypertension, especially treatment-resistant hypertension, and its CV and renal complications. Volume overload and fluid shifts, as well as increases in sympathetic activation, oxidative stress, inflammation, and release of vasoactive substances secondary to intermittent hypoxemia, contribute to BP elevation in patients with OSA.

In hypertensive patients with OSA who are overweight, the cornerstone of treatment is weight loss (see "Nonpharmacologic Therapy" section), which improves sleep efficiency and oxygenation and lowers BP. In the absence of dramatic reductions in etiologic factors for OSA, these patients generally require lifetime treatment with continuous positive airway pressure to reduce the number of hypoxemic events. Addition of the mineralocorticoid receptor antagonist spironolactone to conventional antihypertensive drug regimens has been shown to reduce the severity of OSA and to lower BP in patients with OSA and resistant hypertension.

Pheochromocytomas are rare tumors responsible for 0.5% of secondary hypertension cases and usually present between 30 and 60 years of age. Intracranial tumors in structures close to the glossopharyngeal nerve can lead to baroreceptor failure, which can present as volatile hypertension (abrupt increase in BP, lasting minutes to hours, and tachycardia), hypertensive crisis (severe, unremitting hypertension, tachycardia, and headache), or orthostatic tachycardia (increase in heart rate by 30 beats/min from the supine to upright position).

G. Pseudohypertension

Pseudohypertension is identified when there is a significantly higher peripheral pressure (eg, brachial site) compared with a direct arterial measurement. Arterial rigidity from extensive atherosclerosis is considered to be responsible for this relatively rare phenomenon. Although it can be diagnosed by direct intra-arterial measurement, this invasive technique is usually unnecessary.

Once the above exclusions have been made, a workup for causes of resistant hypertension should be pursued. Assess for organ damage by performing funduscopic exam, echocardiogram, and urinalysis to look for proteinuria and assess for peripheral artery disease with ankle-brachial index. Table 41–4 lists the common causes of resistant hypertension.

▶ Treatment

A. Treatment Goals

The general objective of hypertension management for both community-dwelling and nursing home patients is to reduce morbidity and mortality by early diagnosis and treatment with the least invasive and most cost-effective methods. The clinical benefit of treating hypertension in older adults appears within a year of treatment. However, the treatment goal for BP in older adults is controversial and differs among guidelines, as shown in Table 41–5. Initiation of antihypertensive medications should reflect the clinical goals of the individual, ensuring that the expected benefits of achieving BP targets are achievable for that specific individual.

Table 41–4. Common causes of resistant hypertension.

- Improper technique of blood pressure measurement
- Nonadherence
- White coat effect
- Primary aldosteronism
- Renal artery stenosis
- Pheochromocytoma
- Cushing syndrome
- Obstructive sleep apnea
- Coarctation of aorta

Table 41–5. BP treatment goals for older adults.

Guidelines	Population	Recommended BP Goal (mm Hg)
2013 Joint National Committee (JNC 8)	Adults ≥60 years old without diabetes or CKD	BP <150/90
	Individuals with diabetes	BP <140/90
	Individuals with CKD	BP <140/90
2017 American College of Cardiology and the American Heart Association Task Force	Noninstitutionalized, ambulatory, community-dwelling adults >65 years old	SBP <130
2018 European Society of Cardiology and the European Society of Hypertension	Adults 65–80 years old	SBP 130–139 DBP <80
	Adults >80 years old	SBP 130–139, if tolerated DBP <80

BP, blood pressure; CKD, chronic kidney disease; DBP, diastolic blood pressure; SBP, systolic blood pressure.

Newer evidence supports targeting lower BP goals to provide greater reduction in fatal and nonfatal major CV events as well as mortality.

In 2015, the Systolic Blood Pressure Intervention Trial (SPRINT) published its results, which largely influenced current guideline recommendations. SPRINT compared standard BP treatment (SBP <140 mm Hg) to intensive treatment (SBP <120 mm Hg). SPRINT included adults >50 years old with increased risk of CV events. Exclusion criteria included individuals with diabetes, prior stroke, or dementia; residents of nursing homes; those with reduced left ventricular ejection fraction (<35%); those with an expected survival of <3 years; and those with a 1-minute standing SBP <110 mm Hg. It should also be noted that BP was monitored using an automated measurement system after the patient had been seated with 5 minutes of rest, which is often not done in the outpatient setting. SPRINT was stopped early after approximately 3 years due to its positive outcomes. When compared to standard treatment (average SBP, 136.2 mm Hg), individuals with intensive treatment (average SBP, 121.4 mm Hg) had a lower rate of the combined outcomes of myocardial infarction, other acute coronary syndromes, stroke, heart failure, or death from CV cause (1.65% vs 2.19% per year). However, the rate of serious adverse events was higher in the intensive treatment group for hypotension, syncope, electrolyte abnormalities, and acute kidney injury. SPRINT found no increased risk of falls resulting in injury in the intensive treatment group.

Although there may be benefit to treating some older community-dwelling individuals with more strict BP control, strict BP targets may not be appropriate for all older adults, especially very frail older adults, nursing home residents, and those with orthostatic hypotension, who are not typically included in randomized controlled trials. The SPRINT-Senior trial analyzed the results of the SPRINT trial for patients ≥75 years old. The approximate average age of these individuals was 80 years, and approximately one in three participants were considered to be frail (frailty index >0.21). SPRINT-Senior found that there was still a significantly lower rate of combined primary outcomes for the intensive therapy group with no difference in the overall rate of serious adverse events. However, in the INVEST substudy on outcomes of treatment of hypertension in individuals with CAD age >80 years when compared with individuals age <80 years, there was persistence of a J-curve relationship between lower BP (especially DBP) and increased all-cause mortality, nonfatal myocardial infarction, and nonfatal strokes in individuals >80 years old (Figure 41–1). Additionally, there may be an increased risk for mortality in those individuals >80 years old residing in nursing facilities with an SBP <130 mm Hg treated with two or more BP medications.

Therefore, treatment of hypertension in older adults requires a patient-centered approach.

BP goals should always be patient centered with consideration of functional status, CV risk, chronic conditions, life expectancy, and tolerability to medications. More strict BP control should be considered for community-dwelling, ambulatory patients at higher CV risk, whereas less strict BP control should be considered for patients with limited life expectancy, with orthostatic hypotension, or in nursing facilities.

B. Nonpharmacologic Therapy

Nonpharmacologic interventions should be included in any plan for management of hypertension. Several interventions have been well studied and have demonstrated significant impact in reduction of BP. As more of these interventions are implemented by the hypertensive patient, the aggregate impact of multiple interventions can be substantial. Although many randomized control trials have been conducted to

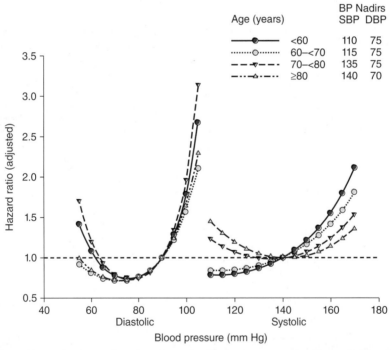

▲ **Figure 41–1.** Adjusted hazard ratio as a function of age (in 10-year increments) and systolic blood pressure (SBP) and diastolic blood pressure (DBP). Reference SBP and DBP for hazard ratio: 140 and 90 mm Hg, respectively. Blood pressures are the on-treatment average of all postbaseline recordings. The quadratic terms for both SBP and DBP were statistically significant in all age groups (all $P < .001$, except for DBP in 60- to 70-year-olds, for whom $P < .006$). The adjustment was based on sex, race, history of myocardial infarction, heart failure, peripheral vascular disease, diabetes, stroke/transient ischemic attack, renal insufficiency, and smoking. (Reproduced with permission from Denardo SJ, Gong Y, Nichols WW, et al. Blood pressure and outcomes in very old hypertensive coronary artery disease patients: an INVEST substudy, *Am J Med* 2010 Aug;123(8):719-726.)

bolster the level of evidence for these interventions, the trials conducted suffer the same limitation of trials for pharmacologic interventions, including lack of a representative cohort of older individuals who are age 70 years or older to demonstrate the interventions' true impact in this population. Nevertheless, the risk associated with these interventions is generally limited but still should be considered. Additionally, implementation of these recommendations can be difficult, particularly in frailer community-dwelling or nursing home-bound older persons. In these individuals, physical and cognitive impairment may be barriers to their ability to follow instructions, and the goals of care of the individual may preclude the necessity to implement these recommendations.

1. Dietary sodium—The US Department of Agriculture recommends reducing dietary sodium intake to 2.3 g (6 g of sodium chloride) per day for adults 50 years or younger and <1.5 g for adults >51 years and those at high risk for vascular diseases. The trials that demonstrated long-term benefits of dietary salt reduction excluded very old subjects, but the strongest evidence for dietary sodium recommendations for hypertension in older adults resulted from lowering dietary sodium to a mean of 2.3 g daily in adults up to the age of 70 years. There are no data in older adults supporting a 1.5-g sodium restriction. Restricting sodium in frail elders may worsen or precipitate anorexia, malnutrition, sarcopenia, and orthostatic hypotension, particularly in individuals in whom caloric intake is already limited. Some data exists showing an association between low-sodium diet and higher mortality risk in older persons.

2. Diet plan—The Dietary Approaches to Stop Hypertension (DASH) diet includes whole-grain products, fish, poultry, and nuts, with reduction in lean red meat, sweets, added sugars, and sugar-containing beverages. It is rich in potassium, magnesium, calcium, protein, and fiber. Although the DASH diet has shown reductions in BP in short-term studies (with up to 8 weeks of follow-up) in middle-aged adults, long-term follow-up data are lacking in older adults. The Mediterranean diet has been shown to reduce all-cause mortality and mortality as a result of cancer and CV disease in older adults, but clinical trials demonstrating its impact on hypertension are limited. As with dietary sodium restriction, implementation of the Mediterranean diet or any other "heart-healthy" diet should be weighed against the potential for reduced caloric intake related to an individual's reduced selection from limited available choices.

3. Alcohol—Heavy alcohol intake (>300 mL/wk or 34 g/day) is strongly, significantly, and independently related to elevation in SBP and DBP. It is also associated with higher risk of CV events, strokes, and all-cause mortality compared with occasional drinking. Moderate alcohol consumption (one standard drink, or 14 g of pure alcohol, per day) is associated with reduced risk of CV disease. A standard drink is 12 oz of beer with 5% alcohol, 5 oz of wine with 12% alcohol, or 1.5 oz of hard liquor with 40% alcohol. Abstinence from alcohol intake should be weighed against the potential benefits associated with moderate consumption.

4. Exercise—CV and resistance exercises have the best clinical evidence demonstrating positive impact in reducing BP. Gradually increasing physical activity to a minimum of 30 minutes of aerobic activity 5 or more days per week should be a primary goal. If this is not attainable, any increase in physical activity is likely to be beneficial. Avoidance of prolonged periods of sedentary behavior may also confer benefit on BP. Any movement is better than no movement at all.

5. Weight reduction—An obese older adult has a body mass index >30 kg/m². Reduction in BP occurs with weight loss through physical exercise and dietary restrictions, but this benefit is less clear for individuals >80 years old and those with chronic diseases who were often excluded from clinical trials with these interventions, and long-term follow-up has not shown mortality benefit between the weight loss and non–weight loss groups. Population data in older adults suggest that being underweight poses as great a threat to physical disability as being excessively obese. Intentional moderate weight loss should be encouraged in obese older adults, only if consistent with functional and nutritional goals.

6. Smoking cessation—Older adults should be encouraged to quit smoking with the assistance of nicotine patches, gums, and other methods. Bupropion and varenicline may be prescribed while monitoring for adverse effects.

7. Polypharmacy—Medications that can potentially impair BP control (eg, venlafaxine, nonsteroidal anti-inflammatory drugs) should be stopped if clinically possible, weighing benefits and risks of such treatments. Table 41–1 lists many medications that could contribute to poorer BP control.

Table 41–6 summarizes the interventions that currently have the best evidence of positive effect on hypertension. A number of other nonpharmacologic interventions could potentially provide benefit in controlling hypertension, but additional clinical trials are needed to demonstrate effectiveness; these are included in Table 41–7.

C. Pharmacologic Therapy

Per current guidelines, recommended first-line agents are an angiotensin-converting enzyme (ACE) inhibitor or an angiotensin receptor blocker (ARB), calcium channel blocker (CCB), or thiazide diuretic due to their effectiveness in preventing CV disease. However, initial therapy selection will also depend on compelling indications, adverse effects, and patient preference. The first-line agent in African Americans with uncomplicated hypertension should be a thiazide diuretic or CCB. Renin-angiotensin-aldosterone system inhibitors appear less effective than other drug classes in decreasing BP in older African Americans, unless combined with diuretics or CCB.

Table 41–6. Nonpharmacologic interventions with the best evidence.

Nonpharmacologic Intervention		Recommended Dose	Caveat in Older Persons
Weight loss		Loss of 1 kg for most overweight adults. Associated with −1 mm Hg for each 1 kg of body weight lost	Benefit only with intentional weight loss in overweight/obese individuals. Risk may exceed benefit in normal weight/underweight individuals or in unintentional weight loss.
Healthy diet: DASH diet		Dietary intake of predominantly fruits, vegetables, whole grains, and low-fat dairy products (reduced saturated and total fat)	Dietary limitations in individuals at risk for malnutrition may further exacerbate their poor nutritional status.
Dietary adjustments	Low sodium	Guideline optimal goal: <1500 mg/day; reduction of 1000 mg/day recommended for most adults	Very low sodium intake may be associated with higher mortality. Lower salt in meals may affect food flavor and lead to reduction in overall calorie intake, with associated weight loss, sarcopenia, and advancing frailty.
	Higher potassium	Guideline recommendation of 3500–5000 mg/day achieved through consuming diet rich with potassium as opposed to supplementation	Caution in older persons taking medications that can increase serum potassium levels or with renal impairment.
Physical activity	Cardiovascular/aerobic	90–150 min/wk at 65%–75% of heart rate reserve	Would start slow and increase duration and intensity to goal as tolerated. Supervised exercise (eg, cardiac rehabilitation) may be appropriate in selected individuals.
	Dynamic resistance	90–150 min/wk; 6 exercises, 3 sets per exercise; 10 reps per set; 1 rep = 50%–80% of 1 rep maximum	Osteoarthritis may limit ability to participate regularly in exercises; consider appropriate analgesia to help improve participation in exercise; referral to physical therapy may initially be needed for patients to learn how to perform exercises properly.
	Isometric resistance	Four 2-minute sessions of handgrip (1-minute rest period between sessions); 8–10 times a week	
Moderation of alcohol consumption		Targets for moderate alcohol consumption: men ≤2 drinks/day; women ≤1 drink/day	Consider abstinence in individuals taking anticoagulants, platelet inhibitors, or psychotropic medications.

DASH, Dietary Approaches to Stop Hypertension.

The key to achieving maximal benefit and minimal risk in older adults is to "start low and go slow" when initiating and titrating BP medications. Lower initial doses of antihypertensives minimize the risk of postural and postprandial hypotension as well as ischemic symptoms, especially in frail older adults.

Special attention should be paid to frail patients and octogenarians when initiating a new antihypertensive medication. They should be seen frequently, with updated medical history and assessment for any new adverse effects, especially dizziness or falls. Standing BP should always be checked to identify excessive orthostatic decline.

Table 41–7. Additional nonpharmacologic interventions.

- Dietary additives: probiotics, increased protein intake, fiber, flaxseed, fish oil, dark chocolate, tea, coffee
- Dietary changes: low-carb, vegetarian, Mediterranean diet
- Supplementation: calcium, magnesium
- Behavioral therapies: yoga, meditation, biofeedback

Route of administration may be an issue in nursing home residents with dysphagia and those who are unwilling to take pills. A low dose clonidine or nitroglycerin patch may be beneficial in BP management in these situations, while monitoring for potential adverse effects. Because orthostatic and postprandial hypotension may contribute to the risk of falling, it may be appropriate to titrate antihypertensives based on readings obtained in standing posture. Also, BP tends to be highest before breakfast in the nursing home resident, and falls after breakfast. So titration of antihypertensives should be done based on multiple readings during various times of the day. Table 41–8 summarizes side effects and considerations for commonly used antihypertensive agents in older adults. In general, most antihypertensive medications are available as generics, although some combination products may not yet have a generic available.

1. Thiazide diuretics—Thiazide and related diuretics are a preferred first-line treatment and have proved particularly effective in African Americans and in salt-sensitive

Table 41–8. Blood pressure medications.[a]

First-Line Therapy				
Drug Class	Drug	Initial Dose (mg/day)	Typical Range (mg/day)	Daily Frequency	Side Effects/Comments
Thiazide and related diuretics	Chlorthalidone	6.25–12.5	12.5–25	1	Hypokalemia, hyponatremia, hyperuricemia, hypercalcemia, metabolic alkalosis, increased urinary frequency (all less likely at low doses) Use caution in patients with history of gout Chlorthalidone preferred agent based on CVD outcomes
	Hydrochlorothiazide (HCTZ)	12.5			
Calcium channel blockers: dihydropyridines	Amlodipine	2.5	2.5–10	1	Peripheral edema (dose dependent and more common in women)
	Felodipine				
Calcium channel blockers: nondihydropyridines	Verapamil IR	120	120–360	3	Constipation (more common with verapamil), AV block, transaminase elevation Should not be routinely used with β-blockers due to risk of bradycardia and heart block Avoid in patients with reduced ejection fraction
	Verapamil SR			1 or 2	
	Verapamil ER	100	100–300	1 (administer in evening)	
	Diltiazem ER	120–180	240–360	1 or 2 (depending on formulation)	
ACE inhibitors	Captopril	12.5–25	25–150	2 or 3	Cough, hyperkalemia, increase in serum creatinine, rash, loss of taste; rarely leukopenia and angioedema Do not use with ARBs or direct renin inhibitor Avoid in patients with bilateral renal artery stenosis due to risk for acute renal failure
	Enalapril	2.5	5–40	1 or 2	
	Lisinopril	5	10–40	1	
ARBs	Losartan	25	50–100	1	Hyperkalemia, increase in serum creatinine; rarely angioedema Do not use with ACE inhibitors or direct renin inhibitor Avoid in patients with bilateral renal artery stenosis due to risk for acute renal failure
	Valsartan	80	80–320	1	
Second-Line Therapy				
β-Blockers	Bisoprolol	2.5–5	2.5–10	1	Bradycardia, AV block, fatigue, insomnia Preferred agent if patient has a compelling indication for use such as reduced ejection fraction or ischemic heart disease Avoid abrupt discontinuation Caution using carvedilol with bronchospastic airway disease
	Metoprolol	25	100–200	1 or 2 (depending on formulation)	
	Carvedilol	6.25	12.5–50	2	
Aldosterone antagonist	Spironolactone	25	25–100	1	Hyperkalemia, renal dysfunction, gynecomastia, impotence Preferred agent in resistant hypertension
Loop diuretics	Bumetanide	0.5	0.5–2	2	Hypokalemia, hyponatremia, renal dysfunction Preferred agent if patient has symptomatic HF Preferred over thiazide in patients with moderate to severe CKD
	Furosemide	20	20–80	2	
	Torsemide	5	5–10	1	

(continued)

Table 41–8. Blood pressure medications.[a] (continued)

Drug Class	Drug	Initial Dose (mg/day)	Typical Range (mg/day)	Daily Frequency	Side Effects/Comments
Potassium-sparing diuretic	Triamterene	37.5[b]	50–100	1 or 2	Not recommended as monotherapy Consider in combination with thiazide if concern for hypokalemia Avoid in patients with poor renal function
α₁-Blockers	Terazosin	1–2	1–20	1 or 2	Per 2019 Beers criteria, not recommended as first-line treatment or for routine use in older adults due to high risk of orthostatic hypotension
	Doxazosin	1–2	1–16	1	
	Prazosin	2	2–20	2 or 3	
α₂-Adrenergic agonist	Clonidine oral	0.1	0.1–0.8	2	Per 2019 Beers criteria, not recommended as first-line treatment or for routine use in older adults due to high-risk CNS adverse effects, bradycardia, and orthostatic hypotension Needs to be tapered to avoid rebound hypertension
	Clonidine patch (TTS)	0.1	0.1–0.3	Weekly	
Direct vasodilator	Hydralazine	30	100–200	2 or 3	Headache, reflex tachycardia, drug-induced lupus-like syndrome at higher doses, fluid retention
Direct renin inhibitor	Aliskiren	150	150–300	1	Hyperkalemia; rarely angioedema Do not use with ACE inhibitors or ARBs Avoid in patients with bilateral renal artery stenosis due to risk for acute renal failure

ACE, angiotensin-converting enzyme; ARBs, angiotensin II receptor blockers; AV, atrioventricular; CKD, chronic kidney disease; CNS, central nervous system; CVD, cardiovascular disease; ER, extended release; HF, heart failure; IR, immediate release; SR, sustained release.

[a]This table is not an all-inclusive list of the available medications to treat hypertension, but rather serves to provide information regarding some of the most commonly used medications.

[b]This dose is only available in combination with hydrochlorothiazide and the lowest starting dose for triamterene monotherapy is 50mg.

hypertensive patients. Diuretics have been shown to lower cerebrovascular and CV morbidity and mortality, decrease left ventricular mass, and prevent heart failure. Thiazides may be ineffective in patients with a creatinine clearance of <30 mL/min and can be replaced by loop diuretics (eg, furosemide) when a diuretic agent is necessary. Chlorthalidone is a preferred agent based on its demonstrated CV disease reduction, although it may have more incidence of hypokalemia compared to hydrochlorothiazide.

2. ACE inhibitors & ARBs—Both classes are considered first-line therapy, although these classes should not be used in combination due to concern for hyperkalemia and renal dysfunction. Older adults are more prone to hyperkalemia with these agents due to reduced renal tubular mass and thus fewer transport pathways for potassium excretion. Although both classes are cost-effective options, ARBs are often used when there is intolerance to ACE inhibitors due to persistent cough. Aliskiren is the only available drug in the class of direct renin inhibitors. It is not included in the guidelines as a recommended agent and should not be used in combination with ACE inhibitors or ARBs due to increased risk for

hyperkalemia and kidney injury with no additional reduction in CV events.

3. CCBs—CCBs are a heterogeneous group, and the benefits of one class of CCBs may not necessarily be extrapolated to another. Nitrendipine (not currently available in United States), a dihydropyridine CCB, significantly decreased the risk of cerebrovascular morbidity and mortality. Dihydropyridine CCBs are available in the United States and include amlodipine, felodipine, and nifedipine. Per the 2019 Beers criteria, nifedipine immediate release is a potentially inappropriate medication for older adults due to risk for hypotension and myocardial ischemia.

Diltiazem and verapamil, two commonly used nondihydropyridine CCBs, have negative inotropic and chronotropic effects on left ventricular systolic function compared with amlodipine or felodipine. They may be used as adjunctive agents in patients with renal parenchymal disease and resistant hypertension but should be used with caution in systolic dysfunction.

4. β-Blockers—Older adults are less responsive than younger adults to β-blockers and are less likely to have BP control with β-blocker as a sole agent. In addition, compared with diuretics, β-blockers may offer less reduction in cerebrovascular and CV events in older antihypertensive patients. However, they are effective in older adults with CAD for secondary prevention of myocardial infarction, for rate control in AF, and for reducing mortality and hospital readmission in patients with left ventricular systolic dysfunction. Atenolol is a less preferred β-blocker given its association with long-term mortality in older community-dwelling adults when used to treat isolated hypertension.

5. α$_1$-Blockers—Low doses of selective α$_1$-adrenergic antagonists (eg, terazosin, doxazosin) may be useful for managing hypertension in the setting of benign prostatic hypertrophy. The findings of slightly increased risk of stroke and CV events and a doubled risk of heart failure in the doxazosin arm compared with chlorthalidone in the ALLHAT trial suggest that the α$_1$-blockers should not be chosen as a first-line antihypertensive agent. If these agents are needed for treatment of benign prostatic hypertrophy rather than hypertension, consider using tamsulosin, which is more selective to the prostate α$_{1a}$-blockers with less incidence of hypotension.

6. Aldosterone antagonists—Aldosterone antagonists (spironolactone and eplerenone) are recommended for treatment of resistant hypertension due to primary hyperaldosteronism and OSA, including in African Americans.

7. Combination drugs—The guidelines recommend that combination drug therapy be considered for individuals with BP >20/10 mm Hg above goal. In the ALLHAT trial, approximately half of the high-risk older adults with hypertension required combination therapy. However, given concern for hypotension or orthostasis in older adults, it may be reasonable to start with one medication initially.

Combination drugs potentiate antihypertensive activity by acting at different sites simultaneously. Formulations that combine low doses of different classes of drugs improve BP control while minimizing the adverse effects of either drug. These medications may, in some cases, be priced competitively with either of the combination agents, reducing the patient's out-of-pocket expenses as well. Lower cost, increased ease of compliance, and potential for fewer side effects make combination drugs attractive for use in older adults once the need for more than one agent is established.

▶ Chronic Condition Considerations

A. Diabetes & Hypertension

BP goals for individuals with diabetes are less clear as there is limited evidence for this population. The ACCORD-BP trial (age range, 40–79 years) failed to show any reduction in fatal and nonfatal major CV events with lowering SBP to <120 mm Hg, when compared with target SBP <140 mm Hg, in patients with diabetes at high risk for CV events. Consistent

with difficulties in finding data for the oldest adults, the ACCORD-BP trial excluded those aged >79 years. A BP goal of <140/90 mm Hg is reasonable for older adults with both diabetes and hypertension.

ACE inhibitors, ARBs, thiazides, and CCBs are all considered first-line therapies in individuals with both diabetes and hypertension. An ACE inhibitor or ARB should be used as the first-line agent in patients with diabetes with albuminuria ≥300 mg/day to slow progression of kidney disease.

B. Hypertension & Chronic Kidney Disease

Treatment with an ACE inhibitor or ARB is recommended in the presence of albuminuria ≥300 mg/day to slow progression of chronic kidney disease.

C. Hypertension & Heart Failure

All older adults with hypertension and heart failure with reduced ejection fraction (HFrEF) should be treated with maximally tolerated doses of a β-blocker as well as an ACE inhibitor, ARB, or angiotensin receptor-neprilysin inhibitor. Of the β-blockers, carvedilol, metoprolol succinate, and bisoprolol have demonstrated a mortality benefit in this population. Additional BP medications could include an aldosterone antagonist, which can further reduce risk for mortality and hospitalizations in this population. Older African American patients with hypertension and HFrEF may also benefit from combination of hydralazine and isosorbide dinitrate. Symptomatic HFrEF should be treated with a loop diuretic, which can provide additional BP reduction. If heart failure is refractory to conventional therapy, workup for renal artery stenosis should be pursued as renal revascularization may improve heart failure in hypertensive patients. In the PARADIGM-HF trial, the combination of sacubitril, a neprilysin inhibitor, and valsartan, an ARB, resulted in fewer combined hospitalizations and CV deaths when compared to enalapril monotherapy but caused more hypotension. Cost may be a limiting factor for sacubitril-valsartan (Entresto), and it should not be used to treat hypertension in patients without heart failure. Additionally, it should not be used in combination with ACE inhibitors or ARBs due to concern for hyperkalemia, renal impairment, and angioedema.

Heart failure with preserved ejection fraction is very common in older adults. Fluid retention should be adequately treated with loop diuretics, hypertension should be controlled, and chronic conditions should be treated. No specific drug class demonstrates superior clinical outcomes at this time, but as previously mentioned, nondihydropyridine CCBs may worsen clinical outcomes and should be avoided in these individuals.

D. Hypertension & Stroke

In those with a stroke history, it is reasonable to target an SBP <130 mm Hg if tolerated, especially in individuals with a recent ischemic stroke. ACE inhibitors, ARBs, and thiazides have all shown benefit in patients with hypertension and a prior transient ischemic attack or stroke and may be preferred agents in patients without other compelling indications. The SPS-3 trial found that in patients with a recent symptomatic lacunar stroke, an SBP goal of <130 mm Hg, compared to 130 to 149 mm Hg, resulted in reduced rates of intracerebral hemorrhage.

E. Resistant Hypertension

If the patient's hypertension remains resistant, other medications can be added to the triple therapy. However, it is important to consider if the adverse effects of multiple BP medications will outweigh the benefit of additional BP reduction. If hydrochlorothiazide is included in triple therapy, consider switching to chlorthalidone, which may offer greater BP reduction. Spironolactone should be considered an initial add-on therapy as long as serum potassium and renal function are appropriate. Eplerenone can be used instead of spironolactone if there is concern for gynecomastia or erectile dysfunction, although it requires twice-daily dosing. If an additional agent is still needed, β-blockers are recommended if there is no concern for bradycardia. Hydralazine can then be considered and combined with a nitrate if heart failure is present. Minoxidil and clonidine are alternative options, although minoxidil is not well tolerated, and clonidine could cause rebound hypertension with nonadherence.

ACCORD Study Group, Cushman WC, Evans GW, et al. Effects of intensive blood-pressure control in type 2 diabetes mellitus. *N Engl J Med.* 2010;362(17):1575-1585.

Carey RM, Calhoun DA, Bakris GL, et al. Resistant hypertension: detection, evaluation, and management: a scientific statement from the American Heart Association. *Hypertension.* 2018;72(5):e53-e90.

Doroszko A, Janus A, Szahidewicz-Krupska E, et al. Resistant hypertension. *Adv Clin Exp Med.* 2016;25(1):173-183.

Duan Y, Xie Z, Dong F, et al. Effectiveness of home blood pressure telemonitoring: a systematic review and meta-analysis of randomised controlled studies. *J Hum Hypertens.* 2017;31(7):427-437.

Dzeshka MS, Shantsila A, Shantsila E, Lip GYH. Atrial fibrillation and hypertension. *Hypertension.* 2017;70(5):854-861.

Gibbons CH, Schmidt P, Biaggioni I, et al. The recommendations of a consensus panel for the screening, diagnosis, and treatment of neurogenic orthostatic hypotension and associated supine hypertension. *J Neurol.* 2017;264(8):1567-1582.

James PA, Oparil S, Carter BL, et al. 2014 evidence-based guideline for the management of high blood pressure in adults: report from the panel members appointed to the eighth Joint National Committee (JNC 8). *JAMA.* 2014;311(5):507-520.

Kalogeropoulos AP, Georgiopoulou VV, Murphy RA, et al. Dietary sodium content, mortality, and risk for cardiovascular events in older adults: the Health, Aging, and Body Composition (Health ABC) Study. *JAMA Intern Med.* 2015;175(3):410-419.

Knoops KT, de Groot LC, Kromhout D, et al. Mediterranean diet, lifestyle factors, and 10-year mortality in elderly European men and women: the HALE project. *JAMA.* 2004;292(12):1433-1439.

McManus RJ, Mant J, Franssen M, et al. Efficacy of self-monitored blood pressure, with or without telemonitoring, for titration of antihypertensive medication (TASMINH4): an unmasked randomised controlled trial. *Lancet.* 2018;391(10124):949-959.

SPRINT MIND Investigators for the SPRINT Research Group. Effect of intensive vs standard blood pressure control on probable dementia. *JAMA.* 2019;321(6):553-561.

SPRINT Research Group. A randomized trial of intensive versus standard blood-pressure control. *N Engl J Med.* 2015;373(22):2103-2116.

SPS3 Study Group. Blood-pressure targets in patients with recent lacunar stroke: the SPS3 randomised trial. *Lancet.* 2013;382(9891):507-515.

Walker KA, Power MC, Gottesman RF. Defining the relationship between hypertension, cognitive decline, and dementia: a review. *Curr Hypertens Rep.* 2017;19(3):24.

Welton PK, Carey RM, Aronow WS, et al. 2017 ACC/AHA/APPA/ABC/ACPM/AGS/APhA/ASH/ASPC/NMA/PCNA guideline for the prevention, detection, evaluation, and management of high blood pressure in adults: a report of the American College of Cardiology/American Heart Association task force on clinical practice guidelines. *Hypertension.* 2018;71:e13-e115.

Wheeler MJ, Dunstan DW, Ellis KA, et al. Effect of morning exercise with or without breaks in prolonged sitting on blood pressure in older overweight/obese adults. *Hypertension.* 2019;73(4):859-867.

Williams B, Mancia G, Spiering W, et al. 2018 ESC/ESH guidelines for the management of arterial hypertension. *Eur Heart J.* 2018;39(33):3021-3104.

Williamson JD, Supiano MA, Applegate WB, et al. Intensive vs standard blood pressure control and cardiovascular disease outcomes in adults aged ≥ 75 years: a randomized clinical trial. *JAMA.* 2016;315(24):2673-2682.

USEFUL WEBSITES

American College of Cardiology. www.acc.org. Accessed April 2, 2020.

American Heart Association. www.americanheart.org. Accessed April 2, 2020.

Centers for Disease Control and Prevention. Hypertension. www.cdc.gov/nchs/fastats/hypertension.htm. Accessed April 2, 2020.

National Heart, Lung, and Blood Institute. www.nhlbi.nih.gov. Accessed April 2, 2020.

Valvular Disease

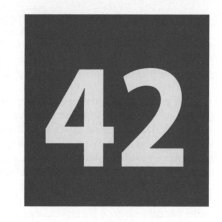

Margarita M. Sotelo, MD
Michael W. Rich, MD

▶ General Principles

Degenerative valvular heart disease (VHD) is expected to grow in prevalence as the population ages. Based on pooled US population studies of adults who underwent echocardiography from 1989 to 1996, the prevalence of VHD is 2.5% and the burden of moderate or severe left-sided VHD increases with age: <1% in those aged 18 to 44 years, 9.9% in those aged >65 years, and 13.2% in those aged >75 years. A more contemporary cross-sectional study of 2500 individuals ≥65 years old enrolled from a primary care population in the United Kingdom and published in 2016 estimates the prevalence of moderate or severe VHD at 11.3%. Mitral regurgitation (MR) and aortic stenosis (AS) are the most common VHDs in older adults.

A standard framework adopted by the American College of Cardiology (ACC)/American Heart Association (AHA) guidelines for staging the severity of VHD highlights the progressive nature of VHD:

1. Stage A: At risk based on structural abnormalities of the valves, myocardium, and vessels

2. Stage B: Progressive disease based on the hemodynamic effects of the VHD

3. Stage C: Asymptomatic severe disease

4. Stage D: Symptomatic severe disease

The emergence of transcatheter techniques, particularly transcatheter aortic valve replacement (TAVR) for treatment of symptomatic severe AS, has transformed the management of VHD in older adults.

The appropriate management of VHD in this population, including the decision to intervene and the choice of intervention, requires complex decision making. The patient's preference is the foremost consideration after detailed discussion of risks, benefits, and goals of care. Weighing the projected benefit and potential risks of any valve intervention against the natural course of untreated disease is crucial. The patient's life expectancy and quality of life (QOL) independent of the valve disease influence the potential benefit derived from any intervention (see Chapter 4, "Goals of Care & Consideration of Prognosis"). A multidisciplinary approach with input from members of an integrated heart valve team is key to achieving desired outcomes.

Improving QOL is an important outcome of surgical treatment for VHD, particularly in older patients. A systematic review of 44 studies (predominantly retrospective) measured QOL and functional outcomes in octogenarians following cardiac surgery (coronary artery bypass grafting [CABG] and valve surgery). Although the majority of patients described improvement in symptoms, 8% to 19% experienced deterioration in QOL. In one study, 43% would not recommend surgery at 1 month following surgery, which improved to 14% at 1 year. A tool for predicting postoperative QOL is needed to enhance the informed consent process.

Validated risk stratification models are used to evaluate and counsel patients on the risks and benefits of surgical interventions and transcatheter options. The most commonly used risk calculators are the EuroSCORE and Society of Thoracic Surgeons (STS) score. The 2008 STS score comprises a portfolio of risk models developed and validated using data from patients who underwent cardiac surgery in the United States from 2002 to 2006. The STS models provide risk estimates of hospital mortality and selected postprocedural complications (eg, stroke and acute kidney injury) for specific cardiac surgery populations. Because of temporal changes in patient characteristics, evolution of perioperative care, and new techniques, the prognostic ability of the models may lag behind current outcomes, and periodic revisions to the models are required. The STS models were last updated in 2018. Other clinical variables, such as anatomic (porcelain aorta, radiation injury) and hemodynamic factors, chronic conditions (severe liver disease, severe chronic obstructive pulmonary disease, chronic kidney disease), disability, and frailty, portend increased surgical risk but are not captured in these prediction models. The ACC/AHA guidelines recommend combining STS risk estimate, frailty index, major organ system dysfunction, and procedure-specific barriers to classify the patient into low, intermediate, high, or prohibitive surgical risk.

The presence of limiting symptoms referable to the valve disease is the clearest rationale for intervening in older persons with AS, MR, mitral stenosis (MS), or aortic regurgitation (AR). In asymptomatic patients with severe AR, the ACC/AHA guidelines recommend operation when the left ventricular (LV) dimension and ejection fraction reach specific parameters. The goal is to prevent further deterioration. Preventive operations such as these may be justified in the older patient with good life expectancy (minimum of 1 year) when the perioperative risks of stroke, acute renal failure, cognitive dysfunction, and other complications that affect QOL are low relative to the anticipated benefit. In general, older patients are at increased risk for major complications following valve surgery (both aortic and mitral), including atrial fibrillation (AF), heart failure (HF), prolonged mechanical ventilation, worsened renal function, bleeding, and delirium. As a result, length of stay tends to be longer and convalescence slower.

Factors that influence the choice between mechanical and bioprosthetic valves are the expected hemodynamics and durability of the valve, procedural risk, need for long-term anticoagulation, and patient preferences. For patients older than 65 years, bioprosthetic valves are usually favored because the 15-year risk of bioprosthetic structural deterioration is low (<10%) and the need for long-term anticoagulation with mechanical valves poses greater challenges and risks. In general, a bioprosthesis is considered appropriate for patients with multiple chronic conditions and a shorter life expectancy. For patients aged 50 to 65 years, the optimum type of prosthesis is uncertain, and shared decision making with the patient is recommended.

Direct oral anticoagulants (DOACs) are not licensed for use in patients with mechanical valves, and vitamin K antagonists are indicated in all cases.

AORTIC STENOSIS

ESSENTIALS OF DIAGNOSIS

► Chest pain, shortness of breath, dizziness, syncope.

► Harsh systolic ejection murmur at the right upper sternal border radiating to the carotid arteries.

► Echocardiography demonstrates a calcified aortic valve with increased systolic velocities and reduced orifice area.

▶ General Principles

The prevalence of AS increases with age. In a systematic review of cross-sectional studies from 1989 to 2009, the pooled prevalence of AS and severe AS in the general population ≥75 years of age was 12.4% and 3.4%, respectively. AS is the most common indication for valve replacement.

The most common cause of AS in the older adult is calcific VHD. Aortic valve (AV) sclerosis represents an earlier stage of the disease. About a third of patients with aortic sclerosis in one study developed some degree of AS over 4 years of follow-up. More than just a "wear-and-tear" process, evidence exists that calcific valve disease shares a common pathogenesis with atherosclerosis and common risk factors including age, male gender, hypertension, tobacco use, and increased lipoprotein(a) and low-density lipoprotein cholesterol levels. Mechanical injury to the endothelium initiates the process that leads to lipid deposition, inflammation, neoangiogenesis, calcification, and sclerosis. Bicuspid AV is the most common cause of severe AS in adults <60 years, and it accounts for 10% to 20% of severe AS in patients ≥70 years.

▶ Prevention

There are no effective strategies to prevent AS. A large trial that randomized patients with asymptomatic mild or moderate AS to intensive cholesterol-lowering treatment with simvastatin and ezetimibe or placebo found no difference in clinical or hemodynamic progression of AS over a median follow-up of 52 months. Statins are not currently recommended for the prevention or treatment of AS in the absence of other indications, such as coronary artery disease (CAD).

The renin-angiotensin system is thought to play a role in the pathogenesis of calcific AV disease as in atherosclerosis; however, evidence that angiotensin-converting enzyme (ACE) inhibitors modify AS progression is lacking.

▶ Clinical Findings

A. Symptoms & Signs

AS is a progressive disease with a prolonged asymptomatic phase and a shorter symptomatic phase. Symptoms usually manifest in the sixth decade or later. Early symptoms are dyspnea on exertion or decreased exercise tolerance. Syncope, angina, and HF indicate a late stage of AS. AS in the older adult is often occult until it reaches an advanced stage because sedentary older persons may experience few symptoms or may attribute their symptoms to another disease or to old age (see Chapter 16, "Atypical Presentations of Illness").

Significant AS is almost invariably associated with a grade II or greater systolic ejection murmur that is usually harsh and best heard in the right second intercostal space with radiation to the carotid arteries. The murmur may be difficult to hear in obese patients and in those with increased chest diameter because of chronic lung disease, whereas in others, it may be heard best at the apex. Murmurs that peak in late systole tend to be associated with more severe AS, but the intensity of the murmur often diminishes in patients with severe LV failure. Other physical findings include an LV heave, S_4 gallop, and reduced intensity or absence of the A_2 component of the second heart sound. A normally split S_2 excludes severe AS. Classically, the carotid upstroke is delayed in patients with severe AS, but this finding may be masked in older patients with stiff, noncompliant vessels.

B. Special Tests

1. Electrocardiography and radiography—The electrocardiogram (ECG) often demonstrates LV hypertrophy, and the chest radiograph frequently reveals LV prominence.

2. Echocardiography—Echocardiography is the noninvasive procedure of choice for diagnosing AS and grading severity. Typical echocardiographic features include a moderately or severely thickened and calcified valve with restricted opening. Doppler examination measures mean gradient and peak velocity across the valve and allows for calculation of the effective AV area. Table 42–1 classifies AS severity.

3. Cardiac catheterization—Because approximately 50% of older patients with severe AS have obstructive CAD, cardiac catheterization with coronary angiography is indicated for all patients in whom AV replacement (AVR) is being considered. Catheterization can also provide definitive information about the severity of AS when the echocardiogram is nondiagnostic.

4. Pre-TAVR imaging—Pre-TAVR imaging requirements can be extensive and include gated contrast-enhanced computed tomography (CT) of the thorax for annular and aortic root measurements and vascular access imaging of peripheral vessels.

5. Dobutamine stress testing—Lower AV velocity and gradient can be seen in severe AS with reduced LVEF. Dobutamine stress testing is useful for differentiating severe AS causing LV systolic dysfunction due to afterload mismatch from moderate AS and primary LV dysfunction causing restricted AV opening due to low transvalvular flow.

▶ Differential Diagnosis

The symptoms of AS may mimic many other cardiac and noncardiac diseases, including CAD, HF, arrhythmia, and chronic lung disease. Likewise, the physical findings, ECG, and chest radiograph are often nonspecific. Consequently, the clinician must maintain a high index of suspicion in patients with symptoms possibly attributable to AS in association with a systolic ejection murmur.

Table 42–1. Classification of aortic stenosis (AS) severity.

AS Stage and Definition	Valve Hemodynamics
A: at risk for AS	• Aortic V_{max} <2 m/s
B: progressive AS	Mild: • Aortic V_{max} 2.0–2.9 m/s or mean ΔP <20 mm Hg Moderate: • Aortic V_{max} 3.0–3.9 m/s or mean ΔP 20–39 mm Hg
C: asymptomatic severe AS	
C1: asymptomatic	• Aortic V_{max} ≥4 m/s or mean ΔP >40 mm Hg • AVA ≤1.0 cm²
C2: asymptomatic with LV dysfunction	• LVEF <50%
D: symptomatic severe AS	
D1: symptomatic severe, high gradient	• Aortic V_{max} ≥ 4 m/s or mean ΔP ≥40 mm Hg • AVA ≤1.0 cm², may be larger with mixed AS/AR
D2: symptomatic severe low-flow/low-gradient with reduced LVEF	• AVA ≤1.0 cm² with resting aortic V_{max} <4 m/s or mean ΔP <40 mm Hg • Dobutamine stress echocardiography shows AVA ≤1.0 cm² with V_{max} ≥4 m/s
D3: symptomatic severe low-gradient AS with normal LVEF or paradoxical low-flow severe AS	• AVA ≤1.0 cm² with aortic V_{max} <4 m/s or mean ΔP <40 mm Hg • Indexed AVA ≤0.6 cm²/m² and stroke volume index <35 mL/m²

Aortic V_{max}, maximum aortic valve velocity; AR, aortic regurgitation; AS, aortic stenosis; AVA, aortic valve area; LV, left ventricular; LVEF, left ventricular ejection fraction; ΔP, pressure gradient.

Data from Nishimura RA, Otto CM, Bonow RO, et al. 2014 AHA/ACC guideline for the management of patients with valvular heart disease: a report of the American College of Cardiology/American Heart Association Task Force on Practice Guidelines, *J Am Coll Cardiol* 2014 Jun 10;63(22):e57-185.

▶ Treatment

There is no effective medical therapy for severe AS. Because AS is generally a disease of older age, hypertension is a frequent comorbidity and contributes to the load on the LV. There are no clear recommendations for antihypertensive therapy in these patients. When used, vasodilators, including nitrates and ACE inhibitors, should be administered at a low dose and titrated cautiously in patients with moderate to severe AS because of the risk of hypotension. Diuretics should also be used with caution if the LV chamber is small because a fall in cardiac output can result from reductions in preload.

Table 42–2. American College of Cardiology/American Heart Association guidelines for VHD interventions.

Valvular Disease	Class I Indications for Valve Interventions and Choice of Interventions
Aortic stenosis	• AVR is recommended in patients who meet an indication for AVR with low or intermediate surgical risk. • An integrated heart valve team should provide care for patients in whom TAVR or SAVR is being considered. • TAVR is recommended in patients who meet an indication for AVR and who have a prohibitive surgical risk and a predicted post-TAVR survival >12 months. • SAVR or TAVR is recommended for symptomatic patients with severe aortic stenosis and high risk for surgical AVR, depending on patient-specific procedural risks, values, and preferences.
Aortic regurgitation (AR)	AVR • Symptomatic severe AR regardless of LV systolic function • Asymptomatic chronic severe AR and LVEF <50% • Chronic severe AR and undergoing cardiac surgery for other indications
Mitral stenosis (MS)	• PBMC is recommended for symptomatic patients with severe MS and favorable valve morphology in the absence of contraindications (left atrial thrombus despite anticoagulation, moderate to severe MR). • MV surgery is indicated in severe MS patients with NYHA class III/IV symptoms who are not high risk for surgery and who are not candidates for or have failed PBMC. • Concomitant MV surgery is indicated for patients with symptomatic and asymptomatic severe MS undergoing other cardiac surgery.
Chronic primary MR	MV replacement or repair (preferred) • Symptomatic chronic severe primary MR and LVEF >30% • Asymptomatic chronic severe primary MR and LV dysfunction (LVEF 30%–60% and/or LVESD ≥40 mm) • Chronic severe primary MR and undergoing cardiac surgery for other indications
Tricuspid regurgitation (TR)	Severe TR at time of left-sided valve surgery

AVR, aortic valve replacement; LV, left ventricular; LVEF, left ventricular ejection fraction; LVESD, left ventricular end-systolic diameter; MR, mitral regurgitation; MS, mitral stenosis; MV, mitral valve; NYHA, New York Heart Association; PBMC, percutaneous mitral balloon commissurotomy; SAVR, surgical aortic valve replacement; TAVR, transcatheter aortic valve replacement; VHD, valvular heart disease.

Data from Nishimura RA, Otto CM, Bonow RO, et al. 2014 AHA/ACC guideline for the management of patients with valvular heart disease: a report of the American College of Cardiology/American Heart Association Task Force on Practice Guidelines, *J Am Coll Cardiol* 2014 Jun 10;63(22):e57-185.

Once symptoms develop, patients with severe AS should be referred for AVR because the prognosis is poor in the absence of definitive therapy. AVR is the procedure of choice for patients with severe symptomatic AS, and the results of valve replacement are excellent in properly selected candidates. Table 42–2 lists other Class I indications for AVR.

Surgical AVR (SAVR) was the only effective treatment for symptomatic severe AS prior to the development of TAVR. Randomized trials have established the noninferiority of TAVR compared to SAVR and the superiority of TAVR compared to medical treatment in patients with symptomatic severe AS who are at high operative risk (≥8% risk of perioperative mortality based on the STS score) or are inoperable because of a 50% or greater likelihood of dying or suffering serious complications from SAVR. In the latter group, TAVR resulted in 20% reduction in absolute mortality at 1 year compared with medical therapy in one trial. Prior to the advent of TAVR, over one-third of patients were deemed inoperable, primarily due to older age and chronic conditions. TAVR has transformed the management of severe symptomatic AS in older patients.

From 2009 to 2015, the number of Medicare beneficiaries (MBs) who underwent isolated AV procedures increased from 48 to 89 per 100,000. The incidence rate of SAVR peaked at 54 per 100,000 MBs in 2011, then fell to 48 per 100,000 by 2015, whereas the incidence of TAVR increased from 11 per 100,000 MBs in 2012 to 41 per 100,000 in 2015. TAVR accounted for 46% of all isolated AVR. The outcomes of isolated AV procedures showed improvement during this period with declines in in-hospital mortality and cumulative 30-day mortality.

TAVR involves implanting a bioprosthetic valve delivered on a catheter, preferably via a femoral approach, inside the native valve. Short-term benefits of TAVR over SAVR include shorter intensive care unit (ICU) and hospital stays. In contrast to reductions in health-related QOL (HRQOL) scores 30 days after SAVR, the less invasive TAVR has been associated with more immediate improvements in HRQOL. TAVR-specific complications include the need to convert to an open surgical procedure (1.4%), valve embolization (0.3%–7.5%), and need for reintervention to correct valve regurgitation (0.7%). Moderate or severe AR after TAVR has been associated with increased 5-year risk of mortality. Cognitive performance was preserved in 91% of 111 patients followed for 2 years after TAVR.

Guidelines recommend TAVR for symptomatic severe AS and a prohibitive surgical risk in patients who have a predicted post-TAVR survival >12 months. In the PARTNER (Placement of Aortic Transcatheter Valve) study, patients with symptomatic severe AS deemed inoperable (mean age, 83.1 years; 53.6% women) were randomized to transfemoral TAVR or medical therapy. Only six patients remained in the control group at 5 years, after crossovers and withdrawals. There were significant differences in median survival (31 months in the TAVR arm and 11.7 months in the control arm) and 5-year mortality (71.8% and 93.6%, respectively). Among survivors, 83.1% in the TAVR group and 42.5% in the control group were asymptomatic or had mild (New York Heart Association [NYHA] class I or II) symptoms at 2 years of follow-up.

For patients with severe symptomatic AS who are at high surgical risk, the choice between SAVR and TAVR is made based on patient-specific procedural risks, values, and preference. Long-term follow-up in randomized trials has shown similar rates of survival. The PARTNER IA trial reported similar 5-year risk of death.

TAVR has not been evaluated for asymptomatic patients with severe AS and high surgical risk; guidelines recommend continued monitoring for symptom onset. However, because disease progression occurs in nearly all patients with severe asymptomatic AS and the additive risk of AVR at the time of cardiac surgery is less than the risk of reoperation, SAVR is recommended for patients with symptomatic and asymptomatic severe AS when undergoing another cardiac surgery, most commonly CABG.

A meta-analysis of randomized controlled trials and propensity-matched observational studies comparing TAVR to SAVR in intermediate-risk patients reported no difference in mortality at a median follow-up of 1.5 years. TAVR was associated with a higher risk of pacemaker implantation and aortic insufficiency. Early stroke, atrial fibrillation, acute kidney injury, cardiogenic shock, and major bleeding were more common in the SAVR group.

The PARTNER 3 trial randomized 1000 low-risk patients (mean age, 73 years; mean STS risk score, 1.9%) to TAVR or surgery and found TAVR to be superior in the primary composite end point of death, stroke, or rehospitalization at 1 year. The duration of index hospitalization was shorter and TAVR was superior to surgery with respect to several secondary end points (stroke, stroke or death, new-onset AF, and QOL). Rates of major vascular complications, new pacemaker insertions, or moderate or severe paravalvular regurgitation were not significantly different between the two groups. Long-term studies of TAVR durability and outcomes are needed for younger, lower risk recipients.

A. SAVR in Older Adults

Age alone is not a contraindication to surgery. In an observational study of patients who underwent isolated SAVR or SAVR combined with CABG in a single institution in the Netherlands from November 2007 to August 2011,

octogenarians (163 or 762 patients) had a higher predicted risk of operative mortality than patients <80 years old, but actual operative mortality was 1.9% in octogenarians compared to 2.9% in those <80 years old. Octogenarians suffered higher rates of postoperative delirium and lengthier hospitalizations. HRQOL transiently worsened 1 month after surgery but improved significantly to levels of age-matched Dutch reference population by 1 year. In another cohort of octogenarians who underwent isolated AVR, nearly 75% survived at 5 years: 81% enjoyed favorable NYHA functional classes, 91% were free of angina, and 68% were living at home. With advances in perioperative management, postoperative mortality rate has declined through the years. Factors predictive of operative mortality in octogenarians are urgent procedure, concurrent CABG, and NYHA class IV HF. Reduced LV ejection fraction (LVEF) <30% and low-gradient severe AS due to LV systolic dysfunction are also associated with worse postoperative outcomes. Another higher risk subgroup consists of patients, mostly older women, who develop excessive LV hypertrophy in response to AS.

B. AVR Assessment

Choosing among SAVR, TAVR, or no intervention requires individualized risk-benefit assessment with consideration of life expectancy, surgical risk, frailty, comorbid conditions, and patient preferences. Guidelines recommend that patients who have an indication for AVR and are expected to derive survival and/or QOL benefit from an intervention be evaluated by a multidisciplinary heart valve team. Patients with life expectancies of <1 year or who have a <25% probability of surviving 2 years with improvement in symptoms and function are unlikely to benefit from any intervention. Medical management focused on palliation of symptoms is recommended.

The heart valve team estimates the risk of mortality and morbidity with SAVR using validated risk calculators, such as the STS Predicted Risk of Mortality (PROM) and EuroSCORE. Coexisting cardiac and noncardiac comorbidities influence the choice between TAVR or SAVR. Patients with comorbid severe multivessel coronary disease may be best managed surgically with concomitant SAVR and CABG, especially if diabetes is also present.

Frailty is a significant risk factor for death and functional decline following either SAVR or TAVR. A prospective cohort study of older adults undergoing TAVR or SAVR compared the incremental predictive value of seven frailty indices in predicting 12-month all-cause mortality, 30-day all-cause mortality, and a composite of death or worsening disability at 12 months. The prevalence of frailty ranged from 26% to 68% depending on the scale used. Death or worsening disability at 1 year occurred in 35% of the cohort. The scale found to be most strongly associated with the outcomes and that contributed the greatest incremental value when added to a predictive model containing the procedure type and STS-PROM score was the Essential Frailty Toolset (EFT).

The EFT score is based on the presence of preprocedural anemia, hypoalbuminemia, lower extremity weakness, and cognitive impairment.

Aortic balloon valvuloplasty, a procedure where a balloon is placed across a stenotic AV and inflated, frequently results in a moderate reduction in transvalvular gradient and early symptom improvement. However, it is not recommended as definitive therapy in older adults because of frequent acute complications, and restenosis occurs within 6 to 12 months in most patients. However, it may be considered as a bridge to SAVR or TAVR.

Prognosis

When aortic velocity is ≥4 m/s or mean pressure gradient is ≥40 mm Hg, symptom onset is likely within 2 to 5 years. Onset of symptoms heralds increased mortality risk. In a recent study, the 2-year survival rate after onset of symptoms was approximately 50%. HF was the cause of death in 50% to 60% of patients, and sudden cardiac death (SCD) occurred in 15% to 20% of patients. SCD is rare in asymptomatic patients and is almost always preceded by symptoms. After AVR, survival is similar to that for persons of comparable age and health status in the general population.

AORTIC REGURGITATION

ESSENTIALS OF DIAGNOSIS

▸ Dyspnea, fatigue, palpitations, chest pain.

▸ Decrescendo diastolic murmur in the left third and fourth intercostal spaces.

▸ Echocardiography demonstrates AR.

General Principles

The prevalence of AR increases with advancing age, and AR of moderate or greater severity has been documented in 1.6% of individuals ≥65 years in a community-based study. Pure AR is uncommon in the older adult population; the majority with AV disease have combined AS and AR. Common causes of chronic AR in older adults are calcific AV disease and ascending aorta dilation from hypertension, bicuspid AV, or primary diseases of the aorta. Moderate to severe periprosthetic AR is an uncommon complication of TAVR but is associated with worse short- and long-term survival.

Chronic AR leads to LV remodeling with progressive LV dilation and hypertrophy. With progression, the LV end-systolic diameter (LVESD) and wall stress increase until, eventually, LV function declines. Older patients develop symptoms or LV dysfunction earlier and suffer worse operative

mortality. Concomitant CAD complicates the evaluation of symptoms, LV dysfunction, and indication for surgery.

Prevention

Therapies directed at preventing the various disorders that cause chronic AR may reduce its prevalence. Effective blood pressure control may lessen AR severity and/or slow the rate of progression.

Clinical Findings

A. Symptoms & Signs

Patients with mild or moderate chronic AR are usually asymptomatic, and those with chronic severe AR report progressive exercise intolerance, shortness of breath, orthopnea, and fatigue.

In patients with mild to moderate chronic AR, a short, early diastolic decrescendo murmur is often the only physical finding, although it has poor sensitivity (21% in one study). In those with chronic severe AR, the diastolic murmur becomes louder, occasionally reaching grade V or VI, and longer, often persisting throughout diastole with presystolic accentuation. The LV apical impulse is often diffuse and displaced laterally and inferiorly. An S_3 gallop may be present and may be palpable. Blood pressure is characterized by a widened pulse pressure and especially by a low diastolic pressure. Peripheral manifestations of severe chronic AR include bounding pulses, head bobbing, Quincke pulses (capillary pulsations), and femoral bruits with light compression of the artery.

B. Special Tests

1. Chest radiography—In patients with acute severe AR, the chest radiograph reveals pulmonary edema, often in association with a normal cardiac silhouette. In patients with chronic severe AR, the heart size is usually markedly increased.

2. ECG—ECG findings are nonspecific, but LV hypertrophy may be evident in patients with severe chronic AR. Table 42–3 classifies AR severity.

3. Echocardiography—Transthoracic and transesophageal echocardiography, CT, and magnetic resonance imaging (MRI) are useful noninvasive techniques for evaluating AR. In most cases, transthoracic echocardiography is the initial procedure of choice for assessing the cause, severity, LV size, and systolic function and for guiding management. In mild to moderate chronic AR, the AR jet is visualized but the echocardiogram may be normal otherwise. In chronic severe AR, the left ventricle is usually dilated and there is a prominent AR jet. Echocardiography provides valuable insight into the cause of AR, such as calcific AV disease, infective endocarditis, flail AV leaflet, or aortic root aneurysm or dissection. If data from echocardiography are suboptimal or are

Table 42–3. Classification of aortic regurgitation (AR) severity.

Stage and Definition	Valve Hemodynamics
A: at risk for AR	• ≤ trace AR
B: progressive AR	Mild AR • Jet width <25% of LVOT • Vena contracta <0.3 cm • RVol <30 mL/beat • ERO <0.10 cm² Moderate AR • Jet width 25%–64% of LVOT • Vena contracta 0.3–0.6 cm • RVol 30–59 mL/beat • RF 30%–49% • ERO 0.10–0.29 cm²
C: asymptomatic severe AR	Severe AR • Jet width ≥65% of LVOT • Vena contracta >0.6 cm • RVol ≥60 mL/beat • RF ≥50% • ERO ≥0.3 cm² • LV dilation
D: symptomatic severe AR	Jet width ≥65% of LVOT • Vena contracta >0.6 cm • RVol ≥60 mL/beat • RF ≥50% • ERO ≥0.3 cm² • LV dilation

ERO, effective regurgitant orifice; LVOT, left ventricular outflow tract; RF, regurgitant fraction; RVol, regurgitant volume; vena contracta, narrowest area of the AR jet.

Data from Nishimura RA, Otto CM, Bonow RO, et al. 2014 AHA/ACC guideline for the management of patients with valvular heart disease: a report of the American College of Cardiology/American Heart Association Task Force on Practice Guidelines, *J Am Coll Cardiol* 2014 Jun 10;63(22):e57-185.

discordant with clinical assessment, cardiac MRI may add useful information.

4. Cardiac catheterization—In most cases, cardiac catheterization is not necessary to diagnose and quantify AR. Older patients who require surgery for AR should first undergo coronary angiography.

▶ Differential Diagnosis

Other causes of chronic HF must be considered in the differential diagnosis of severe chronic AR.

▶ Complications

The course of chronic severe AR is insidious and gradually progressive over many years, ultimately leading to severe HF.

In asymptomatic patients with normal LVEF, the annual rate of progression to symptoms and/or LV dysfunction is <6%; to asymptomatic LV dysfunction, 1.2%; and to SCD, <0.2%. Initial LVESD and rate of change in end-systolic dimension and LVEF during serial studies predict symptoms or death in asymptomatic AR with normal LVEF. An LVESD >50 mm is associated with a risk of death, symptoms, and/or LV dysfunction of 7% to 19% per year. Asymptomatic patients with LV systolic dysfunction (LVEF <50%) develop symptoms that indicate need for AVR within 2 to 3 years.

The onset of angina, dyspnea, or HF heralds greater mortality, with annual rates of 10% in patients with angina and 20% in those with HF. Severity of HF symptoms correlates with mortality risk; annual mortality in a cohort of patients with symptomatic severe AR followed without surgery was 6% in those with NYHA class II and 25% in those with NYHA class III to IV HF symptoms.

▶ Treatment

Mild chronic AR requires no specific treatment. Serial clinical evaluation and echocardiography are recommended at 2- to 3-year intervals. Annual echocardiography is recommended for patients with moderate to severe AR and minimal ventricular dilation if appropriate given prognosis and treatment goals. When the degree of ventricular enlargement approaches surgical indication, echocardiography is recommended every 6 months.

Treatment of hypertension in asymptomatic AR patients is recommended using vasodilators (dihydropyridine calcium antagonist or ACE inhibitor/angiotensin receptor blocker) as first-line agents. New hypertension guidelines suggest a goal of lowering systolic blood pressure to <130 mm Hg, but a goal of <140 mm Hg is generally appropriate in more frail geriatric patients. In the absence of hypertension, vasodilator therapy has not been conclusively shown to alter the natural course of the disease and is not generally recommended in patients with chronic asymptomatic AR and normal LV systolic function. Vasodilators may prolong the compensated phase of asymptomatic patients who have an enlarged LV but normal systolic function. Chronic vasodilator therapy is also recommended in patients with severe AR who are symptomatic or have LV dysfunction but are not considered candidates for surgery.

β-Blockers may potentially worsen AR by prolonging diastole and increasing the volume of regurgitation. On the other hand, β-blockers may be cardioprotective through their effect on LV remodeling. Observational data suggest that β-blocker use is associated with improved survival in patients with chronic severe AR independent of comorbid hypertension and CAD.

Table 42–2 lists Class I indications for surgical treatment of AR. Current guidelines recommend delaying surgery until the appearance of symptoms and/or LV dysfunction or severe LV dilation (Class II recommendation). Results of a prospective observational study that showed similar 10-year overall and cardiovascular survival with early surgery and watchful waiting in propensity-matched patients with asymptomatic severe AR support this recommendation. Lower NYHA classification at the time of surgery predicts better long-term postoperative survival independently of LV function. LV systolic function and LVESD at the time of surgery also predict survival and functional outcomes following SAVR. LV function is more likely to improve following surgery in those with minimal symptoms, milder LV systolic dysfunction, lower LVESD at time of surgery, and a shorter duration of LV dysfunction. In older adults, symptoms and patient preferences should guide the decision of whether or not to consider AVR for chronic severe AR, particularly in octogenarians.

Almost all patients who require surgery for chronic severe AR will undergo valve replacement because the durability of valve repair has not been established. An estimated 3% to 5% of valve surgeries in older adults are for pure primary AR (defined as the absence of concurrent AS and dilated ascending aorta).

A. TAVR

The Euro Heart Survey on Valvular Heart Disease reported that 7.8% of patients with severe AR who met indications for valve surgery had prohibitive perioperative mortality risk and underwent no intervention. Although TAVR has been employed in symptomatic patients with pure native AR, randomized studies are needed to evaluate long-term outcomes and guide patient and device selection. At the present time, TAVR for AR is investigational.

MITRAL STENOSIS

ESSENTIALS OF DIAGNOSIS

▶ History of rheumatic fever or prior streptococcal infection.

▶ Exertional fatigue, hemoptysis, symptoms of HF.

▶ Opening snap and apical mid-diastolic rumbling murmur.

▶ Echocardiogram demonstrating thickened mitral valve with restricted motion and a diastolic pressure gradient between the left atrium and left ventricle.

▶ General Principles

Based on pooled data from US population-based studies, the prevalence of MS is 0.2% in those >65 years old.

MS is an obstruction to the LV inflow caused by a structurally abnormal mitral valve (MV). Normal valve area is 4 to 6 cm². Transvalvular pressure gradient rises when the area

is reduced to <2 cm² and symptoms develop when <1.5 cm². The pathophysiology of MS is associated with the volume of flow through the valve and the duration of diastole. Consequently, patients with severe MS may be intolerant to conditions that result in tachycardia and increased flow, such as exercise, anemia, AF, and infection.

In developed nations, rheumatic fever has become rare while degenerative MV disease is common. MS can occur in patients with prior MV replacement, especially those with bioprosthetic valves. Mitral annular calcification (MAC) is a degenerative process characterized by the deposition of calcium along the valve annulus with extension of the calcification into the leaflets but without fusion of the commissures. The prevalence ranges from 8% to 15% and increases with age. MAC can cause functional MS by impairing the annular dilatation that normally occurs during diastole. In addition to age, chronic kidney disease, chronic inflammatory states, and atherosclerosis risk factors are associated with MAC. Studies support shared pathogenesis between vascular atherosclerosis and MAC. Data on the natural progression of mean MV gradient in calcific MS is limited.

▶ Prevention

Rheumatic MS can be prevented by prompt identification and treatment of group A β-hemolytic streptococcal infections. No interventions have been shown to prevent or delay the development of MAC.

▶ Clinical Findings

A. Symptoms & Signs

The latency period from acute rheumatic fever to symptomatic VHD is two to four decades in developed countries, and the mean age at presentation is in the fifth to sixth decades. Classic symptoms include exertional fatigue, a gradual decline in exercise tolerance, hemoptysis, dyspnea, and orthopnea.

Rheumatic MS is characterized by an opening snap in early diastole followed by a mid-diastolic rumbling murmur. The murmur is low pitched, best heard at the apex in left lateral decubitus position, and intensified by tachycardia. An earlier opening snap and longer duration of the diastolic murmur are associated with more severe stenosis. All of these features may be absent in patients with MS secondary to MAC. Additional findings associated with MS may include evidence for pulmonary hypertension (right ventricular [RV] heave, augmented P$_2$) and evidence for biventricular failure (pulmonary rales, elevated jugular venous pressure [JVP], and peripheral edema).

B. Special Tests

1. Chest radiography—The chest radiograph may demonstrate calcification in the region of the MV, evidence for left atrial or RV enlargement, and increased vascular markings in the lower lung fields.

2. ECG—The ECG demonstrates left atrial enlargement or AF; right axis deviation and signs of RV hypertrophy may also be present.

3. Echocardiography—Echocardiography is the diagnostic procedure of choice because it can reliably determine the presence of MS, assess disease severity, estimate left atrial size, assess suitability for percutaneous balloon mitral commissurotomy (PBMC), and evaluate for rheumatic or calcific involvement of other valves. Transesophageal echocardiography allows better anatomic visualization for further evaluating MS severity and excluding left atrial clot; it is necessary before PBMC. Table 42–4 classifies MS severity.

4. Cardiac catheterization—In older patients with severe MS who are being considered for cardiac surgery, coronary angiography is indicated to evaluate for obstructive CAD.

▶ Differential Diagnosis

Differential diagnosis includes other cardiac and pulmonary conditions that produce left- or right-sided HF, AF, or pulmonary hypertension.

▶ Complications

In minimally symptomatic patients, 10-year survival is >80%. Once limiting symptoms develop, the 10-year survival drops to <15% and is inversely proportional to symptom severity.

After onset of severe pulmonary hypertension, the average survival is 3 years. Increased pulmonary arterial resistance

Table 42–4. Classification of mitral stenosis (MS) severity.

Stage and Definition	Valve Hemodynamics
A: at risk for MS	• Normal transmitral flow velocity
B: progressive MS	• Increased transmitral flow velocity • MVA >1.5 cm² • Diastolic pressure half-time <150 ms
C: asymptomatic severe MS	• MVA ≤1.5 cm² • Diastolic pressure half-time ≥150 ms
D: symptomatic severe MS	• MVA ≤1.5 cm² • Diastolic pressure half-time ≥150 ms

Diastolic pressure half-time, time required for the left atrioventricular *pressure* gradient to decrease to *half* of maximal early diastolic gradient; MVA, mitral valve area.

Data from Nishimura RA, Otto CM, Bonow RO, et al. 2014 AHA/ACC guideline for the management of patients with valvular heart disease: a report of the American College of Cardiology/American Heart Association Task Force on Practice Guidelines, *J Am Coll Cardiol* 2014 Jun 10;63(22):e57-185.

may protect from pulmonary edema and allow patients to be asymptomatic for a prolonged period. Eventually, pulmonary hypertension leads to impaired RV function and adversely affects prognosis.

AF complicates one-third of symptomatic MS cases and affects older patients more frequently. Because atrial contraction helps maintain LV filling, the onset of AF reduces cardiac output, precipitates symptoms, and increases the risk of thromboembolism (approaches 20% per year in the absence of anticoagulation).

Among untreated patients with severe MS, 60% to 70% die from progressive HF, 20% to 30% from systemic embolism, and 10% from pulmonary embolism.

▶ Treatment

Anticoagulation and rate or rhythm control are indicated for AF complicating MS (refer to Chapter 40, "Heart Failure & Heart Rhythm Disorders," for a discussion of AF management). Anticoagulation is also indicated in the setting of sinus rhythm with the presence of a left atrial thrombus or a history of embolism. The efficacy of DOACs for preventing embolic events in MS has not been adequately studied, and vitamin K antagonists are the only approved agents in this setting. Maintenance of sinus rhythm has been shown to improve exercise capacity; however, maintenance may be difficult to achieve, even after commissurotomy, particularly if duration of AF is >1 year and atrial diameter is >45 mm. Injury to the sinoatrial node by the rheumatic process also contributes to difficulty in achieving rhythm control. Anticoagulation should be continued in patients with persistent AF after PBMC. Salt restriction and diuretics are useful to manage vascular congestion. Vasodilator therapy has not been shown to be beneficial in the absence of LV systolic dysfunction.

PBMC involves placing a balloon across the valve and inflating it under pressure to split the fused commissures. PBMC is recommended for symptomatic patients with severe rheumatic MS, a favorable valve morphology (mobile, relatively thin, minimal calcification), and the absence of LA clot or moderate to severe MR. Although PBMC is the mainstay of treatment for MS in younger patients, most older adults are not suitable candidates due to unfavorable valve morphology or concomitant moderate or severe MR. Nonetheless, among older patients without contraindications, PBMC can be performed safely with salutary effects on symptoms and may be considered as a palliative option in selected older adults who are not candidates for surgical treatment. Long-term outcomes after PBMC are less favorable in older compared to younger patients. In one study, 87% of those <40 years compared to 19% of those >70 years were in NYHA class I or II at 5-year follow-up, and mortality rates were 0% and 59%, respectively. Advanced NYHA class and the presence of AF are other predictors of poor outcomes.

In MAC, the annulus and base of the leaflets are calcified but commissures are not fused; therefore, commissurotomy plays no role in the management.

Guidelines recommend MV surgery in severely symptomatic severe MS (NYHA class III/IV) for patients who are not high risk for surgery and who are not candidates for or have failed PBMC. Surgical options include commissurotomy, repair (for MAC), or replacement. Patients with moderate to severe TR may benefit from surgical treatment with concomitant TV repair. The presence of severe MAC can pose technical problems for the surgeon performing valve replacement or repair. Furthermore, patients with MAC are often frail, have multiple comorbidities, and are at high risk for surgery. In older patients with comorbid medical problems or severe pulmonary hypertension, perioperative mortality may be up to 10% to 20%. Patients with markedly elevated pulmonary pressure show reduced RV function and persistent pulmonary hypertension following PBMC or valve replacement.

Concomitant MV surgery is recommended for patients with severe asymptomatic or symptomatic MS who are undergoing cardiac surgery for other indications. Factors to consider when contemplating concomitant MV surgery for patients with moderate MS include presence of AF, rate of progression, and suitability of the valve for subsequent PBMC. In addition, since combining MV surgery with another procedure, such as CABG, increases perioperative risk and may slow recovery, the patient's overall prognosis and goals of care should be taken into account when planning surgery.

MITRAL REGURGITATION

ESSENTIALS OF DIAGNOSIS

▶ Exertional dyspnea or fatigue, orthopnea, peripheral edema.

▶ Holosystolic murmur at the apex radiating to the axilla.

▶ Echocardiography demonstrates MR, increased left atrial size, and ventricular dilation (in chronic severe MR).

General Principles

The prevalence of mild or greater severity MR in the Framingham Heart Study was 19%. MR prevalence increases with advancing age and is the most common valvular disorder in the older adult population.

The mechanisms responsible for MR are classified as primary and secondary. Primary MR results from intrinsic abnormalities in one or more components of the valve apparatus causing incomplete coaptation of leaflets, backflow of blood into the left atrium, and LV volume overload. Eventually, LV dysfunction and symptoms of HF develop. Causes of primary MR include degenerative processes (eg, MV prolapse and annular calcification), ischemia (eg, chordal rupture), rheumatic heart disease, or endocarditis.

In contrast to primary MR, the valve structure is normal in secondary MR; LV remodeling secondary to myocardial infarction or other causes of dilated cardiomyopathy results in papillary muscle and leaflet displacement. Frequent causes of MR in older adults are degenerative processes, ischemia, and nonischemic cardiomyopathy.

Prevention

Therapies directed at preventing the various disorders that cause acute or chronic MR may reduce the prevalence of this condition.

Clinical Findings

A. Symptoms & Signs

Chronic mild or moderate primary MR is usually asymptomatic, and chronic severe MR is often well tolerated as long as LV function is preserved. Once LV dysfunction develops, patients with severe chronic MR typically experience symptoms and signs of left-sided HF, including exertional dyspnea, orthopnea, an S_3 gallop, and pulmonary rales. The onset of symptoms signals worsening prognosis independent of LV function. As the disease progresses, signs of right-sided HF, including elevated JVP and peripheral edema, may ensue. Chronic MR is characterized by an apical holosystolic murmur radiating to the axilla, back, or across the precordium and, in some cases, a diastolic rumble due to high-volume flow across the MV. In patients with MV prolapse, a midsystolic click may be heard, followed by the MR murmur. In patients with severe chronic MR, the apical impulse is laterally displaced, an S_3 gallop may be present, and S_1 and S_2 are blunted.

The presence of symptoms in secondary MR is often confounded by the underlying LV disease, and the associated murmur is often unremarkable, even when MR is severe.

B. Special Tests

1. Chest radiography—The most common finding is cardiomegaly from LV and left atrial enlargement. Annular calcification may be seen. In the absence of pulmonary hypertension, the RV size is normal.

2. ECG—In chronic severe MR, the ECG reveals left atrial enlargement or AF; in advanced stages, there may be evidence of RV hypertrophy.

3. Echocardiography—Echocardiographic findings depend on the cause, chronicity, and severity of primary and secondary MR. A regurgitant MR jet is invariably present, and color Doppler techniques permit a qualitative and semiquantitative assessment of MR severity. The preload is increased and after-load is reduced in MR, resulting in a greater than normal LVEF. LV function may be hyperdynamic (eg, acute severe MR resulting from chordal rupture), normal (eg, moderate chronic MR), or impaired (eg, MR resulting from ischemic or dilated cardiomyopathy). The left atrial size is often normal in acute MR but becomes progressively dilated in severe chronic MR. The MV may appear structurally normal, or there may be evidence of myxomatous degeneration, rheumatic involvement, endocarditis, or a flail leaflet. In secondary MR, the LV is usually dilated with reduced global function and focal LV wall motion abnormalities (WMAs) may be present.

For patients in whom the cause or severity of MR remains in doubt after transthoracic echocardiography, the transesophageal approach provides excellent visualization of MV anatomy and function. Serial measurements of LV size and ejection fraction and pulmonary artery pressure by echocardiography play a crucial role in management and timing of intervention. Follow-up echocardiograms every 3 to 5 years are advised for mild MR, every 1 to 2 years for moderate MR, at time of symptom onset, and with new onset of AF. The echocardiogram is also useful for determining feasibility of valve repair.

4. Cardiac catheterization—Cardiac catheterization with hemodynamic measurement may be helpful in assessing MR severity, and it is essential for defining the coronary anatomy in older adults for whom cardiac surgery is being considered. Table 42–5 classifies MR severity.

▶ Differential Diagnosis

The differential diagnosis of MR includes numerous other conditions that may result in the clinical findings of left- or right-sided HF. Often, multiple such chronic conditions coexist in older patients, and it may be difficult to determine the extent to which the patient's symptoms are a result of MR or other causes.

▶ Treatment

The mechanism of chronic MR influences outcomes with medical therapy. No medical therapy has been shown to delay the need for surgery in primary chronic MR with degenerative causes. Vasodilators are used in acute MR to increase forward flow by reducing impedance to LV ejection; however, there are no conclusive studies of ACE inhibitors, angiotensin receptor blockers, or other vasodilators for primary chronic MR, and they are not recommended for nonhypertensive asymptomatic patients with normal LVEF. For symptomatic patients with severe primary MR and LVEF <60% for whom surgery is not planned, standard treatment for systolic dysfunction is recommended, although with limited supporting evidence.

Table 42–5. Classification of primary mitral regurgitation (MR) severity.

Grade and Definition	Valve Hemodynamics
A: at risk for MR	• MR jet <20% of LA • Vena contracta <0.3 cm
B: progressive MR	• Central jet MR 20%–40% of LA • Vena contracta <0.7 cm • RVol <60 mL • RF <50% • ERO <0.40 cm²
C: asymptomatic severe MR	• Central jet MR >40% LA • Vena contracta ≥0.7 cm • RVol ≥60 mL • RF ≥50% • ERO ≥0.40 cm²
D: symptomatic severe MR	• Central jet MR >40% LA • Vena contracta ≥0.7 cm • RVol ≥60 mL • RF ≥50% • ERO ≥0.40 cm²

ERO, effective regurgitant orifice; LA, left atrium; RF, regurgitant fraction; RVol, regurgitant volume; vena contracta, narrowest area of the MR jet.

Data from Nishimura RA, Otto CM, Bonow RO, et al. 2014 AHA/ACC guideline for the management of patients with valvular heart disease: a report of the American College of Cardiology/American Heart Association Task Force on Practice Guidelines, *J Am Coll Cardiol* 2014 Jun 10;63(22):e57-185.

Optimal medical therapy of systolic dysfunction HF can lead to reverse ventricular remodeling and reduce secondary MR (see Chapter 40, "Heart Failure & Heart Rhythm Disorders").

See Table 42–2 for ACC/AHA Class I recommendations for surgery.

MV repair is the surgical treatment of choice for primary MR to prevent further deterioration of LV function. When there is progressive increase in LV size or decrease in ejection fraction on serial studies, surgery is reasonable if there is a high likelihood of success and low operative risk. Compared with watchful waiting in registry patients with asymptomatic severe degenerative MR, LVEF >60%, and LVESD ≤40 mm, early surgery within 3 months of diagnosis was associated with greater long-term survival and lower risk of HF during a mean follow-up of 10 years.

Improvement in surgical techniques in recent years has yielded better outcomes in all age groups, although it remains worse in the oldest group. Overall operative mortality declined from 16% in 1980 to 3% in 1995. Improvement in cardiac output and length of hospitalization were also observed in all age groups during this period. Patients older than 75 years who underwent MR surgery had more severe disease with NYHA class III or IV symptoms and more comorbidities but experienced similar restoration in life expectancy compared with younger patients when adjusted to expected survival. More recent data of outcomes following isolated primary MV repair in a cohort of 14,604 older adults, performed between January 1991 to December 2007, reported an overall operative mortality of 2.59%. Survival over a mean follow-up period of 5.9 years was 74.9%. The 10-year rates for mitral reoperation, HF, bleeding, and stroke were 6.2%, 30.1%, 15.3%, and 16.4%, respectively, and the 10-year actuarial survival was equivalent to the matched US population (57.4%).

In 31,688 patients who underwent MV replacement alone or in combination with CABG or tricuspid surgery, operative mortality increased from 4% in those aged <50 years to 17% in those aged >80 years, and major operative complications increased from 13.5% to 35.5%, respectively.

Although surgery is recommended for young patients with asymptomatic MR and early LV dysfunction, the presence of symptoms is often the recommended surgical indication in octogenarians. However, MV surgery before onset of LV dysfunction has also been associated with greater freedom from cardiovascular mortality and hospitalization in octogenarians with isolated, nonischemic, nonrheumatic MR. In observational studies, 7-year survival is excellent and no difference between younger and older patients with LVEF >40% and NYHA class I or II symptoms at the time of surgery. Delay in surgery likely contributes to poor outcomes from MV surgery in older adults. Older patients with severe LV dysfunction (LVEF <30%) or markedly dilated left ventricles respond poorly to surgery and should be managed medically.

MV repair is preferred over replacement as treatment of primary MR because it:

1. Preserves the native valve without prosthesis and, in the absence of AF, obviates the need for chronic anticoagulation

2. Preserves LV geometry and function, reducing risk of LV dilatation and HF

3. Is associated with improved survival

Furthermore, mitral repair is associated with lower postoperative stroke and shorter ICU and hospital stay in patients age 75 years and older. However, because of unfavorable valve morphology and the concomitant need for other cardiac surgery, MV repair may be a more complicated procedure in older adults.

Surgical treatment is less straightforward in secondary MR, which is primarily a disease of the ventricle. Outcome of surgery for secondary MR remains suboptimal with high operative and long-term mortality, recurrent MR, and HF rates. For severe nonischemic secondary MR, no evidence supports valve intervention to improve survival or prevent progression of LV dysfunction. For patients with severe ischemic MR from LV systolic dysfunction and evidence of viable myocardium on noninvasive testing, revascularization with CABG improves long-term prognosis, although the effect on MR varies. The benefit of any MV surgery for octogenarians with severe ischemic MR is questionable; in one study, fewer than half of patients who underwent either type of MV surgery were alive at 1 year.

QOL is considered a key indicator of surgical success, particularly in older adults. Two hundred twenty-five patients ≥70 years who underwent surgery for primary MR were surveyed at 3 years; 91% were alive, but greater than half had suboptimal QOL scores, defined as a Minnesota Living with Heart Failure score of >30. Increased age, preoperative AF, diabetes, renal disease, residual MR, and pulmonary hypertension predicted less favorable scores.

A. Transcatheter MV Repair

Percutaneously placed clips (MitraClip) that approximate the anterior and posterior leaflets have been used to treat primary degenerative and secondary MR. Current guidelines recommend limiting transcatheter MV repair (TMVR) to patients with chronic primary MR who remain severely symptomatic despite optimal HF medical treatment, have favorable anatomy for the repair, and a reasonable life expectancy, but prohibitive operative risk.

The Endovascular Valve Edge-to-Edge Repair Study randomized patients with moderate to severe degenerative and secondary MR to MitraClip or MV surgery; patients were followed for the composite end point of freedom from death, MV surgery, and 3+ or greater MR. At 1 year, the rates of the primary end point were 55% in the percutaneous repair group and 73% in the surgery group ($P = .007$), with the difference driven solely by an increased need for surgery in the MitraClip group. At 6 months, few patients experienced worsening MR or surgery indicating long-term durability of the device. Major adverse events occurred within 30 days in 15% of patients in the percutaneous repair group and 48% of patients in the surgery group ($P < .001$). Both groups experienced improvements in LV dimension, NYHA functional class, and QOL measures at 1 year. At 5 years, there was no difference in mortality between surgery and percutaneous repair. NYHA functional class III/IV symptoms were significantly more frequent at 12 months with surgery, a trend that reversed at 5 years, with 8.6% of percutaneous repair patients and 2.5% of surgery patients classified as having severe HF symptoms. Treatment effect heterogeneity was observed, with surgery performing better in patients younger than 70 years and in patients with degenerative MR. Superior results were also seen with surgery in those with LVEF ≥60%. Patients older than 70 years, with secondary MR, or LVEF <60% had similar outcomes with percutaneous repair compared with surgery.

Based on registry data from patients (median age, 83 years) who underwent TMVR from November 2013 to August 2014, early US community experience with TMVR has yielded favorable short-term outcomes. Degenerative MV disease was the cause of MR in 91% of cases, NYHA class III to IV symptoms were present in 86%, and frailty was an indication for the percutaneous procedure in 57%. In-hospital mortality was 2.3%, and 84% of patients were discharged directly home after a median hospital stay of 3 days. At 30 days, mortality rate was 5.8%, stroke rate was 1.8%, and readmission for HF was 3.1%. Overall, 86% were alive at 30 days and were discharged from the hospital with MR grade ≤2 without cardiac surgery. Substantial improvement in HF-specific health status scores were reported at 30 days, which remained stable at 1 year. Although the mortality rate was high (23.0% at 1 year), particularly in subgroups with advanced kidney or lung disease and those with baseline very poor health status, most surviving patients experienced improvements in symptoms, functional status, and QOL.

The COAPT trial, which randomized 614 patients (mean age, 72 years) with HFrEF and moderate or severe secondary MR who remained symptomatic despite the use of maximal medical therapy, demonstrated significantly lower rates of hospitalization for HF (number needed to treat [NNT] = 3.1), lower mortality (NNT = 5.9), and better QOL and functional capacity within 24 months with TMVR plus medical therapy compared with optimal medical therapy alone. Thus, TMVR offers a viable option for appropriately selected older patients with severe MR due to various causes.

B. Cardiac Resynchronization Therapy

WMAs often contribute to secondary MR. Left bundle branch block (LBBB) is one cause of WMA, and in selected patients with severe HF, LVEF <35%, and LBBB with QRS duration ≥150 milliseconds, cardiac resynchronization therapy (CRT) may lead to long-term improvements in MR, cardiac output, symptoms, and reverse remodeling. One-year survival with improvement in NYHA class and without HF hospitalization in older persons who received CRT was comparable with that seen in patients younger than 75 years old (see Chapter 40, "Heart Failure & Heart Rhythm Disorders"). In addition, there was significant reduction in the presence of grade 2 or greater MR in both groups. CRT may be considered for symptomatic patients with chronic severe secondary MR who meet indications for device therapy.

▶ Prognosis

Complications of chronic severe MR include progressive LV failure, eventually leading to AF, pulmonary hypertension, worsening symptoms, and death. Determinants of 5-year adverse events (death, HF, new AF) in asymptomatic persons with primary MR are an effective regurgitant orifice >0.4 cm^2

by echocardiography, increased age, diabetes mellitus, increased LV size, and decreased LV function.

Patients with severe MR from flail leaflet frequently develop symptoms, LV dysfunction, or AF within 2 to 3 years, and mortality related to MR is estimated at 6% to 7% per year. Sudden death occurs in up to 25% of patients with MR due to flail leaflet who are receiving medical treatment.

The presence of MR is associated with worse prognosis in ischemic and nonischemic cardiomyopathy. In older patients, the degree of MR is independently and directly associated with 1-year mortality. Compared to no MR, 1-year mortality rates associated with functional MR from systolic HF in outpatients age 70 years and older with regurgitant severity ranging from 1+ to 4+ were 7%, 15%, 45%, and 57%, respectively.

TRICUSPID REGURGITATION

 ESSENTIALS OF DIAGNOSIS

▶ Symptoms and signs of right-sided HF, including elevated JVP with prominent V wave, enlarged pulsatile liver, ascites, and lower extremity edema.

▶ Holosystolic, high-pitched murmur best heard at the left lower sternal border, increasing during inspiration.

▶ Doppler echocardiography allows visualization of tricuspid regurgitation jet into the right atrium during systole.

▶ General Principles

The tricuspid valve (TV) apparatus consists of three leaflets, chordae tendineae, and papillary muscles. While tricuspid stenosis is rare, tricuspid regurgitation (TR) is frequently encountered. When present in older adults, tricuspid stenosis is usually due to rheumatic heart disease or carcinoid heart disease. In the Framingham Heart Study, the prevalence of moderate to severe TR was 2% in men and 6% in women older than 70 years.

The structural integrity of the TV is intimately linked with RV size and function. In >80% of cases, TR is secondary in nature, arising from chronic volume overload states that lead to RV remodeling, TV annulus dilation, and tethering of the leaflets. The valve apparatus itself is structurally normal in secondary TR. Major causes are left-sided valve (especially mitral) and myocardial disease, AF, pulmonary hypertension from noncardiac conditions, and RV infarction with remodeling. AF, which results in biatrial enlargement and dilation of atrioventricular valve rings, is a common cause in older adults. Primary TR occurs as a result of congenital or acquired causes and is much less prevalent in older adults.

Acquired causes of primary TR include rheumatic disease, TV prolapse, carcinoid, endocarditis, cardiac device, radiation, and trauma. RV pacing can lead to TR through leaflet injury during insertion or intra-annular lead placement.

The management of primary TR should focus on the underlying disease process. The remainder of this section focuses on secondary TR.

► Prevention

Therapies directed at preventing the various disorders that cause TR may reduce its prevalence.

► Clinical Findings

A. Symptoms & Signs

TR typically does not manifest clinically until it has progressed to advanced stages. In severe stages, it is associated with symptoms and signs of right-sided HF including fatigue from low cardiac output, enlarged pulsatile liver due to hepatic congestion with right upper quadrant discomfort, ascites, and edema. Patients may present with palpitations, particularly with concomitant AF. The V wave of TR merges with the C wave, and a large systolic c-V wave may be detected on examination of the JVP. The classic TR murmur is holosystolic, high pitched, best heard at the left lower sternal border, and accentuates during inspiration.

B. Special Tests

The transthoracic echocardiogram is the first-line diagnostic test for differentiating between primary and secondary TR, establishing the cause and severity, defining associated left-sided cardiac disease, assessing RV size and function, and estimating pulmonary artery pressure.

Less commonly, transesophageal echocardiography may be needed to evaluate for vegetations if endocarditis is suspected.

Right heart catheterization is less frequently employed for measuring TR severity, although invasive hemodynamic measurement remains important for diagnosing pulmonary hypertension and assessing response to vasodilator challenge.

► Severity and Stages

Clinically nonsignificant mild TR is commonly seen in structurally normal valves. Grading the severity of TR requires the assessment of hemodynamic parameters measured by echocardiography. The diameter of the TV annulus correlates directly with regurgitant volume. A diastolic diameter of >40 mm is considered significant. TV annuloplasty repair is recommended at the time of left-sided valve surgery with this degree of annular dilation, even in mild to moderate TR,

because of increased risk of progressive TR after isolated MV surgery.

► Treatment

There are no established effective medical therapies for the treatment of severe secondary TR. Diuretics are used to optimize RV preload and treat clinical sequelae of right-sided HF. Medical therapy for RV afterload includes optimizing treatment for left-sided cardiac causes. Pulmonary vasodilators reduce RV afterload and TR in the subgroup of patients with pulmonary hypertension who demonstrate vasoreactive response during right heart catheterization.

A. Surgical & Transcatheter Repair & Replacement

Surgical treatment for secondary TR is aimed at correcting the underlying left-sided valve disease and reducing annular dilation, with the latter often accomplished through an annuloplasty procedure. Annuloplasty, through suture or prosthetic ring implant, improves leaflet coaptation by reducing annulus diameter and correcting annular geometry. TV replacement is considered the primary surgical option when repair is not technically feasible, such as in secondary TR with severe RV remodeling and leaflet tethering.

Isolated TV surgery is rarely performed and is associated with the highest mortality among valve operations. In a large contemporary US registry, only 5005 of these operations were performed over a 10-year period. Factors associated with increased in-hospital mortality include prior left-sided valve surgery, advanced age and NYHA class, RV failure, and pulmonary hypertension.

Surgical management of secondary TR at the time of left-sided valve surgery is recommended because valve regurgitation does not predictably improve following relief of RV overload. Furthermore, concomitant TV repair does not significantly increase the operative risk, whereas reoperation for severe TR after left-sided valve surgery is associated with significant perioperative mortality.

Progression of mild to moderate secondary TR, if uncorrected at the time of left-sided valve surgery, is estimated to occur in 25% of cases. TV annulus diastolic diameter >40 mm or >21 mm/m² is a risk factor for progression. Observational studies and a randomized controlled trial lend support to recommendations for tricuspid repair at the time of MV surgery for stage B secondary TR (mild to moderate TR with impaired leaflet coaptation) and TV annular dilatation. Concurrent TV repair is also recommended for stage B secondary TR in patients with prior evidence of right HF at the time of left-sided valve surgery.

B. Transcatheter Procedures

Transcatheter procedures to treat TV disease are in the early stages of development and clinical application. Several anatomic features of the TV pose challenges to transcatheter interventions. Three types of TV transcatheter procedures are emerging: implantation of a valve at the level of the vena cava; annuloplasty devices to reduce tricuspid annular dimensions; and devices to improve TV leaflet coaptation. Larger trials are needed to evaluate the safety and efficacy of these procedures.

Prognosis

TR of moderate or greater severity was independently associated with increased mortality after adjusting for age and LV and RV function in a study of 5223 ambulatory patients in the Veteran's Administration system who were followed for 4 years. The 1-year survival rate was 65% in patients with severe TR compared with 90% in those without TR.

Prevention of Infective Endocarditis

High-velocity flow through abnormal heart valves is associated with damage to endothelium causing platelet-fibrin deposition, which may be a nidus for infective endocarditis (IE). The estimated proportions of the US population at high and moderate risk of IE are 0.83% and 7.21%, respectively. Older adults are at higher risk for IE due to a greater burden of degenerative valvular disease and implantable devices, as well as increased prevalence of predisposing conditions, such as dental disorders, bacteremia, invasive procedures, and malignancy.

The 2007 AHA guidelines for prevention of IE, updated in 2017, include the following points:

1. Very few cases of IE are prevented by antibiotic prophylaxis, even if it is 100% effective.
2. Prophylaxis is reasonable for dental procedures in the setting of valvular conditions at highest risk for adverse outcome from IE, including those with a prosthetic heart valve, history of IE, cardiac valvulopathy after cardiac transplantation, and certain patients with congenital heart disease.
3. Dental procedures that involve manipulation of gingival tissue, the periapical region of teeth, or oral mucosa perforation warrant prophylaxis in the highest-risk persons.
4. IE prophylaxis prior to a genitourinary or gastrointestinal procedure (eg, cystoscopy, colonoscopy) is not recommended.

Studies of IE trends following the 2007 guideline revision that limited the indications for prophylaxis have reported inconsistent findings. In an interrupted time-series analysis of data from the 2000 to 2007 and 2008 to 2011 National Inpatient Sample, there was a steady increase in the incidence of IE hospitalizations from 2000 to 2011, and the rates were similar in both periods. The rates of valve replacement for IE steadily increased from 2000 to 2007 and plateaued from 2007 to 2011. The effect of the 2007 recommendations on antibiotic prescribing and IE incidence, stratified by IE risk, was investigated in another longitudinal study from May 2003 to August 2015. By the end of the study period, there were significant reductions in antibiotic prescribing for moderate-risk and low/unknown-risk individuals. Of concern was a decrease of 20% in antibiotic prescriptions for those at high risk. These changes in antibiotic prophylaxis prescribing behavior were associated with an increase in the incidence of IE, with the greatest increase seen in high-risk individuals, intermediate increase in moderate-risk patients, and unchanged incidence in the low/unknown-risk group. These findings support the 2017 ACC/AHA guideline, which offers a Class 2a recommendation for antibiotic prophylaxis to highest-risk individuals undergoing high-risk dental procedures. Notably, although older adults are at increased risk for IE, the guideline does not consider age in recommending antibiotic prophylaxis.

In summary, the incidence of heart valve disease increases significantly with age, and the burden of VHD is expected to increase with the aging of the population in the United States and around the world. The emergence of transcatheter valve technology, particularly TAVR for treatment of symptomatic severe AS, has transformed the management of VHD in this population. The appropriate management of VHD in older adults, including the decision to intervene and the choice of intervention, requires complex shared decision making between patients and an integrated multidisciplinary heart valve team in order to achieve desired patient-centered outcomes.

Afilalo J, Lauck S, Kim D, et al. Frailty in older adults undergoing aortic valve replacement: the FRAILTY-AVR study. *J Am Coll Cardiol.* 2017;70(6):689-700.

d'Arcy JL, Coffey S, Loudon MA, et al. Large-scale community echocardiographic screening reveals a major burden of undiagnosed valvular heart disease in older people: the OxVALVE Population Cohort Study. *Eur Heart J.* 2016;37: 3515-3522.

Jansen Klomp WW, Nierich AP, Peelen LM, et al. Survival and quality of life after surgical aortic valve replacement in octogenarians. *J Cardiothorac Surg.* 2016;11:38.

Kapadia SR, Leon MB, Makkar RR, et al. 5-year outcomes of transcatheter aortic valve replacement compared with standard treatment for patients with inoperable aortic stenosis (PARTNER 1): a randomised controlled trial. *Lancet.* 2015;385: 2485-2491.

Mack MJ, Leon MB, Smith CR, et al. 5-year outcomes of transcatheter aortic valve replacement or surgical aortic valve replacement for high surgical risk patients with aortic stenosis (PARTNER 1): a randomised controlled trial. *Lancet.* 2015;385:2477-2484.

Nishimura RA, Otto CM, Bonow RO, et al. 2014 AHA/ACC guideline for the management of patients with valvular heart disease: a report of the American College of Cardiology/American Heart Association Task Force on Practice Guidelines. *J Am Coll Cardiol.* 2014;63:e57-e185.

Nishimura RA, Otto CM, Bonow RO, et al. 2017 AHA/ACC focused update of the 2014 AHA/ACC guideline for the management of patients with valvular heart disease: a report of the American College of Cardiology/American Heart Association Task Force on Clinical Practice Guidelines. *Circulation.* 2017;135:e1159-e1195.

Pant S, Patel NJ, Deshmukh A, et al. Trends in infective endocarditis incidence, microbiology, and valve replacement in the United States from 2000 to 2011. *J Am Coll Cardiol.* 2015;65:20170.

Rodés-Cabau J, Taramasso M, O'Gara PT. Diagnosis and treatment of tricuspid valve disease: current and future perspectives. *Lancet.* 2016;388:2431-2442.

Sabbagh AE, Reddy YNV, Nishimura RA. Mitral valve regurgitation in the contemporary era insights into diagnosis, management, and future directions. *J Am Coll Cardiol.* 2018;11:628-643.

Peripheral Arterial Disease & Venous Thromboembolism

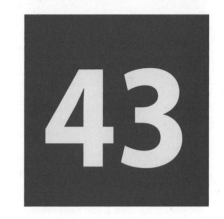

Sik Kim Ang, MB, BCh, BAO
James C. Iannuzzi, MD, MPH

PERIPHERAL ARTERIAL DISEASE

 ESSENTIALS OF DIAGNOSIS

▶ Common symptoms of leg discomfort with ambulation, rest pain, nonhealing ulcers, or gangrene.

▶ Abnormal pulse exam in most patients.

▶ Abnormal ankle-branchial index is diagnostic.

▶ Evidence of systemic atherosclerosis is common.

▶ History of diabetes mellitus, tobacco use, hypertension, or hyperlipidemia may be present.

▶ General Principles

Peripheral vascular disease broadly defines any vascular disease of the extracranial carotid arteries, the aorta and its branches, and the extremities. However, peripheral arterial disease (PAD) is usually used to refer to atherosclerotic disease of the lower extremities. Atherosclerotic PAD is the most common form of PAD in older adults, but the differential diagnosis for arterial vascular disease is quite broad (Table 43–1).

The prevalence of PAD is >10% in individuals older than age 60 years and increases to >25% in people older than 75 years. Although PAD is associated with cardiovascular risk factors such as smoking, hypertension, diabetes mellitus, and hypercholesterolemia, a prevalence of approximately 9% has been documented in patients without traditional risk factors. Nontraditional risk factors, including ethnicity, also influence disease prevalence. Recently, the US Preventive Services Task Force concluded there is insufficient evidence to recommend PAD screening in asymptomatic adults.

In evaluating older adults for PAD, it is important to perform a comprehensive clinical history, review of symptoms, and physical examination. There are two management issues in patients with PAD that are important to successful patient care. First is the need to adequately address underlying cardiovascular risk factors. Atherosclerosis is a systemic process where concomitant cerebrovascular or coronary disease has been demonstrated in up to 30% of patients. The second issue, which is usually more concerning to the patient, is the symptoms related to the vascular occlusive disease. Although most patients with PAD are asymptomatic or present with atypical lower extremity symptoms, intermittent claudication, exertional muscle pain that is consistent in onset and rapidly relieved with rest, is the most common symptom clinically identified with PAD. A minority present with critical limb ischemia (CLI), including ulceration, tissue loss, or gangrene, and are at risk for limb loss. Given this risk for limb loss, CLI is increasingly being referred to as chronic limb-threatening ischemia (CLTI).

▶ Clinical Findings

A. Signs & Symptoms

Intermittent claudication (IC) is recognized as the hallmark of PAD. However, it may be difficult for patients to adequately describe the symptoms of IC. IC is caused by the inability of the arterial supply to meet the metabolic demands of the muscles. Symptoms have been described as muscle pain, cramping, fatigue, tiredness, or even weakness associated with exertion. The symptoms should be reproducible with a constant workload and resolve within 5 to 10 minutes of rest. Most importantly, the symptoms do not occur at rest or with standing alone.

Most patients with PAD do not have symptoms of IC. Only 10% of adults with PAD will have classic IC symptoms, whereas 40% are asymptomatic and the remaining 50% have nonspecific lower extremity exertional symptoms or even have resting symptoms that are difficult to relate to PAD. In many cases, patients are asymptomatic because they

Table 43–1. Peripheral arterial disease.

Vascular etiology
- Atherosclerotic disease—including the carotid, renal, aortomesenteric, and extremities
- Embolic disease—including cardioembolic disease, paradoxical embolism, and artery-to-artery embolism
- Dissection
- Thrombotic disease—related to inherited and acquired thrombophilic processes

Inflammatory
- Vasculitis—may affect any vessel, including large, medium, and small arteries
- Segmental medial arteriolysis—arteriopathy demonstrating necrosis of the media of unknown etiology

Infectious
- Mycotic aneurysm—syphilis, *Salmonella*, and multiple other organisms have been reported

Neoplastic disease
- Primary arterial vascular neoplasm—angiosarcoma and similar malignancies
- Secondary thromboembolic disease—malignancy or myeloproliferative disease related

Drugs
- Culprit agents may include cocaine, amphetamine, ephedrine, intravenous immunoglobulin, pressors (eg, epinephrine, norepinephrine, and phenylephrine), ergotamine, and heparin when associated with heparin-induced thrombocytopenia

Iatrogenic
- Closure devices
- Catheter-related arterial injury
- Small-vessel atheroembolism following instrumentation

Traumatic
- Compression syndromes—popliteal artery entrapment and thoracic outlet syndrome
- Endoluminal iliac artery fibrosis
- Cystic adventitial disease
- Hypothenar hammer syndrome
- Vibration-induced injury

Environmental
- Raynaud disease
- Frost nip
- Frost bite
- Trench foot
- Thromboangiitis obliterans (Buerger disease)—usually in patients younger than age 50 years; related to tobacco use and occasionally to cannabis use

Endocrine
- Calciphylaxis—may be uremic or nonuremic in nature

have altered their lifestyle, becoming more sedentary and/or eliminating symptom-producing activities. Others have nonspecific lower extremity symptoms, both with exertion and at rest, potentially related to comorbid musculoskeletal or neuropathic conditions. The IC history should specifically include an estimate of the walking distance because this can be used to track changes over time.

CLI/CLTI is a more severe presentation of PAD with symptoms of rest pain, nonhealing ulcers or tissue loss, or gangrene. Patients may complain of coldness, numbness, or pain in the foot or toes. This can often be misdiagnosed as neuropathic pain related to diabetes, which is a common comorbidity. A more specific finding is that these symptoms worsen at night when the patient is supine—so-called nocturnal rest pain. These patients may prefer to sleep in a chair or hang the limb over the bed side to improve blood flow and reduce the symptoms through the additional perfusion provided by gravity. Rest pain generally is experienced as pain or cramping in the forefoot in contrast to neuropathy associated with diabetes that is experienced as pins and needles along the entire sole of the foot.

There are nonspecific but common findings of skin changes, including loss of hair elements and dystrophic nail changes. Dependent rubor followed by pallor or blanching of the extremity with elevation may be easily assessed in the office. This physical exam finding of blanching with elevation is important to help distinguish dependent rubor from cellulitis, which will not blanch with elevation. The feet should be regularly inspected at office visits for ulcers between the toes—so-called "kissing ulcers"—and ulcers related to ill-fitting footwear. Ulceration in PAD is a particularly ominous sign because many of these patients ultimately require revascularization for healing.

Pulse examination should include both palpation and grading of the peripheral pulses. Pulses are graded as absent (grade 0), present but diminished (grade 1), normal (grade 2), or bounding (grade 3). In addition to the routine palpation and inspection of the feet, patients should be examined for vascular disease involving other vascular beds. Patients with confirmed diagnosis of PAD are at increased risk for subclavian artery stenosis. Blood pressure should be recorded in both arms. An interarm blood pressure differential of >15 to 20 mm Hg is suggestive of subclavian artery stenosis. The higher of the two extremities should be used for monitoring hypertension and medication titration. The aorta and carotid and femoral arteries should be auscultated for the presence of bruits. The aorta should be palpated for the presence of an abdominal aortic aneurysm. However, the absence of a bruit or inability to palpate the aorta does not exclude disease. Coexistent compromise in cardiopulmonary function, neuropathy, arrhythmia, and severe anemia should be identified because these conditions may negatively impact PAD-related outcomes.

B. Laboratory Findings

There are no laboratory markers to identify patients with atherosclerotic PAD. Patients with PAD should have a fasting lipid profile to assist in the management of dyslipidemia. Fasting blood glucose or hemoglobin A1c (glycosylated hemoglobin) should be measured for detection and treatment of diabetes mellitus. Laboratory evaluation to exclude other nonatherosclerotic vascular disease (see Table 43–1) should be performed as indicated. This may include complete blood count, erythrocyte sedimentation rate, C-reactive protein, and a complete metabolic panel.

C. Diagnostic Testing

Along with pulse assessment, patients with a clinical suspicion of PAD should have baseline evaluation of their perfusion. The ankle-brachial index (ABI) can be used to determine the presence and severity of perfusion (Table 43–2). The ABI is a ratio of systolic arterial pressures recorded in the upper and lower extremities. It can easily be performed in the office or by a vascular laboratory. The required equipment includes a continuous-wave handheld Doppler and a blood pressure cuff. To perform an ABI, the blood pressure cuff is placed sequentially over both upper extremities followed by both lower extremities. With the handheld Doppler positioned sequentially over the brachial, dorsalis pedis (DP), and posterior tibial (PT) arteries, the blood pressure cuff is inflated to suprasystolic pressure and then slowly deflated. The pressure at which the systolic signal is audible is recorded. The ABI is calculated by dividing the highest pressure of the limb, either the DP or PT, by the highest brachial pressure. An ABI ≤0.90 is considered abnormal.

Table 43–2. Classification of the ABI.

ABI	Clinical Significance	Recommendations
>1.4	Consistent with calcified arteries	TBI should be used to determine presence of disease; PVR may be used to determine levels of disease.
1.0–1.4	Normal	With high clinical suspicion for PAD based on symptoms, consider treadmill exercise testing.
0.91–0.99	Borderline	With high clinical suspicion for PAD based on symptoms, consider exercise testing.
0.71–0.9	Mild disease—many patients are asymptomatic but may present with claudication	PVR may be useful if there a need to determine level of disease.
0.41–0.7	Moderate disease—usual claudication range	PVR may be useful if there a need to determine level of disease.
<0.4	Severe disease Usually associated with poor wound-healing potential	Angiographic imaging is warranted for patients with nonhealing wounds or gangrene to determine reperfusion options.

ABI, ankle-brachial index; PAD, peripheral arterial disease; PVR, pulse volume recording; TBI, toe-brachial index.

The current American College of Cardiology and American Heart Association guidelines recommend ABI measurement in patients with exertional leg symptoms suspicious for PAD, who have nonhealing wounds and are older than age 65 years. Patients who experience exertional symptoms but have a normal resting ABI should undergo exercise testing using a treadmill. The ABI should increase with exercise due to increased blood flow; in cases of PAD, the ABI will drop. Treadmill testing also allows documentation of what is stopping the patient from walking and how far they can walk before symptoms begin. Standardized protocols are used, and the patient must be able to safely walk on a treadmill without assistance. A history of significant cardiopulmonary disease, nonhealing ulcers or CLI, and gait abnormalities are contraindications for exercise testing.

In patients with calcified arteries caused by advanced age, diabetes, renal disease, or other processes, the ABI will often be artificially elevated, and an ABI >1.4 is nondiagnostic. When the ABI is nondiagnostic, the toe-brachial index (TBI) should be used. A TBI <0.7 is consistent with PAD. When patients have toe lesions, it is also important to measure the toe pressure because a pressure >55 mm Hg is required for wound healing.

D. Additional Testing

When intervention is considered for lifestyle-limiting symptoms or for CLI, additional testing to determine the anatomical level of disease and plan for revascularization is warranted. Segmental arterial limb pressures and pulse volume recording with or without exercise testing can localize disease as well as provide hemodynamic information. Arterial duplex ultrasound may also be used to localize disease. Duplex imaging provides anatomic information regarding stenosis, occlusion, and calcification within the atherosclerotic lesions. The use of ultrasound avoids contrast and radiation associated with other angiographic imaging. Angiographic imaging, including computed tomographic angiography (CTA), magnetic resonance angiography (MRA), and conventional digital subtraction angiography, is not a diagnostic tool but is used to determine the anatomic levels of disease and plan surgical or endovascular revascularization.

▶ Differential Diagnosis

Patients will not typically complain of lower extremity pain with ambulation. Many patients attribute leg pain to arthritis or part of the aging process. The differential diagnosis of exertional leg symptoms may be quite broad, including a variety of musculoskeletal, neurogenic, and inflammatory conditions. A thorough history, including questions to determine the timing, onset, exacerbating and relieving factors, and a complete physical examination, can help distinguish PAD and IC from other vascular and nonvascular causes of lower extremity exertional symptoms. It can be difficult to

Table 43–3. Characteristics of intermittent claudication and neurogenic claudication.

Clinical Characteristic	Intermittent Claudication	Neurogenic Claudication
Location	Typically calf; may be thigh or buttock with aortoiliac disease	May involve the thigh, buttock, or calf
Description	Aching, cramping, weakness, or fatigue of the muscle	Symptoms may be the same but also include burning, numbness, sharp shooting pain, or tingling
Exercise related	Onset and distance are reproducible	Variable in onset, duration, and reproducibility
Related to standing alone	Never	Frequently
Relief	Standing alone relieves the pain in 3–5 minutes	Usually required to sit or change position; pain may last for up to 30 minutes

distinguish IC from neurogenic claudication (Table 43–3). History demonstrating variability of the symptoms, symptom onset at rest or with standing, and improvement when walking with a shopping cart or when bending forward increases suspicion for neurogenic claudication. PAD and other vascular disorders causing lower extremity ischemia are included in the differential diagnosis of IC (Table 43–1). Magnetic resonance imaging of the spine is indicated when there is a high index of suspicion for neurogenic claudication.

▶ **Treatment**

A. General Considerations

Patients should be educated regarding appropriate foot hygiene and supportive footwear with socks. It is important for patients or a caregiver to inspect their feet for wounds to allow for prompt recognition of toe infections. Minor trauma may be associated with a limb- or life-threatening event in patients with PAD. Diabetic patients should have routine podiatric nail care and daily foot inspection. Shoe gear and devices to offload pressure points and boney prominences are recommended. Patients who are hospitalized, in a nursing home, or otherwise immobile are prone to pressure injury and should be protected.

B. Cardiovascular Risk Reduction

The Reduction of Atherosclerosis for Continued Health (REACH) registry has confirmed the undertreatment of risk

factors in PAD, as well as the risk for primary and recurrent cardiovascular events in this at-risk population. Aggressive cardiovascular risk factor modification is required to slow the progression of PAD and decrease future cardiovascular and cerebrovascular morbidity and mortality. Patients should be treated to achieve risk-reduction goals similar to patients with diagnosed coronary artery disease.

Patients should be advised to stop smoking and offered counseling or pharmacologic therapy. There is emerging evidence for lower and tighter blood pressure control in older adults. In general, blood pressure should be treated to a target of <140/90 mm Hg or <130/80 mm Hg in patients with diabetes or chronic kidney disease. Diabetes should be managed to maintain an HbA1c of approximately 7% to 9% depending on comorbidities and life expectancy. A high-intensity statin such as atorvastatin 40 to 80 mg should be prescribed in all PAD patients regardless of their low-density lipoprotein level. All patients should be on antiplatelet therapy. Aspirin 75 to 325 mg daily is recommended. In aspirin-intolerant individuals, clopidogrel 75 mg daily should be considered.

C. Exercise Therapy

A dedicated walking program can improve pain-free walking distance and maximal walking distance. Structured and supervised exercise programs are more beneficial than self-directed programs. Medicare beneficiaries with symptomatic PAD are eligible for supervised exercise therapy in addition to cardiovascular and PAD risk reduction treatment. Motivated patients may benefit from self-directed walking programs. Patients should be instructed to perform a minimum of three walking sessions weekly. They should walk at a pace to induce symptoms within 5 minutes. After symptom onset, they should rest until the symptoms abate and then resume walking. Each exercise session should last for 30 to 45 minutes using walk-rest-walk cycles. Most patients will see improvement in their walking capacity within 4 to 8 weeks of participation, and significant benefits are usually obtained by 12 to 26 weeks. Patients should be advised that acquired benefits are quickly lost once they stop exercising.

D. Pharmacotherapy

The common pharmacotherapy for patients with PAD includes antiplatelet and statin agents and treatment for underlying hypertension and diabetes mellitus. Cilostazol is a phosphodiesterase-3 inhibitor. The mode by which it improves walking performance in IC is not well understood. The usual dose for cilostazol is 100 mg twice a day. Cilostazol is contraindicated in patients with a history of heart failure. Frequent side effects include headache, palpitations, feeling lightheaded or dizzy, and gastrointestinal effects including nausea and diarrhea. These are more common in older adults. Most side effects are self-limited or are better tolerated by initiating therapy at a reduced dose and escalating to full therapy, and a 50-mg tablet is available for dose initiation.

Pentoxifylline is a hemorrheologic agent thought to improved red blood cell distensibility. The usual dose is 400 mg three times daily. Although there are few side effects associated with pentoxifylline, it has not demonstrated benefit for patients with IC.

E. Revascularization

Revascularization is indicated in patients with CLI and may be considered in those with lifestyle-limiting IC despite optimal medical therapy and participation in an exercise regimen. Angiography, MRA, or CTA is used to determine the optimal revascularization strategy. In patients with CLI, including rest pain, ischemic ulceration, or gangrene, revascularization may be limb saving. For patients with IC, revascularization is generally elective.

A complete discussion of revascularization is beyond the scope of this chapter. The tools, strategies, and options for revascularization continue to evolve and may include endovascular approaches that are minimally invasive using a combination of balloon angioplasty and stent placement, open surgical repair using endarterectomy or lower extremity bypass, or a hybrid approach using a combination of all of the above. Patients should be educated about the expected risks and benefits of revascularization. In the CLEVER (Claudication: Exercise Versus Endoluminal Revascularization) trial comparing supervised exercise programs, stent revascularization, and optimal medical therapy, patients had improved walking times and ABI with supervised exercise and stenting compared to optimal medical therapy. Patients in the stenting arm, however, had better quality of life scores. Patients in exercise programs are required to walk until symptom onset, and this effort and pain tolerance may drive this difference in quality of life. Operators and patients alike usually prefer endovascular procedures to surgical management due to the high complication rates and disability associated with open surgical management, although durability may be decreased in endovascular interventions compared to open repair. Today, more patients are candidates for less invasive procedures. The options and choice for revascularization should be individualized to patient preferences and goals of care, and patients should be referred to specialists who are experienced in both open and endovascular approaches to ensure individualized care is provided.

▶ Prognosis

As mentioned, the overwhelming risk to patients with PAD is the morbidity and mortality associated with secondary cardiovascular and cerebrovascular events. The overall limb prognosis in PAD is good. Approximately 75% of patients with IC remain stable or will improve under the influence of pharmacotherapy and exercise. Only approximately 25% of patients will deteriorate with respect to walking capacity.

A minority of these patients will require an intervention or surgery to improve walking capacity. Less than 4% of patients will suffer limb loss. Most of these patients will be diabetic or continue to smoke. In contrast to PAD, CLI is associated with a poor prognosis; at 1 year, 25% of patients with CLI will be dead and 30% will have undergone amputation. The 5-year survival in CLI patients is <40%. Despite the elevated risk CLI confers, it often goes unrecognized, where >70% of primary care physicians were unaware of the presence of CLI in their patients.

Bhatt DL, Eagle KA, Ohman EM, et al. Comparative determinants of 4-year cardiovascular event rates in stable outpatients at risk or with atherothrombosis. *JAMA.* 2010;304(12):1350-1357.

Curry SJ, Krist AH, Owens DK, et al. Screening for peripheral artery disease and cardiovascular disease risk assessment with the ankle-brachial index: US Preventive Services Task Force recommendation statement. *JAMA.* 2018;320(2):177-183.

Davies MG. Critical limb ischemia: epidemiology. *Methodist Debakey Cardiovasc J.* 2012;8(4):10–14.

Gerhard-Herman MD, Gornik HL, Barrett C, et al. 2016 AHA/ACC guideline on the management of patients with lower extremity peripheral artery disease: executive summary: a report of the American College of Cardiology/American Heart Association Task Force on Clinical Practice Guidelines. *Circulation.* 2017;135(12): e686-e725.

Murphy TP, Cutlip DE, Regensteiner JG, Mohler ER, Cohen DJ, Reynolds MR. Supervised exercise, stent revascularization, or medical therapy for claudication due to aortoiliac peripheral artery disease the clever study. *J Am Coll Cardiol.* 2015;65(10):999-1009.

Peters CML, de Vries J, Lodder P, et al. Quality of life and not health status improves after major amputation in the elderly critical limb ischemia patient. *Eur J Vasc Endovasc Surg.* 2019;27:pii: S1078-5884(18)30799-8.

Treat-Jacobson D, McDermott MM, Bronas UG, et al; American Heart Association Council on Peripheral Vascular Disease; Council on Quality of Care and Outcomes Research; and Council on Cardiovascular and Stroke Nursing. Optimal exercise programs for patients with peripheral artery disease: a scientific statement from the American Heart Association. *Circulation.* 2019;139(4):e10-e33.

VENOUS THROMBOEMBOLISM

ESSENTIALS OF DIAGNOSIS

▶ Surgery (especially orthopedic), immobility, and malignancy are common risk factors.

▶ Typical complaints include acute limb pain and swelling for deep venous thrombosis and pleuritic chest pain and shortness of breath for pulmonary embolism.

▶ Physical findings are nonspecific and often absent.

▶ Confirmation with diagnostic imaging is required.

General Principles

Venous thromboembolism (VTE), including deep vein thrombosis (DVT) and pulmonary embolism (PE), is the third leading cause of cardiovascular death in the United States. More than 400,000 deaths annually are attributed to VTE. VTE risk increases with age. Older adults account for 60% of VTE events. VTE risk for patients older than age 70 years is approximately 1% per year, with a higher mortality and morbidity rate than in younger patients. Table 43–4 lists the inherited and acquired risk factors for VTE. Despite a known association between VTE and inherited thrombophilias, testing for these disorders is rarely indicated in older adults. Patients with idiopathic VTE, without an identifiable etiology, should undergo age- and gender-appropriate cancer screening. Following a complete history, physical examination, and basic laboratory testing, additional testing may include computed tomography (CT) scans, bronchoscopy, and bone marrow evaluation to investigate underlying abnormalities.

Table 43–4. Risk factors for venous thromboembolism (VTE).

Commonly Identified VTE Risk Factors	Less Commonly Recognized VTE Risk Factors
Inherited	Myeloproliferative disorders
Factor V Leiden	Chemotherapy drugs
Prothrombin gene mutation	Inflammatory bowel disease
Protein C deficiency	Multiple myeloma
Protein S deficiency	Infection/inflammation
Antithrombin deficiency	Sepsis
Hyperhomocysteinemia	Paroxysmal nocturnal hemoglobinuria
Elevated lipoprotein(a)	Heparin-induced thrombocytopenia
	Vasculitis
Acquired	Factor VIII excess
Antiphospholipid antibodies	Nephrotic syndrome
Hyperhomocysteinemia	Dysplasminogenemia
Malignancy	Dysfibrinogenemia
Obesity	
Travel	
Immobilization	
Surgery	
Trauma	
Prior VTE	
Hormone therapy and oral contraceptives	
Indwelling lines and devices	

Clinical Findings

A. Signs & Symptoms

The signs and symptoms of VTE are nonspecific, especially in older adults. Therefore, a clinical diagnosis is not acceptable. Patients may present with nonspecific constitutional, limb, or cardiopulmonary complaints. High clinical suspicion and imaging are required to exclude VTE.

Up to 50% of DVTs are asymptomatic. Clinical symptoms include limb pain, swelling, erythema, and increased warmth. Superficial thrombophlebitis may present with localized erythema and tenderness associated with a palpable superficial venous cord. The Homan sign—pain on squeezing the calf or with passive dorsiflexion of the foot—is commonly referred to and noted on examination. However, it lacks sensitivity or specificity for diagnosing DVT and is unreliable for clinical diagnosis.

The symptoms of PE are equally nonspecific. Patients may present with tachycardia and tachypnea without associated complaints. When present, chest pain may be pleuritic in nature. Dyspnea, cough, near syncope, and palpitations are common. Hemoptysis is uncommon and usually associated with pulmonary infarction. Syncope is a common admitting complaint, and PE is frequently overlooked in the differential diagnosis, leading to delays in diagnosis and management.

B. Laboratory Findings

No laboratory test is specific to diagnosis VTE. In the appropriate clinical setting, a negative D-dimer may be used to exclude VTE from the differential diagnosis. D-dimer is frequently positive following surgery, trauma, hospitalization, and pregnancy and in older adults. Therefore, it is best used in the outpatient ambulatory setting in patients at low risk for VTE. A positive D-dimer is not helpful.

VTE patients should have complete blood count, comprehensive metabolic panel, and urinalysis performed to identify underlying disorders associated with VTE. Abnormalities on the initial laboratory testing should be used to direct additional testing or imaging that may be warranted. Antiphospholipid antibody testing may be helpful in the geriatric population. Testing for lupus anticoagulant and anticardiolipin antibodies may influence the duration of therapy and the choice of anticoagulation. Testing for other thrombophilias is less likely to be helpful. Protein C, protein S, and antithrombin deficiency testing are virtually never warranted in older adults.

Patients with acute PE should have biomarker assessment, including troponin and B-type natriuretic peptide (BNP) or N-terminal proBNP (NT-proBNP), to look for evidence of myocardial injury. Both troponin and BNP, when normal, have a high negative predictive value for in-hospital and 30-day postdischarge mortality. When the biomarkers are normal, they may be used to risk stratify patients for accelerated hospital discharge.

C. Diagnostic Testing

Venography is rarely required but remains the gold standard for diagnosing DVT. Duplex ultrasound has become the test of choice to diagnose or exclude DVT. It is widely available, noninvasive, and well tolerated. Duplex ultrasound relies on the inability to completely compress the lumen of the vein using externally applied pressure. Intraluminal echogenicity is less specific for DVT. Secondary changes in the venous waveforms are also evaluated. Normal waveforms are phasic with respiration and augment with calf compression. The failure to augment or loss of phasicity, monophasic waveforms, may indicate proximal obstruction. Only venous segments that are adequately visualized can be assessed for DVT. This is a limitation that is frequently misunderstood. If a venous segment is not fully evaluated, DVT cannot be excluded. The sensitivity and specificity of duplex ultrasound for DVT diagnosis are approximately 98%. If there is negative testing but high clinical suspicion, especially for iliac, inferior vena cava (IVC), or calf vein DVT, repeat duplex imaging in 5 to 7 days is likely warranted.

CT venography (CTV) and magnetic resonance venography (MRV) may be used for diagnosis, especially when imaging the IVC and pelvic veins. CTV can easily be added to CT PE imaging. This does not require additional contrast, but the radiation exposure is significant. MRV does not use radiation and does not necessarily require contrast. Furthermore, the contrast used in MRV (usually gadolinium) has a much lower incidence of nephrogenic systemic fibrosis and, in general, is safe even in patients with reduced kidney function. Imaging may be helpful in evaluating patients with acute and chronic DVT. However, imaging may not be readily available, and claustrophobia may limit some patients' ability to perform testing. CTV and MRV may be used as an alternative to venography to confirm the diagnosis of DVT when duplex imaging is nondiagnostic.

Up to 50% of patients with DVT may have clinically asymptomatic PE. Clinical suspicion for PE should prompt appropriate testing, which may include electrocardiogram, chest x-ray, ventilation-perfusion scan, CT with pulmonary angiogram, or pulmonary angiography. Chest x-ray may be normal and is frequently nonspecific. When abnormal, findings of volume loss, atelectasis, effusions, or infiltrates predominate. The classically described Westermark sign (focal oligemia), Hampton hump (wedge-shaped pleural-based density), and pulmonary artery enlargement are uncommon. Electrocardiogram findings are also frequently nonspecific. The most common finding is sinus tachycardia. The classically described $S_1Q_3T_3$ changes may be seen with large PE and right ventricular strain.

Ventilation-perfusion lung scanning is still used to diagnose acute PE. However, in many centers, availability is limited. The testing should be performed in the setting of a normal chest x-ray and when there is high clinical pretest probability for PE. Nondiagnostic intermediate or indeterminant scans are common. Only scans that are read as normal or near normal or high probability are helpful to exclude or diagnose PE.

CT pulmonary angiogram (CTPA) is the most widely available and commonly used test for diagnosing PE. It is readily available and well tolerated. PE is diagnosed as an intraluminal filling defect within the pulmonary arteries. With advanced technology, scanners can complete imaging to the level of the subsegmental pulmonary arteries in a single breath-hold. It requires contrast and may be limited in patients with renal insufficiency. Timing of the contrast bolus is essential, and in some patients may limit the sensitivity and specificity of the examination, especially for more peripheral emboli. CTPA can also be used to evaluate for radiographic signs of right heart strain associated with large PE. A right ventricle to left ventricle ratio >0.9 measured on a four-chamber view is consistent with right heart strain.

Pulmonary angiography remains the gold standard for diagnosing PE, although it has been essentially replaced by CTPA imaging. The contrast and radiation exposure are similar, and CTPA is less invasive. If CTPA imaging is nondiagnostic and there is a need to diagnose or exclude PE, then angiography is the test of choice. Despite widely held beliefs that angiography is too invasive to use regularly, complications related to angiography are infrequent. Angiography may be indicated in cases of massive PE where pulmonary vein thrombectomy may also be indicated as a treatment modality for patients who are hemodynamically unstable.

Echocardiography is not a diagnostic test for PE, although echocardiographic information may be helpful to risk stratify patients for thrombolytic therapy or for accelerated hospital discharge. Echocardiography is used to evaluate right heart dysfunction. Right heart strain portends a worse in-hospital outcome compared to patients without evidence for right ventricle volume overload. Findings on echocardiogram include right ventricle dilation, septal flattening or deviation toward the left ventricle, tricuspid regurgitation, and elevated right ventricle systolic pressure.

▶ Differential Diagnosis

Unilateral leg pain, erythema, and swelling are common symptoms. Within the differential diagnosis, one must consider superficial thrombophlebitis, popliteal cyst with or without rupture, traumatic injury such as a sprain or ruptured calf muscle, cellulitis, chronic regional pain syndrome, and acute inflammation associated with chronic venous insufficiency. In patients with a low pretest clinical probability, a negative D-dimer excludes DVT and eliminates the need for additional testing.

The signs and symptoms associated with PE are also nonspecific. Other cardiopulmonary, vascular, and inflammatory etiologies must be excluded. Included in the differential diagnosis are myocardial injury, pericarditis, congestive heart failure, pneumonia, pleuritis, pneumothorax, aortic dissection, and musculoskeletal sprain, strain, or contusion.

Complications

The risk of postthrombotic syndrome (PTS) after DVT is significant. Many patients develop symptoms within 2 years following the initial event. Extensive DVT and recurrent events increase PTS risk. Compression stockings can be used for symptomatic PTS. A minority of patients (<5%) will develop chronic thromboembolic disease (CTED) after PE. There are no clinical factors, biomarkers, or other strategies to determine which patients are at risk. Patients presenting with progressive dyspnea or right heart dysfunction following PE should be evaluated for CTED.

Treatment

A. General Considerations

Anticoagulation is the mainstay of treatment for VTE. Appropriate therapy should be started when the diagnosis of VTE is considered. In patients at low risk for complications from anticoagulation, data collection and diagnostic testing should not delay the initiation of anticoagulation. Intravenous unfractionated heparin (UFH), low-molecular-weight heparin (LMWH), and fondaparinux are appropriate initial therapies for VTE. Longer term options include vitamin K antagonists (VKAs), direct oral anticoagulants (DOACs), and LMWH. Anticoagulant choice may be informed by the underlying mechanism of the VTE (see Chapter 44, "Anticoagulation").

Patients with DVT without signs or symptoms of PE can frequently be treated either solely or at least partially as an outpatient. Arranging home therapy, self-injection teaching, and patient education require staff time and dedication, but many patients are able to successfully perform the necessary tasks. Clinically stable patients with PE can frequently be assessed using echocardiography and biomarkers such as troponin and BNP. When these tests are normal, patients can be treated either as an inpatient or using an accelerated discharge plan. Close clinical follow-up after discharge should be arranged for all VTE patients.

Patients with a contraindication to anticoagulation should be managed by IVC filter insertion. However, appropriate anticoagulation should be initiated once the anticoagulation risk has resolved and the IVC filter is removed.

B. Pharmacotherapy

Please see Chapter 44, "Anticoagulation," for more in-depth discussion. In the acute inpatient setting, UFH should be administered using weight-based bolus and infusion dosing. The activated partial thromboplastin time (aPTT) should be titrated to keep the patient within the appropriate therapeutic range. It is important to recognize that the aPTT therapeutic range is institution specific and awareness of local protocols is necessary. In patients in whom thrombolysis may be considered, UFH is the drug of choice because of its short half-life and the ability to easily monitor therapy.

Alternative therapy, such as LMWHs, provides the opportunity for once- or twice-daily dosing. Ease of administration also facilitates accelerated discharge or home therapy for appropriate patients. The available LMWHs are all renally excreted. In older adults with creatinine clearance <30 mL/min, the clinician should consider using LMWH with doses adjusted for renal function as recommended in product labeling or switching to an alternative anticoagulant with lower renal clearance. Patients who develop VTE in the setting of an underlying malignancy are best managed with LMWH.

Fondaparinux is a pentasaccharide molecule approved for treating both DVT and PE when therapy is initiated in the hospital. Dosing is weight based. Patients who weigh <50 kg should receive 5 mg daily; patients who weigh 50 to 100 kg should receive 7.5 mg daily; and patients who weigh >100 kg should receive 10 mg daily. Fondaparinux is renally excreted. It should be used cautiously with renal insufficiency and is not appropriate with a creatinine clearance <30 mL/min. The half-life is approximately 17 hours. The drug should be avoided when there is a need for intervention or a high risk of bleeding. There is no antidote to reverse the effects of fondaparinux.

VKA has been the long-term drug of choice for most patients. In general, the first dose of VKA may be started on the day of admission. Warfarin, a vitamin K antagonist, interrupts the terminal carboxylation of vitamin K–dependent proteins. Therefore, a minimum 4- to 5-day overlap between the parenteral drug and warfarin is required to ensure the premade vitamin K–dependent proteins have been adequately depleted. For most patients, the target international normalized ratio (INR) is 2.5, with an acceptable range being between 2 and 3. After the minimum 4- to 5-day overlap, the INR should be >2 on 2 consecutive days before stopping the parenteral drug and maintaining warfarin therapy.

DOACs are the newer oral anticoagulants such as the oral direct thrombin inhibitor dabigatran, and the oral anti-Xa agents rivaroxaban, apixaban, and edoxaban. Potential advantages of these agents are the once- or twice-daily oral administration. These drugs do not require monitoring. There are newly developed antidotes for DOAC, which are discussed in Chapter 44. If specific antidotes are unavailable, activated charcoal (100 g orally or via nasogastric tube if ingestion time is <6 hours) or a four-factor prothrombin complex concentrate (50 units/kg intravenously, single dose not to exceed 5000 units) can be given. Overall, the cost of DOACs is still considerably higher than VKA.

C. Intervention

Patients with extensive DVT or massive PE who are unstable at the time of admission should be assessed for thrombolysis. The use of pharmacomechanical thrombolysis (PMT) or catheter-directed thrombolysis (CDT) is not confined to patients with phlegmasia cerulean dolens (PCD) or venous gangrene. PCD is a life-threatening complication of acute DVT presenting as marked swelling of the extremities with pain and cyanosis due to obstruction of venous outflow. This can progress to phlegmasia alba dolens, where the arterial flow itself is compromised, and can lead to gangrene if not treated promptly. Patients with proximal DVT in the common femoral and iliac veins may benefit from PMT to help clear the thrombus in an effort to preserve valve function, improve mobility, and decrease symptoms associated with the acute DVT. It remains unclear who benefits from PMT and the role that timing from DVT onset plays in preservation of valve function.

Patients with massive unstable PE should also be considered for thrombolysis, either systemic infusion or catheter-based therapies. Patients with submassive PE with significant cardiopulmonary dysfunction may be appropriate for thrombolytic therapy, but the bleeding risks may outweigh the benefits in these patients. The risk for major bleeding in thrombolysis is approximately 15%. The risk for intracranial bleeding is often cited as 1% to 2%. Bleeding risk is increased in patients older than age 70 years. Recent surgery or trauma, gastrointestinal bleeding, uncontrolled hypertension, and recent stroke are contraindications to thrombolysis.

IVC filter insertion is appropriate in patients with a contraindication to anticoagulation or in whom anticoagulation is complicated by bleeding or thrombosis despite adequate therapeutic anticoagulation. Many IVC filters deployed today are used for relative indications, including underlying cardiopulmonary disease, significant PE, free-floating DVT visualized on duplex ultrasound, and patients at high risk for noncompliance with anticoagulation. It is important to realize that IVC filters help manage patients with DVT and prevent massive PE. However, IVC filters do not treat DVT or prevent PE, and anticoagulation is required to stop propagation of the DVT, prevent recurrent DVT, and prevent embolism. Once the absolute or relative risk for anticoagulation has resolved, appropriate anticoagulation should be initiated. Patients with an optionally retrievable IVC filter should be assessed for filter retrieval prior to stopping anticoagulation. There is sufficient data to suggest that retained filters may contribute to subsequent DVT. Once they are no longer required, they should be removed if possible.

D. Additional Considerations

Bed rest used to be frequently advised in patients with DVT and PE, but this is actually detrimental to recovery. Studies demonstrate that ambulation is not associated with increased risk for PE but does improve venous patency. Clinically stable patients should be encouraged to ambulate while hospitalized and return to normal activities after discharge. Patients should be considered for compression stockings after DVT when symptoms include leg swelling. Compression stockings with pressure of 20 to 40 mm Hg have been shown to improve quality of life and may help prevent PTS. Compression stockings have not been associated with any adverse events.

E. Duration of Therapy

The optimal duration of therapy for VTE is unknown. Decisions regarding continuing or discontinuing anticoagulation should take into account the underlying etiology of the VTE, patient comorbidities, patient preference for anticoagulation, and the estimated risk for recurrence. In general, a situational event following surgery, hospitalization, or other limited risk factors should be treated for a minimum of 3 months and until the attributable risk factor is no longer present. Patients with idiopathic VTE require a minimum of 6 to 12 months of initial anticoagulation. Patients with recurrent VTE, underlying high-risk thrombophilias, or cancer likely require indefinite therapy. However, to determine the optimal duration of therapy, the benefits of anticoagulation need to be weighed against the risk.

▶ Prognosis

Older adults with VTE have significantly higher mortality and mortality than younger patients. During the first 3 months of VTE treatment, older adults may die of their underlying cancer, PE, infections, or bleeding complications. Close follow-up after VTE in this group of frail population is recommended because >20% will have recurrent VTE within 5 years. PTS is the major long-term complication of DVT and occurs in over a third of patients. Complaints may include subjective leg symptoms (pain, cramps, pruritis, and paresthesias), signs of stasis (pretibial edema, redness, induration, hyperpigmentation, and venous ectasia), and leg ulceration.

Gould MK, Garcia DA, Wren SM, et al. Prevention of VTE in nonorthopedic surgical patients: Antithrombotic Therapy and Prevention of Thrombosis, 9th ed: American College of Chest Physicians evidence-based clinical practice guidelines. *Chest.* 2012;141(suppl 2):e227S-277S.

Kearon C, Akl EA, Ornelas J, et al. Antithrombotic therapy for VTE disease: CHEST Guideline and Expert Panel report. *Chest.* 2016;149(2):315-352.

Lim W, Le Gal G, Bates SM, et al. American Society of Hematology 2018 guidelines for management of venous thromboembolism: diagnosis of venous thromboembolism. *Blood Adv.* 2018;2(22):3226-3256.

Merli GJ. Pathophysiology of venous thromboembolism, thrombophilia and the diagnosis of deep vein thrombosis-pulmonary embolism in the elderly. *Clin Geriatr Med.* 2006;22(1):75-92.

Prandoni P, Noventa F, Ghirarduzzi A, et al. The risk of recurrent venous thromboembolism after discontinuing anticoagulation in patients with acute proximal deep vein thrombosis or pulmonary embolism. A prospective cohort study in 1,626 patients. *Haematologica.* 2007;92:199-205.

Tritschler T, Aujesky D. Venous thromboembolism in the elderly: a narrative review. *Thromb Res.* 2017;155:140-147.

Tritschler T, Kraaijpoel N, Le Gal G, Wells PS. Venous thromboembolism: advances in diagnosis and treatment. *JAMA.* 2018;320(15):1583-1594.

Anticoagulation

Anita Rajasekhar, MD, MS

Rebecca J. Beyth, MD, MSc

General Principles

Anticoagulants are a class of drugs essential for the optimal management of many thromboembolic and vascular disorders that are highly prevalent among older patients. Anticoagulants are unique compared to most pharmacologic agents because even small deviations from "therapeutic levels" place patients at risk for life-threatening complications. While older patients with multimorbidity are particularly susceptible to thrombosis, they also have higher risks of bleeding than the general population. With the approval of direct oral anticoagulants (DOACs) for thrombotic conditions, these agents are being used more frequently than traditional anticoagulants in the older patient due to convenience and lower bleeding risk in the general population. This chapter briefly reviews current anticoagulant therapy and focuses on the newer agents and recommendations for their use in older patients.

AVAILABLE CLASSES OF ANTICOAGULANT THERAPY

Current anticoagulants that are available for use in the United States include unfractionated heparin (UFH), vitamin K antagonists (VKAs), low-molecular-weight heparins (LMWHs), indirect selective factor Xa inhibitor, and the direct thrombin (parental and oral) and factor Xa inhibitors. Tables 44–1 and 44–2 summarize the specific pharmacologic characteristics of these agents.

Oral Vitamin K Antagonists

Concerns about the use of anticoagulants in older patients arise from their increased risk for anticoagulant-related bleeding. The major determinants of oral VKA-induced bleeding are the intensity of the anticoagulant effect, as measured by the international normalized ratio (INR); patient characteristics; concomitant use of drugs that interfere with hemostasis or vitamin K metabolism; and the length of therapy. Of these, the INR is the most important risk factor, and this is especially true for intracranial hemorrhage (ICH), the most feared site of major bleeding. The risk of ICH increases seven-fold with increasing INR levels >4.0. Patient characteristics, including age and specific comorbid conditions (ischemic stroke, diabetes, renal insufficiency, malignancy, hypertension, liver disease, or alcoholism), also are associated with increased risk of major bleeding. In general, older patients have approximately a two-fold increase in major bleeding compared to their younger counterparts. Decision making around the use of anticoagulants is complex because the risk factors that are associated with anticoagulant-related bleeding are similar to those associated with increased risk of thrombosis. The use of anticoagulant medications in older patients is an area where applying the principles of shared decision making is critical. The choice of whether to prescribe anticoagulants and which specific medication to use should be individualized, considering not only evidence-based medicine, but also patients' goals and preferences to ensure adherence.

The clinical utility of pharmacogenetic-based warfarin dosing in older patients is not clear. In a cohort of patients ≥65 years old (mean age, 81 years) that included nursing home and long-term care residents on warfarin with stable therapeutic INRs, Schwartz et al noted that the addition of genotype information helped to explain a significantly greater proportion of the INR variability when compared to those without genotype information. However, when comparing estimated warfarin doses to actual warfarin doses in patients requiring <2 mg/day of warfarin, the addition of genotype information did not improve the dosing management. Because earlier studies observed that increasing age is associated with increasing response to the effects of warfarin as manifested by lower daily doses, the applicability of pharmacogenetic dosing algorithms to older patients requiring lower warfarin dosing is somewhat limited. Thus, the adage of "start low and go slow" still remains applicable to warfarin dosing in older patients.

Table 44–1. Available classes of parenteral anticoagulant therapy.

Properties	Heparin and Derivatives		Specific Indirect Anti-Xa Inhibitor	Parental Direct Thrombin Inhibitors		
	UFH	LMWH	Fondaparinux	Argatroban	Desirudin	Bivalirudin
Subtype		Enoxaparin, dalteparin, tinzaparin	Fondaparinux			
Elimination	Reticuloendothelial system	Renal	Renal	Hepatic	Renal	Enzymatic, 20% renal
Time to peak concentration	IV: immediate SQ: 20–60 minutes	~1.5 hours	~2 hours	Immediate	Immediate	Immediate
Half-life	~1.5 hours	~2–5 hours	~17–21 hours	~45 minutes	~120 minutes	~25 minutes
Lab monitoring	aPTT, anti-Xa heparin levels	Not required; can measure anti-Xa LMWH levels	Not required; can measure anti-Xa fondaparinux levels	aPTT, ACT	Not required; can monitor aPTT	aPTT, ACT
Prolongation of INR at therapeutic concentrations	No	No	No	Significant	Minor	Minor
Reversible (antidote)	Complete with protamine	Partial with protamine	No	No	No	No
Dose adjustments	None	Renal impairment, extremes of weight: titrate to desired anti-Xa level	Renal impairment: titrate to desired anti-Xa level	Moderate hepatic impairment: 0.5 µg/kg/min in HIT Severe HF: CI	CrCl <31–60 mL/min: DR unnecessary	CrCl 15–60 mL/min: 15%–50% DR CrCl <15 mL/min: CI
FDA indications	• AF with embolization • DIC • Thrombosis prevention in extracorporeal circulation and dialysis procedures • Prophylaxis and treatment of VTE and peripheral arterial embolism • Treatment of unstable angina and NSTEMI	Varies according to subtype of LMWH Includes: • Prophylaxis and treatment of VTE • Prevention of thrombus in hemodialysis circuit • Treatment of unstable angina, NSTEMI, and STEMI	Prophylaxis of DVT in: • Hip fracture surgery • Hip replacement surgery • Knee replacement surgery • Abdominal surgery Treatment of: • Acute VTE when administered with warfarin	• Prophylaxis or treatment of thrombosis complicating HIT • HIT with or without thrombosis undergoing PCI	• DVT prevention after hip replacement surgery	• Unstable angina undergoing PTCA • PCI with provisional use of GPI • HIT with or without thrombosis

ACT, activated clotting time; AF, atrial fibrillation; aPTT, activated partial thromboplastin time; CI, contraindicated; CrCl, creatinine clearance; DIC, disseminated intravascular coagulation; DR, dose reduction; DVT, deep vein thrombosis; FDA, US Food and Drug Administration; GPI, glycoprotein inhibitor; HF, heart failure; HIT, heparin-induced thrombocytopenia; INR, international normalized ratio; IV, intravenous; LMWH, low-molecular-weight heparin; NSTEMI, non–ST-segment elevation myocardial infarction; PCI, percutaneous coronary intervention; PTCA, percutaneous transluminal coronary angioplasty; SQ, subcutaneous; STEMI, ST-segment elevation myocardial infarction; UFH, unfractionated heparin; VTE, venous thromboembolism.

Table 44–2. Available classes of oral anticoagulant therapy.

Properties	Vitamin K Antagonist	New Oral Anticoagulants				
Type	Warfarin	Dabigatran	Rivaroxaban	Apixaban	Edoxaban	Betrixaban
Mechanism of action	Inhibits synthesis of vitamin K–dependent clotting factors	Direct thrombin inhibitor	Direct factor Xa inhibitor	Direct factor Xa inhibitor	Direct factor Xa inhibitor	Direct factor Xa inhibitor
Time to peak concentration	90 minutes (peak anticoagulant effect 5–7 days)	~1.5 hours	~3 hours	~3–4 hours	~1–2 hours	~3–4 hours
Half-life (normal CrCl)	36–42 hours	12–14 hours	4–9 hours Up to 13 hours in older patients	~12 hours	~10–14 hours	~19–27 hours
Clearance	Hepatic	80% renal	33% renal	25% renal	35% renal	11% renal
	Avoid in hepatic insufficiency Lower maintenance doses may be required in patients with the CYP2C9*2, CYP2C9*3, and VKORC1 A variants	CrCl 15–30 mL/min: 75 mg BID CrCl <15 mL/min, severe hepatic disease: contraindicated 110 mg BID if >80 years old	CrCl 15–50 mL/min: caution CrCl <15 mL/min: contraindicated	For atrial fibrillation: in patients with at least 2 of the following characteristics: age ≥80 years, body weight ≤60 kg, or serum creatinine ≥1.5 mg/dL, the recommended dose is 2.5 mg orally BID	For atrial fibrillation: CrCl >95 mL/min: do not use CrCl 15–50 mL/min: 30 mg QD For VTE: CrCl 15–50 mL/min or body weight ≤60 kg or who use certain P-glycoprotein inhibitors: 30 mg QD	CrCl 15–30 mL/min: dose reduction recommended
Lab monitoring	INR	Not required; TT/TCT or aPTT	Not required; anti-Xa assay calibrated to rivaroxaban	Not required; anti-Xa assay calibrated to apixaban	Not required; anti-Xa assay calibrated to edoxaban	Not required; anti-Xa assay calibrated to rivaroxaban
Reversible (antidote)	Vitamin K, fresh-frozen plasma, prothrombin complex concentrates, rFVIIa	Idarucizumab	Andexanet alfa	Andexanet alfa	No FDA-approved reversal	No FDA-approved reversal

(continued)

Table 44–2. Available classes of oral anticoagulant therapy. (continued)

Properties	Vitamin K Antagonist	New Oral Anticoagulants				
	Warfarin	Dabigatran	Rivaroxaban	Apixaban	Edoxaban	Betrixaban
Type						
FDA-approved indications as per package inserts	1. Prophylaxis and treatment of venous thrombosis and its extension, PE 2. Prophylaxis and treatment of thromboembolic complications associated with atrial fibrillation and/or cardiac valve replacement 3. Reduction in the risk of death, recurrent myocardial infarction, and thromboembolic events such as stroke or systemic embolization after myocardial infarction	1. Prevention of stroke and systemic embolism in nonvalvular atrial fibrillation 2. Treatment of DVT and PE patients who have been treated with a parenteral anticoagulant for 5–10 days 3. Prevention of recurrent DVT or PE in patients who have been previously treated 4. Prophylaxis of DVT or PE in patients who have undergone hip replacement surgery	1. Prevention of stroke and systemic embolism in nonvalvular atrial fibrillation 2. Treatment of DVT and PE 3. Reduction in the risk of recurrence of DVT and/or PE in patients at continued risk for recurrent VTE after completion of initial treatment lasting at least 6 months 4. Prophylaxis of DVT or PE in patients who have undergone hip and knee replacement surgery 5. To reduce risk of major cardiovascular events in combination with aspirin in patients with chronic coronary artery disease or peripheral artery disease 6. For the prophylaxis of VTE in acutely ill medical patients at risk for thromboembolic complications not at high risk of bleeding	1. Prevention of stroke and systemic embolism in nonvalvular atrial fibrillation 2. Treatment of DVT and PE 3. Prevention of recurrent DVT or PE in patients who have been previously treated 4. Prophylaxis of DVT or PE in patients who have undergone hip and knee replacement	1. Prevention of stroke and systemic embolism in nonvalvular atrial fibrillation 2. Treatment of DVT and PE in patients who have been treated with a parenteral anticoagulant for 5–10 days	1. Prophylaxis of VTE in adults hospitalized for an acute medical illness who are at risk for thromboembolic complications due to moderate or severe restricted mobility and other risk factors for VTE

aPTT, activated partial thromboplastin time; BID, twice daily; DVT, deep vein thrombosis; DVT, deep vein thrombosis; FDA, US Food and Drug Administration; CrCl, creatinine clearance; INR, international normalized ratio; PE, pulmonary embolism; QD, once daily; rFVIIa, recombinant activated factor VII; TT/TCT, thrombin time/thrombin clotting time; VTE, venous thromboembolism.

Table 44–3. Common warfarin drug interactions.

Drug	Effect on Warfarin	Mechanism
Metronidazole	Potentiates	Inhibition of vitamin K synthesis by intestinal flora and CYP2C9 inhibition
Macrolides	Potentiates	Inhibition of vitamin K synthesis by intestinal flora and CYP2C9 inhibition
Fluoroquinolones	Potentiates	Inhibition of vitamin K synthesis by intestinal flora and CYP2C9 inhibition
Trimethoprim-sulfamethoxazole	Potentiates	CYP2C9 inhibition
Fluconazole	Potentiates	CYP2C9 inhibition
Selective serotonin reuptake inhibitors	Potentiates	CYP2C9 inhibition
Amiodarone	Potentiates	CYP2C9 inhibition
Levothyroxine	Potentiates	Increased vitamin K–dependent clotting factor catabolism
Garlic	Potentiates	Not well understood
Ginger	Potentiates	Not well understood
Gingko biloba	Potentiates	Not well understood
Ginseng	Potentiates	Not well understood
Carbamazepine	Inhibits	CYP2C9 inducer
Phenytoin	Inhibits	CYP2C9 inducer
Phenobarbital	Inhibits	CYP2C9 inducer
St. John's wort	Inhibits	CYP2C9 inducer

CYP2C9, cytochrome P450 2C9.

Many drugs are known to interact with VKAs, and because the majority of older patients are prescribed more than one drug, there is ample opportunity for adverse drug reactions to occur in older patients. Drugs that potentiate the anticoagulant effect (increase the INR) increase the risk of bleeding. Other drugs increase hepatic metabolism, resulting in decreased anticoagulant effect and increased dosage requirements (Table 44–3). When these drugs are discontinued, there can be an increase in INR and bleeding. Additional monitoring with potential dosage adjustment is required when these drugs are either added to or removed from the medication profile of older patients on warfarin therapy.

Despite its efficacy in treatment and prophylaxis, warfarin has several limitations that make its use cumbersome.

These include its slow onset of action, narrow therapeutic window, lack of predictability in anticoagulant effect by drug dose, many dietary and drug interactions, and need for routine INR monitoring. Some of this burden may be lessened with less frequent INR monitoring (up to every 12 weeks vs every 4 weeks), which has been shown to be safe in patients with stable INRs. Older patients who are motivated and can demonstrate competency can self-manage and/or self-test. Best practices for ensuring safety include using a coordinated monitoring system with patient education, systematic INR testing, tracking and follow-up, and good communication. (For travel recommendations for older adults on warfarin, see Chapter 77, "Older Travelers.") Despite the burden of warfarin management, this drug may be the anticoagulant of choice in devices that require anticoagulation (eg, mechanical heart valves), thrombosis in unusual locations (eg, cerebral vein or splanchnic vein thromboses), and pulmonary hypertension.

Coumadin (warfarin sodium) tablet and injection. Safety Labeling Changes Approved by FDA Center for Drug Evaluation and Research (CDER)—January 2010. Accessed May 8, 2012.

Heneghan C, Ward A, Perera R, et al. Self-monitoring of oral anticoagulation: systematic review and meta-analysis of individual patient data. *Lancet.* 2012;379(9813):322-334.

Higashi MK, Veenstra DL, Kondo LM, et al. Association between CYP2C9 genetic variants and anticoagulation-related outcomes during warfarin therapy. *JAMA.* 2002;287(13):1690-1698.

Hutten BA, Lensing AW, Kraaijenhagen RA, Prins MH. Safety of treatment with oral anticoagulants in the elderly. A systematic review. *Drugs Aging.* 1999;14(4):303-312.

Hylek EM, Singer DE. Risk factors for intracranial hemorrhage in outpatients taking warfarin. *Ann Intern Med.* 1994;120(11):897-902.

James AH, Britt RP, Raskino CL, Thompson SG. Factors affecting the maintenance dose of warfarin. *J Clin Pathol.* 1992;45(8):704-706.

Robinson A, Thomson RG; Decision Analysis in Routine Treatments Study (DARTS) Team. The potential use of decision analysis to support shared decision making in the face of uncertainty: the example of atrial fibrillation and warfarin anticoagulation. *Qual Health Care.* 2009;9(4):238-244.

Schwartz JB, Kane L, Moore K, Wu AHB. Failure of pharmacogenetic-based dosing algorithms to identify older patients requiring low daily doses of warfarin. *J Am Med Dir Assoc.* 2011;12(9):633-638.

Witt DM, Nieuwlatt R, Clark NP, et al. American Society of Hematology 2018 guidelines for management of venous thromboembolism: optimal management anticoagulation therapy. *Blood Adv.* 2018;2(22):3257-3291.

▶ Injectable Anticoagulants

LMWH and selective indirect anti-Xa inhibitor (fondaparinux) are also used in older patients. The two major concerns in older patients that must be considered are dose adjustment for renal impairment and lower body weight. Reduced renal clearance occurs with age and increases the susceptibility to major bleeding, as both LMWHs and fondaparinux are primarily renally eliminated. The risk of LMWH accumulation and bleeding is dependent on the severity of renal impairment and the dose (prophylactic or therapeutic) and type of LMWH. Among LMWHs, only enoxaparin has approved dose reduction in older patients with renal impairment. Reduced-dose fondaparinux appears to have good safety and efficacy in older patients with mild renal impairment, but this has not been validated in those with severe renal impairment. Renal function should not be solely assessed by the serum creatinine as this leads to underestimation of renal failure in older patients, and measurement of the glomerular filtration rate is preferred. Thus, it is prudent to test LMWH or fondaparinux anti–factor Xa levels in older patients with renal impairment or low body weight to avoid supratherapeutic doses.

Cohen AT, Davidson BL, Gallus AS, et al. Efficacy and safety of fondaparinux for the prevention of venous thromboembolism in older acute medical patients: randomised placebo controlled trial. *BMJ.* 2006;332(7537):325-329.

Lim W. Low-molecular-weight heparin in patients with chronic renal insufficiency. *Intern Emerg Med.* 2008;3(4):319-323.

Turpie AG, Lensing AW, Fuji T, et al. Influence of renal function on the efficacy and safety of fondaparinux 1.5 mg once daily in the prevention of venous thromboembolism in renally impaired patients. *Blood Coagul Fibrinolysis.* 2009;20(2):1141-1121.

▷ New Oral Anticoagulants

For the first time since the introduction of warfarin in 1954, five new oral anticoagulants have been approved by the US Food and Drug Administration (FDA). Although clinical trials that led to the approval included older patients, those with significant renal and hepatic disease were systematically excluded from these trials. These new oral anticoagulants overcame several of the limitations of warfarin, including slow onset of action, narrow therapeutic window, drug and dietary interactions, and the need for routine laboratory monitoring. As a result of the increased use of these agents in the geriatric population, clinicians should be aware of the indications, pharmacology, methods for monitoring anticoagulant activity, and recommendations for management of bleeding with these new oral anticoagulants (Table 44–2 and Table 44–4).

Although the characteristics of a more rapid onset of action and a more predictable anticoagulant effect make these newer oral agents an attractive alternative to warfarin, caution is still needed when used in older patients. The convenience of no regular laboratory monitoring of coagulation also means there is no readily available and accurate mechanism to objectively assess adherence to therapy or anticoagulant activity in scenarios of life-threatening bleeding. This may be more problematic for older patients in whom a fixed-dose regimen may not universally apply because of variations in their renal function and body weight, where the safety and efficacy of these agents is uncertain. Additionally, the lack of monitoring may potentially lead to missed opportunities for early detection of a complication due to a lack of regular patient-provider interaction. Finally, the comparative drug costs of these DOACs compared to warfarin (including INR monitoring) must be considered, especially in older patients who are often on multiple medications with limited financial resources.

Despite these cautions, more data are emerging of the safety and efficacy of these drugs in the older population. The overall efficacy of DOACs compared to warfarin in the older patient seems to be at least similar to the general population and perhaps safer, specifically with lower incidence of ICH. The results of a meta-analysis of real-world data were similar to those of clinical trials. The differences in study populations between the individual DOAC trials and lack of head-to-head comparisons between DOACs prevent definitive recommendations on which DOAC to choose in the older patient requiring anticoagulation. Choice of one DOAC over another depends on individual patient preference, prior treatment failures, cost, and organ function.

A. Dabigatran

Dabigatran is a novel competitive direct thrombin inhibitor. Dabigatran is FDA approved for the prevention of stroke and systemic embolism in nonvalvular atrial fibrillation (NVAF), treatment of deep vein thrombosis (DVT) and pulmonary embolism (PE), prevention of recurrent DVT or PE in patients who have been previously treated, and prophylaxis of DVT or PE in patients who have undergone hip and knee replacement surgery. Of note, dabigatran is the most dependent on renal clearance (~80%). Consideration should be given to age-related changes in kidney function that lead to increased concentration and greater exposure to the drug resulting in potential bleeding complications. The RELY study showed dabigatran at two different doses to be as effective as warfarin without a difference in bleeding for prevention of stroke or systemic embolism. However, a subset analysis by age groups revealed that among the 39% of patients older than age 75 years, bleeding was increased in the high-dose dabigatran (150 mg) arm. This effect occurred regardless of renal function. In the RECOVER trial, dabigatran was noninferior to warfarin for the primary efficacy outcome of recurrent venous thromboembolism (VTE) and for the safety outcome of major bleeding. At the 2019 World Stroke Congress, two trials were presented studying dabigatran for new indications including embolic stroke of undetermined sources (ESUS) and cerebral vein thrombosis (CVT); both trials failed to show a benefit over standard treatment (aspirin in the RE-SPECT ESUS trial and warfarin in the RE-SPECT CVT trial). However, a post hoc subgroup analysis

Table 44–4. Management of life-threatening bleeding on anticoagulants.

Anticoagulant	Drug/Blood Product Options	Laboratory Monitoring of Reversal	Special Considerations
Unfractionated heparin	Protamine	PTT or anti-Xa activity	Consider only amount of heparin administered in the 3 hours prior to protamine for dose calculation Risk for allergic/hypersensitivity reactions in patients with fish allergy or previous protamine exposure Cap protamine at 50 mg/dose Reversal effect in 5–10 minutes Repeat doses may be necessary
Warfarin	(1) Four- factor prothrombin complex concentrates (PCCs) and vitamin K IV (preferred) OR (2) Fresh-frozen plasma (FFP) and vitamin K IV	PT/INR	Dose of PCC should be based on INR; consider FEIBA instead of PCC if documented heparin allergy FFP has the potential for volume overload, TRALI, and delays related to preparation and delivery of FFP; FFP not recommended with use of PCC PT/INR check 10–30 minutes after PCC dose to assess efficacy Repeat PT/INR every 6 hours for 24 hours; short half-life of PCCs
LMWHs • Enoxaparin • Dalteparin • Tinzaparin	(1) Protamine (preferred) OR (2) rFVIIa for life-threatening bleeding	Anti-Xa activity	Protamine only partially reverses LMWHs (~60%) 1 mg protamine/mg of LMWH if anticoagulant given <8 hours prior to protamine; 0.5mg protamine/mg of LMWH if anticoagulant given 8–12 hours prior to protamine Repeat protamine dose at 0.5 mg/mg LMWH if bleeding persists or elevated anti-Xa activity after 4 hours Risk for allergic/hypersensitivity reactions in patients with fish allergy or previous protamine exposure Cap protamine at 50 mg/dose If anti-Xa activity is undetectable, reversal is not needed
Indirect parenteral factor Xa inhibitor • Fondaparinux	(1) PCC OR (2) rFVIIa	Anti-Xa activity	rFVIIa if no clinical response to PCC or if documented heparin allergy If anti-Xa activity is undetectable, reversal is not needed
Parenteral direct thrombin inhibitors • Argatroban • Bivalirudin • Desirudin	(1) DDAVP (2) Cryoprecipitate (3) Antifibrinolytics	aPTT, PT	These anticoagulants have short half-lives
Oral direct thrombin inhibitor • Dabigatran	(1) Idarucizumab (preferred) OR (2) rFVIIa OR (3) PCCs Oral charcoal if last known drug ingestion within 3 hours	aPTT, TT/TCT	Hemodialysis can remove dabigatran If PTT, TT, or TCT is normal, reversal is not needed
Oral direct factor Xa inhibitor • Rivaroxaban • Apixaban • Edoxaban • Betrixaban	(1) Andexanet alfa; FDA approved for reversal of apixaban and rivaroxaban only (preferred) OR (2) PCC Oral charcoal if last known drug ingestion within 3 hours	Anti-Xa activity	rFVIIa or FEIBA (if no clinical response to PCC or documented heparin allergy) If anti-Xa activity is undetectable, reversal is not needed

aPTT, activated partial thromboplastin time; DDAVP, desmopressin; FDA, US Food and Drug Administration; FEIBA, factor VIII bypassing agent; INR, international normalized ratio; IV, intravenous; LMWH, low-molecular-weight heparin; PCC, prothrombin complex concentrates; PT, prothrombin time; PTT, partial thromboplastin time; rFVIIa, recombinant factor VIIa; TRALI, transfusion-related acute lung injury; TT/TCT, thrombin time/thrombin clotting time.

of the RE-SPECT ESUS trial suggested that patients aged 75 and older may benefit from dabigatran compared with aspirin therapy alone, possibly because this group has the highest incidence of atrial fibrillation.

B. Rivaroxaban

Rivaroxaban is a reversible direct factor Xa inhibitor. Rivaroxaban is FDA approved for the prevention of stroke and systemic embolism in NVAF, treatment of DVT and PE, prevention of recurrent DVT or PE in patients who have been previously treated, prophylaxis of DVT or PE in patients who have undergone knee replacement surgery, and reduction of risk of major cardiovascular events in combination with aspirin in patients with chronic coronary artery disease or peripheral artery disease. Rivaroxaban was investigated in four large phase III trials for prevention of VTE after total hip and knee arthroplasty (RECORD 1–4 trials). In all four trials, rivaroxaban prophylaxis was superior to enoxaparin for the composite end point of total VTE and all-cause mortality without significant differences in major bleeding. In the ROCKET AF study, rivaroxaban was noninferior to warfarin for prevention of stroke or systemic embolism in patients with NVAF. In all of these trials, a representative number of older patients were included, adding to the external validity of the findings. A prespecified subgroup analysis compared outcomes in older and younger patients enrolled in the ROCKET AF study. Patients ≥75 years on rivaroxaban had higher absolute hemorrhagic stroke and major bleeding rates than those <75 years on rivaroxaban. Thus, caution is still needed in using rivaroxaban in older patients with atrial fibrillation.

Rivaroxaban was noninferior to warfarin for the treatment of acute VTE in the EINSTEIN-DVT and EINSTEIN-PE trials in terms of efficacy and safety; however, there was a trend toward lower recurrent VTE events in those aged 65 years and older receiving rivaroxaban. In the EINSTEIN-PE study, in patients aged ≥75 years old or with creatinine clearance of 50 to <80 mL/min and fragility, there was a trend toward lower rates of recurrent VTE with rivaroxaban, with a similar nonsignificant trend in the primary bleeding outcome. Older patients were well represented in these rivaroxaban trials.

Rivaroxaban has recently been evaluated in prevention of arterial events specifically in older patients. In the COMPASS trial, patients aged 65 or older with stable coronary artery disease, peripheral arterial disease, or both randomized to low-dose rivaroxaban (2.5 mg twice a day) plus aspirin (100 mg once a day) had a lower risk of the composite outcome of myocardial infarction, stroke, or cardiovascular death compared to patients receiving aspirin alone. A similar comparison in patients with stable peripheral arterial disease or carotid artery disease revealed a reduction in the composite outcome of myocardial infarction, stroke, or cardiovascular death by nearly 50% in those receiving rivaroxaban plus aspirin versus aspirin alone. Perhaps as expected, the risk of bleeding was increased in patients receiving rivaroxaban compared to aspirin alone. Notably, because the trial was terminated early due to efficacy, reported bleeding rates with rivaroxaban may be underestimated.

New data are now emerging for the efficacy of DOACs in the treatment of cancer-associated VTE. The SELECT-D trial showed that rivaroxaban was noninferior to dalteparin in the treatment of symptomatic or incidental PE or symptomatic lower extremity DVT in patients with cancer. Major bleeding was no different, whereas critically relevant nonmajor bleeding (CRNMB) was higher in patients who received rivaroxaban. Several other studies have investigated rivaroxaban's efficacy for new populations, including chronic heart failure with coronary artery disease, stroke prevention after an embolic stroke, extended-duration thromboprophylaxis in hospitalized medically ill patients, and patients with ESUS (see Table 44–4).

C. Apixaban

Apixaban, like rivaroxaban, is a reversible direct factor Xa inhibitor. Apixaban is FDA approved for prevention of stroke and systemic embolism in NVAF, treatment of DVT and PE, prevention of recurrent DVT or PE in patients who have been previously treated, and prophylaxis of DVT or PE in patients who have undergone knee replacement surgery. Of all the DOACs, it is the least dependent on renal clearance (~25%). In patients with NVAF on apixaban for prevention of stroke and systemic embolism, a dose reduction is recommended if patients have at least two of the following characteristics: age ≥80 years, body weight ≤60 kg, or serum creatinine ≥1.5 mg/dL. Many older patients could meet this dose reduction criteria. For treatment of VTE, no dose reduction is required regardless of age, weight, or creatinine per the package insert.

Apixaban was investigated for prevention of stroke and systemic embolism in NVAF in the ARISTOTLE (apixaban vs warfarin) and AVERROES trials (apixaban vs aspirin in patients deemed unsuitable for warfarin clinical trials). In both studies, apixaban was superior to the comparator. In the ARISTOTLE study, less major bleeding and lower mortality were reported. The AVERROES study is particularly relevant to the older patient because >50% of patients ≥75 years old at risk for stroke due to atrial fibrillation are not anticoagulated in real-world practices. Based on the ADVANCE 1–3 studies, apixaban was FDA approved for prevention of VTE after total knee arthroplasty. Apixaban was FDA approved for the treatment of acute VTE and for extended therapy in patients who have completed 6 to 12 months of anticoagulation for VTE based on favorable results from the AMPLIFY and AMPLIFY-Ext trials, respectively. In all the above studies, older patients were well represented (30%–70% over the age of 65 and approximately 15% over the age of 75). In the AMPLIFY and AMPLIFY-Ext studies, no clinically significant differences in safety or efficacy were observed when comparing subjects in older versus younger age groups.

In the AVERT study, patients with cancer at intermediate or high risk of VTE benefited from apixaban prophylaxis compared to placebo with lower rates of VTE but higher rates of major bleeding. This study may be less generalizable to the older patient with cancer because few patients with colorectal and prostate cancer were included and only 5.9% of patients had renal dysfunction. In the ADOPT study evaluating extended-duration apixaban versus enoxaparin in hospitalized medically ill patients with congestive heart failure or respiratory failure and at least one additional VTE risk factor, older patients were well represented (~30% over the age of 75 years). In all comers, apixaban was associated with significantly more major bleeding than enoxaparin without any evidence of superiority in reducing VTE outcomes. Therefore, current evidence-based guidelines do not recommend extended VTE prophylaxis in acutely ill hospitalized medical patients after hospital discharge.

D. Edoxaban

Edoxaban is an oral direct factor Xa inhibitor. Edoxaban is FDA approved for the prevention of stroke and systemic embolism in NVAF and treatment of DVT or PE. Dose recommendations are given for renal insufficiency, and it is not recommended in patients with creatinine clearance >95 mL/min due to increased risk of ischemia in these patients, presumably due to lower edoxaban levels.

Edoxaban has been evaluated in three large randomized controlled trials for the following indications: prevention of stroke or systemic embolism in NVAF, treatment of acute VTE, and treatment of cancer-associated VTE. In the ENGAGE-AF TIMI trial, edoxaban was noninferior to warfarin in preventing stroke or systemic embolism and was associated with lower rates of bleeding and death from cardiovascular causes. As expected, stroke and systemic embolism events, as well as major bleeding events, were more frequent in older patients; however, in those aged ≥75 years, thrombotic outcomes were similar and major bleeding rates were reduced with edoxaban compared to warfarin. In the HOKUSAI study, edoxaban was noninferior to warfarin for treatment of acute VTE, whereas edoxaban was superior to warfarin in terms of major or CRNMB. In patients with cancer-associated VTE, the HOKUSAI-Cancer VTE study showed that edoxaban was noninferior to LMWH (dalteparin) in prevention of recurrent VTE. However major bleeding was higher with edoxaban, specifically in patients with gastrointestinal cancer, a common tumor type in older patients.

E. Betrixaban

Betrixaban is a direct oral factor Xa inhibitor. Betrixaban is FDA approved for prophylaxis of VTE in adults hospitalized for an acute medical illness who are at risk for thromboembolic complications due to moderate or severe restricted mobility and other risk factors for VTE. Betrixaban has the longest half-life (19–27 hours) of the DOACs, allowing for stable and predictable once-daily dosing that presumably minimizes anticoagulant variability. Betrixaban has only been studied in the setting of acutely hospitalized medically ill patients for prevention of VTE in the APEX trial. The mean age of the study population was higher than other DOAC trials (76 years old). When extended-duration betrixaban (40 mg daily for 35–42 days) was compared to limited-duration enoxaparin (40 mg daily for 10 ± 4 days), no significant difference in asymptomatic proximal DVT and symptomatic VTE or major bleeding was found. However, in a prespecified exploratory analyses of patients with elevated D-dimer and age >75 years old, betrixaban did have a benefit over enoxaparin for the primary efficacy outcome, albeit at increased risk of major bleeding or CRNMB.

Burnett AE, Mahan CE, Vazquez SR, et al. Guidance for the practical management of the direct oral anticoagulants (DOACs) in VTE treatment. *J Thromb Thrombolysis.* 2016;41:206-232.

Jacobs JM, Stessman J. New anticoagulant drugs among elderly patients is caution necessary? Comment on "The use of dabigatran in elderly patients." *Arch Intern Med.* 2011;171(14):1287-1288.

Mitchell AP, Conway SE. Rivaroxaban for treatment of venous thromboembolism in older adults. *Consult Pharm.* 2014;29(9):627-630.

Mitchell A, Watson MC, Welsh MC, McGrogan A. Effectiveness and safety of direct oral anticoagulants versus vitamin K antagonists for people aged 75 years and over with atrial fibrillation: a systematic review and meta-analyses of observational studies. *J Clin Med.* 2019;8(4):554.

Ng KH, Hart RG, Eikelboom JW. Anticoagulation in patients aged ≥ 75 years with atrial fibrillation: role of novel oral anticoagulants. *Cardiol Ther.* 2013;2:135-149.

Ntaios G, Papavasileiou V, Makaritsis K, et al. Real-world setting comparison of nonvitamin-K antagonist oral anticoagulants versus vitamin-K antagonists for stroke prevention in atrial fibrillation: a systematic review and meta-analysis. *Stroke.* 2017;48(9):2494-2503.

Schunemann HJ, Cushman M, Burnett AE, et al. American Society of Hematology 2018 guidelines for management of venous thromboembolism: prophylaxis for hospitalized and nonhospitalized medical patients. *Blood Adv.* 2018;2:3198-3225.

Stangier J, Stahle H, Rathgen K. Pharmacokinetics and pharmacodynamics of the direct oral thrombin inhibitor dabigatran in healthy elderly subjects. *Clin Pharmacokinet.* 2008;47(1):47-59.

MANAGEMENT OF MAJOR BLEEDING AND PERIOPERATIVE MANAGEMENT OF ANTICOAGULANTS IN OLDER PATIENTS

Bleeding is the primary complication of anticoagulation therapy. Older patients are particularly susceptible to anticoagulant-related bleeding complications as a result of their inherent risk for falls; chronic conditions such as renal failure, hepatic dysfunction, malnutrition, malignancy, and amyloid angiopathy; concomitant use of antiplatelet agents; and noncompliance with drug regimens. Although reversal of older therapeutic agents such as UFH and warfarin is possible, many of the newer anticoagulants, including LMWHs, fondaparinux, and parenteral direct thrombin inhibitors, do not have a complete and specific antidote that has been studied in controlled trials. Recently idarucizumab and andexanet alfa have been FDA approved for reversal of dabigatran and the oral anti–Xa inhibitors, respectively. Idarucizumab is a humanized mouse monoclonal antibody that binds dabigatran with higher affinity compared to endogenous thrombin and neutralizes the drug's anticoagulant activity. Idarucizumab is subsequently rapidly cleared with bound dabigatran by the kidney.

In the REVERSE-AD study, patients on dabigatran presenting with life-threatening bleeding or those requiring emergent surgery who received idarucizumab had rapid cessation of bleeding and, in those who needed emergent surgery, achieved normal intraoperative hemostasis. Andexanet alfa is a recombinant human factor Xa decoy that binds with high affinity to factor Xa inhibitors, thereby blocking inhibition of factor Xa. Similarly, in the ANNEXA-4 trial, administration of andexanet alfa to patients on anti-Xa inhibitors with life-threatening bleeding led to substantial reversal of anti–factor Xa activity with clinical hemostasis. The mean age of patients was 77 years, and a significant portion of patients had underlying cardiovascular or cerebrovascular disease. Clinical hemostasis was similar in those aged 75 or older compared to younger patients. Of note, rebound thrombotic events occurred in 18% and included one myocardial infarction, five strokes, seven DVTs, and one PE. Based on these results, andexanet alfa is FDA approved for reversal of rivaroxaban and apixaban when reversal of anticoagulation is needed due to life-threatening or uncontrolled bleeding.

While management of anticoagulant-related major bleeding associated with VKA, UFH, and LMWH is well known, the ideal method to manage bleeding in patients receiving DOACs is not known. Furthermore, accurate and widely available laboratory tests to measure anticoagulant activity may not be available for these newer oral agents. Although laboratory monitoring is not routinely required for patients on DOACs, special clinical scenarios, such as clinically significant bleeding, may call for measurement of anticoagulant effect. Even though the thrombin time/thrombin clotting time (TT/TCT), activated partial thromboplastin time (aPTT) (for dabigatran), and anti-Xa activity (for rivaroxaban, apixaban, and edoxaban) are the most effective available coagulation assays to determine anticoagulant activity, the therapeutic range of these tests is not well defined, and these tests are best used to determine the presence or absence of the drug. Clinicians should not routinely use these laboratory tests to monitor and adjust DOAC doses or assess the degree of bleeding risk for surgical procedures. Commercially

available anti–factor Xa assays specific for rivaroxaban, apixaban, or edoxaban or drug concentration assays for any DOAC would be ideal for determining plasma drug levels. In their absence, a normal TT/TCT and aPTT essentially excludes dabigatran activity, whereas normal anti-Xa activity (eg, heparin or LMWH level) rules out anticoagulant activity of not only standard parenteral anticoagulants, such as UFH and LMWH, but also oral direct factor Xa inhibitors (rivaroxaban, apixaban, and edoxaban). However recent evidence-based guidelines do not recommend measuring DOAC anticoagulant effect during management of life-threatening bleeding. Instead of delaying interventions for major bleeding while awaiting DOAC test results, a comprehensive approach to assessing bleeding is recommended. Suggestions for the management of bleeding complications in patients on anticoagulation are described in Table 44–4.

Interruption of anticoagulation before interventions with a risk of bleeding must be weighed carefully against thrombotic risk. Renal and hepatic impairment, which can prolong clearance of anticoagulants, and the long half-life of the drug need to be considered prior to discontinuation of the drug. Recommendations for interruption of the newer anticoagulants, including LMWHs, fondaparinux, parenteral direct thrombin inhibitors, and the DOACs, are provided in Table 44–5. Clearly, some procedures are very low risk for bleeding and may not require anticoagulation interruption (eg, superficial skin surgeries, cataract surgery, simple endoscopy without biopsy, and minor dental procedures). Pacemaker or cardioverter-defibrillator devices can be safely implanted without stopping VKA, but more evidence is needed in patients on DOACs. Surgeries associated with high-risk bleeding include neuraxial anesthesia, intracranial surgery, cardiothoracic surgery, major abdominopelvic surgery, major orthopedic surgery, liver and kidney biopsy, and transurethral prostate and bladder resection, among others. Bridging therapy with parenteral anticoagulation is rarely performed now due to increased risk of bleeding and minimal reduction in perioperative thrombosis rates. However, in certain patients at high risk for thrombosis perioperatively, bridging therapy should be considered (eg, in those with last VTE or stroke within 3 months, mechanical heart valve, high-risk thrombophilias such as antiphospholipid syndrome, prior thrombotic event during temporary interruption of anticoagulation). Restarting anticoagulation in a timely manner postoperatively depends on individualized assessment of risks of bleeding from the procedure and thrombosis for underlying hypercoagulable state. Postoperatively, it is critical to note that, unlike warfarin, the DOACs have more immediate onsets of action. Therefore, if these drugs are interrupted for surgery, they should not be reintroduced until hemostasis is assured.

Anticoagulants are among the most common drugs used to prevent and treat thrombotic and vascular disorders prevalent in the geriatric population. Special attention must be

Table 44-5. Recommendations for interruption and restarting of anticoagulants.

	UFH	LMWH	Warfarin	Dabigatran	Apixaban/Rivaroxaban/Edoxaban
Preoperative interruption					
CrCl >80 mL/min	Hold UFH infusion 4 hours prior to procedure given short half-life of UFH	Last dose of LMWH to be given 24 hours before the procedure	Hold warfarin 5 days to ensure INR <2 before procedure Preoperative bridging when INR <2 should be considered in high thromboembolic risk patients	High risk: Hold ≥48 hours Low risk: Hold ≥24 hours Bridging with LMWH/UFH should be avoided with DOACs given short half-life and quick time to peak concentration	High risk: Hold ≥48 hours Low risk: Hold ≥24 hours Bridging with LMWH/UFH should be avoided with DOACs given short half-life and quick time to peak concentration
CrCl 50–80 mL/min	Same as above	Same as above	Same as above	High risk: Hold ≥72 hours Low risk: Hold ≥36 hours	High risk: Hold ≥48 hours Low risk: Hold ≥24 hours
CrCl 30–50 mL/min	Same as above	Same as above	Same as above	High risk: Hold ≥96 hours Low risk: Hold ≥48 hours	High risk: Hold ≥48 hours Low risk: Hold ≥24 hours
CrCl 15–30 mL/min	Same as above	Same as above	Same as above	N/A	High risk: Hold ≥48 hours Low risk: Hold ≥36 hours prior to surgery
Postoperative management	Restart within 8–24 hours depending on bleeding risk	Restart within 8–24 hours depending on bleeding risk	Restart home dose of warfarin on evening of procedure Postoperative bridging back to warfarin should be considered in high thromboembolic risk patients (last VTE or stroke within 3 months, mechanical heart valve, high-risk thrombophilias such as APLS, prior thrombotic event during temporary interruption of anticoagulation); all others do not need bridging, which as associated with increased bleeding risk	No bridging required Low bleeding risk: 8–24 hours High bleeding risk and low TE risk: resume 48–72 hours postoperatively High bleeding risk and high TE risk: resume prophylactic dose LMWH or DOAC evening after surgery and then resume therapeutic dose DOAC within 48–72 hours	No bridging required Low bleeding risk: 8–24 hours High bleeding risk and low TE risk: resume 48–72 hours postoperatively High bleeding risk and high TE risk: resume prophylactic or intermediate-dose LMWH 6–8 hours postoperatively; resume DOACs when hemostasis controlled (within 48–72 hours)

APLS, antiphospholipid syndrome; CrCl, Creatine Clearance; DOAC, direct oral anticoagulant; INR, international normalized ratio; LMWH, low-molecular-weight heparin; N/A, not applicable; TE, thromboembolic; UFH, unfractionated heparin; VTE, venous thromboembolism

High bleeding risk procedures: major abdominopelvic, orthopedic, or cardiothoracic surgery; central nervous system surgery/neuraxial procedure; transjugular intrahepatic portosystemic shunt; and renal biopsy.

Very low bleeding risk (does not require interruption of anticoagulant): superficial skin surgeries, cataract surgery, simple endoscopy without biopsy, and minor dental procedures.

paid to the unique characteristics of older patients that may affect type, dose, monitoring, and management of bleeding of the anticoagulant chosen. Randomized controlled trials specifically addressing geriatric patients are needed to make evidence-based recommendations on the use of anticoagulants in this population.

Burnett AE, Mahan CE, Vazquez SR, et al. Guidance for the practical management of the direct oral anticoagulants (DOACs) in VTE treatment. *J Thromb Thrombolysis.* 2016;41:206-232.

Crowther M, Warkentin T. Bleeding risk and the management of bleeding complications in patients undergoing anticoagulant therapy: focus on new anticoagulant agents. *Blood.* 2008;111(10):4871-4879.

Dubois V, Dincq A, Douxfils J, et al. Perioperative management of patients on direct oral anticoagulants. *Thromb J.* 2017;15:14

Heidbuchel H, Verhamme P, Alings M, et al. Updated European Heart Rhythm Association practical guide on the use of non-vitamin K antagonist anticoagulants in patients with non-valvular atrial fibrillation. *Europace.* 2015;17:1467-1507.

Chronic Venous Insufficiency

45

Samira Ghaniwala, MD

Teresa L. Carman, MD

ESSENTIALS OF DIAGNOSIS

▶ Symptoms including heaviness, aching, swelling, throbbing, or itching.

▶ Skin changes include hemosiderin staining, lipodermatosclerosis, and atrophie blanche.

▶ Varicose veins may range from telangiectasia to ropey varicosities.

▶ Edema, which may be soft and pitting or brawny and fibrotic, usually increases throughout the day with dependency and improves with elevation.

▶ Ultrasound imaging demonstrates venous reflux or chronic postthrombotic changes.

▶ Severe disease presents with ulceration typically located above the medial malleolus.

General Principles

Chronic venous disease (CVD) is a broad term that refers globally to anatomic or functional changes affecting the venous system that prompts an individual to seek medical attention. At one end of the spectrum, patients with CVD may present with no apparent clinical signs but report symptoms of heaviness, aching, or late-day leg fatigue. At the other end of the spectrum is chronic venous insufficiency (CVI). CVI refers to a more advanced form of CVD that is associated with apparent clinical signs such as trophic skin changes, edema, lymphedema, or venous stasis ulcers. From recent epidemiologic studies, the prevalence of CVD may be as high as 70% to 80% of the general population. When followed longitudinally, the incidence of CVD is approximately 1% to 2% annually. However, once an individual is affected, CVD progression is common and estimated at 30% to 50% over a 5-year period. CVI is costly; in the United States,

approximately $2 to $3 billion is spent annually on CVI and related treatments.

Despite its high prevalence, CVD is underrecognized and clinically underappreciated. In part, this is due to the nonspecific nature of the presenting symptoms. Leg pain or aching, swelling, nocturnal cramping, and nonspecific complaints such as burning, itching, or throbbing may be attributed to many different etiologies. Frequently the disease is overlooked until it becomes more severe, presenting with advanced skin changes including venous stasis ulcers. CVD is more common in women than in men, with a ratio of approximately 3:1. Men tend to present with more advanced venous disease, whereas women are more likely to present with superficial venous disease such as spider veins and varicose veins. Risk factors for CVD and CVI include advancing age, obesity, pregnancy, history of lower extremity injury, and prolonged standing or dependency. Patients with limited mobility or a history of stroke or those who are using walking aids or ankle-foot orthoses will frequently have decreased calf muscle pump function and secondary CVI. It is important to ask about sleeping habits. Chair or recliner sleeping is common in older adults because of back or joint pain, limited mobility, cardiopulmonary disease, or poor sleep habits. Sleeping in a chair or recliner predisposes older adults to secondary venous hypertension, which can progress to CVD and even CVI.

Pathogenesis

The venous system is made up of (1) deep veins within the subfascial, muscular compartment of the limbs; (2) superficial veins, which are located in the epifascial, subcutaneous compartment; and (3) perforator veins, which communicate between the two compartments. Normal venous physiology depends on vein patency, intact venous valves, and a functional calf muscle pump to return blood from the periphery to the right side of the heart. In addition, normal right-sided cardiac function, intact vascular endothelium, and intact functioning lymphatics are required for tissue fluid management.

Although edema may result from an abnormality of venous physiology or any of the components related to fluid management, CVI is specifically related to ambulatory venous hypertension or sustained venous pressure within the deep or superficial venous system. Venous hypertension may be related to failure of any of the required components: (1) abnormal or damaged venous valves and associated reflux or retrograde flow; (2) venous outflow obstruction either as a result of intrinsic or extrinsic venous injury or compression; or (3) loss of the normal calf muscle pump. Venous insufficiency may be primary or secondary. Primary CVD is venous dysfunction without a related secondary etiology or identifiable mechanism of venous injury. The underlying pathology responsible for primary venous disease and varicose veins is unknown. Primary venous disease (ie, varicose veins) are more common in women. Associated risk factors include advancing age, pregnancy, obesity, and a family history of varicose veins. Despite identifying a familial component, a genetic risk has yet to be identified.

Postthrombotic syndrome (PTS) is the most common form of secondary venous insufficiency. PTS is related to valve damage or venous obstruction due to incomplete recanalization of the veins following deep vein thrombosis or superficial thrombophlebitis. Since many venous thromboses are asymptomatic, patients may not report a venous thromboembolic episode, and the findings of chronic venous injury are often only identified when duplex ultrasound is performed to investigate associated symptomatology.

Another increasingly common cause of CVD is central obesity. Patients with obesity-related CVD may present with advanced CVD even in the absence of underlying venous changes. When associated with severe skin changes and secondary lymphedema, this syndrome is referred to as phlebolymphedema.

▶ Prevention

Reducing risk factors possibly causing or contributing to CVD must first be addressed. Body weight has an impact on venous function. Hence, weight loss or maintaining ideal weight is recommended for all CVD patients. While compression is a mainstay of treatment for CVD, there is insufficient evidence to suggest that compression prevents CVD progression. Using appropriate hospital prophylaxis and preventing deep vein thrombosis is the most important intervention to prevent PTS and secondary CVD.

▶ Clinical Findings

A. Signs & Symptoms

History and physical examination are frequently sufficient to make the diagnosis of CVD and CVI. CEAP (clinical,

Table 45–1. Clinical classification of venous disease.

C0	No visible sign of venous disease
C1	Telangiectasias (spider vein) or reticular veins
C2	Varicose veins
C3	Edema
C4	Trophic skin changes including pigmentation, eczema, lipodermatosclerosis, or atrophie blanche
C5	Healed venous ulcer
C6	Active venous stasis ulcer

etiology, anatomy, and pathophysiology) classification is used to describe CVD and allow practitioners to communicate disease severity. The clinical staging of CVD using the CEAP classification is noted in Table 45–1. Varicose veins are a prominent feature of CVD. Varicosities may range from small venous telangiectasias or spider veins to subdermal reticular veins (that are 1–3 mm in size) to ropey, bulging varicosities. Another prominent clinical feature of CVI is edema. Early in the disease, the edema is usually soft and pitting; however, as the disease progresses, many patients will develop thickening and fibrosis of the subcutaneous tissue termed *lipodermatosclerosis*. Unlike lymphedema, the edema of CVI usually involves the ankle and lower calf and typically spares the dorsum of the foot. Patients will frequently report minimal swelling upon awakening but increasing edema as the day progresses. In CVI, skin changes are prominent. Patients may have dry, flakey, or hyperkeratotic skin. In advanced stages inflammation or stasis dermatitis, hyperpigmentation or hemosiderin staining, lipodermatosclerosis, and atrophie blanche or white atrophic scarring of the subcutaneous tissue are common. Venous ulceration is the most severe complication of CVI. Venous ulceration may be differentiated from arterial ulceration by the characteristics of the ulcer (Table 45–2). It is important to recognize that mixed venous and arterial disease is common, especially in older adults, and may impact venous ulcer healing.

Clinical symptoms of CVD are nonspecific and variable. Patients with CVI range from virtually asymptomatic to having severe disease associated with painful venous ulceration. Common symptoms associated with CVI include heaviness, aching, swelling, throbbing, and itching—the so-called HASTI symptoms. In addition, patients frequently endorse nocturnal cramps, restlessness, and leg fatigue with walking. Similar to the edema, symptoms may worsen during the day and are relieved with rest and elevation of the leg. Many women report worsening symptoms during their menstrual cycle.

B. Laboratory Findings

There are no laboratory findings required for the diagnosis or evaluation of CVI. However, patients with significant edema

Table 45–2. Differentiation between venous and arterial ulceration.

Characteristic	Venous	Arterial
Location	Medial malleolus or calf	Distal over the toes, foot, or heels
Base	Minimal fibrous slough Granular and healthy	Dry, fibrous, or necrotic Painful skin fissure Punched out appearance
Pain	Usually absent or minimal	Painful, may require narcotic therapy
Associated findings	Warm limb Edema, hemosiderin staining, and skin fibrosis	Cool limb Pallor on elevation and dependent rubor Edema from limb dependency
Color	Brown, violet, or blue from venous congestion	Erythematous dependent rubor
Pulses	Usually normal	Absent
Treatment	Compression, elevation, and moist wound dressing	Requires revascularization

should be fully evaluated for systemic conditions that may be related to or worsen swelling. This includes a complete metabolic panel to exclude significant renal disease, liver disease, and low protein or albumin levels. Thyroid-stimulating hormone should be evaluated because myxedema may be considered in the differential of the skin changes. Brain natriuretic peptide or the local laboratory equivalent may be helpful to exclude concomitant heart failure and volume overload.

C. Imaging Studies

Duplex ultrasonography for venous insufficiency is considered the "gold standard" for diagnosis of CVI. Performed by the vascular laboratory, the testing is usually done standing or in steep reverse Trendelenburg to augment valvular incompetency and reflux. In addition to compression ultrasound to exclude deep vein thrombosis, both Valsalva maneuvers and distal calf compression may be used to elicit reflux during imaging. Given the prevalence of peripheral arterial disease (PAD) in the aging population, the vascular laboratory should also be used to exclude PAD in patients with absent or diminished pulses prior to initiating compression therapy. Patients with an ankle-brachial index (ABI) <0.6 require care and caution when using compression for managing edema or venous ulcer healing.

D. Special Tests

The most basic office assessment for CVD includes having the patient stand and examining the patient for bulging varicosities. Holding your hand over the groin at the saphenofemoral junction while the patient performs a Valsalva maneuver will confirm reflux if the vein pressurizes. This clinical finding has a high specificity but overall low sensitivity for diagnosis of CVI. Photoplethysmography and air plethysmography are simple noninvasive tests that can evaluate for reflux, obstruction, and the calf muscle pump. However, this testing is not widely performed and has largely been supplanted by venous insufficiency ultrasound.

E. Special Examinations

Nonthrombotic iliac vein lesions or May-Thurner syndrome usually presents in younger patients; however, in patients with unilateral limb swelling especially when associated with advanced CVD, this may be a consideration. Ascending phlebography or contrast venography using pressure measurements and intravascular ultrasound may be warranted. This permits intraluminal assessment and, when combined with pressure measurement, may provide the most definitive evaluation for extrinsic venous obstruction and intraluminal webs or synechia.

In patients with unilateral limb swelling or bilateral symmetrical swelling, especially if it is of recent onset or rapidly progressive, abdominal and pelvic CT imaging may be required to exclude intrinsic or extrinsic injury from tumor or fibrosis. Pelvic congestion syndrome may present with gluteal, vulvar, and/or thigh varices. Additional symptoms such as pelvic pain, postcoital pain, dysmenorrhea, urinary urgency, and/or deep dyspareunia are also usually present. In patients with varicosities that extend from the buttocks or are over the perineum or anterior abdominal wall, further evaluation with magnetic resonance venography or CT venography to exclude pelvic reflux through the ovarian veins may be warranted.

► Differential Diagnosis

When faced with a patient with lower extremity swelling and suspected CVD, systematic evaluation is required. The history, physical examination, and supportive noninvasive testing will frequently be sufficient to establish a diagnosis and exclude other causes of edema. However, in older adults, most edema is multifactorial with contributions from systemic illness, CVD, loss of the calf muscle pump, and medications. A thorough history and physical examination are required to exclude other secondary causes of edema apart from CVI or lymphedema. Contributing systemic conditions include heart failure, increased right heart pressures from pulmonary hypertension or valvular heart disease, sleep apnea, protein loss related to renal or enteric disease, decreased protein from cirrhosis, other liver disease or malnutrition, and endocrine disorders, such as Cushing disease. Myxedema related to thyroid disease may also be confused with edema and, in the appropriate clinical setting, should be excluded by biopsy.

Identifying the use of ankle-foot orthoses and mobility aids such as a cane or walker and clinical evaluation of ankle range of motion or gait disturbance are essential to exclude calf muscle pump dysfunction. Chronic dependent edema from sleeping in a chair is also surprisingly common. All patients should be questioned regarding sleeping habits.

Medications are a frequent cause for lower extremity edema. Hormone therapy, steroids, dihydropyridine calcium channel blockers, thiazolidinediones, and nonsteroidal anti-inflammatory agents are all associated with edema. In addition, gabapentin, pregabalin, and pramipexole are common offenders.

▶ Complications

Pain, swelling, impaired mobility, and skin changes are typical complications experienced with CVI. The most problematic complication is that of venous stasis ulceration. Conservative estimates suggest that 20,000 patients are diagnosed with venous stasis ulcers annually. Ulcer care requires frequent office or home health care visits. Patients may experience pain associated with debridement and dressing changes. Some patients may feel isolated because of the appearance of the dressings or odor associated with active wounds. Bleeding from superficial varicosities, while dramatic, usually responds well to light compression and limb elevation. Secondary sclerotherapy may prevent recurrent bleeding.

▶ Treatment

A. General Considerations

Patients with no visible signs of CVD but who complain of venous symptoms should be treated conservatively. The goals for treating CVI are to reduce edema, alleviate pain, and improve the overall condition of the skin. In patients with venous stasis ulcers, wound healing and preventing ulcer recidivism are the goals of care. Thorough evaluation will allow patients to be approached with a comprehensive plan of care including interventional management when appropriate (Table 45–3). Skin care, elevation, and compression therapy are the mainstay of treatment for CVI. Patients with demonstrable reflux who have persistent symptoms despite conservative care or venous stasis ulcers may be considered for endovascular or surgical interventions.

B. Medical Management

1. Skin care—Stasis dermatitis, contact dermatitis, and venous ulcers are associated with CVI. Venous eczema or stasis dermatitis may present with intense itching, blisters, and/or oozing and requires skin cleaning, emollients, and/or preparations that maintain skin barrier. Water-based emollients improve the skin texture and prevent dryness and cracking that may promote ulceration. Mild or

Table 45–3. Therapeutic modalities for chronic venous insufficiency.

Skin Care
Water-based or petroleum-based emollients
Lactic acid– or urea-based emollients for debriding hyperkeratotic skin
Low- or medium-potency steroids as needed for dermatitis
Compression: Initial Decongestion
Tubular elastic compression
Medium- or low-stretch elastic bandaging
Multilayer compression systems
Compression: Maintenance
Graded compression stockings
Velcro compression wraps
Adjunctive Pharmaceuticals
Horse chestnut seed extract
Micronized purified flavonoid fraction (MPFF)
Pentoxifylline for ulcer healing
Venous Ablation
Endovenous laser ablation
Radiofrequency ablation
Sclerotherapy
Mechanochemical ablation (MOCA)
Cyanoacrylate glue closure
Surgical Therapy
Vein stripping
Phlebectomy or avulsion

intermediate-potency topical steroids may be used for a short duration to reduce itching, manage the inflammation, and promote healing. Tinea pedis is a common source of cellulitis. If there is maceration and breakdown in the web spaces between one's toes, an antifungal powder twice daily should be recommended. Venous ulcer management consists of basic wound care including debridement as well as dressings to manage exudate and keep the base moist along with high-grade compression.

2. Elevation—As previously noted, patients should be questioned about their sleeping habits. Chair or recliner sleeping maintains the venous hypertension; patients should be strongly advised to return to the bed. Lower extremity elevation should be used to provide passive decongestion of the legs. Elevation decreases the venous hypertension and reduces swelling and pain. Patients should be advised to elevate their legs above the level of the right atrium several times a day. Patients should be encouraged to elevate the foot of their bed using a 3- to 4-inch brick under the bed posts. This provides approximately 10 degrees of elevation of the foot of the bed and supports passive decongestion of their legs while they are sleeping. Using pillows to elevate is not as efficient or as well tolerated as elevating the foot of the bed. When using pillows, patients are required to maintain a still sleeping position on their back lest the pillows are kicked off the bed. Elevating the foot of the bed allows the patient to sleep comfortably in any position and maintain elevation. In addition, the use of pillows may be associated with hip pain, knee pain, and even back pain over time. Unless the patient has significant esophageal reflux, most patients and spouses tolerate this change in sleeping position without much difficulty.

3. Compression therapy—Depending on the etiology of CVI, committing to compression may be a lifelong endeavor. Compression decreases venous capacitance, decreases capillary exudate, and improves the ejection fraction and ejection volume of calf muscle pump function with ambulation. The type of compression garment and the amount of compression or strength of the garment need to be individually tailored to the patient. It is imperative that compression is measured to fit appropriately. Using a knee-high garment instead of thigh-high compression increases compliance and acceptance. Most patients are sufficiently managed with a knee-high garment.

In general, patients with C0 to C1 disease will usually see improvement with low-grade 15 to 20 mm Hg compression. Patients with C2 to C3 disease typically are best managed with 20 to 30 mm Hg compression. Patients with more severe disease including venous ulcers or healed ulceration (ie, C5–C6 disease) are best managed with 30 to 40 mm Hg compression. In reality, most older persons cannot apply stockings in excess of 20 mm Hg. Compression is recommended to alleviate symptoms in CVD (Grade IB); improve the quality of life (Grade IB); prevent and reduce edema associated with flights and occupational swelling (Grade IB); and improve skin changes (Grade IC) and lipodermatosclerosis (Grade IB) in patients with CVD.

Caregivers or family members may be required to assist with the stocking application. Compression should always be tailored to the patient with respect to tolerance and ability to don and doff the compression. In addition, patients with moderate or severe PAD should also not be in higher grades of compression. The compression must be matched to the severity of the PAD. In general, compression should be avoided with an ABI <0.4.

Patients who are limited by osteoarthritis, limited mobility, prior hip replacement, or obesity frequently cannot reach their feet to apply the garments. Stocking-donning aids may be helpful. In addition, for patients with arthritis of their hands or decreased hand strength, using a cotton-based stocking and rubber gloves may be helpful for donning and doffing the garments. Patients should be advised to lose weight, if needed. Central obesity increases pressure in the venous system and further limits compliance with stockings. Morbidly obese patients may require a higher grade of compression for symptomatic relief. Exercise is helpful to increase venous return. If possible, patients should walk on a regular basis to improve venous circulation. Pool exercise or walking may be helpful for patients with arthritis who find weight-bearing exercise uncomfortable. Regular foot and ankle exercises that augment the calf muscle pump action can be used to improve venous return.

Stockings are measured and fitted to the extremity. Therefore, prior to prescribing compression stockings, the edema should be optimally controlled. Tubular elastic compression, medium stretch elastic wraps, and multilayered compression wraps may be used for decongestion and ulcer management. However, these devices may not be ideal for long-term use. Velcro-based inelastic compression devices may be a useful alternative to compression stocking, especially in the elderly. Velcro compression tends to require less dexterity and strength for donning. Stocking care is very important. Stockings should be gently washed without fabric softener, and excess water should be removed by squeezing and not wringing the garment. They should be hung to dry and never placed in a dryer. With good care, stockings will last 4 to 6 months.

4. Systemic therapy—Venotonic drugs such as flavonoids and saponosides are more commonly used in Europe than in the United States. Some patients will benefit from escin, which is a horse chestnut seed extract and available as an over-the-counter supplement. The only US Food and Drug Administration–approved agent for CVD is diosmiplex (Vasculera). Diosmiplex contains purified diosmin and is classified as a medical food. It is a micronized purified flavonoid fraction (MPFF). Current guidelines suggest MPFF may be used as an adjunctive therapy in CVD. Pentoxifylline is recommended as an adjunct for venous ulcer healing.

C. Endovenous Therapy

Symptomatic patients with demonstrable superficial reflux who are refractory to conservative treatment with compression and elevation for 3 to 6 months may be considered for ablation or surgery. Endovenous ablation can improve symptoms and appearance of veins that are dilated, cosmetically displeasing, or causing pain. In addition, laser ablation has been shown to help improve ulcer healing and delay ulcer recidivism. Typically, these procedures can be performed in an ambulatory setting, and patients experience little pain or bruising. Many patients return to normal activities the day after the procedure. The goal of endovenous therapy is to create a chemical or heat-induced injury to the endothelium and incite a thrombo-inflammatory reaction that ends with fibrosis and obliteration of the pathologic vein. The most common techniques use laser or radiofrequency thermal energy to injure the endothelium and promote thrombosis, fibrosis, and venous occlusion. Nonthermal ablative techniques are increasing. Liquid sclerotherapy is frequently used for symptomatic telangiectasias or reticular veins. Ultrasound-guided foam sclerotherapy is being used with increasing frequency, even for larger varicose veins. Other nonthermal, nontumescent ablation techniques, including mechanochemical ablation and polymerizing glue, are also available. Determining the best procedure is dependent on clinical factors, venous anatomy and imaging, and operator and patient preference. The surgeon or operator should choose the procedure most likely to offer the best opportunity for successful venous closure.

D. Surgical Intervention (Phlebectomy)

For large axial varicose veins, venous stripping was historically used for most patients. Although still used in some clinical settings, traditional vein stripping has been largely replaced by endovenous ablation. Some patients will still benefit from other minor surgical procedures including power phlebectomy or stab phlebectomy. Decisions regarding the optimal endovascular and/or surgical approach should be made by the managing physician.

▶ Prognosis

CVI is rarely life or limb threatening. It is a chronic disease characterized by progression if left unmanaged and potential for improvement in the signs and symptoms with successful management.

Belramman A, Bootun R, Lane TRA, Davies AH. Endovenous management of varicose veins. *Angiology.* 2019;70(5):388-396.

Carman TL, Al-Omari A. Evaluation and management of chronic venous disease using the foundation of CEAP. *Curr Cardiol Rep.* 2019;21(10):114.

Garcia R, Labropoulos N. Duplex ultrasound for the diagnosis of acute and chronic venous diseases. *Surg Clin North Am.* 2018;98:201-218.

Gloviczki P, Comerota AJ, Dalsing MC, et al. The care of patients with varicose veins and associated chronic venous disease: clinical practice guidelines of the Society for Vascular Surgery and the American Venous Forum. *J Vasc Surg.* 2011;53(suppl):2S-48S.

Rabe E, Partsch H, Hafner J, et al. Indications for medical compression stockings in venous and lymphatic disorders: an evidence-based consensus statement. *Phlebology.* 2018;33: 163-184.

Wittens C, Davies AH, Bækgaard N, et al. Management of chronic venous disease. Clinical practical guidelines of the European Society for Vascular Surgery. *Eur J Vasc Endovasc Surg.* 2015;49:678-737.

Chronic Lung Disease

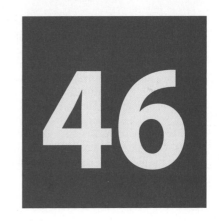

Brooke Salzman, MD

Danielle Snyderman, MD

Michael Weissberger, MD

Gillian Love, MD

Chronic lung diseases are common in older adults and can significantly impact overall health, function, and quality of life. However, older adults often have other comorbidities and complicating factors that play a role in pulmonary disease processes and treatments. When assessing older adults, clinicians must consider and possibly differentiate between the normal physiologic changes of aging and disease pathology.

As people age, chest wall compliance and respiratory muscle strength both decrease. Age and diseases such as osteoporosis are associated with thoracic spine changes that structurally affect lung function. It has been shown that the forced expiratory volume in 1 second (FEV_1) decreases with advancing age, more quickly after 70 years of age. Within the lungs, the alveolar dead space increases, diffusing capacity for carbon monoxide (DLCO) decreases, and receptors become less sensitive to medications. The respiratory response to hypoxia and hypercapnia also decreases; this contributes to reduced awareness symptoms and leaves older patients at greater risk for respiratory decompensation. Because of pulmonary changes associated with aging, pulmonary function tests may need to be interpreted differently for older patients. When treating older adults with chronic lung disease, functional ability, cognitive status, and polypharmacy must all be taken into account.

CHRONIC OBSTRUCTIVE PULMONARY DISEASE

ESSENTIALS OF DIAGNOSIS

▶ Symptoms: dyspnea, cough, sputum production, and wheeze.

▶ Risk factors: tobacco smoke, air pollution.

▶ Spirometry: airflow obstruction, FEV_1/forced vital capacity (FVC) ≤0.7.

▶ General Principles

Chronic obstructive pulmonary disease (COPD) is a common pulmonary condition characterized by persistent respiratory symptoms and airflow obstruction. COPD is a major cause of morbidity and mortality in the United States and worldwide. In the United States, COPD affects approximately 5% to 10% of the adult population, depending on the population studied. COPD is of special concern to older adults, as its prevalence rises steeply with age. Over the past 30 years, mortality from COPD has increased substantially in the United States, and the number of women dying from COPD has surpassed the number for men. COPD is now the fourth leading cause of death in the United States, accounting for >154,000 deaths in 2016. Worldwide, COPD is currently the fourth leading cause of death but is projected to be the third leading cause of death by 2020.

COPD represents a major public health challenge, as it is largely preventable and treatable, and, yet, it is the only common chronic illness where morbidity and mortality continue to climb. It is a significant cause of hospitalization, particularly in the older population. Rates of hospitalization for COPD increased >30% between 1992 and 2006. In 2010, COPD accounted for approximately 715,000 hospital discharges in the United States, up from 672,000 in 2006. Approximately 65% of discharges were in the population aged 65 years and older. The hospitalization rate for those 65 years of age and older was four times higher than for those in the 45- to 64-year age group. According to the National Heart, Lung, and Blood Institute, the national projected annual cost for COPD in 2010 was $49.9 billion, including $29.5 billion in direct health care expenditures, $8 billion in indirect morbidity costs, and $12.4 billion in indirect mortality costs. The economic burden of COPD is projected to increase in the coming decades as a result of continued exposure to COPD risk factors and the aging of the population.

COPD is defined as an inflammatory respiratory disease involving persistent respiratory symptoms and airflow limitation. The airflow obstruction is usually progressive and associated with an abnormal chronic inflammatory response of the lungs to noxious particles or gases, primarily associated with cigarette smoking. Current definitions of COPD no longer include the terms *emphysema* and *chronic bronchitis*, although such terms are still used clinically. Emphysema is defined pathologically and refers to the destruction of the alveoli, the gas-exchanging surfaces of the lung, resulting in the enlargement of the airspaces distal to the terminal bronchioles. Chronic bronchitis is a clinical term that is used to describe the presence of cough and sputum production for at least 3 months during each of 2 consecutive years.

Pathogenesis

Estimates of the prevalence of COPD depend on the definition and criteria used and vary widely throughout the world, ranging from 5.5% to 20%. It is estimated that between 12.7 and 14.7 million US adults aged 18 years and older are known to have a clinical diagnosis of COPD. However, prevalence data may greatly underestimate the true prevalence of COPD due to its widespread underrecognition and underdiagnosis. It is estimated that up to 24 million adults in the United States may have COPD.

The prevalence of COPD, as well as mortality from COPD, rises considerably with age, with the highest prevalence among those older than age 65 years. Patients younger than age 35 years rarely have COPD, as the disease develops over years of inhalational exposure to a causative agent. In the past, studies showed that COPD prevalence and mortality were greater among men than women. However, this has generally been a consequence of differences in rates of smoking between men and women. More recent data suggest that the prevalence of COPD is now almost equal in men and women and that women may be more susceptible to the effects of tobacco than men. Beginning in 2000, women have exceeded men in the number of deaths attributable to COPD in the United States.

COPD develops as a result of a complex interplay of genetic and environment factors. Tobacco smoke is by far the most important risk factor for COPD, with an estimated 80% to 90% of COPD attributable to cigarette smoking. Smokers are 12 to 13 times more likely to die from COPD than nonsmokers. It is commonly stated that only 15% to 20% of smokers develop clinically significant COPD. However, experts propose that this statistic greatly underestimates the true burden of COPD. A 10-pack-year history of smoking is considered to be the threshold for development of COPD. After 25 years of age, a nonsmoking adult's FEV_1 decreases by an average of 20 to 40 mL per year. In smokers who are susceptible to COPD, the FEV_1 decreases two to five times the normal rate of decline. Smoking cessation can give a former smoker the same average ongoing loss of lung function as a never-smoker.

Besides cigarette smoking, other types of tobacco (eg, pipes, cigars) and marijuana are also risk factors for COPD. Additional risk factors for COPD include advancing age, secondhand smoke exposure, reduced lung growth during gestation, chronic exposure to environmental or occupational pollutants, α_1-antitrypsin deficiency, a childhood history of recurrent respiratory infections, a family history of COPD, and low socioeconomic status. Occupational pollutants associated with COPD include mineral dust from coal and hard rock mining, tunnel work, concrete manufacturing, and silica exposure; organic dust from cotton, flax, hemp, or other grains; and noxious gases, including sulfur dioxide, isocyanates, cadmium, and welding fumes. The percentage of COPD attributable to occupational exposures was estimated as 19.2% overall and 31.1% in never-smokers.

High levels of indoor air pollution resulting from the burning of wood, animal dung, crop residues, or coal for cooking or heating may predispose individuals, particularly women, to develop COPD in developing countries. High levels of outdoor air pollution may be harmful to individuals with existing heart or lung disease, but its role as a risk factor for the development of COPD is unclear.

α_1-Antitrypsin deficiency is a rare hereditary cause of COPD and accounts for only about 2% to 4% of cases. The deficiency is caused by a genetic anomaly of chromosome 14 that leads to premature hepatic and pulmonary disease because of increased tissue damage from neutrophil elastase. However, smoking significantly increases the risk for the progressive development of emphysema associated with α_1-antitrypsin deficiency. This rare recessive trait is most commonly seen in individuals of Northern European origin. Testing for the inherited deficiency is indicated for patients presenting at an early age for COPD, including those younger than age 45 years.

Clinical Findings

A. Symptoms & Signs

The diagnosis of COPD should be suspected in any patient who has a history of tobacco use or exposure to risk factors for COPD and any of the following: chronic cough, chronic sputum production, or dyspnea on exertion or rest. The presence of a productive cough is usually the initial presenting symptom of COPD. The cough associated with COPD is typically worse in the morning but can be present throughout the day, whereas an isolated nocturnal cough is less consistent with COPD. Sputum production also initially occurs in the morning and tends to occur more frequently as the disease progresses. A change in sputum color or volume may suggest an infectious exacerbation. Dyspnea is often associated with exertion or exercise early in the disease course and may be evaded by avoiding physical activities. However, dyspnea may develop at rest as the disease progresses. Wheezing can also be the presenting symptom in patients with COPD. The relationship between the severity of symptoms related to

COPD and the degree of airflow obstruction is highly variable. Some patients with advanced airflow limitation may be relatively asymptomatic. Less commonly reported symptoms associated with COPD include fatigue, edema, chest tightness, weight loss, and increased nocturnal awakenings.

The assessment for COPD should evaluate for the presence of the aforementioned symptoms, as well as their frequency, magnitude, and impact on daily life. The Modified British Medical Research Council (MRC) dyspnea index is a validated tool for quantifying dyspnea and assessing the severity of COPD. Using the MRC, dyspnea can be graded on a 5-point scale, with 1 being not being bothered by dyspnea except during strenuous activities, and 5 being too short of breath to leave the house or breathless with activities of daily living. Other comprehensive assessment tools that measure the symptomatic impact of COPD include the COPD Assessment Test (CAT) and the COPD Control Questionnaire (CCQ).

Important elements in the initial evaluation of COPD include assessing for risk factors, particularly smoking; prior medical history of asthma, allergies, or recurrent respiratory illnesses; and family history of COPD. Because COPD often coexists with other conditions such as coronary artery disease, heart failure, depression, and anxiety that may have a significant impact on symptoms as well as prognosis, clinicians should aim to identify and address comorbidities. For instance, approximately 30% of patients with COPD have congestive heart failure (CHF), and approximately 30% of patients with CHF have COPD. Each condition is commonly implicated as causing an exacerbation or acute flare of the other. Other important elements in the medical history include the pattern of symptom development, history of exacerbations and hospitalizations, and impact of symptoms on the patient's daily life.

While deteriorating airflow limitation as measured by spirometry is associated with an increasing prevalence of COPD exacerbations, the best predictor of having frequent COPD exacerbations is having a history of earlier exacerbations. Therefore, a history of moderate or severe COPD exacerbations should be a part of a comprehensive COPD assessment.

The physical examination may be unremarkable early in the disease. With more advanced disease, patients with COPD may have diminished or distant breath sounds and hyperresonance on percussion and may demonstrate a prolonged expiratory phase and expiratory wheezing. Additional findings associated with COPD include an increased anteroposterior chest diameter or "barrel chest," use of accessory muscles of respiration including suprasternal retractions, and pursed lip breathing. The latter refers to learning forward and supporting oneself using the elbows to relieve dyspnea. The presence of jugular venous distension suggests elevated right heart pressures. Lower extremity edema, central cyanosis, and a widened split second heart sound may indicate right-sided heart failure and cor pulmonale. Pulse oximetry at rest and with exertion should be performed to evaluate for hypoxemia and the need for supplemental oxygen.

COPD commonly manifests systemically, not only affecting the pulmonary system, but also often involving the cardiovascular, muscular, and immune systems, particularly in patients with severe disease. In addition, COPD is associated with chronic weight loss and may lead to cachexia, which is an independent predictor of mortality. Therefore, body mass index (BMI) should be measured and monitored in patients with COPD. Other systemic findings include peripheral muscle wasting and weakness as a result of increased apoptosis and muscle disuse. Individuals with COPD have an increased likelihood of having osteoporosis, depression, chronic anemia, and cardiovascular disease.

B. Laboratory Findings

Suspected COPD should be confirmed by spirometry. Spirometry is a pulmonary function test that measures the presence and severity of airflow obstruction. The diagnosis of COPD is supported when spirometry demonstrates airflow obstruction. The key spirometric measurements related to COPD are FEV_1 and FVC. The FEV_1 is the volume of air that a patient can expire in 1 second following a full inspiration. The FVC is the total maximum volume of air that a patient can exhale after a full inspiration. A postbronchodilator FEV_1-to-FVC ratio of <0.7 is diagnostic of airflow limitation and confirms the diagnosis of COPD. Although postbronchodilator spirometry is required for the diagnosis and assessment of COPD, assessing the degree of reversibility of airflow limitation is no longer recommended because the degree of reversibility has not been shown to augment the diagnosis of COPD, differentiate COPD from asthma, or predict the response to long-term treatment.

The classification of airflow limitation severity in COPD is shown in Table 46–1. However, the degree of airflow limitation alone is insufficient for staging COPD. Current Global Initiatives for Chronic Obstructive Lung Disease (GOLD) guidelines suggest using the Refined ABCD Assessment Tool

Table 46–1. Classification of airflow limitation severity in COPD.

Grade: Degree of Airflow Limitation in Patients with FEV_1/FVC <0.70	Spirometric Findings: Based on Postbronchodilator FEV_1
Grade 1: Mild	$FEV_1 \geq 80\%$ of predicted
Grade 2: Moderate	FEV_1 between 50% and 80% of predicted
Grade 3: Severe	FEV_1 between 30% and 50% of predicted
Grade 4: Very severe	$FEV_1 < 30\%$ of predicted or $FEV_1 < 50\%$ of predicted plus chronic respiratory failure

COPD, chronic obstructive pulmonary disease; FEV_1, forced expiratory volume in 1 second; FVC, forced vital capacity.

Table 46–2. The Refined ABCD Assessment Tool for COPD.

Moderate or Severe Exacerbation History	COPD Group	
≥2 or ≥1 leading to hospital admission	C	D
0 or 1 (not leading to hospital admission)	A	B
Symptoms	mMRC 0–1 CAT <10	mMRC ≥2 CAT ≥10

CAT, COPD Assessment Test; COPD, chronic obstructive pulmonary disease; mMRC, Modified British Medical Research Council dyspnea index.

for COPD, shown in Table 46–2, which incorporates assessment of symptoms and history of moderate to severe COPD exacerbations to categorize patients into COPD groups A to D. The US Preventive Services Task Force (USPSTF) currently recommends against screening asymptomatic adults for COPD using spirometry because there is no evidence of benefit in this population regardless of a patient's age, smoking status, or family history of COPD. Furthermore, nonselective use of spirometry can lead to substantial overdiagnosis of COPD in never-smokers older than age 70 years. Nor is it recommended to use periodic spirometry after initiation of therapy to routinely monitor disease status or to modify therapy. However, spirometry can be helpful to perform if there is a substantial change in symptoms or functional capacity.

Although spirometry is the major diagnostic test used to diagnose COPD, other tests may be helpful for ruling out other conditions or concomitant disease. A chest radiograph should be performed to evaluate for lung masses or nodules, interstitial or fibrotic changes, and pulmonary edema. Radiologic changes associated with COPD include signs of lung hyperinflation, hyperlucency of the lungs, and raid tapering of the vascular markings. A computed tomography (CT) scan of the chest is not routinely recommended except for the detection of bronchiectasis and COPD patients who meet the criteria for lung cancer risk assessment. A complete blood count should be performed to rule out anemia or polycythemia. An electrocardiogram and/or echocardiograph may be useful if there is suspicion for cardiac ischemia or CHF or in patients with signs of cor pulmonale.

▶ Differential Diagnosis

The differential diagnosis of COPD includes asthma, CHF, bronchiectasis, bronchiolitis obliterans, diffuse panbronchiolitis, lung cancer, interstitial lung disease, pulmonary fibrosis, sarcoidosis, cystic fibrosis, tuberculosis, and bronchopulmonary dysplasia. The clinical history, physical examination, and diagnostic testing, such as spirometry, can help diagnose COPD. However, good evidence indicates that history and physical examination are not accurate predictors of airflow limitation. Studies suggest that the single best variable for identifying adults with COPD is a history of >40 pack-years of smoking. A combination of all three of the following findings—>55-pack-year history of smoking, wheezing on auscultation, and patient self-reported wheezing—is highly predictive of COPD. In contrast, the best combination of factors to exclude COPD is absence of a smoking history, no patient-reported wheezing, and no wheezing on physical examination.

▶ Treatment

The goals of COPD treatment are manifold and include reducing long-term decline in lung function, preventing and treating exacerbations, decreasing hospitalizations and mortality, relieving symptoms, improving exercise tolerance, and enhancing health-related quality of life. All patients diagnosed with COPD should receive immunizations, including pneumococcal vaccine and yearly influenza vaccinations. Because smoking is usually the cause of COPD, smoking cessation is the most important component of therapy for patients who still smoke. Quitting smoking can prevent or delay the development of COPD, reduce its progression, and have a substantial impact on mortality. The rate of decline in lung function approaches that of a nonsmoker when a patient quits smoking. "Treating Tobacco Use and Dependence" is a comprehensive, evidence-based guideline published in 2008 by the US Department of Health and Human Services.

Smoking cessation is paramount for patients with COPD at any age, and advanced age does not diminish the benefits of quitting smoking. Treatments shown to be effective for smoking cessation in the general population also have been shown to be effective in older smokers. Specifically, research has demonstrated the effectiveness of counseling interventions, physician advice, buddy support programs, age-tailored self-help materials, telephone counseling, and the nicotine patch in treating tobacco use in adults age 50 years and older. Unfortunately, smokers older than age 65 years may be less likely to receive smoking cessation medications. Use of nicotine replacement products (eg, nicotine gum, inhaler, nasal spray, transdermal patch, sublingual tablet or lozenge) increases long-term smoking quit rates, as does pharmacologic treatment with varenicline and bupropion. Legislative smoking bans are also effective in increasing quit rates and reducing harm from secondhand smoke exposure.

A. Pharmacologic Therapy

Pharmacologic therapy for patients with COPD depends on the severity of symptoms, the degree of lung dysfunction, and response to, as well as tolerance of, specific medications.

A stepwise approach is often employed to provide symptomatic relief, improve exercise tolerance and quality of life, and possibly decrease mortality. However, none of the existing medications for COPD have been shown to conclusively modify the progressive decline in lung function that is characteristic of COPD. Therefore, pharmacotherapy for COPD is generally used to decrease symptoms, reduce the frequency and severity of exacerbations, and improve exercise tolerance and health status. Table 46–3 provides a summary of pharmacologic treatments for COPD, and Table 46–4 presents treatment recommendations based on COPD ABCD groups.

Evidence suggests that there is no benefit to treating asymptomatic persons with evidence of airflow obstruction on spirometry as there is no difference in the progression of lung dysfunction or development of symptoms in treated asymptomatic patients.

When treatment for COPD is delivered by an inhaled method, it is essential to train and evaluate patients regarding inhaler technique. Some older patients with COPD cannot effectively use a metered-dose inhaler (MDI), either because of difficulties with grip strength or coordination or because of cognitive impairment, and may benefit from using a spacer or nebulizer. Use of a spacer or nebulizer can allow caregivers to more easily assist with medication administration. Some studies have shown dry powder inhalers (DPIs) to be easier to handle than MDIs, but DPIs have not demonstrated superior health outcomes.

B. Nonpharmacologic Therapy

1. Oxygen—Guidelines recommend that clinicians prescribe continuous oxygen therapy in patients with COPD who have severe resting hypoxemia (partial pressure of arterial oxygen [PaO_2] of 55 mm Hg or oxygen saturation as measured using pulse oximetry [SpO_2] of 88%). Studies have shown that the use of supplemental oxygen for 15 or more hours daily can help improve survival and quality of life in patients with COPD who have severe resting hypoxemia. Supplemental oxygen has not been shown to benefit outcomes for those with stable COPD or moderate oxygen desaturation.

2. Noninvasive ventilation—Noninvasive positive-pressure ventilation (NPPV) is used to decrease morbidity and mortality in patients hospitalized with a COPD exacerbation and acute respiratory failure. The benefits of using NPPV chronically at home for patients with acute-on-chronic respiratory failure following hospitalization remain undetermined, but studies suggest improved survival and reduced readmissions, particularly for those with persistent hypercapnia. For patients with both COPD and obstructive sleep apnea, the use of continuous positive airway pressure has clear benefits on survival and hospitalizations.

3. Lung volume reduction—Bullectomy, lung volume reductive surgery (LVRS), and lung transplantation have all been used to treat patients with COPD. However, research regarding use and benefit of these procedures for older adults is limited. Bullectomy can be used for a rare subset of patients with COPD who have giant bullous emphysema, where single or multiple large bullae encompass 30% or more of a hemithorax. Surgical resection of these bullae can restore significant pulmonary function and improve symptoms. LVRS is considered in patients with severe emphysema and disabling dyspnea who are refractory to optimal medical management. A variety of surgical approaches and reduction techniques have been used. Overall, LVRS has not demonstrated a survival benefit over medical therapy. LVRS has shown a survival advantage and improved quality of life only for a small subgroup of patients with upper lobe emphysema and low baseline exercise capacity. Unilateral or bilateral lung transplantation is a treatment option in highly selected patients with severe COPD. Studies demonstrate improvements in quality of life after lung transplantation; the effect on survival is less clear. However, age >60 years is considered a relative contraindication for a double-lung transplant. Less invasive bronchoscopic approaches to reduce lung volumes may have benefits for select patients with advanced emphysema.

4. Pulmonary rehabilitation—Pulmonary rehabilitation programs are effective in improving exercise capacity, quality of life, dyspnea, and health status, regardless of age. Pulmonary rehabilitation also reduces hospitalization among patients who have had a recent exacerbation. Pulmonary rehabilitation uses an interdisciplinary approach, including education, self-management support, and exercise training. It is appropriate for most patients with COPD, although the evidence is strongest for those with moderate to severe COPD.

▶ Prognosis

As pharmacologic therapy has not been shown to slow or reverse the progressive loss of lung function that occurs, it remains difficult to prognosticate in COPD because of its variable history and individual heterogeneity. Data from both patients and their physicians demonstrate that advance care planning in COPD is rarely done well, if at all. Patients often have a poor understanding that COPD is a life-limiting illness. In the month prior to their death, less than one-third of patients with severe COPD, CHF, or cancer estimated their life expectancy to be <1 year. Clinicians themselves report their shortcomings when it comes to discussing end-of-life care with patients who have advanced COPD, often waiting until patients are too sick to make care decisions. The landmark study designed to improve end-of-life decision making, Study to Understand Prognoses and Preference for Outcomes and Risks of Treatments (SUPPORT), failed to influence end-of-life care. Specifically, SUPPORT showed that COPD patients who expressed a preference for care focused

Table 46–3. Pharmacologic therapy for COPD.

	Principal Action	Benefits	Indication	Adverse Effects
Bronchodilators				
β$_2$-Agonists Short-acting β-agonists (SABAs; albuterol, levalbuterol) Long-acting β-agonists (LABAs; formoterol, salmeterol)	Promote smooth muscle relaxation by stimulating β$_2$-adrenergic receptors and increasing cyclic adenosine monophosphate (AMP)	SABAs: improve FEV$_1$ and symptoms LABAs: improve FEV$_1$ and lung volumes, dyspnea, and health status; reduce exacerbations and number of hospitalizations	SABAs: first-line initial therapy for mild intermittent symptoms as needed LABAs: for patients with persistent symptoms at a dose of 1 or 2 puffs BID	Resting tachycardia, cardiac rhythm disturbances, tremor, sleep disturbances, hypokalemia
Anticholinergics Short-acting antimuscarinics (SAMAs; ipratropium, oxitropium) Long-acting antimuscarinics (LAMAs; tiotropium, umeclidinium)	Promote smooth muscle relaxation by blocking muscarinic receptors	SAMAs: small benefits in lung function, health status, and requirement for oral steroids LAMAs: improve symptoms and health status, decrease exacerbations and hospitalizations	Short-acting: can be used for symptoms as needed, less rapid onset than β$_2$-agonists but effect lasts longer Long-acting: first-line therapy for patients with persistent symptoms at a dose of 1 puff daily	Dry mouth, bitter or metallic taste, Closed-angle glaucoma using solutions with a facemask
Methylxanthines (theophylline)	Promote smooth muscle relaxation by acting as a nonspecific phosphodiesterase inhibitor that increases intracellular cyclic AMP	Less effective than long-acting bronchodilators, improved FEV$_1$ and symptoms when added to salmeterol	Third-line agent for patients with persistent symptoms	Toxicity is dose related, clearance declines with age, atrial and ventricular arrhythmias, grand mal convulsions, headaches, insomnia, nausea, heartburn, significant interactions with medications including warfarin and digoxin
Anti-inflammatory Agents				
Inhaled corticosteroids (ICS)	Reduce inflammation	Possible slower decline in FEV$_1$	For patients with stage III–IV COPD or for those with repeated exacerbations, blood eosinophil counts may predict the effect of ICS	Increased likelihood of oral candidiasis, hoarseness, bruising, and pneumonia, possibly associated with decreased bone mineral density
PDE4 inhibitors (roflumilast)	Reduce inflammation through inhibition of the breakdown of intracellular AMP	Improves lung function and reduces exacerbations	For patients with stage III or IV COPD and history of exacerbations	Cannot give with theophylline, nausea, anorexia, abdominal pain, diarrhea, sleep disturbances, headache

Antibiotics	Antimicrobial agents	For COPD exacerbations, reduces risk of treatment failure and death	Not generally recommended for use in chronic COPD management. May consider azithromycin (250 mg three times a week) in patients who have optimized other therapies with frequent hospitalizations. Use for COPD exacerbations	Increased incidence of bacterial resistance, tinnitus, and hearing impairment
Mucolytic agents (erdosteine, carbocysteine, and N-acetyl cysteine)	Decrease sputum viscosity and adhesiveness to facilitate expectoration	Reduces exacerbations in select populations		
Oral glucocorticoids	Reduce inflammation	Use for COPD exacerbations to increase the time to subsequent exacerbations, decrease rate of treatment failure, shorten hospital stays, and improve hypoxemia and FEV_1	Avoid for chronic COPD management. Use for COPD exacerbations	Hypertension, hyperglycemia, osteoporosis, myopathy, delirium
Combination Treatments				
SABAs + SAMAs	Combination of short-acting bronchodilators with different mechanisms of action	Combination more effective than either component alone in improving FEV_1 and symptoms		
LABAs + LAMAs	Combination of long-acting bronchodilators with different mechanisms of action	Combination more effective than either component alone in improving lung function and quality of life, and possibly reducing exacerbations		
ICS + LABAs	Combination of inhaled corticosteroid with long-acting bronchodilator	Combination more effective than either component alone in improving lung function and health status and reducing exacerbations	For patients with moderate to severe COPD and exacerbations	
LABA + LAMA + ICS	Combination of long-acting bronchodilators with different mechanisms of action, with an inhaled corticosteroid	May improve lung function and reduce exacerbations		

COPD, chronic obstructive pulmonary disease; FEV_1, forced expiratory volume in 1 second.

Table 46–4. Treatment of COPD.

COPD Group	Initial Pharmacologic Treatment	Nonpharmacologic Treatment (not related to group)
Group A	SABA or SAMA	Active reduction of risk factors including smoking cessation
Group B	LABA or LAMA	Influenza and pneumococcal vaccination
Group C	LAMA	
Group D	LAMA, or LAMA + LABA, or LABA + ICS	Consider pulmonary rehabilitation Add long-term oxygen if chronic hypoxia

COPD, chronic obstructive pulmonary disease; ICS, inhaled corticosteroid; LABA, long-acting β-agonist; LAMA, long-acting antimuscarinic; SABA, short-acting β-agonist; SAMA, short-acting antimuscarinic.

on comfort, rather than life-prolonging measures, were much more likely than patients with lung cancer to receive invasive mechanical ventilation, cardiopulmonary resuscitation, or tube feeding.

Although making a prognosis may be difficult, several tools have been developed to help clinicians stratify severity of disease. For example, the GOLD guidelines classify grades of COPD from I to IV based on the degree of airflow obstruction as measured by spirometry, as well as ABCD groups based on symptom severity and exacerbation history. The GOLD guidelines make accompanying treatment recommendations for each stage of severity (see Table 46–4). The BODE index, which includes BMI, 6-minute walking distance, FEV_1, and the Modified MRC dyspnea scale, has been shown to predict mortality and may provide the clinician with a practical tool to classify how severity of disease may impact life expectancy. The score provides an approximate 4-year survival rate, with low scores (0–2 points) suggesting 80% surviving 4 years and high scores (7–10) suggesting 18% surviving 4 years.

Although the BODE index has been helpful to predict survival over a 1- to 3-year period, it is not validated to predict a 6-month survival. The current National Hospice and Palliative Care Organization Criteria for hospice admission for COPD include disabling dyspnea at rest resulting in decreased functional capacity and progression of end-stage pulmonary diseases, as evidenced by increasing visits to the emergency department or hospitalizations for pulmonary infections and/or respiratory failure. An FEV_1 of 30% and/or a decrease of 40 mL per year provide objective evidence for disease progression but are not necessary for certification. Additionally, the presence of any of the following support certification of the hospice benefit: hypoxemia (partial pressure of oxygen [PO_2] of 55 mm Hg or pulse oximetry of 88% on supplemental oxygen) or hypercapnia (partial pressure of carbon dioxide [PCO_2] of 55 mm Hg), right heart failure as a result of pulmonary disease (cor pulmonale), unintentional weight loss of 10% in the preceding 6 months,

and resting tachycardia of 100/min. Certainly, these criteria serve as a rule of thumb that may guide clinicians to think more actively about increasing services available to patients with end-stage COPD, but studies show they have not been accurate in predicting survival time. Although epidemiologists and researchers have begun to identify characteristics of COPD patients who are most at risk to die in the next 6 to 12 months, perhaps a common sense approach is most practical when considering advance care planning for patients with COPD.

Factors associated with a poorer prognosis in COPD include FEV_1 30% of predicted, declining performance status and emerging dependence in the activities of daily living, more than one acute hospitalization in the past year, additional comorbid illness, older age, depression, and single marital status. Clinicians' identification of many of these in their patients should prompt a discussion about advance care planning. Identification of a medical proxy is a meaningful first step. Ideally, an outpatient discussion between the clinician, patient, and designated proxy during a visit for this specific purpose could be scheduled. Topics that may be discussed at the meeting include the patient's understanding of their illness and its trajectory, discussion of patient preferences for initiation and termination of life-prolonging measures including aggressive mechanical ventilation, and identification of the most appropriate setting (home vs institutional) for end-of-life care. SUPPORT demonstrated that preferences for life-sustaining treatments may change during the course of an illness; therefore, reassessments of patient preferences are particularly important after recent hospitalization, new decline in functional status, and/or new oxygen dependence.

With the chronic nature and severity of COPD, it has become clear that COPD is a major contributor to health care utilization and costs. The Centers for Medicare and Medicaid Services (CMS) requires health plans to conduct performance improvement initiatives focusing on reducing readmissions. Specifically, beginning in 2014, CMS has reduced payments to hospitals with high rates of COPD readmissions within 30 days of discharge. Performance improvement programs have focused on the medication management, discharge planning, and transitional care aspects of COPD management with the goal of reducing readmissions. Using GOLD guidelines, an individualized medication regimen should be optimized with particular emphasis on teaching the correct administration of inhalers, medication reconciliation after hospitalization, and patient education about the purpose of each medication. In addition to proper medication reconciliation, discharge planning should focus on oxygen therapy when needed, coordination of follow-up appointments as needed, and pulmonary rehab. Transitional planning is essential for all chronic disease management and should focus on sound communication between health providers, family members, and home care agencies.

American Lung Association Epidemiology and Statistics Unit. Trends in COPD (Chronic bronchitis and emphysema): morbidity and mortality. 2013. https://www.lung.org/assets/documents/research/copd-trend-report.pdf. Accessed October 29, 2019.

Criner GJ, Bourbeau J, Diekemper RL, et al. Prevention of acute exacerbations of COPD: American College of Chest Physicians and Canadian Thoracic Society Guideline. *Chest*. 2015;147(4):894-942.

Department of Veterans Affairs, Department of Defense. VA/DoD clinical practice guideline for the management of chronic obstructive pulmonary disease, version 3.0, 2014. https://www.healthquality.va.gov/guidelines/CD/copd/VADoDCOPDCPG2014.pdf. Accessed October 29, 2019.

Global Initiative for Chronic Lung Disease (GOLD). Global Strategy for the Diagnosis, Management, and Prevention of Chronic Obstructive Pulmonary Disease (2019 Report). https://goldcopd.org/wp-content/uploads/2018/11/GOLD-2019-v1.7-FINAL-14Nov2018-WMS.pdf. Accessed October 29, 2019.

Jin J. Screening for obstructive pulmonary disease. *JAMA*. 2016;315(13):1419.

Karner C, Chong J, Poole P. Tiotropium versus placebo for chronic obstructive pulmonary disease. *Cochrane Database Syst Rev*. 2014;7:CD009285.

National Institute of Clinical Excellence. Chronic obstructive pulmonary disease in over 16s: diagnosis and management, 2018. https://www.nice.org.uk/guidance/ng115/resources/chronic-obstructive-pulmonary-disease-in-over-16s-diagnosis-and-management-pdf-66141600098245. Accessed October 29, 2019.

Papi A, Rabe KF, Rigau D, et al. Management of COPD exacerbations: a European Respiratory Society/American Thoracic Society guideline. *Eur Respir J*. 2017;49:1600791.

Puhan MA, Gimeno-Santos E, Cates CJ, Troosters T. Pulmonary rehabilitation following exacerbations of chronic obstructive pulmonary disease. *Cochrane Database Syst Rev*. 2016;12:CD005305.

Van Eerd EA, van der Meer RM, van Schayck OC, Kotz D. Smoking cessation for people with chronic obstructive pulmonary disease. *Cochrane Database Sys Rev*. 2016;8:CD010744.

Walters JA, Tang JN, Poole P, Wood-Baker R. Pneumococcal vaccines for preventing pneumonia in chronic obstructive pulmonary disease. *Cochrane Database Syst Rev*. 2017;1:CD001390.

ASTHMA

ESSENTIALS OF DIAGNOSIS

▶ Symptoms: cough, shortness of breath, wheeze.

▶ Risk factors: childhood asthma, smoking, allergen exposure.

▶ Diagnosis: airflow obstruction, $FEV_1/FVC \leq 0.7$.

▶ General Principles

Studies have shown the lifetime prevalence of asthma in individuals >65 years of age approaches 13%, whereas that of children <18 years of age is 14%. Although these rates are similar despite age, the consequences of asthma in older adults may be farther reaching than in young patients. From 2007 to 2009, the asthma-related death rate of patients >65 years was four times higher than the general average population. Studies have shown that the rates of hospitalization, medical costs, and mortality are higher among older populations with asthma.

Further, current reported rates of asthma among older adults may be falsely low. Asthma may be underdiagnosed in older adults for a variety of factors. As patients age, they are less likely to report their symptoms. The misdiagnosis of COPD is common. Finally, health care providers may attribute symptoms to the presence of normal aging changes of lung structure or comorbid conditions.

▶ Pathogenesis

Forty percent of adults over 60 years of age with asthma report their symptoms began after age 40. Asthma in older adults may be due to a different etiology than that in younger patients. In 2017, Baptist and colleagues studied 180 adults over age 55 who had persistent asthma. Cluster analysis study showed that distinct asthma phenotypes exist in older adults. Differing features among the phenotypes included the presence of other medical comorbidities, duration of asthma ≥40 years, and fixed airway obstruction; these were found to be more pronounced among older adults. This study suggests the importance of further research evaluating appropriate management for varying phenotypes of asthma in older patients.

Asthma in older adults has been differentiated into two categories: long-standing asthma and late-onset asthma. The former represents asthma that developed before age 12, while the latter developed later in life. Although both versions have varying severity, it has been suggested that long-standing asthma is more closely linked to atopy and family history while late-onset asthma is correlated with obesity and tobacco use. Long-standing asthma is associated with more airway hyperinflation. Late-onset asthma has a higher baseline FEV_1 with better response to bronchodilators. Obesity rates are rising faster in older adults than most other age groups, pointing to a concern for an increased incidence of late-onset asthma in the future.

Asthma is considered a heterogeneous disease that has a strong environmental element. Although a link between atopy and asthma exists, this link is not as clear in older adults as it is in children. Although asthma in older adults was previously considered nonallergic, more recent research shows that atopy may be linked with asthma in older patients. Studies have identified cats, dust mites, and cockroaches as the most common allergens in older patients. However, the impact of these allergens on the severity of disease has not been clearly established.

In 2017, Busse and colleagues guided a prospective study comparing older and younger inner-city asthmatics. This study showed that older patients had higher sputum neutrophil and eosinophil numbers and decreased rates of asthma control and lower FEV_1 on spirometry. Further, this study showed a correlation between increased sputum cytokines and decreased asthma control and increased hospitalization rates.

Differential Diagnosis

As with patients of any age, there is a broad differential diagnosis for asthma in older patients. Because cough is the most common symptom, gastroesophageal reflux disease (GERD), postnasal drip, CHF, and other lung pathology must be considered. Although a decreased FEV_1/FVC ratio is normal for aging, this may lead to a misdiagnosis of COPD in older patients.

Clinical Findings

The presenting symptoms of asthma in older adults are similar to those findings of younger patients and include shortness of breath, wheeze, and cough. In fact, cough may be the only symptom for some older patients, as they may be less likely to notice dyspnea.

Cavallazzi and colleagues looked at individuals 60 years of age and older who had clinically suspected asthma despite a negative postbronchodilator response on spirometry. These patients were then given a methacholine challenge test. Patients who reported wheezing or allergic coughing were more likely to have a positive methacholine challenge test. Thus, questioning older adults about these specific symptoms may be helpful to predict an asthma diagnosis.

However, as with clinical findings, interpretation of diagnostic tools must also be taken into special consideration when diagnosing asthma in older adults. Frailty should be taken into account when performing spirometry, as frail patients may have difficulty with such tests. As age increases, the FEV_1/FVC ratio decreases and bronchial hyperresponsiveness to methacholine increases. Thus, age-adjusted spirometry values must be used to prevent overdiagnosing obstruction and methacholine challenges may be less accurate as patients age. In older patients with poor lung function or cardiac conditions, bronchoprovocation testing may be contraindicated.

Complications

Although patients may report their asthma symptoms less frequently and providers may not always recognize the diagnosis, the importance of diagnosing asthma in an older population remains. Asthma in older adults significantly decreases their quality of life, and depression has been linked with poor asthma outcomes. Older patients account for >50% of annual asthma fatalities. In 2012, a study showed that asthmatic patients over age 55 had more emergency department visits,

hospitalizations, and near-fatal events than younger patients. In fact, older patients are more than five times more likely to die from asthma complications than younger patients, and the mortality rate of older adults has not decreased, as it has in other age groups.

Treatment

There have not been sufficient studies evaluating the treatment of asthma specifically in older populations; thus, the treatment usually parallels that of asthma for younger patients. However, the treatment of asthma in older adults may be complicated by a variety of factors. Over 50% of adults with asthma report coexisting medical conditions, and 36% of adults over age 60 take five or more prescription medications daily. In addition to comorbidities and polypharmacy, other factors include decreased cognition or physical ability, improper medication use, and adverse effects. Decreased physical ability of inhalation can lead to only 10% to 40% of the inhaled dose to be deposited in the lungs. Although nebulizer treatments require less coordination and may increase medication delivery, they are less portable and efficient. Studies have shown that older patients also recorded more severe airflow obstruction and more frequently required high doses of medications.

Eliminating modifiable factors is an important step in asthma control. Decreasing smoke exposure may decrease asthma exacerbations and increase patients' responses to inhaled corticosteroids (ICS). Environmental allergen exposure control and IgE sensitization contribute to asthma treatment. As the obesity epidemic is growing at the fastest rate in aged populations and obesity is associated with late-onset asthma, weight loss may also help patients control their asthma.

A careful medication reconciliation is necessary in older patients with asthma because polypharmacy may contribute to worsening asthma. Because both oral and topical ocular formulations of β-blockers may cause worsening bronchospasm, cardioselective β-blockers are recommended for patients with asthma. In addition to the polypharmacy of multiple medications, the cost of many medications can also affect a patient's asthma control.

Many frequently used asthma medications have increased adverse effects in older patients. β-Agonists may cause tremor, tachycardia, and dysrhythmias. Prolonged use of ICS in older patients is associated with cataracts, open-angle glaucoma, increased intraocular pressure, and lower bone mineral density in postmenopausal women. The risk of fracture related to ICS has been shown to be dose related.

Leukotriene antagonists may be used as second-line treatment, after ICS. However, these medications have been shown to have less effect on pulmonary function and symptom improvement in older populations. More recent studies have shown that adding montelukast to a low-dose ICS regimen led to fewer asthma exacerbations in older asthmatics than ICS alone. It has been shown to reduce rescue medication use in older patients with severe asthma.

Like salmeterol, tiotropium is a safe and tolerable bronchodilator that can be added to ICS. Tiotropium plus ICS has been shown to reduce airway obstruction and improve asthma control. It has also been shown to reduce the risk of asthma exacerbations requiring oral steroids when added to a regimen of ICS and long-acting β-agonists.

Similar to those of younger age, older patients may have severe asthma exacerbations triggered by viral upper respiratory infections. Influenza and pneumonia are also known triggers of asthma exacerbations. The Centers for Disease Control and Prevention recommends patients 65 years of age or older receive both pneumococcal conjugate vaccine-13 and pneumococcal polysaccharide vaccine-23 to decrease risk of pneumonia.

Baptist AP, Hao W, Karamched KR, et al. Distinct asthma phenotypes among older adults with asthma. *J Allergy Clin Immunol Pract.* 2017;6:244-249.

Blackwell DL, Villarroel MA. Tables of summary health statistics for U.S. adults: 2015 National Health Interview Survey. National Center for Health Statistics. 2016. https://www.cdc.gov/nchs/nhis/shs/tables.htm. Accessed April 6, 2020.

Busse PJ, Birmingham JM, Calatroni A, et al. The effect of aging on sputum inflammation and asthma control. *J Allergy Clin Immunol.* 2017;129(6):1808-1818.

Cavallazzi R, Jorayeva A, Beatty B, et al. Predicting asthma in older adults on the basis of clinical history. *Respir Med.* 2018;142:36-40.

Dunn RM, Busse PJ, Wechsler ME. Asthma in the elderly and late-onset adult asthma. *Allergy.* 2018;73:284-294.

Herscher ML, Wisnivesky JP, Busse PJ, et al. Characteristics and outcomes of older adults with long-standing versus late-onset asthma. *J Asthma.* 2017;54:223-229.

Kerstjens HA, Casale TB, Bleecker ER, et al. Tiotropium or salmeterol as add-on therapy to inhaled corticosteroids for patients with moderate symptomatic asthma: two replicate, double-blind, placebo-controlled, parallel-group, active-comparator, randomized trials. *Lancet Respir Med.* 2015;3:367-376.

Pasha MA, Sundquist B, Rownley R. Asthma pathogenesis, diagnosis, and management in the elderly. *Allerg Asthma Proc.* 2017;38:184-191.

Trinh HK, Ban GY, Lee JH, Park HS. Leukotriene receptor antagonists for the treatment of asthma in elderly patients. *Drugs Aging.* 2016;33:699-710.

US Department of Health and Human Services. Centers for Disease Control and Prevention. National Center for Health Statistics. National Surveillance of Asthma: United States. 2001-2010. Centers for Disease Control and Prevention. Most Recent Asthma Data; 2016. https://www.cdc.gov/nchs/data/series/sr_03/sr03_035.pdf. Accessed April 6, 2020.

Vaz Fragoso CA, McAvay G, Van Ness PH, et al. Phenotype of normal spirometry in an aging population. *Am J Resp Crit Care Med.* 2015;192:817-825.

Vercelli D. Does epigenetics play a role in human asthma? *Allergol Int.* 2016;65:123-126.

INTERSTITIAL LUNG DISEASE

ESSENTIALS OF DIAGNOSIS

▶ Risk factors: smoking, occupational exposures, exposure to radiation, family history of interstitial lung disease (ILD) or connective tissue disease (CTD).

▶ Symptoms: cough (typically dry), wheezing, dyspnea, chronic exercise intolerance.

▶ Physical findings: Velcro-like/"rice crispy"-like rales; lymphadenopathy, hepatosplenomegaly, uveitis, and skin rashes in sarcoidosis or CTD-ILD; right heart failure with lower extremity edema.

▶ Spirometry: usually restrictive pulmonary function test pattern. Varies depending on the etiology of ILD in a particular patient.

▶ Radiographic findings: honeycombing or ground glass opacity on high-resolution CT.

▶ General Principles

ILD describes a spectrum of chronic, progressive parenchymal lung conditions including fibrotic, inflammatory, and occupational insults. There are >100 separate, largely unrelated disease processes that are in this spectrum. These diseases are all commonly diagnosed in the older adult population with typical symptom onset in the sixth or seventh decade of life, and very rarely earlier in life. Of this spectrum of diseases, ILD is most commonly classified as one of idiopathic interstitial pneumonia (the most common being idiopathic pulmonary fibrosis [IPF]), CTD-related ILD (CTD-ILD), hypersensitivity/occupational pneumonitis, and sarcoidosis-related ILD. Prevalence estimates for the ILDs vary depending on the population studied; however, they are on the order of 1000 per 100,000. IPF, generally the entity with one of the worst prognoses, has a significantly lower prevalence, on the order of 10 to 70 per 100,000. Significantly more common are ILD due to sarcoidosis and CTD, which are typically less morbid and have a better overall prognosis with the exception of ILD secondary to rheumatoid arthritis (RA).

The unifying characteristics between these different diseases are that they all typically present with chronic dyspnea and progressive exercise intolerance, with characteristic patterns on chest radiography and high-resolution CT (HRCT) and, when obtained, interstitial fibrosis on lung biopsy. Often comorbidities like COPD/emphysema, asthma, lung malignancies, sleep apnea, CHF, and pulmonary hypertension cloud the diagnosis or contribute to the clinical findings of ILD. Smoking is a particular unifying risk factor among all of the ILDs. In patients with clinical findings and radiography suspicious for ILDs, consultation is best made with a respiratory clinician for firm diagnosis. There is evidence that diagnosis of IPF is best made with a multidisciplinary group of physicians including radiologists, pathologists, and pulmonologists. Up to 30% of diagnoses made by single clinicians or single specialty decision makers may differ from those made by a multidisciplinary group. Diagnosis of ILD should be more strongly suspected in patients with suspicious clinical findings and preexisting CTDs (RA, systemic lupus erythematosus, Sjögren syndrome, mixed connective tissue disorder) and sarcoidosis and must involve a thorough exploration of occupational exposures and drug toxicities. The diagnosis of ILD is often putative, especially in the older adult population, as the risks of surgical lung biopsy often outweigh the benefits of firm diagnosis.

Pathogenesis

The precise pathophysiologic mechanism of fibrosis in many of the ILD spectrum disorders is not well understood. This is particularly the case with IPF and the other idiopathic interstitial pneumonias, where inflammation is not typically thought of as playing a major role, and instead, disordered epithelial cell and fibroblast function leads to progressive fibrosis of the parenchyma of the lung. There is likely an interplay of genetic susceptibility, environmental exposures, and drug toxicities in IPF. In the CTD-ILD and sarcoidosis subtypes, it is likely that the underlying defect in autoimmunity and its associated chronic inflammatory states result in lung fibrosis. Hypersensitivity pneumonitis, also called allergic alveolitis, generally involves disordered immune response to chemicals, pathogens, and other agents. These offending agents are often tied to occupational exposures, for instance, bird fancier's lung, farmer's lung, hot tub lung, and mushroom picker's disease. The pneumoconioses, on the other hand, are the lung's gradual accumulation of inflammation and fibrosis in reaction to inhaled organic dusts or minerals and the lung's tissue response and remodeling in the face of this insult. The most common are asbestosis, silicosis, and coal pneumoconiosis.

Smoking is a unique and particular risk factor for all of the ILDs. More than 50% to 70% of patients diagnosed with an ILD are either current or past smokers. The role that smoking plays in some disease subtypes is better understood than in others. For instance, in RA-ILD, it is thought that smoking leads to deposition of citrullinated proteins in the lung interstitium, which in turn leads to an autoimmune inflammatory response. The mechanism for the marked increase in risk that smoking conveys to the other ILDs is not well understood, but it is a common unifying factor among all of these otherwise dissimilar diseases. Finally, chronic microaspirations also may play a role in ILD and the idiopathic interstitial pneumonias specifically, as patients with esophageal reflux diseases are more likely to develop these conditions later in life.

Clinical Findings

A. Symptoms & Signs

An ILD should be suspected in any patient with progressive dyspnea and exercise intolerance. Sometimes present are wheezing and coughing, typically without mucus production. Classically these patients also present with dry, Velcro-like rales and crackles in the bilateral bases of the lungs on exam. In patients with CTD-ILD, pulmonary symptoms typically occur later in the disease process than articular or musculoskeletal symptoms. Findings associated with these diseases can include lymphadenopathy, hepatosplenomegaly, uveitis and skin rashes, arthralgias, myalgias, or diffuse chronic pain syndromes. Finally, many of these ILDs and their restrictive lung pathology lead to pulmonary hypertension, which eventually causes symptoms of right heart failure (cor pulmonale). These include hepatic congestion and ascites, hepatojugular reflex, widened second heart sound split, lower extremity edema, central cyanosis, and symptoms of portal hypertension.

Spirometry is an important component in the diagnosis of the ILDs. Lung function testing often shows restrictive patterns, often with decreased FVC and FEV_1 (with a preserved FEV_1/FVC ratio); however, in concomitant COPD or sarcoidosis, an obstructive pattern may also manifest. Lung function testing is also useful in monitoring disease progression; however, this is mostly well studied in IPF and less well studied in the other ILDs. Patients with poorer lung function on diagnosis of IPF tend to have more rapidly progressive disease courses with worsened prognosis.

B. Radiologic & Laboratory Findings

Radiography is typically abnormal if the disease is clinically significant. Noncontrast HRCT with specific protocols for IPF with typical "honeycombing," bronchiectasis, and ground-glass opacities with or without mediastinal adenopathy are generally highly suggestive in the right clinical setting. HRCT shows several patterns of fibrosis that cut across these diverse ILD etiologies. These include usual interstitial pneumonia, with honeycombing and traction bronchiectasis; cryptogenic organizing pneumonia, with consolidation and linear opacities; nonspecific interstitial pneumonia, with ground-glass and linear opacities; and lymphocytic interstitial pneumonia, with centrilobular and subpleural nodes, cysts, and ground-glass opacities. Each typically portends different courses and prognoses, with usual interstitial pneumonia carrying a worse prognosis. Any of these radio-histologic patterns may be present in the idiopathic interstitial pneumonias, as well as across the CTD-ILDs.

The laboratory workup leading to a diagnosis of ILD typically involves the exclusion of other etiologies and the diagnosis of diseases that may cause ILD. A urine dipstick, complete blood count with differential, serum electrolytes, creatinine, and liver function tests are often undertaken to rule out vasculitides and malignancies. Inflammatory markers such as C-reactive protein, erythrocyte sedimentation rate (ESR), antinuclear antibodies, rheumatoid factor and anti-cyclic citrullinated peptide (CCP) antibodies, myositis panels including creatinine phosphokinase and myoglobin, and anti-SS-A and anti-SS-B are indicated to diagnose ILD related to RA, Sjögren syndrome, systemic lupus erythematosus (SLE), mixed connective tissue disorder, and scleroderma. Patients who have positive serologies and clinical signs suggestive of CTD or demographically nontypical patients (younger women) should be referred to rheumatology. In sarcoidosis, a serum angiotensin-converting enzyme, serum and urinary calcium, and an electrocardiogram (ECG) are often indicated. Finally, in hypersensitivity or occupational pneumonitis, a careful history may indicate serum IgG specific to a possible exposed antigen (eg, bird fancier's lung may be precipitated by certain avian antigens). Unfortunately, these serum immunologic tests often have high false-positive rates. For patients with positive RA studies, there is an association between positive rheumatoid factor, higher ESR titers, and anti-CCP positivity (94% vs 55%) in the development of ILD in RA patients, and these laboratory abnormalities should raise suspicion for current or future development of lung disease.

Finally, in the correct clinical scenario, select other studies are indicated to rule out alternative diagnoses, including ECG, cardiac troponins, pro-B-type natriuretic peptide, studies to rule out pulmonary embolism, echocardiography to rule out CHF and valvular abnormalities, and sleep polysomnography.

▶ Differential Diagnosis

The differential diagnosis of the ILDs is broad and includes COPD, CHF, cystic fibrosis, acute infectious diseases such as bacterial pneumonia, pulmonary aspergillosis, *Pneumocystis* pneumonia in HIV patients, tuberculosis, viral influenza and other acute viral syndromes, acute respiratory distress syndrome, and asthma and reactive airway disease. Acute exacerbations of ILD can mimic acute pulmonary embolism, myocardial infarction, pleural effusion, and pneumothorax. Finally, primary and metastatic lung malignancies are also alternative diagnoses that must be considered. The diagnosis of ILD is made by characteristic historical and clinical findings, fibrosis on HRCT, and, less often, lung biopsy.

▶ Management

It is unfortunate that many of the ILDs have very limited effective management options. In fact, for IPF and those ILDs with imaging or histopathologic similarities to IPF, there is no evidence that any current treatments increase survival. All patients who are diagnosed with an ILD should have baseline spirometry and DLCO recorded as both a prognostic indicator and to guide treatment. Possibly the single most effective recommendation is for tobacco cessation therapy in patients who continue to smoke tobacco. Smoking cessation is crucial not only to reduce the risk of developing lung cancer, but also to improve lung function and reduce comorbid lung conditions such as COPD, which will worsen prognosis. In advanced IPF and other ILDs, symptomatic treatment includes oxygen for patients with dyspnea or desaturation with exertion, oral opiates for breathlessness, and cough medications. Physicians must balance a patient's symptom burden with the increased adverse effects of opioids in the older population. Pulmonary rehabilitation, a multidisciplinary intervention, can increase quality of life and decrease dyspnea in severely affected patients. Proton pump inhibitors should be prescribed in patients with symptomatic and possibly asymptomatic GERD because chronic gastric microaspiration may be involved in the pathogenesis of the disease.

Pirfenidone (a transforming growth factor-β inhibitor and antifibrotic) and nintedanib (a nonspecific receptor tyrosine kinase inhibitor) are considered disease-modifying treatments and are useful in patients who have FVC between 50% and 80%. There is modest evidence that these two medications significantly slow the reduction in FVC in these diseases; however, multiple studies have failed to show a significant decrease in all-cause mortality as well as respiratory illness–associated mortality. These two agents are also largely similar to each other in efficacy. They should be started early in the course of IPF as they seem to have a larger effect size in patients with mild to moderate disease activity. In IPF, there is no role for azathioprine, bosentan, mycophenolate mofetil, oral glucocorticoids, warfarin, or sildenafil.

For the CTD-ILD subtypes, immunosuppressives and disease-modifying antirheumatic drugs are first-line agents. Glucocorticoids, high dose if acutely ill, and maintenance with mycophenolate, cyclophosphamide, azathioprine, or mycophenolate are used in the management of RA-ILD, SLE-ILD, and Sjögren syndrome–associated ILD, as well as tumor necrosis factor-α blockade with biologics and anti-CD20 treatment with rituximab. Biologics and methotrexate, however, may exacerbate lung disease in this population. An important caveat is that in all of these ILD subtypes, the presence of usual interstitial pneumonia heralds a lack of response to these immunosuppressive therapies.

In sarcoidosis, hypersensitivity, and occupational pneumonias and pneumoconioses, supplemental oxygen and systemic glucocorticoids are useful. Definitive management of the latter includes avoidance of exposure or reduction to lowest possible level of offending agent. Finally, lung transplantation remains an option in patients with advanced ILD.

Prognosis

For IPF and all ILD subtypes with IPF-like features (usual interstitial pneumonia on imaging and histopathology), mean survival is 3 years from diagnosis, and only 20% survive to 5 years. This reality is important to convey to patients, as many will be relieved they "do not have cancer," while in reality, IPF carries a worse prognosis than many malignancies. Similarly, RA-ILD carries a mean survival of 3 years from diagnosis of RA-ILD to death, which is uniquely poor among the CTD-ILDs. Sjögren syndrome–associated ILD similarly has a poorer prognosis, with up to 50% of patients having recovery after exacerbation, with the rest experiencing a stabilization or worsening of respiratory symptoms. Patients with Reynaud phenomenon and esophageal involvement show a worse prognosis in Sjögren syndrome–associated ILD. Pulmonary sarcoidosis, SLE-ILD, and mixed CTD enjoy a better prognosis, with pulmonary symptoms typically responsive to immunotherapy. Finally, hypersensitivity and occupational pneumonia and pneumonitis generally have a spectrum of prognoses related to the duration and severity of exposure to the offending agent, underscoring the importance of exposure reduction therapy.

Canestaro WJ, Forrester SH, Raghu G, Ho L, Devine BE. Drug treatment of idiopathic pulmonary fibrosis: systematic review and network meta-analysis. *Chest*. 2016;149(3):756-766.

Kelly CA, Saravanan V, Nisar M, et al. Rheumatoid arthritis-related interstitial lung disease: associations, prognostic factors and physiological and radiological characteristics—a large multicentre UK study. *Rheumatology (Oxford)*. 2014;53(9):1676-1682.

Litow FK, Petsonk EL, Bohnker BK, et al. Occupational interstitial lung diseases. *J Occup Environ Med*. 2015;57(11):1250-1254.

Medlin JL, Hansen KE, Mccoy SS, Bartels CM. Pulmonary manifestations in late versus early systemic lupus erythematosus: a systematic review and meta-analysis. *Semin Arthritis Rheum*. 2018;48(2):198-204.

Moua T, Zamora Martinez AC, Baqir M, Vassallo R, Limper AH, Ryu JH. Predictors of diagnosis and survival in idiopathic pulmonary fibrosis and connective tissue disease-related usual interstitial pneumonia. *Respir Res*. 2014;15:154.

National Clinical Guideline Centre (UK). Diagnosis and management of suspected idiopathic pulmonary fibrosis: idiopathic pulmonary fibrosis [internet]. London: Royal College of Physicians; 2013 (NICE Clinical Guidelines, no. 163). https://www.ncbi.nlm.nih.gov/books/nbk247530/. Accessed April 6, 2020.

Patterson KC, Shah RJ, Porteous MK, et al. Interstitial lung disease in the elderly. *Chest*. 2017;151(4):838-844.

Raghu G, Remy-Jardin M, Myers JL, et al. Diagnosis of idiopathic pulmonary fibrosis. An official ATS/ERS/JRS/ALAT clinical practice guideline. *Am J Respir Crit Care Med*. 2018;198(5):e44-e68.

Roca F, Dominique S, Schmidt J, et al. Interstitial lung disease in primary Sjögren's syndrome. *Autoimmun Rev*. 2017;16(1):48-54.

Skeoch S, Weatherley N, Swift AJ, et al. Drug-induced interstitial lung disease: a systematic review. *J Clin Med*. 2018;7(10):E356.

PULMONARY HYPERTENSION

ESSENTIALS OF DIAGNOSIS

▶ Symptoms: fatigue, angina, exertional dyspnea, exercise intolerance, syncope, and concomitant diagnoses associated with pulmonary hypertension.

▶ Risk factors: chronic lung diseases and sleep disorders, high cardiac output states, hypertension, left heart disease, obesity, volume overload, chronic kidney disease, end-stage renal disease, and connective tissue diseases.

▶ Diagnosis: echocardiogram: estimated systolic pulmonary arterial pressure of 35 to 40 mm Hg (usually higher in older adults) is suggestive of pulmonary hypertension; right cardiac catheterization if suspicious for pulmonary arterial hypertension.

General Considerations

Pulmonary hypertension is an umbrella term for a myriad of complex medical conditions that causes the pulmonary artery pressure to be >25 mm Hg upon right heart catheterization. This is a challenging diagnosis in senior adults due to its vague, nonspecific symptomatology, which is often attributed to comorbid conditions in this population. Pulmonary hypertension and pulmonary arterial hypertension are not synonymous. Many diseases such as obstructive sleep apnea, chronic lung diseases, and heart failure can lead to increased pressure in the pulmonary arteries. Whereas in pulmonary arterial hypertension, the blood vessels are constricted, causing increased pressure in the pulmonary arteries.

There are five different categories of pulmonary hypertension, which are classified based on pathophysiology and treatment options; these are as follows: group 1, pulmonary arterial hypertension; group 2, pulmonary hypertension due to left heart disease; group 3, pulmonary hypertension due to lung disease or hypoxia; group 4, chronic thromboembolic pulmonary hypertension; and group 5, multifactorial pulmonary hypertension. See Table 46–5.

Pathogenesis

Although age-related increased vascular stiffening is known to contribute to systolic hypertension in the systemic circulation, less is understood about the impact of age on the pulmonary artery systolic pressure (PASP). It is likely that age-associated pulmonary artery remodeling may lead to pulmonary vascular stiffening and an increase in PASP. Age-related left ventricular heart failure with preserved ejection fraction can lead to increased left heart filling pressures, which can have a downstream effect on pulmonary artery pressure. There is evidence to support some genetic

Table 46–5. World Health Organization (WHO) pulmonary hypertension groups.

Group 1: Pulmonary arterial hypertension	Idiopathic, heritable, and HIV-associated; systemic sclerosis and other connective tissue disease; congenital heart disease; schistosomiasis; drug and toxin induced
Group 2: Pulmonary hypertension due to left heart disease	HFrEF, HFpEF and valvular heart disease
Group 3: Pulmonary hypertension due to lung diseases and/or hypoxia	Chronic obstructive pulmonary disease, sleep-disordered breathing, and interstitial lung disease
Group 4: Chronic thromboembolic pulmonary hypertension	
Group 5: Multifactorial pulmonary hypertension	Metabolic, systemic, and hematologic disorders (sickle cell disease), and others

HFpEF, heart failure with preserved ejection fraction; HFrEF, heart failure with reduced ejection fraction.

associations such as *BMPR*2, yet the gene alone does not appear to explain the disease process in the absence of other contributing risk. Given the wide range of causes of pulmonary hypertension, there are multiple potential mechanisms contributing to its pathophysiology. Ultimately, the consequence of increased pulmonary arterial pressure is strain on the right ventricle, which is unable to sustain cardiac output. Therefore, the most common cause of death in patients with pulmonary hypertension is right ventricular failure.

Clinical Findings and Differential Diagnosis

Patients with pulmonary hypertension often present with fatigue and dyspnea on exertion that is insidious and ultimately may present as overt right heart failure when the disease becomes severe. Commonly, patents are impacted by nonspecific symptoms for 2 years prior to receiving a diagnosis. It is not recommended to screen the general population for pulmonary hypertension, thus increasing the likelihood that the disease is not diagnosed until it is more severe in its course. Guidelines recommend annual echocardiogram and pulmonary function tests to screen for asymptomatic pulmonary hypertension in all patients with scleroderma, given the increased likelihood of pulmonary hypertension in CTDs. For patients who continue to have suggestive symptoms out of proportion to already known chronic diseases or are not responding to first-line treatments, pulmonary hypertension

should be kept high in the differential, thus prompting the clinician to pursue diagnostic testing. Physical exam signs may include hypoxia, elevated jugular venous pressure, ascites, lower extremity edema, a right ventricular heave, and a pansystolic murmur at the left lower sternal border, characteristic of tricuspid regurgitation.

Diagnosis

Depending on the patient's clinical presentation, multiple tests can be used to work up a patient for pulmonary hypertension. An ECG can be instrumental in showing signs of right ventricular strain or hypertrophy. The next best test is a transthoracic echocardiogram. The tricuspid regurgitant jet velocity can be a proxy to measure the PASP (ePASP). Additionally, the right ventricle should be assessed to determine its size, thickness, and function. Signs of left heart disease may also be identified on echocardiogram and are a key determinant of group 2 pulmonary hypertension. An echocardiogram can be suggestive of pulmonary hypertension, but it is insufficient to determine disease severity or to assess possible response to therapy if the clinician is trying to rule in pulmonary artery hypertension (PAH) as the cause of pulmonary hypertension. Right heart catheterization plays an essential role in making a definitive diagnosis of PAH but may not be required in patients whose pulmonary hypertension is clearly attributed to left heart disease or an underlying lung disease.

Treatment

Accurate diagnosis and classification of the type of pulmonary hypertension are critical to management. PAH or chronic thromboembolic pulmonary hypertension are the only two specific diagnoses of pulmonary hypertension for which targeted therapies are recommended. Treatment for pulmonary hypertension due to left heart disease should be focused on the underlying cause. Standard of care for treatment of heart failure with reduced ejection fraction includes angiotensin-converting enzyme inhibitors, β-adrenergic antagonists, and diuretics. Aggressive treatments may include placement of implantable cardioverter-defibrillators when appropriate and consistent with the patient's goals of care. Treatment of heart failure with preserved ejection fraction relies on control of systemic blood pressure, heart rate, and diuretics when necessary. Treatment of pulmonary hypertension associated with chronic lung disease is aimed at correcting hypoxia and optimal management of the underlying etiology. When appropriate, patients should be tested for obstructive sleep apnea and treated if indicated. Vasodilators should be avoided in chronic lung disease as they may worsen the ventilation/perfusion mismatch. For appropriate surgical candidates, a pulmonary endarterectomy is the potentially curative treatment of choice for patients with chronic thromboembolic pulmonary hypertension. Although less effective, targeted therapies

Table 46–6. Advanced therapies for PAH.

Class	Mechanism	Notes
Endothelin receptor antagonists (bosentan, ambrisentan)	Antagonize endothelin-1, which is a potent endogenous vasoconstrictor and mitogen present at high levels in patients with PAH	Improve exercise capacity, functional class, time to worsening Monitor LFTs and hemoglobin
Phosphodiesterase type 5 inhibitors (sildenafil, tadalafil)	Potentiate vasodilatory effects of cyclic guanosine monophosphate by inhibiting its breakdown	TID dosing of sildenafil; once daily dosing of tadalafil Concomitant nitrates can lead to systemic hypotension
Prostacyclins (epoprostenol)	Act as potent vasodilatory, antiplatelet, and antiproliferative properties	Most potent therapy Given IV or SC

IV, intravenous; LFTs, liver function tests; PAH, pulmonary artery hypertension; SC, subcutaneous; TID, three times a day.

for PAH may be offered to patients who are not able to undergo surgery. For all patients with chronic thromboembolic hypertension, lifelong anticoagulation is indicated. For patients diagnosed with PAH, referral to a specialized center is appropriate to confirm diagnosis and explore options of advance therapies (Table 46–6). Additionally, appropriate patients referred to a specialized center may realize opportunities to participate in clinical trials and undergo evaluation for lung transplantation, when appropriate.

Prognosis

Prognosis for patients with pulmonary hypertension varies depending on the underlying etiology. No matter the cause, the presence of pulmonary hypertension is generally considered a poor prognostic indicator, especially in diseases such as heart failure or COPD. More is understood about the prognosis for PAH as a result of the Registry to Evaluate Early and Long-Term PAH Disease Management (REVEAL) trial. The goal of this trial was to design a clinically relevant and accurate model to predict outcomes in patients with World Health Organization group 1 PAH. This multicenter study concluded PAH associated with CTD, functional class III, mean right atrial pressure, systolic blood pressure and heart rate at rest, 6-minute walk distance, brain natriuretic peptide level, percent predicted carbon monoxide diffusing capacity, and pericardial effusion all predicted increased 1-year mortality. Data from this study were used to inform a tool that has been validated to use as a prognostic calculator.

Al Danaf J, Harry J, Catino A. Pulmonary hypertension: better or for worse. *J Am Coll Cardiol.* 2018;71:A2443-A2443.

Harari S, Elia D, Humbert M. Pulmonary hypertension in parenchymal lung diseases: any future for new therapies? Any future for new therapies? *Chest.* 2018;153:217-223.

Kolte D, Lakshmanan S, Jankowich MD, et al. Mild pulmonary hypertension is associated with increased mortality: a systematic review and meta-analysis. *J Am Heart Assoc.* 2018;7(18):e009729.

Maron BA, Galiè N. Diagnosis, treatment, and clinical management of pulmonary arterial hypertension in the contemporary era: a review. *JAMA Cardiol.* 2016;1(9):1056-1065.

Pugh ME, Sivarajan L, Wang L, et al. Causes of pulmonary hypertension in the elderly. *Chest.* 2014;146(1):159-166.

Taichman DB, Ornelas J, Chung L, et al. Pharmacologic therapy for pulmonary arterial hypertension in adults: CHEST guideline and expert panel report. *Chest.* 2014;146(2):449-475.

Gastrointestinal Diseases

Annsa Huang, MD

Priya Kathpalia, MD

General Principles

Gastrointestinal (GI) conditions are commonly seen in older adults and can present in various forms and severity, ranging from mild bouts of constipation to life-threatening episodes of bowel ischemia. Certain conditions have a higher prevalence in older people, such as vascular disease and neoplasia. In addition, older adults often have multiple chronic illnesses and use concomitant medications, such as nonsteroidal anti-inflammatory drugs (NSAIDs) and anticoagulants, which can both predispose them to GI diseases and complicate their management. Endoscopic procedures can be safely performed in older patients but require careful consideration of their medical multimorbidity, cardiopulmonary status, and overall ability to tolerate procedural sedation.

DYSPHAGIA

ESSENTIALS OF DIAGNOSIS

▶ Dysphagia can be oropharyngeal or esophageal.

▶ Alarm features such as unintentional weight loss, anemia, and odynophagia should be solicited and warrant endoscopy for evaluation.

▶ A modified barium swallow test evaluates oropharyngeal swallow function but does not extend distally to evaluate the entire esophagus, unlike a barium esophagram, which also evaluates the distal esophagus.

▶ Successful management of dysphagia requires an interprofessional approach, with medical and endoscopic therapies, as well as behavioral modifications.

General Principles

Dysphagia, or difficulty swallowing, is a common complaint in older adults. Dysphagia can be classified as either oropharyngeal or esophageal. Oropharyngeal dysphagia refers to impaired movement of liquids or solids from the oral cavity to the upper esophagus. Esophageal dysphagia occurs in the esophagus distal to the upper esophageal sphincter. Both types of dysphagia are common, with an estimated 20% of community-dwelling adults experiencing dysphagia of any type over a 1-year period. Various disorders can adversely affect swallow function, particularly in older people, such as neurologic causes (stroke, dementia) and malignancy involving the aerodigestive tract. The aging process itself, associated with decrease in muscle mass and connective tissue elasticity, also predisposes to presbyesophagus, which can impair the swallowing process in older adults.

Clinical Findings

A. Symptoms & Signs

Patients with oropharyngeal dysphagia typically cough, choke, or regurgitate their food during the initiation of a swallow. Those with esophageal dysphagia often feel food getting "caught" or "stuck" in the esophagus and may identify discomfort in the throat or substernal area. Patients may also complain of painful swallowing, known as odynophagia. Dysphagia to solids can often reflect an underlying structural disorder, such as a mechanical obstruction, whereas progressive dysphagia to both solids and liquids is more typical of an underlying motility problem. Alarm features that may indicate underlying serious pathology, such as malignancy, should be solicited and include unintentional weight loss, anemia, and odynophagia.

B. Diagnostic Evaluation

There are a variety of diagnostic tests that evaluate dysphagia, including modified barium swallow, barium esophagram, upper endoscopy, and esophageal manometry.

The modified barium swallow test is useful for evaluation of oropharyngeal dysphagia. This is a swallowing study that is carried out by both speech-language pathologists and radiologists to assess the phases of swallowing in real time. Patients are observed while swallowing food of different consistencies (thin and thick liquids, as well as solid), which allows for an assessment of oropharyngeal coordination and the presence and extent of aspiration. It is important to note that the modified barium swallow test does not evaluate the esophagus more distally and is not sufficient to rule out more distal esophageal pathology, such as an obstructive mass or lesion.

A barium esophagram is a noninvasive test of the esophagus, during which a food bolus is viewed as it passes from the oropharynx into the stomach, allowing for assessment of the upper and lower esophageal sphincters. A barium esophagram is able to detect anatomic abnormalities throughout the entire esophagus, such as strictures, rings, or mass lesions. It is more sensitive in detecting esophageal webs and rings than endoscopy.

Although the modified barium swallow test and barium esophagram can provide a significant amount of information, endoscopy should be performed, if possible, in all patients with dysphagia. Upper endoscopy allows for direct visualization of the esophagus to assess for mucosal inflammation, masses, lesions, and other structural abnormalities. In addition to serving as a diagnostic procedure, endoscopy also allows for therapeutic interventions such as esophageal dilation if a stricture is found.

In patients with ongoing dysphagia despite a normal upper endoscopy, esophageal manometry should be performed to evaluate for a motility disorder. Manometry is the gold standard test for the diagnosis of achalasia.

Differential Diagnosis

The differential diagnosis for esophageal dysphagia is broad and can be characterized as structural or related to dysmotility (Table 47–1). There are many benign causes of dysphagia, including gastroesophageal reflux disease (GERD) and its complications (peptic stricture), Schatzki ring, esophageal web, eosinophilic esophagitis, and cricopharyngeal bar. Esophageal malignancy should always be ruled out, as above. Common motility disorders include achalasia, distal esophageal spasm, and absent contractility. Cardiopulmonary causes for chest or retrosternal pain should be ruled out well before any GI evaluation, given the potential life-threatening nature of diseases such as acute coronary syndrome, aortic dissection, or pulmonary disease.

Table 47–1. Causes of esophageal dysphagia.

Benign	Malignant	Motility
Gastroesophageal reflux disease	Esophageal squamous cell carcinoma	Achalasia
Peptic stricture	Esophageal adenocarcinoma	Distal esophageal spasm
Schatzki ring	Extrinsic compression	Jackhammer esophagus
Esophageal web		Absent contractility
Eosinophilic esophagitis		Ineffective esophageal motility
Infectious esophagitis		Fragmented peristalsis
Medication-induced esophagitis		
Cricopharyngeal bar		

Treatment

Treatment of dysphagia is directed toward addressing the underlying causative disorder, in addition to preventing aspiration and ensuring adequate nutrition. Successful management of dysphagia requires an interprofessional approach, involving physicians (both geriatricians and subspecialists such as gastroenterologists and otolaryngologists), nurses, nutritionists, and speech-language pathologists. Behavioral modifications are often the primary manner to improve symptoms of dysphagia. This includes dietary modification and changing consistency of foods, postural adjustments during swallowing, and proper swallowing techniques. Medical therapy is determined by the underlying etiology. For example, GERD should be treated with proton pump inhibitor (PPI) or histamine-2 receptor antagonists (H_2 blockers) and lifestyle modifications, and achalasia should be treated with endoscopic pneumatic balloon dilation, botulinum toxin injection, or even via endoscopic or surgical myotomy in carefully and appropriately selected patients.

Cho SY, Choung RS, Saito YA, et al. Prevalence and risk factors for dysphagia: a U.S. community study. *Neurogastroenterol Motil.* 2015;27(2):212-210.

Firth M, Prather CM. Gastrointestinal motility problems in the elderly patient. *Gastroenterology.* 2002;122(6):1688-1700.

Kuo P, Holloway RH, Nguyen NQ. Current and future techniques in the evaluation of dysphagia. *J Gastroenterol Hepatol.* 2012;27(5):873-881.

Nawaz S, Tulunay-Ugur OE. Dysphagia in the older patient. *Otolaryngol Clin North Am.* 2018;51(4):769-777.

GASTROESOPHAGEAL REFLUX DISEASE

ESSENTIALS OF DIAGNOSIS

▶ GERD is defined as experiencing heartburn and/or acid regurgitation at least once weekly.

▶ GERD can be complicated by esophagitis, peptic strictures, and Barrett esophagus.

▶ Upper endoscopy should be performed in patients with alarm features or who have persistent symptoms despite medical management.

▶ Acid suppression with PPI or H₂ blocker therapy along with lifestyle modifications should be used to treat GERD.

▶ PPI therapy should be used only when clinically indicated, which includes patients with symptomatic GERD who require PPI for long-term symptom control, patients with acid-related complications such as erosive esophagitis and Barrett esophagus, and those at high risk for ulcer bleeding due to chronic NSAID use.

▶ General Principles

GERD is a common GI disorder. The prevalence of GERD, defined as experiencing heartburn and/or acid regurgitation at least once weekly, is estimated to range from 18% to 28% in the United States. The severity of GERD has been found to increase with age, with increasing prevalence of more severe erosive esophagitis in older adults. Despite the predisposition to more severe disease, population-based studies demonstrate that, paradoxically, symptoms tend to become less intense and more nonspecific with age.

▶ Clinical Findings

A. Symptoms & Signs

Common symptoms of GERD include heartburn, regurgitation, and epigastric pain. Patients often describe the sensation of substernal burning with radiation to the mouth and throat. They may also present with atypical symptoms, including chronic cough, difficult to control asthma, and recurrent chest pain. Erosive esophagitis can lead to iron deficiency anemia or manifest more prominently as melena or hematemesis. Untreated or poorly controlled GERD can lead to complications such as GI bleeding secondary to esophagitis or ulceration, peptic esophageal strictures, and Barrett esophagus, a premalignant condition with increased risk of esophageal adenocarcinoma.

B. Diagnostic Evaluation

Upper endoscopy is the test of choice to evaluate for significant upper GI tract findings associated with GERD, such as erosive esophagitis, peptic strictures, and malignancy. An initial trial of empiric medical therapy with PPI, prior to endoscopy, is appropriate for most patients if their history is consistent with uncomplicated GERD without alarm features. However, esophagogastroduodenoscopy should be performed in all patients who have persistent symptoms despite medical therapy, in addition to those with red flag symptoms such as dysphagia, odynophagia, unintentional weight loss, anemia or evidence of GI bleeding, or concern for mass or stricture on imaging studies. Upper endoscopy should also be performed in the preoperative evaluation for patients being considered for antireflux surgery.

Other diagnostic modalities for GERD include ambulatory pH monitoring and impedance testing. These tests assess the presence and frequency of abnormal esophageal acid exposure and symptom association with reflux events. They can be effective in distinguishing between true acid-related and nonacid reflux episodes.

▶ Treatment

The treatment of GERD in older adults is the same as that in younger patients. Lifestyle modifications to decrease symptom burden include eating smaller, more frequent meals; avoiding trigger foods; waiting 3 to 4 hours after eating before going to bed; and sleeping with the head of the bed elevated. PPI therapy is indicated for symptomatic GERD, acid-related complications such as erosive esophagitis and Barrett esophagus, and those at high risk for ulcer bleeding due to chronic NSAID use. In those with erosive esophagitis, PPI therapy has been found to have improved healing rates and decreased relapse rates compared with H₂ blockers.

Long-term PPI use has been associated with a variety of potential side effects over time, although the evidence supporting these claims is of overall low quality, with the majority of data from retrospective and observational studies that are often methodologically limited. The potential risks of chronic PPI use that have been reported include dementia, chronic kidney disease, coronary artery disease, and osteoporosis, but these have not been validated in controlled studies. Higher quality evidence does support that PPI therapy is a risk factor for *Clostridium difficile* and other diarrheal illnesses, likely due to alteration of gut microbial flora from acid suppression. Although further research is needed in this area, these existing studies on chronic PPI use shed light that this class of medication should be used thoughtfully to minimize the risk of long-term side effects. The dose of long-term PPI therapy should be periodically reevaluated so that the lowest effective dose can be used.

Patients with refractory GERD despite medical therapy with maximal acid suppression should be considered for endoscopic interventions or antireflux surgery. These modalities aim to tighten the lower esophageal sphincter to treat GERD. Underlying esophageal motility disorders should be excluded prior to consideration of antireflux surgery.

El-Serag HB, Sweet S, Winchester CC, Dent J. Update on the epidemiology of gastro-oesophageal reflux disease: a systematic review. *Gut.* 2014;63(6):871-880.

Katz PO, Gerson LB, Vela MF. Guidelines for the diagnosis and management of gastroesophageal reflux disease. *Am J Gastroenterol.* 2013;108(3):308-328.

Scholl S, Dellon ES, Shaheen NJ. Treatment of GERD and proton pump inhibitor use in the elderly: practical approaches and frequently asked questions. *Am J Gastroenterol.* 2011;106(3):386-392.

DYSPEPSIA

ESSENTIALS OF DIAGNOSIS

▶ Dyspepsia is defined as epigastric pain that can be associated with other GI symptoms such as nausea, heartburn, and bloating.

▶ Functional dyspepsia occurs in patients without organic pathology and is chronic and fluctuating in nature.

▶ *Helicobacter pylori* infection can contribute to dyspepsia and should be tested for and treated if positive.

▶ Upper endoscopy is indicated in patients over age 60 or with alarm features.

▶ PPI therapy and neuromodulators are therapeutic options for functional dyspepsia.

▶ General Principles

Dyspepsia is defined as epigastric pain lasting at least 1 month. It can be associated with other upper GI tract symptoms, such as nausea, vomiting, heartburn, and bloating, although epigastric pain is the predominant symptom. Functional dyspepsia occurs in patients without organic pathology to explain their symptoms, as evaluated by lab testing, imaging, and upper endoscopy. Dyspepsia is a very common complaint, with an estimated global prevalence of around 20%. Population-based studies have shown that, in the United States, a greater proportion of older adults >65 years of age seek care for dyspepsia compared to the general population. Functional dyspepsia is chronic in nature, and often patients will experience fluctuating episodes of symptom relapse.

▶ Clinical Findings

A. Signs & Symptoms

Patients may complain of epigastric abdominal pain, nausea, vomiting, bloating, early satiety, or reflux symptoms. Given its broad definition and nonspecific associated symptoms, the presentation and evaluation of dyspepsia often overlap with other common GI complaints, such as dysphagia, GERD, peptic ulcer disease (PUD), and irritable bowel syndrome.

B. Diagnostic Evaluation

Evaluation of dyspepsia begins with a thorough history and physical exam to determine whether symptoms arise in the GI tract or elsewhere (heart, lungs, musculoskeletal system). Patients should be asked about unintentional weight loss, dysphagia, odynophagia, prior PUD, pancreatitis, or biliary tract disease.

H pylori infection, as a risk factor for PUD, can contribute to dyspepsia. The presence of active *H pylori* infection can be evaluated in a variety of ways. Two sensitive, noninvasive tests are the stool antigen and urease breath tests, but patients must be off PPI therapy for at least 2 weeks before testing.

Patients with new-onset dyspepsia over the age of 60 years should be evaluated with upper endoscopy to evaluate for organic pathology and to rule out malignancy. In addition, upper endoscopy is indicated in patients with alarm features suggestive of more serious disease, such as dysphagia, odynophagia, unintentional weight loss, and anemia. Endoscopy should also be performed in those under the age of 60 who do not respond to maximal acid suppressive therapy after 6 to 8 weeks. Therefore, in clinical practice, dyspepsia in older adults should be evaluated endoscopically as part of the initial evaluation.

Finally, if upper endoscopy is normal, ambulatory pH monitoring and impedance testing, while the patient is off PPI therapy, may confirm presence or absence of true acid reflux. Imaging with abdominal ultrasound or abdomen and pelvis computed tomography (CT) scans allows for evaluation for alternative causes of dyspepsia such as pancreatic or biliary pathology.

▶ Treatment

If an organic cause of dyspepsia is identified by endoscopy, treatment should be guided by the specific diagnosis. However, patients with functional dyspepsia (by definition, normal evaluation without specific organic pathology identified) can be challenging to treat. These patients should be tested for *H pylori* infection and treated if positive. If symptoms persist despite *H pylori* eradication, empiric acid suppression therapy should be initiated with a PPI. The effect of *H pylori* eradication on symptom improvement in dyspepsia is often modest, at best, as there is some thought that the bacterial infection may in fact have a protective effect on decreasing gastric acid production. Antidepressants may be used as second- or third-line agents to target the possible role of the brain-gut axis in functional dyspepsia. These neuromodulators include tricyclic antidepressants, selective serotonin reuptake inhibitors, serotonin-norepinephrine reuptake inhibitors, and other classes of medications such as bupropion and mirtazapine. For similar reasons, hypnosis therapy and acupuncture may also be useful if dyspeptic symptoms do not improve with conventional medical therapies.

Ford AC, Marwaha A, Sood R, Moayyedi P. Global prevalence of, and risk factors for, uninvestigated dyspepsia: a meta-analysis. *Gut.* 2015;64(7):1049-1057.

Moayyedi PM, Lacy BE, Andrews CN, Enns RA, Howden CW, Vakil N. ACG and CAG clinical guideline: management of dyspepsia. *Am J Gastroenterol.* 2017;112(7):998-1013.

Talley NJ, Ford AC. Functional dyspepsia. *N Engl J Med.* 2015;373(19):1853-1863.

PEPTIC ULCER DISEASE

 ESSENTIALS OF DIAGNOSIS

▶ PUD refers to both gastric and duodenal ulcers.

▶ The most common etiologies of PUD are *H pylori* and NSAID use.

▶ *H pylori* should be tested for and treated if positive.

▶ PPI therapy should be initiated for treatment of PUD.

▶ General Principles

PUD refers to both gastric ulcers and duodenal ulcers. The most common causes of PUD are *H pylori* and NSAID use, although PUD can be idiopathic as well. In older adults, the use of NSAIDs, aspirin and other antithrombotic agents, and anticoagulants are important risk factors for the development of PUD. The lifetime prevalence of PUD is around 5% in the general population, although the incidence and prevalence are thought to be declining over time, due to the decreasing prevalence of *H pylori* infection, more thoughtful use of NSAIDs, and widespread availability of acid suppression therapy.

▶ Clinical Findings

A. Symptoms & Signs

Patients may present with epigastric pain, in addition to related symptoms of abdominal fullness, bloating, nausea, and vomiting. They may also develop symptoms of GI bleeding, such as hematemesis, coffee-ground emesis, or melena. Chronic ulcers can be asymptomatic. Older patients are frequently asymptomatic or have mild symptoms. Complications of PUD include significant ulceration, hemorrhage, perforation, and even gastric outlet obstruction.

Patients should be asked about history of PUD, risk factors for *H pylori*, and use of aspirin, NSAIDs, and anticoagulation.

B. Diagnostic Evaluation

In patients suspected of having PUD, a complete blood cell count, prothrombin time, blood urea nitrogen, and creatinine should be obtained. Rectal exam should be done to evaluate for signs of active GI bleeding.

There are various modalities to test for *H pylori*. The stool antigen test and urea breath tests are noninvasive tests for active infection, but patients must be off PPI therapy for at least 2 weeks preceding testing. Serologic testing for *H pylori* IgG does not distinguish between active infection and prior infection, as antibodies can persist for several years, but this result is not affected by the use of PPIs.

Finally, upper endoscopy should be performed in older patients suspected of having PUD to identify the lesion, perform gastric biopsies to test for *H pylori*, rule out a malignancy, and perform endoscopic therapy for a bleeding ulcer, if indicated.

▶ Treatment

If a peptic ulcer is diagnosed, PPI therapy should be initiated for at least 8 weeks for mucosal healing. NSAIDs and aspirin should be stopped, if possible. National guidelines recommend that idiopathic PUD (non–*H pylori*, non–NSAID related) should be treated with long-term daily PPI therapy because the likelihood of recurrent ulcer bleeding in these patients is high.

PUD related to *H pylori* should be treated with triple or quadruple therapy to eradicate *H pylori*. There are a multitude of treatment regimens available for *H pylori* eradication, which involves a combination of two to three antibiotics along with a PPI, often taken for 14 days. Table 47–2 describes a few first-line regimens available, although there are many

Table 47–2. First-line therapies for *Helicobacter pylori* infection.

Regimen	Medications	Duration (days)
Clarithromycin triple	PPI (standard or double dose) BID Clarithromycin 500 mg BID Amoxicillin 1 g BID or metronidazole 500 mg TID	14
Bismuth quadruple	PPI (standard dose) BID Bismuth subcitrate 420 mg QID Tetracycline 500 mg QID Metronidazole 250 QID or 500 mg TID to QID	10–14
Levofloxacin triple	PPI (standard dose) BID Levofloxacin 500 mg QD Amoxicillin 1 g BID	10–14

BID, twice a day; PPI, proton pump inhibitor; QD, once a day; QID, four times a day; TID, three times a day.

other possible regimens. Selection of an appropriate treatment regimen depends on local geographic resistance profiles and patient-specific factors, such as prior *H pylori* treatment, antibiotic exposure, and penicillin allergy. It is recommended to test for cure once treatment has been completed, at least 4 weeks after antibiotic therapy, assuming the patient has also been off PPI therapy for 2 weeks preceding testing.

Follow-up upper endoscopy is warranted in patients with gastric ulcers to document mucosal healing after 8 to 12 weeks of PPI therapy and to rule out malignant causes of ulceration. Repeat endoscopy is not indicated for duodenal ulcers because the risk of malignancy is much lower compared with gastric ulcers.

Certain patients may benefit from prophylactic PPI therapy to prevent development of PUD and its complications. This includes patients with prior NSAID-associated ulcers who need to remain on NSAIDs, aspirin, or anticoagulants long term. Prophylactic PPI use is also indicated in patients taking medications that impair the gastric mucosal barrier, such as glucocorticoids.

Crowe SE. Helicobacter pylori infection. *N Engl J Med.* 2019;380 (12):1158-1165.

Laine L, Jensen DM. Management of patients with ulcer bleeding. *Am J Gastroenterol.* 2012;107(3):345-360.

Lanas A, Chan FKL. Peptic ulcer disease. *Lancet.* 2017;390(10094): 613-624.

DIARRHEA

ESSENTIALS OF DIAGNOSIS

▶ Acute diarrhea is defined as symptom duration for ≤4 weeks, whereas chronic diarrhea occurs when persistent for >4 weeks.

▶ Causes of chronic diarrhea are broad and include infectious, inflammatory, malabsorptive, and malignant etiologies.

▶ Evaluation should include infectious stool studies, as well as other targeted stool and blood testing based on patient history. Endoscopy may be considered in the evaluation of chronic diarrhea.

General Considerations

Patients with diarrhea complain of frequent stools (more than three times per day) or change in consistency (loose or liquid stools). It is important to note that many older adults will also use the term diarrhea to describe fecal incontinence or fecal urgency. Diarrheal illness can have significant morbidity in older adults, who may be more affected by shifts in fluid balance and changes in nutritional status compared

to younger patients. In general, acute diarrhea is defined as symptom duration for ≤4 weeks, and chronic diarrhea is when diarrhea is persistent for >4 weeks. It is important to differentiate between acute and chronic diarrhea because the causes, evaluation, and management may vary drastically between the two types.

Clinical Findings

A. Symptoms & Signs

A thorough history and physical exam, including a rectal exam, may provide information on cause and direct further evaluation. Medication history may reveal a causative agent for the diarrhea, and recent antibiotic use or hospitalization should trigger an evaluation for *C difficile*. A history of recent weight loss raises the concern for malignancy, inflammatory bowel disease (IBD), malabsorption, or endocrinopathy. Bloating and gas may indicate small intestinal bacterial overgrowth (SIBO). Fluid status should be assessed in all older patients with diarrhea as they are particularly susceptible to dehydration.

B. Diagnostic Evaluation

For acute diarrhea, infectious stool studies should be obtained to exclude infection. *C difficile* testing should be obtained, particularly if there is a history of recent antibiotic use, although the prevalence is increasing in the community in patients without risk factors. Endoscopy should not be performed in the initial evaluation of acute diarrhea, as symptoms often resolve spontaneously.

The workup for chronic diarrhea can be extensive and should be targeted to the patient's history and exam. In addition to infectious stool studies, it may also include other stool studies such as fecal elastase (to evaluate for pancreatic insufficiency) and fecal calprotectin (as an intestinal inflammatory marker). Serologic testing with tissue transglutaminase IgA antibody should be sent when suspicious for celiac disease. Breath testing may be done for small intestinal bacterial overgrowth, although the sensitivity and specificity of this test are poor.

Endoscopy is appropriate in patients with persistent, chronic diarrhea despite empiric therapy or concerning symptoms such as bloody diarrhea or unintentional weight loss. It is also the next diagnostic step if routine blood and stool testing are inconclusive. Colonoscopy with or without upper endoscopy may be considered. Even if the findings are endoscopically normal, biopsies should be taken as many disorders are evident only by histology, such as microscopic colitis, Celiac disease, or early stages of IBD.

Differential Diagnosis

Most cases of acute diarrhea are related to bacterial or viral infections, but medication effects should also be considered.

Table 47–3. Causes of chronic diarrhea.

Type	Disorders
Secretory	Endocrinopathies Microscopic colitis Medications Bile acid malabsorption Postsurgical (eg, cholecystectomy, gastrectomy, vagotomy)
Osmotic	Carbohydrate malabsorption (eg, lactose, fructose) Osmotic laxatives (ie, magnesium) Sugar substitutes (eg, sorbitol, xylitol)
Inflammatory	IBD Infection Malignancy (eg, colorectal cancer, lymphoma)
Malabsorption	Celiac disease SIBO Pancreatic exocrine insufficiency Postsurgical (eg, gastric bypass, short bowel syndrome)
Functional	IBS

IBD, inflammatory bowel disease; IBS, irritable bowel syndrome; SIBO, small intestinal bacterial overgrowth.

C difficile colitis is an important cause of acute diarrhea in older adults; it is more prevalent in this population due to more frequent hospitalizations, increased antibiotic use, and higher numbers of patients in communal residencies or nursing homes. Diarrhea related to tube feeding is another important cause of both acute and chronic diarrhea in older patients.

There is a broad differential diagnosis for chronic diarrhea, which can be categorized as secretory, osmotic, inflammatory, or malabsorptive in etiology. Malignancy, including both colorectal cancer and small bowel lymphoma, is also an important etiology of chronic diarrhea that should be considered and ruled out (Table 47–3). Secretory diarrhea, related to decreased intestinal fluid absorption, can be caused by various endocrinopathies (hyperthyroidism), microscopic colitis, and medications. Microscopic colitis is characterized by watery diarrhea without overt abnormalities seen on colonoscopy. There are two forms diagnosed by biopsy: lymphocytic colitis and collagenous colitis. Osmotic diarrhea is caused by ingestion of a substance that is poorly absorbed by the gut, such as lactose intolerance. Inflammatory causes of diarrhea include IBD, infection, ischemia, and neoplasia. Diarrhea due to malabsorption can be due to celiac disease, SIBO, and pancreatic insufficiency. Celiac disease is an immune-based reaction to dietary gluten, leading to injury of the small bowel and impaired absorption of nutrients. It is increasingly recognized as a cause of diarrhea and other GI complaints in older adults. SIBO occurs when small bowel transit is slowed or when the normal flora of the colon is altered with antibiotic treatment. The resulting dysbiosis leads to premature fermentation of carbohydrates by bacteria in the small bowel, which produces bloating and gas production. Finally, a functional etiology of diarrhea such as irritable bowel syndrome must also be considered.

▶ Treatment

Treatment of diarrhea is based on the underlying cause and whether or not symptoms are acute or chronic. Because the clinical course is often self-limited in acute diarrhea, expectant management with supportive care is often sufficient in older adults. Routine antibiotics for acute diarrhea are not necessary, although they should be considered if the patient is immunocompromised.

In those with no evidence of acute infection, antidiarrheal medications are generally effective for symptom management. Care must be exercised in older adults with commonly used antimotility agents, such as diphenoxylate-atropine, given the opioid (diphenoxylate) and anticholinergic (atropine) components of this medication. Similarly, tincture of opium is also opioid based and therefore should be used with caution in patients who fail to respond to other treatments.

C difficile is treated with oral vancomycin or fidaxomicin for 10 days as first-line therapy, which is recommended over metronidazole for the initial episode of *C difficile*. Patients who have had multiple recurrences of *C difficile* infection who have failed antibiotic therapy may be considered for fecal microbiota transplantation (FMT). FMT can be administered by colonoscopy or oral capsules, although what is available varies by institution. While there are no age restrictions on FMT, the procedural risks of undergoing a colonoscopy should be taken into consideration in older adults who otherwise meet criteria for FMT.

Budesonide, a locally active and topical corticosteroid with low systemic bioavailability, is the first-line treatment for microscopic colitis. This often requires at least 8 weeks of induction therapy, after which budesonide should be tapered. Recurrence of symptoms can occur after discontinuation of budesonide, and many patients may require maintenance therapy for 6 to 12 months, although effort should be made to avoid prolonged use.

Antibiotics are the primary treatment for SIBO. A variety of antibiotics, taken for a 14-day course, have been shown to be effective, including ciprofloxacin, metronidazole, neomycin, and rifaximin. Rifaximin is well tolerated and preferable as it is not absorbed systemically and has minimal interactions with other medications, but the high cost of this medication often limits its use.

Elimination of gluten is imperative in the treatment of celiac disease. Gluten is found in wheat, barley, and rye. Successful maintenance of a lifelong gluten-free diet requires patient knowledge and motivation, which is best supported with a referral to a dietitian. For most patients with celiac disease, a gluten-free diet will lead to symptom resolution and healing of intestinal injury.

Krajicek EJ, Hansel SL. Small intestinal bacterial overgrowth: a primary care review. *Mayo Clin Proc.* 2016;91(12):1828-1833.

McDonald LC, Gerding DN, Johnson S, et al. Clinical practice guidelines for Clostridium difficile infection in adults and children: 2017 update by the Infectious Diseases Society of America (IDSA) and Society for Healthcare Epidemiology of America (SHEA). *Clin Infect Dis.* 2018;66(7):987-994.

Nguyen GC, Smalley WE, Vege SS, Carrasco-Labra A. American Gastroenterological Association Institute guideline on the medical management of microscopic colitis. *Gastroenterology.* 2016;150(1):242-246.

Rubio-Tapia A, Hill ID, Kelly CP, Calderwood AH, Murray JA. ACG clinical guidelines: diagnosis and management of celiac disease. *Am J Gastroenterol.* 2013;108(5):656-676.

Shen B, Khan K, Ikenberry SO, et al. The role of endoscopy in the management of patients with diarrhea. *Gastrointest Endosc.* 2010;71(6):887-892.

DIVERTICULAR DISEASE

ESSENTIALS OF DIAGNOSIS

▶ Diverticular disease can present as diverticulitis or bleeding.

▶ CT of the abdomen and pelvis is the test of choice to diagnose acute diverticulitis.

▶ Colonoscopy should be performed for diverticular bleeding as a diagnostic and possibly therapeutic test.

▶ Diverticulitis should be treated with supportive care and 7 to 10 days of antibiotics.

▶ General Principles

Colonic diverticulosis is defined by the presence of thin-walled outpouchings of the colonic mucosa and serosa. They are thought to develop from increased colonic luminal pressures, particularly from constipation and straining. Diverticula are most commonly found on the left side of the colon. The prevalence of diverticulosis increases with age, occurring in about 30% of patients ≥50 years old and rising to around 60% in those ≥80 years old.

▶ Clinical Findings

A. Symptoms & Signs

The majority of diverticula are asymptomatic and are often detected incidentally by colonoscopy or imaging.

Symptomatic diverticular disease can present as either inflammation (diverticulitis) or diverticular bleeding.

Diverticulitis presents as acute abdominal pain and can be associated with nausea, vomiting, anorexia, and a change in bowel habits. Fever and leukocytosis are also often present. Patients with acute diverticulitis can also have complicated disease, defined by the presence of abscess, perforation, fistula, or colonic obstruction.

Diverticular bleeding is characterized by the sudden onset of painless hematochezia, sometimes in large volume. History should be obtained regarding prior episodes of lower GI bleeding and NSAID use, which are associated with increased risk of diverticular bleeding.

B. Diagnostic Evaluation

The evaluation for diverticulitis begins with basic laboratory tests to evaluate for leukocytosis, elevated inflammatory markers, and signs of end-organ damage as an indication of disease severity. A CT scan of the abdomen and pelvis is the test of choice to diagnose acute diverticulitis, with high sensitivity and specificity, and also allows for evaluation for complications of diverticular disease, such as abscess or perforation. Colonoscopy should not be performed in the setting of acute diverticulitis due to concern for perforation and other procedural complications in the setting of acute colonic inflammation. A colonoscopy, however, is recommended approximately 6 to 8 weeks after resolution of acute diverticulitis to exclude an underlying colon cancer.

If a patient presents with diverticular hemorrhage that does not cease on its own, colonoscopy should be performed as both a diagnostic and therapeutic procedure. If the bleeding diverticulum is found during colonoscopy, various endoscopic techniques can be applied to help control the bleeding. Colonoscopy also helps exclude other sources of lower GI bleeding, such as arteriovenous malformations (AVMs), ischemic colitis, IBD, and malignancy. If colonoscopy cannot be performed or bleeding continues despite endoscopic therapy, radiographic modalities such as a tagged red blood cell scan, CT angiography, and angiography are alternative ways to identify the source of active bleeding.

▶ Differential Diagnoses

The differential diagnosis for diverticulitis includes IBD, ischemic colitis, appendicitis, and infectious gastroenteritis, all of which can present with the symptoms of acute abdominal pain, fever, and change in bowel habits. Conditions that present with bleeding include AVMs, ischemic colitis, IBD, malignancy, and hemorrhoids.

▶ Treatment

The management of diverticulitis is determined by the patient's clinical status and the presence or absence of complicated disease. For acute, uncomplicated diverticulitis, without signs of systemic toxicity, treatment should generally be initiated in the outpatient setting. Antibiotics that cover gram-negative organisms and anaerobes should be used selectively, depending on the patient's presentation and risk profile, for approximately 7 to 10 days. Patients with complicated diverticulitis should be hospitalized for bowel rest, intravenous fluids, and antibiotic therapy. If abscess is present, drainage should be performed either percutaneously or surgically. Surgical resection for acute diverticulitis should be limited to those with severe, complicated disease, such as those who present with septic shock, diffuse peritonitis, or failure to respond to medical therapy or percutaneous drainage.

Acute diverticular bleeding usually requires inpatient management, particularly in older patients, as resuscitation with intravenous fluids and blood products is often needed for initial stabilization. Colonoscopy should be performed for diverticular bleeding once the patient has been adequately resuscitated. If a source of bleeding is found, it should be treated endoscopically using various modalities such as hemostatic clips, epinephrine injection, or thermal contact coagulation. Around 80% of diverticular bleeding episodes stop spontaneously without treatment.

Prevention of recurrent diverticular disease should be a priority once the acute episode, whether inflammatory or hemorrhagic, has resolved. Unfortunately, preventative medical therapies are limited, but include a high-fiber diet and avoiding NSAID use if bleeding has occurred. A fiber-rich diet is recommended in patients with a history of acute diverticulitis. In addition, studies now show that consumption of nuts and popcorn is not associated with increased risk of diverticulitis, so patients do not need to be routinely advised against eating these items to prevent recurrent diverticular disease. Surgical resection has historically been performed in patients with recurrent episodes of diverticulitis, but antibiotics have been shown to be as effective in those with uncomplicated disease. In addition, surgical resection carries substantial postoperative risks that are increased in older patients. Therefore, elective surgery for recurrent diverticulitis should not be routinely performed in older patients; rather, it should be an individualized decision based on patient-specific factors and preference.

Morris AM, Regenbogen SE, Hardiman KM, Hendren S. Sigmoid diverticulitis: a systematic review. *JAMA*. 2014;311(3): 287-297.

Stollman N, Smalley W, Hirano I. American Gastroenterological Association Institute guideline on management of acute diverticulitis. *Gastroenterology*. 2015;149(7):1944-1949.

Strate LL, Gralnek IM. ACG clinical guideline: management of patients with acute lower gastrointestinal bleeding. *Am J Gastroenterol*. 2016;111(4):459-474.

COLONIC ISCHEMIA

 ESSENTIALS OF DIAGNOSIS

► Colonic ischemia (CI) presents as abdominal pain followed by hematochezia. It occurs in "watershed" areas of the colon located in between two vascular supplies.

► Most cases of CI will improve spontaneously with supportive care.

► A 7-day course of antibiotics should be considered in patients with moderate to severe CI. Patients with severe CI, such as massive bleeding or acute peritonitis, should be evaluated for surgical intervention.

General Principles

CI occurs in the setting of a sudden reduction in mesenteric blood flow, which could be due to hypoperfusion, vasospasm, or vascular occlusion. Therefore, the causes of CI are broad, ranging from thrombotic or embolic disease of the mesenteric vasculature, congestive heart failure, hypotension and shock, vasculitis, medication effect (vasoconstrictive medications, constipation-inducing medications), illicit substance use (cocaine, amphetamines), or aortoiliac surgery (abnormal aortic aneurysm repair). The typical locations for CI occur in "watershed" areas, which are regions of the colon that are located between two vascular supplies, making them susceptible to ischemia. For example, the splenic flexure and rectosigmoid junction are common sites of ischemic insult due to limited collateral blood flow in these areas. The rectum is supplied by both splanchnic and systemic vascular systems and therefore is usually spared from ischemic injury.

Clinical Findings

A. Symptoms & Signs

Patients with acute CI present with crampy abdominal pain, followed by hematochezia or bloody diarrhea. Physical examination often reveals abdominal tenderness of variable severity over the location of the affected portion of bowel. Peritoneal signs suggest transmural infarction and mandate surgical exploration, as these patients have a rare, severe variant of CI known as universal fulminant colitis that can be rapidly progressive.

A targeted history should be performed to evaluate for history of cardiovascular disease, culprit medications, and illicit substances. Common chronic medical conditions in patients with CI include hypertension, diabetes mellitus, coronary artery disease, congestive heart failure, atrial fibrillation, peripheral vascular disease, and renal disease.

B. Diagnostic Evaluation

Initial evaluation of symptoms suspicious of CI should include basic laboratory tests and infectious stool studies. Labs help predict severity of ischemia and should include a complete blood count, comprehensive metabolic panel, and serum lactate. Imaging with CT of the abdomen and pelvis with contrast should also be performed, which assesses the extent and distribution of colon involved. The presence of colonic pneumatosis or portal venous gas on imaging suggests transmural infarction and warrants urgent surgical evaluation.

Colonoscopy with biopsy should be performed if the diagnosis of CI is in question or if there is no clinical improvement with empiric management. Colonoscopy should only be performed in patients without signs of peritonitis, perforation, or irreversible ischemic injury.

▶ Differential Diagnosis

The differential diagnosis for abdominal pain and bloody diarrhea is broad. It includes infectious diarrhea, IBD, and colorectal cancer.

▶ Treatment

Most patients with CI will improve with supportive management, which includes intravenous fluids, bowel rest, and addressing the underlying etiology of disease. The majority of symptoms will resolve spontaneously within 2 to 3 days, although colonic healing can take place over weeks to months depending on the severity of injury. Antibiotics should be considered in patients with moderate to severe disease, as they presumably decrease colonic bacterial translocation, although the data supporting antibiotic therapy are overall limited. Antibiotics should have gram-negative and anaerobic organism coverage to account for gut flora. The optimal duration of antibiotics has not been rigorously studied, but general clinical practice suggests a 7-day course of therapy. Surgical intervention should be considered for patients with severe presentation of CI, such as those with acute peritonitis or peritoneal signs, massive bleeding, portal venous gas, or pneumatosis intestinalis.

Brandt LJ, Feuerstadt P, Longstreth GF, Boley SJ. ACG clinical guideline: epidemiology, risk factors, patterns of presentation, diagnosis, and management of colon ischemia (CI). *Am J Gastroenterol.* 2015;110(1):18-44.

INFLAMMATORY BOWEL DISEASE

ESSENTIALS OF DIAGNOSIS

▶ The prevalence of IBD is rising in older adults and should be considered in the differential for symptoms of abdominal pain and diarrhea.

▶ Colonoscopy should be performed to diagnose disease severity and extent.

▶ There are many treatment options available for IBD, including biologic agents, that are generally deemed safe for use in older adults.

▶ General Principles

Although IBD is generally considered a disease of younger patients, the prevalence of IBD is rising in older adults. Incidence rates for IBD peak in the third and fourth decades of life, although some studies suggest a bimodal distribution with incidence again rising around age 60. In addition, many older IBD patients were initially diagnosed at a younger age but have now transitioned into older age. The management of IBD is rapidly evolving as new biologic agents have become available to successfully treat both Crohn disease (CD) and ulcerative colitis (UC). CD is characterized by transmural inflammation of the GI tract. It can affect the GI tract anywhere from the mouth to the perianal area, often in a patchy distribution. UC is defined by inflammation limited to the mucosal layer of the colon. It involves the rectum and can extend proximally to other parts of the colon in a continuous fashion.

▶ Clinical Findings

A. Symptoms & Signs

Clinical manifestations of both CD and UC include symptoms of abdominal pain, diarrhea with or without blood, fecal urgency, and tenesmus. Systemic symptoms such as weight loss, fever, and fatigue are also common. Patients with CD are more likely than those with UC to develop fistulas, strictures, and perianal disease. There are also extraintestinal manifestations of IBD, such as oral ulcers, arthritis, ocular involvement (uveitis), and dermatologic changes (erythema nodosum, pyoderma gangrenosum). IBD patients have an increased risk of venous thromboembolism due to a hypercoagulable state, especially if their disease is not well controlled.

Several conditions can mimic IBD, such as infectious diarrhea, diverticular disease, and ischemic colitis. Obtaining the correct diagnosis is often delayed in older patients given the high prevalence of these alternative diagnoses in this population. In older patients with UC, the initial presentation tends to be more severe than in younger patients; however, after resolution of this first acute episode, the disease course tends to be less severe overall. Older adults with CD more commonly have colonic disease rather than small bowel or ileocolonic involvement; they are also less likely to have fistulizing or stricturing disease compared to younger patients. Longitudinal, prospective cohort studies suggest that the clinical course of IBD diagnosed at an older age is generally less aggressive than reported in younger patients.

B. Diagnostic Evaluation

Infectious stool studies should be sent to rule out infectious diarrhea in all patients with suspected IBD. Laboratory evaluation should also include a complete blood count, metabolic panel, albumin, and inflammatory markers (erythrocyte sedimentation rate and C-reactive protein). Diagnosis of IBD is determined primarily by endoscopic evaluation. Colonoscopy should be performed to determine the extent and severity of disease, as well as to determine chronicity of inflammation by biopsy. Some endoscopic findings that can be seen in IBD include mucosal erythema, edema, loss of vascularity, friability, erosions, and ulcerations.

▶ Treatment

There are many treatment options for IBD, which now include a vast array of biologic therapies to induce and maintain remission. In general, the approach to choosing a treatment regimen for IBD in older patients should be similar to that in younger patients. Medication options include corticosteroids (to be used temporarily in the setting of an acute flare), 5-aminosalicylates (mesalamine, sulfasalazine), immunomodulators (6-mercaptopurine, azathioprine), and biologic agents (anti–tumor necrosis factor inhibitors, interleukin inhibitors, and integrin receptor antagonists). In general, it is safe to initiate biologic therapy in older adults. If a biologic agent is used, the type depends on a variety of patient-specific factors, including multimorbidity and disease extent and severity. This requires careful shared decision making between the patient and his or her gastroenterologist.

Charpentier C, Salleron S, Savoye G, et al. Natural history of elderly-onset inflammatory bowel disease: a population-based cohort study. *Gut.* 2014;63(3):423-432.

Katz S, Pardi DS. Inflammatory bowel disease of the elderly: frequently asked questions. *Am J Gastroenterol.* 2011;106(11):1889-1897.

Shergill AK, Lightdale JR, Bruining DH, et al. The role of endoscopy in inflammatory bowel disease. *Gastrointest Endosc.* 2015;81(5):1101-1121.e1-13.

Sturm A, Maaser C, Mendall M, et al. European Crohn's and Colitis Organisation topical review on IBD in the elderly. *J Crohns Colitis.* 2017;11(3):263-273.

FECAL INCONTINENCE

ESSENTIALS OF DIAGNOSIS

▶ Fecal incontinence is common in older patients and can greatly impact quality of life.

▶ Impairment in vision, speech, and gait can contribute to fecal incontinence, as well as neurologic and cognitive conditions such as stroke or dementia.

▶ Constipation can paradoxically lead to fecal incontinence.

▶ Treatment of fecal incontinence includes behavioral modifications, addressing underlying diarrhea or constipation, and optimizing physical mobility and strength.

▶ General Principles

Fecal incontinence is the involuntary passage of or inability to control passage of fecal material. Fecal incontinence occurs commonly in older patients, particularly those with chronic illnesses. The prevalence of fecal incontinence increases with age; in community-dwelling adults, the prevalence is approximately 8%, rising to as high as 16% in those over the age of 90. Fecal incontinence is particularly prevalent in nursing home populations; in one survey, approximately 42% of nursing home residents have experienced fecal incontinence. Despite its significant adverse impact on patients, including quality of life, fecal incontinence is often underreported to physicians.

There are many conditions common in older adults that predispose to fecal incontinence. Fecal incontinence is associated with neurologic and cognitive disease, such as stroke, dementia, and diabetes mellitus. Loss of physical mobility can also impact anorectal control. Importantly, fecal incontinence can also be a result of fecal impaction caused paradoxically by constipation.

▶ Clinical Findings

A. Symptoms & Signs

There are different types of fecal incontinence, including urge incontinence, passive incontinence, and fecal seepage. Urge incontinence occurs when patients experience the desire to defecate but are unable to reach the toilet in time. Passive incontinence, on the other hand, occurs when patients experience involuntary loss of stool without awareness of the need to defecate. Fecal seepage involves having a normal bowel movement, but with subsequent leakage of stool afterward into undergarments. Incontinence of semi-formed or liquid stools suggests pelvic floor dysfunction, whereas involuntary loss of solid stool points toward sphincter weakness as the primary mechanism of incontinence.

Careful history should be taken to assess the patient's cognitive status, circumstances of incontinent episodes, multimorbidity, and any disturbances in vision and gait that can impair mobility. Patients may describe diarrhea as their chief complaint, rather than labeling their symptoms as fecal incontinence. Conversely, chronic constipation can also lead to fecal incontinence, either related to overflow incontinence from fecal impaction or constipation-inducing medications. Physical examination with a rectal exam should be performed, which allows for evaluation of anal sphincter tone and distal structural pathology, such as a rectal mass. The absence of anal sphincter tone ("anal wink") may suggest damage to the pudendal nerve (S2–4).

B. Diagnostic Evaluation

After careful history and exam, further formal testing of fecal incontinence may be pursued with imaging, endoscopy, or more dedicated structural and functional testing of the anal sphincter. An abdominal plain film is helpful when fecal impaction is suspected. Endoscopic evaluation with either flexible sigmoidoscopy or colonoscopy should be considered for all patients to evaluate for malignancy or proctitis, either of which can manifest as fecal incontinence. Specialized modalities of testing, such as anorectal manometry, anal ultrasound, and rectal compliance studies, can be performed at the discretion of a gastroenterologist.

▶ Treatment

The treatment of fecal incontinence requires identifying the underlying etiology and other contributing factors. This requires an interprofessional approach that may involve caregivers, physicians, nurses, dietitians, and physical therapists. The primary management of fecal incontinence should include behavioral modification, including bowel habit training, scheduled toileting, and use of a bedside commode if decreased mobility is implicated. Physical activity and exercise are encouraged to maintain patient mobility and function as much as possible. Medications should be used to treat diarrhea (antidiarrheal agents) or constipation depending on the underlying mechanism. Fiber supplements bulk up stools to minimize fecal incontinence, whether driven by diarrhea or constipation. Biofeedback and pelvic floor rehabilitation are also treatment options aimed at retraining the pelvic floor muscles, although these exercises require intact cognition and cooperation.

Ng KS, Sivakumaran Y, Nassar N, Gladman MA. Fecal incontinence: community prevalence and associated factors: a systematic review. *Dis Colon Rectum*. 2015;58(12):1194-1209.

Shah BJ, Chokhavatia S, Rose S. Fecal incontinence in the elderly: FAQ. *Am J Gastroenterol*. 2012;107(11):1635-1646.

Wald A, Bharucha AE, Cosman BC, Whitehead WE. ACG clinical guideline: management of benign anorectal disorders. *Am J Gastroenterol*. 2014;109(8):1141-1157.

COLORECTAL CANCER SCREENING

ESSENTIALS OF DIAGNOSIS

▶ The prevalence of colorectal cancer (CRC) rises with age.

▶ When to stop CRC screening should be an individualized decision and depends on life expectancy, prior endoscopic evaluation, multimorbidity, and overall functional status.

▶ General Principles

CRC disproportionately affects older adults. The incidence of CRC increases with age, nearly doubling between the ages of 40 and 80 years. While it is well established that CRC screening should begin at age 50, there is significant debate as to what age screening should be discontinued. Part of this deliberation relates to the fact that the older adult population is diverse, which is not reflected by chronologic age. Although some older patients are relatively healthy, others of similar age may have significant chronic illnesses that add complexity to the decision on screening. In addition, there are potential risks associated with screening with colonoscopy that should also be taken into consideration, particularly in older adults.

The decision to stop screening is influenced by a variety of patient-specific factors, including life expectancy, polyp profile from prior colonoscopies, and multimorbidity. The benefit of CRC screening is to detect adenomas and malignancy with the goal of extending life expectancy. However, this gain in life years diminishes with age, especially for patients over the age of 80. The risks of CRC screening in older patients, particularly with colonoscopy, include higher complication rates, risk of inadequate bowel preparation, and lower procedural completion rates.

Bowel preparation for colonoscopy itself also carries potential risks and should be tailored to the individual patient. Polyethylene glycol electrolyte lavage solution (PEG) and oral sodium phosphate (OSP) are two common agents available for bowel preparation. PEG is the preferred bowel preparation solution as it has an excellent safety profile in older adults. OSP, on the other hand, is a smaller-volume solution but has been associated with kidney injury and electrolyte disturbances given more rapid fluid shifts. Therefore, small-volume preparations are not recommended in older adults, especially in the presence of renal or cardiac dysfunction.

Current national societal guidelines generally agree that CRC screening should be continued until age 75. From age 76 to 85, the decision to stop screening should be individualized and take into account the patient's overall health status and prior screening history. The US Multi-Society Task Force on Colorectal Cancer (MSTF), which represents the three national GI societies, recommends that patients who are up to date with screening, with negative prior screening tests, may stop screening at age 75 or when life expectancy is <10 years. The MSTF also suggests that patients without prior screening may be considered for initial screening up to age 85.

Ultimately, the decision to stop CRC screening at any age should be individualized and must consider the patient's life expectancy, concurrent chronic illnesses, and potential risks associated with a screening colonoscopy.

Bibbins-Domingo K, Grossman DC, Curry SJ, et al. Screening for colorectal cancer: US Preventive Services Task Force recommendation statement. *JAMA*. 2016;315(23):2564-2575.

Day LW, Velayos F. Colorectal cancer screening and surveillance in the elderly: updates and controversies. *Gut Liver*. 2015;9(2):143-151.

Rex DK, Boland CR, Dominitz JA, et al. Colorectal cancer screening: recommendations for physicians and patients from the U.S. Multi-Society Task Force on Colorectal Cancer. *Am J Gastroenterol*. 2017;112(7):1016-1030.

Travis AC, Pievsky D, Saltzman JR. Endoscopy in the elderly. *Am J Gastroenterol*. 2012;107(10):1495-1501.

CONCLUSION

There is a wide range of GI diseases that affect older adults and significantly impact their quality of life. Management of GI disorders in older adults requires careful consideration of their multimorbidity, life expectancy, and overall goals of care.

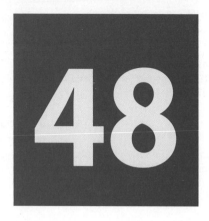

Fluid & Electrolyte Abnormalities

Anna Malkina, MD

Lesca Hadley, MD

ESSENTIALS OF DIAGNOSIS

▶ Hyponatremia is commonly defined as a serum sodium concentration <135 mEq/L (135 mmol/L).

▶ Hypernatremia is commonly defined as a serum sodium >145 mEq/L (145 mmol/L).

▶ Hypokalemia is typically defined as a serum potassium concentration of <3.5 mEq/L.

▶ Hyperkalemia is typically defined as a serum potassium concentration >5.0 mEq/L.

▶ Nocturnal polyuria is present when urine production during 8 hours of sleep is >33% of 24-hour urine production; nighttime urine production rate is >0.9 mL/min *or* 7 PM to 7 AM urine volume is >50% of total 24-hour volume.

General Principles

Fluid and electrolyte abnormalities are common among older adults as a consequence of age-related functional changes in the kidney in addition to multiple comorbidities and polypharmacy. This chapter discusses concepts of sodium disorders, potassium disorders, and nocturnal polyuria as they relate to older adults.

HYPONATREMIA

General Principles

Older adults are more vulnerable to developing sodium disorders as a result of age-related changes in water and sodium metabolism. Older adults may have an impaired ability to excrete water and to dilute urine due to reductions in the number of functioning nephrons and decreased renal blood flow with age, predisposing them to water overload and possible hyponatremia. Geriatric patients also tend to take multiple medications that are associated with sodium disorders, such as diuretics and psychotropic medications (Table 48–1). Reviewing all medications is an integral part of evaluating patients with sodium disorders.

Hyponatremia is commonly defined as a serum sodium concentration <135 mEq/L (135 mmol/L). In the community setting, hyponatremia occurs in 7% to 11% of older patients, and it occurs in up to 50% of older hospitalized patients.

▶ Pathogenesis

A. Hypervolemic Hyponatremia

In older adults with impaired cardiac, renal, or hepatic function, a common etiology of hyponatremia is excessive water retention. This type of hyponatremia is commonly described as dilutional or hypervolemic hyponatremia. These patients typically exhibit edematous states, resulting from conditions such as congestive heart failure, cirrhosis, or nephrotic syndrome. These conditions decrease effective circulating blood volume, leading to increased antidiuretic hormone (ADH) secretion, which results in water retention. Dilutional hyponatremia can also be iatrogenic, as a result of administration of excess hypotonic intravenous (IV) fluids, especially in hospitalized patients.

B. Hypovolemic Hyponatremia

Salt depletion with or without loss of extracellular fluid can cause depletional or hypovolemic hyponatremia. Hypovolemic hyponatremia can be caused by renal losses (eg, diuretic use) or from extrarenal losses, such as vomiting, diarrhea, laxative abuse, ostomies, or the presence of large burns. A particular etiology to consider in geriatric patients is restricted sodium intake, especially in the setting of tube feedings.

Table 48–1. Medications associated with hyponatremia.

Class of Drug	Examples
Antipsychotics	Fluphenazine, thiothixene, phenothiazine, haloperidol
Antidepressants	TCAs, MAOIs, SSRIs (especially fluoxetine)
Anticonvulsants	Carbamazepine
Diuretics	Loop diuretics, thiazides
ACE inhibitors	Lisinopril, enalapril, ramipril
Chemotherapeutic agents	Vincristine, vinblastine, cyclophosphamide, cisplatin, methotrexate

ACE, angiotensin-converting enzyme; MAOI, monoamine oxidase inhibitor; SSRI, selective serotonin reuptake inhibitor; TCA, tricyclic antidepressant.

Data from Liamis G, Milionis H, Elisaf M. A review of drug-induced hyponatremia, *Am J Kidney Dis* 2008 Jul;52(1):144-153.

C. Euvolemic Hyponatremia

The syndrome of inappropriate secretion of ADH (SIADH) is a disorder in which water excretion is partially impaired due to the inability to suppress the secretion of ADH. Patients with SIADH will generally appear euvolemic. Many diseases that are common in older adults are associated with SIADH such as central nervous system disorders and malignancies (Table 48–2). In addition, although rare, older age itself may be a risk factor for SIADH. Medications (Table 48–1) are also an important cause of SIADH. As a result of multi-morbidity, older adults are at higher risk for polypharmacy, typically defined as the use of five or more medications. In

Table 48–2. Diseases associated with syndrome of inappropriate antidiuretic hormone (SIADH).

Central nervous system diseases	Stroke, hemorrhage, vasculitis, tumor, trauma, infection
Malignancies	Small cell carcinoma of the lung (most commonly associated), cancers of the pancreas and bowel, lymphoma
Inflammatory lung diseases	Infection (eg, pneumonia, lung abscesses, tuberculosis), bronchiectasis, atelectasis, acute respiratory failure, positive-pressure ventilation
Endocrine	Hypothyroidism, adrenal insufficiency
Others	Acute psychosis, pain, postoperative state, severe hypokalemia
Idiopathic	Advanced age can be a risk factor for SIADH

Data from Fried LF, Palevsky PM. Hyponatremia and hypernatremia, *Med Clin North Am* 1997 May;81(3):585-609.

older patients, careful medication review is imperative. Other causes of euvolemic hyponatremia include hypothyroidism and adrenal insufficiency. An elevated serum potassium level in conjunction with hyponatremia and hypotension should increase suspicion for adrenal insufficiency. Lastly, it is important to include pseudohyponatremia in the differential, which can occur in the setting of hyperlipidemia or hyperproteinemia.

▶ Clinical Findings

A. Symptoms & Signs

The primary symptoms of sodium disorders (hyper- or hyponatremia) are neurologic. Slow changes in serum sodium concentration (chronic hyponatremia) are more likely to be asymptomatic as the brain has had time to adapt to osmotic changes. Symptoms associated with hyponatremia include anorexia, nausea, vomiting, headache, weakness, loss of coordination, muscle cramps, agitation, tremors, disorientation, psychosis, delirium, seizures, and coma. Patients with chronic hyponatremia are more prone to have marked gait and attention impairments leading to an increased risk of falls.

B. Evaluation of Volume Status

After obtaining the history, the next step in the evaluation of a patient with hyponatremia is to evaluate the volume status. Hypovolemic patients may have dry mucous membranes and tachycardia in addition to relative or true orthostatic hypotension. On the other hand, hypervolemic patients may have increased jugular venous pressures, bibasilar pulmonary rales, ascites, and peripheral edema.

C. Laboratory Findings

Serum osmolality, urine osmolality, and urine sodium should be obtained. Hyponatremia secondary to pseudohyponatremia or hyperglycemia will have a normal serum osmolality, whereas all other etiologies will demonstrate a low serum osmolality. Urine osmolality of >100 mOsm/kg is consistent with an inability to normally excrete water, which is generally caused by SIADH or low effective circulating volume states, such as true hypovolemia, heart failure, and cirrhosis. Urine sodium is useful in differentiating between SIADH and a low effective circulating volume. A urine sodium of <25 mEq/L suggests hypovolemia, and a value of >40 mEq/L suggests SIADH.

▶ Treatment

Treatment methods for hyponatremia are based on the presence of symptoms, the severity of symptoms, and the acuity of the condition. The goal of hyponatremia treatment even in the absence of symptoms is to reduce associated mortality and morbidity (eg, gait disturbances, falls, and cognitive impairment).

A. Acute Hyponatremia

Acute hyponatremia develops in <48 hours, and it is typically found in the hospital setting with frequent lab monitoring. It is associated with neurologic complications due to cerebral edema, and it warrants prompt therapy. If symptomatic, then 3% hypertonic IV saline is administered to rapidly raise serum sodium by 4 to 6 mEq/L from its nadir to alleviate the symptoms over a few hours. If asymptomatic, then causes of underlying hyponatremia are identified and treated, while closely monitoring for an appropriate rise in serum sodium. Hypertonic saline (3%) should be considered to prevent further decline.

B. Chronic Hyponatremia

Chronic hyponatremia develops over >48 hours, or its duration is unknown. Rapid correction can lead to a severe and often irreversible neurologic complication, osmotic demyelination syndrome (ODS), formerly known as central pontine myelinolysis. ODS symptoms (dysarthria, dysphagia, paresis, seizures, encephalopathy, and coma) typically present 2 to 6 days after the rapid elevation of serum sodium. Highest risk factors for ODS are serum sodium concentration ≤105 mEq/L, hypokalemia, alcohol use disorder, malnutrition, and liver disease. If chronic hyponatremia is severe (serum sodium <120 mEq/L), symptomatic, or asymptomatic moderate (serum sodium <130 mEq/L) in a patient with known intracranial pathology, then the treatment of choice is 3% hypertonic saline infusion calculated to raise serum sodium by 4 to 6 mEq/L in the first few hours and maintained for the next 24 hours. Then the rate of correction should not exceed 8 mEq/L per 24-hour period until normalization.

The rate of infusion for each patient based on the desired change in the serum sodium can be calculated using the following formula:

Change in serum sodium (Na) in older men
= (infusate Na – serum Na)/[(0.50 × body weight in kg) + 1]

Change in serum sodium (Na) in older women
= (infusate Na – serum Na)/[(0.45 × body weight in kg) + 1]

These equations have limitations, and thus the actual change in serum sodium may differ. The equations should be used to guide the initial infusion rate, which should then be adjusted by obtaining frequent serum sodium levels to avoid rapid overcorrection.

Treatment of mild hyponatremia (>130 mEq/L) in a patient with intracranial pathology or asymptomatic mild to moderate hyponatremia (120–135 mEq/L) in a patient without intracranial pathology should be aimed at the underlying etiology. For example, patients who are hyponatremic due to

volume depletion secondary to diuretic use should hold their diuretics while receiving volume repletion with fluids such as IV isotonic saline. In contrast, patients with SIADH will not benefit from IV isotonic saline as the infused salt will be excreted in the concentrated urine, resulting in the net retention of water and worsening of their hyponatremia. In these patients, long-term water restriction may be needed. Use of salt tablets or vasopressin receptor antagonists in patients who do not respond to water restriction is also an option.

HYPERNATREMIA

▶ General Principles

Older adults have a decreased ability to concentrate urine and a reduced sensation of thirst, which, if combined with limited access to fluids, may predispose older adults to water depletion and hypernatremia. Hypernatremia is commonly defined as a serum sodium >145 mEq/L (145 mmol/L). Hypernatremia is associated with high mortality. In hospitalized patients aged 65 years and older, the prevalence is approximately 1%, and the mortality rate is seven times that of age-matched hospitalized patients. In a study of patients with hypernatremia in short-term and long-term geriatric care units, the mortality was roughly 40%.

▶ Pathogenesis

Four clinical conditions can lead to hypernatremia in older patients. In many patients, an overlap of these conditions will exist. Hypernatremia usually results from the excessive loss of body water relative to the loss of sodium, and in older patients, hypernatremia is most often associated with inadequate hypotonic fluid (eg, water, juice, tea, coffee, milk) intake. Hypernatremia secondary to excess salt intake is rare.

A. Insufficient Intake

Multiple reasons exist for inadequate fluid intake in the older adult. Many older adults have impaired thirst or hypodipsia. Cognitive impairment and delirium especially in the hospital setting present barriers to adequate hydration. Another common cause of insufficient fluid intake in older adults is impaired mobility or dependence on caregivers for access to water. Older adults with dysphagia may also have inadequate fluid intake.

B. Loss of Water

The loss of water is seen with increased insensible losses (eg, from fever) and in diabetes insipidus (DI). DI is a syndrome characterized by hypotonic polyuria from either inadequate ADH secretion (central DI) or inadequate renal response to ADH (nephrogenic DI). Nephrogenic DI can be induced by medications such as lithium and cisplatin. Patients with DI usually compensate by increasing their fluid intake; thus, when they have adequate access to water, most patients maintain normal sodium concentrations. Hypernatremia develops when they have limited access to water or have an inadequate intake.

C. Water Deficiency in Excess of Salt Deficiency

Water deficiency in excess of a salt deficiency can be caused by gastrointestinal losses, such as vomiting and diarrhea; or renal losses, such as osmotic diuresis secondary to hyperglycemia, solute load with parenteral nutrition, or tube feeding. Diuretics can lead to excess renal loss as well. Skin losses can occur from burns and severe dermatitis.

D. Salt Excess

Salt excess is usually iatrogenic, for example, from the administration of excess saline or sodium bicarbonate.

▶ Clinical Findings

Symptoms of hypernatremia include confusion, restlessness, hyperreflexia, progressive obtundation, coma, and, in severe cases, death.

▶ Treatment

The main goal of treatment is to administer dilute fluids to replace the water deficit and to limit further water loss. The first step is the calculation of the total body water deficit.

Water deficit in older men = body weight in kg
$\times$ 0.50(serum Na – 140)/serum Na

Water deficit in older women = body weight in kg
$\times$ 0.45(serum Na – 140)/serum Na

This estimation formula is based on the assumption of lean body weight. Additionally, it tends to overestimate the water deficit in volume-depleted patients and underestimate it in edematous states. Furthermore, ongoing free water losses (eg, dilute urine, stool, gastric fluid, and sweat) must be replaced. When the collection of urine is feasible, the amount of urinary free water losses could be measured. However, the contribution of other bodily fluid losses may have to rely on estimates due to practical limitations. Therefore, the above calculations provide an initial guide to therapy, which must be reassessed with repeat serum sodium measures.

Acute hypernatremia (onset <48 hours) should be corrected within 24 hours, whereas chronic hypernatremia (onset >48 hours or unknown) should be corrected slowly at a rate of 10 mEq/L per 24 hours. Replacement should be with hypotonic fluids (0.5% normal saline or 5% dextrose water), with oral route preferable to IV if feasible.

Treatment of DI differs in that (in addition to the correction of water deficit, as discussed earlier) efforts must be made to reduce the excessive urinary water loss. In central DI, intranasal or oral desmopressin is used. In nephrogenic DI, treatment includes liberal dietary water intake, dietary sodium restriction, and administration of a thiazide diuretic plus a prostaglandin synthesis inhibitor such as indomethacin or ibuprofen.

POTASSIUM DISORDERS

▶ General Principles

Although less common than disorders of sodium balance, disorders of potassium balance can have serious consequences. Older adults are susceptible to disorders of potassium balance for several reasons, including underlying changes in the structure and function of the kidney that occur with aging, common chronic medical conditions that disrupt potassium homeostasis, and polypharmacy that affects potassium regulation.

HYPOKALEMIA

Hypokalemia is typically defined as a serum potassium concentration of <3.5 mEq/L.

▶ Pathogenesis

Hypokalemia is usually a result of depletion of serum potassium from extrarenal losses, intrarenal losses, or iatrogenic causes. Rarely, hypokalemia can result from an acute shift of potassium from the extracellular compartment into cells.

A. Extrarenal Losses

Extrarenal losses of potassium occur in the GI tract. Chronic diarrhea can cause a loss of serum potassium due to an increase in stool volume. Among older adults, diarrhea is associated with many commonly prescribed medications, including antibiotics, proton pump inhibitors, allopurinol, neuroleptics, serotonin reuptake inhibitors, and angiotensin II receptor blockers. More rarely, diarrhea may occur due to malabsorptive disorders or GI infections. Habitual laxative use can also result in loss of potassium. As many as one-third of older adults suffer from chronic constipation and thus resort to chronic use of laxatives.

Although a rare cause of potassium depletion, decreased nutritional intake of potassium can potentiate the hypokalemia caused by other losses. Older adults may have a limited intake of potassium-rich foods (eg, bananas, potatoes) as a result of impaired access due to financial constraints, institutionalization, poor dentition, or swallowing disorders.

Table 48–3. Intrarenal causes of hypokalemia.

	Mechanism of Action	Etiology in Older Adults
Renal tubular acidosis type I	Distal effects on collecting tubules leading to inappropriate secretion of hydrogen into the urine	Obstructive uropathy from benign prostatic hyperplasia, prostate cancer Autoimmune disease
Renal tubular acidosis type II	Proximal tubules are affected, resulting in failed bicarbonate reabsorption	Malignancies associated with proximal tubular dysfunction (eg, amyloidosis, multiple myeloma) Medications such as carbonic anhydrase inhibitors
Increased mineralocorticoid activity	Increased sodium reabsorption and potassium secretion in collecting tubule of nephron under influence of aldosterone	Aldosterone-producing adrenal adenoma
Postobstructive diuresis	Decreased ability to reabsorb sodium in the distal tubules; inability to concentrate urine; increased tubular transit flow that reduces the time for reabsorption of sodium and water	Hospitalized patients after treatment for obstructive uropathy

Table 48–4. Medications associated with hypokalemia.

Medication Class	Mechanism of Action
Thiazide and loop diuretics	Increased sodium delivery to distal nephron causing increased potassium secretion
Mineralocorticoids and glucocorticoids	Increased potassium secretion via aldosterone effect on collecting tubules
β-Agonists	Translocation of potassium into cells
Xanthines	Translocation of potassium into cells
Insulin	Translocation of potassium into cells

with reversibility within several hours of administration. Selective β_2-sympathomimetic agonists such as pseudoepinephrine and albuterol, xanthines (including theophylline), and insulin can cause transient shifts of potassium into cells (Table 48–4).

Clinical Findings

Although mild hypokalemia is generally asymptomatic, more severe hypokalemia (<3 mEq/L) can result in neuromuscular weakness, including paralysis and respiratory muscle dysfunction, rhabdomyolysis, GI disruption including constipation and ileus, and cardiac dysregulation evidenced by electrocardiogram (ECG) changes (eg, increase in amplitude of U wave, prolongation of QT interval) and cardiac arrhythmias (eg, premature atrial and ventricular beats).

Treatment

Because only a small portion of total-body potassium is present in the extracellular space, estimation of potassium deficiency from serum potassium levels is crude. In chronic hypokalemia, each 1 mEq/L decrease is equivalent to between 150 and 400 mEq/L in total-body potassium deficit. For older adults with decreased muscle mass, the lower estimates are most appropriate.

Treatment of hypokalemia involves the replacement of potassium. However, excessive supplemental administration of potassium can be dangerous due to the high risk of severe hyperkalemia, particularly in hospitalized patients and those with underlying chronic kidney disease. IV potassium is associated with the highest risk of hyperkalemia, as well as pain and phlebitis of peripheral veins, and it should be avoided if possible. Oral potassium supplementation is preferable. Generally, potassium chloride is the preferred choice for potassium repletion because it effectively treats most causes of hypokalemia. Potassium phosphate may be used in situations where phosphate replacement is also required. Potassium bicarbonate may be used in the setting of metabolic acidosis.

B. Intrarenal Losses

Intrarenal losses of potassium occur as a result of conditions that directly affect the kidney. These include renal tubular acidosis (types I and II), hypomagnesemia, malignancies associated with proximal tubular dysfunction (eg, multiple myeloma), medications, increased mineralocorticoid activity, and postobstructive and osmotic diuresis (Table 48–3). Other conditions that may result in intrarenal losses of potassium, although less common in older adults, include diabetic ketoacidosis and ureterosigmoidostomy.

C. Iatrogenic Causes

The most common cause of hypokalemia among older adults is medications. Thiazide and loop diuretics are commonly prescribed to older adults for the management of blood pressure, congestive heart failure, and edema. Medications that cause transcellular shifts in potassium are generally transient

For older patients taking diuretics, instruction in adequate potassium intake is important. Examples of fresh fruits and vegetables with a high potassium content include bananas, oranges, squash, and avocados. Combining a potassium-sparing diuretic (amiloride, triamterene, or spironolactone) with a thiazide or loop diuretic may offset potassium loses from the latter. However, caution must be taken to avoid overcorrection that results in hyperkalemia.

HYPERKALEMIA

Hyperkalemia is typically defined as a serum potassium concentration >5 mEq/L.

▶ Pathogenesis

Hyperkalemia is the result of underlying physiologic and pathophysiologic changes that commonly occur in older adults that predispose to elevated potassium levels. Hyperkalemia is commonly augmented by iatrogenic factors. Age-related changes in the kidney include the development of glomerulosclerosis and arteriosclerosis, which lead to a gradual decline in glomerular filtration rate over time. Although these structural and functional changes do not cause hyperkalemia, they do predispose older adults to experience hyperkalemia if also affected by medical conditions or medications that disrupt potassium balance.

Older adults are more likely to experience pathologic changes to the kidney as a result of common comorbidities such as diabetes, hypertension, and urinary obstruction. These comorbidities can lead to disruptions in renin and aldosterone activity, which impair renal tubular potassium secretion into the urine resulting in increased serum potassium levels. The degree of hyperkalemia can be affected by the intravascular volume status, the amount of dietary potassium intake, medications, and presence of chronic kidney disease.

A. Intravascular Volume Status

Older adults are at risk for decreased intravascular volume for several reasons. First, older adults commonly experience dehydration secondary to hypodipsia. Decreased fluid intake leads to increased sodium and water reabsorption (hypernatremia) and decreased potassium secretion with subsequent hyperkalemia. Older adults are also subject to intravascular volume depletion as a result of total body volume overload states, such as congestive heart failure, cirrhosis, or nephrotic syndrome. Persons with hypoaldosteronism (primary adrenal failure caused by autoimmune disease, hemorrhage, or tumor infiltration), hyporeninemic hypoaldosteronism (commonly caused by diabetes), or tubular unresponsiveness to aldosterone (interstitial renal disease) are most vulnerable to the effects of decreased intravascular volume.

B. Potassium Intake

Increased potassium consumption is also a cause of hyperkalemia, especially in the setting of acute or chronic kidney disease. Hyperkalemia may result from increased dietary potassium or potassium supplements. Older adults have higher rates of potassium supplement use as these are commonly prescribed concurrently with loop or thiazide diuretics to prevent hypokalemia. In addition, older adults may use nonprescription supplements that contain potassium either out of concern for potassium deficiency or inadvertently, not realizing that such supplements contain potassium as one of the ingredients. Similarly, older adults may use salt substitutes in their diets to control hypertension or edema. Many of these salt substitutes use potassium rather than sodium, and they can result in a potentially dangerous potassium load to predisposed individuals.

C. Medication-Induced Hyperkalemia

The primary etiology of hyperkalemia in older adults is medication induced. The incidence of hyperkalemia among patients taking offending medications approaches 10%, with older adults at increased risk. Several commonly prescribed classes of medications can cause hyperkalemia (Table 48–5).

D. Kidney Disease

Hyperkalemia occurs in acute and chronic kidney disease because potassium excretion is proportional to glomerular

Table 48–5. Medications associated with hyperkalemia.

Medication Class	Mechanism of Action
Potassium-sparing diuretics	
Spironolactone	Aldosterone antagonism
Triamterene and amiloride	Block sodium reabsorption in distal nephron causing decrease in urinary potassium excretion
Nonsteroidal anti-inflammatory drugs	Decrease renin and aldosterone
Angiotensin-converting enzyme inhibitors	Decrease aldosterone. Decrease renal blood flow and glomerular filtration rate
β-Blocking agents	Decrease potassium movement into cells. Decrease renin and aldosterone
Heparin	Decreases aldosterone synthesis
Digoxin intoxication	Decreases Na-K-ATPase activity in heart and skeletal muscle leading to increased extracellular potassium
Trimethoprim	Blocks sodium channels in distal nephron leading to decreased urinary potassium excretion

filtration rate (GFR). As GFR declines, the ability of the kidney to effectively excrete potassium also declines. The degree of hyperkalemia is dependent on potassium intake, and it is also affected by compensatory kidney potassium secretion mechanisms as well as losses of potassium in the stool.

Clinical Findings

The clinical consequences of hyperkalemia generally occur at severe elevations of serum potassium (>6.5 mEq/L) in chronic hyperkalemia or a lower level in acute potassium rise. The clinical manifestations involve neuromuscular signs including weakness, ascending paralysis, respiratory failure, and muscle cramping in addition to cardiac abnormalities including chest pain and progressive ECG changes (peaked T waves → flattened P waves → prolonged PR interval → idioventricular rhythm → widened QRS with deep S waves → ventricular fibrillation → cardiac arrest).

Treatment

Diagnosis of hyperkalemia is made by laboratory evaluation. Pseudohyperkalemia may be due to hemolysis due to mechanical trauma of venipuncture, transient movement of potassium from muscle cells with repeated fist clenching during the blood draws from the arm, prolonged specimen storage before processing, or severe thrombocytosis (platelet count >500,000) or leukocytosis (white blood cell count >120,000). Potassium levels should then be repeated with a collection process modification prior to treatment. In cases of true hyperkalemia, an expedited ECG should be obtained to determine if there are any changes related to hyperkalemia. The presence of ECG changes elevates the urgency of treatment.

A. Acute Hyperkalemia

Emergency treatment of severe hyperkalemia with associated ECG changes requires temporizing measures with rapidly acting agents.

1. Calcium infusion—Calcium temporarily antagonizes the cardiac effects of hyperkalemia to prevent cardiac complications while potassium shifting and removal therapies are instituted. The effects of calcium on hyperkalemia are immediate but short lived, lasting only 30 to 60 minutes. Calcium gluconate 1000 mg (10 mL of 10% solution) infused over 3 to 5 minutes may be administered peripherally. Calcium chloride 500 to 100 mg (5–10 mL of 10% solution) infused over 3 to 5 minutes should be delivered via a central or deep vein because it can cause peripheral vein irritation and tissue necrosis in the event of extravasation.

2. Insulin with glucose—Insulin temporarily translocates potassium into cells by enhancing the activity of the Na-K-ATPase pump in skeletal muscle. Glucose should be administered simultaneously with insulin to avoid hypoglycemia, both IV. Several regimens are generally used. Ten units of regular insulin in 10% dextrose solution can be infused over 60 minutes. Alternatively, a bolus of 10 units of regular insulin is given followed by 50 mL of 50% dextrose solution (25 g of glucose). Serum glucose should be monitored closely due to the risks of hypoglycemia.

3. β_2-Adrenergic agonists—β_2-Adrenergic agonists also enhance the activity of the Na-K-ATPase pump in skeletal muscle and activate the Na-K-2Cl cotransporter to translocate potassium into cells. Albuterol can be administered as a nebulized solution (10–20 mg in 4 mL of saline) over 10 minutes with a peak effect at 90 minutes or as an IV infusion (0.5 mg) with a peak effect at 30 minutes.

4. Sodium bicarbonate—Sodium bicarbonate raises the systemic pH, resulting in the release of hydrogen ions with the movement of potassium into cells to maintain electroneutrality. Bicarbonate is used to treat hyperkalemia in the setting of acidosis, and it is not recommended as a single-agent therapy. In the acute setting, one 50-mL ampule of sodium bicarbonate (50 mEq) IV over 5 to 10 minutes can be administered.

B. Potassium Removal

The acute treatment of hyperkalemia described earlier is useful in lowering dangerously high serum potassium levels temporarily, but additional therapy is required to remove potassium. Several modalities exist to remove potassium from the body.

1. Loop or thiazide diuretics—Loop and thiazide diuretics increase potassium loss in the urine. These diuretics are particularly effective for patients with normal to moderately impaired kidney function.

2. Cation exchange resins—Patiromer, zirconium cyclosilicate, and sodium polystyrene sulfonate (SPS) are cation exchange resins that bind potassium in the gut for increased fecal excretion. These can be used to control hyperkalemia in patients with chronic kidney disease who are not yet on dialysis as well as patients with end-stage renal disease on dialysis. However, due to delayed onset of action, these should not be used as the only therapies in life-threatening hyperkalemia. SPS, also known as Kayexalate, can be delivered orally (15–30 g every 4–6 hours) or as a retention enema (50 g in 150 mL of tap water) for severe hyperkalemia. Lower doses can be used for chronic hyperkalemia. Patiromer 8.4 g or zirconium cyclosilicate 10 g can be administered orally daily as needed. The main concern with the use of SPS is the potential for intestinal necrosis. The majority of these complication cases involved oral sorbitol suspension, so it is no longer recommended. Intestinal necrosis is a particular concern for older adults with a postoperative ileus or patients who are receiving opiates, as well as patients with active bowel obstruction or bowel disease (eg, ulcerative colitis,

Clostridium difficile colitis). Therefore, all cation exchange resins should be avoided in these high-risk cases.

3. Dialysis—Dialysis is indicated for the treatment of severe hyperkalemia, hyperkalemia not responding to other measures, or conditions where cellular breakdown can release large amounts of potassium, such as crush injuries or tumor lysis syndrome. Hemodialysis is the preferred modality due to the rapid rate of potassium removal.

NOCTURNAL POLYURIA

▶ General Principles

Nocturnal polyuria is a syndrome in which excessive urine is produced at night. Nocturnal polyuria is highly prevalent in older adults, with estimates suggesting that nearly 90% of adults older than age 80 are affected. Nocturnal polyuria causes disruptions in sleep, which can lead to daytime somnolence, cognitive impairment, and a poor quality of life. Nocturia is also associated with a higher risk of injuries due to falls.

Nocturnal polyuria is considered to be present when one of the following criteria are met: (1) urine production during 8 hours of sleep is >33% of the 24-hour urine production; (2) nighttime urine production rate is >0.9 mL/min; or (3) 7 PM to 7 AM urine volume is >50% of total 24-hour volume.

▶ Pathogenesis

The cause of nocturnal polyuria is usually multifactorial. First, age-related changes in the diurnal pattern of ADH secretion lead to increased urine flow at night, sometimes exceeding that during the day. Structural and functional changes in the urinary tract commonly occur with age, such as decreased functional bladder capacity, bladder outlet obstruction caused by benign prostatic hypertrophy, and detrusor overactivity. These structural and functional changes in the urinary tract can predispose older adults to infections, which can cause nocturnal polyuria. In addition, many medical conditions that affect older adults, such as diabetes mellitus, DI, congestive heart failure, chronic kidney disease, and chronic severe hypokalemia and hypercalcemia, may also cause nocturnal polyuria. Finally, many common medications, such as diuretics, calcium channel blockers, lithium, selective serotonin reuptake inhibitors, caffeine, and alcohol, may also contribute to nocturnal polyuria.

▶ Treatment

A careful history and review of medical conditions and medications are important in identifying the etiology and recommending treatment. If a urinary tract infection is present, then treatment with antibiotics is indicated, and reevaluation is necessary to determine if the nocturnal polyuria has resolved. If no evidence of infection exists, then nonpharmacologic treatments, such as the reduction of fluid intake and avoidance of diuretics and caffeine before bedtime, should be attempted. In patients with edema, the use of compression stockings and elevation of the legs during the day are recommended. In women with urge incontinence, Kegel exercises and scheduled voiding during the day may be helpful. In patients with chronic illnesses contributing to nocturia, managing the underlying disease is the primary treatment.

Several pharmacologic treatments exist for nocturnal polyuria. Diuretics taken 6 to 8 hours prior to bedtime may decrease a patient's overall volume status, thus decreasing nocturnal urine production. If benign prostatic hypertrophy is present, α-blockers and 5α-reductase inhibitors can be used. In women with detrusor overactivity and urge incontinence, medications such as oxybutynin, propantheline, and solifenacin may be useful. However, caution should be exercised when prescribing anticholinergic medications to older adults due to the increased risk of falls and cognitive impairment. Starting with low doses and slowly escalating to the minimal effective dose is recommended. Women with concurrent genitourinary symptoms of menopause may also benefit from topical vaginal estrogen therapy, provided no contraindication exists from estrogen-dependent malignancies. Finally, diagnosis and treatment of sleep disorders (eg, obstructive sleep apnea, restless legs syndrome) may ameliorate nocturia.

Filippatos TD, Makri A, Elisaf MS, Liamis G. Hyponatremia in the elderly: challenges and solutions. *Clin Intervent Aging.* 2017;12:1957-1965.

Liamis G, Milionis H, Elisaf M. A review of drug-induced hyponatremia. *Am J Kidney Dis.* 2008;52(1):144-153.

Passare G, Viitanen M, Törring O, Winblad B, Fastbom J. Sodium and potassium disturbances in the elderly: prevalence and association with drug use. *Clin Drug Investig.* 2004;24(9):535-544.

Pilotto A, Franceschi M, Vitale D, et al. The prevalence of diarrhea and its association with drug use in elderly outpatients: a multicenter study. *Am J Gastroenterol.* 2008;103(11):2816-2823.

Vaughan CP, Bliwise DL. Sleep and nocturia in older adults. *Sleep Med Clin.* 2018;13:107-116.

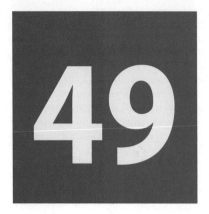

Chronic Kidney Disease

49

C. Barrett Bowling, MD, MSPH

Laura Perry, MD

ESSENTIALS OF DIAGNOSIS

- ▶ Evaluation of chronic kidney disease (CKD) includes a thorough medical history, physical exam, and specific laboratory measures.
- ▶ Symptoms related to CKD may not occur until disease is advanced and include sleep disturbance, decreased attentiveness, nausea, vomiting, weight change, dyspnea, lower extremity edema, fatigue, muscle cramps, peripheral neuropathy, and pruritus.
- ▶ Reduced estimated glomerular filtration rate (eGFR) (<60 mL/min/1.73 m^2) should be interpreted in the context of the medical history and other lab abnormalities (eg, history of diabetic retinopathy, rate of eGFR decline, presence of elevated albumin-to-creatinine ratio) before a diagnosis of CKD is made.

General Principles

CKD is defined as the presence of reduced glomerular filtration rate (GFR) or evidence of kidney damage for at least 3 months. The prevalence of CKD is highest among older adults. The vast majority of older adults with CKD will die without progressing to end-stage renal disease (ESRD); however, even mild to moderate CKD is associated with functional decline, cognitive impairment, frailty, and multimorbidity.

The Kidney Disease: Improving Global Outcomes (KDIGO) Clinical Practice Guidelines were established to direct the evaluation and management of patients with CKD; however, because of the substantial heterogeneity in life expectancy, functional status, and health priorities among older adults with CKD, an individualized, patient-centered approach is appropriate. Among older adults with advanced CKD, a shared decision-making approach should be used to

facilitate decisions about dialysis. Geriatric assessment may be helpful to identify older adults who are vulnerable to functional decline and poor outcomes after initiation of dialysis. Palliative and supportive care should be offered to those who experience a high symptom burden regardless of disease stage and dialysis decision.

Diagnosis and Staging

The KDIGO Clinical Practice Guidelines provide standardized terminology for the evaluation and stratification of CKD. Based on these guidelines, CKD is defined as abnormalities of kidney structure or function for at least 3 months with implications for health. Abnormalities in kidney function include decreased GFR or other markers of kidney damage (albuminuria, urine sediment abnormalities, electrolyte abnormalities due to tubular disorders, and histologic evidence of abnormalities). After diagnosis of CKD is made, the guidelines recommend staging of CKD using the CGA classification, which stands for cause of kidney disease, GFR level, and albuminuria level.

Among older adults, serum creatinine is a poor marker of kidney function. However, because measuring GFR is not clinically feasible, GFR should be determined using estimating equations based on the serum creatinine and other factors affecting creatinine production including age and gender. Although multiple estimating formulas are available, current guidelines recommend the use of the Chronic Kidney Disease Epidemiology Collaboration (CKD-EPI) equation because it has been validated in large populations. Estimation of GFR assumes a stable serum creatinine, and therefore, estimated GFR (eGFR) may not be accurate among patients with acute kidney injury (AKI). Cystatin C has been identified as a biomarker for kidney disease and can be used alone or with serum creatinine to estimate GFR. There is currently no consensus on when to use cystatin C–based GFR equations in place of serum creatinine–based GFR equations.

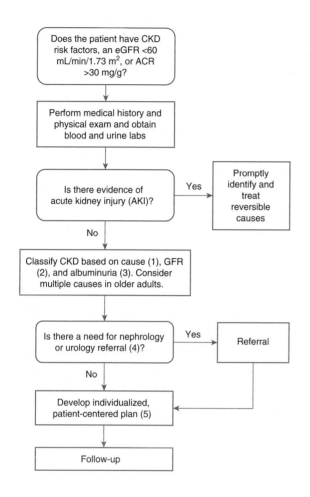

1. Common causes of CKD in older patients
Hypertension, diabetes, renal vascular disease, chronic urinary obstruction, systemic vasculitis, multiple myeloma, or intrinsic kidney disorders such as glomerulonephritis or nephrotic syndrome.

2. GFR categories		3. ACR categories	
	GFR, mL/min/1.73m^2		
G1	>90		ACR, mg/g
G2	60–89		
G3a	45–59	A1	<30
G3b	30–44	A2	30–299
4	15–29	A3	≥300
5	<15		

4. Indications for referral
Nephrology –
- eGFR <30 mL/min/1.73 m^2
- Unexplained, rapid decline in kidney function
- Abnormal urine microscopy – cells, casts, or crystals
- Proteinuria without underlying diabetes
- Possible underlying systemic diseases
Urology –
- Gross hematuria or microscopic hematuria with a negative nephrologic workup or with risk factors for bladder cancer

5. Patient-centered approach
- Informed by patient preferences and health goals
- Emphasizes modifiable outcomes that matter to the patient
- Addresses symptoms, even if not directly related to CKD
- Recognizes heterogeneity in health status, life expectancy, treatment efficacy among older adults with CKD
- Encourages a shared decision-making approach for decisions about dialysis treatment

▲ **Figure 49–1.** Recommendations for evaluation and management of chronic kidney disease (CKD) among older adults. ACR, albumin-to-creatinine ratio; eGFR, estimated glomerular filtration rate; GFR, glomerular filtration rate.

After estimating GFR, categories should be assigned corresponding to prognosis. The eGFR categories range from G1 to G5, with higher levels indicating more severe CKD (Figure 49–1). Additionally, the classification system incorporates the urinary albumin-to-creatinine (ACR) ratio, categorized as A1, A2, and A3 (ACR: normal <30, high 30–300, and very high >300 mg/g), with prognostic implications depending on the level of ACR. The guidelines include a clinical action plan based on the CKD prognosis. Early in the course of kidney disease (eg, G3a, G3b, A2), the focus is on diagnosis of CKD, treatment of comorbid conditions, and slowing CKD progression. As kidney disease progresses (eg, G4, G5, A3), guidelines recommend preparation and initiation of renal replacement therapy.

The prevalence and incidence of CKD increase markedly with age. In a large analysis of data from a US population-based study of >30,000 participants, the prevalence of CKD, defined as an eGFR <60 mL/min/1.73 m^2, was 1%, 10%, 27%, and 51% among those <60, 60 to 69, 70 to 79, and ≥80 years old, respectively. The prevalence of albuminuria, defined as an ACR (ie, A2) ≥30 mg/g, was 7%, 14%, 21%, and 33% among those <60, 60 to 69, 70 to 79, and ≥80 years old, respectively.

Among older adults, CKD is associated with adverse health outcomes, including mortality, cardiovascular disease (CVD), and ESRD. The natural history of CKD has traditionally been described as a progressive, linear decline in kidney function with an expectation that a significant proportion of these patients will develop ESRD and require renal replacement therapy. Accordingly, a priority of CKD management is to identify and treat patients with early-stage CKD to slow disease progression. However, among older adults, trajectories of decline in kidney function are often nonlinear, many have no progression, and >95% of older adults with CKD die without experiencing kidney failure.

Clinical Findings

A. Common Risk Factors

Risk factors for new-onset CKD include older age, obesity, smoking history, diabetes, and hypertension. Other important risk factors include history of CVD, family history of CKD or ESRD, history of urinary tract infection or urinary obstruction, and systemic illnesses that may affect the kidney (eg, systemic lupus erythematosus, multiple myeloma). CKD may also develop as a consequence of AKI.

B. Screening for Chronic Kidney Disease

Because of the age-related decline in kidney function, poor correlation between eGFR and pathologic findings on kidney biopsy, and concerns about the validity of GFR estimating equations in older populations, using eGFR to screen all older adults for CKD is not recommended. For an older patient, reduced eGFR (<60 mL/min/1.73 m^2) should be interpreted in the context of the medical history and other lab abnormalities (eg, history of diabetic retinopathy, rate of eGFR decline, presence of elevated ACR) before a diagnosis of CKD is made.

C. Medical History & Physical Exam

Evaluation of CKD includes a thorough medical history, physical exam, and specific laboratory measures. The goal of this evaluation is to identify the underlying cause or causes, as multifactorial disease is common among older adults. A further goal is to identify CKD-related complications.

The medical history should include information on diabetes, hypertension, CVD, lower urinary tract disease, and an evaluation for symptoms suggestive of vasculitis. Patients should be asked if they have a family history of CKD or ESRD. Typically, symptoms related to CKD do not occur until disease is advanced (eGFR <15 mL/min/1.73 m^2) and include sleep disturbance, decreased attentiveness, nausea, vomiting, weight change, dyspnea, lower extremity edema, fatigue, muscle cramps, peripheral neuropathy, and pruritus. A review of medications should also be performed to assess for medications that may be exacerbating kidney injury, such as nonsteroidal anti-inflammatory drugs (NSAIDs), or medications that may be contraindicated or require dose reductions in CKD, such as hypoglycemic agents, oral and intravenous antimicrobials, antihypertensive agents, and opioids.

Because of the disproportionately higher rates of geriatric syndromes among older adults with CKD, a comprehensive geriatric assessment of functional status, cognition, depression, and impaired mobility should be considered in this population.

The physical exam should include vital signs, orthostatic blood pressure and pulse, evaluation of volume status, and evaluation of lower extremities to evaluate for edema.

D. Lab Evaluation

Diagnostic testing should include urinalysis and random/spot ACR. Twenty-four-hour urine collections for protein and creatinine clearance can be considered but are often difficult to collect, and errors in collection may lead to misleading results, particularly in individuals with urinary incontinence. Blood work includes sodium, potassium, chloride, bicarbonate, blood urea nitrogen, creatinine, glucose, calcium, phosphorus, albumin, total protein, lipid profile, and complete blood count with differential. Additional tests may be indicated if the differential diagnosis includes causes other than diabetes or hypertension.

E. Evaluation for Underlying Causes

Prior to attributing reduced eGFR to CKD, an evaluation for reversible conditions causing AKI should be considered. In addition, a rapid reduction in eGFR in a patient with known CKD should be considered AKI and evaluated promptly (see Figure 49–1).

Hypertension and diabetes are the two most common causes of CKD. However, multiple factors may contribute to the risk for CKD in the older population, including renal vascular disease, chronic urinary obstruction, systemic vasculitis, multiple myeloma, or intrinsic kidney disorders such as glomerulonephritis or nephrotic syndrome. High levels of proteinuria, abnormal urinary sediment with red or white blood cells, or rapidly progressive loss of kidney function should prompt workup for causes other than diabetes or hypertension and referral to a nephrologist.

Complications

CKD-related complications include fluid and electrolyte abnormalities, bone and mineral disease, anemia, and poor nutrition. Many of these complications can be treated by a primary care physician, but as kidney disease progresses and complications become more complex, referral to a nephrologist may be helpful. There are also special considerations for treating CKD-related complications among older adults (Table 49–1). As CKD progresses, the likelihood of developing concomitant CVD also increases, and patients should be evaluated for risk factors such as hyperlipidemia, smoking, and diabetes, and treated accordingly.

Treatment

A. In the Primary Care Setting

Because of the large number of older adults with mild to moderate CKD, care for these patients is often provided by

Table 49–1. Treatment recommendations and special considerations for CKD-related comorbidities and complications in geriatric patients.

	Treatment Recommendations	Special Considerations for Geriatric Patients
Comorbidities		
Hypertension	• Goal ≤130/80 mm Hg • ACEIs or ARBs are first-line treatment in patients with proteinuria with goal urine protein-to-creatinine ratio of <0.2 or ACR <30 mg/g	• Orthostatic hypotension is common • BP should be checked while standing • Evidence for BP goals for older CKD patients is limited to community-dwelling adults and may not be generalizable to those living in nursing homes, frail older adults, those with dementia, or others with limited life expectancy • Older adults underrepresented in clinical trials of ACEIs and ARBs in CKD
Diabetes	• Goal HgbA1c ~7% • Oral hypoglycemic agents and insulin may need to be dose reduced or are contraindicated	• In frail older adults, hypoglycemia may be dangerous (avoid glyburide and use caution with insulin) • Patients with limited life expectancy are unlikely to benefit from tight glucose control • Consider higher HgbA1c target
Cardiovascular disease	• Goal LDL <100 mg/dL • Low-dose aspirin unless contraindicated • Smoking cessation	• No change in goals, but must weigh risk-to-benefit of polypharmacy • Greater risk of GI bleeding, particularly with concomitant anticoagulants or other antiplatelet agents
Complications		
Fluid and electrolyte abnormalities	• Use loop diuretics and dietary restriction to maintain euvolemia and normal electrolyte ranges	• Burden of treatment (ie, worsening urinary incontinence) vs benefit must be considered • Older adult patients often decrease dietary intake; restrictions may not be necessary
Bone and mineral disease	• Check levels of 25-hydroxyvitamin D, calcium, phosphorus, intact PTH, alkaline phosphatase • Maintain 25-hydroxyvitamin D in normal range with repletion • Maintain normal calcium and phosphorus with dietary restriction or phosphate binders • Check labs every 3–12 months depending on stage of CKD	• Burden of frequent serologic assessment, dietary restriction, and polypharmacy should be considered with patient input • Older adults are at risk for concurrent osteoporosis • Bone densitometry may be less accurate in advanced CKD • Bisphosphonates are contraindicated if GFR <30 mL/min/1.73 m²
Anemia	• Check CBC with differential, iron saturation, ferritin, folate, B_{12}, and rule out other causes • Consider ESA in patients with adequate iron stores and symptomatic anemia with Hgb <10 mg/dL • Treatment with ESA to Hgb >12 mg/dL associated with risk of stroke and cardiovascular mortality	• Anemia in older adults is often multifactorial • ESA use requires self-injections and frequent lab draws and clinic visits • Burden of treatment must be weighed against benefits
Nutrition	• Dietary sodium <2000 mg/day • Limit dietary potassium and phosphorus if serum levels elevated • Consider daily protein restriction in advanced CKD: 0.8–1.0 g/kg body weight	• Older adults often decrease oral intake • Encourage adequate nutrition • Evaluate dentition when making nutrition recommendations • Hypoalbuminemia is associated with increased risk of death in patients initiating dialysis

ACEIs, Angiotensin-converting enzyme inhibitors; ACR, albumin-to-creatinine ratio; ARBs, angiotensin receptor blockers; BP, blood pressure; CBC, complete blood count; CKD, chronic kidney disease; ESA, erythrocyte-stimulating agents; GFR, glomerular filtration rate; GI, gastrointestinal; Hgb, hemoglobin; HgbA1c, glycosylated hemoglobin; LDL, low-density lipoprotein; PTH, parathyroid hormone.

the primary care physician. Routine treatment of CKD in the primary care setting includes monitoring of kidney function, managing CKD-related complications, treating CVD risk factors, preventing additional kidney injury, and promoting general health.

Medical optimization of hypertension and diabetes may improve kidney function and prevent progression of kidney disease (see Table 49–1). Preferred medications for blood pressure control in patients with CKD include diuretics, angiotensin-converting enzyme inhibitors (ACEIs) or angiotensin receptor blockers (ARBs), and β-blockers. Achieving blood pressure and hemoglobin A1c goals often require multiple medications, and the benefits of aggressive medical treatments to reach recommended targets should be considered in the context of the patient's health goals and balanced against the risks of treatment, particularly in frail older patients.

Proteinuria is an independent risk factor for progression of kidney disease as well as for mortality. ACEIs or ARBs are recommended as first-line treatment for proteinuria. However, older adults are underrepresented in the clinical trials used to develop CKD guidelines and evidence on the benefits of ACEIs and ARBs in this population is limited. Furthermore, many older adults with reduced eGFR do not have proteinuria, and the effectiveness of angiotensin blockade in these patients is limited. Finally, older adults are at risk for adverse drug events; therefore, after initiation or dose increase of an ACEI or ARB, the serum creatinine and potassium should be measured.

In addition to treatment of high blood pressure and hyperglycemia, optimization of other risk factors to prevent CKD progression include smoking cessation and avoidance of nephrotoxins and additional kidney injury. However, there is limited evidence of the effectiveness of these interventions specifically among older adults with CKD.

B. Patient-Centered Approach

There are several unique challenges to caring for older adults with CKD for which an individualized, patient-centered approach to CKD management is appropriate. The majority of older patients with CKD have additional unrelated chronic conditions, many of which have opposing or unrelated treatment goals (ie, CKD-discordant conditions). The presence of discordant conditions is associated with higher health care utilization. Patients report that having CKD-discordant conditions results in conflicting treatment plans from different providers. Recognizing CKD-discordant conditions and reconciling conflicting treatment advice may be one way to provide individualized care to these patients (see Figure 49–1).

Another challenge to CKD management is the high prevalence of geriatric conditions in this population. The risk for cognitive impairment, falls, mobility limitations, and polypharmacy is higher at lower levels of kidney function.

However, routine care for CKD does not include assessment for these conditions. Brief geriatric assessment has been shown to be feasible and may be helpful for developing appropriate care plans based on cognitive or physical limitations.

C. Referral

The KDIGO guidelines recommend referral of patients with stage 4 CKD (eGFR <30 mL/min/1.73 m^2) to a nephrologist for co-management (see Figure 49–1). Indications for earlier nephrology referral include an unexplained, rapid decline in kidney function, the presence of active urinary sediment, proteinuria without underlying diabetes, or possible underlying systemic diseases such as multiple myeloma, hepatitis, or HIV. Additionally, patients with significant metabolic derangements may benefit from earlier evaluation and management by a nephrologist. Patients with gross hematuria or microscopic hematuria with a negative nephrologic workup or with risk factors for bladder cancer should be considered for urologic referral.

D. Dialysis

Older adults represent the fastest growing group with ESRD. Decisions about whether or not to start dialysis can be challenging. While it is ideal to make decisions about dialysis initiation well in advance of a patient's reaching ESRD, because of the difficulty in predicting CKD progression and the competing risk for death, this is often not possible. Qualitative research in this area suggests that uncertainty about the expected course of CKD appears to be an important concern among both patients and nephrologists. Because of this uncertainty, nephrologists have also reported avoiding discussions with patients about the future and prognosis.

Overall, progression to ESRD carries a poor prognosis. The benefits of dialysis in geriatric patients are less well studied and highly variable, depending on the patient's baseline functional status and other medical conditions. Among patients 80 to 84 years old who initiate dialysis, the average life expectancy is 16 months; however, survival ranges from as short as 5 months to as long as 36 months (interquartile range). Older adults starting dialysis are at increased risk for persistent functional decline and increased hospitalizations and are more likely to die in the hospital than at home. In one study of patients ≥80 years of age, within 6 months of initiating dialysis, >30% had a decline in functional ability and required increased caregiver support or nursing home care. Often dialysis is initiated during a hospitalization, and patients may require postacute care in a skilled nursing facility. Studies have shown that up to a third of these patients may transition to needing long-term care in a nursing home and the majority never return to predialysis function. Factors associated with death within 1 year of initiating dialysis in octogenarian patients were poor nutritional status, late referral to a nephrologist, and functional dependence. Factors associated with loss of independence include cognitive impairment, low mobility, history of falls, depression, symptoms of exhaustion, and polypharmacy.

A shared decision-making approach should be used that includes the patient, their family and caregivers, and the nephrologist and primary care physician. It may be helpful to elicit the patient's and family's values, preferences, and health goals and then use these to guide decision making. Discussions of dialysis should include consideration of peritoneal dialysis and home hemodialysis, which may be preferable in functionally impaired or frail patients. However, these modalities may require higher levels of caregiver support. Because of the likelihood of functional decline after dialysis initiation, geriatric assessment before initiation of dialysis that includes measures such as gait speed, functional assessment for basic and instrumental activities of daily living, and cognitive testing may be helpful to identify those at highest risk for poor outcomes. Clinicians may also use prognostic calculators (see www.eprognosis.org) to inform these discussions. Patients for whom a poor outcome is likely can be offered a time-limited trial of dialysis, with a prespecified time to revisit the decision and determine whether to continue or terminate dialysis. Advance care planning, including end-of-life care planning, should be discussed as part of the conversation regardless of what decision is made regarding renal replacement therapy.

E. Withdrawal of Dialysis

Particularly for older adults with multimorbidity and geriatric syndromes, any early benefit of dialysis may quickly become a burden to the patient and family or may fail to improve symptoms that were attributed to ESRD, such as cognitive deficits. Withdrawal of dialysis is best done with the support of hospice or palliative care teams, as patients are likely to live for several days after stopping dialysis and have high symptom burden.

F. Kidney Transplant

Transplant is the best option for long-term renal replacement therapy. Advanced age alone should not be a contraindication to consideration for transplantation; several studies have demonstrated comparable outcomes among younger and older transplant patients. However, potential candidates must be selected carefully because of the competing risk of death and high complexity of posttransplant care. Predictive models may help determine which older patients may be appropriate for consideration.

G. Palliative & Supportive Care

Regardless of whether patients decide to pursue or forgo dialysis, patients with advanced CKD experience a high symptom burden, and palliative and supportive care that addresses physical, emotional, and social suffering should be considered. For patients not on dialysis, fluid overload can be managed with diuretics if the patient still produces urine. Uremia commonly manifests as nausea and can be managed with antiemetics. Hyperkalemia can be managed to some extent with diuretics. Potassium-excreting agents such as Kayexalate (sodium polystyrene sulfonate) may be used with caution, as these carry a risk of bowel necrosis that may increase with age. The improvement of metabolic parameters achieved with these therapies must be balanced with the burden of treatment (eg, urinary incontinence, diarrhea). Patients with ESRD often report symptom burdens and reductions in quality of life similar to patients with terminal malignancy. Pain is a common symptom and should be treated aggressively; however, caution is needed when using renally cleared opioids such as morphine. Patients nearing the end of life may benefit from hospice or palliative care referral.

Bowling CB, O'Hare AM. Managing older adults with CKD: individualized versus disease-based approaches. *Am J Kidney Dis.* 2012;59(2):293-302.

Bowling CB, Plantinga L, Phillips LS, et al. Association of multimorbidity with mortality and healthcare utilization in chronic kidney disease. *J Am Geriatr Soc.* 2017;65(4):704-711.

Bowling CB, Vandenberg A, Phillips L, McClellan W, Johnson II TM, Echt KV. Older patients' perspectives on managing complexity in CKD self-management. *Clin J Am Soc Nephrol.* 2017;12(4):635-643.

Coresh J, Selvin E, Stevens LA, et al. Prevalence of chronic kidney disease in the United States. *JAMA.* 2007;298(17):2038-2047.

Galla JH. Clinical practice guideline on shared decision-making in the appropriate initiation of and withdrawal from dialysis. The Renal Physicians Association and the American Society of Nephrology. *J Am Soc Nephrol.* 2000;11(7):1340-1342.

Hall RK, Haines C, Gorbatkin SM, et al. Incorporating geriatric assessment into a nephrology clinic: preliminary data from two models of care. *J Am Geriatr Soc.* 2016;64(10):2154-2158.

KDIGO CKD Work Group. KDIGO 2012 clinical practice guidelines for the evaluation and management of chronic kidney disease. *Kidney Int Suppl.* 2013;3(1):1-150.

O'Hare AM, Choi AI, Berenthal D, et al. Age affects outcomes in chronic kidney disease. *J Am Soc Nephrol.* 2007;18(10):2758-2765.

50

Thyroid, Parathyroid, & Adrenal Gland Disorders

Steven R. Gambert, MD

Ravi Kant, MD

Myron Miller, MD

▼ DISEASES OF THE THYROID GLAND

SUBCLINICAL HYPOTHYROIDISM

▶ General Principles

Subclinical hypothyroidism, defined as serum thyroid-stimulating hormone (TSH) level above the upper limit of normal with normal concentrations of free thyroxine (T_4), affects a relatively large number of older persons. It is most common in older women, affecting 15% to 20% of women over the age of 75 years, most of whom will demonstrate elevated serum levels of antithyroid antibodies. Older women with serum TSH >6 mU/L and the presence of antimicrosomal and antithyroid peroxidase antibodies will progress to overt clinical hypothyroidism at a rate of 5% to 7% per year. Conversely, older women with a modest increase in serum TSH who are antithyroid antibody negative may undergo spontaneous reversion to a euthyroid state. Several studies have observed beneficial effects of T_4 therapy on measures of cardiovascular function and general well-being in patients with subclinical hypothyroidism. However, there remain questions as to the benefits of T_4 treatment in patients with minimal clinical symptoms.

▶ Clinical Findings

Older patients with subclinical hypothyroidism may present with few or no complaints. Studies have demonstrated reduced cognitive function, increased intestinal transit time, increased intraocular pressure, higher low-density lipoprotein cholesterol levels, an increased risk for coronary artery and peripheral vascular atherosclerosis, decreased systolic and left ventricular diastolic contractility, and increased risk of congestive heart failure. Subclinical hypothyroidism has been associated with an increased risk of ischemic heart disease, cardiovascular mortality, and all-cause mortality. Older women with atherosclerosis, and an even higher percentage of those with a history of myocardial infarction, have a higher incidence of subclinical hypothyroidism.

Some older patients with severe illness may have transient elevation of serum TSH along with decrease in T_4 and T_3 due to lowered serum thyroid-binding proteins. Among the illnesses is traumatic brain injury. These findings have been termed *sick euthyroid syndrome* and can be confused with subclinical hypothyroidism, but the changes in thyroid function tests will usually normalize over several weeks as the patients recover from their underlying illness.

▶ Treatment

Treatment with L-thyroxine compared with placebo results in an overall improvement in general well-being, memory, psychomotor speed, and serum lipid levels. Many studies have documented that L-thyroxine treatment will improve systolic and diastolic ventricular function, left ventricular ejection fraction, and endothelial function while decreasing systolic vascular resistance. L-Thyroxine treatment of subclinical hypothyroidism has recently been shown to be effective in reducing ischemic heart disease events in persons aged 40 to 70 years but not in those over the age of 70 years. Other studies have also shown little benefit of treatment in older persons on cardiovascular events and mortality.

Although some physicians advocate thyroid replacement therapy for all persons with subclinical hypothyroidism, current guidelines recommend that treatment is best reserved for individuals with TSH levels >10 mU/L or for those with serum TSH levels between 5 and 10 mU/L with coexisting high levels of antimicrosomal and antithyroid peroxidase antibodies. If treatment is not initiated, careful follow-up is essential because 5% to 7% of these individuals will progress to develop overt hypothyroidism each year. The goal of treatment, when initiated, is to normalize serum TSH values as long as the dose of thyroid hormone that is required produces no adverse clinical effects. Most experts recommend targeting a normal TSH range in older patients, although it should be noted that serum TSH concentrations increase with age. One study examining individuals with "extreme longevity" noted serum TSH to be significantly higher in centenarians, with 7.5 mU/L considered to be the true upper limit of normal for those aged 80 years and older.

Atzmon G, Barzilai N, Hollowell JG, Surks MI, Gabriely I. Extreme longevity is associated with increased serum thyrotropin. *J Clin Endocrinol Metab.* 2009;94(4):1251-1254.

Biondi B, Cooper DS. The clinical significance of subclinical thyroid dysfunction. *Endocr Rev.* 2008;29:76-131.

Bremner A, Feddema P, Leedman PJ, et al. Age-related changes in thyroid function: a longitudinal study of a community-based cohort. *J Clin Endocrinol Metab.* 2012;97(5):1554-1562.

Canaris GJ, Manowitz NR, Mayor G, Ridgway EC. The Colorado thyroid disease prevalence study. *Arch Intern Med.* 2000;160(4):526-534.

Garber JR, Cobin RH, Gharib H, et al. American Association of Clinical Endocrinologists and American Thyroid Association Task Force on Hypothyroidism in Adults. Clinical practice guidelines for hypothyroidism in adults. *Thyroid.* 2012;22:988-1028.

Ravzi S, Weaver JU, Butler TJ, et al. Levothyroxine treatment of subclinical hypothyroidism, fatal and nonfatal cardiovascular events, and mortality. *Arch Intern Med.* 2012;172:811-817.

Rodondi N, den Elzen WPJ, Bauer DC, et al. Subclinical hypothyroidism and the risk of coronary heart disease and mortality. *JAMA.* 2010;304:1365-1374.

Somwaru LL, Rariy CM, Arnold AM, Cappola A. The natural history of subclinical hypothyroidism in the elderly: the cardiovascular health study. *J Clin Endocrinol Metab.* 2012;97:1962-1969.

Stott DJ, Rodondi PM, Kearney I, et al. Thyroid hormone therapy for older adults with subclinical hypothyroidism. *N Engl J Med.* 2017;376:2534-2544.

SUBCLINICAL HYPERTHYROIDISM

General Principles

Subclinical hyperthyroidism is defined as a serum TSH value below the lower limit of normal with a normal level of circulating thyroid hormones. Epidemiologic data suggest that this condition affects 1% to 4% of persons older than age 60 years and appears to be more common in women than in men. Over time, some persons with subclinical hyperthyroidism will undergo spontaneous reversion to normal thyroid function. However, approximately 30% will have persistent abnormal thyroid function tests and a small number will progress to overt hyperthyroidism. Underlying causes include mild Graves disease, functioning thyroid nodules, and overreplacement with L-thyroxine in patients with hypothyroidism. Since the thyroid hormone half-life increases with advancing age, elderly persons with hypothyroidism who had been on a stable dose of thyroid hormone replacement for a long period of time may be at risk for now developing subclinical hyperthyroidism.

Clinical Findings

Persons with subclinical hyperthyroidism may have no overt clinical symptoms. However, a number of cardiovascular alterations have been identified. These include increased heart rate, increased prevalence of atrial premature contractions, shorter isovolumetric contraction time, shorter pre-ejection period, impaired left ventricular diastolic filling, increased left ventricular mass index, and reduced peak oxygen uptake. These changes can lead to reduced exercise performance. The incidence of peripheral vascular disease is also increased. Several large studies have shown an increased risk for onset of atrial fibrillation. Assessment of thyroid function in older patients with new-onset atrial fibrillation has revealed approximately 4% with values characteristic of subclinical hyperthyroidism. Persons with subclinical hyperthyroidism are at increased risk for development of congestive heart failure. Subclinical hyperthyroidism is associated with increased risk of both cardiovascular mortality and all-cause mortality. In addition to cardiovascular adverse effects, subclinical hyperthyroidism has been associated with accelerated bone loss, leading to increased risk for developing or worsening of osteopenia and osteoporosis.

Treatment

Treatment should be initiated if there are clearly associated symptoms, such as a worsening of cardiovascular function, development of cardiac arrhythmias, excessive muscle wasting, or significant osteopenia or osteoporosis. Individuals receiving excessive thyroid hormone replacement therapy that suppresses TSH should have their dose of thyroid hormone reduced. For persons who are asymptomatic, treatment decisions are more complex since the clinical course is highly variable and difficult to predict. A consensus panel of endocrinologists has recommended treatment for all persons aged >65 years who have a TSH of <0.1 mU/L. However, 47% to 61% of patients will have normal serum TSH levels on retesting within 1 year without any intervention, whereas 1.5% to 13% will progress to develop overt hyperthyroidism. A reasonable approach for asymptomatic persons is to follow them at 6- to 12-month intervals clinically and with serum TSH, free T_4, and free triiodothyronine (T_3). If symptoms develop or there is progression to overt hyperthyroidism, then therapy can be initiated, preferably with iodine-131 (^{131}I) thyroid ablation. For patients with significant osteopenia or osteoporosis, treatment may improve bone mineral density.

Collet T-H, Gussekloo J, Bauer DC, et al. Subclinical hyperthyroidism and the risk of coronary heart disease and mortality. *Arch Intern Med.* 2012;172:799-809.

Cooper DS. Approach to the patient with subclinical hyperthyroidism. *J Clin Endocrinol Metab.* 2007;92:3-9.

Nanchen D, Gussekloo J, Westendorp RG, et al. PROSPER Group. Subclinical thyroid dysfunction and the risk of heart failure in older persons at high cardiovascular risk. *J Clin Endocrinol Metab.* 2012;97(3):852-861.

Parle JV, Maisonneuve P, Sheppard MC, Boyle P, Franklyn JA. Prediction of all-cause and cardiovascular mortality in elderly people from one low serum thyrotropin result: a 10-year cohort study. *Lancet.* 2001;358(9285):861-865.

Ross DS, Burch HB, Cooper DS, et al. 2016 American Thyroid Association guidelines for diagnosis and management of hyperthyroidism and other causes of thyrotoxicosis. *Thyroid.* 2016;10:1343-1421.

Sawin CT, Geller A, Wolf PA, et al. Low serum thyrotropin concentrations as a risk factor for atrial fibrillation in older persons. *N Engl J Med.* 1994;331(19):1249-1252.

Seimer C, Olesen JB, Hansen ML, et al. Subclinical and overt thyroid dysfunction and risk of all-cause mortality and cardiovascular events: a large population study. *J Clin Endocrinol Metab.* 2014;99:2372-2382.

HYPOTHYROIDISM

General Principles

Hypothyroidism is a common disease of older adults, especially of older women, with a reported prevalence of 15% to 20% in women over the age of 75 years and 4% to 7% of older men. Consequently, the American Thyroid Association recommends screening for hypothyroidism in persons older than 65 years. Hypothyroidism in older adults most commonly results from an autoimmune thyroiditis with increased serum levels of antithyroid peroxidase and antimicrosomal antibodies. Prior radioiodine treatment of hyperthyroidism and subtotal thyroidectomy are also potential causes. The risk of hypothyroidism is >50% after the first year of radioiodine treatment, with an additional annual incidence of 2% to 4% each year thereafter. Hypothyroidism may also be the natural end point to previous Graves disease. Medications may also lead to hypothyroidism, particularly in persons with autoimmune thyroiditis. The most common medications associated with hypothyroidism include iodine-containing radiographic contrast agents, lithium, amiodarone, and iodine-containing cough medicines. Hypothyroidism may also be secondary to either pituitary or hypothalamic abnormality in production or release of TSH.

Clinical Findings

Many of the presenting complaints are confused with other age-prevalent disorders. This problem is further compounded by the often-insidious onset of illness. Fatigue and weakness are common. Whereas younger patients commonly present with weight gain, cold intolerance, paresthesia, and muscle cramps, older patients may not, or they may have these or other classic symptoms such as constipation in the absence of a thyroid disorder. Many persons who are later discovered to be hypothyroid are unable to identify exactly when the symptoms actually began. Neurologic findings may include cognitive impairment, ataxia, and carpal tunnel syndrome, and a delay in the relaxation of deep tendon reflexes, which may not be easily apparent in a person of advancing age. Hypercholesterolemia may be more common in both circumstances as well. For these reasons, the examining physician should maintain a high index of suspicion of hypothyroidism when evaluating any older person, especially women and those with a personal or family history of some form of thyroid disease.

A major impact of hypothyroidism is on cardiovascular function with associated symptoms of easy fatigue and dyspnea on exertion. Functionally, there is a decrease in heart rate and reduction in myocardial contractility and ejection fraction. Systemic vascular resistance is increased and can lead to diastolic hypertension and increased risk for adverse cardiovascular events. There is an increased risk for congestive heart failure, atrial fibrillation, ischemic heart disease, myocardial infarction, and mortality. The electrocardiogram often shows bradycardia, prolonged QT interval, low-amplitude QRS complex, and flattening or inversion of T waves. Peripheral vascular disease is also increased in patients with hypothyroidism. Primary hypothyroidism is associated with an elevated serum TSH concentration. Changes in protein binding may reduce the level of total T_4; T_3 may be reduced in persons with significant medical illness or malnutrition. Even measures of free T_4 may be misleading; T_4 may be suppressed in individuals with T_3 toxicosis. For these reasons, an increase in serum TSH remains the best way to detect primary failure of the thyroid gland regardless of age. During the recovery phase after an acute nonthyroidal illness, however, an elevation of serum TSH level may not represent true clinical hypothyroidism; in this case, the serum TSH returns to the range of normal within 4 to 6 weeks. Although uncommon in older adults, hypothyroidism can be secondary to pituitary or hypothalamic failure, with low serum TSH and T_4 levels. TSH >10 mU/L, female sex, and positive antithyroid antibodies are associated with an increased risk of progression from subclinical hypothyroidism to overt hypothyroidism. In patients with TSH <10 mU/L, testing for antithyroid antibodies can be helpful and favors the treatment with L-thyroxine. TSH screening is indicated in older patients with cognitive problems, goiter or history of thyroid abnormality, hypercholesterolemia, or family history of thyroid illness.

Differential Diagnosis

Many of the presenting signs and symptoms of hypothyroidism in persons of any age resemble findings common to many other age-prevalent disorders, notably congestive heart failure and unexplained ascites resulting from cardiac or hepatic abnormalities. A thick tongue may result from primary amyloidosis. Anemia may result from vitamin B_{12}, folate, or iron deficiency or volume expansion. Depression may be present, and other alterations in cognition may be caused by medication toxicity or dementia.

Treatment

L-Thyroxine is the preferred medication to treat hypothyroidism and results in improvement of clinical symptoms, cardiovascular function, and lipid profile. In general, consistent use of one of the brand name preparations is suggested to minimize variability that may occur with generic preparations. It is also easier for the older person to identify medication with a consistent color and shape. Older patients generally require a smaller amount of L-thyroxine to normalize their thyroid status. Because of the age-related increase in T_4 half-life, approximately 9 days in persons aged 80 years or older, it will take longer to reach a steady state. A longer time between dose increases is necessary to reduce unwanted side effects.

The commonly used adage of "start low and go slow" should be followed when starting any older patient on thyroid hormone replacement therapy. Because many older patients with hypothyroidism may have underlying cardiovascular disease, therapy should start with 25 µg/day, with gradually increasing increments of 25 µg every 4 to 6 weeks. The final dose required is the amount of L-thyroxine that reduces the serum TSH into the range of normal and does not have associated side effects. Individuals with significant cardiac disease may require dose changes as low as 12.5 µg and should even be started at that dose. Achievement of a euthyroid state may exacerbate cardiac symptoms in some patients with significant coronary artery disease. In this circumstance, the use of a β-adrenergic blocking agent may allow a clinically euthyroid state to be reached without induction of symptoms of myocardial ischemia. Monitoring of TSH is necessary to avoid inducing iatrogenic subclinical hyperthyroidism from excessive doses of replacement thyroid hormone.

Prognosis

With effective treatment, return to a normal state of health is expected. Complete response to thyroid treatment, however, may take months, and patients will require replacement therapy with thyroid hormone and periodic monitoring with thyroid function tests for life.

Calsolaro V, Niccolai F, Pasqualetti G, et al. Hypothyroidism in the elderly: who should be treated and how. *J Endocr Soc.* 2019;3:146-158.

Cappola AR, Ladenson PW. Hypothyroidism and atherosclerosis. *J Clin Endocrinol Metab.* 2003;88:2438-2444.

Jonklaas J, Bianco AC, Bauer AJ, et al. Guidelines for the treatment of hypothyroidism. *Thyroid.* 2014;24:1670-1751.

Journy NMY, Bernier M-O, Doody MM, et al. Hyperthyroidism, hypothyroidism, and cause-specific mortality in a large cohort of women. *Thyroid.* 2017;27:1000-1010.

Thvilum M, Brandt F, Brix TH, Hegedus L. A review of the evidence for and against increased mortality in hypothyroidism. *Nat Rev Endocrinol.* 2012;8:417-424.

MYXEDEMA COMA

General Principles

Myxedema coma is a serious life-threatening consequence of untreated or inadequately treated hypothyroidism. Although rare, it almost exclusively occurs in older patients. Coma is seen in the most severe cases; more common features include alteration in cognition, lethargy, seizures, psychotic symptoms, and confusion and disorientation. In most cases, the affected individual has had a precipitating event such as a severe infection, cold exposure, alcoholism, or the use of psychoactive medications, sedatives, or narcotics. Early recognition and treatment are essential.

Clinical Findings

A history of increased fatigue and somnolence is common, as is a history of prior treatment of a thyroid disorder or use of narcotic, sedative, or antipsychotic medication. Infections, particularly pneumonia and urosepsis, are common. Physical examination may demonstrate classic signs and symptoms of hypothyroidism, including dry, scaly skin, bradycardia, and edema. Profound hypothermia, as well as hypoventilation and hypotension, may exist. Headaches, ataxia, nystagmus, psychotic behavior, muscle spasms, and sinus bradycardia may precede the coma. There may also be a pericardial effusion, ileus, megacolon, and easy bruising.

Laboratory findings classically include a markedly elevated serum TSH and reduced total and free serum T_4. Hypoglycemia and hyponatremia are common. Autoimmune deficiency states, including diabetes mellitus and adrenal insufficiency, are sometimes associated with hypothyroidism and other autoimmune disorders. Creatine phosphokinase of muscle origin is often elevated as a result of muscle breakdown. Myocardial infarction can occur in the presence of myxedema coma or may even be the precipitating event, and may complicate the initiation of thyroid hormone therapy. In rare circumstances, myoglobinuria and rhabdomyolysis may occur. Arterial blood gases usually demonstrate a decrease in partial pressure of oxygen and an increase in partial pressure of carbon dioxide, indicating acute or impending respiratory failure. Anemia is also a common finding and is often normochromic, normocytic, or macrocytic. Cardiomegaly is often seen on chest x-ray film. Evoked potentials may have abnormal amplitude or latency, and electroencephalogram may demonstrate triphasic waves that disappear with thyroid replacement.

Differential Diagnosis

Included in the differential diagnosis are dementia, sepsis, intracranial bleed or tumor, hepatic encephalopathy, congestive heart failure, and hypothyroidism.

Treatment

Patients should be cared for in an intensive care unit. Suspicion of possible myxedema coma requires immediate treatment with L-thyroxine given intravenously, even before confirmatory laboratory studies are available. When deciding on therapy, the following principles are important:

1. Myxedema coma has a very high mortality rate if treatment is delayed or is inadequate.

2. The suspicion of possible diagnosis of myxedema coma mandates treatment even before receiving laboratory results since empiric therapy can be discontinued if the patient is later found not to be hypothyroid.

3. Supportive therapy must be provided and includes ventilatory support for respiratory failure, antibiotics for infection as indicated, and management of hypothermia by external rewarming. Hypotension is treated with fluid replacement, although dopamine infusion might also be required. Severe hyponatremia must be treated initially until thyroid hormone replacement results in a decrease in antidiuretic hormone (ADH) and produces a brisk diuresis. Hypoglycemia and anemia will need to be monitored carefully and treated as needed. Care must be taken to prevent aspiration, fecal impaction, pressure sores, and urinary retention.

4. Prompt initiation of thyroid hormone replacement is essential. The initial dose for treatment of myxedema coma is between 300 and 500 µg of L-thyroxine given intravenously. This high dose is necessary to occupy thyroid hormone–binding sites that have been left free as a result of significant and prolonged hormone deficiency. In addition, precipitating factors, such as infection, may increase the turnover of T_4, and thus warrant a higher initial replacement dose. High doses can increase myocardial oxygen consumption and the potential for myocardial infarction. Once there is evidence of a clinical response, usually noted by a diuresis and increase in body temperature and heart rate, the daily dose of L-thyroxine should be reduced to 25 to 50 µg and can be given orally and adjusted upward as necessary based on clinical response and serum TSH level. The use of T_3 or a combination of T_4 and T_3 has been suggested by some clinicians because of the shorter onset of action of T_3 and reduced ability to deiodinate T_4 to the more active T_3 in persons with significant illness and/or malnutrition. Data are not available upon which to make a more definitive recommendation.

5. Because adrenal insufficiency may coexist with myxedema coma, suspicion of cortisol deficiency should be high. A suggestive history, physical examination, and electrolyte abnormalities call for administration of stress doses of intravenous glucocorticoids. Initiating glucocorticoid therapy for all patients with myxedema coma is controversial. In life-threatening situations, blood for measurement of plasma cortisol should be drawn, and intravenous stress doses of corticosteroids should be administered and continued until there is laboratory confirmation of adrenal status and a decision can then be made to continue, taper, or stop the corticosteroids.

Prognosis

Myxedema coma is a serious condition that occurs largely in older hypothyroid persons. Aggressive supportive therapy and thyroid hormone therapy are essential while possible contributing factors are evaluated and treated as necessary. Close monitoring is required when treatment is initiated to avoid toxicity from the relatively large starting doses of thyroid hormone. Even under the best of circumstances, there is considerable mortality related to delay in diagnosis and presence of coexisting morbidities.

Dutta P, Bhansali A, Masoodi SR, Bhadada S, Sharma N, Rajput R. Predictors of outcome in myxoedema coma: a study from a tertiary care centre. *Crit Care*. 2008;12(1):R1.

Kwaku MP, Burman KD. Myxedema coma. *J Intensive Care Med*. 2007;22(4):224-231.

Yamamoto T, Fukuyama J, Fujiyoshi A. Factors associated with mortality of myxedema coma: report of eight cases and literature survey. *Thyroid*. 1999;9(12):1167-1174.

HYPERTHYROIDISM

General Principles

Hyperthyroidism is the result of an excessive amount of circulating thyroid hormone either from endogenous production or iatrogenic sources. Clinically, this disorder is accompanied by a broad spectrum of signs and symptoms that vary among individuals and can differ markedly between young and old persons. A greater percentage of affected individuals are older than age 60 years. Several studies of prevalence indicate the presence of hyperthyroidism in 1% to 3% of community-residing older persons. Hyperthyroidism is far more common in women than in men, with estimates ranging from 4:1 to 10:1.

Graves disease remains the most common cause of hyperthyroidism in young persons and may still be present in older patients. With increasing age, however, more cases of hyperthyroidism result from multinodular toxic goiter. Although multinodular goiters are commonly found in older persons and are not usually associated with clinical disease, they may evolve into toxic multinodular thyroid goiters. A toxic adenoma may also be a cause of hyperthyroidism and is usually identified on thyroid scan as a solitary hyperfunctioning nodule with suppression of activity in the remaining portion of the thyroid gland.

Rarely, hyperthyroidism may result from ingestion of iodide or iodine-containing substances. Iodine may be introduced from seafood, although this problem is more common after exposure to iodinated radiocontrast agents and to amiodarone. Up to 40% of patients taking amiodarone will have serum T_4 levels above the normal range as a result of the drug's effect on T_4 metabolism; far fewer (5%) will develop clinically apparent thyrotoxicosis. The hyperthyroidism can be of rapid onset and severe in magnitude.

Hyperthyroidism must always be considered in the older person who is already receiving thyroid hormone therapy. This is particularly important if the dose is >0.15 mg of L-thyroxine daily, although even smaller doses may be excessive, especially in small individuals of advanced age. Persons taking the same dose of thyroid hormone for many years may become hyperthyroid simply because of an age-associated decline in the body's ability to degrade T_4.

Although extremely rare, a TSH-producing pituitary tumor may be the cause of hyperthyroidism. Nonsuppressed levels of serum TSH in the presence of increased amounts of circulating thyroid hormone are seen with these tumors. Hyperthyroidism may also rarely result in overproduction of thyroid hormone from a widespread metastatic follicular carcinoma.

Transient hyperthyroidism may occur in patients with silent or subacute thyroiditis as a result of increased release of thyroid hormone into the circulation during the inflammatory phase of the illness. Radiation injury, which may be caused by radioactive iodine therapy for hyperthyroidism, may also result in an outpouring of thyroid hormone.

Hyperthyroidism is usually accompanied by elevated levels of both T_4 and T_3. However, a subgroup of older hyperthyroid individuals has isolated elevations of T_3 alone. T_4 is either within the normal range or may, in fact, be suppressed. This circumstance is referred to as T_3 toxicosis. Although it can occur with any type of hyperthyroidism, it is most commonly seen in older patients with toxic multinodular goiter or solitary toxic adenomas. The diagnosis is made on clinical grounds and measurements demonstrating an elevated level of serum T_3 and a suppressed level of serum TSH. T_4 toxicosis, or an isolated increase in serum T_4 without an elevation in serum T_3, most commonly occurs in a sick older person with hyperthyroidism. Disease or malnutrition interferes in the normal removal of iodine from the 5′ position of T_4 and thus results in a decreased ability to convert T_4 to T_3.

▶ Clinical Findings

A. Symptoms & Signs

Clinical findings associated with hyperthyroidism in the older adult vary greatly. In general, the clinical presentation of hyperthyroidism at this time of life differs from the more classic findings noted earlier in life (Table 50–1). The presenting feature may be a decline in functional capacity. There may be increased fatigue, heat intolerance, muscle weakness, cognitive changes, loss of appetite, weight loss, cardiac arrhythmias, atrial fibrillation, and congestive heart failure. New onset of atrial fibrillation in an older person warrants testing for the possible presence of hyperthyroidism. Exophthalmos associated with the hyperthyroidism is less commonly noted in older adults. Rather than frequent bowel movements, more commonly there is a resolution of preexisting constipation. Anemia and hyponatremia are often noted and thought to be caused by other coexisting illnesses. Although this relative lack of the classic findings of hyperthyroidism does not occur in every older person with hyperthyroidism, a subgroup develops an apathetic hyperthyroid state. In this circumstance, the patient lacks the hyperactivity, irritability, and restlessness common to young patients who are hyperthyroid and presents instead with severe weakness, lethargy, listlessness, depression, and the appearance of a chronic wasting illness. Often the person is incorrectly diagnosed as having a malignancy or severe depression.

Symptoms less common in older patients include nervousness, increased diaphoresis, increased appetite, and increased frequency of bowel movements. More common symptoms include marked weight loss (present in >80% of older patients), poor appetite, worsening angina, agitation, confusion, and edema.

Similarly, physical findings differ in older patients. Hyperreflexia, palpable goiter, and exophthalmos are usually absent, although lid lag and lid retraction may be present. The pulse rate tends to be slower. Cardiac manifestations are particularly important in the older person who may

Table 50–1. Frequency of signs and symptoms of hyperthyroidism in young versus elderly patients.

Symptom/Sign	Young (%)	Elderly (%)[a]
Palpitation	100	61.5
Goiter	98	61.0
Tremor	96	63.0
Excessive perspiration	92	52.0
Weight loss	73	77.0
Eye signs	71	42.0
Arrhythmias	4.6	39.0

[a]Data represent a compilation of several studies.

have coexisting heart disease. An increased heart rate with a related increase in myocardial oxygen demand, stroke volume, cardiac output, and shortened left ventricular ejection time underlie the clinical consequences of palpitations. There is also an increased risk of atrial fibrillation (often with slow ventricular response), exacerbation of angina in patients with preexisting coronary artery disease, and precipitation of congestive heart failure that responds less readily to conventional therapy.

Gastrointestinal problems may occasionally include abdominal pain, nausea, and vomiting. Diarrhea and increased frequency of bowel movements resulting from the effect of the thyroid hormone on intestinal motility can occur, but these symptoms are often absent, and constipation is still common. There may be an alteration in liver enzymes, including elevation of alkaline phosphatase and γ-glutamyltranspeptidase levels, which become normal after a return to the euthyroid state. Weakness, especially of proximal muscles, is a major feature of hyperthyroidism in older persons and is often accompanied by muscle wasting and functional decline. Disorders of gait, postural instability, and falling may be noted. Tremor is noted in >70% of older persons with hyperthyroidism. The tremor is usually coarser than in other common tremors. A rapid relaxation phase of the deep tendon reflex is difficult to identify in the older thyrotoxic individual. Central nervous system (CNS) manifestations may be prominent and include confusion, depression, changes in short-term memory, agitation and anxiety, and a decreased attention span. Other findings associated with hyperthyroidism include worsening of glucose tolerance, mild increases in serum calcium, and osteoporosis resulting from increased bone turnover.

B. Laboratory Tests

The altered and often atypical presentation of hyperthyroidism in the older patient warrants a high degree of suspicion among clinicians and the initiation of appropriate laboratory studies. Serum free T_4 and a measurement of serum TSH are the preferred tests for diagnosing thyroid dysfunction. The findings of a normal or low serum free T_4 with a suppressed serum TSH raises the possibility of T_3 toxicosis and warrants a measurement of serum T_3 by radioimmunoassay. Although the finding of anti-TSH receptor antibodies confirms the diagnosis of Graves disease, it is rarely necessary to obtain this test.

C. Special Tests

Thyroid scanning with technetium and measurement of 24-hour ^{131}I uptake can be useful in distinguishing Graves disease from toxic multinodular goiter. Scanning may also demonstrate the presence of a small, diffusely active goiter that could not be detected on physical examination. Very low ^{131}I uptake in a patient with elevated circulating thyroid hormone levels suggests exogenous thyroid hormone ingestion,

the hyperthyroid phase of painless or subacute thyroiditis, or iodine-induced hyperthyroidism.

▶ Differential Diagnosis

Patients with hyperthyroidism in later life commonly have coexisting illness, and it is important not to attribute all presenting signs and symptoms to the hyperthyroid state itself. The most common differential diagnoses to consider include anxiety, malignancy, depression, diabetes mellitus, menopause, and pheochromocytoma.

▶ Treatment

Therapy should be directed at the specific cause of the hyperthyroid state. Therefore, the underlying cause must be determined to exclude the possibility of one of the transient forms of illness, such as excessive hormone ingestion, iodine exposure, or subacute thyroiditis. The majority of older patients with either Graves disease or multinodular toxic goiter can be treated with antithyroid medications, radioactive iodine, or surgery. The preferred treatment, however, is radioactive iodine in order to avoid hospitalization and associated anesthesia and surgery risks.

A useful initial step in treating suspected hyperthyroidism is to administer a β-adrenergic blocking agent such as long-acting propranolol, metoprolol, nadolol, or atenolol. These agents quickly control associated palpitations, angina, tachycardia, and agitation. Caution is advised, however, in persons with congestive heart failure, chronic obstructive pulmonary disease, or diabetes mellitus being treated with insulin.

Once a diagnosis of Graves disease or toxic nodular goiter is confirmed, treatment should be initiated with one of the antithyroid drugs: propylthiouracil or methimazole. These agents impair biosynthesis of thyroid hormone, thus depleting intrathyroidal hormone stores and ultimately leading to decreased hormone secretion. A decline in serum T_4 concentration is usually seen within 2 to 4 weeks after initiation of antithyroid drug therapy, and the dose should be tapered once thyroid hormone levels reach the normal range to avoid hypothyroidism. In 1% to 5% of patients, the antithyroid medications may result in fever, rash, and arthralgias. A drug-induced agranulocytosis may be more common in older patients and will most likely occur within the first 3 months of treatment, especially in those who receive >30 mg/day of methimazole. Periodic white blood cell count monitoring should be considered, with discontinuation of the antithyroid medication if there is evidence of neutropenia.

Long-term antithyroid medication use can be effective in patients older than age 60 years with Graves disease, who appear to respond fairly quickly and have a greater likelihood of a long-lasting remission. Because these medications rarely will provide a long-lasting effect for those with a toxic multinodular goiter, more definitive therapy is needed once the patient returns to a euthyroid state on medication. The recommended treatment in most older persons with hyperthyroidism is thyroid gland ablation with [131]I. Once the patient achieves a euthyroid status on antithyroid medication, these agents should be stopped for 3 to 5 days, after which ^{131}I is given orally. Therapy with β-blockers can be maintained and antithyroid agents restarted 5 days after radiotherapy and should be continued for 1 to 3 months until the major effect of radioiodine is achieved. Although some physicians attempt to calculate a specific dose that will render the patient euthyroid without subsequently developing hypothyroidism, many patients will still develop permanent hypothyroidism. For this reason, most clinicians now advocate treating the older person with hyperthyroidism with a relatively large dose of ^{131}I to ensure ablation of thyroid tissue and thus avoid the possibility of hyperthyroidism recurrence.

After treatment, the patient is closely monitored in order to start replacement doses of thyroid hormone, because hypothyroidism may develop in as few as 4 weeks after treatment. Regardless of radioiodine dosing regimen used, 40% to 50% of patients will be hypothyroid within 12 months of ^{131}I administration, with 2% to 5% developing hypothyroidism each year thereafter.

Prior treatment with antithyroid medication prevents the possibility of radiation-induced thyroiditis after ^{131}I therapy. However, in some circumstances, when clinical and laboratory features suggest a mild case of hyperthyroidism and no cardiac problems are noted, it may be appropriate to treat the hyperthyroid patient with ^{131}I without antithyroid medication pretreatment. When this option is chosen, the patients should be started on a β-blocker and continue with it until thyroid hormone levels return to normal.

Surgery is not recommended as a primary treatment for hyperthyroidism in older patients. Coexisting illness, particularly cardiac, increases operative risk. In addition, postoperative complications of hypoparathyroidism and recurrent laryngeal nerve damage are significant risks. Surgery may be indicated in the rare patient with tracheal compression secondary to a large goiter.

Atrial fibrillation occurs in 10% to 15% of hyperthyroid patients. Treatment of the underlying disease is essential; cardioversion and anticoagulation are considered on an individual basis. The longer the hyperthyroid period, the less likely is the return to normal sinus rhythm; most benefit is found in those who become euthyroid within 3 weeks. Cardioversion is usually reserved for patients who still remain in atrial fibrillation after 16 weeks of euthyroidism. Many older individuals with hyperthyroidism who develop atrial fibrillation are at greater risk of thromboembolic events, especially those with a history of thromboembolism, hypertension, or congestive heart failure and those with evidence of left atrial enlargement or left ventricular dysfunction. In the absence of contraindications, anticoagulant therapy should be given with the oral anticoagulants dabigatran, rivaroxaban, and apixaban, which do not require blood monitoring. Hyperthyroidism increases sensitivity to the anticoagulant effect of warfarin, resulting in greater lowering of coagulation factors II and VII so that smaller than usual doses will likely be needed to achieve an international normalized ratio of 2.0 to 3.0. Consequently, warfarin is no longer the anticoagulant of choice.

Allahabadia A, Daykin J, Holder RL, Sheppard MC, Gough SC, Franklyn JA. Age and gender predict the outcome of treatment for Graves' hyperthyroidism. *J Clin Endocrinol Metab.* 2000;85(3):1038-1042.

Boelaert K, Torlinska B, Holder RL, et al. Older subjects with hyperthyroidism present with a paucity of symptoms and signs: a large cross-sectional study. *J Clin Endocrinol Metab.* 2010;95:2715-2726.

Ryodi E, Almi J, Jaatinen, et al. Cardiovascular morbidity and mortality in surgically treated hyperthyroidism: a nation-wide cohort study with a long-term follow-up. *Clin Endocrinol* 2014;80:743-750.

Seimer C, Olesen JB, Hansen ML, et al. The spectrum of thyroid disease and risk of new onset atrial fibrillation: a large population cohort study. *BMJ.* 2012;345:e7985.

Trivalle C, Doucet J, Chassagne P, et al. Differences in the signs and symptoms of hyperthyroidism in older and younger patients. *J Am Geriatr Soc.* 1996;44(1):50-53.

Zhou Z, Ma L-L, Wang L-X. Risk factors for persistent atrial fibrillation following successful hyperthyroidism treatment with radioiodine therapy. *Intern Med.* 2011;50:2947-2951.

NODULAR THYROID DISEASE & NEOPLASIA

▶ General Principles

The incidence of thyroid nodules increases with advancing age and female gender. By age 50 years, ultrasonography will identify at least 50% of women with one or more thyroid nodules. Multinodular thyroid glands occur more commonly in individuals who have lived in areas of iodine deficiency. Often there is a history of goiter dating to childhood or young adulthood. Very large multinodular goiters, particularly those with a significant substernal component, may compress the trachea and lead to problems of dyspnea and wheezing or problems with swallowing. All patients with thyroid nodules should be questioned regarding prior exposure to external radiation of the head, neck, and upper thorax. Radiation to these areas markedly increases the risk of thyroid malignancy. Radiation increases the risk of thyroid malignancy as well as benign nodules and parathyroid adenomas. Approximately 16% to 29% of persons who received low-dose radiation to the head and neck as children will develop palpable thyroid nodules; approximately 33% become malignant and clinically detected only after 10 to 20 years, reaching a peak incidence 20 to 30 years after radiation exposure.

▶ **Clinical Findings**

A. Symptoms & Signs

Thyroid nodules often remain asymptomatic, being discovered by the patient inadvertently or by the physician during a routine physical examination. On occasion, a thyroid nodule may result in an acute onset of neck pain and neck tenderness. This may be an acute or subacute thyroiditis or hemorrhage into a preexisting nodule. Although a single thyroid nodule is more commonly associated with malignancy than is a multinodular thyroid gland, only 5% of clinically apparent solitary nodules will be malignant. The vast majority of thyroid nodules are benign and include follicular and colloid adenomas, Hashimoto thyroiditis, and thyroid cysts.

Malignant thyroid neoplasms may be papillary, follicular, medullary, or anaplastic carcinomas; lymphoma; or, in rare cases, metastatic disease to the thyroid. Nonthyroid lesions may appear as nodules on physical examination; these include lymph nodes, aneurysms, parathyroid cysts and adenomas, and thyroglossal duct cysts. The risk that a solitary thyroid nodule will prove to be malignant is increased by a history of radiation exposure, age >60 years, rapid increase in size, hoarseness of the voice suggesting an impingement of the recurrent laryngeal nerve, and hardness on palpation. Age is also a factor in predicting the histologic type of malignancy. The overall histologic distribution of all thyroid cancer is 79% papillary, 13% follicular, 3% Hürthle cell, 3.5% medullary, and 1.7% anaplastic. In patients older than 60 years, papillary carcinoma accounts for 64% of thyroid cancers. Follicular carcinoma peaks in frequency between the fourth and sixth decades of life (mean age at diagnosis, 44 years). Together with Hürthle cell carcinoma, these cancers account for 20% of thyroid malignancies in the population older than age 60 years. Medullary carcinoma has a peak incidence during the fifth and sixth decades of life and represents approximately 5% of thyroid cancers in the older adult (Table 50–2). Anaplastic carcinomas occur almost exclusively in older populations and account for approximately 6% of thyroid cancers in older patients. Anaplastic carcinoma is characterized by rapid growth, rock-hard consistency, and local invasiveness. Involvement of the recurrent laryngeal nerve and compression of the trachea are common. Lymphoma and metastatic cancers occur infrequently in the older patient. Lymphoma usually presents with a rapidly enlarging painless neck mass that may cause compressive symptoms. Coexisting Hashimoto thyroiditis is common.

B. Laboratory Tests

The major objective in evaluating an older person with a thyroid nodule is to rule out the presence of a malignancy. Blood tests of thyroid function will usually be normal unless there is a hyperfunctioning adenoma or toxic multinodular goiter. An elevated serum TSH may be noted in persons with subclinical hypothyroidism and nodular disease, as may result from longstanding Hashimoto thyroiditis. Serum thyroglobulin is often elevated in the setting of thyroid cancer but cannot differentiate malignancy from benign nodules or thyroiditis with any degree of certainty. It is, therefore, more commonly used as a marker for recurrence or metastasis in patients with papillary or follicular carcinoma who have undergone total thyroidectomy. An elevation of serum calcitonin concentration is indicative of a medullary carcinoma but is not part of the initial evaluation, unless there is a family history of multiple endocrine neoplasia.

C. Special Tests

Fine-needle aspiration (FNA) of the thyroid remains the best way to obtain tissue for cytologic or histologic examination. FNA is indicated in any patient with a solitary nodule and in patients with multinodular goiter when there is suspicion of thyroid malignancy based on clinical evaluation, ultrasonography, or thyroid scan. This procedure, when performed by a skilled clinician, has proven to be safe, inexpensive, and capable of determining the presence or absence of malignancy with an accuracy of close to 95%, and even greater accuracy with sonographic guidance. In general, cytopathologic findings from FNA are divided into four categories: positive for malignancy, suspicious for malignancy, negative for malignancy, and nondiagnostic. A repeat FNA is indicated for a nondiagnostic but clinically suspicious nodule. Malignant cells found on FNA indicate the need for surgery. The combination of suspicious cytology by FNA and a cold-appearing nodule on thyroid scan also indicates the need for surgical excision of the suspicious nodule. Benign cytology in either a solid or cystic nodule warrants observation. If the FNA is suggestive of a lymphoma, a repeat biopsy using a large needle or even a surgical biopsy is indicated. For persons whose FNA is nondiagnostic, testing for genetic variants can be done on the sample to see if *BRAF, RET/PTC*, or other genes are mutated. Panels are now available that can search simultaneously for multiple genetic variants. Finding these changes makes thyroid cancer much more likely and thus may also play a role in determining the best treatment for the cancer. A majority of nodules with indeterminate cytology will prove to be benign on postoperative histopathology. Thus, tests that

Table 50–2. Thyroid malignancy in the older patient.

Cancer Type	Patients Affected (%)		10-Year Survival
	Age >40	Age >60	Age >60
Papillary/mixed	79	64	<65
Follicular	13	20	<57
Medullary	3	5	<63
Anaplastic	2	6	0
Lymphoma	3	5	99+

use genomic profiling to rule out cancer with high sensitivity have demonstrated clinical utility in the management of cytologically indeterminate nodules. Isotopic scanning is no longer considered the initial diagnostic test in evaluating a suspicious nodule because of its relatively high false-positive and false-negative rates and high cost. Isotope imaging is best used when evaluating a patient with a thyroid nodule who has had a nondiagnostic result from FNA.

Because malignant tissue is more likely unable to take up iodine, the identification of a nodule as hot on ^{123}I or technetium scanning makes malignancy in the nodule less likely, although clearly still possible. Scanning may also reveal an apparent single nodule that is, in fact, part of a multinodular thyroid gland, again decreasing the risk of malignancy. The presence of a nonfunctioning or a cold nodule is not proof of a malignancy because 95% of thyroid nodules will prove to be cold; the frequency of malignancy in cold nodules is 5%. Hot nodules associated with normal circulating levels of thyroid hormone and no compressive symptoms should be observed with repeat examinations performed at 6- to 12-month intervals. These nodules may eventually result in hyperthyroidism; thus, clinical correlation is also warranted.

High-resolution ultrasonography can detect thyroid lesions as small as 2 mm and can also permit classification of a nodule as solid, cystic, or mixed solid-cystic. It will often identify multiple nodules in a gland even when only a single nodule is palpated clinically. This technique cannot be used to distinguish with certainty malignant from benign nodules because there is a great deal of overlap in the characteristics identified using ultrasonography. However, ultrasonography features common in malignant nodules are as follows: (1) size >1 cm in diameter; (2) solid rather than cystic; (3) hypoechoic; (4) central hypervascularity; (5) presence of microcalcifications; and (6) irregular borders. Ultrasonography is used to detect recurrent or residual thyroid cancer in previously treated patients as well as to screen persons with a history of radiation exposure earlier in life.

Computed tomography (CT) and magnetic resonance imaging (MRI) are expensive and add little to the initial assessment of malignancy. They may be useful in evaluating the extent of disease in patients found to have anaplastic carcinoma or lymphoma and may provide useful information regarding compression of neck structures and the size and substernal extent of nodules and goiters.

Medullary carcinoma of the thyroid gland can be monitored using blood calcitonin measurements, both in the basal state and after stimulation. Blood levels of carcinoembryonic antigen may also be elevated in patients with residual or recurrent medullary carcinoma.

Differential Diagnosis

The differential diagnosis includes thyroid duct cysts, benign adenomas, toxic thyroid nodule, thyroid malignancy, hemorrhage, and multinodular thyroid gland.

Treatment

Although the basic principles for treating thyroid cancer do not differ significantly between the young and old, older individuals need to be more carefully evaluated for comorbid conditions and risk of surgery. Surgery for thyroid cancer should be performed only by an experienced surgeon. Papillary or follicular carcinoma is usually treated with near-total thyroidectomy because of the high frequency of multicentricity of malignancy and the need to remove functional thyroid tissue in order to monitor the patient with total-body radioiodine scanning postoperatively. Thyroid remnants detected postoperatively are ablated with ^{131}I. At 6 months, and subsequently at yearly intervals, scanning should be obtained and serum thyroglobulin measured to determine whether residual functional tissue exists. If active tissue is found, large ablative doses of ^{131}I should be administered. This approach has reduced the recurrence rate of both papillary and follicular carcinomas and prolonged survival.

Patients who have been treated for malignancy are judiciously given suppressive doses of L-thyroxine as tolerated with the desired objective of reducing serum TSH to below normal as measured by third-generation TSH assays. The administration of suppressive doses of L-thyroxine carries a substantial risk of precipitating or aggravating ischemic heart disease and arrhythmias as well as accelerating bone turnover. The older patient will need to be monitored closely and the dose of thyroid hormone reduced if cardiac symptoms develop. Since acceleration of bone loss is likely to occur, treatment with bone antiresorptive agents may be necessary in some circumstances (eg, in osteopenic women). Medullary carcinoma of the thyroid gland is best treated with a total thyroidectomy because the disease is often multicentric. The majority of medullary carcinomas do not respond to ^{131}I treatment; therefore, palliative therapy is recommended using external irradiation if residual thyroid tissue or recurrent disease is detected. Thyroid lymphoma should be clinically staged using CT or MRI. External irradiation in combination with chemotherapy has been associated with a survival rate close to 100%.

Prognosis

Age at diagnosis is an important factor in predicting cancer aggressiveness and mortality from differentiated thyroid cancer. Individuals diagnosed after age 50 years have a higher rate of recurrence and death (see Table 50–2). The 10-year survival for patients with papillary carcinoma is approximately 97% in those younger than 45 years and <65% for those older than 60 years at diagnosis. The 10-year survival rate for persons with follicular carcinoma is 98% for those younger than 45 years and <57% for those older than 60 years at diagnosis. The older the person is when a follicular carcinoma is diagnosed, the greater is the risk of recurrence and death.

The 10-year survival rate for persons with medullary carcinoma is 84% for individuals younger than 45 years and decreases with advancing age. Persons in the seventh decade of life have a high rate of persistent disease even after surgery. Anaplastic carcinoma of the thyroid gland is rarely associated with more than a 1-year survival after diagnosis because of its rapid progression and high propensity to metastasize. Palliative treatment of compressive symptoms may be achieved by surgery followed by high-dose external radiation. Chemotherapy with doxorubicin or cisplatin, or a combination, may be beneficial in combination with surgery and external irradiation.

Burman KD, Wartofsky L. Thyroid nodules. *N Engl J Med.* 2015;373:2347-2355.

Fagin JA, Wells SA. Biologic and clinical perspectives in thyroid cancer. *N Engl J Med.* 2016;375:1054-1067.

Ferris RL, Baloch Z, Bernet V, et al. American Thyroid Association statement on surgical application of molecular profiling for thyroid nodules: current impact on perioperative decision making. *Thyroid.* 2015;25(7):760-768.

Gharib H, Papini E, Garber JR, et al. American Association of Clinical Endocrinologists, American College of Endocrinology, and Associazione Medici Endocrinologi medical guidelines for clinical practice for the diagnosis and management of thyroid nodules – 2016 Update Appendix. *Endocr Pract.* 2016;22(suppl 1): 1-60.

Grani G, Lamartina L, Ascoli V, et al. Reducing the number of unnecessary thyroid biopsies while improving diagnostic accuracy: toward the "right" TIRADS. *J Clin Endocrinol Metab.* 2019;104:95-102.

Haugen BR, Alexander EK, Bible KC, et al. 2015 American Thyroid Association management guidelines for adult patients with thyroid nodules and differentiated thyroid cancer. *Thyroid.* 2015;26(1):1-251.

DISEASES OF THE ADRENAL CORTEX

Advancing age is associated with a reduced metabolic clearance rate of cortisol, but with a compensatory decrease in secretion rate. Consequently, basal levels of serum cortisol are unaffected over the life span. Basal adrenocorticotropic hormone (ACTH) levels are unchanged or slightly increased with age in healthy individuals. Diurnal cortisol rhythm is reported to show a significant age-related phase advance (earlier peak and nadir level) similar to that observed in depressed patients. This is thought to be related to changes in sleep patterns.

The adrenal androgen precursor dehydroepiandrosterone (DHEA) reaches peak blood levels in both men and women by age 20 to 30 years, and then declines steadily, so that, after age 70 years, levels are <20% of the peak. Although early reports and popular lay literature have attributed a number of antiaging properties to DHEA, more recent studies in which DHEA has been administered for 6 to 12 months have shown little or no effect on objective measures of physiologic function. Some studies, however, suggest a beneficial effect on mood and sense of general well-being.

The hypothalamic-pituitary-adrenal axis response to known major stimuli remains intact with increasing age. Stimulation tests of this axis using insulin-induced hypoglycemia or metyrapone administration result in a normal or slightly longer period of cortisol and ACTH secretory response in older persons. Peak cortisol response to stress is also greater, and both cortisol and ACTH levels remain elevated for a longer period in older compared with younger persons. Moreover, dexamethasone causes less inhibition of cortisol in older patients. It is unknown whether this age-related hyperresponsiveness of the pituitary-adrenal axis to stressful situations contributes to age-prevalent illness, including osteoporosis, glucose intolerance, muscle atrophy, and immunosuppression. Adrenal cortical response to exogenous ACTH, measured by circulating cortisol levels, is unaffected by aging.

ACUTE ADRENAL INSUFFICIENCY

▶ General Principles

Acute adrenal insufficiency results from a deficiency in cortisol secretion and, in older people, occurs most often as a result of failure of the adrenal gland rather than a pituitary gland disorder. The adrenal gland may be unable to produce an adequate amount of corticosteroids and mineralocorticoids because of an autoimmune process involving the entire adrenal gland or from a replacement of healthy adrenal tissue with tumor or infection, such as in tuberculosis. Adrenal crisis may also result from an increased demand for glucocorticoids in an individual unable to increase output sufficiently. This occurs most commonly as a result of chronic adrenal suppression from exogenous corticoid use and less often from stress from trauma, surgery, hemorrhage, or infection. Rarely, this may result from a sudden increase in the metabolic turnover of corticosteroids, as can occur when a patient with both adrenal insufficiency and hypothyroidism is treated with thyroid hormone. Corticosteroid-induced adrenal suppression can occur after as few as 3 to 4 weeks of exogenous steroid treatment with doses >15 mg of prednisone daily or the equivalent dose of other glucocorticoids. In general, individuals on long-term glucocorticoid therapy who have stopped treatment before the return of function of the suppressed adrenal glands or who need a higher dose will have a less clear picture because of the ability of renin and angiotensin to maintain aldosterone function despite suppression of glucocorticoid activity in the adrenal gland.

▶ Clinical Findings

A. Symptoms & Signs

Patients with adrenal insufficiency often have nausea and vomiting and abdominal pain and may have an altered mental state and fever. In general, blood pressure is low. Signs of primary adrenal insufficiency may include hyperpigmentation and evidence of dehydration. Older persons commonly have sparse or absent pubic and axillary hair; therefore, this is less commonly noted as a presenting sign in older patients.

B. Laboratory Tests

Laboratory findings may include hyponatremia or hyperkalemia. Hypoglycemia and elevation of blood urea nitrogen (BUN) and creatinine are common. Eosinophilia may be noted as well. Cultures may be positive if there is an underlying infection. The cosyntropin (ACTH 1–24) stimulation test is abnormal, and plasma ACTH is usually elevated in persons with primary failure of the adrenal gland. With this test, patients are given 0.25 mg of cosyntropin intravenously over 2 to 3 minutes, and serum cortisol is measured immediately before and 30 and 60 minutes after administration. Under normal circumstances, serum cortisol rises to a peak of ≥18 to 20 µg/dL after either 30 or 60 minutes of cosyntropin administration. Hydrocortisone administration will interfere with the test results, but dexamethasone does not interfere with the specific assay for cortisol.

▶ Differential Diagnosis

Although adrenal insufficiency should be considered in any patient who presents with hyperkalemia and hypotension, other possible causes for these findings should be considered.

Other causes of hypotension in particular include sepsis, hemorrhage, and cardiogenic diseases. Renal insufficiency may cause hyperkalemia, as may gastrointestinal bleeding, rhabdomyolysis, and medications such as spironolactone and angiotensin-converting enzyme inhibitors. Hyponatremia may occur in hypothyroidism, with diuretic use, in drug and disease states associated with inappropriate ADH secretion, and with malnutrition, cirrhosis, and vomiting. Eosinophilia may be associated with blood dyscrasias, allergies, medication reactions, and parasitic infections. The associated gastrointestinal findings of nausea, vomiting, and abdominal pain may, in fact, be caused by other gastrointestinal tract disorders common during later life. Hyperpigmentation may not be noted in older persons of dark complexion or who have sun-induced skin damage.

▶ Treatment

Replacement of both glucocorticoids and mineralocorticoids is needed in severe cases of adrenal insufficiency. Because hydrocortisone has some mineralocorticoid activity, it is the corticosteroid of choice for patients with mild cases and is effective in doses of 10 to 12 mg/m²/day orally; two-thirds

of the dose is given in the morning and one-third in the late afternoon or evening. If salt-retaining effects from this therapy are insufficient, fludrocortisone is added to the daily regimen in dosages of 0.05 to 0.3 mg orally each day or every other day. The exact dose required varies with the individual and, therefore, should be clinically adjusted in relation to postural blood pressure changes, level of potassium, and body weight. The dose is reduced if hypokalemia, hypertension, or edema occurs, especially when fluid and electrolyte management is complicated by cardiac disease or renal insufficiency. Underlying factors that may have contributed to the onset of adrenal insufficiency, particularly infections, should be sought. The dosage of hydrocortisone may need to be adjusted upward to a stress dosage as high as 300 mg/day, although usually 50 mg intravenously or intramuscularly every 6 hours will be sufficient, even for the most stressful situations.

▶ Prognosis

With adequate replacement therapy, adrenal insufficiency is a treatable illness. When accompanied by other illnesses, the risk mortality is increased. If the underlying cause is an autoimmune disease, other endocrine problems, such as diabetes mellitus and hypothyroidism, as well as pernicious anemia, may be present.

Bornstein SR, Allolio B, Arlt W, et al. Diagnosis and treatment of primary adrenal insufficiency: an Endocrine Society clinical practice guideline. *J Clin Endocrinol Metab.* 2016;101:364.

Parker CR Jr, Slayden SM, Azziz R, et al. Effects of aging on adrenal function in the human: responsiveness and sensitivity of adrenal androgens and cortisol to adrenocorticotropin in premenopausal and postmenopausal women. *J Clin Endocrinol Metab.* 2000;85(1):48-54.

CUSHING SYNDROME

▶ General Principles

Cushing syndrome is caused by an excessive amount of circulating corticosteroids. In older patients, it most commonly results from exogenous exposure to corticosteroids given for a variety of medical disorders. The most frequent endogenous cause is ectopic production of ACTH by neoplasms, especially small cell carcinoma of the lung and carcinoid tumor. Cushing disease (ie, oversecretion of ACTH by a pituitary tumor) is less common in older than in younger patients, is usually associated with a small benign pituitary adenoma, and occurs more often in women than in men. Approximately 15% of cases of endogenous Cushing syndrome are non–ACTH dependent and result from an adrenal adenoma, carcinoma, or bilateral nodular adrenal hyperplasia. Although adrenal adenomas are generally small and produce mostly glucocorticoids, carcinomas tend to be larger on presentation and more commonly produce excessive amounts of both glucocorticoids and androgens, often resulting in virilization and hirsutism.

Clinical Findings

A. Symptoms & Signs

Although central obesity, thin arms and legs, and a round "moon face" are classic findings, these may be harder to detect in older patients. For example, the "buffalo hump" deposition of fat at the back of the neck may, in older women, be confused with kyphosis resulting from osteoporosis. Thin, transparent skin, bruising, muscle atrophy and weakness, diabetes mellitus, and hypertension are other common findings easily confused with many other age-prevalent disorders. Thirst is less often reported by older adults compared with younger patients. Polyuria may result from increases in blood sugar from glucocorticoid-induced diabetes. Blood glucose is often elevated, and glycosuria may be present. Occasionally, there is a leukocytosis and hypokalemia. Wound healing may be impaired, and changes in mental function, including anxiety, psychosis, and depression, may occur.

B. Laboratory Tests

A 1-mg overnight dexamethasone suppression test, urine free cortisol, late-night salivary cortisol (two measurements), or longer low-dose dexamethasone suppression test (2 mg/day for 48 hours) can be used to screen for hypercortisolism, based on its suitability for a given patient. In a 1-mg overnight dexamethasone suppression test, dexamethasone 1 mg is given orally at 11 PM, and serum is collected at 8 AM the next morning for cortisol. A cortisol level <1.8 μg/dL is considered normal and excludes a diagnosis of Cushing syndrome. If there is failure of suppression, further evaluation should include a 24-hour urine collection for free cortisol and creatinine and late-night salivary cortisol (two measurements). A 2-mg dexamethasone suppression test using 0.5 mg of dexamethasone administered orally every 6 hours for 48 hours can also be used as a screening test. Serum cortisol is measured 6 hours after the last dose of dexamethasone, and cortisol level <1.8 μg/dL is considered normal suppression. The longer low-dose dexamethasone suppression test excludes hypercortisolism with improved specificity compared to a 1-mg dexamethasone suppression test.

Once hypercortisolism is confirmed, plasma ACTH should be determined. A level of ACTH below the normal range indicates a probable adrenal tumor; an elevated or high normal level indicates overproduction by either the pituitary or an ectopic ACTH-secreting tumor. MRI of the pituitary can identify a pituitary adenoma with considerable accuracy. Selective inferior petrosal venous sampling for ACTH can be done to confirm a pituitary source of ACTH and to help distinguish its origin from other sites. A CT or MRI scan of the chest and abdomen to look for ectopic sources of ACTH is indicated and can localize a tumor of the adrenal glands.

Differential Diagnosis

Hypercortisolism can result from iatrogenic use of steroid medications. Alcoholic patients and those with depression may also have increased levels of cortisol. Abnormal dexamethasone suppression tests have been described in patients with morbid obesity, depression, and a variety of CNS disorders. In these patients, urine free cortisol should be measured and an attempt made to assess diurnal variation in cortisol secretion because these tests are usually within normal limits in the setting of obesity. Hypertension resulting from other causes is common in the older adults, and estrogen replacement therapy may alter normal dexamethasone suppressibility.

Treatment

Cushing disease is best treated by removing the pituitary adenoma responsible for the increase in ACTH secretion. After its removal, the adrenal gland remains unable to respond to normal stimulation for a prolonged time, and there is an altered ability to respond under conditions of stress. Hydrocortisone replacement therapy is necessary until normal pituitary-adrenal axis function returns, often taking as long as 6 to 24 months. Radiation therapy has also been used to treat Cushing disease, with cortisol excess biochemically controlled in 30% to 85% of patients.

For patients who are not surgical candidates or have persistent disease after pituitary surgery, medical treatment for inhibition of adrenal steroid biosynthesis with or without radiation therapy can be useful. Cabergoline and pasireotide act directly on pituitary tumor to inhibit ACTH production. Hyperglycemia is a common adverse effect of pasireotide, and most patients experience it soon after initiating pasireotide. Therefore, it should be avoided in patients with uncontrolled diabetes mellitus.

Mifepristone can be used for the control of diabetes due to hypercortisolism. Mifepristone is a glucocorticoid receptor antagonist. Therefore, cortisol level cannot be used to monitor treatment response. Mifepristone is initiated at a dose of 300 mg/day, and dose is adjusted based on clinical parameters such as serum glucose level and weight reduction. Inhibition of steroidogenesis can also be achieved by metyrapone, 500 mg/day to 6 g/day in three to four divided doses, in combination with ketoconazole, 200 mg every 6 hours. Physiologic replacement doses of a glucocorticoid may be necessary to avoid drug-induced adrenal insufficiency.

Adrenal neoplasms secreting cortisol should be resected when possible and often can be removed laparoscopically.

Because the nonaffected adrenal gland is usually suppressed, once again hydrocortisone replacement is indicated until the gland returns to normal function. Metastatic adrenal carcinoma can be managed with the medications just mentioned or with mitotane, 2 to 10 mg daily in divided doses. Ectopic ACTH-secreting tumors should be surgically resected. If this is not possible, once again, medications may be used to suppress the high levels of cortisol.

Patients with Cushing syndrome should be offered age-appropriate vaccinations due to an increased risk of infection.

▶ Prognosis

Patients who have hypercortisolism as a result of iatrogenic use of corticosteroids can usually expect a return to normal after discontinuation of the steroid therapy. In hypercortisolism, the best prognosis for total recovery is seen when a benign adrenal adenoma is easily removed. Pituitary adenomas are more difficult to treat and, even in the best of hands, have a failure rate of 10% to 20%. Patients with pituitary macroadenoma have a lower remission rate of approximately 43%. Even those who respond have a 15% to 20% recurrence rate over the next decade. Patients should be screened for hypercortisolism after surgery to assess for recurrence. The prognosis of patients with ectopic ACTH-producing tumors depends on the underlying type and degree of tumor involvement.

Nieman LK, Biller BM, Findling JW, et al. Treatment of Cushing's syndrome: an Endocrine Society clinical practice guideline. *J Clin Endocrinol Metab.* 2015;100(8):2807-2831.

Papanicolaou DA, Yanovski JA, Cutler GB Jr, Chrousos GP, Nieman LK. A single midnight serum cortisol measurement distinguishes Cushing's syndrome from pseudo-Cushing states. *J Clin Endocrinol Metab.* 1998;83(4):1163-1167.

ADRENAL NODULES

▶ General Principles

The incidence of incidentally discovered adrenal masses, or incidentaloma, increases with age. CT scans incidentally discover adrenal masses in 0.2% of young adults between ages 20 and 29 years and in 7% of older adults over 70 years of age. Most of the adrenal masses are benign and clinically nonfunctioning. Types of malignant adrenal masses include malignant pheochromocytoma, adrenocortical carcinoma, and metastasis to the adrenal. In patients without a known diagnosis of cancer, malignant adrenal masses are rare. Given higher prevalence of cancers known to metastasize to adrenal gland (lung cancer, melanoma, renal cancer), older adults are more likely to be diagnosed with malignant adrenal masses. Up to 15% of adrenal masses can be hormonally active. Therefore, patients with adrenal incidentaloma should be evaluated for excess cortisol, aldosterone, and catecholamine production.

▶ Clinical Findings

A. Symptoms & Signs

The majority of adrenal masses are asymptomatic and are detected incidentally on imaging done for evaluation of diagnoses unrelated to the adrenal glands. Patients with hyperaldosteronism have hypertension and may have hypokalemia on laboratory evaluation. Most patients with pheochromocytoma have elevated blood pressure, but approximately 12% of cases may be normotensive. Pheochromocytoma presents with a typical triad of sweating, headaches, and palpitations in only 10% of patients. Clinical features and diagnosis of Cushing syndrome are discussed in detail earlier in the section on Cushing syndrome. Symptoms and signs of hormone hypersecretion may be atypical and/or masked due to polypharmacy in older patients. Due to high prevalence of essential hypertension in the older population, diagnosis of subtle cases of hyperfunctioning adrenal masses may be challenging.

B. Laboratory Tests & Imaging Studies

CT characteristics are useful to differentiate lipid-rich adenomas from lipid-poor adrenal nodules. Precontrast enhancement of <10 Hounsfield units (HU) is consistent with benign adenoma and rules out malignant pathology. Precontrast enhancement to >10 HU and <40% contrast washout after 15 minutes are considered indeterminate and could represent lipid-poor adenomas or malignant pathology. Other CT characteristics suggestive for malignancy are large size (>4–6 cm), inhomogeneity, and irregular borders. Precontrast enhancement of less than –20 HU on CT scan is consistent with myelolipoma, and further diagnostic evaluation is not required.

Because patients with functioning adrenal nodules may be asymptomatic and normotensive, each patient should be screened for hormone hypersecretion. Either urine fractionated metanephrines or plasma free metanephrines can be used for screening for pheochromocytomas. Plasma free metanephrines are more sensitive but less specific compared to urine fractionated metanephrines. All patients with hypertension should also be evaluated for hyperaldosteronism. Plasma aldosterone-to-renin ratio (ARR) of >20 is recommended for initial case detection. ARR >20 with plasma aldosterone concentration >10 to 15 ng/dL is suspicious for primary hyperaldosteronism and should be further evaluated by one of the confirmatory tests such as saline infusion, oral sodium loading, or fludrocortisone suppression test. Once diagnosis of primary hyperaldosteronism is confirmed, adrenal venous sampling is recommended in older adults to distinguish bilateral adrenal hyperplasia from unilateral adrenal adenoma as etiology for excess aldosterone production.

FNA of adrenal nodules is usually not indicated because cytology cannot discriminate adrenal cancer from adenoma. FNA can be considered if metastatic adrenal disease is suspected in patients with known diagnosis of cancer. It is advisable to rule out pheochromocytoma through laboratory testing prior to adrenal nodule FNA because biopsy of undiagnosed pheochromocytoma could result in life-threatening complications.

Treatment

Functional adrenal nodules and malignant adrenal nodules are best treated with surgical resection. Most experts also recommend resection of any adrenal mass measuring >4 cm. Patients with pheochromocytoma should be treated medically with α-blockers prior to surgery, whenever possible, to decrease intraoperative and postoperative mortality and morbidity. Medical management with spironolactone is an option for patients with hyperaldosteronism, if potential risks of the surgery outweigh the benefits. Patients with Cushing syndrome due to adrenal mass require hydrocortisone replacement for a short period of time after adrenalectomy until the unaffected adrenal gland returns to normal function. Asymptomatic myelolipomas are followed conservatively and rarely need surgical intervention.

For patients with adrenal adenomas who do not need surgery or who are not good surgical candidates, continued surveillance is recommended. Nonfunctioning benign nodules should undergo repeat biochemical and imaging evaluation at 1 year, but indeterminate nodules should have repeat imaging at 3 to 6 months to reassess the growth.

Prognosis

Laparoscopic adrenalectomy has shown 0.2% mortality at 1 month and a 9% morbidity rate. Morbidity and mortality are greater with pheochromocytoma. Previous open abdominal surgeries in older patients may further complicate laparoscopic surgery. Frail older patients are at higher risk for pulmonary embolism and cardiopulmonary failure. Prognosis is best with benign nonfunctioning adenoma.

Fassnacht M, Arit W, Bancos I, et al. Management of adrenal incidentalomas: European Society of Endocrinology clinical practice guideline in collaboration with the European Network for the study of adrenal tumors. *Eur J Endocrinol.* 2016;175:G1-G34.

Kapoor A, Morris T, Rebello R. Guidelines for the management of the incidentally discovered adrenal mass. *Can Urol Assoc J.* 2011;5:241-247.

Mayo-Smith WW, Song JH, Boland GL, et al. Management of incidental adrenal masses: a white paper of the ACR Incidental Findings Committee. *J Am Coll Radiol.* 2017;14:1038-1044.

Nieman LK. Approach to the patient with an adrenal incidentaloma. *J Clin Endocrinol Metab.* 2010;95(9):4106-4113.

HYPERPARATHYROIDISM

General Principles

Hyperparathyroidism is a common disorder that affects predominantly postmenopausal women, with an incidence of approximately 2 per 1000 women. At least 50% of patients have no or minimal nonspecific symptoms or signs. Although a primary abnormality in one or all of the parathyroid glands may be responsible (primary hyperparathyroidism), suboptimal levels of vitamin D are associated with elevated parathyroid hormone (PTH) levels, although usually with normal or low levels of calcium. PTH concentrations are also influenced by a number of other factors and are higher in older individuals, especially older women; in blacks relative to whites; in those with low calcium; and in obese individuals.

Primary hyperparathyroidism (PHPT) is caused by the inappropriate secretion of PTH, which results in hypercalcemia. The most frequent underlying disease is a single benign parathyroid adenoma. Less commonly, there may be multiple adenomas, or four-gland hyperplasia may be present. With the availability and more widespread usage of PTH assays, normocalcemic hyperparathyroidism is being increasingly identified. In making the diagnosis of normocalcemic hyperparathyroidism, it is critical to exclude other causes of elevated PTH and normal serum calcium (secondary hyperparathyroidism). These individuals may have isolated hypercalciuria and are predisposed to renal calculi.

Secondary hyperparathyroidism (SHPT) is the result of the parathyroid gland's response to hypocalcemia in an attempt to maintain calcium homeostasis. The common causes of SHPT are chronic renal failure, vitamin D insufficiency, malabsorption syndromes, drugs (bisphosphonates, furosemide, anticonvulsants, phosphorus), hypercalciuria caused by renal calcium leak, and pseudohypoparathyroidism type 1b. Tertiary hyperparathyroidism (THPT) occurs because of prolonged hypocalcemia, leading to parathyroid gland hyperplasia and autonomous oversecretion of PTH, resulting in hypercalcemia.

Clinical Findings

A. Symptoms & Signs

The most common clinical circumstance is an unanticipated finding of hypercalcemia during a routine blood test. Mild nonspecific complaints may include fatigue and generalized weakness. CNS symptoms of depression or mild cognitive impairment may be present. Questioning may disclose increased thirst and polyuria thought to be caused by the antagonistic effect of hypercalcemia on the renal action of ADH. A history of renal calculi, fracture, loss of height, and/or disproportionately low-for-age bone mineral density on dual energy x-ray absorptiometry scan call for measurement of serum calcium. In SHPT and THPT, patients may have symptoms from the primary disease process. Even if asymptomatic, PHPT patients with calcium stones and/or nephrocalcinosis are categorized as having symptomatic disease.

B. Laboratory Findings

When serum calcium is minimally or only intermittently increased, measurement of ionized calcium can establish the presence of hypercalcemia. Vitamin D deficiency and insufficiency in patients with PHPT may mask hypercalcemia, and calcium levels will increase in most cases after repletion of vitamin D. It is recommended that 1,25-dihydroxyvitamin D_3 [1,25(OH)2] levels be measured in all patients with PHPT. The diagnosis is confirmed by measuring serum intact PTH and correlating to levels of serum calcium. Levels of PTH are almost always elevated above the upper limit of normal or within the normal range but inappropriately high for the level of hypercalcemia. Renal imaging by ultrasound is recommended if kidney stones are suspected. Serum BUN and creatinine should be measured because SHPT is often found in the presence of renal insufficiency. PTH levels tend to rise steadily with the progression of renal disease. A rise in PTH up to the three-fold normal range is generally accepted as a "physiologic" mechanism of compensating for low 1,25(OH)2, but should revert to normal when vitamin D is repleted.

Once the diagnosis of PHPT is confirmed biochemically, bone mineral density should be measured. Parathyroid adenomas can be localized with a high degree of sensitivity and specificity by means of isotopic scanning with technetium-99m sestamibi. Selective sampling of veins draining the parathyroid glands for step-up in PTH levels can be done in patients who have had previous parathyroid surgery with failure to identify abnormal parathyroid tissue or if the sestamibi scan is nondiagnostic.

Differential Diagnosis

The finding of hypercalcemia along with low-normal or low serum phosphorus levels suggests the diagnosis of PHPT. Elderly patients with renal insufficiency or failure may present with normal or even high phosphorous levels. Other causes of hypercalcemia are usually associated with a lowered level of PTH and include a number of malignancies with or without bone metastases (squamous cell carcinoma of the lung, breast cancer, renal cell carcinoma, multiple myeloma, lymphoma). Hypercalcemia in many of these malignancies may be mediated by tumor-secreted PTH-related protein. Other causes of hypercalcemia include thiazide diuretics, vitamin D toxicity, sarcoidosis, hyperthyroidism, and familial hypocalciuric hypercalcemia (FHH). FHH has traditionally been diagnosed in families by the presence of hypercalcemia and relative hypocalciuria. The calcium-to-creatinine clearance ratio is of particular value and is usually <0.01 in FHH; this ratio is usually >0.01 in typical PHPT. It is important to

ensure that other causes of hypercalcemia and relative hypocalciuria are excluded, including concurrent treatment with thiazide diuretics or lithium.

Treatment

Parathyroidectomy should be offered to patients who meet the criteria for surgery established by the 2008 National Institutes of Health consensus panel (Table 50–3) or who are symptomatic. Older patients are at risk for sudden elevation of serum calcium if they become dehydrated or immobile for whatever reason. The increased risk of fracture in the older woman with significant osteoporosis can be reduced by correction of the hyperparathyroidism. Calcimimetic cinacalcet may be used as a therapeutic trial to determine the effect of lowering serum calcium and the potential benefits of parathyroidectomy in complex cases with significant comorbidity. In the case of parathyroid adenoma, identification and removal of the adenoma will be curative. If parathyroid hyperplasia is found, 3.5 of 4 identified glands must be removed. Intraoperative rapid PTH assay, if available, can confirm that the surgeon has successfully removed the abnormal tissue.

When surgery is not recommended, medical monitoring is critical. Recommended surveillance includes annual measurement of serum calcium and creatinine levels and annual or biannual bone density testing. Vitamin D replacement in patients with suboptimal vitamin D is associated with reductions in serum PTH and has not resulted in further increases in serum calcium. It would be appropriate to consider vitamin D supplementation in all individuals with PHPT if serum levels are <50 nmol/L (20 ng/mL) before making any medical or surgical management decisions. Guidelines for calcium intake should be the same as for patients without PHPT.

Medical options for patients unable to undergo parathyroidectomy include antiresorptive treatments, such as bisphosphonates; raloxifene; and calcimimetic cinacalcet. Several randomized controlled trials have reported that bisphosphonate therapy and estrogen replacement therapy in PHPT decrease bone turnover and increase bone mineral density (BMD), but fracture outcomes have not

Table 50–3. Indications for surgical treatment of primary hyperparathyroidism.

Symptomatic primary hyperparathyroidism
Asymptomatic primary hyperparathyroidism
a. Serum calcium level >1.0 mg/dL (0.25 mmol/L) above the upper limits of normal
b. Creatinine clearance (calculated) reduced to <60 mL/min
c. Bone mineral density with T-score less than −2.5 at any site and/ or previous fragility fracture
d. Patient age <50 years
e. Medical surveillance not desirable or possible

been evaluated. Very limited data are available in regard to the biochemical and skeletal effects of raloxifene in post-menopausal women with PHPT. If skeletal protection is the primary reason for intervention, bisphosphonates are the drug of choice. If present, vitamin D deficiency should be corrected first, as it increases the risk of hypocalcemia with bisphosphonate therapy. Bisphosphonates should be used cautiously in the presence of renal insufficiency. Only cal-cimimetic cinacalcet effectively lowers serum calcium and PTH levels during long-term therapy in PHPT but has not been shown to alter bone turnover or increase BMD. At pres-ent, use of this agent in PHPT is limited to management of symptomatic hypercalcemia in patients who are unable to undergo corrective surgery and in whom bisphosphonates are ineffective or are contraindicated.

Goals of medical management in SHPT are the normal-ization of calcium and skeletal protection. Medical therapy starts with prevention of the development of severe SHPT with close monitoring of serum calcium, phosphate, PTH, and vitamin D_3. Principles of managing SHPT in end-stage renal disease include normalization of hyperphosphatemia, regulation of serum calcium, and lowering PTH secretion (calcitriol and calcimimetic administration). Whenever pos-sible, the underlying cause of SHPT should be treated. THPT should be managed by parathyroidectomy, especially in the presence of severe metabolic bone disease.

Marx SJ. Hyperparathyroid and hypoparathyroid disorders. *N Engl J Med.* 2000;343(25):1863-1875.

Silverberg SJ, Shane E, Jacobs TP, Siris E, Bilezikian JP. A 10-year prospective study of primary hyperparathyroidism with or without parathyroid surgery. *N Engl J Med.* 1999;341(17): 1249-1255.

Wu B, Haigh PI, Hwang R, et al. Underutilization of parathyroid-ectomy in elderly patients with primary hyperparathyroidism. *J Clin Endocrinol Metab.* 2010;95(9):4324-4330.

HYPOPARATHYROIDISM

▶ General Principles

Hypoparathyroidism is rarely diagnosed later in life. The four parathyroid glands produce and secrete PTH. Along with the hormone vitamin D, PTH regulates the body's cal-cium and phosphate levels and activates the conversion of 25-hydroxyvitamin D to 1,25-dihydroxyvitamin D, the active form of vitamin D that stimulates calcium and phosphate absorption in the gastrointestinal tract. When the parathy-roid glands fail to secrete sufficient quantities of PTH, hypo-parathyroidism develops and may result in a low calcium level paired with a high phosphorus level. In patients with hypo-parathyroidism, PTH is either undetectable or inappropriately normal in the setting of low serum calcium levels. This helps to distinguish this entity from pseudohypoparathyroidism, a

rare familial disorder with target tissue resistance to PTH, in which hypocalcemia is associated with hyperphosphatemia and elevated PTH levels.

Hypoparathyroidism can occur sporadically or from a primary disorder caused by a genetic mutation that is auto-somal dominant (Barakat syndrome), autosomal recessive (Wilson disease), or X-linked with or without other poly-glandular failure. Activating mutations of the parathyroid and renal calcium-sensing receptor lead to inhibition of PTH secretion and, hence, hypocalcemia and hypercalciuria. The hypocalcemia is usually mild and asymptomatic and may escape detection until later in life. Autoimmune hypopara-thyroidism may occur in isolation or in patients with one or more other autoimmune disorder, such as autoimmune poly-endocrine syndrome type 1. Idiopathic hypoparathyroidism is an uncommon condition characterized by the absence of, fatty replacement of, or atrophy of the parathyroid glands. It may be familial or sporadic. To diagnose idiopathic hypo-parathyroidism, the following criteria are necessary: low or normal levels of PTH; low serum calcium levels; high serum phosphorous levels; and absence of renal insufficiency, ste-atorrhea, chronic diarrhea, and alkalosis. Rickets and osteo-malacia must also be excluded, and patients must not have recently received a transfusion or chelating agents. While idiopathic or autoimmune hypoparathyroidism is usu-ally diagnosed earlier in life, it may not be diagnosed until maturity is reached and should always be considered if other causes of hypocalcemia have not been identified. With proper treatment, individuals may attain normal levels of serum cal-cium and be able to lead normal lives. Hypoparathyroidism may also occur after injury to or removal of the parathyroid glands during neck surgery, particularly following thyroidec-tomy. This is the most common cause of hypoparathyroid-ism in the elderly. Postsurgical hypoparathyroidism is usually transient, but it can be permanent due to irreversible dam-age to the parathyroid glands or their inadvertent removal. Other possible etiologies of hypoparathyroidism include immune-mediated destruction of parathyroid glands; defec-tive regulation of PTH secretion; activating mutations of cal-cium-sensing receptors; infiltration of the parathyroid glands by iron, copper, amyloid protein, or metastasis; defects in the PTH molecule; reduced parathyroid function due to chemi-cal or drug toxicity; sarcoidosis; radiation or mechanical injury; or infection. Hypoparathyroidism may exist for many years without any clinical signs or symptoms and may only be diagnosed after another condition further lowers the patient's calcium level.

▶ Clinical Findings

A. Symptoms & Signs

Hypocalcemia results whenever there is a net efflux of cal-cium from the extracellular fluid in greater quantities than the intestine or bones can replace. Symptoms are primarily neurologic with the inadequate calcium levels causing hyper-excitability of neuronal membranes. Neurologic symptoms may include an altered mental status, confusion, depression, psychosis, gait disturbances, muscle twitching, paresthesias, tremors, seizures, muscle rigidity, or tetany. Clinical signs of latent tetany may include the Trousseau sign, in which a carpopedal spasm occurs when an inflated blood pressure cuff is left on the arm for several minutes, thereby creating ischemia of the nerves in the upper arm. A Chvostek sign may also be noted due to a contraction of the muscles of the eye, mouth, and nose when one taps on the facial nerve in front of the ear. Tetany may occur with numbness, cramps, carpopedal spasm, laryngeal stridor, and generalized convulsions. Hypocalcemia may also cause cardiac effects including prolongation of the QT interval. Subcapsular cataracts and calcification in areas of the brain may also be noted.

B. Laboratory Findings

Classically, a low ionized serum calcium and elevated serum phosphorus are identified in association with a low PTH level.

▶ Differential Diagnosis

Hypocalcemia is a common occurrence in older persons. Most commonly, it is wrongly assumed based on measurement of total calcium, and the low value reflects low binding proteins. Measurement of ionized calcium is the only accurate way to assess true serum calcium values. That said, many other factors may lower ionized calcium in the elderly other than hypoparathyroidism including vitamin D deficiency; hyperphosphatemia; hungry bone syndrome following successful parathyroidectomy in patients with primary or tertiary hyperparathyroidism; blood transfusions; and magnesium metabolism disorders.

▶ Treatment

It is first essential to make sure true hypocalcemia exists by verifying with a measurement of ionized calcium. Any causative medication should be discontinued and treatment initiated guided by symptoms and the acuity of the hypocalcemia. The main treatment is to use calcium salts and vitamin D. The goal of treatment is to maintain serum calcium levels within normal range with the calcium-phosphate product <55 mg/dL. Patients who have hypoparathyroidism may have hypercalciuria and an increased risk of forming kidney stones with renal complications. This is most common in persons with hypocalcemia due to activating mutations in the calcium-sensing receptor. A 24-hour urine calcium should be monitored at least biannually in these patients, and thiazide should be used when the 24-hour calcium is 250 mg or higher.

Treatment with calcium and vitamin D is recommended in patients with symptoms of hypocalcemia. Patients with chronic hypocalcemia may be asymptomatic or have only subtle symptoms. That said, even an acute mild reduction in serum calcium may precipitate severe symptoms. The presence of severe hypocalcemic symptoms or a prolongation of the QT interval in association with hypocalcemia may warrant hospital admission with consideration of intravenous calcium therapy.

Serum creatinine, serum phosphate, and 24-hour urine calcium should be routinely monitored in patients with hypoparathyroidism. There is no value in monitoring PTH in these patients. Thiazide diuretics and a low-salt diet should be added if 24-hour urine calcium is ≥250 mg to decrease the risk of renal complications. An electrocardiogram is recommended in all patients with hypocalcemia even in the absence of symptoms, and it is important to maintain serum magnesium levels in the normal range because both hypomagnesemia and hypermagnesemia can cause functional hypoparathyroidism.

Unfortunately, hypoparathyroidism is one of the few endocrinopathies for which no hormone replacement therapy has as yet been approved. Two formulations of PTH are currently under investigation and may become standard therapy for hypoparathyroidism in the future.

Cusano NE, Rubin MR, Sliney J Jr, Bilezikian JP. Mini-review: new therapeutic options in hypoparathyroidism. *Endocrine.* 2012;41(3):410-414.

Kant R, Zelesnick B, Saini B, Gambert SR. Hypocalcemia in the older adult: pathophysiology, diagnosis, and treatment. *Clin Geriatr.* 2013;21(4):24-28.

Shoback D. Hypoparathyroidism. *N Engl J Med.* 2008;359(4): 391-403.

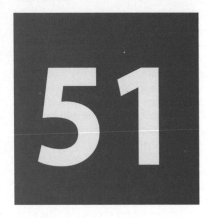

Diabetes

Nami Safai Haeri, MD

Sei Lee, MD, MAS

Audrey K. Chun, MD

ESSENTIALS OF DIAGNOSIS

▶ Hemoglobin A1c ≥6.5, *or*

▶ Fasting (no caloric intake for ≥8 hours) plasma glucose ≥126 mg/dL (7.0 mmol/L), *or*

▶ Symptoms of hyperglycemia plus random plasma glucose ≥200 mg/dL (11.1 mmol/L), *or*

▶ Two-hour plasma glucose ≥200 mg/dL (11.1 mmol/L) during a 75-g oral glucose tolerance test.

General Principles

Diabetes mellitus (DM) is a common condition in older adults and is associated with increased risk of morbidity and mortality. The prevalence of DM (diagnosed and undiagnosed) in the US population of older adults has been estimated at 9.9 million, or 25.2% of people older than age 65 years. If current trends continue, 16.8 million adults older than age 65 will have diabetes by 2050. There are many reasons for the increasing prevalence of diabetes in older adults, including decline in β cell function, increased obesity, lack of physical activity, and loss of muscle mass. Compared to younger people with diabetes, people older than age 65 years tend to have longer duration of diabetes, with a median duration of 10 years, higher rates of diabetic complications and comorbid disease, and more functional dependence.

The population of older adults with diabetes is incredibly diverse. Some older adults have had type 1 diabetes for many decades and reach old age with significant end-organ complications. Others develop insulin resistance and diabetes in their 70s or 80s and have no clear evidence of related complications. Some are able to effectively self-manage their disease, whereas others cannot because of cognitive, visual, or functional impairments. Thus, the management of an older patient with diabetes must account for this tremendous heterogeneity, and decision making should be individualized, focusing on patient factors such as the duration of diabetes, presence of complications, comorbid conditions, life expectancy, patient goals and preferences, and functional abilities.

Boyle JP, Honeycutt AA, Narayan KM, et al. Projection of diabetes burden through 2050: impact of changing demography and disease prevalence in the U.S. *Diabetes Care.* 2001;24(11):1936-1940.

Centers for Disease Control and Prevention (CDC). *National Diabetes Fact Sheet: National Estimates and General Information on Diabetes and Prediabetes in the United States, 2017.* Atlanta, GA: Centers for Disease Control and Prevention US Department of Health and Human Services, 2017.

Pathogenesis

Most patients older than 65 years with diagnosed DM have type 2 DM, and a small minority has type 1 DM. Type 1 DM is an autoimmune disease in which pancreatic β cells are destroyed, resulting in absolute insulinopenia, subsequent hyperglycemia, and risk for ketoacidosis. Exogenous insulin is required for survival and glucose control.

In contrast, type 2 DM results from insulin resistance, increased insulin requirements to maintain euglycemia, and ultimately, relative insulin deficiency when the pancreatic beta cells are unable to meet the higher insulin requirements. Aging is associated with reduced capacity for β-cell regeneration. In older patients, impaired β-cell adaptation to insulin resistance can be the predominant factor in the pathogenesis of type 2 DM.

Saisho Y, Butler AE, Manesso E, Elashoff D, Rizza RA, Butler PC. β-Cell mass and turnover in humans: effects of obesity and aging. *Diabetes Care.* 2013;36:111-117.

Stumvoll M, Goldstein BJ, van Haeften TW. Type 2 diabetes: principles of pathogenesis and therapy. *Lancet.* 2005;365(9467): 1333-1346.

Prevention

Numerous studies show that, for adults with obesity and impaired glucose tolerance who are at high risk for developing type 2 DM, lifestyle modification that focuses on diet, exercise, and weight loss can delay or prevent progression to diabetes. The largest of these trials was the Diabetes Prevention Program (DPP), a nationwide multicenter trial that examined whether metformin or lifestyle modification decreases progression to diabetes in high-risk adults. In older adults (>60 years), lifestyle modification was especially powerful, decreasing the incidence of diabetes 49% compared to usual care in the 10 years of follow-up. Metformin, however, reduced the incidence of diabetes by 18% regardless of age.

Knowler WC, Barrett-Connor E, Fowler SE, et al. Diabetes Prevention Program Research Group. Reduction in the incidence of type 2 diabetes with lifestyle intervention or metformin. *N Engl J Med.* 2002;346(6):393-403.

Saito T, Watanabe M, Nishida J, et al. Zensharen Study for Prevention of Lifestyle Diseases Group. Lifestyle modification and prevention of type 2 diabetes in overweight Japanese with impaired fasting glucose levels: a randomized controlled trial. *Arch Intern Med.* 2011;171(15):1352-1360.

Complications

A. Acute Complications

Acute complications of DM are primarily metabolic and infectious.

Diabetic ketoacidosis (DKA) is characteristic of type 1 DM, but can also occur in type 2 DM, particularly among Hispanic and African American individuals. Insulin deficiency, most commonly a result of inadequate insulin therapy in type 1 DM, leads to decreased glucose metabolism, resulting in increased lipolysis, free fatty acid metabolism, and subsequent ketoacidosis. Common precipitating factors for DKA, such as pneumonia, myocardial infarction, and stroke, contribute to DKA by invoking a systemic stress response with increased cortisol, glucagon, and catecholamines that counteracts some of the effects of insulin. Typically, patients present with symptoms of dyspnea, acidosis, dehydration, abdominal pain, nausea, and vomiting. Mental status alteration and coma may be present. Effective management focuses on identifying and treating the precipitating factors as well as treating the metabolic derangements with insulin and volume repletion.

Hyperglycemic hyperosmolar state occurs predominantly in older patients with type 2 DM and results in marked hyperglycemia (often glucose >600 mg/dL), hyperosmolarity, severe volume depletion, and associated acute kidney injury. Patients typically have a several-week history of hyperglycemia and osmotic diuresis, leading to dehydration and altered mental status. As with DKA, precipitating factors include serious infection, stroke, and myocardial infarction. Besides identifying and treating the precipitating condition, volume resuscitation with fluids can lead to rapid, dramatic improvements in hyperglycemia and hyperosmolarity. Mental status alterations often take longer to normalize.

Older patients with diabetes are at increased risk of infections. Hyperglycemia is associated with worse outcomes in common infections such as pneumonia, and diabetes is a potent risk factor for unusual infections such as malignant otitis externa that are uncommon in patients without diabetes. A number of causes for increased infection risk have been proposed, including impaired immune function caused by decreased neutrophil chemotaxis, phagocytosis, and opsonization. Lower extremity soft-tissue and bone infections are common, because of vascular insufficiency and repeated trauma that is unrecognized by the patient as a result of neuropathy. Urinary tract infections are more common in patients with diabetes because of glucosuria and urinary retention from autonomic neuropathy.

Kitabchi AE, Umpierrez GE, Miles JM, Fisher JN. Hyperglycemic crises in adult patients with diabetes. *Diabetes Care.* 2009;32(7):1335-1343.

Rajagopalan S. Serious infections in elderly patients with diabetes mellitus. *Clin Infect Dis.* 2005;40(7):990-996.

B. Chronic Complications

Older adults are at high risk for all of the chronic complications of diabetes seen in younger adults including microvascular (retinopathy, neuropathy, and nephropathy) and macrovascular disease (coronary artery disease, stroke, and peripheral vascular disease). Because vascular pathology plays a central role in diabetes-related complications, prevention and treatment should focus on vascular risk factors, such as smoking cessation, and blood pressure, lipid, and glycemic control.

1. Macrovascular complications—Cardiovascular disease (CVD) is the major cause of morbidity and mortality for older adults with diabetes. Diabetes imparts a two-fold risk in coronary heart disease and stroke and increases the risk of amputation 10-fold. Diabetes often co-occurs with other CVD risk factors, such as hypertension and hyperlipidemia, and studies suggest a multifaceted approach addressing multiple risk factors is most effective in decreasing cardiovascular risk. Currently, the American Diabetes Association (ADA) recommends aspirin (75–162 mg/day) for patients with diabetes and known CVD. Furthermore, the ADA also recommends consideration of high-intensity statin therapy in all patients with diabetes and CVD, and moderate intensity statin therapy in older adults with diabetes but without CVD. Blood pressure target in patients with diabetes and lower risk for CVD (10-year risk <15%) is <140/90 mm Hg, and in patients with higher risk for CVD (10-year risk >15%), it is < 130/80 mm Hg. For frail older adults at higher risk for complications of treatment such as orthostatic hypotension, less aggressive goals may be more appropriate.

American Diabetes Association. Standards of medical care in diabetes—2019. *Diabetes Care.* 2019;42(suppl 1):S103-S123.

2. Microvascular complications: retinopathy—Diabetes is a leading cause of blindness in the United States. Early detection and treatment of proliferative retinopathy with laser photocoagulation have been shown to decrease the risk of visual loss by >50% at 6 years. Further, because visual compromise is insidious, most patients do not recognize declining visual acuity, and regular screening to detect retinopathy at an early, treatable stage is especially important. The ADA currently recommends a dilated eye exam by an ophthalmologist at diagnosis, with regular follow-up exams every 1 to 2 years, depending on the individual patient's risk factors and initial exam results. In addition to retinopathy, older patients with diabetes also have a two-fold risk of cataracts and a three-fold risk of glaucoma compared to older patients without diabetes.

Solomon SD, Chew E, Duh EJ, Sobrin L, Sun JK, VanderBeek BL, Wykoff CC, Gardner TW. Erratum. Diabetic retinopathy: a position statement by the American Diabetes Association. *Diabetes Care.* 2017;40:412-418. *Diabetes Care.* 2017;40(9):1285.

3. Microvascular complications: neuropathy—Diabetic neuropathy is generally classified by the types of nerves that are affected. The most common type of neuropathy is the sensory distal symmetric polyneuropathy, or "glove-and-stocking" neuropathy. Common symptoms include numbness and burning pain of the hands and feet. Because sensory neuropathy predisposes patients to unrecognized lower extremity trauma, which can ultimately progress to infection and amputation, annual screening with a 10-g monofilament at the plantar aspect of the hallux and metatarsal joint is recommended. Autonomic diabetic neuropathies include diabetic gastroparesis, which can cause nausea and vomiting after eating as a result of impaired gastric emptying, as well as erectile dysfunction and neurogenic bladder. Unlike many other microvascular complications, diabetic gastroparesis can improve quickly and dramatically with improved glycemic control.

Pop-Busui R, Boulton AH, Feldman EL, et al. Diabetic neuropathy: a position statement by the American Diabetes Association. *Diabetes Care.* 2017;40(1):136-154.

4. Microvascular complications: nephropathy—Diabetic nephropathy is the most common cause of end-stage renal disease and is strongly associated with cardiovascular mortality. Diabetic nephropathy is also more common in older diabetic patients than younger patients; however, the association between severity of nephropathy and mortality appears to be weaker in older adults. Compared to other common causes of kidney disease, diabetic nephropathy leads to more albuminuria and less early declines in glomerular filtration rate. This is reflected in the diagnostic criteria for diabetic nephropathy, which is albuminuria >300 g/day in a patient with known diabetes without other potential causes of albuminuria. Many studies have shown that treatment with angiotensin-converting enzyme inhibitors or angiotensin receptor blockers slows the progression of diabetic nephropathy and decreases the risk of cardiovascular events. Thus, the ADA recommends annual screening for microalbuminuria, which can be accomplished by measuring the urinary albumin-to-creatinine ratio on a spot urine specimen.

Tuttle KR, Bakris GL, Bilous RW, et al. Diabetic kidney disease: a report from an ADA Consensus Conference. *Diabetes Care.* 2014;37(10):2864-2883.

C. Geriatric Syndromes

Geriatric syndromes are common, serious conditions in older adults that often present similarly in different patients despite disparate causes. For example, delirium may present as an acute confusional state with a fluctuating level of consciousness in patients with urinary tract infections as well as a myocardial infarction. DM appears to increase the risk of many geriatric syndromes, including cognitive impairment, depression, urinary incontinence, falls, and functional decline.

American Geriatrics Society Expert Panel on Care of Older Adults with Diabetes Mellitus, Moreno G, Mangione CM, et al. Guidelines abstracted from the American Geriatrics Society Guidelines for improving the care of older adults with diabetes mellitus: 2013 update. *J Am Geriatr Soc.* 2013;61(11):2020-2026.

Araki A, Ito H. Diabetes mellitus and geriatric syndromes. *Geriatr Gerontol Int.* 2009;9(2):105-114.

1. Cognitive impairment—In epidemiologic studies, DM appears to increase the subsequent risk of Alzheimer dementia by 50% to 100% and vascular dementia by 100% to 150%. This could be due to the role of insulin in glucose metabolism and also its effect on modulation of acetylcholine and other neurotransmitters in the brain. Although some studies suggest that poor glycemic control and hyperglycemia may lead to elevated risk of dementia, there is also evidence that hypoglycemia may increase the risk of subsequent dementia.

Cognitive impairment is an especially important comorbidity in patients with diabetes, because patient activation and self-management is a cornerstone of effective diabetes treatment. Patients with even mild cognitive impairment may be less able to manage their diet, exercise, and medication regimen and less able to identify symptoms of early hypoglycemia. Thus, the American Geriatrics Society (AGS) recommends screening for cognitive impairment during the initial evaluation of the older adult with diabetes and repeating the screening if increased difficulty with self-care or self-management is suspected.

Biessels GJ, Staekenborg S, Brunner E, Brayne C, Scheltens P. Risk of dementia in diabetes mellitus: a systematic review. *Lancet Neurol.* 2006;5(1):64-74.

Munshi MN. Cognitive dysfunction in older adults with diabetes: what a clinician needs to know. *Diabetes Care.* 2017;40(4): 461-467.

2. Depression

Depression is a common condition in older adults and is associated with adverse outcomes, including poor health-related quality of life, functional decline, and increased all-cause mortality. Diabetes and depression commonly co-occur, with 30% of older adults with diabetes reporting depressive symptoms and 5% to 10% of older adults with diabetes meeting criteria for major depressive disorder. Like cognitive impairment, depression may interfere with an older adult's ability to self-manage their diabetes care, leading to worse diabetes control. Thus, the AGS recommends screening for depressive symptoms with a validated instrument. Repeat screening may be warranted if an older patient with diabetes has new difficulty with self-management.

Kimbro LB, Mangione CM, Steers WN, et al. Depression and all-cause mortality in persons with diabetes mellitus: are older adults at higher risk? Results from the Translating Research Into Action for Diabetes Study. *J Am Geriatr Soc.* 2014;62:1017-1022.

Wu CY, Terhorst L, Karp JF, Skidmore ER, Rodakowski J. Trajectory of disability in older adults with newly diagnosed diabetes: role of elevated depressive symptoms. *Diabetes Care.* 2018;41(10):2072-2078.

3. Urinary incontinence

Urinary incontinence is very common in older women with diabetes, with studies reporting a prevalence of >50%. Studies suggest a strong relationship between DM and urinary incontinence, with diabetes associated with a three-fold increased prevalence of urge incontinence and a two-fold increased prevalence of stress incontinence. Body mass index appears to be an important risk factor for incontinence, and weight loss reduces the incidence of new incontinence. Some studies have suggested poor glycemic control may lead to worse incontinence through glycosuria. Very little data exist for incontinence in older men with diabetes.

Brown JS, Wing R, Barrett-Connor E, et al; Diabetes Prevention Program Research Group. Lifestyle intervention is associated with lower prevalence of urinary incontinence: the Diabetes Prevention Program. *Diabetes Care.* 2006;29(2):385-390.

Wang R, Lefevre R, Hacker MR, Golen TH. Diabetes, glycemic control, and urinary incontinence in women. *Female Pelvic Med Reconstr Surg.* 2015;21(5):293-297.

4. Falls and fractures

Falls are common in older adults and associated with increased morbidity and mortality. Overweight patients are more likely to have a higher bone mass and diabetes, leading some to initially hypothesize that patients with diabetes may be less susceptible to injurious falls. However, subsequent studies have shown nearly a two-fold increased risk of injurious falls in older adults with diabetes compared to older adults without diabetes. Insulin use, poor vision, and peripheral neuropathy appear to further increase the risk of falls. The AGS recommends screening for falls risk in older adults with diabetes to identify potentially modifiable risk factors for falls and fractures.

Schwartz AV, Vittinghoff E, Sellmeyer DE, et al. Diabetes-related complications, glycemic control, and falls in older adults. *Diabetes Care.* 2008;31(3):391-396.

Vinik AI, Camacho P, Reddy S, et al. Aging, diabetes, and falls. *Endocr Pract.* 2017;23(9):1117-1139.

5. Functional decline

Functional limitations are strongly associated with quality of life, as well as mortality and nursing home admission. Diabetes increases the risk of functional limitations, with increased rates of difficulty with activities of daily living (bathing, transferring, toileting, dressing, and eating), as well as walking and shopping. The association between diabetes and functional limitations persisted even after accounting for other chronic conditions.

Sinclair AJ, Conroy SP, Bayer AJ. Impact of diabetes on physical function in older people. *Diabetes Care.* 2008;31(2):233-235.

► Treatment

A. Glycemic Treatment

Hyperglycemia is the core pathologic finding in DM, and control of hyperglycemia is a cornerstone of diabetes treatment. However, it is important to recognize that blood pressure control and lipid control appear to be as important (if not more important) in preventing and minimizing most end-organ complications of diabetes. Thus, when prioritizing interventions in medically complex older adults with diabetes, focusing first on blood pressure is a reasonable approach in most patients.

1. Glycemic control targets—Hemoglobin A1c (HbA1c) has been shown to correlate closely with average glucose levels and is strongly predictive of microvascular complications. A reasonable rule of thumb is that each 1% increase or decrease in HbA1c is equivalent to a corresponding approximately 30 mg/dL change in average glucose levels, as shown in Table 51–1.

The goals of glycemic treatment differ in healthy and frail older patients, resulting in different recommended glycemic targets. Studies suggest that tight glycemic control to HbA1c

Table 51–1. Change in average glucose level by HbA1c.

HbA1c (%)	Average Glucose in mg/dL (95% CI)
5	97 (76–120)
6	126 (100–152)
7	154 (123–185)
8	183 (147–217)
9	212 (170–249)
10	240 (193–282)
11	269 (217–314)
12	298 (240–347)

HbA1c, hemoglobin A1c.

≤7% decreases the rates of microvascular complications over 8 years. Thus, the ADA recommends HbA1c <7% for healthy older adults with an extended life expectancy.

However, tighter glycemic control has also been associated with increased rates of hypoglycemia and mortality. For older patients with limited life expectancy, tight glycemic control exposes them to a higher risk of adverse events with little chance that they would survive to benefit from decreases in microvascular complications. Because very poor glycemic control can lead to immediate symptoms such as fatigue, older patients with limited life expectancy should receive glycemic treatment that is aimed at avoiding symptomatic hyperglycemia while minimizing the risk of hypoglycemia. A recent guideline from the AGS suggests an HbA1c target of 7.5% to 8% for older adults. For older adults who are healthy, with a few chronic conditions, few functional limitations, and extended life expectancy, HbA1c target of 7% to 7.5% is appropriate. Conversely, for older adults with extensive comorbidities, functional limitations, and limited life expectancy, HbA1c target of 8% to 9% is appropriate (Table 51–2).

Table 51–2. Guideline recommendations for HbA1c targets for older patients with limited life expectancy.[a]

	Year	HbA1c Target
American Diabetes Association (ADA)	2019	8.0–8.5
American Geriatrics Society (AGS)	2013	8.0–9.0
Veterans Affairs and Department of Defense (VA/DoD)	2017	8.0–9.0

HbA1c, hemoglobin A1c.

[a]Multiple coexisting chronic conditions or functional or cognitive impairment.

American Geriatrics Society Expert Panel on Care of Older Adults with Diabetes Mellitus, Moreno G, Mangione CM, Kimbro L, Vaisberg E. Guidelines abstracted from the American Geriatrics Society guidelines for improving the care of older adults with diabetes mellitus: 2013 update. *J Am Geriatr Soc.* 2013;61(11):2020-2026.

Davies MJ, D'Alessio DA, Fradkin J, et al. Management of hyperglycemia in type 2 diabetes, 2018. A consensus report by the American Diabetes Association (ADA) and the European Association for the Study of Diabetes (EASD). *Diabetes Care.* 2018;41(12):2669-2701.

Lee SJ, Eng C. Goals of glycemic control in frail older patients with diabetes. *JAMA.* 2011;305(13):1350-1351.

Management of Diabetes Mellitus Update Working Group. *VA/DoD Clinical Practice Guideline for the Management of Type 2 Diabetes Mellitus in Primary Care. Version 5.0.* Washington, DC: Veterans Health Administration and Department of Defense; 2017.

Nathan DM, Kuenen J, Borg R, Zheng H, Schoenfeld D, Heine RJ; A1c-Derived Average Glucose Study Group. Translating the A1c assay into estimated average glucose values. *Diabetes Care.* 2008;31(8):1473-1478.

Ray KK, Seshasai SR, Wijesuriya S, et al. Effect of intensive control of glucose on cardiovascular outcomes and death in patients with diabetes mellitus: a meta-analysis of randomised controlled trials. *Lancet.* 2009;373(9677):1765-1772.

2. Glycemic control targets in hospitalized patients— Many older patients with diabetes are admitted to the hospital, most often for conditions other than diabetes. The goals for glycemic control in older hospitalized patients are to maintain euglycemia, avoid adverse events, and return to a stable outpatient regimen as soon as feasible. However, the stress of acute illness and frequent preprocedural fasting can make maintaining euglycemia challenging in hospitalized patients.

Although initial studies suggested improved outcomes in critically ill surgical patients with tight glycemic control (glucose levels of 80–110 mg/dL), subsequent studies have shown that tighter glycemic control is associated with more risk for hypoglycemia and does not improve outcomes such as death from any cause, length of hospital stay, and cardiovascular and infectious complications. The ADA recommends glucose levels between 140 and 180 mg/dL in both critically ill and noncritically ill patients.

American Diabetes Association. Diabetes Care in the Hospital: Standards of Medical Care in Diabetes—2019. *Diabetes Care.* 2019;42(suppl 1):S173-S181.

Buchleitner AM, Martínez-Alonso M, Hernández M, Solà I, Mauricio D. Perioperative glycaemic control for diabetic patients undergoing surgery. *Cochrane Database Syst Rev.* 2012;9:CD007315.

Moghissi ES, Korytkowski MT, DiNardo M, et al. American Association of Clinical Endocrinologists; American Diabetes Association. American Association of Clinical Endocrinologists and American Diabetes Association consensus statement on inpatient glycemic control. *Diabetes Care.* 2009;32(6):1119-1131.

3. Glycemic control in long-term care (LTC) patients—There is high prevalence of DM in nursing home facilities, and DM is associated with remarkable increase in geriatrics syndromes and health care costs. Risk of hypoglycemia is the major factor in determining targets for glycemic control, as many of these patients have higher risk for hypoglycemia due to their multimorbidities and polypharmacy. For residents in LTC, an HbA1c target of 8% to 9% and fasting blood sugar between 100 and 200 mg/dL are reasonable. A basal/bolus insulin regimen is preferred in this population, and guidelines discourage sole use of sliding scale insulin as it may lead to wide fluctuations of blood glucose.

Munshi MN, Florez H, Huang ES, et al. Management of diabetes in long-term care and skilled nursing facilities: a position statement of the American Diabetes Association. *Diabetes Care.* 2016;39(2):308-318.

Pandya N, Thompson S, Sambamoorthi U. The prevalence and persistence of sliding scale insulin use among newly admitted elderly nursing home residents with diabetes mellitus. *J Am Med Dir Assoc.* 2008;9(9):663-669.

4. Glycemic control in patients at end of life—Management of DM at the end of life needs to emphasize providing care focused on comfort by relaxing glycemic goals, avoiding hypoglycemia or symptomatic hyperglycemia, and simplifying complex regimens. For patients nearing the end of life, there is little benefit to monitor HbA1c. Since the decline preceding death often includes anorexia, weight loss, and worsening renal function, it is often necessary to decrease glucose-lowering therapies to avoid hypoglycemia. Anticipatory guidance to patients and families about reducing glucose-lowering therapies should begin as the patient declines and at hospice enrollment.

Lee SJ, Jacobson MA, Johnston CB. Improving diabetes care for hospice patients. *Am J Hosp Palliat Care.* 2016;33(6):517-519.

Munshi MN, Florez H, Huang ES, et al. Management of diabetes in long-term care and skilled nursing facilities: a position statement of the American Diabetes Association. *Diabetes Care.* 2016;39(2):308-318.

B. Nonpharmacologic Treatments

1. Diet—Dietary intervention is an integral component of diabetes treatment. A recommended lifestyle intervention for the appropriate patients with DM is caloric restriction with the goal of at least 7% loss of body weight. A wide variety of diets with varying macronutrient (carbohydrates, proteins, fats) proportions have been studied, but there are few data to suggest one diet is superior to another. Current ADA dietary recommendations mirror the American Heart Association recommendations and suggest (1) limiting saturated fat (<7% of total calories), (2) minimizing trans fats, and (3) limiting cholesterol intake (<200 mg/day). Medical nutritional therapy provided by a registered dietician is a covered Medicare benefit.

It is important to recognize that for some older adults with diabetes, caloric or dietary restriction may be especially difficult or even harmful. First, changes in diet may be especially challenging for older patients who have established dietary habits over a lifetime. Second, older adults with functional difficulties who have difficulty shopping for groceries and preparing food are at risk for undernutrition; recommending a restricted range of foods may lead to weight loss or micronutrient deficiencies. Third, older adults with diabetes are at higher risk for periodontal disease and xerostomia, which may limit their ability to adapt to a new diet. Fourth, for many older adults, presence of multimorbidity may lead to even more restrictions in dietary options. Thus, dietary modifications should be approached with caution in older patients who have diabetes without obesity.

Klein S, Sheard NF, Pi-Sunyer X, et al. American Diabetes Association; North American Association for the Study of Obesity; American Society for Clinical Nutrition. Weight management through lifestyle modification for the prevention and management of type 2 diabetes: rationale and strategies: a statement of the American Diabetes Association, the North American Association for the Study of Obesity, and the American Society for Clinical Nutrition. *Diabetes Care.* 2004;27(8):2067-2073.

2. Exercise—Regular exercise has been shown to improve glycemic control, blood pressure, and lipids and contribute to weight loss. The ADA recommends that older adults with diabetes should strive to achieve 150 minutes per week of moderate-intensity exercise including both aerobic activity and resistance training. For older patients with functional impairments who are unable to accomplish this, the ADA recommends maximizing their physical activity to reap some of the benefits of exercise. Because older patients with diabetes are at high risk for CVD, exercise regimens should start with low-intensity physical activity and gradually increase in intensity and duration.

Colberg SR, Sigal RJ, Fernhall B, et al. American College of Sports Medicine; American Diabetes Association. Exercise and type 2 diabetes: the American College of Sports Medicine and the American Diabetes Association: joint position statement executive summary. *Diabetes Care.* 2010;33(12):2692-2696.

C. Pharmacologic Therapy (Table 51–3)

1. Biguanides—Most guidelines recommend metformin as first-line oral therapy for type 2 DM because it is efficacious (decreasing HbA1c approximately 1.5%) and is not associated with weight gain or hypoglycemia. In addition, metformin appears to be associated with decreased cardiovascular complications compared to sulfonylureas. Large registry-based observational data suggest that patients taking metformin were at 15% to 21% decreased hazard of cardiovascular complications compared to patients taking glyburide or glipizide. Furthermore, a 5-year randomized trial showed 46% decreased risk of cardiovascular outcomes in patients treated with metformin versus glipizide.

Table 51-3. Noninsulin therapies for hyperglycemia.

Class	Drug	Action	Expected Decrease in HbA1c (%)	Advantages	Disadvantages	Cost
Biguanides	Metformin	Decrease hepatic glucose production	1–2	No weight gain No hypoglycemia Decreased cardiovascular mortality	Nausea, diarrhea Lactic acidosis (rare)	$
Sulfonylureas	Glyburide Glipizide Gliclazide Glimepiride	Stimulate insulin secretion	1–2	Generally well tolerated	Hypoglycemia (especially with glyburide) Weight gain	$
Meglitinides	Repaglinide Nateglinide	Stimulate insulin secretion	1–2	Decrease postprandial hyperglycemia	Hypoglycemia Weight gain Frequent preprandial dosing	$$
α-Glucosidase inhibitors	Acarbose Miglitol	Decrease intestinal carbohydrate absorption	0.5–1	Not absorbed, limiting possibility of drug-drug interactions	Gastrointestinal side effects	$$
Thiazolidinediones	Pioglitazone Rosiglitazone	Increase peripheral insulin sensitivity	1–2	Little hypoglycemia	Weight gain Heart failure exacerbation Increased fractures	$$$
GLP-1 agonists	Exenatide Liraglutide Dulaglutide Lixisenatide Semaglutide	Increase glucose-dependent insulin secretion Delay gastric emptying	1–2	Weight loss Improve cardiovascular risk factors	Nausea, vomiting, diarrhea Acute pancreatitis Medullary thyroid carcinoma	$$$
DPP-4 inhibitors	Sitagliptin Saxagliptin Linagliptin Alogliptin	Accentuates GLP-1 activity Decrease glucagon	0.5–1	No weight gain No hypoglycemia	Acute pancreatitis Modest potency May be associated with severe joint pain Increased hospitalization for decompensated heart failure (saxagliptin)	$$$
Amylin mimetics	Pramlintide	Delays gastric emptying Promotes satiety Decreases postprandial glucagon secretion	0.5	Generally well tolerated Weight loss	Frequent injections Gastrointestinal side effects Cannot be mixed with insulin	$$$
SGLT-2 inhibitors	Canagliflozin Dapagliflozin Empagliflozin Ertugliflozin	Blocks renal glucose reabsorption	0.5–1	No hypoglycemia Weight loss Decrease in blood pressure and cardiovascular risks	Increased urogenital infections Hypotension Increased risk for amputation and fracture with canagliflozin	$$$

Severe renal dysfunction (creatinine clearance <30 mL/min/1.73 m²) has been a contraindication to metformin because of the concern for lactic acidosis. However, lactic acidosis appears to be exceedingly rare with metformin, with an incidence of <1 per 10,000 person-years of treatment.

Davies MJ, D'Alessio DA, Fradkin J, et al. Management of hyperglycemia in type 2 diabetes, 2018. A consensus report by the American Diabetes Association (ADA) and the European Association for the Study of Diabetes (EASD). *Diabetes Care.* 2018;41(12):2669-2701.

Hong J, Zhang Y, Lai S, et al. SPREAD-DIMCAD Investigators. Effects of metformin versus glipizide on cardiovascular outcomes in patients with type 2 diabetes and coronary artery disease. *Diabetes Care.* 2013;36(5):1304-1311.

Maruthur NM, Tseng E, Hutfless S, et al. Diabetes medications as monotherapy or metformin-based combination therapy for type 2 diabetes: a systematic review and meta-analysis. *Ann Intern Med.* 2016;164(11):740-751.

Qaseem A, Barry MJ, Humphrey LL, Forciea MA; Clinical Guidelines Committee of the American College of Physicians.

Oral pharmacologic treatment of type 2 diabetes mellitus: a clinical practice guideline update from the American College of Physicians. *Ann Intern Med.* 2017;166(4):279-290.

2. Sulfonylureas

2. Sulfonylureas—The commonly used sulfonylureas include glipizide, glyburide, glimepiride, and gliclazide. Because sulfonylureas act predominantly by increasing pancreatic insulin secretion, weight gain is common and hypoglycemia may occur. Studies suggest that the risk of hypoglycemia is 1.5 to 2 times higher with glyburide than other sulfonylureas, possibly as a result of active metabolites; thus, glyburide should be avoided in older adults. Generally, most of the therapeutic effect occurs with half of the maximum recommended dose, and sulfonylureas can reduce HbA1c by 1% to 2%. Starting doses should be low, perhaps half that used for younger patients, and education regarding hypoglycemia provided. Sulfonylureas should be used with caution in patients with kidney disease since active metabolites are excreted slowly. Increased risk of hypoglycemia and growing evidence for poor cardiovascular outcomes make sulfonylureas a less desirable choice compared with other hypoglycemic agents.

Azoulay L, Suissa S. Sulfonylureas and the risks of cardiovascular events and death: a methodological meta-regression analysis of the observational studies. *Diabetes Care.* 2017;40(5):706-714.

Bain S, Druyts E, Balijepalli C, et al. Cardiovascular events and all-cause mortality associated with sulphonylureas compared with other antihyperglycaemic drugs: a Bayesian meta-analysis of survival data. *Diabetes Obes Metab.* 2017;19(3):329-335.

3. α-Glucosidase inhibitors

3. α-Glucosidase inhibitors—The α-glucosidase inhibitors, acarbose and miglitol, inhibit the absorption of carbohydrates in the gut and decrease postprandial hyperglycemia. Consequently, they do not cause hypoglycemia or weight gain. Because α-glucosidase inhibitors are not systemically absorbed at usual doses (especially acarbose), they generally can be safely used in older adults and in patients with either renal or hepatic insufficiency. The primary drawbacks of α-glucosidase inhibitors are gastrointestinal discomfort, including flatulence and diarrhea, and lower reduction of HbA1c by approximately 0.5% to 1%.

Sherifali D, Nerenberg K, Pullenayegum E, Cheng JE, Gerstein HC. The effect of oral antidiabetic agents on A1C levels: a systematic review and meta-analysis. *Diabetes Care.* 2010;33(8):1859-1864.

4. Thiazolidinediones

4. Thiazolidinediones—The thiazolidinediones rosiglitazone and pioglitazone act as insulin sensitizers. Thiazolidinediones have fallen out of favor as mounting evidence suggests increased heart failure, bone loss, and hepatotoxicity, especially with rosiglitazone, and bladder cancer with pioglitazone.

Home PD, Pocock SJ, Beck-Nielsen H, et al; RECORD Study Team. Rosiglitazone evaluated for cardiovascular outcomes in oral agent combination therapy for type 2 diabetes (RECORD): a multicenter, randomised, open-label trial. *Lancet.* 2009;373(9681):2125-2135.

Nissen SE, Wolski K. Rosiglitazone revisited: an updated meta-analysis of risk for myocardial infarction and cardiovascular mortality. *Arch Intern Med.* 2010;170(14):1191-1201.

Zhu ZN, Jiang YF, Ding T. Risk of fracture with thiazolidinediones: an updated meta-analysis of randomized clinical trials. *Bone.* 2014;68:115-123.

5. Meglitinides

5. Meglitinides—Meglitinides are short-acting insulin secretagogues that can decrease postprandial hyperglycemia. Repaglinide and nateglinide are the meglitinides available in the United States. Nateglinide appears to have a faster onset and shorter duration of action than repaglinide. There is limited experience with these drugs in older adults, but they may be effective for patients with fasting euglycemia and postprandial hyperglycemia. Both medications should be taken before each meal, which may make medication adherence more difficult.

Black C, Donnelly P, McIntyre L, Royle PL, Shepherd JP, Thomas S. Meglitinide analogues for type 2 diabetes mellitus. *Cochrane Database Syst Rev.* 2007;2:CD004654.

6. Incretin modulators: glucagon-like peptide-1 (GLP-1) analog and dipeptidyl peptidase-4 (DPP-4) inhibitors

6. Incretin modulators: glucagon-like peptide-1 (GLP-1) analog and dipeptidyl peptidase-4 (DPP-4) inhibitors—Incretins, such as GLP-1 and DPP-4, are gastrointestinal hormones that modulate postprandial glucose homeostasis. Incretin modulators can decrease postprandial hyperglycemia by increasing glucose-dependent insulin secretion and slowing gastric emptying. Although these medications do not cause hypoglycemia when used alone, they may aggravate hypoglycemia when used with insulin or sulfonylureas.

Exenatide, liraglutide, dulaglutide, lixisenatide, and semaglutide are the injectable GLP-1 analogs available in the United States. Exenatide is a synthetic analog of exendin-4, a component of Gila monster saliva. Exendin-4 is structurally similar to GLP-1 (which decreases postprandial hyperglycemia) but is resistant to DPP-4 degradation, leading to more prolonged action. GLP-1 analogs appear to decrease HbA1c by approximately 1% to 2%. Liraglutide and semaglutide have been associated with improved cardiovascular benefits. Because of delayed gastric emptying, nausea and weight loss are common.

Sitagliptin, saxagliptin, linagliptin, and alogliptin are the DPP-4 inhibitors available in the United States. They lead to HbA1c decreases of approximately 0.5% to 1%. They are generally well tolerated, with less nausea and weight loss than GLP-1 analogs. Acute pancreatitis is a rare but serious complication. Some of these agents have been associated with increased heart failure in older adults.

LeRoith D, Biessels GJ, Braithwaite SS, et al. Treatment of diabetes in older adults: an Endocrine Society clinical practice guideline. *J Clin Endocrinol Metab.* 2019;104(5):1520-1574.

Marso SP, Daniels GH, Brown-Frandsen K, et al. Liraglutide and cardiovascular outcomes in type 2 diabetes. *N Engl J Med.* 2016;375(4):311-322.

Shyangdan DS, Royle P, Clar C, Sharma P, Waugh N, Snaith A. Glucagon-like peptide analogues for type 2 diabetes mellitus. *Cochrane Database Syst Rev.* 2011;10:CD006423.

7. Sodium-glucose cotransporter 2 (SGLT2) inhibitors—SGLT2 inhibitors such as canagliflozin, dapagliflozin, empagliflozin, and ertugliflozin are oral medications that reduce renal reabsorption of glucose by enhancing its urinary excretion. Efficacy of SGLT2 inhibitors is highly dependent on patients' renal function. As the renal function worsens, these medications become less effective. All SGLT2 inhibitors are associated with decrease in weight, blood pressure, and cardiovascular risks. The primary drawbacks of these drugs include increased risk for acute kidney injury, dehydration, hypotension, and urogenital infections. In some studies, canagliflozin has been associated with increased risk for fracture and lower limb amputation. SGLT2 inhibitors can reduce HbA1c by 0.5% to 1%.

Neal B, Perkovic V, Mahaffey KW, et al; CANVAS Program Collaborative Group. Canagliflozin and cardiovascular and renal events in type 2 diabetes. *N Engl J Med.* 2017;377(7):644-657.

Wu JH, Foote C, Blomster J, et al. Effects of sodium-glucose cotransporter-2 inhibitors on cardiovascular events, death, and major safety outcomes in adults with type 2 diabetes: a systematic review and meta-analysis. *Lancet Diabetes Endocrinol.* 2016;4(5):411-419. Erratum in: *Lancet Diabetes Endocrinol.* 2016;4(9):e9.

8. Insulin—Insulin is required in all patients with type 1 diabetes and in many patients with moderate or severe type 2 diabetes. There is more than 80 years of clinical experience with insulin. With proper dosing, it can be used safely in cases of renal or hepatic insufficiency, as well as in the hospital, nursing home, or ambulatory care settings. Disadvantages of insulin include the risk of hypoglycemia, weight gain, and patient psychological barriers to injection.

Different types of insulin have been developed to provide flexible treatment options for different patterns of hyperglycemia (Table 51–4). Commonly used longer-acting insulins include glargine, degludec, detemir, and neutral protamine Hagedorn (NPH), which are used once or twice daily, to provide basal insulin for control of fasting glucose levels. Commonly used shorter-acting insulins such as lispro, aspart, glulisine, and regular and inhaled insulin are used before meals to provide bolus insulin to control postprandial glucose levels. For many older patients with type 2 diabetes, once-daily long-acting insulin at nighttime, often in addition to metformin, may be a reasonable starting regimen.

Starting dose for basal insulin is 0.1 to 0.2 units/kg/day depending on the level of hyperglycemia. In most cases, titration of basal insulin is based on fasting blood glucose levels. Patients with persistent elevation in their HbA1c despite

Table 51–4. Commonly used insulin products in the United States.

Type	Onset of Action	Peak Action	Duration	Cost
Aspart	15 min	30–90 min	3–5 h	$$
Glulisine	15 min	30-90 min	3–4 h	$$
Inhaled insulin	15 min	30-90 min	3–4 h	$$
Lispro	15 min	30–90 min	3–4 h	$$
Regular	30–60 min	2–3 h	4–6 h	$
NPH	2–4 h	6–10 h	10–16 h	$
Detemir	1–2 h	Minimal	Up to 24 h	$$
Glargine	1–2 h	Minimal	Up to 24 h	$$
Degludec	1–2 h	–	>24 h (up to 42 h)	$$$

having fasting blood glucose within target range may require additional shorter-acting premeal insulin. The starting dose for premeal insulin is determined by target glucose levels and carbohydrate content of the meal.

Other insulin options such as premixed insulin (70/30 NPH/regular, 70/30 aspart mix, 75/25 or 50/50 lispro mix) may help simplify insulin regimens for many patients and are also less costly. However, they are not recommended as a first step due to their unpredictable pharmacodynamics, which may increase the risk for blood glucose excursions, especially in patients with irregular meal patterns.

American Diabetes Association. 9. Pharmacologic approaches to glycemic treatment: standards of medical care in diabetes-2019. *Diabetes Care.* 2019;42(suppl 1):S90-S102.

Wallia A, Molitch ME. Insulin therapy for type 2 diabetes mellitus. *JAMA.* 2014;311(22):2315-2325.

9. Amylin mimetic—Amylin is a peptide that is co-secreted with insulin and modulates glucose homeostasis by delaying gastric emptying, promoting satiety, and decreasing postprandial glucagon secretion. Pramlintide is the only amylin mimetic available in the United States; it is approved for subcutaneous use for patients with type 1 or 2 diabetes taking insulin. Although generally well tolerated, its effect is modest, decreasing HbA1c approximately 0.5%. Pramlintide must be injected separately from insulin, complicating medication adherence.

Riddle M, Pencek R, Charenkavanich S, Lutz K, Wilhelm K, Porter L. Randomized comparison of pramlintide or mealtime insulin added to basal insulin treatment for patients with type 2 diabetes. *Diabetes Care.* 2009;32(9):1577-1582.

Anemia

Thomas Reske, MD
Paul D. Zito, MBBS

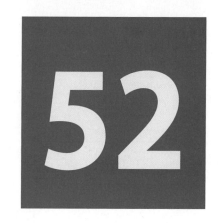

52

General Principles

Anemia is the most common hematologic abnormality in older adults. Overall prevalence of anemia in community-dwelling older adults ranges from 10% to 24%. The prevalence in long-term care or hospitalized older adults is close to 40%. The age distribution of anemia is shown in Figure 52–1. Race appears to also influence hemoglobin levels. In the longitudinal National Health and Nutrition Examination Survey (NHANES) III, the prevalence of anemia was found to be three times higher in non-Hispanic blacks compared with non-Hispanic whites. Anemia is recognized as a contributor to increased morbidity and mortality, and therefore, it is important to properly diagnose and treat anemia.

The NHANES III study revealed that there are three broad categories of anemia in older adults: one-third of cases are secondary to nutritional deficiencies (iron, folic acid, or vitamin B_{12}); one-third are secondary to inflammation; and one-third are unexplained. Unexplained anemia is commonly multifactorial and includes bone marrow failure and nutritional and inflammatory syndromes. There has been extensive literature and research on the increased proinflammatory cytokines and impact on bone marrow function (defined as inflammaging), as well as literature on the gradual degradation of the immune system, called immunosenescence.

Definition of Anemia

Similar to younger patients, anemia in older adults is most commonly defined according to the 1968 World Health Organization criteria of a hemoglobin (Hgb) <13 g/dL in men and <12 g/dL in women.

Symptoms of Anemia in Older Adults

Clinical symptoms of anemia are dependent on the severity and acuity of the anemia and the patient's oxygen demand. Symptomatic anemia typically reflects impaired oxygen delivery to tissues as a consequence of decreased Hgb concentration. This may lead to increased cardiac output states and increased tissue hypoxia and progressive decline in organ function. In general, anemia that develops slowly over time tends to present with fewer symptoms than acute-onset anemia, regardless of the underlying etiology. As in younger adults, rapidly developing anemia may additionally cause symptoms because of the effects of hypovolemia. Such symptomatic illness may be more profound and poorly tolerated in older adults because of increased frailty and decreased performance status often related to the presence of multiple chronic comorbidities. The primary symptoms of anemia may include:

1. Varying degrees of fatigue
2. Dyspnea on exertion or dyspnea at rest
3. Some combination of tachycardia, palpitations, and sensation of bounding pulses reflecting a hyperdynamic cardiac state

More severe anemia may additionally present with:

1. Lethargy and loss of drive
2. Confusion
3. Severe cardiac symptoms, including congestive heart failure, arrhythmias, angina, or myocardial infarction

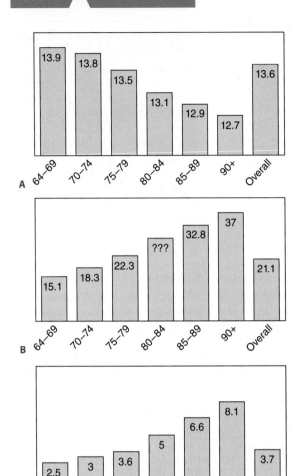

▲ **Figure 52–1.** Age distribution of anemia.
(**A**) Hemoglobin values by age. (**B**) Prevalence (%) of anemia by age. (**C**) Prevalence (%) of severe anemia (hemoglobin <10 g/dL) by age. (Data from Bach V, Schruckmayer G, Sam I, Kemmler G, Stauder R. Prevalence and possible causes of anemia in the elderly: a cross-sectional analysis of a large European university hospital cohort, *Clin Interv Aging* 2014 Jul 22;9:1187-96.)

Anemia as a result of acute blood loss or severe acute hemolysis may initially present with the following symptoms that reflect physiologic hypovolemia:

1. Lightheadedness
2. Orthostatic hypotension
3. Syncope
4. Symptoms associated with hypovolemic shock, including coma and death

Many epidemiologic studies have associated anemia with a number of clinically relevant conditions, including cardiovascular diseases, cognitive impairment, insomnia, impaired mood, and quality of life. Anemia is also associated with decreased executive function, decreased physical performance, an increased risk of falls and fractures, and hence more frequent hospitalization and longer hospital stays. It has been recognized that even mild forms of anemia are associated with increased morbidity, mortality, and frailty in older adults.

It is unclear whether the anemia itself causes unfavorable outcomes or if anemia is a surrogate marker for underlying processes that cause unfavorable outcomes. The highest mortality has been found in those who have anemia with concurrent nutritional disorders, chronic renal disease, and chronic inflammation as compared to unexplained anemia.

▶ Pathophysiology of Anemia in Older Adults

The pathophysiology of anemia still lacks complete detailed understanding. Multiple signaling cascades are involved in the complex regulatory framework. Figure 52–2 provides an overview of these suggested interactions. Key contributors to anemia include clonal stem cell changes, an altered microenvironment including inflammation, alterations in the reticuloendothelial system and kidney, and nutrition.

Hematopoietic stem cells retain the ability to replicate freely and terminally differentiate into any type of cell usually produced in the bone marrow. The precise molecular mechanisms by which a cell becomes committed to a specific cell line are complex and still not fully defined but involve epigenetic silencing and adoptive gene expression. Erythropoietin (EPO) is one of the most important regulatory hormones, as it responds to hypoxia and anemia to stimulate the development of red blood cells (RBCs) in the marrow. RBCs start as nucleated cells in the marrow before beginning the process of losing their nucleus to form reticulocytes. Reticulocytes are released from the marrow to circulate and fully mature into mature RBCs. Once in circulation, an RBC has a life span of approximately 120 days before being removed from circulation as a senescent red cell. Numerous vitamins and cofactors are required for the growth and maturation of hematopoietic stem cells into RBCs, and various other factors including microenvironmental change, free radical damage, mechanical disruption, and immunologic and inflammatory changes may affect the life span and durability of the RBC in circulation.

Impaired EPO responsiveness of hematopoietic stem cells has been implicated in the pathophysiology of anemia in older adults, with some studies showing increased EPO levels with age, even in healthy adults. The Baltimore Longitudinal Study on Aging demonstrated that EPO levels rose with age

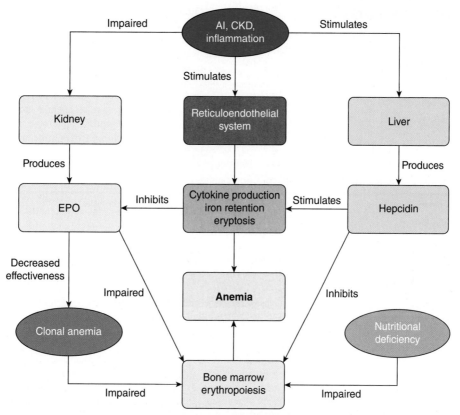

▲ **Figure 52–2.** Proposed interactions in anemia of older age. Possible mechanism for anemia in elderly patients with chronic kidney disease (CKD) or inflammation. Inflammatory cytokines stimulate hepcidin production, with increased iron storage in the reticuloendothelial system. Aging kidneys and inflammation affect erythropoietin (EPO) production and effectiveness. Increased red cell phagocytosis occurs (eryptosis) in response to these cascades further exacerbating anemia. These elements combined with impaired production from nutritional deficiency result in decreased bone marrow erythropoiesis. AI, anemia of chronic disease or inflammation.

in healthy, nonanemic individuals and that the slope of the rise was greater for individuals without diabetes or hypertension. Those with anemia had a lower slope of rise, suggesting that anemia reflected a failure of a normal age-related compensatory rise in EPO levels.

In addition to the altered EPO responsiveness, clonal abnormalities in the bone marrow are increasingly being recognized as contributing to unexplained anemia. Clonal hematopoietic abnormalities are associated with an increased prevalence of myeloid hematologic malignancies such as myelodysplastic syndromes (MDS), myeloproliferative neoplasms, and acute leukemia.

Inflammation has a direct negative effect on cytokine pathways. Tumor necrosis factor-α, interleukin-1, and transforming growth factor-β can influence proliferation and differentiation of erythroid progenitor cells. This inflammation can lead to downregulation of EPO receptor expression on erythroid progenitors and a net effect of reduced erythropoiesis. Inflammation appears to also influence and regulate uptake and retention of iron (in the form of senescent/damaged erythrocytes) within the reticuloendothelial system, leading to an iron-restricted erythropoiesis.

The hepcidin pathway is another important regulatory pathway. An acute phase protein produced by the liver, hepcidin reduces both duodenal iron absorption and iron release from macrophages. In the presence of increased hepcidin, ongoing iron restriction will lead to increased ferritin levels and decreased transferrin saturation, resulting in a relative iron-deficient erythropoiesis. Increased hepcidin production is seen in inflammatory disease, infections, and malignancy. In mouse models, transgenic upregulation of hepcidin resulted in mild to moderate anemia and impaired response to EPO, mimicking key features of anemia of inflammation.

Laboratory Testing and Evaluation

When beginning the workup to identify the underlying cause of anemia, it is clinically useful to consider whether one of three processes is at work. These three processes are discussed in detail below:

1. Destruction of red cells
2. Production deficits
3. Blood loss

Often more than one factor may be contributing to anemia in the older adult; hence, a workup must be comprehensive. Mild anemia should not be ignored, as it may be the warning sign of an underlying disorder. Table 52–1 is a summary of conditions associated with anemia in the older adult.

In addition to a complete history and physical examination, the basic workup of anemia includes a complete blood count (CBC) with differential, peripheral smear, mean corpuscular volume (MCV), mean corpuscular Hgb,

Table 52–1. Anemia categories and subtypes with common causes.

Category and Subtypes	Specific Examples
Chronic inflammatory diseases • Rheumatologic diseases • Chronic infectious diseases • Inflammaging • Miscellaneous	• RA, polymyalgia rheumatica, SLE • Chronic hepatitis, osteomyelitis, HIV • Frailty, cachexia, geriatric syndromes • Chronic leg ulcers, recurrent infections, UTI/PNA
Nonhematopoietic neoplasms • Gastrointestinal tumors • Multiorgan metastasis or bone marrow metastasis	• Colorectal cancer, gastric cancer • End-stage cancer including breast cancer, prostate cancer, melanoma
Endocrinologic and metabolic causes • Low production of EPO • Thyroid dysfunction • Insulin deficiency	• Renal failure or pure EPO deficiency • Hypothyroidism or hyperthyroidism • Diabetes mellitus
Blood loss • Gastrointestinal tract bleeding • Surgical procedures • Alternate bleeding sites	• Peptic ulcer disease, ulcerative colitis, diverticular, variceal, angiodysplasia, hemorrhoidal, mesenteric ischemia, anticoagulant related • Hip and orthopedic procedures, colectomy, cardiothoracic, postcolonoscopy with biopsy • Epistaxis, genitourinary, retroperitoneal
Increased consumption or destruction of erythrocytes • Chronic nonmechanical hemolysis • Mechanical destruction of red cells • Hypersplenism • Acute destruction of red cells	• Autoimmune hemolytic anemia, PNH, sickle cell, chronic TTP • Heart valve–mediated red cell lysis • Hepatomegaly/splenomegaly • TTP/HUS, DIC, sepsis, G6PD deficiency
Nutrient deficiency • Vitamin deficiency • Trace element deficiency • Iron deficiency	• Vitamin B_{12}/pernicious anemia, folate, vitamin B_6 • Copper deficiency • Blood loss, dietary deficiency
Drug-induced anemia • Chemotherapy • Antimetabolites, anticonvulsants • Toxic drug reactions/drug-induced hemolysis	• Chemotherapy-induced pancytopenia • Methotrexate, phenytoin • β-Lactams, cephalosporins, cotrimoxazole, ciprofloxacin, fludarabine, lorazepam, diclofenac, alcohol
Bone marrow/impaired production • Hematologic malignancy • Myelodysplasia • Premalignant • Infectious	• AML, ALL, CML, CLL • MDS, MPN, aplastic anemia, myelofibrosis • ICUS, CCUS • Parvovirus, HIV, tuberculosis, Q fever, brucellosis, ehrlichiosis, EBV, CMV

ALL, acute lymphoblastic leukemia; AML, acute myeloid leukemia; CCUS, clonal cytopenia of undetermined significance; CLL, chronic lymphocytic leukemia; CML, chronic myelogenous leukemia; CMV, cytomegalovirus; DIC, disseminated intravascular coagulation; EBV, Epstein-Barr virus; EPO, erythropoietin; G6PD, glucose-6-phosphate dehydrogenase; HUS, hemolytic uremic syndrome; ICUS, idiopathic cytopenia of undetermined significance; MDS, myelodysplastic syndrome; MPN, myeloproliferative neoplasm; PNA, pneumonia; PNH, paroxysmal nocturnal hemoglobinuria; RA, rheumatoid arthritis; SLE, systemic lupus erythematosus; TTP, thrombotic thrombocytopenic purpura; UTI, urinary tract infection.

reticulocyte count, ferritin, iron studies, EPO level, C-reactive protein, fibrinogen, creatinine, vitamin B_{12}, serum folate, thyroid-stimulating hormone, lactate dehydrogenase (LDH), haptoglobin, aspartate transaminase, alanine transaminase, and serum electrophoresis. Clinical red flags, such as myelopathy and neuropathy, should trigger considering copper deficiency. Symptoms of cheilosis, glossitis, and mental status changes suggest vitamin B_6 deficiency. The morphologic changes on a peripheral blood smear help to exclude life-threatening causes of anemia such as microangiopathic hemolytic anemia (thrombotic thrombocytopenic purpura [TTP]/hemolytic uremic syndrome [HUS]) or an acute leukemia.

The MCV helps classify anemia as either microcytic, normocytic, or macrocytic, and review of the absolute reticulocyte count or reticulocyte index will help determine whether anemia is hyper- or hypoproliferative. Given the increased prevalence of monoclonal gammopathy in older adults, serum and urine protein electrophoresis with immunofixation is warranted in patients with normocytic anemia to evaluate for the presence of an underlying plasma cell dyscrasia.

Although the diagnostic approach to nutritional anemia is similar to that in younger adults, there are some special circumstances to consider in older adults. For example, iron deficiency typically presents with microcytic and hypochromic red cells. However, when found in combination with macrocytic causes of anemia, such as MDS or vitamin B_{12} deficiency, the MCV may be in the normocytic range.

Iron deficiency anemia is commonly diagnosed by the presence of low serum iron, increased total iron-binding capacity, and decreased serum ferritin, with serum ferritin <12 μg/L being the most sensitive peripheral blood laboratory measure of reduced iron stores. However, ferritin also functions as an acute phase reactant, and serum levels may be falsely elevated in the presence of chronic inflammatory conditions, making it difficult to identify iron deficiency in the backdrop of underlying anemia of inflammation. Ferritin levels may also increase with age, but it remains to be determined whether this occurs in healthy older adults or whether it reflects increases in age-related inflammatory comorbidities.

At least one-third of anemic patients older than 65 years have a diagnosis of anemia of chronic disease or inflammation (AI). It is classically characterized biochemically by the presence of low serum iron and low iron-binding capacity in the setting of an elevated serum ferritin. AI is the result of complex biochemical and inflammatory feedback processes, which are referred to as inflammaging.

It may be difficult at times to delineate iron deficiency in the setting of chronic inflammation. A bone marrow biopsy remains the gold standard for measuring total-body iron stores and evaluate the presence or absence of iron in erythroid progenitors. Because a bone marrow biopsy is often not wanted or tolerated by older adults, the soluble transferrin receptor (sTfR)/log ferritin index can be used. This index is calculated dividing sTfR by the log ferritin. The transferrin receptor is the major mediator for iron uptake, and its concentration is elevated in iron deficiency.

▷ Destruction

A. Mechanical Causes of Hemolysis

Destruction of red cells through mechanical destruction and shear stress in the vasculature can be found in patients with intravascular stenosis or foreign bodies, such as metallic heart valves. A sudden worsening of hemolysis in these patients should prompt an exploration for either inadequate anticoagulation or a perivalvular leak.

B. Autoimmune Hemolytic Anemia

In autoimmune hemolytic anemia (AHA), RBC survival is shortened by autoantibodies. AHAs can be temperature sensitive and induced by temperature changes that promote antibody binding, leading to the distinction between warm AHA (>37°C; warm antibodies) and cold AHAs (<37°C; cold antibodies) (Table 52–2). Some patients exhibit both warm and cold reactive autoantibodies, and this is termed mixed AHA. Patients present with anemia and have a mixture of positive findings on lab work including elevated LDH, elevated bilirubin, decreased haptoglobin, and direct antiglobulin test (DAT) or Coombs positivity. These disorders can be idiopathic or primary or secondary to an underlying disorder. Treatment of the primary disorder is indicated to help resolve the hemolytic process.

1. Warm AHA—Warm AHA is primarily an IgG-related phenomenon that promotes Fc receptor–mediated removal of RBCs from circulation by macrophages in the spleen. Peripheral smear may display spherocytes as a result of partial phagocytosis.

2. Cold AHA—Cold reactive autoantibodies bind primarily at temperatures below 37°C. The binding is usually mediated by IgM antibodies with large pentamers spanning the distance between numerous RBCs. The pentamers have a tendency to activate complement with C3b-coated cells attaching to complement receptors on macrophages and being removed in the liver and spleen. Cold AHA is often associated with infectious agents such as *Mycoplasma* or Epstein-Barr virus (EBV).

3. Mixed AHA—Mixed AHA is usually associated with both IgG and IgM antibodies and tends to be more severe. IgA antibodies in this condition are rare.

C. Drug-Induced Immune Hemolytic Anemias

These reactions present similarly to the other hemolytic anemias, and a careful drug history and timeline is important.

Table 52–2. Etiology and classification of hemolytic anemias.

Warm autoantibody type: Autoantibody maximally activated at 37°C

A. Primary or idiopathic warm AHA
B. Secondary warm AHA; associated with:
   1. Lymphoproliferative diseases (eg, Hodgkin disease, lymphoma)
   2. Rheumatologic disorders (eg, SLE)
   3. Nonlymphoid neoplasms (eg, ovarian neoplasms)
   4. Chronic inflammatory diseases (eg, Crohn disease)
   5. Ingestion of certain drugs (eg, methyldopa)

Cold autoantibody type: Autoantibody optimally activated below 37°C

A. Mediated by cold agglutinins
   1. Idiopathic cold agglutinin disease (usually associated with clonal B-lymphocyte proliferation)
   2. Secondary cold agglutinin hemolytic anemia
      a. Postinfectious (eg, *Mycoplasma*, infectious mononucleosis)
      b. Associated with malignant B-cell lymphoproliferative disorder
B. Mediated by cold hemolysins
   1. Idiopathic paroxysmal cold hemoglobinuria
   2. Secondary
      a. Donath-Landsteiner hemolytic anemia (usually after acute viral illness in children)
      b. Associated with congenital or tertiary syphilis in adults

Mixed warm and cold autoantibodies

A. Primary or idiopathic mixed AHA
B. Secondary mixed AHA
   1. Associated with rheumatic disorders, primarily SLE

Drug-induced immune hemolytic anemia

A. Hapten or drug absorption mechanism
B. Ternary (immune) complex mechanism
C. True autoantibody mechanism
D. Nonimmunologic protein adsorption (probably does not cause hemolysis)

AHA, autoimmune hemolytic anemia; SLE, systemic lupus erythematosus.

Reproduced with permission from Kaushansky K, Lichtman MA, Prhal JT, et al: *Williams Hematology*, 9th ed. New York, NY: McGraw Hill; 2016.

Second- and third-generation cephalosporins are thought to reflect >80% of drug-induced immune hemolytic anemias. A list of medications associated with immune hemolytic anemias can be found in Table 52–3. There are various mechanisms by which drugs may induce hemolysis, as follows:

1. Hapten or drug adsorption mechanism in which a drug may bind directly to RBC membranes.
2. Ternary or immune complex mechanism in which a drug or drug metabolite binds to an RBC membrane or antigen and a drug-dependent antibody binds these to form a ternary complex.

Table 52–3. Drugs associated with immune injury to red blood cells or a positive direct antiglobulin test likely to be relevant to a geriatric population.

Hapten or drug adsorption mechanism	• Oxaliplatin
• Oxaliplatin	• Pentostatin
• Cephalosporins	• Fludarabine
• Penicillins	• Procainamide
• Tetracycline	• Teniposide
• Hydrocortisone	• Tolmetin
• Tolbutamide	Nonimmunologic protein
• 6-Mercaptopurine	adsorption
Ternary immune complex mechanism	• Carboplatin
• Amphotericin B	• Cisplatin
• Oxaliplatin	• Cephalosporins
• Cephalosporins	• Oxaliplatin
• Pemetrexed	Uncertain mechanism of
• Chlorpropamide	immune injury
• Probenecid	• Acetaminophen
• Diclofenac	• Melphalan
• Quinine	• P-Aminosalicylic acid
• Diethylstilbestrol	• Mephenytoin
• Quinidine	• Carboplatin
• Doxepin	• Chlorpromazine
• Rifampicin	• Omeprazole
• Etodolac	• Efavirenz
• Hydrocortisone	• Phenacetin
• Metformin	• Erythromycin
• Tolmetin	• Streptomycin
Autoantibody mechanism	• Fluorouracil
• Cephalosporins	• Sulindac
• Lenalidomide	• Ibuprofen
• Mefenamic acid	• Temafloxacin
• Cladribine	• Insecticides
• α-Methyldopa	• Thiazides
• Diclofenac	• Isoniazid
• Levodopa	• Triamterene

3. Autoantibody mechanism in which the drug stimulates production of an autoantibody most likely by dysregulation of T lymphocytes.
4. Nonimmunologic protein adsorption in which multiple plasma proteins, including immunoglobulins, complement, albumin, fibrinogen, and others, may be detected on RBC membranes; this does not in itself cause hemolytic anemia but may complicate cross-matching blood and will result in a positive DAT.
5. Associations with uncertain mechanisms for hemolysis also exist for some drugs.

D. TTP, HUS, & Atypical HUS

An in-depth discussion of TTP and HUS is beyond the scope of this chapter. Most important is to rule out TTP and HUS, as those are medical emergencies. The pathophysiology is different, although both present as microangiopathic hemolytic anemia with varying degrees of thrombocytopenia, anemia, renal dysfunction, neurologic symptoms, and fever. TTP and HUS are usually preceded by an infection such as diarrheal illness or pneumonia. Prompt evaluation includes CBC, LDH, serum creatinine, and complete metabolic panel, as well as haptoglobin, fibrinogen, and coagulation studies. Peripheral smear demonstrates schistocytes. In acquired TTP, an autoantibody is responsible for removing the ADAMTS13 molecule from circulation. ADAMTS13 functions normally to cleave von Willebrand from large multimers to smaller proteins. In the absence of ADAMTS13, the large von Willebrand multimers persist and cause platelet adhesion and microangiopathic thrombosis, eventually leading to hemolytic anemia. If TTP is suspected, an ADAMTS13 level should be ordered before any blood or plasma products are given as this result will be affected by exogenous plasma products.

Plasma exchange serves two purposes; it helps to remove any antibodies that are facilitating the depletion of the ADAMTS13 molecule, and it replenishes the patient's ADAMTS13 levels with exogenous plasma. Steroids and rituximab, a CD20 antibody, are also often used, especially in refractory cases. These agents work by slowing the production of the autoantibodies responsible for attacking ADAMTS13. Newer medicines are soon to be approved including caplacizumab, which is an antibody that binds to von Willebrand factor to inhibit platelet adhesion, effectively halting the microangiopathic hemolytic process.

As HUS is primarily initiated by an infectious process, the treatment is usually supportive in nature and should also be aimed at treating any concurrent infection. Plasma exchange is less likely to be of benefit but may have been initiated during the acute phase of illness when TTP was a possibility.

In a geriatric population, it is possible to encounter both of these disorders; however, the peak incidence for HUS is in childhood, with its lowest incidence in older age. TTP conversely has its peak incidence after the age of 40 years, but it can be seen in the older adult.

▶ Production

A. Nutritional Deficiency, Vitamin B$_{12}$, & Folate Deficiency

Malnutrition, particularly in association with alcohol abuse, may result in folate deficiency. Drugs like anticonvulsants and methotrexate can also cause folate deficiency. Pernicious anemia, the classic vitamin B$_{12}$ deficiency anemia, is relatively rare; however, we would caution that severe vitamin B$_{12}$ deficiency must be monitored after initiating high-dose oral vitamin B$_{12}$ to ensure the anemia and deficiency are improving. *Helicobacter pylori* infections, acid-reducing agents, and

atrophic gastritis may cause hypochlorhydria, leading to a food-cobalamin malabsorption syndrome.

Prompt treatment of these reversible causes of anemia often results in meaningful resolution of the clinical syndrome including neurologic issues related to vitamin B$_{12}$ deficiency. Copper and vitamin B$_6$ deficiency are other rarer causes of nutrient deficiency anemias. Copper deficiency can present with anemia (microcytic, normocytic, or macrocytic), neutropenia, and dysmorphic changes on bone marrow biopsy mimicking MDS. Common causes of copper deficiency include malabsorption, especially in patients with a history of gastric surgeries, enteropathies, use of copper chelators, zinc supplement overuse, denture cream ingestion, chronic TPN, or simple dietary deficiency.

Vitamin B$_6$ is another potentially reversible cause of anemia. One cross-sectional study identified vitamin B$_6$ deficiency in half of nursing home residents. Routine supplementation should be considered in nursing home residents or those with unexplained anemia.

B. Iron Deficiency

Iron deficiency is by far the most frequent nutritional deficiency anemia. Similar to folate deficiency, iron depletion is often associated with malnutrition. However, it is highly uncommon in the industrialized world for iron deficiency to be caused by inadequate dietary intake of iron. With iron deficiency anemia, one must consider blood loss, especially given the prevalence of malignancy and anticoagulant medicines in this age group.

Gastrointestinal and genitourinary blood loss remains the most likely cause of iron deficiency in older adults. Because of the increased incidence of malignancies in older adults, a genitourinary and gastrointestinal evaluation in patients diagnosed with iron deficiency anemia is recommended in patients clinically well enough to tolerate diagnostic evaluation and who may be candidates for therapeutic interventions.

C. Hemoglobinopathy

Hemoglobinopathies, such as sickle cell disease or thalassemia, are usually diagnosed earlier in life, but patients may eventually end up in the care of a geriatrician due to lack of access or choice of avoiding health care. The shortened life expectancy of patients with these conditions precludes many of them from surviving to geriatric age, but improvements in care are prolonging survival in these patients, and they are at risk for iron overload if supplementation is given.

1. Sickle cell & Hgb C—Sickle cell anemia is a qualitative hemoglobinopathy, resulting from a mutation in the hemoglobin β gene, which produces sickling of red cells in a hypoxic environment. It is a disease of the young, with most of these patients having a decreased life expectancy due to the progressive detrimental effects of this disease. Sickle cell trait is essentially a normal carrier state, and these patients should

Table 52–4. Summary of β-thalassemias, complications, and life expectancy.

Common Genotypes	Name	Phenotype	Life Expectancy
β/β	Normal	None	Normal
β/β°, β/β+	β-Thalassemia trait	Thalassemia minor; asymptomatic, mild, microcytic anemia	Normal
β+/β+ β+/β° β^E/β+ β^E/β+	β-Thalassemia intermedia	Variable severity Mild to moderate anemia Possible extramedullary hematopoiesis Iron overload	Historically <75 years but improving with aggressive therapy
β°/β°	β-Thalassemia major (Cooley anemia)	Severe anemia Transfusion dependence Extramedullary hematopoiesis Iron overload	Historically <60 years but improving with aggressive therapy

have no sequelae from this condition. In the older adult population, these patients are more likely to be encountered.

Hgb C is the result of a mutation in the hemoglobin β molecule, which decreases solubility; hence, RBCs become less deformable with a predilection for entrapment in the spleen. Hgb C can also coexist with β-thalassemia. In both conditions, these patients will have a chronic microcytic hemolytic anemia and may develop cholelithiasis. A CBC will show microcytosis with a high mean corpuscular Hgb concentration due to cellular dehydration and a slightly elevated reticulocyte count.

2. Thalassemia—Thalassemias are quantitative hemoglobinopathies. In older patients, thalassemia traits are diagnosed quite frequently. Finding a low MCV and adequate iron stores on workup should prompt investigation into an underlying thalassemia trait. A family history is very important in these cases, noting ancestry and country of origin and other family members who may have been diagnosed or given spurious diagnoses of iron deficiency.

Hgb electrophoresis may be helpful in some cases in consultation with a hematologist; however, with some thalassemia traits, it is necessary to obtain genetic studies to obtain the final diagnoses. A summary of the investigations and results for the most common thalassemias likely to be seen as well as the varying indices for sickle cell conditions can be found in Tables 52–4 and 52–5.

a. β-Thalassemia—This condition is prevalent in populations in the Mediterranean region, the Middle East, India, Pakistan, and Southeast Asia. It is rarely encountered in Northern European Caucasian populations.

β-Thalassemia results in impaired synthesis of one or both of the β-globulin molecules, leading to relative excess of α-chain globulin. This condition is variable in presentation and severity due to a multitude of mutations that can lead to a spectrum of deficiency. Patients who suffer from β-thalassemia major have deletion of both of their β gene

alleles, leading to β°/β° genotype. These patients traditionally did not survive long into adulthood; however, with improvement in transfusions, iron chelation, aggressive treatment of infections, and cardiac complications, some studies have shown that survival is beginning to match that of β-thalassemia intermedia.

β-Thalassemia intermedia encompasses the full spectrum of deficiency. These patients may have clinical presentations ranging from severe anemia and transfusion dependence to moderate anemia with infrequent transfusions during

Table 52–5. α-Thalassemia variants and clinical presentation.

Variant	Chromosome 16	Signs and Symptoms
α-Thalassemia silent carrier	One of four gene deletion -α/αα	Asymptomatic
α-Thalassemia trait	Two of four gene deletion --/αα (cis) -α/-α (trans)	Asymptomatic
Hemoglobin constant spring	Reduced output of A globin (--/α^{CS}α)	Silent or mildly symptomatic
α-Thalassemia intermedia with significant hemoglobin H	Three of four gene deletion --/-α	Moderate to severe hemolytic anemia, modest degree of ineffective erythropoiesis, splenomegaly, variable bone changes
α-Thalassemia with hemoglobin Barts	Four of four gene deletion --/--	Causes nonimmune hydrops fetalis, usually fatal

intercurrent illness. Clinical findings may include hepato-splenomegaly, extramedullary hematopoietic pseudotumors, leg ulcers, thrombotic events, pulmonary hypertension, gallstones, bone deformities, leg ulcers, silent infarcts, and iron overload.

β-Thalassemia trait is the most likely condition to be seen in the aging population. These patients have a relative deficiency of their β gene with genotypes such as β/β+ or β/β° and only mild microcytic anemia that does not require regular transfusions.

All conditions will have a tendency toward iron retention as persistent anemia will stimulate iron uptake and storage throughout life. This may be exacerbated by misdiagnosis and inappropriate iron supplementation, which is why assessing iron stores in a microcytic anemia is essential to avoid this potentially damaging intervention.

b. α-Thalassemia—This condition is more prevalent in the African, Mediterranean, and Southeast Asian populations and, to a lesser extent, in the Middle East.

The α-thalassemia gene has two copies on each chromosome 16; hence, a normal cell carries four copies of this gene. The silent carrier state (-α/αα) exists in one in three African Americans. Hgb constant spring is an α+ gene variation common in Southeast Asia that affects termination of translation and results in an abnormally long α-chain. α-Thalassemia trait involves two different genotypes. The --/αα (cis) genotype is more common in those of Asian descent and involves deletion of both genes from one chromosome 16. The -α/-α (trans) genotype is more common in individuals from the Mediterranean or Africa. The silent carrier states are clinically normal and result in a lifelong mild microcytic anemia.

More severe forms of α-thalassemia include Hgb H (--/-α) and Hgb constant spring (--/α^{CS}α). These patients may suffer mild to more severe anemia with splenomegaly and transfusion requirements.

Hgb Barts or homozygous α^0 (--/--) results in hydrops fetalis and is incompatible with life.

Similar to β-thalassemia, sufferers from these clinically relevant disorders, Hgb H and Hgb constant spring, may have shortened life expectancy but would be expected to survive longer in the future due to advances in care, which may make them relevant to the geriatric clinician.

Likewise, α-thalassemia trait patients may be undiagnosed or misdiagnosed. There are usually no management changes for trait patients other than recognizing that iron supplementation may be inappropriate in these patients and iron stores should be assessed. Adults with this condition will have a normal Hgb electrophoresis and may require genetic testing to confirm the diagnosis.

Hematologic indices for iron deficiency and α- and β-thalassemia are shown in Table 52–6.

D. Anemia of Chronic Kidney Disease

The body's oxygen-sensing mechanism in the kidney responds to increased hypoxia associated with decreased Hgb concentrations and results in a logarithmic increase in EPO levels that corresponds to anemia severity. Renal disease leads to a blunted EPO response, with lower serum EPO levels seen in patients with declining renal function.

Because aging is associated with a decline in renal function, anemia associated with chronic renal disease is an important consideration in older adults. However, the required degree of renal disease to promote the development of anemia remains in question. In the InCHIANTI Study, a creatinine clearance (CrCl) of <30 mL/min was significantly associated with an increased risk of anemia, as well as age- and Hgb-adjusted serum EPO levels, in 1005 participants age 65 years or older. In contrast, a cross-sectional study involving 3222 subjects with a mean age of 65 years found that estimated CrCl levels of <50 mL/min were associated with three- and five-fold increased risks of anemia in women and men, respectively. These differences highlight the fact that the overall impact of moderate degrees of renal disease on the risk of anemia and decline in EPO synthesis requires more rigorous determination. It is important to note that measurement of serum EPO levels is often diagnostically equivocal, unless the Hgb drops below <10 g/dL.

Table 52–6. Hematologic indices for iron deficiency and α- and β-thalassemia.

Test	Iron Deficiency	β-Thalassemia	α-Thalassemia
MCV (abnormal if <80 fL in adults; <70 fL in children age 6 months to 6 years; and <76 fL in children 7–12 years of age)	Low	Low	Low
RDW	High	Normal; occasionally high	Normal
Ferritin	Low	Normal	Normal
Hb electrophoresis	Normal (may have reduced HbA2)	Increased HbA2, reduced HbA, and probably increased HbF	Adults: normal Newborns: may have HbH or Hb Barts

Hb, hemoglobin; HbF, fetal hemoglobin; MCV, mean corpuscular volume; RDW, red blood cell distribution width.

E. Infectious & Drug Induced

As displayed in Tables 52–2 and 52–3, there are numerous infectious and drug-related causes of anemia. An exhaustive discussion of each of these is beyond the scope of this chapter.

1. HIV—HIV, due to its chronic nature with the availability of potent therapy, is likely to factor heavily in the care of older adults in the future. Anemia is the most common hematologic complication of HIV infection. The etiology of anemia in the setting of HIV infection is multifactorial and includes opportunistic infections, decreased EPO levels, effects on the kinetics of hematopoietic cell differentiation, nutritional deficiency, and associated malignancy and medications. Even young patients with active HIV infection will present with clinically relevant anemias and cytopenias, suggesting a direct effect on marrow either due to the virus itself or the chronic inflammatory state that arises from the infection, which can also predispose patients to venous thromboembolism and other complications.

We recommend that patients presenting with HIV and anemia receive a full workup for reversible causes including consultations with infectious disease and hematology to evaluate for infiltrative diseases such as histoplasmosis, tuberculosis, cytomegalovirus, EBV, Q fever, and ehrlichiosis.

▶ Loss

This topic has been covered to some extent in the iron deficiency section, and some possible causes of blood loss are listed in Table 52–1. In a postoperative patient, a clinician must focus on the particulars of the surgery itself such as duration and expected blood loss. Early and late complications from procedures should also be considered, such as retroperitoneal or psoas bleeds following spinal procedures or renal biopsies.

Besides postoperative blood loss, older adults are more likely to use higher doses of over-the-counter pain medicines, which may predispose them to bleed from peptic ulcer disease, varices, angiodysplasia, or diverticulosis. They are also much more likely to be on chronic anticoagulation for conditions such as stroke, atrial fibrillation, venous thromboembolism/pulmonary embolism, and coronary artery disease. Investigation should begin with history and exam, followed by further testing such as esophagogastroduodenoscopy, colonoscopy, or cystoscopy as appropriate for the clinical situation.

▶ Prevention

There are presently no recommended or agreed upon strategies for the prevention of anemia in older populations.

▶ Treatment

In general, effective management of anemia in older adults should be based on identification of treatable causes of anemia. Monitoring of treatment should focus on the individual's response to therapy and the impact of anemia on clinical status, with therapeutic adjustments made as clinically indicated. Treatable causes of anemia in older adults include the following.

A. Nutritional Deficiencies of Iron, Vitamin B_{12}, & Folic Acid

Nutritional supplementation for folate and B_{12} is a routine procedure. Folate is supplemented orally and vitamin B_{12} is given orally or intramuscularly according to patient preference and underlying cause of deficiency. We suggest maintaining vitamin B_{12} levels in the high normal range.

In most patients with iron deficiency, oral substitution appears to be adequate. It is recommended to give iron with vitamin C to help with oral iron absorption.

If oral application is intolerable or unable to correct the iron deficiency, intravenous iron may be of benefit. There are different intravenous iron formulations available, including iron sucrose, ferric gluconate, ferumoxytol, ferric carboxymaltose, and iron isomaltoside. Ferric carboxymaltose has the benefit of containing 750 mg of iron in a single dose, allowing for sufficient replacement in one to two treatments. Ferric carboxymaltose and iron isomaltoside may rarely lead to severe hypophosphatemia with subsequent osteomalacia and bone fractures.

B. Unexplained Anemia & MDS

The majority of older adults with unexplained anemia present with mild anemia that does not require initiation of therapy. For symptomatic patients, currently available therapies are limited to red cell transfusions and erythropoiesis-stimulating agents (ESAs). There is no absolute Hgb level that requires the initiation of therapy, and therapeutic intervention should be based on the individual patient, with consideration placed on performance status, clinical impact of disease comorbidities, and quality-of-life assessment. The benefits of red cell transfusions must be weighed against the associated risks of iron overload, infectious complications, anaphylaxis, and red cell alloimmunization.

The use of ESAs in older adults with unexplained anemia is not currently approved by the US Food and Drug Administration (FDA), and there are few studies that have evaluated their use in this population. In one exploratory, randomized trial examining the impact of epoetin-α in a cohort of 62 predominantly black older women with AI or unexplained anemia, 69% receiving epoetin-α achieved a >2 g/dL increase in Hgb compared with those taking placebo ($P < .001$) and demonstrated improvement in their assessment of fatigue. However, the target Hgb in this study was 13.0 to 13.9 g/dL, which represents a level above current FDA guidelines and one associated with adverse effects in numerous studies. Future randomized controlled studies are needed to effectively determine the safety and efficacy of ESA therapy in older patients with unexplained anemia and to determine whether there exists appropriate and safe target Hgb levels.

ESAs are approved for treatment of anemia of chronic kidney disease and in European Union countries in patients with MDS. Data on application of ESAs in other subtypes of anemia are limited. In general, the risk of thrombotic complications increases with higher Hgb levels, so that the current recommendation is to maintain Hgb levels between 9 and 11.5 g/dL.

C. Hypothyroidism & Hyperthyroidism

Hypothyroidism and hyperthyroidism must be corrected.

D. Acute Blood Loss

As discussed previously, the most important treatment of acute or chronic blood loss is identifying the etiology and treating the underlying cause. Supportive measures such as transfusion may be indicated. General consensus guidelines currently seem to support transfusion for a stricter threshold of Hgb <7 g/dL, with a more liberal transfusion goal of <9 g/dL only appearing to be indicated in life-threatening situations such as acute myocardial infarction or if bleeding is so brisk that recorded Hgb level may be unreliable. Following acute treatment, oral or intravenous iron may be indicated to replete iron stores.

E. Anemia of Chronic Disease or Inflammation

Because there are no currently proven therapies that directly target inflammatory pathways in patients with AI, management of AI should be targeted to the underlying disorder.

F. Anemia of Chronic Renal Disease

For treatment of anemia caused by chronic renal disease, the FDA has approved the use of ESA therapy. Guidelines for use of ESAs in older adults with both hemodialysis-dependent and -independent renal disease are similar to those in younger adults. However, recent studies have highlighted the potential for adverse cardiovascular outcomes, such as thrombosis and stroke, with the use of ESAs in anemic patients with renal disease. The Trial to Reduce Cardiovascular Events with Aranesp Therapy (TREAT) evaluated the effect of darbepoetin alfa in 1872 patients with anemia, diabetes, and non–dialysis-dependent chronic kidney disease and found that the risk of stroke was double in patients receiving darbepoetin alfa compared with placebo. The etiology of these adverse cardiovascular outcomes is unclear but may involve attempts to normalize Hgb levels in resistant subpopulations of patients. For this reason, the FDA recently placed a black box warning on the use of ESAs in patients with anemia caused by renal disease, with recommendations targeting Hgb levels between 10 and 12 g/dL.

▶ Complications

Complications may arise as a result of the chronic impact of anemia or may be associated with specific therapeutic interventions. Chronic anemia may predispose to symptoms associated with high-output congestive heart failure. Common complications of therapy include the following:

1. Adverse effects of oral iron therapy include abdominal pain, constipation, diarrhea, nausea, and vomiting.

2. Adverse effects of parenteral iron administration include allergic reactions, back pain, generalized muscle aches, dizziness, skin rash or erythema, fever, dizziness, headache, hypotension, or anaphylaxis. Anaphylaxis is rare, especially with newer iron formulations, and typically occurs within several minutes of administration.

3. Folic acid therapy may mask coexisting vitamin B_{12} deficiency, allowing for progression of unrecognized neurologic symptoms of vitamin B_{12} deficiency.

4. ESAs may worsen underlying hypertension.

Adamson JW. Renal disease and anemia in the elderly. *Semin Hematol.* 2008;45(4):235-241.

Agnihotri P, Telfer M, Butt Z, et al. Chronic anemia and fatigue in elderly patients: results of a randomized, double-blind, placebo-controlled, crossover exploratory study with epoetin alfa. *J Am Geriatr Soc.* 2007;55(10):1557-1565.

Berenson JR, Anderson KC, Audell RA, et al. Monoclonal gammopathy of undetermined significance: a consensus statement. *Br J Haematol.* 2010;150(1):28-38.

Carmel R. Nutritional anemias and the elderly. *Semin Hematol.* 2008;45(4):225-234.

den Elzen WP, Willems JM, Westendorp RG, de Craen AJ, Assendelft WJ, Gussekloo J. Effect of anemia and comorbidity on functional status and mortality in old age: results from the Leiden 85-plus Study. *CMAJ.* 2009;181(3-4):151-157.

Ershler WB, Sheng S, McKelvey J, et al. Serum erythropoietin and aging: a longitudinal analysis. *J Am Geriatr Soc.* 2005;53(8):1360-1365.

Ferrucci L, Guralnik JM, Bandinelli S, et al. Unexplained anaemia in older persons is characterised by low erythropoietin and low levels of pro-inflammatory markers. *Br J Haematol.* 2007;136(6):849-855.

Ferrucci L, Semba RD, Guralnik JM, et al. Proinflammatory state, hepcidin, and anemia in older persons. *Blood.* 2010;115(18):3810-3816.

Fishbane S, Besarab A. Mechanism of increased mortality risk with erythropoietin treatment to higher hemoglobin targets. *Clin J Am Soc Nephrol.* 2007;2(6):1274-1282.

Gaskell H, Derry S, Moore RA, McQuay HJ. Prevalence of anaemia in older persons: systematic review. *BMC Geriatr.* 2008;8:1.

Guralnik JM, Eisenstaedt RS, Ferrucci L, Klein HG, Woodman RC. Prevalence of anemia in persons 65 years and older in the United States: evidence for a high rate of unexplained anemia. *Blood.* 2004;104(8):2263-2268.

Liu K, Kaffes AJ. Iron deficiency anaemia: a review of diagnosis, investigation and management. *Eur J Gastroenterol Hepatol.* 2012;24(2):109-116.

Lucca U, Tettamanti M, Mosconi P, et al. Association of mild anemia with cognitive, functional, mood and quality of life outcomes in the elderly: the "Health and Anemia" study. *PLoS One.* 2008;3(4):e1920.

Price EA, Mehra R, Holmes TH, Schrier SL. Anemia in older persons: etiology and evaluation. *Blood Cells Mol Dis.* 2011;46(2):159-165.

Roy CN, Andrews NC. Anemia of inflammation: the hepcidin link. *Curr Opin Hematol.* 2005;12(2):107-111.

Skikne BS, Punnonen K, Caldron PH, et al. Improved differential diagnosis of anemia of chronic disease and iron deficiency anemia: a prospective multicenter evaluation of soluble transferrin receptor and the sTfR/log ferritin index. *Am J Hematol.* 2011;86(11):923-927.

Solomon SD, Uno H, Lewis EF, et al. Erythropoietic response and outcomes in kidney disease and type 2 diabetes. *N Engl J Med.* 2010;363(12):1146-1155.

Stauder R, Thein SL. Anemia in the elderly: clinical implications and new therapeutic concepts. *Haematologica.* 2014;99(7):1127-1130.

Stauder R, Valent P, Theurl I. Anemia at older age: etiologies, clinical implications, and management. *Blood.* 2018;131:505-514.

Tettamanti M, Lucca U, Gandini F, et al. Prevalence, incidence and types of mild anemia in the elderly: the "Health and Anemia" population-based study. *Haematologica.* 2010;95(11):1849-1856.

Common Cancers

Melisa L. Wong, MD, MAS

Kah Poh Loh, MBBCh, BAO

Mina S. Sedrak, MD, MS

Grant R. Williams, MD

YaoYao G. Pollock, MD

William Dale, MD, PhD

▶ General Principles

With the rapidly growing number of older adults in the United States, an estimated 70% of all new cancer diagnoses will be in adults age 65 and older by 2030. Similarly, by 2040, the number of older cancer survivors is expected to increase to 19.1 million. Caring for older adults with cancer provides a unique challenge for clinicians, whether the goals of care are curative or palliative. Curative therapy may require more aggressive and potentially morbid treatment with surgery, radiation, systemic therapy (eg, chemotherapy, immunotherapy, targeted therapy), or a multimodality approach. Such aggressive approaches are often more likely to cause toxicity in older patients, who tend to be less tolerant of current therapies.

Older adults, especially those who are frail, remain underrepresented in cancer clinical trials, resulting in a lack of robust data on the safety, tolerability, and efficacy of cancer treatments in this vulnerable population. While most cancer clinical trials no longer have a formal upper age limit for participation, persistent barriers to enrollment include strict performance status and organ function eligibility criteria (eg, creatinine clearance >60 mL/min in a trial of a drug that is not renally excreted), physician bias (ie, ageism) in not presenting trial options based on chronologic age, and patient lack of social support or ability to travel to meet rigorous trial requirements. The 2017 American Society of Clinical Oncology (ASCO) and Friends of Cancer Research joint research statement outlines consensus recommendations to safely broaden trial eligibility criteria to optimize the generalizability of results. The need for alternative trial end points to capture more than the gold standard of overall survival and to focus on issues important to older adults such as quality of life and the maintenance of functional capacity is detailed in a 2013 joint position paper from two cancer cooperative groups (the European Organization for Research and Treatment of Cancer and Alliance for Clinical Trials in Oncology) and the International Society for Geriatric Oncology.

In 2018, ASCO published its first guidelines on the practical assessment and management of vulnerabilities in older patients receiving chemotherapy. An expert panel developed these clinical practice guidelines through a systematic review of the medical literature. While the guidelines primarily focused on older adults receiving chemotherapy, many of the recommendations are applicable to a broad range of therapies and cancer care issues. ASCO recommends that all patients age 65 and older receiving chemotherapy undergo a geriatric assessment (GA; see Chapter 2: "Overview of Geriatric Assessment") to identify impairments that are often missed in traditional oncology assessments. The feasibility of conducting GAs in older adults with cancer has been well established in both routine clinical care and the clinical trial setting. Assessment of physical function, falls, multimorbidity, medications, psychological health, cognition, nutrition, and social support can help risk-stratify older adults to determine their risk of treatment toxicity, inform shared decision making, and provide an opportunity to implement GA-guided interventions to optimize non–cancer-related chronic conditions and functional impairments. Randomized clinical trials of GA-guided interventions in oncology on patient-centered outcomes such as cancer patient and caregiver quality of life, communication, and physical function are ongoing.

There are two validated risk prediction models for older adults receiving chemotherapy. Both tools predict the risk of serious adverse events graded according to the National Cancer Institute Common Terminology Criteria for Adverse Events (1 = mild, 2 = moderate, 3 = severe, 4 = life-threatening, 5 = death related to adverse event). Developed and validated in studies of patients age 65 and older with a solid tumor, the Cancer and Aging Research Group (CARG) Hurria Tox Tool incorporates GA characteristics (ie, falls, limitations with hearing, medication administration, walking one block, social activities), age, cancer type and chemotherapy information, and laboratory results (ie, hemoglobin, creatinine clearance) to predict the risk of developing a grade 3 or higher adverse event during chemotherapy. The CARG Hurria Tox Tool predicts chemotherapy toxicity with better discrimination than the commonly used clinician-rated Karnofsky Performance Status scale. The Chemotherapy Risk Assessment Scale for High-Age Patients (CRASH) score includes patients age 70 and older with a solid tumor or hematologic malignancy. The CRASH score incorporates GA characteristics (ie, instrumental activities of daily living [IADL], cognition, nutrition), Eastern Cooperative Oncology Group (ECOG) performance status, diastolic blood pressure, lactic dehydrogenase, and an adjustment for the specific chemotherapy regimen called the MAX2 index to predict grade 3 or 4 nonhematologic toxicity and grade 4 hematologic toxicity. Of note, both models only included older adults receiving chemotherapy and did not include patients receiving other types of systemic therapy (eg, immunotherapy, targeted therapy) or other modalities of treatment (eg, radiation, surgery).

Furthermore, the ASCO guidelines recommend the use of validated tools, such as those found at ePrognosis, to estimate life expectancy to evaluate competing risks of mortality (see Chapter 4, "Goals of Care & Consideration of Prognosis"). Understanding non–cancer-related life expectancy is especially pertinent when considering treatment for an indolent cancer or decisions regarding adjuvant therapy, where the patient has completed definitive therapy and is considering additional treatment to decrease the recurrence risk.

To move beyond traditional measures of cancer treatment toxicity, several studies have examined changes in physical function in older adults during chemotherapy. In a French study of patients age 70 and older receiving first-line chemotherapy, factors associated with functional decline in activities of daily living (ADL) after one cycle of chemotherapy included high baseline depression score and dependence in IADL. In a Belgian study, abnormal nutrition status on the Mini Nutritional Assessment–Short Form was associated with functional decline in ADL 2 to 3 months after initiation of chemotherapy. In contrast, patients receiving chemotherapy for a new cancer diagnosis had a higher risk of decline in IADL than those receiving chemotherapy for disease progression or relapse. Importantly, decline in ADL was strongly associated with worse overall survival. In a US study of patients age 65 and older with a new cancer diagnosis or progressive disease receiving chemotherapy, higher baseline morning fatigue was associated with functional decline over two cycles.

Treatment

Diagnosis-specific therapies are described in the sections that follow. In addition to disease-specific guideline recommendations on treatment options, several factors including functional status, life expectancy, and the patient's preferences, values, and goals of care should be taken into consideration for shared decision making regarding cancer screening and treatment in the older population. If it has been determined that the cancer is not curable or that the patient is unable to tolerate aggressive therapy, the goal becomes palliation of cancer-related symptoms such as nausea, dyspnea, and pain. Cancer pain management should be tailored to the individual patient's pain needs and may require nonpharmacologic interventions such as radiation therapy. Attention should be paid to the effective management of potential complications of pain management such as constipation and delirium (see Chapter 22, "Geriatric Palliative Care"; Chapter 36, "Delirium"; Chapter 61, "Constipation"; and Chapter 63, "Persistent Pain"). ASCO recommends that all patients with advanced cancer receive early palliative care concurrent with their oncologic care.

LUNG CANCER

▶ General Principles

With a median age at diagnosis of 70 years, lung cancer is the leading cause of cancer death. Over 50% of patients with lung cancer have metastatic disease at diagnosis. Lung cancers are categorized as either non–small cell lung cancer (NSCLC) or small cell lung cancer (SCLC), with the majority of lung carcinomas being adenocarcinomas. Tissue confirmation for histologic type provides important diagnostic, prognostic, and therapeutic information. Prognosis is also related to stage, performance status, gender, and the patient's ability to tolerate adequate treatment. Although age is not an independent prognostic factor, older patients can experience more side effects from lung cancer treatment.

▶ Screening

Since 2013, the US Preventive Services Task Force (USPSTF) has recommended that adults between the ages of 55 and 80 who have at least a 30-pack-year smoking history and currently smoke or have quit within the past 15 years receive annual low-dose CT chest scans to screen for lung cancer. Older adults with a limited life expectancy or who would not want or tolerate definitive lung cancer treatment should not be screened. While the Centers for Medicare and Medicaid Services requires shared decision making using a decision aid to discuss the benefits and harms of screening as part of lung cancer screening coverage, a qualitative analysis of these visits showed minimal discussion of potential harms. For a more detailed approach to decision making regarding cancer screening, see Chapter 4, "Goals of Care & Consideration of Prognosis," and Chapter 20, "Prevention & Health Promotion."

▶ Treatment

Treatment options are determined by tumor histology, stage, and predictive biomarkers including genomic alterations and programmed death-ligand 1 (PD-L1) tumor proportion score. Staging workup should include a fluorodeoxyglucose positron emission tomography (FDG-PET) scan and magnetic resonance imaging of the brain.

A. NSCLC

1. Localized disease—For older adults with localized NSCLC, appropriate staging includes a mediastinoscopy or bronchoscopy for nodal sampling before resection of the primary tumor. If there is no nodal involvement, then surgical resection is recommended for fit patients. For frail patients or patients who prefer to avoid a surgical approach, stereotactic body radiation is an alternative option. Adjuvant chemotherapy may be recommended if high-risk pathologic features or nodal involvement are identified at surgery. For locally advanced NSCLC, the optimal multimodality approach including chemotherapy, radiation, and/or surgery should be discussed as part of a multidisciplinary tumor board. If concurrent chemoradiation is pursued for inoperable, locally advanced NSCLC, adjuvant durvalumab (anti–PD-L1 monoclonal antibody) improves overall survival compared to no adjuvant therapy. Of note, existing chemotherapy toxicity risk models (CARG Hurria Tox Tool, CRASH score) excluded patients receiving radiation. In a study of patients age 75 years or older with inoperable, locally advanced NSCLC, GA and the Vulnerable Elders Survey (VES-13)—a brief frailty screening tool that assesses age, self-rated health, limitations in physical function, and functional disabilities—were independently prognostic and should be performed to inform clinical decision making.

2. Metastatic disease—Patients with metastatic lung adenocarcinoma should undergo molecular testing to determine if actionable genomic alterations, which include mutations and gene rearrangements, are present to guide therapy. To minimize tissue use, which is often scarce from lung biopsies, the National Comprehensive Cancer Network (NCCN) recommends testing as part of broad molecular profiling to assess multiple genes simultaneously to identify alterations including mutations in *EGFR*, *BRAF*, and *NTRK* and rearrangements in *ALK* and *ROS1* (please see online NCCN NSCLC guidelines for updated list of actionable alterations). Peripheral blood testing for cell-free DNA is an additional option for molecular testing when biopsy tissue samples are exhausted or the risk of biopsy is high. Molecular testing should be considered for patients with metastatic squamous cell carcinoma if they are never-smokers, had a small biopsy specimen, or had mixed histology. Patients with metastatic NSCLC should also undergo PD-L1 testing to guide first-line therapy.

Immunotherapy has revolutionized the treatment of metastatic NSCLC without an actionable mutation. For metastatic NSCLC, first-line treatment has changed from chemotherapy alone to chemoimmunotherapy. For metastatic NSCLC, guideline-recommended first-line treatment is combination pembrolizumab (anti–PD-1 monoclonal antibody), carboplatin, and pemetrexed (if adenocarcinoma) or (nab)-paclitaxel (if squamous cell carcinoma). Additional treatment options include carboplatin, paclitaxel, bevacizumab (anti-VEGF monoclonal antibody), and atezolizumab (anti–PD-L1 monoclonal antibody); doublet chemotherapy (for patients with a contraindication to immunotherapy); or single-agent chemotherapy for patients with a vulnerable performance status. For patients with a high PD-L1 score (≥50%), pembrolizumab alone is an effective, more tolerable option. Of note, for patients with a low PD-L1 score (<50%), first-line pembrolizumab monotherapy is not currently approved by the US Food and Drug Administration (FDA). Geriatricians and primary care clinicians caring for patients receiving immunotherapy should be aware that immune-related adverse events (eg, rash, colitis, pneumonitis, nephritis, hepatitis) can develop any time during treatment or after immunotherapy has been discontinued. ASCO and NCCN both have published guidelines on the management of immune-related adverse events.

In the preimmunotherapy era of NSCLC treatment, the landmark Elderly Selection on Geriatric Index Assessment (ESOGIA) phase III randomized trial compared a standard chemotherapy allocation strategy based on age and ECOG performance status with a GA-driven chemotherapy allocation strategy. The GA-driven chemotherapy allocation strategy resulted in similar overall survival but lower rates of treatment discontinuation for toxicity and better quality of life scores during follow-up. A GA-driven treatment allocation strategy in the era of chemoimmunotherapy has not yet been conducted.

B. SCLC

Approximately 10% to 15% of all lung cancers are SCLCs. Among patients with limited-stage SCLC (stage I–III that can be safely treated with definitive radiation doses), concurrent chemoradiation is the standard of care. A subset of limited-stage disease can be treated with resection followed by adjuvant chemotherapy and, if nodal involvement is present, adjuvant radiation as well. Older patients are more likely to require delays in chemotherapy or dose reductions as a result of toxicity. Yet, despite these modifications, the likelihood of response to treatment and overall survival are similar to those for younger patients. Prophylactic cranial irradiation can be considered for patients with a good response to initial therapy but can be associated with significant morbidity. For patients with extensive-stage SCLC, chemoimmunotherapy with carboplatin, etoposide, and atezolizumab is the new standard of care.

BREAST CANCER

► General Principles

Breast cancer is the most common cancer among women worldwide. Women age 65 and older account for approximately 40% of all breast cancer diagnoses, and age is an independent risk factor for developing breast cancer. Multiple studies have demonstrated that older adults with breast cancer are less likely to be offered or receive guideline-recommended treatment, even after adjusting for confounding factors such as comorbidity, social support, and functional status. Consequently, undertreatment of older adults leads to an increased risk of breast cancer–specific mortality, and several studies have shown that older patients are more likely to die of their breast cancer compared to younger patients.

Screening

The USPSTF recommends biennial screening mammography for women age 50 to 74 years and concludes that there is insufficient evidence to assess the benefits and harms of mammography in women age 75 and older. However, shared decision making for cancer screening decisions for older women should not be based on chronologic age alone and should incorporate life expectancy, goals of care, functional status, and comorbidities (see Chapter 4, "Goals of Care & Consideration of Prognosis," and Chapter 20, "Prevention & Health Promotion"). Shared decision making must be informed by weighing both the potential benefits (eg, early detection, early treatment, and reduced mortality) and harms (eg, false positives, unnecessary biopsies, and anxiety).

Treatment

A. Early-Stage Breast Cancer

1. Surgery—Surgical resection is the standard of care for the treatment of early-stage breast cancer. However, in older patients, clinicians may have concerns about higher rates of anesthetic and/or surgical complications. As a result, there remains a fundamental question of whether surgery can be omitted and replaced with primary endocrine therapy alone in older patients with estrogen receptor (ER)–positive breast cancer. Several studies compared surgery with or without adjuvant tamoxifen and primary endocrine therapy with tamoxifen alone. Findings demonstrated no significant differences in overall survival between these approaches. However, in terms of local disease control, tamoxifen alone was inferior to surgery with tamoxifen. Therefore, primary endocrine therapy is a reasonable alternative for a select group of patients who are frail with a limited life expectancy (<2–3 years). In contrast, older women who are medically fit and have a favorable life expectancy (estimated survival of at least several years) should be treated with standard of care surgical approaches, including sentinel lymph node biopsy.

2. Radiation—Although adjuvant radiation is generally well tolerated, the absolute benefit may be less in older women. This finding has been demonstrated in randomized clinical trials, which support the omission of adjuvant radiation in patients age 70 and older with small, ER-positive,

node-negative tumors on endocrine therapy. Despite higher rates of local recurrence, data show that there is no survival advantage for additional radiation following breast-conserving surgery in this population. Informed decisions about adjuvant radiation after breast-conserving surgery should be individualized to each patient's goals, values, and priorities. For patients who do choose to undergo radiation, hypofractionated treatment courses (higher dose of radiation administered over a shorter time frame) have demonstrated similar efficacy and improved toxicity at reduced costs. Ongoing studies examining techniques to deliver radiation more effectively, including partial breast irradiation, brachytherapy, and intraoperative radiotherapy, may be of particular relevance to older patients.

3. Systemic therapy—Limited prospective data exist about the efficacy and toxicity of adjuvant chemotherapy in older adults with breast cancer. Existing studies, however, suggest that adjuvant chemotherapy can result in an improved survival for older patients but at the risk of higher rates of treatment-related toxicity including cardiotoxicity and bone marrow disorders. The most pronounced benefits were experienced in patients with positive lymph nodes or other high-risk features such as large tumor size. Therefore, for medically fit patients, the same principles that guide the use of adjuvant systemic therapy in younger individuals should also apply to older adults.

Identifying who is at high risk of developing chemotherapy toxicity can help guide treatment strategies for older women with early-stage, high-risk breast cancer. To determine which clinical factors predict severe grade 3 or higher chemotherapy-related toxicities, Hurria and colleagues from CARG performed a prospective, multicenter study of approximately 500 women age 65 and older with stage I to III breast cancer receiving neoadjuvant or adjuvant chemotherapy. Findings revealed key factors associated with an increased risk of chemotherapy toxicity, including stage II/III breast cancer, planned duration of chemotherapy >3 months, anthracycline use, baseline anemia, abnormal liver function tests, more than one fall in the past 6 months, limited ambulatory abilities, and decreased social support. These factors were then used to construct and validate a predictive model for toxicity risk, known as CARG–Breast Cancer (CARG-BC) Chemotherapy Toxicity Tool. This is the first predictive model developed specifically for the geriatric breast cancer population. Utilization of this tool can help oncologists and patients estimate chemotherapy risk and potentially identify interventions to minimize toxicity.

4. Endocrine therapy—Compared to younger patients, older patients are more likely to have low-grade, ER-positive tumors. As a consequence, endocrine therapy has been the mainstay of adjuvant systemic therapy in geriatric breast oncology. The efficacy of adjuvant endocrine therapy, with tamoxifen or an aromatase inhibitor, in older patients is well established. In women with ER-positive breast cancer, tamoxifen for a duration of 5 years reduces the annual risk of recurrence and mortality by 39% and 31%, respectively, irrespective of age. Additionally, several studies have demonstrated a small benefit of aromatase inhibitors over tamoxifen across all age groups. Older patients on aromatase inhibitors should be evaluated for osteopenia or osteoporosis with a baseline dual x-ray absorptiometry scan given the well-described increased bone loss during treatment coupled with the age-related decline in bone mineral density. In contrast, patients on tamoxifen need to be counseled about the risk of cerebrovascular and thromboembolic events and endometrial cancer.

B. Metastatic Disease

Given that the majority of breast cancers in older adults are ER-positive, endocrine therapy is the mainstay of treatment for metastatic breast cancer. In particular, aromatase inhibitors have achieved a higher rate of tumor regression and a longer duration of efficacy and have a more favorable toxicity profile relative to tamoxifen. The addition of targeted therapy, such as CDK4/6 inhibitors, to endocrine therapy can significantly improve progression-free survival. Pooled retrospective analysis of the targeted therapies demonstrates that both efficacy and adverse events are similar for older and younger patients. However, prospective trials to assess the safety and tolerability of these drugs in older patients are ongoing.

In ER-negative disease and ER-positive breast cancers that are hormone resistant, chemotherapy may provide effective palliation. Single-agent cytotoxic therapy is recommended given the increased toxicity associated with combination chemotherapy. In women with HER2-positive breast cancer, anti-HER2 therapy alone can be given to older adults or in combination with an aromatase inhibitor or chemotherapy depending on the hormone receptor status. Anti-HER2 therapy (trastuzumab and pertuzumab) combined with chemotherapy has been shown to further improve survival compared to trastuzumab and chemotherapy alone. Additionally, single-agent ado-trastuzumab emtansine has also been shown to decrease recurrence risk compared to trastuzumab alone and has a favorable toxicity profile.

PROSTATE CANCER

▶ General Principles

Prostate cancer is the second most common nonskin malignancy in men after lung cancer. More than 2 million men are currently living with the disease, and 1 million over the age of 75. It is an especially important cancer in older adults as the incidence and mortality rise steadily with age. Approximately 60% of those diagnosed with and 90% who die from prostate cancer are over the age of 65. Given the heterogeneity of prostate cancer, ranging from indolent to aggressive phenotypes, a risk-adopted approach is used to manage prostate cancer.

It categorizes prostate cancer into several clinical states: (1) localized, (2) biochemical recurrence, (3) metastatic castration-sensitive disease, and (4) castration-resistant disease. Each clinical state has a distinct prognosis and therapeutic objectives that balance an individual's risk of developing metastasis or death from prostate cancer with their overall health and competing comorbidities. Thus, using this model, some patients may not require treatment, while others would benefit from immediate intervention.

▶ Screening

Screening modalities include serum prostate-specific antigen (PSA) measurement and digital rectal exams (DRE). Due to the heterogeneity of prostate cancer, the risk of overdiagnosis and overtreatment with routine screening are major concerns, especially among older adults. With routine screening among average-risk men, a large proportion of men are diagnosed with low-risk prostate cancer that would otherwise not progress to clinically significant disease during their lifetime. Thus, most organizations recommend against routine screening for prostate cancer in asymptomatic older men with either PSA or DRE, including the USPSTF, the Canadian Task Force on Preventive Health Care, the European Society for Medical Oncology, and the NCCN. ASCO recommends a discussion with men with over a 10-year life expectancy. In general, the overall health status and life expectancy of an individual must be incorporated into the decision to screen. Average-risk, asymptomatic patients with a life expectancy of <10 years are unlikely to benefit from routine screening given competing comorbidities, and many can be harmed from unnecessary procedures and emotional distress. Screening should not be offered if a patient would not be an appropriate candidate for treatment. For those with a life expectancy >10 years, it is important to weigh the risks, benefits, and current uncertainties of scientific evidence on screening, alongside the patient's preferences and the potential effects of treatment on the patient's quality of life. For a more detailed approach to decision making regarding cancer screening, see Chapter 4, "Goals of Care & Consideration of Prognosis," and Chapter 20, "Prevention & Health Promotion."

▶ Clinical Approach

A. Symptoms & Signs

Prostate cancer in its earlier stages is typically asymptomatic. As it becomes more advanced, symptoms develop, including urinary urgency, frequency, hesitancy, and nocturia. Prostate cancer can also present as new-onset erectile dysfunction or with the presence of blood in the urine or semen. Patients may present when the cancer has already metastasized to distant sites. The most common site is bone, presenting with pain or a pathologic fracture.

On physical exam, prostate cancer can sometimes be detected through abnormalities on the DRE. These changes include asymmetry, distinct areas of induration, and frank nodules on the prostate gland.

B. Laboratory Findings

Elevations in serum PSA can be associated with prostate cancer. A general rule is that the higher the PSA and the faster the rise in PSA over time, the higher is the likelihood of detecting cancer on biopsy. Biopsy is usually recommended if the PSA level is >10 ng/mL or if there is a persistent rise in PSA.

C. Diagnostics

A histologic biopsy is required to confirm the diagnosis of prostate cancer. Biopsies are obtained via transrectal ultrasonography to increase accuracy. Biopsies can have substantial associated morbidities, including pain, hematuria, infection, urinary obstruction, and anxiety from a positive result that may not require treatment.

▶ Treatment

Biopsy results, along with TNM (tumor, node, metastasis) and clinical staging, will guide the selection of initial therapy. It is important to assess older adults with a GA, including assessment for comorbidities, functional status, cognition, falls, nutrition, frailty, mood, and social support. Equally important is balancing a patient's stated goals and preferences with the risks and benefits of each therapeutic option being considered. Involvement of an interdisciplinary team, including the primary care provider, oncologist, and urologist, along with nursing, social work, and physical therapy will allow formulation of a comprehensive, patient-centered treatment plan.

A. Localized Prostate Cancer

For localized, organ-confined prostate cancer, the goal of therapy is to balance the risk of metastasis and death from prostate cancer with adverse effects from treatment and competing comorbidities. Pathologic grading is central, as low-grade disease (Gleason scores of ≤6) is often managed with observation or active surveillance, whereas high-grade disease (Gleason scores of ≥8) should be treated with definitive prostate-directed therapy. Definitive treatment options include surgical resection (prostatectomy), radiation via external beam radiation therapy, or brachytherapy. There is no evidence of the superiority of any of these options in otherwise similar patients. Active surveillance is an important option for patients with a favorable phenotype (small tumor, low Gleason score). The goal of active surveillance is to monitor closely with PSA measurements and repeat biopsy; curative treatment is only pursued for disease progression. For fit older adults with high-risk features (large tumor and

Gleason score of ≥8), short-term androgen-deprivation therapy (ADT) can be considered as adjuvant therapy to lower the risk of future metastasis.

B. Biochemical Recurrence

Biochemical recurrence is a disease state where PSA rises without detectable metastatic disease on imaging after definitive treatment for localized disease. Depending on the rate of increase in PSA, Gleason score, and the amount of time from definitive local therapy to biochemical recurrence, patients are treated with either observation or ADT. If ADT is used, intermittent ADT should be considered over continuous ADT given similar survival rates, less toxicity, and lower risk of developing castration resistance with intermittent ADT.

C. Advanced Prostate Cancer

For advanced prostate cancer, an important treatment distinction is between castrate-sensitive and castrate-resistant disease, as the latter has the shortest survival. Castrate levels of serum testosterone (<50 ng/dL) are used to distinguish between these two disease states. Continuous ADT is considered the backbone treatment for all advanced prostate cancer. It is accomplished with either surgical castration through bilateral orchiectomy or chemical castration with gonadotropin-releasing hormone agonists or antagonists. For castrate-sensitive disease, ADT alone is reasonable for frail older adults who are symptomatic from their prostate cancer. In a fit older adult, ADT can be combined with chemotherapy (eg, docetaxel) or another therapeutic agent that intensifies androgen blockade (eg, abiraterone, enzalutamide, or apalutamide). It is important to note that while survival is improved in combination therapy compared to ADT alone, the survival benefit is less in older men, who are also at higher risk for toxicity.

Treatment options for castrate-resistant prostate cancer in a man with optimal health include intensified androgen blockade (eg, ADT with either abiraterone or enzalutamide) or ADT in combination with chemotherapy (eg, docetaxel or cabazitaxel). All have similar impact on survival, so the choice of therapy is based on the toxicity profile. For patients who have symptomatic bone metastasis and are castrate resistant, palliative treatment with radium-223 is recommended, as it has been shown to prolong life and decrease complications. Immunotherapy with Sipuleucel-T, an autologous cellular vaccine, is another FDA-approved treatment for patients with metastatic castration-resistant prostate cancer; however, the overall survival benefit is only 4 months.

▶ Complications

Older men have higher surgical complication rates. Urinary incontinence and erectile dysfunction are common. Gastrointestinal (colitis) and genitourinary (proctitis) symptoms are the most common adverse effects of localized radiation.

ADT for the treatment of advanced prostate cancer also has several potential complications, including osteoporosis and fractures, metabolic syndrome, diabetes, cardiovascular disease, hot flashes, gynecomastia, testicular atrophy, fatigue, sarcopenia, and depression. With such an extensive side effect profile, the prescribing provider must consider the potential interactions with already present underlying comorbidities, as these may be exacerbated during treatment. Sexual dysfunction is a common adverse effect that can result from all treatment options, with incidence rates between <5% and 60%. This potential adverse outcome should be discussed with patients prior to initiation of therapy.

COLORECTAL CANCER

▶ Colorectal Cancer Screening

Colonoscopy has been established as a cost-effective screening tool. The initial screening should begin at age 50 years and is repeated every 10 years until age 75 years. If polyps are identified, the procedure should be repeated every 3 to 5 years. As with any screening test, the decision to screen should weigh life expectancy and goals of care with the potential risks and benefits of screening. For a more detailed approach to decision making regarding screening, see Chapter 4, "Goals of Care & Consideration of Prognosis," and Chapter 20, "Prevention & Health Promotion."

▶ Rectal Cancer Treatment

The natural history of rectal cancer differs from colon cancer. Because the rectum lies in close proximity to the sacral plexus, uterus, bladder, and prostate, a wide radial margin is often difficult to obtain with surgery, and local recurrences are more common. To prevent local disease recurrence, fluorouracil (5-FU; as infusion or in the form of oral capecitabine) is given in conjunction with radiation therapy prior to surgical resection. Among older adults, the advantages of combined-modality treatment of rectal cancer are similar to those observed in younger patients.

▶ Adjuvant Colon Cancer Treatment

Older adults who have undergone colonic resection for stage II or III colon cancer require a careful consideration of adjuvant chemotherapy that should include an assessment of an individual's risk of recurrence, estimated risk of chemotherapy toxicity, and estimated life expectancy (without recurrence). For fit older adults with high-risk stage II or III colon cancer and life expectancies >5 years, single-agent treatment with either 5-FU or oral capecitabine chemotherapy is recommended. The additional benefit of adding oxaliplatin to 5-FU is unclear and was not found to improve survival in patients older than 70 years in clinical trials in stage III colon cancers, as was demonstrated in younger patients (Adjuvant Colon Cancer Endpoints [ACCENT] trial). A large population-based analysis of real-world data suggests a marginal improvement in survival with the addition of oxaliplatin in patients older than age 75 years with stage III colon cancer. Thus, the addition of oxaliplatin could be considered but should be reserved only for the healthiest subset of older patients. Although recent data have suggested similar benefits of adjuvant 5-FU plus oxaliplatin (FOLFOX) for lower risk stage III colon cancers (T3N1 disease) with 3 versus 6 months of therapy, these data do not readily apply to single-agent therapy, and 6 months of treatment remains the standard duration for single-agent adjuvant chemotherapy.

▶ Metastatic Colorectal Cancer

Although most large bowel cancers metastasize to the liver, the pattern of disease recurrence differs somewhat depending on whether the primary tumor arises from the colon or rectum. The drainage of the colon is via the portal vein, and the liver is the most common site, and possibly the only site, of metastasis. Because the inferior mesenteric vein receives drainage from the rectum, systemic metastasis to sites in addition to the liver may develop.

The treatment of colorectal cancers in older patients does not differ substantially from that for younger individuals; however, clinically relevant comorbid conditions, functional impairments, and geriatric syndromes are more prevalent in older patients and, combined with age-related declines in organ function, can alter the tolerability of systemic chemotherapy. In determining the risk and benefits of systemic treatment, a GA can be beneficial in gauging treatment tolerability. Metastatic colorectal cancer is generally incurable. However, resection of liver metastases may provide long-term disease-free survival and potential cure for select oligometastatic patients.

5-FU–based regimens are the mainstay of chemotherapy and provide prolongation of survival and often improve or maintain quality of life. The addition of irinotecan or oxaliplatin to 5-FU (FOLFIRI or FOLFOX) produces a greater likelihood of tumor regression and a longer survival than is achievable with 5-FU alone. Upfront dose reductions can be used in frail older adults, as performed in the seminal FOCUS2 study that demonstrated the tolerability and efficacy of systemic chemotherapy in frail older adults with metastatic colorectal cancer. Bevacizumab (an antiangiogenic monoclonal antibody) or EGFR inhibitors (cetuximab or panitumumab) are often added to first-line chemotherapy depending on tumor location and the molecular characterization of the tumor. While these agents may lead to some increased risk of chemotherapy toxicities, both appear to be tolerable in fit older adults with metastatic colorectal cancer.

Although the primary tumor may result in potential perforation, bleeding, or obstruction that may require emergency surgical intervention, the majority of patients without symptoms from the primary tumor at presentation do not require upfront resection because these events only occur in a minority of patients (ranging from 9%–29%) treated with 5-FU–based chemotherapy.

LEUKEMIA

▶ Acute Myeloid Leukemia

Acute myeloid leukemia (AML) is the most common type of acute leukemia, and approximately 58% of new AML cases are diagnosed in adults age 65 and older. Median overall survival is generally <1 year, and 5-year overall survival is <5%.

A. Treatment

Treatment for AML is generally based on whether patients are considered "fit" or "unfit," although there are no standard criteria to define fitness. Fitness for therapy is often based on physicians' subjective assessment and is commonly influenced by chronologic age and chronic conditions. Inpatient intensive chemotherapy has been the standard of care for >40 years for older adults who are considered "fit." Given its high associated treatment-related mortality, outpatient chemotherapy such as hypomethylating agents (decitabine or azacytidine) has been increasingly used in the past decade, especially in those who are considered "unfit," due to better tolerability. More recently, combination outpatient regimens have been shown to have better or similar efficacy and better tolerability compared to inpatient intensive chemotherapy. For example, venetoclax (an inhibitor of B-cell lymphoma 2 [Bcl-2]) is approved for use with hypomethylating agents in adults aged 75 years or older or who have chronic conditions that preclude the use of intensive chemotherapy. Because AML is a heterogeneous disease, cancer therapies targeting specific mutations associated with AML are also increasingly available (eg, the isocitrate dehydrogenase-1 inhibitor enasidenib). Allogeneic stem cell transplantation (ASCT) is the only curative option, but age and fitness frequently preclude older adults from receiving ASCT. There has been an increasing effort to use GA to better define fitness for therapy. For example, studies have shown that poor functional status and physical performance are associated with worse outcomes and may better define fitness versus using chronologic age alone. However, these factors are currently not incorporated in therapeutic trials.

▶ Acute Lymphoid Leukemia

Acute lymphoid leukemia (ALL) is less common than AML, with 12% of new ALL cases occurring in adults age 65 and older. ALL is generally divided into Philadelphia chromosome positive (Ph+) and negative (Ph–).

A. Treatment

Patients with Ph+ ALL respond well to tyrosine kinase inhibitors and steroids as initial therapy, but most patients eventually relapse and very few have long-term survival. Ph– ALL is treated with combination chemotherapy regimens, which may be challenging for older adults who are considered "unfit." Like AML, the criteria for fitness are largely based on physicians' subjective assessment and commonly use chronologic age.

▶ Acute Promyelocytic Leukemia

Acute promyelocytic leukemia (APML) is uncommon in older adults, but outcomes are relatively favorable compared to AML and ALL. Depending on the risk, older adults with APML are treated with all-trans retinoic acid (ATRA) with arsenic acid or ATRA with chemotherapy.

LYMPHOMA

Lymphoid malignancies are currently categorized using the 2016 World Health Organization (WHO) classification system. More broadly, lymphomas are categorized into non-Hodgkin (NHL) and Hodgkin lymphoma or indolent and aggressive lymphomas.

▶ Indolent Lymphomas

Common types of indolent lymphomas include follicular lymphoma, marginal zone lymphoma, and lymphoplasmacytic lymphoma (or Waldenström macroglobulinemia).

A. Treatment

Indolent lymphomas are treatable but generally incurable. Treatments include observation, radiation, and systemic therapy such as rituximab and chemoimmunotherapy (eg, bendamustine and rituximab).

▶ Chronic Lymphocytic Leukemia

Chronic lymphocytic leukemia (CLL) or small lymphocytic lymphoma (SLL) constitutes approximately 7% of newly diagnosed NHL and is considered an indolent lymphoma. Approximately 67% of new CLL/SLL cases occur in adults age 65 and older. Many CLL cases are detected incidentally from blood tests.

A. Treatment

Initiation of treatment for CLL is based on severe symptoms (eg, fever, night sweats), cytopenias due to bone marrow failure, bulky lymphadenopathy, and/or rapidly increasing lymphocyte counts. It is worth noting that autoimmune cytopenias occur in <10% of CLLs. Many treatments have been approved for use in CLL, and these include the Bruton tyrosine kinase (BTK) inhibitor ibrutinib and the combination of an alkylating agent (chlorambucil or bendamustine) and an anti-CD20 monoclonal antibody (rituximab or obinutuzumab).

Aggressive Lymphoma

The most common type of aggressive lymphoma is diffuse large B-cell lymphoma (DLBCL). Others include high-grade B-cell lymphoma with *MYC* and *BCL2* and/or *BCL6* translocations (ie, "double-hit" or "triple-hit" lymphomas) and Burkitt lymphoma.

Diffuse Large B-Cell Lymphoma

DLBCL is the most common type of NHL, composing approximately 30% of NHLs. Approximately 58% of new DLBCL cases occur in adults age 65 and older. More than 50% of older adults with DLBCL achieve cure from standard treatment.

A. Treatment

The standard first-line treatment for DLBCL is combination chemoimmunotherapy (rituximab, cyclophosphamide, doxorubicin, vincristine, and prednisone [R-CHOP]). Radiation is also incorporated in the treatment of early-stage DLBCL. Refractory DLBCL occurs in 10% of cases and relapsed DLBCL occurs in 30% to 40% of cases. Options in these patients include a different chemoimmunotherapy typically followed by an autologous hematopoietic stem cell transplantation (HCT). More recently, chimeric antigen receptor T-cell (CAR-T) therapies have become available. Although treatment-related toxicities are of concern in older adults, the development of newer CAR-T therapies with better tolerability will allow older adults to receive this therapy.

Multiple Myeloma

Multiple myeloma (MM) is a plasma cell neoplasm, and approximately 63% of new MM cases occur in adults age 65 and older. The treatment paradigm for MM has drastically changed in the past decade given emerging novel therapeutic agents and combination regimens. Many older adults with MM now receive continuous treatment for many years with or without autologous HCT. Therefore, supportive care for MM and therapy-related toxicities such as osteoporosis, infection, and venous thromboembolism are crucial in this population.

Brahmer JR, Lacchetti C, Schneider BJ, et al. Management of immune-related adverse events in patients treated with immune checkpoint inhibitor therapy: American Society of Clinical Oncology Clinical practice guideline. *J Clin Oncol.* 2018;36(17):1714-1768.

Corre R, Greillier L, Le Caer H, et al. Use of a comprehensive geriatric assessment for the management of elderly patients with advanced non-small-cell lung cancer: the phase III randomized ESOGIA-GFPC-GECP 08-02 study. *J Clin Oncol.* 2016;34(13):1476-1483.

Extermann M, Boler I, Reich RR, et al. Predicting the risk of chemotherapy toxicity in older patients: the Chemotherapy Risk Assessment Scale for High-Age Patients (CRASH) score. *Cancer.* 2012;118(13):3377-3386.

Hoppe S, Rainfray M, Fonck M, et al. Functional decline in older patients with cancer receiving first-line chemotherapy. *J Clin Oncol.* 2013;31(31):3877-3882.

Hurria A, Mohile S, Gajra A, et al. Validation of a prediction tool for chemotherapy toxicity in older adults with cancer. *J Clin Oncol.* 2016;34(20):2366-2371.

Hurria A, Togawa K, Mohile SG, et al. Predicting chemotherapy toxicity in older adults with cancer: A prospective multicenter study. *J Clin Oncol.* 2011;29(25):3457-3465.

Kenis C, Decoster L, Bastin J, et al. Functional decline in older patients with cancer receiving chemotherapy: a multicenter prospective study. *J Geriatr Oncol.* 2017;8(3):196-205.

Kim ES, Bruinooge SS, Roberts S, et al. Broadening eligibility criteria to make clinical trials more representative: American Society of Clinical Oncology and Friends of Cancer Research joint research statement. *J Clin Oncol.* 2017;35(33):3737-3744.

Mohile SG, Dale W, Somerfield MR, et al. Practical assessment and management of vulnerabilities in older patients receiving chemotherapy: ASCO guideline for geriatric oncology. *J Clin Oncol.* 2018;36(22):2326-2347.

Smith BD, Smith GL, Hurria A, Hortobagyi GN, Buchholz TA. Future of cancer incidence in the United States: burdens upon an aging, changing nation. *J Clin Oncol.* 2009;27(17):2758-2765.

USEFUL WEBSITES

Cancer and Aging Research Group (CARG) geriatric assessment tools. http://www.mycarg.org/SelectQuestionnaire. Accessed April 7, 2020.

International Society of Geriatric Oncology (SIOG) guidelines. http://siog.org/content/siog-guidelines-0. Accessed April 7, 2020.

National Cancer Institute Cancer Therapy Evaluation Program. Common Terminology Criteria for Adverse Events (CTCAE) v5.0. https://ctep.cancer.gov/protocolDevelopment/electronic_applications/ctc.htm. Accessed April 7, 2020.

National Cancer Institute's Surveillance Epidemiology, and End Results database. http://seer.cancer.gov/index.html. Accessed April 7, 2020.

National Comprehensive Cancer Network (NCCN). https://www.nccn.org. Accessed April 7, 2020.

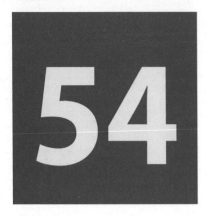

Common Infections

54

Ana Montoya, MD, MPH
Robin Jump, MD, PhD
Lona Mody, MD, MSc

ESSENTIALS OF DIAGNOSIS

► Diagnosing infections in older adults can be challenging because they may present with atypical symptoms and frequently do so in patients with cognitive impairment.

► Atypical symptoms include delirium, falls, or functional decline. Fever and other localizing symptoms may be subtle, absent, or difficult to elicit.

► Hospitalization and death as a consequence of pneumonia, influenza, and other respiratory tract infections are common.

► Urinary tract infection remains the most common over-diagnosed bacterial infection. Asymptomatic bacteriuria is common in older adults and requires no treatment.

► Optimal management of chronic diseases, immunizations, prevention of pressure ulcers, oral hygiene, judicious antibiotic use, and attention to infection prevention practices, including hand hygiene and appropriate gown and glove use, are key preventive measures to reduce infections and enhance quality of care in older adults in skilled nursing facilities.

General Principles

Infections remain a major cause of mortality and morbidity in older adults across all health care settings. Atypical presentations, immunologic changes related to aging, and multiple chronic conditions continue to make diagnosis of infections in older adults challenging. Infections are associated with higher rates of rehospitalization as well as functional decline and increased mortality among older adults. When infections lead to hospitalizations, older adults can be exposed to nosocomial pathogens and resultant complications, such as functional disability, delirium, and pressure ulcers.

Pneumonia and influenza are still among the top 10 causes of death in older adults. Infections common to older adults include the following: urinary tract infections (UTI), upper and lower respiratory tract infections, gastroenteritis including *Clostridioides* (formerly *Clostridium*) *difficile* infection, skin and soft-tissue infections including surgical site infections, osteomyelitis, and prosthetic device–associated infections. HIV/AIDS in aging populations is also a growing concern because those infected as younger adults now have an increasing life expectancy because of the effectiveness of antiretroviral therapy and because the number of new infections in older adults is also on the rise (see Chapter 55).

There are an estimated 1.13 to 2.68 million infections in nursing home residents each year, suggesting a downward trend from previous estimates, particularly for UTIs, wound infections, and infections due to multidrug-resistant organisms. Even so, infections continue to be a major concern. Moreover, about 25% of the short-stay older adults admitted to skilled nursing facilities return to a hospital for treatment of an infection within 30 days, accounting for 325,000 hospital transfers and over $4 billion in additional health care costs annually.

Pathogenesis

The risk of developing an infection and its resultant morbidity and mortality depend on the virulence of the pathogen, its inoculum, and the host's defense system. The ability of a pathogen to attach and replicate in a host environment determines its virulence. Age-related changes in the immune system, known as immunosenescence, result in increased susceptibility to infections, such as influenza and bacterial pneumonia, and in decreased effectiveness of vaccines, such as seasonal influenza and pneumococcal vaccines, to prevent infection. Specific changes include a decrease in the number and delays in activation of both B and T lymphocytes. Due to the involution of the thymus. older adults have few naïve

T cells and their B cells do not produce the same level of antibodies compared to younger adults. Chronic conditions, such as chronic kidney disease, diabetes, congestive heart failure, chronic lung diseases, and malnutrition, may further erode host defense mechanisms.

Atypical or subtle presenting signs and symptoms may lead to delayed recognition of infection, which can result in poor outcomes. Some early signs of infection in older adults are exacerbation of chronic illnesses, such as congestive heart failure, or of functional impairments, such as hemiplegia among those with a history of stroke. Delirium, assessed with specific criteria such as the Confusion Assessment Method (CAM), may also indicate infection. Less dramatic changes in mental status may be caused by many factors besides infection, including dehydration, pain, decreased sleep, or a change in medication, as well as infection, making this neither a specific nor sensitive indicator of potential infection. Since febrile response is often blunted, especially in frail older adults residing in long-term care facilities, the Practice Guidelines Committee of the Infectious Diseases Society of America (IDSA) recommends a clinical evaluation for residents in skilled nursing facilities with a single oral temperature over 100°F (37.8°C), or persistent oral temperatures of over 99°F (37.2°C). Two or more readings of greater than 2°F (1.1°C) over the baseline temperature should also prompt an evaluation by a clinician. Fever of 38.0°C or higher is associated with increased probability of infection.

Commonly used disease severity scores have been found less useful for risk stratification of older adults with sepsis. Criteria used to assess for sepsis (temperature, heart rate, and white blood cell count) may be blunted in older adults. Accordingly, for older adults, clinicians may need to consider atypical signs, such as mental status changes, fatigue, decreased appetite, falls, and unsteady gait as potential early indicators of serious illness. Active monitoring of older adults with these atypical signs may facilitate early initiation of interventions that have a major impact on improving patient outcomes.

Conversely, clinicians must also be cautious not to overdiagnose infections in older adults and pursue excessive or unnecessary testing. The presence of altered mental status or malaise may be due to a variety of reasons and should not be considered as a manifestation of infection in the absence of fever and/or localizing symptoms.

Principles of Antimicrobial Therapy

Similar to younger populations, the general principles of antimicrobial use in older adults include early and accurate diagnosis of infection, prompt decision to initiate broad-spectrum antibiotics, with equal attention to narrowing or discontinuing antibiotics based on clinical progress, and identification of the implicated pathogens. Selection of specific antimicrobial agents depends on the individual risk

factors (eg, chronic health conditions, recent health care exposure, previous microbiological history), as well as local susceptibility patterns and the results of contemporary diagnostic tests and cultures. While pharmacokinetics and pharmacodynamics of older adults differ from those of younger adults, in practice, only reduced glomerular filtration indicated by decreased creatinine clearance is likely to require changes in antibiotic doses given to older adults.

Clinicians faced with diagnostic uncertainty, which is common when caring for institutionalized older adults, may have a low threshold to attribute a change in condition to infection, leading to inappropriate antibiotic use. Use of evidence- and consensus-based criteria may help clinicians not only ascertain the likelihood of infection, but also order and ultimately interpret diagnostic tests as well as initiate appropriate antibiotic therapy. Several definitions of infections in nursing homes have been published, the most commonly used are Loeb minimum criteria and the Centers for Disease Control and Prevention (CDC)'s National Healthcare Safety Network (NHSN) criteria, which are based on the revised McGeer criteria. The Loeb minimum criteria, based on assessment of symptoms and signs for UTI, respiratory infection, skin and soft-tissue infections, and fever of unknown origin, were developed to help clinicians make decisions about initiating antibiotics for nursing home residents. In contrast, the NHSN surveillance definitions are used to identify and track health care–associated infections with the intent of helping individual facilities, networks, states, and the nation identify areas of concern. While the NHSN surveillance definitions have a role in improving the care of older adults with infection, their application is best suited to comparing rates of infection over time and across health care settings or regions.

Prevention

Like cardiovascular disease and cancer, in infection, prevention is key. In addition to judicious use of antibiotics, optimal management of chronic diseases and prevention of pressure ulcers are preventive measures to reduce infections and enhance quality of care in older adults in different health care settings. Adult vaccinations also play an important role in infection prevention. Administration of influenza vaccine to older adults as well as health care workers lowers infection rates, saves lives, and reduces complications. The 2019 CDC's recommended immunization schedule includes pneumococcal, influenza, zoster, and tetanus vaccines for older adults. Influenza vaccine (influenza inactivated or influenza recombinant) must be administered yearly. For pneumococcal vaccine, all adults aged 65 years or older should receive one dose of pneumococcal polysaccharide (PPSV23), regardless of their previous PPSV23 vaccination history. Additionally, the CDC recommends pneumococcal conjugate (PCV13) based on shared clinical decision making for adults aged 65 years or older who do not have an immunocompromising condition, cerebrospinal fluid leak, or cochlear implant. The recommendations are as follows: (1) if the individual has not received previous pneumococcal vaccination and does not want to receive PCV13, administer one dose of PPSV23; (2) if the individual has not received previous pneumococcal vaccination and wants to receive both PPSV23 and PCV13, administer one dose of PCV13 first and then give one dose of PPSV23 at least 1 year later; (3) if the individual has received previous pneumococcal vaccination and wants to receive PPSV23, administer one dose of PPSV23 5 years after previous dose; and (4) if the individual has received previous pneumococcal vaccination and wants to receive PPSV23 and PCV13, administer one dose of PCV13, at least 1 year after the most recent PPSV23 dose and one dose of PPSV23 5 years after previous PPSV23 dose. Zoster vaccine (zoster recombinant) administered in two doses is recommended for adults older than age 60 years. For tetanus vaccine, Tdap once and then a Td booster every 10 years is recommended.

Finally, attention to infection prevention and control practices (eg, hand hygiene compliance, appropriate gown and glove use, early recognition of potential influenza outbreaks) and prompt recognition of pathogens commonly transmitted in institutional settings (eg, multidrug-resistant pathogens, respiratory viruses, C difficile, scabies) are important to preventing infections in older adults. Hand hygiene is the most effective infection control measure. The World Health Organization global campaign to improve hand hygiene among health care workers, "SAVE LIVES: Clean Your Hands," is a major component of the "Clean Care Is Safer Care" program. It advocates the need to improve and sustain hand hygiene practices of health care workers at the right times and in the right way to help reduce the spread of potentially life-threatening infections in health care facilities. Emerging evidence suggests older adults often carry multidrug-resistant organisms on their hands. Thus, engaging older adults in hand hygiene even if, and particularly if, they are functionally disabled becomes important. Health care workers may need to both encourage and assist nursing home residents with application of alcohol hand rub.

Cao J, Min L, Lansing B, Foxman B, Mody L. Multidrug-resistant organisms on patients' hands. *JAMA Intern Med.* 2016;176(5):705.

Clifford KM, Dy-Boarman EA, Haase KK, Maxvill K, Pass SE, Alvarez CA. Challenges with diagnosing and managing sepsis in older adults. *Expert Rev Anti Infect Ther.* 2016;14(2):231-241.

Herzig CTA, Dick AW, Sorbero M, et al. Infection trends in US nursing homes, 2006-2013. *J Am Med Dir Assoc.* 2017;18(7):635. e9-635.e20.

Jump RLP, Crnich CJ, Mody L, Bradley SF, Nicolle LE, Yoshikawa TT. Infectious diseases in older adults of long-term care facilities: update on approach to diagnosis and management. *J Am Geriatr Soc.* 2018;66(4):789-803.

McElligott M, Welham G, Pop-Vicas A, Taylor L, Crnich CJ. Antibiotic stewardship in nursing facilities. *Infect Dis Clin North Am.* 2017;31(4):619-638

Mody L, Foxman B, Bradley S, et al. Longitudinal assessment of multidrug-resistant organisms in newly admitted nursing facility patients: implications for an evolving population. *Clin Infect Dis.* 2018;67(6):837-844.

Stone ND, Ashraf MS, Calder J, et al. Surveillance definitions of infections in long-term care facilities: revisiting the McGeer criteria. *Control Hosp Epidemiol.* 2012;33(10):965-977.

URINARY TRACT INFECTIONS

▶ General Principles

UTI, which most often refers to simple cystitis, remains the most common and overdiagnosed bacterial infection in older adults. In nursing homes, UTI is the most commonly reported infection in nursing homes, with a 30-day prevalence ranging from 5.6% to 8.1%. Confusion between asymptomatic bacteriuria (pyuria and positive urine culture) and UTI (pyuria and positive urine culture in a person with symptoms that localize to the genitourinary tract) is a strong contributor to the overdiagnosis of UTI and overuse of antibiotics in older adults. The prevalence of asymptomatic bacteriuria ranges from 2% to 10% in the community and can be as high as 40% to 50% in skilled nursing facilities, affecting individuals with and without urinary catheters. In fact, since bacterial biofilm formation along the internal and external catheter surfaces is nearly universal after 30 days, most residents with a urinary catheter will have catheter-associated asymptomatic bacteriuria. An older adult who manifests nonlocalizing infectious symptoms, such as fever and malaise, and also has a positive urine culture may create a challenging diagnostic dilemma for clinicians. To help reduce overprescription of antimicrobials, a diagnosis of UTI, and especially catheter-associated UTI (CAUTI), should be a diagnosis of exclusion.

The risk factors for UTIs include prostatic hyperplasia with retention, a history of recurrent UTIs, loss of the protective effect of estrogen on bladder mucosa, functional disability, cognitive impairment, and the presence of a urinary catheter. Approximately 5% to 10% of skilled nursing facility residents have a urinary catheter. The presence of a catheter is associated with greater incidence of symptomatic UTI. Moreover, UTI is a frequent cause of bacteremia in both community-dwelling and institutionalized older adults.

▶ Prevention

Whenever possible, indwelling urinary catheters should be discontinued. If absolutely indicated, indwelling urinary catheters can be replaced with a condom catheter or intermittent straight catheterization when appropriate. Chronic indwelling urinary catheters require diligent health care worker attention to maintain a closed drainage system and to keep the drainage bag positioned below the level of the bladder. Hand hygiene compliance and glove use during any catheter manipulation are important components of infection prevention. Routine urinalysis, bladder irrigations, or catheter changes are not useful in UTI prevention. Indwelling catheter or drainage bag change is recommended only based on clinical indications such as infection, obstruction, or when the closed system has been compromised.

When there is concern for a CAUTIs, for individuals with urinary catheters in place for >2 weeks, the urinary catheter and collection system should be removed and replaced, with a urine sample obtained from the newly placed device. For individuals with a urinary catheter in place for <2 weeks, clinical judgment should be used to determine whether to remove and replace the urinary catheter or to collect a urine sample aseptically by aspirating the urine from the needle-less sampling port with a sterile syringe/cannula adapter after cleansing the port with a disinfectant.

Independence in ambulation reduces the risk of hospitalization from a UTI in skilled nursing facility residents. Increasing mobility and maintaining adequate nutrition and hydration can reduce the frequency and adverse consequences from UTIs. Cranberry products do not decrease the frequency of infection or bacteriuria. It is unclear whether vaginal estrogens decrease the risk of symptomatic UTI in postmenopausal women.

▶ Clinical Findings

Presenting findings of symptomatic UTIs among community-dwelling older adults include dysuria, increased urgency and frequency of urination, new-onset or worsening of incontinence, hematuria, and suprapubic discomfort. Pyelonephritis can present with fever, vomiting, and abdominal and/or flank pain. Frail, cognitively impaired skilled nursing facility residents may not be able to communicate if they are having symptoms and may not manifest robust signs of UTI-specific symptoms. Despite these challenges, a careful history, physical examination, discussion with nursing and other ancillary staff, and rehydration can lead to reduced inappropriate antimicrobial usage in institutionalized older adults. Recent studies show that the triad of dysuria, change in character of urine, and recent mental status change is most predictive of a symptomatic UTI. A change in the character of urine can be caused by dehydration, which may also influence mental status, making hydration of older adults in whom there is a concern for UTI an important consideration.

Because pyuria and positive urine cultures are present among older adults with a true UTI and those with asymptomatic bacteriuria, neither pyuria nor a positive urine culture is sufficient to diagnose UTI. A negative urinalysis and/or a negative urine culture, however, are sufficient to rule out UTI and reduce inappropriate antimicrobial use. Use of

Table 54–1. Minimum criteria for initiation of antibiotics for suspected urinary tract infection.

A. For residents without an indwelling urinary catheter
• Acute dysuria or
• Fever (>37.9°C [100°F] or a 1.5°C [2.4°F] increase above baseline temperature) and at least one of the following:
New or worsening:
• Urgency
• Frequency
• Suprapubic pain
• Gross hematuria
• Costovertebral angle tenderness
• Urinary incontinence

B. For residents with an indwelling urinary catheter
At least one of the following:
• Fever (>37.9°C [100°F] or a 1.5°C [2.4°F] increase above baseline temperature)
• New costovertebral tenderness
• Rigors
• New onset of delirium

Loeb minimum criteria is recommended to guide initiation of antibiotics for presumed UTI (Table 54–1).

▶ Treatment

Treatment of asymptomatic bacteriuria is not recommended and may even be harmful. Asymptomatic bacteriuria should only be treated with antibiotics prior to genitourinary procedures or surgeries during which the bladder mucosa might be damaged in order to prevent bacteremia and sepsis. Treatment of symptomatic UTI requires appropriate antimicrobial therapy, attention to hydration, and efforts to reduce dysuria. Choice of antimicrobial agent usually depends on the organism isolated from urine cultures and local susceptibility patterns. Per IDSA guidelines, if local resistance rates of uropathogens causing acute uncomplicated cystitis do not exceed 20%, nitrofurantoin monohydrate/macrocrystals for 5 days or trimethoprim-sulfamethoxazole for 3 days are appropriate choices and are recommended for empiric antibiotic therapy if resistance rates are unknown. When other recommended agents cannot be used, β-lactam agents, in 3- to 7-day regimens, are appropriate choices for therapy. Amoxicillin or ampicillin should not be used for empirical treatment given the prevalence of antimicrobial resistance. Broad-spectrum antibiotics targeting gram-negative organisms and enterococci may be required if the patient appears significantly ill. Because of their lack of systemic absorption, neither nitrofurantoin nor fosfomycin should be used in people for whom there is a concern for pyelonephritis. Furthermore, although fosfomycin, given as a single dose, is effective for cystitis, it is also a drug that should be reserved for individuals known to have a history of multidrug-resistant organisms, such as those resistant to extended-spectrum β-lactams or carbapenems. Several fluoroquinolones, ofloxacin, ciprofloxacin, and levofloxacin, are highly efficacious in 3-day regimens but should be reserved for when other antimicrobial agents cannot be used. Skilled nursing facility residents with urinary catheters may require a broader spectrum antibiotic regimen to incorporate coverage for resistant gram-positive organisms such as methicillin-resistant *Staphylococcus aureus* (MRSA). Once identification and susceptibility test results are available, appropriate antibiotics can be selected and the treatment period determined.

The duration of antimicrobial therapy usually depends on the risk group. A period of 7 days is the recommended duration of antimicrobial treatment for patients with CAUTI who have prompt resolution of symptoms; 10 to 14 days of treatment are recommended for those with a delayed response, regardless of whether the patient remains catheterized or not. A 5-day regimen of levofloxacin may be considered in patients with CAUTI who are not severely ill. Data are insufficient to make such a recommendation about other fluoroquinolones. A 3-day antimicrobial regimen may be considered for women aged ≤65 years who develop CAUTI without upper urinary tract symptoms after an indwelling catheter has been removed.

Additionally, IDSA guidelines recommend that in men for whom a urinary catheter is indicated and who have minimal postvoid residual urine, condom catheterization should be considered as an alternative to short-term and long-term indwelling catheterization to reduce catheter-associated bacteriuria in those who are not cognitively impaired; moreover, intermittent catheterization should be considered as an alternative to short-term or long-term indwelling urethral catheterization to reduce catheter-associated bacteriuria and CAUTI.

Ashraf MS, Gaur S, Bushen OY, et al. Diagnosis, treatment, and prevention of urinary tract infections in post-acute and long-term care settings: a consensus statement from AMDA's Infection Advisory Subcommittee. *J Am Med Dir Assoc.* 2020;21(1):12-24.

Canales JP, Castro V, Rada G. Are vaginal estrogens effective for preventing urinary tract infection in postmenopausal women? *Medwave.* 2017;17(09):e7093-e7093.

Gupta K, Hooton TM, Naber KG, et al. International clinical practice guidelines for the treatment of acute uncomplicated cystitis and pyelonephritis in women: a 2010 update by the infectious Diseases Society of America and the European Society for Microbiology and Infectious Diseases. *Clin Infect Dis.* 2011;52(5):e103-e120.

Hooton TM, Bradley SF, Cardenas DD, et al. Diagnosis, prevention, and treatment of catheter-associated urinary tract infection in adults: 2009 international clinical practice guidelines from the Infectious Diseases Society of America. *Clin Infect Dis.* 2010;50(5):625-663.

Juthani-Mehta M, Van Ness PH, Bianco L, et al. Effect of cranberry capsules on bacteriuria plus pyuria among older women in nursing homes. *JAMA.* 2016;316(18):1879.

Mody L, Greene MT, Meddings J, et al. A national implementation project to prevent catheter-Associated urinary tract infection in nursing home residents. *JAMA Intern Med.* 2017;177(8):1154-1162.

Nicolle LE. Asymptomatic bacteriuria in older adults. *Curr Geriatr Reports.* 2016;5(1):1-8.

RESPIRATORY TRACT INFECTIONS

▶ General Principles

Hospitalization and death as a consequence of pneumonia, influenza, and other respiratory tract infections are common in older adults. Pneumonia and influenza are among the top 10 most common causes of death in this age group. Pneumonia in older adults can be categorized as community-acquired (CAP), hospital-acquired, or skilled nursing facility–acquired. The annual incidence of pneumonia has been reported at 63 cases per 10,000 adults aged 65 to 79 years and 164.3 cases per 10,000 adults aged ≥80 years. These rates are 9 and 25 times, respectively, higher than the incidence of pneumonia among adults aged 18 to 49 years. In nursing homes, the prevalence of pneumonia ranges from 1.4% to 2.5%. During the 2017 to 2018 influenza season, there were 959,000 hospitalizations and 79,400 deaths, with 70% of hospitalizations in adults aged ≥65 years. Older adults also accounted for 90% of deaths, highlighting that older adults are particularly vulnerable to severe disease with influenza virus infection. Additionally, outbreaks of seasonal influenza are reported frequently, particularly in the skilled nursing facility setting.

Respiratory tract infections are the second most common infection among skilled nursing facility residents. Aspiration pneumonia is common among this population and is often associated with oropharyngeal dysphagia and regurgitation of gastric contents. Poor oral hygiene, including dental plaque, which contains as many as 25,000 species of bacteria, may contribute to the risk of pneumonia following an aspiration event.

There are several risk factors for pneumonia: older age; male gender; history of aspiration; functional disability; history of smoking; chronic bronchitis or emphysema; heart disease; malignancy; neurologic conditions such as cerebrovascular diseases; recent surgery or intensive care unit stay; and the presence of a feeding tube. With age, lung parenchyma loses its elastic recoil and there is reduced chest wall compliance, along with a loss of alveoli and alveolar ducts, all of which can increase the risk of pneumonia in the setting of functional disability and acute illness.

▶ Prevention

The prevention strategies for respiratory tract infections are largely designed to help mitigate risk factors. Pneumococcal vaccine as well as annual influenza vaccines for older adults and their caregivers, especially health care workers, can reduce the incidence and complications related to respiratory tract infections in the older population. A 2018 systematic review found low-quality evidence suggesting that compared to usual care, professional oral care could reduce mortality due to pneumonia in nursing home residents. Although no high-quality evidence was found to determine which oral care measures are most effective for reducing nursing home–acquired pneumonia, oral hygiene is important for good quality of care. Smoking cessation can also reduce bronchitis and respiratory infections.

Clinical Findings

In older adults, pneumonia may manifest with typical (eg, fever, cough, chest congestion, pleuritic chest pain) and atypical signs and symptoms (eg, fatigue, anorexia, functional decline, new confusion). A quarter of older adults with pneumonia may not mount a fever and, in general, are less likely to present with chills or pleuritic chest pain. An increased respiratory rate of >25 breaths/min and hypoxia portend a poor prognosis and are useful objective signs to consider during assessments. Clinical presentation should be confirmed rapidly with diagnostic testing, including chest radiographs, white blood cell count, and blood cultures. The yield from blood cultures may not be high but, if positive, may help drive appropriate antibiotic choice. Although sputum studies are often not feasible in older adults and, when obtained, may not be of sufficient quality to help guide therapy for older adults with a productive cough, a sputum culture may be helpful for similar reasons. Additional diagnostic tests to consider are urinary antigen studies for *Streptococcus pneumoniae* and *Legionella* spp. These can be obtained after antibiotics have been started. Finally, nasopharyngeal samples should be collected to test for influenza, particularly from October through March, and, depending on the setting and circumstances, a respiratory viral panel. Rapid tests that can detect either influenza A or B or both are available; these can detect influenza viruses within 30 minutes. The sensitivity and specificity of these tests increases when they are performed close to the illness onset.

Older adults typically manifest fewer respiratory symptoms compared to younger adults. Cough, fever, and altered mental status predominate as presenting findings in older adults hospitalized with documented influenza. Older adults with influenza may have more gastrointestinal symptoms when compared with other respiratory viruses. Loeb minimum criteria are recommended to guide initiation of antibiotics for presumed lower respiratory tract infections (Table 54–2).

Treatment

Several risk indices have been developed to predict outcomes, particularly mortality, in older adults. These include the pneumonia severity index (PSI; a 20-item two-step system more applicable to younger adults), CURB (four items:

Table 54–2. Minimum criteria for initiation of antibiotics for suspected lower respiratory tract infection.

- Fever >38.9°C [102°F] and at least one of the following:
  - Respiratory rate >25
  - Productive cough

or

- Fever (>37.9°C [100°F] or a 1.5°C [2.4°F] increase above baseline temperature, but ≤38.9°C [102°F]) and cough and at least one of the following:
  - Pulse >100
  - Rigors
  - Delirium
  - Respiratory rate >25

or

- Afebrile resident with COPD and >65 years old and new or increased cough with purulent sputum production

or

- Afebrile resident without COPD and new cough with purulent sputum production and at least one of the following:
  - Respiratory rate >25
  - Delirium

or

- New infiltrate on chest x-ray thought to represent pneumonia and at least one of the following:
  - Fever (>37.9°C [100°F] or a 1.5°C [2.4°F] increase above baseline temperature)
  - Respiratory rate >25
  - Productive cough

COPD, chronic obstructive pulmonary disease.

confusion, urea, respiratory rate, and blood pressure), the modified CURB-65 (confusion, urea, respiratory rate, blood pressure, and age ≥65 years) from the British Thoracic Society (Table 54–3), and SOAR (systolic blood pressure, oxygenation, age ≥65 years, and respiratory rate). The accuracy of CURB-65 and PSI for predicting outcome in CAP decreases with advancing age. The scoring systems can help identify older adults who can potentially be treated as outpatients and

Table 54–3. CURB-65: Risk index to predict mortality from community-acquired pneumonia.

Symptom	Points
Confusion	1
Urea >7 mmol/L	1
Respiratory rate >30 breaths/min	1
Systolic blood pressure <90 mm Hg, diastolic blood pressure <60 mm Hg	1
Age ≥65 years	1
Total (30-day mortality risk)	0 (0.6%), 1 (3.2%), 2 (13%), 3 (17%), 4 (41.5%), 5 (57.5%)

can assist in making treatment recommendations, particularly toward the end of life. Recent studies that seek to develop models specific for assessing pneumonia mortality in older adults combine biomarkers with performance and cognitive status to provide more accurate prognostic information.

Empiric therapy varies and depends on both host and environmental factors. For community-dwelling older adults without chronic conditions and without recent health care exposure (within 90 days), empiric treatment for CAP includes a macrolide or doxycycline. For older adults with chronic conditions such as chronic lung disease, chronic kidney disease, diabetes, or immunosuppression, a respiratory quinolone or β-lactam plus a macrolide are recommended. Recent exposure (within 90 days) to health care settings, including nursing homes and dialysis centers, is considered a risk factor for hospital-acquired pneumonia. Depending on the severity of their presentation, these individuals may require an initial parenteral antibiotic regimen such as piperacillin-tazobactam and vancomycin to cover for *Pseudomonas*, MRSA, and/or other nosocomial gram-negative organisms. In choosing empiric antimicrobial therapy, local antimicrobial susceptibilities should be considered. Empiric therapy can be narrowed to target a specific pathogen once it has been identified. A typical length of therapy for CAP and for hospital-acquired pneumonia is 5 days and 7 days, respectively.

Adherence to the 2007 IDSA/American Thoracic Society guidelines for CAP has a significant beneficial impact on clinical outcomes in older adults. Attention must also be given to nutritional status, fluid administration, early mobilization, and comorbidity-stabilizing therapy in older patients.

Jain S, Self WH, Wunderink RG, et al. Community-acquired pneumonia requiring hospitalization among U.S. adults. *N Engl J Med.* 2015;373(5):415-427.

Liu C, Cao Y, Lin J, et al. Oral care measures for preventing nursing home-acquired pneumonia. *Cochrane Database Syst Rev.* 2018;9:CD012416.

Mandell LA, Wunderink RG, Anzueto A, et al. Infectious Diseases Society of America/American Thoracic Society consensus guidelines on the management of community-acquired pneumonia in adults. *Clin Infect Dis.* 2007;44(suppl 2):S27-S72.

Sanz F, Morales-Suárez-Varela M, Fernández E, et al. A composite of functional status and pneumonia severity index improves the prediction of pneumonia mortality in older patients. *J Gen Intern Med.* 2017;33(4):437-481.

Simonetti AF, Viasus D, Garcia-Vidal C, Carratalà J. Management of community-acquired pneumonia in older adults. *Ther Adv Infect Dis.* 2014;2(1):3-16.

GASTROINTESTINAL INFECTIONS

▷ General Principles

Gastrointestinal infections are fairly common in older adults. Deaths attributable to diarrheal diseases, such as other infections, affect older adults disproportionately. Infection is generally by fecal-oral spread. Hypochlorhydria and achlorhydria, impaired gastric motility, inappropriate use of antibiotics, and waning immunity increase the predisposition to diarrheal illnesses in older adults. Viral gastroenteritis (caused by rotavirus and enteroviruses including Norwalk virus), bacterial gastroenteritis (caused by *C difficile*, *Bacillus cereus*, *Escherichia coli*, *Campylobacter*, *Clostridium perfringens*, or *Salmonella*), and parasites are well-known causes of diarrhea in skilled nursing facilities. Norovirus gastroenteritis is also common among nursing home residents, with 90% of norovirus-associated deaths occurring in adults aged 65 and older.

C difficile infection (CDI) is the most common cause of health care–associated diarrhea. CDI incidence in older adults is at least five times that of younger people. In 2011, >90% of deaths from CDI were among adults aged 65 years and older. In particular, nursing home–onset CDI is associated with substantial morbidity and mortality. In 2012, the incidence of nursing home–onset CDI was 112,800 cases, with 28% of those individuals hospitalized within 7 days of a positive specimen, 19% of whom had recurrent CDI and 8% of whom died within 30 days. The incidence, hospitalization, recurrence, and mortality due to CDI were highest in adults aged 85 years or older.

▷ Prevention

Compliance with hand hygiene guidelines remains key in preventing diarrheal illnesses, particularly CDI and viral gastroenteritis such as norovirus. Yet, hand hygiene compliance rates remain poor in all settings. The use of alcohol-based hand rub has increased hand hygiene rates; however, its effectiveness may be diminished against certain diarrheal pathogens, particularly *C difficile* and norovirus. Nonmodifiable risk factors for CDI in older adults include age-related changes in immunity and the intestinal microbiota, resulting in decreased diversity and numbers of gut bacteria. The primary risk factor for CDI is exposure to antibiotics, which may be modified by reducing inappropriate antibiotic use whenever possible; this may be considered as a quality improvement process measure. Fluoroquinolones, clindamycin, and cephalosporins are particularly associated with an increased risk of CDI. Per the most recent IDSA guidelines, although there is an epidemiologic association between proton pump inhibitor use and CDI, there is insufficient evidence for discontinuation of proton pump inhibitors as a measure for preventing CDI. Furthermore, there are insufficient data at this time to recommend administration of probiotics for primary prevention of CDI outside of clinical trials.

▷ Clinical Findings

Patient history is often an initial guide to appropriate diagnostic evaluation. Information on food history and exposure, travel history, antimicrobial usage, use of immunosuppressive medications, frequency of diarrhea, tenesmus, and presence of blood and mucus in the stool should be obtained at the initial evaluation. History of exposure and symptoms in other family members or close contacts should be obtained as well. The physical exam should initially focus on the severity of the diarrheal illness including symptoms of dehydration, such as dry mucous membranes, fatigue, loss of appetite, change in mentation, reduced blood pressure, and tachycardia. An abdominal exam may be useful, although it can often be misleading because of a paucity of positive findings.

▶ Treatment

Initial laboratory tests should include electrolytes and a complete blood count. Stool studies for white blood cells, stool culture, assessment for ova and parasites, and molecular-based tests for *C difficile* and other pathogens are clinically appropriate. Initial treatment should address dehydration and electrolyte disorders. In severe cases, vital signs should be closely monitored. Antimotility agents (loperamide, diphenoxylate) are frequently overused in older adults, and their use should be generally restricted. Travelers' diarrhea is generally self-limited. Adequate hydration and rest are often sufficient. Due to the risks of resistant bacterial pathogens, prophylactic antibiotics are not recommended for most travelers. Norovirus can present with nausea, vomiting, and diarrhea. Supportive treatment is key to early recovery. In nursing homes, infection prevention and control measures must address residents and health care providers. Affected residents should be placed on contact precautions for at least 48 hours after symptom resolution. Antibiotic-associated diarrhea is common and is usually self-limited.

CDI is the most likely bacterial pathogen to cause diarrhea in older adults and may be associated with severe disease requiring hospitalization with resultant morbidity and mortality. Suspicions of CDI should be followed by prompt diagnosis and treatment that includes volume repletion and, when possible, cessation of precipitating antibiotics. The 2017 IDSA guidelines recommend either oral vancomycin or fidaxomicin over metronidazole for initial and recurrent episodes of CDI. If these medications are not available, metronidazole could be used for an initial episode of nonsevere CDI only. Older adults are at increased risk for recurrent CDI, which may occur weeks to months after recovery from a previous episode. Exposure to antibiotics is the most common reason for CDI recurrence.

Compared to CDI, other bacteria are far less common causes of acute diarrhea in older adults. The following signs and symptoms indicate severe disease, for which antibiotics should be considered: fever, more than six stools per day, grossly bloody or mucoid stools, and volume depletion requiring hospitalization. If indicated, antibiotics should be started promptly, with consideration of azithromycin or fluoroquinolones (ciprofloxacin or levofloxacin) for empiric treatment.

Hunter JC, Mu Y, Dumyati GK, et al. Burden of nursing home-onset *Clostridium difficile* infection in the United States: estimates of incidence and patient outcomes. *Open Forum Infect Dis.* 2016;3(1):ofv196.

McDonald LC, Gerding DN, Johnson S, et al. Clinical practice guidelines for *Clostridium difficile* infection in adults and children: 2017 update by the Infectious Diseases Society of America (IDSA) and Society for Healthcare Epidemiology of America (SHEA). *Clin Infect Dis.* 2018;66(7):e1-e48.

SKIN AND SOFT-TISSUE INFECTIONS

▶ General Principles

In addition to immunosenescence, several chronic medical and skin conditions put older adults at risk for skin and soft-tissue infections (SSTIs): diabetes, peripheral vascular disease, congestive heart failure leading to lower extremity edema, eczema, venous stasis, and minor traumas. Defective cutaneous immunity with aging increases the susceptibility of older adults to SSTIs. Use of antibiotics and corticosteroids contributes to overgrowth of bacteria and fungi. Additionally, older adults have a greater likelihood of being bed-bound and hence are at an increased risk for pressure ulcers.

Common types of SSTIs in older adults include cellulitis, abscesses (ie, furuncles and carbuncles), and infected pressure ulcers. The incidence of each of these SSTIs varies: 1% to 9% for cellulitis and 4% to 6% for infected pressure ulcers among nursing home residents. Compared to younger adults, older adults are at greater risk for surgical site infections as well as necrotizing fasciitis. Older adults with SSTIs have a higher mortality, morbidity, and attributable hospital costs compared to younger adults with SSTIs. Reactivation of herpes virus infections is also problematic in older adults. Shingles (herpes zoster), which will occur in about half of people who reach age 85 years, can be particularly devasting due to chronic pain that lasts weeks to months following the resolution of all skin changes.

SSTIs are the third most common infection diagnosed in nursing home residents. In addition to the bacterial and viral infections mentioned earlier, nursing home residents may experience fungal infections and infestations. *Candida* spp. may cause superficial mucocutaneous infections such as intertrigo, thrush, and vaginal candidiasis. An array of other fungi cause dermatophytosis, more commonly termed *ringworm* or designated with tinea in conjunction with a Latin term to describe the anatomic location involved (eg, tinea pedis or tinea capitis). Scabies (*Sarcoptes scabiei*), lice (*Pediculus humanus capitis, P humanus corporis, Phthirus pubis*), and bedbugs (*Cimex lectularius*) also cause rashes. Scabies has been reported in 3.3% of nursing home residents, with an attack rate of approximately 70%.

▶ Prevention

The prevention of SSTIs varies by type. Cellulitis can be prevented by elevating the limb to aid adequate fluid drainage and prevent edema, using medical stockings, and treating macerated skin with topical antifungals to prevent recurrences due to bacteria gaining entry via skin damaged by fungal infection or concomitant excoriation. *S aureus,* including methicillin-susceptible and methicillin-resistant strains, is the most likely cause of skin abscesses, commonly termed furuncles and carbuncles. Good hand hygiene, using antibacterial soap baths, and not sharing personal items reduce the risk of infections caused by transmission of *S aureus*, particularly MRSA. Prevention strategies for pressure ulcers include frequent turning of bed-bound patients, appropriate use of pressure-relieving devices, good nutrition, and maintaining moist sacral skin. Other principles of preventing SSTIs are glucose control, smoking cessation, preventing hypothermia, and, for those undergoing surgical procedures, appropriate timing and dosing of prophylactic antibiotics.

Prevention is also key to avoiding scabies outbreaks. Transmission of scabies is facilitated by prolonged skin-to-skin contact with an infested individual or their belongings. Major preventive strategies include cleaning of fomites, adequate hand hygiene and personal protective equipment use by staff, and avoiding overcrowding in skilled nursing facilities. Finally, ensuring that affected individuals receive two treatments a week apart reduces the risk of reinfestation.

▶ Clinical Findings

Similar to other infections, SSTIs may manifest differently in older compared to younger adults. Atrophic changes to skin as well as chronic skin changes may confound the clinical exam. Infected pressure ulcers may go unnoticed in chronically bed-bound older adults.

Erysipelas and cellulitis are both infections of the skin, with erysipelas involving more superficial layers and often presenting with a clearly demarcated border. Cellulitis affects deeper skin layers and may involve the dermis, with a less distinct border. Both conditions involve superficial swelling of the skin, accompanied by erythema, heat, and pain, and are usually caused by streptococci species, specifically group A *Streptococcus* (*S pyogenes*), group B *Streptococcus* (*S agalactiae*), and group C *Streptococcus*. *S aureus* is a less common cause of these conditions and, when present, tends to manifest as abscesses.

Pressure ulcer infections are often polymicrobial and most develop in the sacrum, heels, elbows, and lower extremities. Cultures are rarely indicated and should be reserved for detection of frank pus or gross serosanguinous drainage.

Necrotizing fasciitis is an uncommon, severe SSTI that involves deeper subcutaneous tissue, with rapid spread along fascial plains with toxin-mediated tissue destruction. Pathogens that cause necrotizing fasciitis include group A

Streptococcus and *S aureus*, either of which may occur alone or with other bacterial species. Mixed anaerobic organisms, often accompanied by *Enterobacteriaceae* spp., may also cause disease; these are more frequently associated with Fournier gangrene, which is necrotizing fasciitis beginning in the perineum. Regardless of the pathogens involved, the clinical presentation includes an exquisitely tender, hot, swollen region of skin, often a lower extremity, without sharp margins. The patient may describe pain out of proportion with the exam and will likely have a fever and manifest systemic toxicity. Diagnosing necrotizing fasciitis requires a high index of clinical suspicion, early consultation of surgical teams, and imaging with computed tomography.

With fungal and viral infections, the location, distribution, and appearance of skin lesions may help identify potential pathogens. As mentioned earlier, although *Candida* spp. may affect skin and mucosal tissues differently, the characteristics of infections caused by dermatophytes tend to be more specific to the location than the pathogen. Herpes zoster (shingles) typically manifests in a single dermatome and may be preceded by sensations of itching, burning, pin and needles, or severe pain. The involvement of more than one dermatome or any involvement of the eye or ear should prompt evaluation in an acute care setting.

Scabies is a commonly missed diagnosis in older adults and hence responsible for outbreaks in skilled nursing facility residents. Scabies, which may emerge in the webs between fingers, can present as normal scabies or crusted scabies, both of which can be difficult to diagnose in older adults. Normal scabies presents as raised, red, itchy lesions called burrows, typically in interdigital areas and ankles. Crusted scabies, on the other hand, presents more atypically (itching being present in only 50% of patients) in older adults owing to their lack of ability to scratch and to mount an immune response. The burden of mites on the skin is much higher in crusted scabies than in normal scabies; hence, there are more opportunities for outbreaks. Skin scraping and testing help to confirm the diagnosis for crusted scabies as it is often confused with psoriasis or eczema. In nursing homes, scabies should be considered in the differential diagnosis of pruritus and dermatologic disorders because a delay in diagnosis may have implications not only for the patient involved but also for other residents, family members, and health care workers.

▶ Treatment

In the evaluation of SSTIs, the clinical syndrome being addressed is the strongest determinant of the urgency for initiating antimicrobials. Most bacterial infections require prompt (erysipelas, cellulitis) to urgent (necrotizing fasciitis) antibiotics, whereas fungal infections typically follow a slower course, permitting time for consideration of other diagnoses when appropriate. Minimum criteria to initiate an antibiotic for a SSTI include pus in a wound, skin, or soft-tissue site or at least two of the following: fever, new or worsening redness, tenderness, warmth, or swelling at the suspected site.

Both cellulitis and erysipelas are usually caused by streptococci species; hence, antimicrobial choices include cefazolin, cephalexin, amoxicillin, ampicillin, nafcillin, oxacillin, dicloxacillin, and, for those with a true allergy to penicillins, clindamycin. For abscesses or purulent cellulitis, S aureus is a typical pathogen. For abscesses <4 to 5 cm in diameter in people who are otherwise clinically stable, incision and drainage is usually sufficient therapy. For larger abscesses or for individuals with indications of systemic infection or other concerning medical conditions, such as patients with poorly controlled diabetes or people receiving dialysis, antibiotics with activity against MRSA are indicated. The decision between oral versus intravenous therapy generally depends on the severity at presentation and comorbidities. First-line therapy includes doxycycline or trimethoprim-sulfamethoxazole; for sicker individuals, vancomycin, daptomycin, or linezolid should be considered, again reserving clindamycin for individuals with a true penicillin allergy. Culture results collected at the time of abscess incision and drainage will help narrow therapy to cefalexin or a similar narrow-spectrum agent if the pathogen is methicillin-sensitive S aureus. Vancomycin plus either ampicillin-sulbactam or piperacillin-tazobactam is recommended as a reasonable empiric regimen for severe infections.

Necrotizing fasciitis can be especially devastating in older adults. Surgical intervention is the gold standard diagnostic and treatment modality. In addition to surgery, antimicrobial therapy is important in infection management. In addition to the empiric antibiotic treatment options specified earlier for severe infections, the addition of clindamycin offers additional benefit in that it helps prevent toxin production.

Because all pressure ulcers, like the skin, are colonized with bacteria, antibiotic therapy is not appropriate for a positive surface-swab culture without signs and symptoms of infection. True infection of a pressure ulcer (cellulitis, osteomyelitis, or sepsis) is a serious condition, generally requiring broad-spectrum parenteral antibiotics and sometimes surgical debridement in an acute-care facility. Attention to hand hygiene and glove use by health care workers involved in wound care and dressing changes should help to prevent the spread of pathogens.

For surgical site infections, suture removal plus incision and drainage are often sufficient to promote healing. In the absence of systemic signs or symptoms of infection, systemic antimicrobial therapy is not routinely indicated. For surgical site infections following clean operations on the trunk, head and neck, or extremities, a first-generation cephalosporin provides appropriate treatment; if the person is at high risk for MRSA, other options include vancomycin, linezolid, daptomycin, telavancin, or ceftaroline. For surgical site infections following operations on the axilla, gastrointestinal tract, perineum, or female genital tract, coverage against gram-negative bacteria and anaerobes may be achieved

with a cephalosporin, amoxicillin-clavulanate, ampicillin-sulbactam, or, for individuals with a true penicillin allergy, a fluoroquinolone in combination with metronidazole.

Treatment of scabies involves application of topical permethrin from the neck down followed by bathing 8 to 14 hours later. A repeat application 1 week later may be necessary and is recommended for people in institutional settings. Two doses of oral ivermectin, given 1 to 2 weeks apart, is a reasonable option as well. Oral ivermectin in combination with topical permethrin is the treatment of choice for crusted scabies. Depending on the severity of infection, the schedule for ivermectin ranges from three doses (days 1, 2, and 8) up to seven doses (days 1, 2, 8, 9, 15, 22, and 29). Concomitant permethrin is applied every 2 to 3 days for 1 to 2 weeks as well. Confirming the diagnosis of scabies prior to initiating treatment will avoid exposing older adults to the discomfort and side effects associated with these intense treatment regimens. Because scabies can be transmitted by linen and clothing, the environment should be cleaned thoroughly, including inanimate surfaces, hot-cycle washing of washable items (eg, clothing, sheets, towels), and carpets.

Stevens DL, Bisno AL, Chambers HF, et al. Executive summary: practice guidelines for the diagnosis and management of skin and soft tissue infections: 2014 update by the Infectious Diseases Society of America. Clin Infect Dis. 2014;59(2):147-159.

Suwandhi P, Dharmarajan TS. Scabies in the nursing home. Curr Infect Dis Rep. 2015;17(1):453.

PROSTHETIC JOINT INFECTIONS AND OSTEOMYELITIS

▶ General Principles

With the increasing number of total joint arthroplasties in older adults as well as people with prosthetic joints living to an older age, the rate of prosthetic joint infections (PJIs) is increasing. The annual incidence rate of PJIs in the United States is 2% for hip and knee arthroplasties, 1% after shoulder arthroplasties, and 3.3% after elbow arthroplasties. Given multiple comorbidities in older adults, PJIs are commonly associated with potential loss of joint function and mobility. Older adults who develop septic arthritis have a high risk of poor joint-related outcomes, including severe functional deterioration or amputation, with mortality in the range of 10% to 15%. Similar to other infections, septic arthritis in older adults might manifest atypically with poor inflammatory response and is often mistaken for preexisting joint disease.

The incidence of osteomyelitis (OM) also increases with age. Reasons for this are multifactorial and include falls or other injuries with resultant bone trauma, peripheral vascular disease, diabetes, peripheral neuropathy, and prosthetic joints. Data from a population-based study conducted over 40 years reported an annual incidence of OM of <11 cases per 100,000 person-years until the sixth decade of life; thereafter, the incidence increased by 50% per decade of life. The highest incidence was among men aged ≥80 years old, with 128 cases per 100,000 person-years.

Clinical Findings

PJIs may sometimes be difficult to diagnose in older adults due to a subdued inflammatory response, especially in patients with delayed-onset infections. Common signs and symptoms of PJIs include pain, effusion or swelling, and erythema affecting the joint, sometimes accompanied by fever and chills. Occasionally, drainage or presence of a sinus tract communicating with the prosthesis may be the first indication of a PJI. Joint loosening may be an indication of bone infection. Inflammatory markers such as erythrocyte sedimentation rate (ESR) and C-reactive protein (CRP) can help differentiate infection from mechanical loosening. Septic arthritis, even in older adults, tends to have a more acute presentation with a hot, red, painful, and swollen joint and evidence of systemic involvement including fevers, rigors or chills, and malaise. For both PJI and septic arthritis, sending fluid aspirated from the joint for Gram stain, culture, and cell count prior to initiating antibiotics is a key aspect of subsequent diagnosis and treatment decisions. For both PJI and septic arthritis, gram-positive organisms, specifically S aureus followed by coagulase-negative staphylococci, are the most likely pathogens. Group B Streptococcus (S agalactiae) is very common in adults older than age 80, and Cutibacterium (Propionibacterium) acnes is typical in shoulder arthropathies. Although gram-negative pathogens are recovered from <10% of PJIs, they cause on the order of 25% of septic arthritis cases in older adults. Possible reasons for this may relate to hematogenous spread of pathogens that affected the gastrointestinal or urinary tracts.

Just as with younger adults, the presentation of OM in older adults may be acute, subacute, or chronic. Pain is a common presenting finding, whereas fever and chills may or may not be present. For chronic OM, plain films may be sufficient to make a diagnosis, with magnetic resonance imaging or other imaging studies more suited to detecting acute OM. Blood cultures and, when possible, bone biopsy support both diagnosis and treatment decisions. Vertebral OM is typically a subacute presentation that begins with moderate to severe back pain and may progress to fevers and chills. Chronic OM, defined as present for >6 weeks, may develop in association with pressure ulcers, diabetic foot infections, peripheral vascular disease, or dental infections or following sternotomy. Typical pathogens depend on the anatomic location, with S aureus and other gram-positive organisms most likely to cause vertebral or sternal OM. Oropharyngeal bacteria are usually implicated in mandibular OM. Although S aureus and other gram-positive pathogens are still dominant, Pseudomonas spp. may cause OM in the context of diabetic foot infections.

Treatment

Treatment for PJI includes 4 to 6 weeks of intravenous antimicrobial therapy and, depending on the host's goals of care and overall health, the type of prosthesis and available surgical expertise, consideration of surgical debridement, and possible joint removal and replacement. On occasion, usually in concert with an infectious disease physician, older adults with PJI may be put on long-term suppression with oral antibiotics. Treatment for septic arthritis involves close attention to source control through either serial joint aspirations or surgical debridement and long-term intravenous antibiotics (2–4 weeks). Treatment for OM also centers around long-term antibiotics, typically 6 weeks, with surgical debridement used judiciously for OM involving the feet or sacral regions. For all of these infections, trending ESR and CRP over time helps assess the response to antibiotic therapy. In the months following completion of antibiotics, a rise in inflammatory markers may herald recurrence.

Berbari EF, Kanj SS, Kowalski TJ, et al. 2015 Infectious Diseases Society of America (IDSA) clinical practice guidelines for the diagnosis and treatment of native vertebral osteomyelitis in adults. Clin Infect Dis. 2015;61(6):e26-e46.

Kremers HM, Nwojo ME, Ransom JE, Wood-Wentz CM, Melton LJ, Huddleston PM III. Trends in the epidemiology of osteomyelitis: a population-based study. J Bone Joint Surg Am. 2015;97(10):837-845.

Mears SC, Edwards PK. Bone and joint infections in older adults. Clin Geriatr Med. 2016;32(3):555-570.

Nair R, Schweizer ML, Singh N. Septic arthritis and prosthetic joint infections in older adults. Infect Dis Clin North Am. 2017;31(4):715-729.

HIV & AIDS

Amy Baca, MD
Meredith Greene, MD

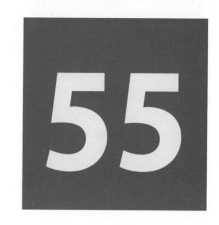

55

ESSENTIALS OF DIAGNOSIS

▶ The proportion of persons living with HIV over age 50 continues to dramatically increase. Globally, older adults represent 20% of persons currently living with HIV.

▶ Infections such as recurrent bacterial pneumonia, thrush, and symptoms such as neurocognitive changes should prompt HIV testing in the older adult.

▶ People living with HIV are at increased risk for other chronic conditions such as cardiovascular disease, osteoporosis, and geriatric syndromes (eg, falls, frailty). They are also at increased risk for polypharmacy, including drug-drug interactions with antiretroviral medications.

General Principles

Currently, 36.9 million individuals are living with HIV worldwide and 5.7 million are age ≥50 years. The Centers for Disease Control and Prevention (CDC) estimates that >1 million people are living with HIV (PLWH) in the United States. Of PLWH in the United States, 50% are aged ≥50 years. In 2017, persons over the age of 50 also accounted for 17% (n = 6640) of all newly diagnosed cases in the United States. Similar to younger adults, most new infections among older adults occurred in men who have sex with men. Heterosexual women accounted for the second largest group of newly diagnosed persons. Given the availability of effective, well-tolerated treatments, the number of older adults living with HIV is expected to grow.

The classification of those aged ≥50 years as "older" has been used since the beginning of the AIDS epidemic, and it is now well established that PLWH have higher rates of multimorbidity and polypharmacy and experience earlier onset of geriatric syndromes including frailty and falls. Ongoing debate exists as to whether this represents accelerated

or accentuated aging in this population. These findings are likely mediated through factors such as chronic inflammation despite treatment of HIV, toxicity from antiretroviral medications, and lifestyle factors that are more common among PLWH such as tobacco and alcohol use. Regardless of the mechanism, providers caring for this rapidly growing population must be prepared to address the complications faced by those aging with HIV.

Screening and Prevention

Older adults are at risk for acquiring HIV due to a number of social and biological factors. The availability of medications to treat erectile dysfunction has led to increased sexual activity in older males. Additionally, older adults are more likely to engage in condomless sex acts, given that unwanted pregnancy is no longer a concern. Moreover, age-related vaginal wall dryness and thinning can increase a woman's risk of contracting HIV. HIV prevention campaigns targeting an older demographic remain scarce, and many older adults are also simply unaware of their risk. Clinicians also often fail to recognize that older adults may be sexually active or using drugs, and hence do not discuss safer sex practices or substance use. As a result, older adults are screened less frequently and diagnosed with advanced HIV at higher rates than their younger counterparts.

The CDC currently recommends opt-out screening for all individuals between the ages of 13 and 64, regardless of risk factors, at least once in their lifetime. The US Preventive Services Task Force (USPSTF) has similar recommendations for those aged 15 to 65 years. Both the CDC and USPSTF recommend that those at high risk receive more frequent screening. The CDC recommends testing at least annually or more frequently (every 3–6 months) based on risk factors and local HIV epidemiology. Given that clinicians frequently underestimate older adults' risks for HIV acquisition, some organizations have recommended routine opt-out screening regardless of age, not ending at age 65.

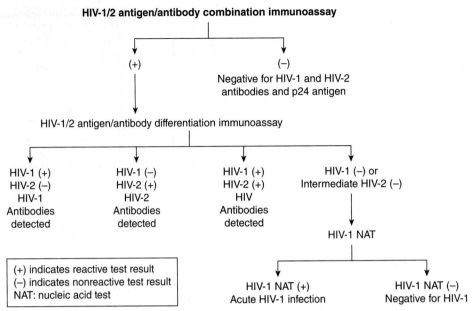

HIV-1/2 antigen/antibody combination immunoassay

(+)

(−)
Negative for HIV-1 and HIV-2
antibodies and p24 antigen

HIV-1/2 antigen/antibody differentiation immunoassay

HIV-1 (+)
HIV-2 (−)
HIV-1
Antibodies
detected

HIV-1 (−)
HIV-2 (+)
HIV-2
Antibodies
detected

HIV-1 (+)
HIV-2 (+)
HIV
Antibodies
detected

HIV-1 (−) or
Intermediate HIV-2 (−)

HIV-1 NAT

(+) indicates reactive test result
(−) indicates nonreactive test result
NAT: nucleic acid test

HIV-1 NAT (+)
Acute HIV-1 infection

HIV-1 NAT (−)
Negative for HIV-1

▲ **Figure 55–1.** Recommended HIV testing algorithm for serum or plasma specimens. (Reproduced with permission from the Centers for Disease Control and Prevention. The 2018 Quick Reference Guide: Recommended Laboratory HIV Testing Algorithm for Serum or Plasma Specimens. January 2018. https://stacks.cdc.gov/view/cdc/50872. Accessed June 15, 2020.)

The CDC recommends that initial screening be conducted using a US Food and Drug Administration (FDA)–approved antigen/antibody (ag/ab) test that detects HIV-1/HIV-2 antibodies as well as the HIV p24 antigen. This combination is favored because it reduces the window period (time from infection to reactive test) to 18 days. Positive results on this initial screen should be confirmed with an antibody immunoassay that differentiates HIV-1 antibodies from HIV-2 antibodies. Positive results on both tests are indicative of HIV infection. Indeterminate results on the second differentiation assay should be followed by an HIV-1 nucleic acid test (NAT) (Figure 55–1). The World Health Organization (WHO) testing guidelines also employ a two-step testing algorithm, with rapid diagnostic tests and point-of-care testing preferred. If acute HIV infection is suspected, an HIV-NAT should be the initial screening test ordered.

Preexposure prophylaxis (PrEP), the daily use of a fixed-dose tablet containing emtricitabine (FTC) and tenofovir-disoproxil fumarate (TDF) to prevent HIV, has been shown to be a highly effective prevention strategy. In 2019, the FDA also approved the use of a fixed-dose tablet of FTC and tenofovir-alafenamide but only for PrEP for cisgender men who have sex with men and transgender women. Unfortunately, there are limited data regarding the safety and efficacy of PrEP in adults over age 50. While older adults can benefit from this intervention, they are potentially at increased risk for renal failure and decreased bone density related to TDF use. In light of this, PrEP in older adults should include

careful consideration of chronic conditions that could predispose them to these conditions.

Evaluation for PrEP initiation should include HIV ag/ab testing (HIV RNA testing if history of recent exposure), hepatitis B serologic testing (surface antigen, surface antibody, and core antibody), serum creatinine, and testing for sexually transmitted infections (STIs) (ie, gonorrhea, chlamydia, and syphilis). Current guidelines recommend repeat HIV testing every 3 months and testing for STIs and estimated creatinine clearance (eCrCl) at least every 6 months. The use of PrEP is contraindicated if the eCrCl is <60 mL/min. Although TDF is associated with bone density loss, current guidelines do not recommend screening with dual-energy x-ray absorptiometry (DEXA) prior to PrEP initiation or while on PrEP. It is recommended that individuals being considered for PrEP who have a history of fragility fractures or risk factors for osteoporosis be referred to an HIV specialist and potentially an endocrinologist for appropriate treatment and management.

▶ Clinical Findings

A. Symptoms & Signs

Clinical presentation will vary based on the stage of disease at time of diagnosis. It is estimated that up to 20% of individuals newly infected with HIV are completely asymptomatic. Symptoms of acute retroviral syndrome include fever, lymphadenopathy, pharyngitis, generalized maculopapular rash, and fatigue. Onset is typically 2 to 4 weeks following HIV exposure, and median duration of symptoms is 14 days. Although rare, acute HIV infection can present with neurologic manifestations including aseptic meningitis or acute demyelinating polyneuropathy. Older adults who present with frequent bacterial pneumonia, thrush, or neurocognitive changes should prompt HIV testing.

B. Initial Testing & Monitoring on Antiretroviral therapy

Baseline laboratory tests should be obtained upon entering HIV care. These initial tests include CD4 T-cell count; plasma HIV RNA level; hepatitis A, B, and C serologic testing; serum chemistries; complete cell count; STI screening; fasting lipid profile; and genotypic testing for antiretroviral (ARV) resistance mutations. If the use of abacavir is being considered, an HLA-5701 test should also be obtained. HIV RNA should be monitored every 4 to 6 weeks after initiating ARV therapy (ART) until the viral load is undetectable. Once viral suppression is achieved, HIV RNA should be checked every 3 months and then every 6 months for those who are clinically stable and adherent to ARTs. CD4 cell count should be monitored every 3 to 6 months for the first 2 years of ART, then annually thereafter in the setting of viral suppression and CD4 T-cell count >300 cells/mm$_3$. STI testing, including syphilis screening, should be offered at least every 3 months (Table 55–1).

▶ Complications

A. Multimorbidity & Polypharmacy

As a result of modern ART, HIV has transformed to a chronic condition. However, even adults with well-controlled disease are at increased risk for developing a number of additional chronic conditions. These include cardiovascular disease, osteoporosis, certain malignancies (eg, anal cancers, cervical cancers, lung cancers), and resultant multimorbidity. Older adults living with HIV also have higher rates of polypharmacy than their HIV-negative counterparts.

The Veteran's Aging Cohort Study (VACS) is a prospective, observational cohort study of HIV-positive veterans examining the role of chronic medical and psychiatric diseases in determining clinical outcomes of adults living with HIV. With regard to polypharmacy, in the VACS cohort, over half of PLWH age ≥50 were taking five or more medications. Potential consequences of polypharmacy in older adults include drug-drug interactions, compounded drug toxicities, and adherence problems with non-ARV medications. Studies have also shown that prescribing issues, including potentially inappropriate medications, may be more common in older HIV-positive adults. In a United Kingdom–based cohort, older (age ≥50 years) PLWH had

a higher prevalence of potential drug-drug interactions (35.1%) compared to younger (<50 years) PLWH (20.3%) and HIV-negative adults age ≥50 (16.4%). In a San Francisco–based study of PLWH age 60 or older, 52% had at least one potentially inappropriate medication defined by the Beers criteria, and 17% had a clinically significant anticholinergic burden of medications. Both of these medication issues were higher than in an HIV-negative control group. Pill burden is common and may be addressed by the use of single-pill ARV regimens when appropriate. Performing frequent medication reconciliations, especially under the guidance of a clinical pharmacist with HIV expertise, may also be beneficial.

B. Cardiovascular Disease

It is well established that persons living with HIV are at increased risk for cardiovascular disease (CVD), even when accounting for other risk factors such as tobacco use and hypertension. The VACS found that PLWH have 1.5 times higher risk of developing an acute myocardial infarction compared to the general population. Despite the increased risk, there are no formal guidelines regarding the use of statins or antithrombotic agents for primary prevention of CVD in PLWH, nor is HIV included in any of the currently available risk stratification tools, including the Atherosclerotic Cardiovascular Disease (ASCVD) calculator. One approach, based on expert consensus, suggests combining information from established CVD risk assessment tools with HIV-related CVD risk factors to determine need for lipid-lowering therapy. A randomized controlled trial to prevent vascular events in HIV (REPRIEVE) is underway examining the effect of pitavastatin on serious cardiovascular events and all-cause mortality in adults living with HIV aged 40 to 75. While PLWH benefit from statins, it is important to recognize that certain ARV medications (eg, protease inhibitors and non-nucleoside reverse transcriptase inhibitors) affect hepatic metabolism of statins. Statins should be selected with careful consideration of the individual's current ARV regimen to avoid significant drug-drug interactions.

C. Osteoporosis & Fractures

Older adults living with HIV are at a three- to four-fold higher risk for bone mineralization disorders and fractures than the general population. Several mechanisms for this process have been proposed, including cytokine activation of osteoclasts secondary to chronic T-cell activation caused by HIV. Certain ARVs have also been associated with bone loss including TDF and stavudine.

Current expert opinion dictates that all HIV-positive men over age 50 and HIV-positive postmenopausal women should receive bone mineral density screening with DEXA. Those with prior history of fragility fractures, at high risk for falls, or on chronic glucocorticoid therapy should also undergo screening with DEXA. All men living with HIV aged 40 to 49

Table 55–1. Lab monitoring schedule for patients with HIV.

Laboratory Test	Entry to Care	ART Initiation or Modification	2–8 Weeks After ART Initiation or Modification	Every 3–6 Months	Every 6 Months	Every 12 Months	Treatment Failure
HIV serology	✔						
CD4 count	✔	✔		✔During first 2 years of ART, or if viremia develops while patient is on ART, or CD4 count <300 cells/mm³		✔During first 2 years of ART, or if viremia develops while patient is on ART, or CD4 count <300 cells/mm³	✔
HIV viral load	✔	✔	✔	✔	✔		✔
Resistance testing	✔	✔					✔
HLA-B*5701		✔If considering ABC					
Tropism testing		✔If considering a CCR5 antagonist					✔If considering a CCR5 antagonist, or for patients experiencing virologic failure on a CCR5 antagonist–based regimen
Hepatitis B serology (HBsAb, HBsAg, HBcAb, total)	✔	✔May repeat if patient is nonimmune and does not have chronic HBV infection				✔May repeat if patient is nonimmune and does not have chronic HBV infection	
Hepatitis C screening (HCV antibody or, if indicated, HCV RNA)	✔					✔Repeat HCV screening for at-risk patients	
Basic chemistry	✔	✔	✔	✔			
ALT, AST, total bilirubin	✔	✔	✔	✔			
CBC with differential	✔	✔		✔If CD4 testing is done	✔		
Fasting lipid profile	✔	✔			✔If abnormal at last measurement	✔If normal at last measurement	
Fasting glucose or hemoglobin A1c	✔	✔		✔If abnormal at last measurement		✔If normal at last measurement	
Urinalysis	✔	✔			✔If on TAF or TDF	✔	

ABC, abacavir; ALT, alanine aminotransferase; ART, antiretroviral therapy; AST, aspartate aminotransferase; CBC, complete blood count; HBV, hepatitis B virus; HCV, hepatitis C virus; TAF, tenofovir-alafenamide; TDF, tenofovir-disoproxil fumarate.

Table 55–2. Frailty measurements used in studies of older adults with HIV.

Frailty Phenotype	Frailty Index	VACS Index
5 criteria: 1. Shrinking (weight loss) 2. Exhaustion (self-report CES-D) 3. Weakness (grip strength) 4. Slowness (gait speed) 5. Low activity (Minnesota Leisure Time Scale) 3/5 criteria = frail, 1–2 criteria = prefrail	Include at least 30 items: • Can be signs, symptoms, disabilities, diseases • Items included must increase with age • Different domains (eg, cognition, function) Example items: lipoatrophy, hepatitis C co-infection, polypharmacy, low physical activity, lab tests	1. Age 2. CD4 count 3. HIV viral load 4. Hemoglobin (anemia) 5. FIB-4 (liver tests, platelets) 6. eGFR (renal function) 7. Hepatitis C co-infection

CES-D, Center for Epidemiologic Studies Depression Scale; eGFR, estimated glomerular filtration rate; FIB-4, Fibrosis-4; VACS, Veterans Aging Cohort Study.

Adapted with permission from Greene M, Justice AC, Covinsky KE. Assessment of geriatric syndromes and physical function in people living with HIV, Virulence 2017 Jul 4;8(5):586-598.

and premenopausal women living with HIV aged 40 and over should be screened for risk of fragility fractures using the Fracture Risk Assessment Tool (FRAX). In settings where DEXA is not readily available, use of the FRAX tool is recommended. Treatment and monitoring of low bone mineral density follow guidelines for the general population.

D. Geriatric Syndromes

An increasing number of studies suggest that geriatric syndromes are common among older HIV-positive adults. Presence of these conditions is associated with both HIV markers including CD4 T-cell count and viral suppression, as well as general risk factors including multimorbidity. Rates of geriatric syndromes in middle-aged adults with HIV are similar to those reported for the general population age 65 and older, suggesting earlier occurrence of these conditions. Similar to the general population, geriatric conditions such as frailty and falls often co-occur.

1. Frailty—Adults living with HIV have a high frequency of frailty, with onset often occurring at a younger age than their HIV-negative counterparts. Frailty in PLWH is associated with increasing age, longer duration of HIV infection, detectable viral load, and lower CD4 T-cell count. Co-occurring conditions such as diabetes, chronic obstructive pulmonary disease, depression, and hepatitis C infection contribute to the severity of frailty seen in this cohort. Social factors including lower income and lower education are also strong predictors of frailty in older adults living with HIV. Furthermore, frailty in this group is associated with poor health-related outcomes including mortality, falls, and fracture risk.

Screening for frailty should be integrated into the clinical care of older adults living with HIV. While there is no consensus on the best method to assess frailty, the Fried phenotype is the most commonly used assessment in research examining frailty among this cohort (Please see Chapter 5 for more information about the frailty phenotype.) The VACS Index, originally designed as a prognostic index, has also been used to assess frailty in PLWH. The Cumulative Deficits Model/

Frailty Index has shown similar ability to predict 5-year mortality as the VACS Index but is less studied in this population. Table 55–2 summarizes the components of each of these indices.

2. Falls—Given the increased risk of osteoporosis and fractures, falls are a particular concern in older HIV-positive adults. Although cohort studies of HIV-positive and uninfected adults have not clearly demonstrated an increased risk of falls among PLWH, studies have indicated that PLWH have higher rates of balance problems. Additionally, across multiple studies, fall rates in middle-aged (aged 50) PLWH are at least 20%, similar to rates in the general population aged ≥65. The American Geriatrics Society/British Geriatrics Society Fall Prevention Guideline and the CDC Stopping Elderly Accidents, Deaths, and Injuries (STEADI) program recommend asking about falls in the prior year, along with a question about unsteadiness with walking as a starting point to screen for falls. (See Chapter 6 for more information on falls.)

3. Neurocognitive disorders—Even in the current ART era, approximately 50% of older adults living with HIV will exhibit symptoms of HIV-associated neurocognitive disorder (HAND). The term HAND refers to a spectrum of cognitive impairment that includes asymptomatic neurocognitive impairment (ANI), mild neurocognitive impairment (MNI), and HIV-associated dementia (HAD). ANI is defined as any degree of neurocognitive impairment in at least two cognitive domains but no functional impairment. MNI is defined as mild to moderate impairment in at least two cognitive domains in conjunction with mild to moderate functional impairment. HAD is severe impairment in at least two cognitive domains with severe impairment in function. Patients with symptomatic cerebrospinal fluid (CSF) escape, where PLWH have a detectable HIV viral load in the CSF, despite having an undetectable plasma HIV viral load, often have rapidly progressing neuropsychiatric symptoms.

HAND tends to have a more fluctuating course compared to other neurodegenerative diseases and follows a more subcortical pattern. This includes deficits in executive dysfunction, attention, and concentration. Determining which short screening tools are best for HAND remains a challenge. The HIV Dementia Scale (HDS) and International HIV Dementia Scale (IHDS) were developed earlier in the HIV/AIDS epidemic and demonstrate poor sensitivity for milder forms of HAND. The Mini-Mental Status Examination (MMSE) also has poor sensitivity. The Montreal Cognitive Assessment (MoCA), which may be the most promising tool, has a sensitivity and specificity of 72% and 67%, respectively, including milder forms of HAND.

For older adults without virologic control, treatment starts with initiating ART. Selecting a more central nervous system (CNS)–penetrating ART regimen, based on CNS penetration effectiveness scores, remains controversial for those without clear CSF escape. The role of exercise as well as other treatment modalities remain an area of active research. As with other geriatric syndromes, neurocognitive symptoms in PLWH are multifactorial and may take a multifaceted management approach.

▶ Treatment

A. Antiretroviral Medications

Except in cases of certain opportunistic infections (eg, cryptococcal meningitis) treatment of HIV should begin at time of diagnosis, regardless of CD4 count, as recommended by the CDC and WHO. Early ART initiation has been shown to reduce the risk of developing HIV-related chronic conditions. This is especially important in older adults, who are at risk for more rapid progression to advanced HIV disease and demonstrate slower rates of CD4 reconstitution, even in the setting of adherence to ARV medications. The goal of ART is to maintain lifelong viral suppression. Studies show that older adults (age ≥50 years) have higher rates of viral suppression than their younger (age <50 years) HIV-positive counterparts.

An initial ARV regimen for a treatment-naïve individual generally contains two nucleoside reverse transcriptase inhibitors (NRTIs) and a third agent from one of the following drug classes: integrase strand transfer inhibitors (INSTIs), nonnucleoside reverse transcriptase inhibitors (NNRTIs), or protease inhibitors (PIs) with a pharmacokinetic booster (ie, cobicistat or ritonavir). Table 55–3 contains the WHO and Department of Health and Human Services preferred initial regimens.

Given the high rates of polypharmacy in older adults living with HIV, they are also at high risk of significant drug interactions related to ARV use. Table 55–4 contains a list of some commonly used medications known to have significant drug interactions with ARVs. The use of an online drug interaction tool, such as the University of Liverpool Interaction Checker (hiv-druginteractions.org), is strongly recommended when starting any new medication.

Table 55–3. Initial antiretroviral recommendations.

Department of Health and Human Services (DHHS) guidelines
INSTI plus 2 NRTIs (in alphabetical order)
• Bictegravir/tenofovir alafenamide/emtricitabine
• Dolutegravir/abacavir/lamivudine (only for patients who are HLA-B5701 negative)
• Dolutegravir plus tenofovir[a]/emtricitabine
• Raltegravir plus tenofovir[a]/emtricitabine
World Health Organization (WHO) guidelines
Tenofovir-disoproxil fumarate/lamivudine or emtricitabine plus one of the following (in alphabetical order)
• Dolutegravir
• Efavirenz
• Raltegravir

INSTI, integrase strand transfer inhibitors; NRTI, nucleoside reverse transcriptase inhibitor.

[a]Tenofovir-alafenamide or tenofovir-disoproxil fumarate.

▶ Prognosis

Since the advent of effective, well-tolerated ART, the mortality associated with HIV/AIDS has declined dramatically. There are approximately 15,000 deaths among PLWH in the United States annually, and 940,000 worldwide. Although AIDS-related complications have drastically declined in high-resource countries, this remains a leading cause of death among PLWH in resource-limited settings. In high-resource areas, comorbid conditions, including CVD, substance use, and non–AIDS-related malignancies, contribute greatly to mortality among PLWH.

Life expectancy is approaching that of the general population, but gaps remain. Identifying vulnerable adults living with HIV is an important component of reducing morbidity in this cohort. The VACS Index (components included in Table 55–2) has been used as a prognostic tool for PLWH. This index predicts 5-year mortality and morbidity including hospitalization, and an easy-to-use calculator is available for free online (https://medicine.yale.edu/intmed/vacs/vacsresources/vacsindexinfo.aspx). An updated version, VACS 2.0, is under development, and adds albumin, white blood cell count, and body mass index. The VACS Index can be used to estimate life expectancy and thus help identify those who may benefit from specific screening tests.

Allavena C, Hanf M, Rey D, et al. Antiretroviral exposure and comorbidities in an aging HIV-infected population: the challenge of geriatric patients. *PLoS One.* 2018;13(9):e0203895.

Autenrieth CS, Beck EJ, Stelzle D, Mallouris C, Mahy M, Ghys P. Global and regional trends of people living with HIV aged 50 and over: estimates and projections for 2000–2020. *PloS One.* 2018;13(11):e0207005.

Table 55–4. Common drug interactions between antiretroviral and other prescribed medications.

Class or Interacting Medication	Interaction with INSTIs	Interaction with NNRTIs	Interaction with PIs	Comment
Rifampin	Decreases INSTI levels	Decreased efavirenz and doravirine levels	Decreases PI levels	Avoid coadministration with PIs or INSTIs, consider rifabutin as alternative agent.
Statins			PIs increase statin levels	Lovastatin/simvastatin contraindicated with PI use. Atorvastatin/rosuvastatin: start with lowest dose. Pitavastatin: least potential for interaction.
Acid-blocking medications (eg, PPIs, H₂ blockers)		Decreased rilpivirine absorption	Decreased atazanavir absorption	PPIs: rilpivirine coadministration contraindicated.
Corticosteroids (systemic, inhaled, or intranasal)	Increased fluticasone and budesonide with boosted INSTI[a]	Dexamethasone can decrease NNRTI levels, especially rilpivirine	Increased fluticasone and budesonide levels with boosted PIs	Beclomethasone/flunisolide preferred alternative with boosted ARVs. Avoid dexamethasone and rilpivirine coadministration.
Warfarin		Increased or decreased warfarin levels with NNRTIs	Decreased warfarin levels with protease inhibitors	Follow INR closely if coadministered with these agents.
DOACs	Increased DOAC levels with boosted INSTIs	NNRTIs lower DOAC levels	Increased DOAC levels with boosted PIs	Edoxaban safe with all NNRTIs.
Phosphodiesterase type 5 inhibitors (sildenafil, tadalafil, vardenafil, avanafil)		Decreased phosphodiesterase type 5 inhibitor effect with etravirine	Increased phosphodiesterase type 5 inhibitor exposure with ritonavir-boosted protease inhibitors	Start with the lowest effective dose with ritonavir-boosted protease inhibitors. Avoid coadministration of avanafil with NNTRIs or protease inhibitors.
Polyvalent cation supplements/antacids (eg, calcium, iron)	Decrease INSTI levels			Avoid or give INSTI 2 hours before or 6 hours after cation.

ARVs, antiretrovirals; DOACs, direct oral anticoagulants; INSTI, integrase strand transfer inhibitors; NNRTI, nonnucleoside reverse transcriptase inhibitor; PIs, protease inhibitors; PPIs, proton pump inhibitors.

[a]Boosted = combined with cobicistat or ritonavir.

Brown TT, Hoy J, Borderi M, et al. Recommendations for evaluation and management of bone disease in HIV. *Clin Infect Dis.* 2015;60(8):1242-1251.

Centers for Disease Control and Prevention. HIV Surveillance Report, 2017; vol. 29. http://www.cdc.gov/hiv/library/reports/hiv-surveillance.html. Published November 2018. Accessed November 26, 2019.

Feinstein MJ, Hsue PY, Benjamin LA, et al. Characteristics, prevention, and management of cardiovascular disease in people living with HIV: a scientific statement from the American Heart Association. *Circulation.* 2019;140(2):e98-e124.

Gandhi M, Glidden DV, Mayer K, et al. Association of age, baseline kidney function, and medication exposure with declines in creatinine clearance on pre-exposure prophylaxis: an observational cohort study. *Lancet HIV.* 2016;3(11):e528.

Greene M, Covinsky KE, Valcour V, et al. Geriatric syndromes in older HIV-infected adults. *J Acquir Immune Defic Syndr.* 2015;69(2):161-167.

Greene M, Justice AC, Covinsky KE. Assessment of geriatric syndromes and physical function in people living with HIV. *Virulence.* 2017;8(5):586-598.

Hellmuth J, Psy M, Valcour V. Interactions between aging and NeuroAIDS. *Curr Opin HIV AIDS.* 2014;9(6):527-532.

Hurt C, Nelson J, Hightow-Weidman L, Miller W. Selecting an HIV test: a narrative review for clinicians and researchers. *Sex Transm Dis.* 2017;44(12):739-746.

Legarth R, Ahlström M, Kronborg G, et al. Long-term mortality in HIV-infected individuals 50 years or older: a nationwide, population-based cohort study. *J Acquir Immune Defic Syndr.* 2016;71(2):213-218.

Maciel RA, Klück HM, Durand M, Sprinz E. Comorbidity is more common and occurs earlier in persons living with HIV than in HIV-uninfected matched controls, aged 50 years and older: a cross-sectional study. *Int J Infect Dis.* 2018;70:30-35.

McNicholl IR, Gandhi M, Hare CB, Greene M, Pierluissi E. A pharmacist-led program to evaluate and reduce polypharmacy and potentially inappropriate prescribing in older HIV-Positive patients. *Pharmacotherapy.* 2017;37(12):1498-1506.

Panel on Antiretroviral Guidelines for Adults and Adolescents. Guidelines for the Use of Antiretroviral Agents in Adults and Adolescents with HIV. Department of Health and Human Services. http://www.aidsinfo.nih.gov/ContentFiles/ AdultandAdolescentGL.pdf. Accessed April 28, 2019.

Pilowsky DJ, Wu L. Sexual risk behaviors and HIV risk among Americans aged 50 years or older: a review. *Subst Abuse Rehabil.* 2015;6:51-60.

Tate J, Sterne J, Justice A. Albumin, white blood cell count, and body mass index improve discrimination of mortality in HIV-positive individuals. *AIDS.* 2019;33(5):903-912.

Common Skin Disorders

56

Daniel Butler, MD
Eleni Linos, MD, DrPH

General Principles

The incidence of dermatologic conditions is increasing in parallel to the aging population. Each year, there are >27 million visits to dermatologists and >5 million new skin cancers diagnosed, most in older adults. While there are many skin conditions that are common in both younger and older adults, there are certain important principles that make geriatric dermatology different from general dermatology. These principles, including consideration of life expectancy, lag time to benefit of interventions, functional status, social support polypharmacy, and medical comorbidities are summarized in Table 56–1. Taken together these principles can guide clinicians in making appropriate treatment decisions for skin diseases that are more likely to help older patients and improve their quality of life. With limited literature, these principles should be the backbone of decision making.

Aging skin is subject to both intrinsic aging processes and many years of environmental insults. With regard to intrinsic changes, as one ages, the skin's barrier function declines, making it much more difficult to maintain moisture. Thus, dry skin in older adults is common. This has multiple consequences, the most common being pruritus. In addition to skin barrier changes, there are also intrinsic changes to the immune system that are believed to play an important role in aging skin.

While intrinsic changes contribute to aging skin pathology, external elements also play crucial role. Dry skin is also more susceptible to environmental insults, which can cause eczematous dermatitis because of an irritant or an allergen. After many years of being subject to oxidative damage from environmental pollution and radiation, skin cells have accumulated many mutations. Thus, skin cancers, are more prevalent in the older population.

The complex interplay between the intrinsic and extrinsic aging holds the key to clinical pathology of aging skin. Increases in certain infections such as herpes zoster and onychomycosis, inflammatory dermatoses, and neoplasms are examples of this complex interplay.

SEBORRHEIC KERATOSIS

 ESSENTIALS OF DIAGNOSIS

► Seborrheic keratosis is the most common benign epithelial tumor in adulthood.

► The trunk is affected more than the extremities, head, and neck.

► Primary lesions are 5- to 20-mm light brown to dark brown–black papules and plaques with a rough, warty surface (Figure 56–1).

► Differential diagnosis includes solar lentigo, melanocytic nevus, verruca vulgaris, and lentigo maligna melanoma.

Complications

Friction, pressure, and trauma to these lesions may cause irritation or inflammation.

Treatment

Irritated or inflamed lesions can be treated with cryotherapy (Box 56–1), curettage, or shave removal. Lesions in cosmetically sensitive areas are best treated with light electrodessication to minimize scarring and dyspigmentation.

Table 56–1. Principles of geriatrics applied to dermatology.

Geriatrics Principle	Relevance to Dermatology	Example
Life expectancy is more than age	Treatment of low-risk basal cell carcinoma (BCC)	A healthy 80-year-old may have a life expectancy of over 10-years, making treatment of low-risk BCC appropriate to prevent future growth. Meanwhile, a frail 80-year-old with many comorbidities may not live long enough to benefit from treatment of a low-risk BCC.
Lag time to benefit	Screening total body skin examination	A patient in the last year of life may not benefit from routine screening total body skin examination.
Polypharmacy and medication adverse effects	Sedating antihistamines	A patient with itch who is prescribed a sedating antihistamine may experience dizziness and fall due to this medication.
Cognition	Ability to tolerate minor procedures	A patient with dementia may not understand why they are having a biopsy procedure performed, and what seems like a simple procedure can induce anxiety and fear. In a patient prone to behavioral symptoms, this risks precipitating agitation, significantly complicating the caregiver's management during and after the procedure. Also a patient with dementia may not keep a bandage on, and may have hard time keeping the wound clean.
Function and mobility	Wound healing, office visits, bandage changes	Pressure ulcers may develop due to immobility, and wound healing may be complicated by difficulties bathing and moving.
Caregivers, social support	Office visits, bandage changes	A clinic visit may be logistically challenging for the family of a patient who needs support during and after visits. Caregiver availability may determine if follow-up visits and bandage changes are possible.
Patient preference matter	Treatment of actinic keratoses (AK)	Regarding a painless but cosmetically visible AK, treatment may not be necessary for a patient who is not bothered by it, but may be necessary for a patient who is bothered by its appearance.

Reproduced with permission from Linos E, Chren MM, Covinsky K. Geriatric Dermatology-A Framework for Caring for Older Patients With Skin Disease, *JAMA Dermatol* 2018 Jul 1;154(7):757-758.

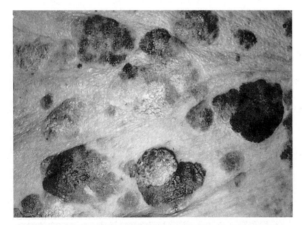

▲ **Figure 56–1.** Seborrheic keratoses. Waxy, stuck-on papules and plaques, with varying shades of brown and a verrucous surface. (Used with permission from Neill Peters, MD.)

EPIDERMAL INCLUSION CYST

 ESSENTIALS OF DIAGNOSIS

▶ This cutaneous cyst is an epithelium-lined sac filled with keratin and located within the dermis.

▶ Distribution is more common on the trunk than the face and extremities.

▶ Primary lesions are 0.5- to 4-cm flesh-colored to yellow dermal to subcutaneous nodules (Figure 56–2).

▶ Cysts are freely mobile on palpation. With pressure, cheese-like keratin can often be expressed through a central punctum.

▶ Differential diagnosis includes lipoma.

▶ **Complications**

Rupture of the cyst wall leads to extrusion of keratin debris into the dermis and a foreign-body inflammatory response. The area becomes tense, tender, and painful.

Box 56–1. Cryotherapy

Indications to use liquid nitrogen

- Actinic keratosis
- Seborrheic keratosis (irritated)
- Warts

A. Dipstick technique
1. Roll extra cotton over the tip of the cotton applicator.
2. Dip tip into liquid nitrogen.
3. Apply tip of applicator to lesion until 1–2 mm of normal surrounding skin turns white.
4. Wait until lesion completely thaws back to normal color.
5. Repeat (number of freeze-thaw cycles depends on the lesion being treated).

B. Open-spray technique (requires hand-held nitrogen unit and C-tip aperture)
1. Nozzle should be 1–2 cm from target lesion and perpendicular to it.
2. Squeeze trigger to emit continuous burst of spray.
3. The lesion and not more than 2 mm of surrounding normal skin should be frosted.
4. Wait until lesion completely thaws back to normal color.
5. Repeat (number of freeze-thaw cycles depends on the lesion being treated).

Adverse Effects

Patients must be informed:
1. During treatment, the treated area will sting or burn followed by throbbing.
2. Treated area will become erythematous and edematous and will vesiculate or blister within hours.
3. Hypopigmentation is common in darkly pigmented individuals.

▶ Treatment

These cysts do not resolve spontaneously. Permanent removal can be achieved only by excising the entire cyst wall. Incision and drainage may temporarily relieve pressure but is not curative. In the case of a ruptured cyst, the use of antibiotics is controversial because this is not a true infection (abscess), but rather an inflammatory reaction to foreign material. However, minocycline and doxycycline have an anti-inflammatory effect, and a dosage of 100 mg twice daily may be helpful. If there is no improvement within a week, incision and drainage followed by infiltration of the area with triamcinolone acetonide 10 mg/mL will provide relief. Surgery of inflamed tissue is not recommended. If any portion of the cyst wall remains after treatment, recurrence is likely.

WARTS (VERRUCA VULGARIS AND VERRUCA PLANTARIS)

 ESSENTIALS OF DIAGNOSIS

▶ These human papillomavirus–induced growths are found most frequently on the hands and feet, followed by arms, legs, and trunk.

▶ Primary lesions are 5- to 15-mm flesh-colored papules and plaques with a verrucous or filiform surface. Reddish-brown punctate dots (thrombosed capillary loops) are diagnostic (Figure 56–3). The lesion may require paring with a No. 15 blade to visualize the capillary loops.

▶ Differential diagnosis includes flat warts, seborrheic keratosis, and squamous cell carcinoma.

▶ Complications

Localized spread and communication to others are the predominant concern with verrucae vulgaris and verrucae plantaris.

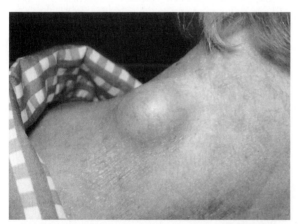

▲ **Figure 56–2.** Epidermal inclusion cyst. This large 4- to 5-cm cyst on the left shoulder is tense but freely mobile over underlying tissues.

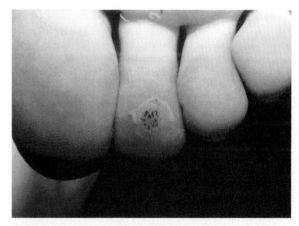

▲ **Figure 56–3.** Plantar wart. The 2- to 3-mm punctate brown papules are thrombosed capillary loops.

Treatment

The decision of whether and how to treat warts should be made based on the number and location of lesions, presence of symptoms, and patient preference. For example, if warts are asymptomatic, treatment may not be needed. Patients should be informed that multiple plantar warts are often stubborn regardless of the treatment modality. Several treatments may be needed before significant improvement occurs. Immunocompromised patients may have widespread involvement and are refractory to standard treatment modalities, in which case, referral to dermatology for advanced therapy is necessary. First-line treatment modalities include the following.

A. Cryotherapy

In addition to the cryotherapy described in Box 56–1, two to three freeze-thaw cycles are recommended to induce blistering. Treatment is repeated every 3 to 4 weeks. Plantar warts are thicker and often require paring with a No. 15 blade before freezing.

B. Cantharidin

Cantharidin 0.7% (Cantharone) is a chemical agent that induces blistering. It must be applied in the office setting because of potential side effects, including blistering, dyspigmentation, and scarring. It is applied to the wart using the wood end of a cotton-tipped applicator, allowed to dry, covered for 8 to 12 hours, and then washed off with soap and water. A blister develops within 1 to 2 days. Treatment is repeated every 3 to 4 weeks. Cantharidin may be used alone or in combination with podophyllin and salicylic acid. Patients are asked to avoid removing the blister roof; however, if the blister is tense and causing discomfort, they may puncture it with a clean needle to relieve some of the pressure.

C. Salicylic Acid

Salicylic acid 40% plasters can be used at home. The plaster is cut to fit over the wart and left in place for 24 hours. This is repeated daily. Between treatments, the superficial macerated debris can be removed with a pumice stone or emery board.

ONYCHOMYCOSIS

ESSENTIALS OF DIAGNOSIS

▶ Characteristic features include distal thickening of the nail plate, yellow discoloration, and subungual debris (Figure 56–4).

▶ Differential diagnosis includes pincer nails, onychogryphosis, psoriasis, lichen planus, and repeated trauma.

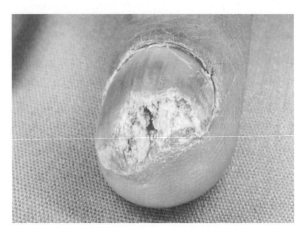

▲ **Figure 56–4.** Onychomycosis. This fingernail demonstrates the characteristic thick subungual hyperkeratosis and debris.

General Considerations

Onychomycosis is very common in older adults, with a prevalence of about 20% after age 60. Most patients do not choose to treat this, especially if it is asymptomatic.

Clinical Findings

If treatment is deemed necessary, yeast or dermatophyte infection of the nail plate requires laboratory confirmation. Nail dystrophy alone is not sensitive or specific for onychomycosis. There are three diagnostic tests, as follows.

A. Direct Microscopy

Trim back the distal edge of the involved nail. Use a small 1-mm curette or No. 15 blade to scrape the undersurface of the nail plate and nail bed. Place the sample on a glass slide and add one drop of potassium hydroxide (KOH) 20% with dimethylsulfoxide (DMSO). Demonstration of hyphae after a few minutes confirms the diagnosis. Sensitivity is highly variable and dependent on experience. This is the preferential method for diagnosis in the aging adult given real-time confirmation and cost efficacy, but if a provider is not versed in microscopy, the below options can be easily used.

B. Culture

Obtain sample as described earlier, and place on Sabouraud dextrose agar containing chloramphenicol and cycloheximide (Mycosel or mycobiotic agar). Nail clippings are poor specimens for culture. If there is no growth within 3 weeks, the test is negative. Sensitivity is 50% to 60%.

C. Pathology

Send a nail clipping in a formalin container for periodic acid-Schiff (PAS) stain. Sensitivity is >90%.

Pathogenesis

Public exercise facilities and pools are common sites for transmission of dermatophytes, usually via the feet. Tinea pedis can spread to the adjacent nail and often precedes onychomycosis. Toenails are affected more often than fingernails.

Prevention

Treatment of tinea pedis with topical antifungals can prevent onychomycosis and decrease risk of recurrence.

Treatment

Treatment can be a difficult decision, particularly in older adults, as efficacy is limited with both topical and oral options. If a patient does not report symptoms from onychomycosis, no treatment is recommended. If patient experiences pain, recurrent swelling, recurrent tinea pedis, or other quality of life impairing symptoms, treatment may be warranted. Given the low efficacy of topical options, when treatment is needed, oral options may be more effective.

Toenails grow very slowly, approximately 1 mm per month. Thus, if half of the nail is involved, it will take 6 to 9 months to clear. If the entire nail is involved, it will take 12 to 15 months to clear. Systemic antifungals maintain an effective concentration in the nail matrix for 6 to 9 months after therapy is discontinued.

A. Systemic Antifungals

Systemic antifungals should be reserved only for older adults with significant symptoms given side effect profiles of the antifungal agents in older adults. Table 56–2 compares dosing regimens and mycologic cure rates.

1. Terbinafine—This is the treatment of choice for dermatophyte onychomycosis, providing superior long-term clinical efficacy and lower rates of relapse compared with pulse itraconazole. Terbinafine may increase levels of theophylline, nortriptyline, and caffeine and decrease the level of cyclosporine. Rifampin, cimetidine, and terfenadine may alter serum levels of terbinafine. Terbinafine is best avoided in patients with active hepatitis B or C, cirrhosis, or other chronic

hepatic disorders. In healthy individuals, baseline liver function tests are optional.

2. Itraconazole—This is the treatment of choice for onychomycosis caused by yeast (*Candida*) or molds. Itraconazole is contraindicated in patients taking astemizole, terfenadine, triazolam, midazolam, cisapride, lovastatin, or simvastatin. Itraconazole may increase drug levels of oral hypoglycemic agents, immunosuppressants, HIV-1 protease inhibitors, and anticoagulants. Anticonvulsants, antituberculosis agents, nevirapine, H_2 antihistamines, proton pump inhibitors, and didanosine may alter serum levels of itraconazole. Itraconazole is best avoided in patients with active hepatitis B or C, cirrhosis, or other chronic hepatic disorders. In healthy individuals, baseline liver function tests are optional.

B. Topical

1. Ciclopirox nail lacquer solution—Nail lacquers are generally ineffective, with the exception of patients with only one to two nails affected and minimal involvement of the distal nail plate. It is brushed onto affected nails daily for 6 months. Nails should be trimmed, with regular removal of the unattached infected nail.

Prognosis

With the use of systemic antifungals, relapse rates range from 20% to 50%. Prophylactic weekend application of topical antifungals may prevent recurrences.

Sigurgeirsson B, Olafsson JH, Steinsson JB, et al. Long-term effectiveness of treatment with terbinafine vs itraconazole in onychomycosis: a 5-year blinded prospective follow-up study. *Arch Dermatol.* 2002;138(3):353-357.

PRURITUS

ESSENTIALS OF DIAGNOSIS

▶ The most common causes of itch in older adults include dry skin, age-related changes in the immune system, and nerve-mediated itch sensations. Symptoms are often multifactorial, and treatment should be tailored to contributing etiologies.

▶ Dry skin is closely related to diminished barrier function. It can present as cracking and dry scaling (Figure 56–5).

▶ Immunologic causes of itch have a broad range of presentations, which include a differential diagnosis of atopic dermatitis, contact dermatitis, and irritant dermatitis, among other immunologic conditions.

▶ Nerve-mediated itch often presents with fixed, localized areas of pruritus and may require further workup for nerve-damaging conditions such as diabetes or spinal arthritis.

Table 56–2. Systemic antifungal treatment of toenails.

Drug	Dosing Regimen	Mycological Cure (18 months)
Terbinafine	Continuous: 250 mg/day × 3 months	76%
Itraconazole	Continuous: 200 mg/day × 3 months	59%
	Pulse: 400 mg/day × 1 week/month × 3 months	63%
Fluconazole	150 mg × 1 day/week × 9 months	48%

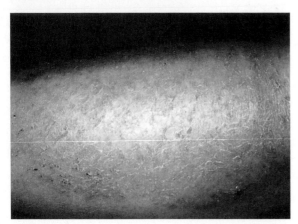

▲ **Figure 56–5.** Asteatotic dermatitis. This plaque on the left lateral shin demonstrates fine crackling or fissuring.

General Considerations

Pruritus in older adults is the result of a variety of dermatologic and systemic conditions, but the most common cause is dry skin.

Clinical Approach to Differential Diagnosis

The most important initial evaluation is to determine if the patient's itch is new onset or longstanding. If acute onset, it may suggest the introduction of modifiable external factors, and further evaluation should focus on new exposures, living situations, or contacts. Beyond the natural history of the itch, it is important to examine the patient to see if a primary rash is appreciated. Often pruritic patients present with secondary changes from scratching rather than a primary rash. A primary rash that is suggestive of a dominant immunologic basis of a patient's itch should be treated by both barrier augmentation (emollients) and immune-targeting agents such as topical steroids.

Diagnostics

With the guidance of a history and physical examination, recommended further testing remains broad because the causes of itch are extensive, particularly in older adults. Suggested workup includes complete blood count with differential, basic metabolic panel, liver function tests, thyroid function tests, erythrocyte sedimentation rate, and imaging studies to look for nerve compression.

Treatment

Initial intervention should include daily use of moisturizers. Skin hydration is essential to help maintain barrier function. Ointments and creams, rather than lotions, should be used after bathing, while the skin is still slightly moist. Ointments and creams have lower alcohol contents and fewer preservatives, which make them more hydrating and less irritating to the skin. Lotions are higher in alcohol content and preservatives, which result in little skin hydration and potential additional irritation. Clinicians should educate patients about preventing dry skin. Counseling recommendations include to shower or bathe with warm, not hot, water; eliminate scented soaps; limit soap use to armpit and groin; and apply hydrophilic petrolatum (Vaseline) to moist skin immediately after bath or shower.

Beyond conservative measures of topical hydration, there are a variety of interventions both topical and systemic. Ideally, treatment should be targeted to the likely etiology (immunologic, neurologic, barrier compromise); however, this is often difficult for even the most well-versed pruritus specialists as the etiology is unclear even with a thorough history and physical examination.

Topical steroids are first-line treatment for immune-mediated processes. Extended use of topical steroids can lead to skin thinning and breakdown; thus, extended use of topical steroids should be approached cautiously with no more than 2 weeks of use without a steroid holiday. Particular areas of concern for skin thinning include the face, axilla, and groin; thus, lower-potency topicals, such as hydrocortisone, should be preferentially used. Multiple steroids of different strengths should be used with caution to avoid polypharmacy and minimize adherence issues. If multiple topical steroids are necessary, deliberate instructions should be put onto the prescription, and the patient should be told to ignore percentage on the tube as these do not reflect strengths. Other steroid-sparing topical immune-targeted treatments include calcineurin inhibitors, tacrolimus and pimecrolimus, and phototherapy. In some cases, systemic immunosuppression is required when a diagnosis is clear and topical options have been exhausted.

Other topical and systemic options target known itch-mediating pathways, including topical anesthetics such as pramoxine, topical desensitizers such as capsaicin, systemic γ-aminobutyric acid (GABA) agonists, antihistamines, antidepressants, and opioid receptor–targeting agents. These medications, particularly antihistamines, can have deleterious effects in older adults and should not be given empirically. In recalcitrant cases, consultation with dermatology should be considered. New agents continue to emerge since pruritus is becoming a focus of medication development. New biologic agents targeting specific pruritus-mediating immunologic pathways such as interleukin (IL)-4, IL-5, IL-13, and IL-31 have shown benefit in clinical trials and in practice. Table 56–3 provides topical steroid potency ratings.

Valdes-Rodriguez R, Stull C, Yosipovitch G. Chronic pruritus in the elderly: pathophysiology, diagnosis, and management. *Drugs Aging.* 2015;32:201-215.

Table 56–3. Steroid cream potency rating.

Class	Trade Name	Generic
1 (Strongest)	Temovate 0.05%	Clobetasol propionate
	Diprolene 0.05%	Betamethasone dipropionate
2	Lidex 0.05%	Fluocinonide
	Psorcon 0.05%	Diflorasone diacetate
3	Aristocort A 0.5%	Triamcinolone acetonide
	Topicort LP 0.05%	Desoximetasone
4	Elocon 0.1%	Mometasone furoate
	Kenalog 0.1%	Triamcinolone acetonide
5	Westcort 0.2%	Hydrocortisone valerate
	Dermatop 0.1%	Prednicarbate
6	Desowen 0.05%	Desonide
	Aristocort A 0.025%	Triamcinolone acetonide
7 (Weakest)	Hytone 1%	Hydrocortisone
	Hytone 2.5%	Hydrocortisone

A. Steroid ranking from
   Class 1 (strongest) → class 7 (weakest)
   1. Most steroids come in both a cream and ointment. For the same concentration, the ointment is slightly more potent than the cream (fluocinonide 0.05% ointment is stronger than fluocinonide 0.05% cream).
   2. Most topical steroids are applied twice daily.
   3. Class 1 steroids should be used in severe inflammatory or pruritic skin conditions (psoriasis, contact dermatitis, scabies).

B. Adverse effects
   1. Atrophy, telangiectasia, and striae may occur with prolonged use of potent topical steroids (classes 1 and 2). For instance, clobetasol cream applied twice daily for >1 month may result in atrophy. The US Food and Drug Administration limits the duration of use of all class 1 steroids to 2 weeks.
   2. The face, genitals, intertriginous areas, and mucosal surfaces absorb steroids more readily and are more prone to these side effects. Potent topical steroids should not be used for >2 weeks on the face, genitals, intertriginous areas, and mucosal surfaces.
   3. Potent topical steroids applied to >50% total body surface area may have systemic effects.

SEBORRHEIC DERMATITIS

 ESSENTIALS OF DIAGNOSIS

▶ The face (especially between the eyebrows and nasolabial folds), scalp, and chest are affected (Figure 56–6).

▶ Primary lesions are erythematous patches and plaques with secondary changes of greasy scales.

▶ Rosacea, eczema, lupus, and photosensitivity disorders must be considered in the differential diagnosis.

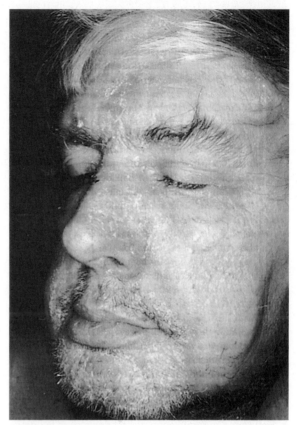

▲ **Figure 56–6.** Seborrheic dermatitis. Abundant scale distributed over the medial eyebrows, nasolabial folds, mustache, and beard.

▶ General Considerations

Overgrowth of commensal yeast and *Malassezia globosa* results in this common dermatitis.

▶ Treatment

A. Shampoos

Nonprescription zinc pyrithione 1%, selenium sulfide 1%, or ketoconazole 1% shampoo should be first-line treatments that can be applied to the scalp every day for 1 week and then tapered to once or twice weekly to prevent recurrence. The lather should be massaged into the skin for a few minutes before rinsing. Ketoconazole 2% shampoo may be more effective.

B. Other Topical Treatment

Other topical treatment may be needed for patients who are unresponsive to shampoos alone.

1. Facial involvement—Apply ketoconazole 2% cream twice daily for 2 to 3 weeks or class 6 steroid cream twice daily for 2 to 3 weeks (see Table 56–3). Sodium sulfacetamide 10%/sulfur 5% cream or wash is also effective when used once or twice daily.

2. Scalp pruritus—A class 5 steroid solution can be applied daily as needed (see Table 56–3).

STASIS DERMATITIS

 ESSENTIALS OF DIAGNOSIS

▶ Chronic venous insufficiency results from pooling of venous blood in the lower extremities and increased capillary pressure.

▶ Chronic venous insufficiency is most commonly associated with varicose veins.

▶ Anterior shins are affected most, followed by calves, dorsal feet, and ankles.

▶ Primary lesions are red-brown to brown hyperpigmented macules and patches (Figure 56–7), often with pedal edema.

▶ Erythematous patches with fine crackling and scales can be seen as secondary changes.

▶ Ulceration may occur in up to 30% of patients.

▶ Pigmented purpuric dermatosis, minocycline hyperpigmentation, and contact dermatitis are included in the differential diagnosis.

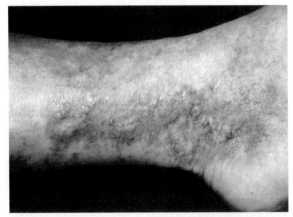

▲ **Figure 56–7.** Stasis dermatitis. Hyperpigmented macules and patches involving the left medial malleolus. (Used with permission from Neill Peters, MD.)

Prevention

Compression stockings and leg elevation in patients with varicose veins may help prevent stasis changes.

Treatment

Compression stockings at 20 to 30 mm Hg can be applied. This can be difficult to tolerate for older adults as well as difficult to put on. It can be helpful to start with lower pressure stockings, and apply them in the morning, while in bed, when the legs are the least swollen. Elastic wraps can also be used instead, but they often require help from a caregiver for application. Elevation of the legs above the level of the heart whenever sitting or lying down will reduce venous pooling. Class 5 steroid ointment applied twice daily can relieve any eczematous patches or plaques.

ROSACEA

 ESSENTIALS OF DIAGNOSIS

▶ Sometimes referred to as adult acne, rosacea is most common in women age 40 to 50 years and is characterized by flushing.

▶ Lesions affect the central face (nose, cheeks, forehead, and chin).

▶ Primary lesions are erythematous papules and pustules (Figure 56–8).

▶ Secondary changes include confluent telangiectasias with erythema.

▶ Differential diagnosis includes acne, perioral dermatitis, and systemic lupus erythematosus.

Pathogenesis

Although the cause of rosacea is unknown, any stimulus that increases skin temperature of the head and neck can trigger flushing, including sunlight, hot showers, exercise, alcohol, hot beverages, and spicy foods. Frequent flushing, in turn, can cause inflammatory and microvascular changes, leading to the development of rosacea.

Complications

Ocular involvement (blepharitis, conjunctivitis) may occur in up to 50% of patients. Some cases can progress to rhinophyma (enlarged bulbous nose).

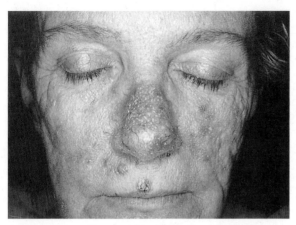

▲ **Figure 56–8.** Rosacea. Papules and pustules of the central face with enlarged nose and telangiectasias.

Treatment

Topical options should always be preferentially used when starting treatment, and combination topical regimens can be more effective than individual use.

A. Sunscreen

Patients may be able to reduce symptoms by avoiding triggers and applying sunscreen with a sun protection factor of 30 daily. Broad-spectrum sunscreens that protect from both ultraviolet A (UVA) and ultraviolet B (UVB) should be recommended.

B. Topical Antibiotics

Topical antibiotics include metronidazole 0.75% cream or gel applied twice daily and sodium sulfacetamide 10%/sulfur 5% lotion applied twice daily.

C. Systemic Antibiotics

Systemic antibiotics are effective for treatment of inflammatory papules or pustules. Minocycline 100 mg orally twice daily or doxycycline 100 mg orally twice daily is most commonly prescribed.

D. Laser Treatment

For telangiectasia, a dermatologist can provide pulsed-dye laser treatment. This is most effective, although it does not prevent development of new telangiectasias.

Draelos ZD. The multifunctionality of 10% sodium sulfacetamide, 5% sulfur emollient foam in the treatment of inflammatory facial dermatoses. *J Drugs Dermatol.* 2010;9(3):234-236.

CONTACT DERMATITIS

 ESSENTIALS OF DIAGNOSIS

▶ Contact dermatitis is a delayed-type hypersensitivity reaction to an antigen (allergen) that contacts the skin and causes severe pruritus.

▶ Symptoms can be acute or chronic:

- Acute contact dermatitis can be localized or generalized and has linear or artificial patterns (Figure 56–9). Primary lesions include vesicles and erythematous, edematous plaques. Secondary changes include erosions, exudates, and crusts.

- Chronic contact dermatitis can be localized or generalized and occurs in linear or artificial patterns (indicative of external contact). Primary lesions appear as lichenified plaques. Secondary changes include hyperpigmentation.

▶ Differential diagnosis: atopic dermatitis, scabies, and irritant dermatitis.

Prevention

Patients should be advised to avoid sources of known allergens. Table 56–4 lists the most frequent contact allergens and their sources.

Complications

Left untreated, dermatitis may spread, causing debilitating pruritus.

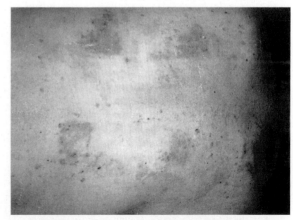

▲ **Figure 56–9.** Contact dermatitis. These square-shaped, itchy plaques resulted from electrode adhesive pads from a transcutaneous electrical nerve stimulation unit.

Table 56–4. Most frequent contact allergens and their sources.

Contact Allergens	Common Sources
Nickel	Jewelry
Gold	Jewelry
Fragrance mix	Skin or hair care products
Thimerosal	Vaccines, eye and nasal medications
Quaternium-15	Cosmetics (preservative)
Neomycin	Antibiotic ointment
Formaldehyde	Nail polish, cosmetics (preservative)
Methylchloroisothiazolinone/ methylisothiazolinone	Cosmetics (preservative)
Bacitracin	Antibiotic ointment
Thiuram	Latex gloves, shoes (rubber products)
Balsam of Peru	Fragrance in cosmetics
Cobalt	Metal-plated objects (buckles, button, zippers)
P-paraphenylenediamine	Hair dye
Carba mix	Rubber elastic of undergarment

▶ **Treatment**

If <10% of the surface area is involved, a class 1 steroid ointment can be applied three times a day for 2 to 3 weeks or until the dermatitis and pruritus resolve. If >10% of body surface area is affected, a prednisone taper is appropriate (Box 56–2).

Box 56–2. Prednisone Taper

A. Indications (severe pruritus from a variety of conditions)
   1. Contact dermatitis >10% surface area
   2. Severe eczema
   3. Drug eruption

B. Dosing
   Start with 1 mg/kg (maximum 60 mg/day) and then taper by 5 mg each consecutive day.
   1. For 60-kg patient, start with 60 mg and taper by 5 mg each day for 12-day course.
   2. Severe cases may require a prolonged taper over 2–3 weeks.
   3. Medrol Dosepaks are inadequate for most adults.

C. Side effects (review patient's medical history for conditions such as cognitive impairment, congestive heart failure, diabetes, hypertension, glaucoma, or mental health disorders)
   1. Water retention
   2. Weight gain
   3. Increased appetite
   4. Mood swings
   5. Restlessness
   6. Avascular necrosis of the hip

For chronic and extensive dermatitis, the patient should see dermatology for patch testing and possibly chronic systemic immunosuppressive therapy.

DRUG ERUPTION (MORBILLIFORM)

ESSENTIALS OF DIAGNOSIS

▶ The most common medications implicated in drug eruptions are penicillins (ampicillin, amoxicillin), sulfonamides (trimethoprim-sulfamethoxazole), nonsteroidal anti-inflammatory medications (naproxen, piroxicam), anticonvulsants (carbamazepine, phenytoin), and antihypertensives (captopril, diltiazem).

▶ Maculopapular eruptions, the most common type of drug eruption, usually occur during the first 2 weeks of a new medication.

▶ Distribution of drug eruptions is bilateral and symmetric, usually beginning on the head and neck or upper trunk and progressing down the limbs.

▶ Primary lesions are erythematous macules and/or papules with areas of confluence (Figure 56–10).

▶ Pruritus is occasionally present.

▶ Differential diagnosis includes viral exanthem, bacterial infection, and collagen vascular disease.

▶ **Complications**

Drug hypersensitivity syndrome is potentially life threatening and presents as a triad of fever, skin eruption

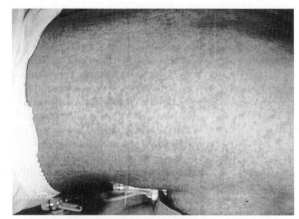

▲ **Figure 56–10.** Morbilliform drug eruption. Macules and papules of the right flank and back with areas of confluence. (Used with permission from Melvin Lu, MD.)

(80% morbilliform), and internal organ involvement, such as hepatitis, nephritis, and lymphadenopathy. Drug hypersensitivity occurs on first exposure to the medication, with symptoms starting 1 to 6 weeks after exposure. Laboratory tests, such as transaminases, complete blood cell count, urinalysis, and serum creatinine, should be obtained to evaluate potential asymptomatic internal organ involvement. Stevens-Johnson syndrome is a severe form of a bullous drug reaction that involves two or more mucosal sites; cutaneous blisters quickly peel off to reveal denuded skin. Hospitalization, close monitoring, and supportive care are required early in the course of the disease.

▶ Treatment

Treatments of drug eruption include discontinuation of the medication that most likely to have caused the drug eruption and deprescribing other unnecessary medications. Topical and oral steroids provide symptomatic relief. Regimens include class 1 steroid cream twice daily for 2 to 3 weeks (see Table 56–3) or prednisone taper (see Box 56–2) if creams are ineffective. Resolution usually occurs within several weeks.

Sullivan JR, Shear NH. Drug eruptions and other adverse drug effects in aged skin. *Clin Geriatr Med.* 2002;18(1):21-42.

HERPES ZOSTER

 ESSENTIALS OF DIAGNOSIS

▶ Herpes zoster is caused by reactivation of varicella-zoster virus in the dorsal root ganglion.

▶ Distribution of grouped vesicular lesions is unilateral (Figure 56–11) and within one to two adjacent dermatomes (ophthalmic branch of trigeminal nerve, thoracic, and cervical are most commonly affected).

▶ Primary lesions are vesicles (Figure 56–12) on an erythematous base. Secondary changes consist of pustules and crusts.

▶ Immunosuppression, especially hematologic malignancy, and HIV infection, substantially increase the risk for herpes zoster as well as dissemination.

▶ Differential diagnosis includes herpes simplex, eczema herpeticum, varicella, and acute contact dermatitis.

▶ General Considerations

Pain precedes the eruption in >90% of cases. Rarely, the eruption does not develop, and neuralgia is the only manifestation of zoster (zoster sine herpete). In most cases, grouped

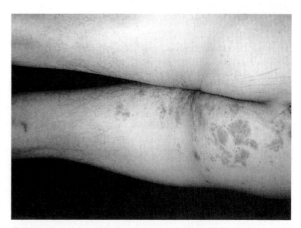

▲ **Figure 56–11.** Herpes zoster. Unilateral S1 and S2 distribution.

vesicles in a dermatomal distribution are enough to establish the diagnosis.

▶ Complications

Patients with cutaneous involvement of the V1 branch of the trigeminal nerve may experience ocular complications (eg, keratitis and acute retinal necrosis), and they need to undergo immediate slit-lamp examination by an ophthalmologist, particularly if skin lesions involve the side and tip of the nose (Hutchinson sign). Immunocompromised patients are at risk for dissemination, defined as >20 vesicles outside the primary and immediately adjacent dermatomes. Cutaneous dissemination may be followed by visceral involvement (lung, liver, brain) in 10% of these high-risk patients.

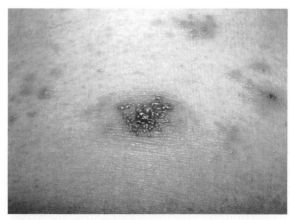

▲ **Figure 56–12.** Herpes zoster. The same patient as in Figure 56–11 has grouped vesicles on an erythematous base.

Postherpetic neuralgia is pain that persists after resolution of the cutaneous eruption. This most common complication is age dependent, affecting at least 50% of patients older than age 60 years, and most frequently involves the face.

Treatment

The systemic antiviral medications (acyclovir, famciclovir, valacyclovir) are effective in the acute phase of zoster and should be started within 48 to 72 hours of rash onset. These medications reduce acute pain, accelerate healing, prevent scarring, and reduce the incidence of postherpetic neuralgia. Systemic corticosteroids (prednisone) may help to reduce acute pain but have no effect on incidence or severity of postherpetic neuralgia. Although the safety profile for the antiviral medications is excellent, headache, nausea, diarrhea, and central nervous system, renal, and hepatic dysfunction can occur. It is important to evaluate renal function as creatinine clearance is often lower in older adults, which can predispose them to nephrotoxicity from antivirals. In more severe cases, especially in disseminated zoster, initial intravenous acyclovir should be considered. Studies indicate that oral therapy is as effective as intravenous therapy in ophthalmic zoster.

Prevention

A new recombinant zoster vaccine (Shingrix) replaced the previous herpes zoster vaccine (Zostavax). This two-part vaccine is recommended for all adults of ≥50 years of age. It is recommended that those who have received Zostavax in the past receive Shingrix 5 years after receiving Zostavax. It is recommended that the recombinant vaccine not be administer while there is acute zoster infection.

Prognosis

The affected dermatome usually heals within 3 to 4 weeks and occasionally may scar. Postherpetic neuralgia (PHN) is the major cause of morbidity. PHN is more common in older adults as incidence rises with age. Although PHN can be difficult to prevent or treat, vaccination and early treatment of shingles lesions with antivirals improve outcomes. Once developed, first-line treatment, although without proven effectiveness in the majority of the cases, includes topical (eg, lidocaine and capsaicin) and oral neurotropic agents (eg, gabapentin or pregabalin).

Dooling KL, Guo A, Patel M, et al. Recommendations of the Advisory Committee on Immunization Practices for Use of Herpes Zoster Vaccines. *MMWR Morb Mortal Wkly Rep.* 2018;67(3):103-108.

SCABIES

ESSENTIALS OF DIAGNOSIS

► The *Sarcoptes scabiei* mite inhabits the human stratum corneum. Characteristic initial lesions are 3- to 8-millimeter linear or serpiginous ridges (burrows; Figure 56–13), often with a gray dot at one end (mite).

► The interdigital web spaces of the hands, volar wrists, penis, and areolas are commonly involved.

► Secondary changes include papules and nodules (nodular scabies), diffuse eczematous dermatitis, thick hyperkeratotic crusted plaques (crusted or Norwegian scabies), and vesicles or bullae (bullous scabies).

► Pruritus is intractable and debilitating.

► Differential diagnosis includes atopic dermatitis, contact dermatitis, drug eruption, and urticarial bullous pemphigoid.

General Considerations

Close body contact is the most common mode of transmission. Fomite transmission is rare because the female mite cannot survive away from the host for >24 to 36 hours. Risk factors include nursing home residence, HIV and AIDS, and crowded living conditions.

Diagnostics

Diagnosis is confirmed (finding mites, eggs [Figure 56–14], or feces) using direct microscopy in a simple bedside test.

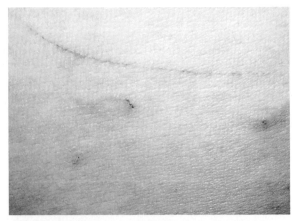

▲ **Figure 56–13.** Scabies. Serpiginous 3- to 8-mm burrows above a linear excoriation.

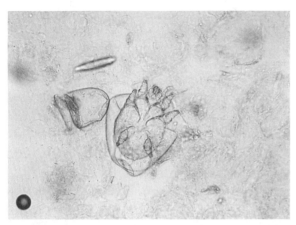

▲ **Figure 56–14.** Direct microscopy. Scabies mite hatched from an egg. (Used with permission from Neill Peters, MD.)

A. Specimen Collection

Place a drop of mineral oil on the center of a glass slide. Touch the sharp part of a No. 15 blade to the drop (so that the specimen will adhere to the blade). Holding the blade perpendicular to the skin, scrape an epidermal burrow to remove the stratum corneum. Pinpoint bleeding indicates the correct depth. Wipe contents onto the center of the glass slide. Choose two other burrows to scrape. Place coverslip over specimen and gently press down.

B. Microscope Settings

Use 4× objective to scan the slide.

▶ Complications

Nodular scabies is a pruritic hypersensitivity reaction to remnants of the mite. The lesions are firm erythematous to red-brown nodules occurring on the genitals and the axillae. Patients who are immunocompromised may develop crusted or Norwegian scabies with extensive yellow crusting. Norwegian scabies is extremely contagious because each crust contains hundreds of mites. Epidemics of scabies in nursing homes are relatively common and often go undetected for long periods.

▶ Treatment

Goals of therapy include mite eradication, alleviation of pruritus, and prevention of transmission. There are unique treatment challenges in older adults who live in group settings, such as nursing homes or assisted living facilities. Older adults living in nursing homes or assisted living facilities may have a difficult time explaining their symptoms if they

also experience cognitive impairment and may require help with application of medications. Clinicians may need to discuss treatment of close contacts and application strategies of needed medications with caregivers. If application of a topical medication is not an option, oral options can be used.

A. Scabicide

The patient and all close contacts should be treated simultaneously, including those who are asymptomatic.

1. Permethrin—Permethrin 5% cream is the most effective topical treatment. Use a 60-g tube for whole-body application. Patients should take a bath or shower and completely dry before application. Cream should be applied to the entire skin surface (from the neck down), with particular attention to finger web spaces, feet, genitals, and intertriginous sites. The cream should be washed off in 8 hours. This regimen is repeated in 1 week. Compliance will result in >90% cure rate.

2. Ivermectin—Ivermectin, 0.2 mg/kg as an oral dose and repeated in 10 to 14 days, is a safe and efficacious alternative to topical treatment. However, two doses 2 weeks apart must be used, as the medication only kills the mite and not the eggs.

B. Pruritus

Even after successful mite eradication, severe pruritus can persist for 3 to 4 weeks, leading to unnecessary discomfort and suffering. Patients may mistakenly receive repeated treatment for scabies because of the belief that infestation persists. Class 1 steroid ointment can be applied two to three times daily for 2 to 4 weeks or until pruritus resolves (see Table 56–3). Prednisone taper (see Box 56–2) may be required to manage patients with debilitating pruritus.

C. Transmission Prevention

All clothes worn within 2 days of treatment, towels, and bedsheets should be machine washed in hot water or dry cleaned. Management of nursing home outbreaks requires clinical and epidemiologic expertise and possibly involvement of public health experts.

▶ Prognosis

Immunocompetent individuals do well with standard therapy. Crusted scabies, usually in the immunosuppressed, may require more than two applications of topical scabicides, oral ivermectin, or a combination.

Currie BJ, McCarthy JS. Permethrin and ivermectin for scabies. *N Engl J Med.* 2010;362(8):717-725.

Walker GJ, Johnstone PW. Interventions for treating scabies. *Cochrane Database Syst Rev.* 2000;2:CD000320.

BULLOUS PEMPHIGOID

ESSENTIALS OF DIAGNOSIS

▶ Bullous pemphigoid is an autoimmune disease in which antibodies target components of skin's basement membrane.

▶ Distribution of lesions may be localized or generalized on the extremities or trunk.

▶ Primary lesions are tense vesicles or bullae filled with serous or serosanguineous fluid (Figure 56–15). Primary lesions in urticarial bullous pemphigoid are wheals and edematous erythematous plaques. The latter presentation is less common (Figure 56–16).

▶ Secondary changes are erosions, ulcers, and crusts.

▶ Pruritus can be debilitating.

▶ Differential diagnosis includes bullous drug reactions, pemphigus, contact dermatitis, scabies, and arthropod bites.

General Considerations

Bullous pemphigoid (BP) is a chronic disease that occurs primarily in older adults and may be associated with significant morbidity. Occasionally BP can be caused by medications, such as diuretics, antibiotics, and angiotensin-converting enzyme inhibitors.

Diagnostics

Diagnosis of BP requires two biopsies to confirm the diagnosis. A 4-mm punch biopsy of the edge of a blister demonstrates a subepidermal split with eosinophils and lymphocytes. A perilesional biopsy for direct immunofluorescence demonstrates binding of immunoglobulin G and C3 in a linear pattern along the basement membrane zone.

Complications

Complications, usually the result of extensive scratching, include erosions and ulcers that can heal slowly and may become secondarily infected and eventually scar.

Treatment

Highly potent topical corticosteroids can be used successfully in localized disease (<5% total body surface area) with significantly lower risks than oral corticosteroids.

Oral corticosteroid therapy has been widely used and is very effective when used in high doses and tapered over

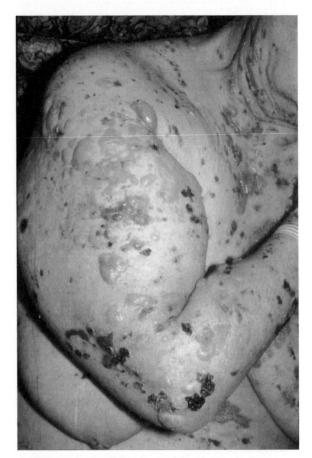

▲ **Figure 56–15.** Bullous pemphigoid. One- to 3-cm tense blisters with secondary erosions and hemorrhagic crusts. (Used with permission from Dana Sachs, MD.)

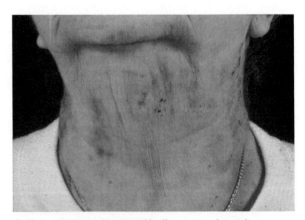

▲ **Figure 56–16.** Urticarial bullous pemphigoid. Erythematous slightly edematous plaques with pinpoint hemorrhagic crusts and excoriations.

a long period of time (eg, prednisone 0.5–1 mg/kg tapered slowly over 6–12 months); however, in older adults, the side effects can be substantial, including osteoporosis, diabetes, hypertension, and delirium. For patients taking >5 mg/day for >3 months, prophylaxis against osteoporosis includes initiation of a bisphosphonate and daily calcium (1500 mg/day) and vitamin D (800 IU/day) supplementation.

Use nicotinamide (1.5 g/day) in combination with minocycline (100 mg twice a day) or tetracycline (2 g/day) in patients who did not adequately respond to topical therapy alone and have contraindications to oral corticosteroids. Difficult-to-treat cases should be referred to a dermatologist for a steroid-sparing immunosuppressive agent, such as methotrexate, cyclosporine, azathioprine, or mycophenolate mofetil.

▶ Prognosis

BP is a chronic disease with multiple remissions and exacerbations. Morbidity and mortality are higher in patients with BP but can be reduced with adequate and prompt treatment.

SKIN CANCER

- There are three common types of skin cancer: basal cell carcinoma (BCC), squamous cell carcinoma (SCC) and malignant melanoma.
- In 2016, the US Preventive Services Task Force (USPSTF) found insufficient evidence to recommend skin examinations for the early detection of skin cancer in adults. As new data emerge, screening may become useful among high-risk populations including immunosuppressed patients, those with a strong family or personal history of skin cancer, or those with excessive ultraviolet (UV) exposure.

ACTINIC KERATOSIS

ESSENTIALS OF DIAGNOSIS

- ▶ Actinic keratoses (AKs) are 3- to 10-mm, rough, adherent, scaly white papules and plaques (Figure 56–17), often on an erythematous base
- ▶ AKs typically occur on sun-exposed areas, including the face, lips, ears, dorsal hands, and forearms.
- ▶ Palpation reveals a gritty, sandpaper-like texture. Lesions are often more readily palpated than visualized.

- ▶ Differential diagnosis includes dry seborrheic keratosis and retention hyperkeratosis.
- ▶ Most AKs remain stable or spontaneously regress, whereas a small proportion may progress to SCC in situ or SCC.

▶ General Considerations

AKs are more common in whites and are directly related to cumulative lifetime sun exposure. Immunosuppressed patients, particularly transplant recipients, are at higher risk for actinic keratoses. Sun protection including wearing long-sleeve shirts, wearing broad-brimmed hats, seeking shade, using sunscreen, and avoiding the sun may prevent these lesions. Recent prospective studies on the natural history of untreated AKs suggest that the majority of these lesions may spontaneously regress. At 1 year of follow up, 55% of AKs were no longer present and 70% were not present at 5-year follow-up. In the same prospective study, the risk of progression of AKs to primary SCCs (invasive or in situ) is 0.6% at 1 year and 2.6% at 4 years.

▶ Treatment

There are several effective treatments for AKs including cryotherapy (see Box 56–1) with two freeze-thaw cycles. For extensive actinic damage, field therapy using a topical treatment, such as imiquimod 5% cream and 5-fluorouracil 5% cream, is recommended. In a recent randomized controlled trial comparing four field-directed therapies for multiple AKs, including 5% 5-fluorouracil cream, 5% imiquimod cream, methyl aminolevulinate photodynamic therapy (MAL-PDT), or 0.015% ingenol mebutate gel, 5% 5-fluorouracil cream was the most effective therapy. Fluorouracil 5% cream is applied

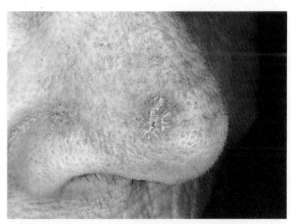

▲ **Figure 56–17.** Actinic keratosis. This is a rough, adherent, scaly papule on the right nasal bridge.

twice a day for 3 to 4 weeks until erythema and crusting are attained. Then, discontinue the treatment to allow the skin to heal. Application of topical corticosteroids may be needed if the reaction is exuberant or the patient experiences extensive pruritus. Imiquimod 5% cream can also be applied twice a week for 16 weeks. Reactions to imiquimod are less predictable than those using 5-fluorouracil as the molecule is an immunomodulator and its action depends on the host's immune status. The main drawbacks of topical treatment are severe inflammatory reactions that may be uncomfortable for patients. Imiquimod may also cause a systemic inflammatory response with flu-like symptoms, fevers, chills, and malaise. The added benefit of topical therapy is treatment of subclinical lesions.

Criscione VD, Weinstock MA, Naylor MF, et al. Actinic keratoses: natural history and risk of malignant transformation in the Veterans Affairs Topical Tretinoin Chemoprevention Trial. *Cancer*. 2009;115(11):2523-2530.

Jansen MHE, Kessels JPHM, Nelemans PJ, et al. Randomized trial of four treatment approaches for actinic keratosis. *N Engl J Med*. 2019;380(10):935-946.

BASAL CELL CARCINOMA

ESSENTIALS OF DIAGNOSIS

▶ BCC, related to chronic UV light exposure, is the most common skin cancer.

▶ The head and neck are most frequently involved; the nose is the most common site.

▶ Primary lesions are translucent or pearly papules or nodules (Figure 56–18), often with visible telangiectasias. Secondary changes include central ulceration or crusting.

▶ Chief complaint is that the lesion "breaks down, bleeds, or does not heal."

▶ Biopsy (shave or punch technique) can confirm the diagnosis.

▶ SCC, keratoacanthoma, and sebaceous hyperplasia are included in the differential diagnosis.

▶ BCC rarely metastasizes, and associated mortality is very low.

General Considerations and Management Approach for Low-Risk BCC

The natural history of BCC is not fully known, but clinical experience suggests these tumors grow slowly, typically over years to decades. One pilot study of the natural history of untreated clinically suspicious BCC revealed that approximately half of these lesions remained stable in size over an

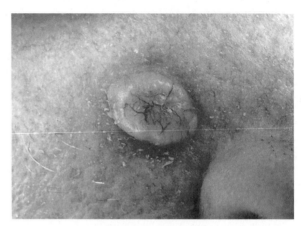

▲ **Figure 56–18.** Basal cell carcinoma. A 1.5-cm shiny nodule with telangiectasias adjacent to the right nasal ala.

average 16-month follow-up period. Among the tumors that grew, they did so at a rate of 8 mm² per month. These findings suggest that the natural history of BCC may be heterogeneous, with some tumors remaining stable over years while others grow slowly. Another study of 200 partially biopsied low-risk BCCs showed that >90% did not recur despite no treatment. Conversely, the potential harms of treatment are immediate. In a prospective study including >800 patients, 27% of patients report complications following treatment. For patients who are near the end of life and who may already be managing multiple serious medical conditions, the risks of BCC treatment may outweigh the potential benefits of treatment, making active surveillance a reasonable option. Although BCC rarely metastasizes, neglected BCCs can invade into underlying cartilage, fascia, muscle, and bone. Therefore, it is important that if patients select active surveillance, they are monitored clinically to ensure the tumors are not growing or becoming locally invasive or symptomatic.

High-Risk BCC

Patients with BCC are more likely to develop a subsequent new skin cancer, and those who have had at least two BCCs are at significantly higher risk. Among those who have had at least two BCCs, the 3-year risk of a new BCC or SCC is 71%. BCC features that predict recurrence and metastasis include recurrent tumors, large tumors >2 cm, immunosuppressed host, and tumors occurring at a site of prior radiation.

Prevention

Although all patients with BCC are assumed to have higher risk for subsequent tumors, a subset may not develop another BCC after their first tumor, suggesting that ongoing screening efforts are likely most effective when directed to patients with highest risk.

Treatment

There are several highly effective treatments for BCC. Electrodesiccation and curettage (ED&C), surgical excision, and Mohs surgery all have cure rates of 90% or higher. Mohs surgery, indicated for high-risk tumors, has the highest cure rate (98%). Treatment for superficial small lesions (<2 cm) located on the trunk and proximal extremities includes either 5-fluorouracil 5% cream or imiquimod 5% cream. Cure rates are around 90% for 5-fluorouracil and 80% for imiquimod 5% cream.

Most BCCs are treated surgically, regardless of a patient's life expectancy. Patient-reported problems following procedures for BCC are common. In one prospective cohort study, 27% of patients perceived a complication, such as bleeding and discomfort, and 10% of patients regarded this as at least moderately serious. Given the potential harms of treatment, the low rates of morbidity and mortality from BCC, and limited life expectancy in some older adults, it is necessary to provide a more thoughtful and individualized approach when making treatment decisions in older adults with low-risk BCCs.

Giesse JK, Rich P, Pandya A, et al. Imiquimod 5% cream for the treatment of superficial basal cell carcinoma: A double-blind, randomized, vehicle-controlled study. *J Am Acad Dermatol.* 2002;47(3):390-398.

Linos E, Schroeder SA, Chren M. Potential overdiagnosis of basal cell carcinoma in older patients with limited life expectancy. *JAMA.* 2014;312(10):997-998.

Wehner M, Dalma N, Landefeld C, et al. Natural history of lesions suspicious for basal cell carcinoma in older adults in Ikaria, Greece. *Br J Dermatol.* 2018;179:767-768.

SQUAMOUS CELL CARCINOMA

 ESSENTIALS OF DIAGNOSIS

▶ SCC is derived from keratinocytes above the basal layer of the epidermis, often with actinic keratoses as precursor lesions.

▶ The head, neck, dorsal hands, and forearms are affected.

▶ Primary lesions are firm indurated papules, plaques, or nodules (Figure 56–19). Secondary changes include rough adherent scale, central erosion, or ulceration with crust.

▶ The lesion does not heal and breaks down or bleeds.

▶ Biopsy with rolled shave or punch technique can confirm the diagnosis.

▶ Differential diagnosis includes BCC, AK, and keratoacanthoma.

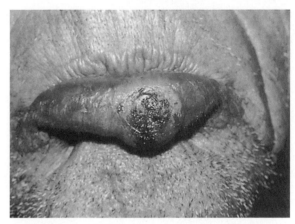

▲ **Figure 56–19.** Squamous cell carcinoma. This hard 2.5-cm nodule with overlying dry hemorrhagic crust is at risk for spread to cervical nodes. (Used with permission from Melvin Lu, MD.)

General Considerations

SCC composes approximately 20% of all skin cancers and has the capacity to metastasize. If SCC is suspected, palpation of regional lymph nodes is recommended. SCC should be suspected in any persistent nodule, plaque, or ulcer, especially when occurring in sun-damaged skin, on the lower lip, in areas of prior radiation, in old burn scars, or on the genitals. Immunosuppressed patients (eg, transplant recipients) are at higher risk for SCC because of impaired cell-mediated immunity.

Complications

SCC on the lips or ears has a 10% to 15% risk of spread to cervical nodes. The overall rate of metastasis from all skin sites ranges from <1% to 5%.

Treatment

ED&C and excision have comparable cure rates of 90% for low-risk tumors. Mohs surgery, indicated for high-risk tumors, is the most effective technique (98%–100% cure rate).

Prognosis

Patients with SCC have high risk for recurrence and metastasis when they have one or more of the following features: recurrent tumor; tumor >2 cm on the trunk and extremities; tumor >1 cm on the head and neck; tumor occurring on the genitals, lips, ears, site of prior radiation, or scar; tumor with poorly defined borders; and tumor in immunosuppressed host. Lifetime recurrence rates with standard modalities (ED&C or excision) are >10%, with most recurrences occurring between 5 and 10 years.

Marcil I, Stern RS. Risk of developing a subsequent nonmelanoma skin cancer in patients with a history of nonmelanoma skin cancer: a critical review of the literature and meta-analysis. *Arch Dermatol.* 2000;136(12):1524-1530.

National Comprehensive Cancer Network. National Comprehensive Cancer Network (NCCN) clinical practice guidelines in oncology. Basal cell and squamous cell skin cancers. Version 2.2013. http://www.nccn.org/professionals/physician_gls/pdf/nmsc.pdf. Accessed April 9, 2020.

US Preventive Services Task Force. Screening for skin cancer: US Preventive Services Task Force recommendation statement. *JAMA.* 2016;316(4):429-435.

Wehner MR, Linos E, Parvataneni R, Stuart SE, Boscardin WJ, Chren M. Timing of subsequent new tumors in patients who present with basal cell carcinoma or cutaneous squamous cell carcinoma. *JAMA Dermatol.* 2015;151(4):382-388.

MELANOMA

ESSENTIALS OF DIAGNOSIS

▶ Melanoma, derived from melanocytes, is the skin cancer type with the greatest potential for metastasis.

▶ The trunk and legs are affected more than the face and neck, although the face and neck are more likely to be affected in older adults.

▶ The primary lesion is a brown-black macule, papule, plaque, or nodule with one of the following features (Figure 56–20): asymmetry, border irregularity, color variegation, diameter >6 mm.

▶ Lentigo maligna is a subtype of melanoma that is almost exclusively found in older adults and occurs in areas of chronic sun exposure.

▶ Lesions should be excised with a margin of clinically normal skin down to subcutaneous fat.

▶ Differential diagnosis includes seborrheic keratosis, solar lentigo, dysplastic nevus, and pigmented BCC.

▶ General Considerations

The incidence of melanoma is increasing. The lifetime probability of developing melanoma in an individual in the United States born in 2012 is estimated at 1 in 36 for a man and 1 in 55 for a woman. Melanoma is the fifth most common cancer in men and the sixth most common cancer in women.

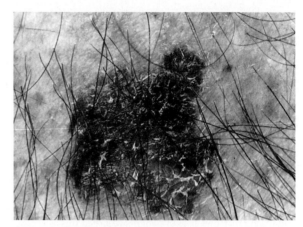

▲ **Figure 56–20.** Melanoma. A 2-cm plaque on the chest with varying shades of brown to black, asymmetry, and irregular borders.

Older men have the highest incidence of melanoma and the highest mortality rates from melanoma. In the United States, the incidence of thick tumors (>4 mm) has continued to increase in men 60 years of age and older. Nearly 50% of all melanoma deaths involve white men 50 years of age and older.

Lentigo maligna (LM) is a type of melanoma in situ that typically occurs in chronically sun-exposed skin. Over time, LM can slowly progress to invasive lentigo maligna melanoma. Risk factors include light complexion (red-blond hair), blistering sunburns during childhood, tendency to tan poorly and sunburn easily, and a positive family history. Additional risk factors in the middle-aged population include age >50 years, male sex, and a history of AKs or nonmelanoma skin cancers.

▶ Complications

Untreated melanoma has the potential risk of metastasis to lymph nodes, liver, lungs, and brain.

▶ Treatment

Melanoma is treated by surgical excision with margins determined by histologic tumor thickness (Breslow depth). Evaluation of nodal involvement with sentinel lymph node biopsy is recommended for primary melanomas deeper than 1 mm and for tumors <1 mm when histologic ulceration or mitoses are present. Frequency of follow-up, laboratory tests, and imaging studies depends on stage of disease.

Prognosis

Tumor thickness and presence or absence of histologic ulceration are the most important prognostic factors. Patients with thin melanomas (<1 mm) have the best prognosis (>90% 5-year survival rate), whereas those with thick tumors (>4 mm) have a 49% 5-year survival rate. For patients with nodal involvement, the number of affected nodes determines the overall prognosis.

Gershenwald JE, Scolyer RA, Hess KR, et al. Melanoma staging: evidence-based changes in the American Joint Committee on Cancer eighth edition Cancer Staging Manual. *CA Cancer J Clin.* 2017;67(6):472-492.

National Comprehensive Cancer Network. National Comprehensive Cancer Network (NCCN) clinical practice guidelines in oncology. Melanoma. Version 3.2014. http://www.nccn.org/professionals/physician_gls/pdf/melanoma.pdf. (Subscription only). Accessed April 9, 2020.

Common Oral Diseases & Disorders

Bonnie Lederman, DDS

Elisa M. Chávez, DDS

Susan Hyde, DDS, MPH, PhD

▷ General Principles

Oral health is essential to the general health and quality of life of older adults. Chronic systemic diseases increase the burden of oral diseases, predisposing older adults to oral microbial infections, pain, dysphagia, difficulty chewing, altered taste, and difficulty speaking.

- Periodontal disease (gum disease) is the sixth leading complication of diabetes and threatens glycemic control.

- Having <21 teeth compromises masticatory function and nutritional status and is associated with smoking, low socioeconomic status, low physical and social activity, frailty, living alone or in a nursing home, poor access to care, and higher mortality rates.

- Xerostomia (dry mouth) seriously impairs oral function, promotes dental caries (tooth decay), and exacerbates periodontal disease. Decreased salivary flow is a side effect of >500 medications, including antidepressants, antihistamines, antihypertensives, and diuretics.

- Bone antiresorptive agents, such as intravenous and oral bisphosphonates and denosumab, are given to treat osteoporosis. These drugs are associated with medication-related osteonecrosis of the alveolar bone. Chronic conditions contributing to increased risk are diabetes, steroid use, smoking, and use of antiangiogenic drugs.

- Oral cancer is the eighth most common cancer in men and is seven times more likely to occur in older adults.

- Aspiration pneumonia is a major reason for hospital admission, a leading cause of death in critically ill patients, and the second most costly of the top five hospital-acquired infections.

- Collaboration of an interdisciplinary team, including dentists, physicians, nurses, therapists, pharmacists, and other health care professionals is critical to individualized and appropriate oral health care planning.

▷ Oral Disease and Access to Care

Although changes in oral health are not inevitable consequences of aging, profound, yet often asymptomatic, untreated oral disease is frequently present in older adults. In the United States, 19% of older adults have untreated dental caries on the crowns of their teeth, 38% have untreated dental caries on the roots of their teeth, and 37% have moderate to severe periodontal disease. Fifteen percent of older adults are fully edentulous. Thirteen percent of older adults experience orofacial pain, including jaw joint and facial pain, oral sores, burning mouth, and toothache. Chronic orofacial pain can be associated with increased frailty, social withdrawal, decreased activities of daily living, and diminished quality of life. Less than half of older adults have had a dental visit during the past year, with even lower access to care for minority, impoverished, or institutionalized elders. Medicare and many state Medicaid programs do not cover preventive or restorative dental treatment for older adults. Dental insurance is often lost after retirement. As a result, older adults pay for a significant portion of their dental expenses out of pocket, limiting their treatment choices and ability to receive care. Many forgo routine and preventive care, which can result in the need for more costly and complicated treatment, often resulting in adverse outcomes as oral health declines in the absence of prevention and treatment of oral disease at earlier stages.

According to the World Health Organization and World Dental Federation, 21 teeth constitute the minimum needed for adequate functional dentition. Having <21 teeth, regardless of the use of partial or complete dentures, results in compromised chewing efficiency, reduced fruit and vegetable consumption, decreased oral health–related quality of life, and increased risk for aspiration pneumonia. Thirty-eight percent of those aged 65 to 74 years and 54% of those aged ≥75 years have <21 remaining teeth. However, those living in poverty, those of Hispanic ethnicity or non-Hispanic black race, and frail older people living in skilled nursing facilities average 15 to 16 remaining teeth.

By addressing oral health needs, health care professionals play a critical role in improving the health and quality of life of older adults. Clinicians should be familiar with normal and pathologic oral morphology. They should also be aware of the risks that systemic diseases and their management present to the oral health of older adults and vice versa. Routine inquiry and screening for oral diseases during routine medical examinations and timely referral for dental consultation following new diagnoses of certain systemic diseases can positively impact total health and well-being for older adults.

▶ Dental Diseases

A. Periodontal Disease

Gingivitis, the earliest and most common form of periodontitis, is limited to the gingiva. This inflammation is associated with plaque, hormonal changes, or a foreign-body response. Gingivitis normally reverses with no lasting damage on effective plaque removal, but it can also progress to periodontitis, resulting in inflammatory destruction of periodontal ligament and bone attached to the tooth root.

Currently there is no way to predict which form of gingivitis will progress to periodontal disease, nor is there a consensus on the definition of disease progression. Periodontal disease and associated pathogens have been linked with diabetes, peripheral vascular disease, cerebrovascular disease, and coronary vascular disease. Causation has not been established. However, inflammatory cytokines produced in periodontitis are implicated in several diseases. Periodontal disease can progress rapidly in those with impaired immune systems. Smoking and poor oral hygiene are the most common risk factors for periodontitis. Periodontal disease is marked by the loss of alveolar bone around teeth. Advanced periodontitis leads to increasing tooth mobility and loss. Routine preventive care, such as good daily home care combined with chemotherapeutics such as triclosan-fluoride toothpaste or chlorhexidine mouth rinse as indicated and regular prophylaxis or root planning by a dental provider, reduces plaque and gingivitis but has no significant effect on attachment loss or resultant tooth loss.

B. Caries

Dental caries are a chronic infection. Oral bacteria colonize exposed tooth surfaces, metabolize carbohydrates, and release acids that demineralize tooth surfaces, potentially leading to a cavity. Older adults have untreated dental caries at a rate exceeding that of children. Root caries are the major cause of tooth loss in older adults, and tooth loss is the most significant oral health–related negative variable of quality of life for older adults. Recurrent caries constitute infection around existing fillings and crowns. Caries can destroy the structural integrity of a tooth before the patient experiences pain, and many patients may not express pain due to a history of prior stroke or cognitive impairment. Such patients are at risk for identification of disease at an acute stage, such as fracture of the tooth or development of an abscess or cellulitis.

Those with active or recurrent dental caries can benefit from silver diamine fluoride and fluoride varnish applications and from prescription-strength high-fluoride toothpaste or acidulated phosphate fluoride gel used at home. Patients can also benefit from a caries risk assessment provided by an oral health clinician to determine their specific risk factors for caries and to establish a plan for treatment and prevention. Preventive plans may require modification as patient needs and risk factors change with their health and level of dependency.

C. Partial & Complete Edentulism

Having <21 teeth compromises masticatory function and nutritional status and is associated with smoking, low socioeconomic status, low physical and social activity, frailty, living alone or in a nursing home, poor access to care, and higher mortality rates. Even with dentures, having <21 teeth leads to decreased blood levels of vitamins and minerals; decreased consumption of vegetables, fruits, and fiber; increased consumption of overprepared and overcooked foods; and a preferential consumption of fats and sugars with a resultant increase in caloric intake.

Maintaining or restoring at least four pairs of posterior teeth is needed to preserve masticatory function. Restorative dentistry offers patients several tooth replacement options.

A complete denture replaces all the teeth in the maxilla and/or mandible. Properly made, well-fitting complete dentures restore only 10% to 15% of masticatory function, and patients may require modifications to their diet as well as counseling to ensure they continue to get proper nutrition. A removable partial denture replaces some teeth and is connected by clasps to remaining natural teeth. Partial dentures may be acrylic if they are transitional appliances leading to complete dentures, or metal if they are to be the definitive restoration. Over time, the alveolus resorbs and remodels, and dentures and partial dentures may require relining periodically to ensure proper fit and function in chewing, speech, and appearance, as well as to avoid pathology that can occur with poorly fitting dentures such as denture sores and epulis formation. Epulis is an overgrowth of the tissues that prevents proper seating of the denture and may require surgical removal. Prostheses must be cleaned daily to prevent denture stomatitis, candidiasis, halitosis, and altered taste and may diminish the risk of aspiration pneumonia in frail older adults.

Fixed bridges replace one or more missing teeth and are connected by crowns to the adjacent teeth. More chewing force can be generated with fixed bridges compared to removable dentures; therefore, regular diets can be maintained more routinely. However, they require significant oral hygiene measures to adequately clean around these fixed prostheses. Patients must have the physical and cognitive ability to maintain these restorations as well as the motivation to do so.

Dental implants are surgically placed into the alveolus and can be used to support individual crowns, fixed bridges, and removable dentures. They require regular examination and preventive measures to ensure proper fit and function and screening for peri-implantitis (periodontal disease of the implant). As with fixed prostheses, significant daily care is required, as well as regular dental visits for evaluation and prevention of future disease.

A decision not to replace missing teeth can also be an appropriate choice. This may occur in cases where patients have advanced dementia or other poorly controlled medical conditions that compromise their ability to tolerate and benefit from replacement of missing teeth. In such cases, dietary modification should be considered to help the patient maintain adequate nutrition in the absence of this dentition. As diets become softer, these patients will need additional help with homecare and a preventive routine to combat the risk these soft foods present to the remaining dentition combined with diminished ability to provide adequate self-care and oral hygiene.

D. Orofacial Pain

Orofacial pain conditions of noninfectious etiology include myofascial pain and neuropathic pain disorders. Parafunctional habits such as clenching and grinding of the teeth may lead to myofascial pain, with or without secondary temporomandibular joint (TMJ) arthralgia. Temporomandibular disorders (TMDs) are experienced frequently and are often debilitating pain disorders. TMDs are the third most commonly reported chronic pain condition in the world and are estimated to affect from 5% to 10% of the adult population. Some estimates suggest women are up to three times more likely than men to develop a TMD, and TMDs occur more frequently in older adults. Patients may complain of a dull, aching pain that is exacerbated with wide opening of the jaw and chewing. Pain may radiate from the TMJ, interfering with the individual's eating and talking abilities. Patient history and physical examination may help to discriminate between tooth and other sources of pain. A toothache can present as acute pain in a localized area of the jaw, and the longer it is left untreated, the more likely it is that pain will radiate throughout the jaw and develop into a chronic condition with systemic signs and symptoms. Toothaches are readily diagnostic and isolated after a thorough dental examination. Medical and dental providers will need to collaborate to appropriately diagnose and manage patients with orofacial pain. This will involve multimodal treatments in addressing simultaneously the cognitive, behavioral, and physiologic dimensions of the condition.

▶ Oral Pathology

A. Fungal Infections (Oral Candidiasis)

Oral candidiasis is the most common fungal infection in humans and is underdiagnosed among older adults. Dentures that worn for excessive periods, without daily removal and oral hygiene, can result in an overgrowth of fungus, which is often asymptomatic but can cause a burning sensation and irritation to the roof of the mouth, denture stomatitis, or papillary hyperplasia. To reduce the likelihood of denture stomatitis, a candidiasis infection, and accelerated bone resorption, dentures should not be worn overnight. Individuals with dentures should be instructed to remove the denture for at least 8 hours daily to allow tissue-bearing areas to rest. To treat oral candidiasis, topical antifungal agents are applied to both the oral tissues and denture. In cases of refractory *Candida*, which can occur in people with underlying systemic diseases or chronic use of some systemic medications such as steroid inhalers, systemic antifungals may be required. These should be used with caution as many interact with several other medications commonly taken by older adults or may impact liver function, even with a short course of treatment.

B. Viral Infections

Herpes simplex virus type 1 (HSV-1), also known as herpes labialis or "cold sore," is the cause of vesicular lesions of the lips, tongue, and oral mucosa. Primary lesions can occur on any mucosal surface. Recrudescence of HSV-1 infection most frequently presents on keratinized tissues as labial ulcerations and, less frequently, intraorally. Intraoral mucosal ulcerations are painful and characterized by shallow irregular margins. The lesions are usually self-limiting, but if treated early with topical antiviral ointments, the course may be slightly shorter. Palliative ointments can be provided for comfort as well as to help maintain nutritional intake.

Medically compromised or immunosuppressed individuals may experience progressive symptomatic oral ulcers lasting >10 days, and these ulcers should be cultured to rule out any other infection.

HSV infections can reoccur at any time; the virus migrates to the trigeminal nerve ganglion, where it can remain in a latent state. Reactivation of virus may follow exposure to cold, exposure to sunlight, stress, trauma, or immunosuppression and cause recurrent infection.

C. Oral Cancer

Oral cancer is the eighth most common cancer in men and is seven times more likely to occur in older adults. Squamous cell carcinoma composes 96% of oral and pharyngeal malignancies. Age is the primary risk factor, along with the use of tobacco and alcohol. Both leukoplakia (white patch) and erythroplakia (red patch) persisting for >2 weeks, particularly those that progress to raised plaques of mixed appearance and ulceration, should be referred for biopsy. A persistent erythroplakia is an early manifestation of oropharyngeal squamous cell cancer. Oral cancer screening is noninvasive, and even in the case of frail individuals who may not be candidates for definitive treatment, diagnosis can allow for palliative measures that encourage nutritional intake and maintain quality of life. All older adults should have annual dental screenings, whether they have dentition or any overt evidence of dental pathology.

D. Oral Facial Trauma

Oral facial trauma, including facial fractures and oral lacerations, is common in older adults due to falls. Decreased coordination of movements, cognitive impairments, decreased muscle tone and strength, changes in vision, and polypharmacy can predispose older adults to falls. Osteoporosis further increases the risk for oral-facial fractures. Trauma and fractures may also occur because of elder abuse and neglect (see Chapter 19, "Detecting, Assessing, & Responding to Elder Mistreatment"). Clinicians should evaluate patients for the following injuries:

- Oral laceration: extraoral/intraoral soft tissue or oral mucosa.
  - Lacerations that do not gape open often heal well without intervention.
  - Larger, gaping oral lacerations benefit from wound closure to reduce infection and bleeding complications.
  - Lacerations should heal rapidly (3–5 days). Patients with risk factors for infections should undergo reevaluations at 48 to 72 hours to ensure proper healing.
- Teeth, crowns, bridges, implant trauma: loose, displaced, fractured, or missing teeth.
- Oral appliances (dentures, partials): fractures, cracks, sharp edges, missing appliance.
- Midface fracture: malocclusion; midface instability; ecchymosis of the cheek, upper lip, alveolar ridge, lateral nose, and lower eyelid. The most frequent site for fracture is the middle third of the face.
- Jaw fracture: suggested by malocclusion, trismus (unable to open >5 cm), TMD, or jaw tenderness.

Suspected fractures warrant additional diagnostic information:

- Midface fractures: computed tomography (CT)
- Mandibular and dental fractures: CT most appropriate, or panoramic x-ray (panorex) to isolate mandibular, dental, or alveolar fractures

Referral should be made immediately for emergency medical care. Consultation with a dental provider will be needed to initiate any reparative or restorative care and to ensure follow-up care. Posttrauma and postoperative instructions may include the following:

- Eat soft foods; may need additional nutritional supplements.
- Rinse mouth with warm salt water after eating.
- Brushing teeth may be suspended temporarily.
- Avoid spicy/salty foods until wound is healed.
- Avoid straws or ice.
- Discontinue use of removable prostheses.

E. Xerostomia or Salivary Gland Hypofunction

Saliva should be free-flowing and watery. Saliva that is normal in content and volume lubricates the intraoral tissues and the lips, facilitating speech, taste, mastication, and swallowing, and is protective against dental caries and periodontal disease. Saliva contains antimicrobial elements that modulate plaque formation, buffer intraoral pH against bacterial acid production, and promote remineralization of tooth surfaces with calcium and phosphate salts to repair incipient caries. In normal aging, the amount of saliva remains stable. However, saliva becomes thicker because of a reduction in serous flow relative to mucus, resulting in decreased lubrication.

Xerostomia, or the sensation of a dry mouth, resulting from decreased salivary flow or changed salivary composition will impair oral function, promote dental caries, and exacerbate periodontal disease. The prevalence of xerostomia is 55% in older adults suffering from systemic diseases such as diabetes, parkinsonism, and cancer. Importantly, many people with diminished salivary flow do not report xerostomia until it has been clinically identified; therefore, a proactive discussion with patients of the risks to their oral health may not occur. Xerostomia and salivary hypofunction are also associated with autoimmune diseases such as rheumatic diseases, Sjögren syndrome, head and neck radiation therapy, and some chemotherapeutics. In addition, decreased salivary flow is a side effect of >500 medications, including many commonly prescribed to older adults including, but not limited to, tricyclic antidepressants, antihistamines, antihypertensives, proton pump inhibitors, and diuretics. Several over-the-counter oral lubricants and salivary substitutes are readily available. Palliative measures such as frequent sips of water or use of xylitol candy or gum to help stimulate salivary flow while protecting against caries may be recommended for use as needed. However, relief is temporary, and these substitutes are without the protective properties of saliva. Salivary stimulants may be prescribed for those with salivary hypofunction resulting from Sjögren syndrome or head and neck radiation. These should be used with caution and patients carefully monitored for adverse side effects and drug-drug interactions.

Table 57–1. Medications and intraoral side effects.

Medications	Oral and Systemic Effects
More than 200 medications	Can alter taste and lead to weight loss, depression, and compensation with sugary foods that promote dental caries.
Phenytoin, methotrexate, and calcium channel blockers	Concomitant poor oral hygiene can cause gingival hyperplasia.
Nifedipine (calcium channel blocker)	Periodontal disease is exacerbated in patients.
Progesterone, nitrates, β-blockers, and calcium channel blockers	Gastric reflux erodes the dentition.
Drug preparations and nutritional supplements containing sugar	Promotes dental caries.
Chemotherapy and head and neck radiation therapy	Can cause mild to severe oral mucositis and stomatitis.
Steroid therapy	Patients on steroid therapy are more susceptible to oral candidiasis and poor healing following surgical procedures.

Pharmacologic Considerations

Many medications prescribed for older adults have oral side effects in addition to xerostomia (Table 57–1).

Referral: When and Why—The Case for Collaboration

Many systemic diseases and the medications or treatments used to manage them can have direct and indirect impacts on oral health. For this reason, when patients receive a new diagnosis, a referral to their dentist for an oral evaluation and risk assessment is appropriate. Some of the most common diseases and conditions with known bidirectional impacts on oral and systemic health are reviewed in the following sections. Patients should be apprised of the importance of informing their dentist of any new diagnosis to discuss the potential implications for their oral health and how maintaining good oral health may be of benefit to their systemic condition.

A. Osteonecrosis of the Jaw or Medication-Related Osteonecrosis of the Jaw

Bone antiresorptive agents currently include intravenous and oral bisphosphonates and denosumab. Both classes of drugs are associated with medication-related osteonecrosis of the alveolar bone (MRONJ). Although most cases have been in patients with cancer or in patients with a compromised immune system (particularly multiple myeloma and metastatic breast cancer) who were treated with high doses of intravenous bisphosphonates, cases have been noted in patients with postmenopausal osteoporosis who are taking oral bisphosphonates.

MRONJ is an adverse drug reaction consisting of progressive bone destruction in the maxillofacial region. The American Association of Oral and Maxillofacial Surgeons defines MRONJ as exposed necrotic bone in the maxillofacial region that has been persistent for >8 weeks in a patient with current or previous bisphosphonate treatment and without history of radiation therapy to the jaw. It can manifest clinically as intraoral bone exposure, delayed healing, inflammation, or pain, especially following dental extraction. MRONJ can present with pain, swelling, exposed bone, local infection, and pathologic fracture of the jaw, a rare complication. MRONJ can be debilitating due to the need for multiple treatments, difficulty eating, and pain. Patients on long-term bisphosphonates and antiresorptive medication (>4 years) are at higher risk for MRONJ. Chronic conditions contributing to increased risk are diabetes, steroid use, smoking, and use of antiangiogenic drugs.

A thorough dental evaluation and completion of all dental treatment prior to initiating therapy for patients with cancer receiving intravenous bisphosphonates or patients diagnosed with osteoporosis who will be prescribed oral bisphosphates or denosumab are indicated to minimize the risk of developing MRONJ.

B. Head & Neck Radiation

All patients who will undergo radiation therapy (RT) for head and neck cancer should have a comprehensive dental evaluation prior to treatment. All dental work should be completed prior to start of RT. Dental extractions of teeth after treatment is associated with an increased risk of nonhealing and osteoradionecrosis.

RT can cause salivary hypofunction and changes in saliva consistency that result in altered oral microflora; extreme caries risk; difficulty using dentures; altered speech, mastication, swallowing, and taste; and overall discomfort and diminished quality of life. Oral hygiene is crucial during treatment and requires long-term maintenance. Oral care should include daily prescription-strength fluoride use for life, palliative treatment to relieve the symptoms of salivary function, and salivary stimulants when appropriate. Frequent routine dental visits are indicated to prevent oral diseases and/or to identify them at early stages in order to achieve the best prognoses for treatment.

C. Dementia

Patients with dementia may suffer both cognitive and functional deficits that impact their ability to maintain their oral hygiene and oral health or their ability to identify and communicate the presence of a dental problem. Those with progressive dementias will require revision of their oral care prevention plan and oral hygiene routines as their dementia advances. Those who have concomitant chewing and swallowing problems may require soft diets or thickened liquids, which further complicate their oral hygiene and place them at increased risk for caries, periodontal disease, and oral *Candida*. Concurrent use of xerostomic mediations can increase the risk for tooth extraction in people with dementia. Diagnoses for patients not able to adequately identify and communicate oral health problems may be delayed until acute stages when more complex treatment and management may be required. For this reason, referral to a dental provider at the time of diagnosis of dementia, from any cause, is critical. Involving and educating family members and caregivers, when appropriate, about the importance of maintaining oral health and seeking regular dental care is as important as providing information about how to recognize signs of oral disease and discomfort, such as refusal to take food or accept oral care or changes in behavior. Untreated oral disease can significantly impact nutritional intake and overall health if diagnosis is delayed.

D. Diabetes

People with poorly controlled diabetes are at greater risk of developing periodontal disease and at risk for more severe disease. A bidirectional relationship between periodontal disease and diabetes is well established. Poorly controlled diabetes increases the risk of periodontal disease, and the presence of periodontal inflammation contributes to poor glycemic control, the risk of developing type 2 diabetes, and diabetic complications. In addition, there is evidence that oral debridement (teeth cleaning), antimicrobial therapy (special mouth rinses or medications), and periodontal surgery can potentially reduce the risks associated with diabetes by improving glycemic control. A meta-analysis of 14 studies demonstrated that periodontal intervention led to a 29% decrease in hemoglobin A1c at 3 to 4 months, which was not sustained at 6 months, suggesting the need for more frequently scheduled professional teeth cleaning than the standard twice-a-year recommendation.

E. Pulmonary Disease

Frail older adults with dysphagia and those who are ventilator dependent are at risk for aspiration pneumonia. Aspiration pneumonia is a major reason for hospital admission, a leading cause of death in critically ill patients and the second most costly of the top five hospital-acquired infections. The mouth harbors >600 known varieties of microorganisms, which colonize on the tooth surface and oral mucosa. Risk of aspiration increases when frail patients are dependent for assistance with feeding and oral hygiene. Patients with poor oral health have an increased risk for aspiration pneumonia because of colonized bacteria in the upper airway that can migrate into the lungs. Mechanical plaque removal and chemical disinfection with agents such as chlorhexidine or povidone-iodine mouth rinse reduce the risk for the development and progression of aspiration pneumonia in frail adults.

F. Sleep Disorders & Obstructive Sleep Apnea

Obstructive sleep apnea (OSA) is a chronic disease requiring long-term, multidisciplinary management. Rates of OSA are increased in association with certain medical conditions commonly diagnosed in older adults such as hypertension, diabetes, metabolic syndrome, depression, end-stage renal disease, congestive heart failure, chronic lung disease, posttraumatic stress disorder, and stroke.

Benefits of successful OSA treatment include improved quality of life, improved systemic blood pressure control, reduced motor vehicle accidents, reduced health care utilization and costs, and possibly decreased cardiovascular morbidity and mortality. For patients who have had a medical assessment and sleep study to confirm their diagnosis, oral appliances should be considered as an alternative therapy for some patients. This may be especially beneficial for patients who cannot tolerate or refuse to use a continuous positive airway pressure machine. Referral to a dentist with appropriate training in sleep medicine and fabrication of such appliances can help further determine if the patient is a candidate for such an appliance. Appropriate outcome measures and long-term multidisciplinary follow-up will be required to further evaluate efficacy of such treatment and better identify candidates who can benefit from such treatment.

G. Anticoagulants

Dental procedures such as dental cleanings, fillings, crown preparations, biopsies, and extractions are invasive and cause bleeding but are performed routinely without interrupting anticoagulation or antiplatelet therapy unless specifically instructed by the physician who must also revise the medication orders. Collaboration between the prescriber and the dental provider is critical to reach international normalized ratio (INR), prothrombin time, and partial thromboplastin time values or bleeding times that are acceptable for a given medication's prescribed purpose and to diminish the risk of excessive bleeding during more complex dental surgical procedures. Patients taking warfarin (Coumadin) need an INR that is current, within 24 hours prior to any invasive dental procedures. For most medical conditions, the expected therapeutic range for anticoagulation as measured by the INR is 2.0 to 3.0 (not to exceed 3.5), and this range is also suitable for many surgical procedures. Because direct oral anticoagulants such as apixaban (Eliquis), rivaroxaban (Xarelto), or dabigatran (Pradaxa) do not have reliable lab tests to determine bleeding risk, providers must work together to evaluate overall risks as they relate to the planned procedures and revise their medical and dental treatment planning accordingly.

H. Antibiotic Premedication Before Dental Treatment

The concept of antibiotic premedication (AP) for the prevention of postoperative infections due to dental procedure has changed considerably since it was first introduced in the American Heart Association (AHA) guidelines of 1955. Recommended AP regimens have become simpler and shorter, and the number of individuals and procedures where AP is recommended has significantly reduced. Medical and dental providers still need to consider the individual's health status and designated invasive procedure to determine the need for AP. All guidelines from world committees recommend AP for high-risk individuals undergoing high-risk invasive dental procedures.

The 2017 AHA and American College of Cardiology (ACC) guidelines require AP only for patients with the following conditions, prior to dental procedures that involve manipulation of gingival tissue or the periapical region of the teeth or perforation of the oral mucosa:

- Prosthetic cardiac valves, including transcatheter-implanted prostheses and homografts
- Prosthetic material used for cardiac valve repair, such as annuloplasty rings and chords
- Previous infective endocarditis
- Unrepaired cyanotic congenital heart disease or repaired congenital heart disease, with residual shunts or valvular regurgitation at the site of or adjacent to the site of a prosthetic patch or prosthetic device
- Cardiac transplant with valve regurgitation due to a structurally abnormal valve

If the patient does not meet these criteria and the medical provider believes the patient requires prophylaxis or that a regimen other than that recommended in the guidelines is indicated, the medical provider should provide the patient with a prescription ahead of their scheduled dental appointments. The dental provider can advise whether the planned procedure meets the invasive criteria as described in the guideline.

In 2014, the American Dental Association updated the American Academy of Orthopedic Surgeons 2012 guidelines to discontinue the routine prescribing of prophylactic antibiotics for all total joint replacement patients undergoing dental procedures and, instead, recommended a shared decision-making tool for patients and their health care providers.

▷ Oral Health Assessment: A Shared Responsibility

Addressing oral health plays a critical role in improving the overall health and quality of life of older adults. Collaboration of an interdisciplinary team, including dentists, physicians, nurses, therapists, pharmacists, and other health care professionals, is critical to individualized and appropriate oral health care planning. Medical providers should perform an oral screening examination as part of the traditional head and neck exam. While there is no gold standard oral health assessment tool for nondentist clinicians, the Kayser-Jones Brief Oral Health Status Examination (BOHSE) is an instrument developed for nurses practicing in long-term care. BOHSE has been validated in a variety of older adult populations, including individuals with cognitive impairment. The 10-item BOHSE reflects oral health, with a higher score indicating more problems. The cumulative score is important, and individuals who score on items with an asterisk should be referred for an immediate dental examination. The BOHSE does not replace clinical oral examinations and dental radiographs for diagnosis, but it is a good tool to help determine the need for referral. Refer patients with suspected oral disease to a dental provider for comprehensive evaluation and diagnosis.

Older adults who are medically complex and those with functional limitations are in particular need of care coordination. Timely referrals for patients diagnosed with systemic diseases or prescribed medications that place oral health at risk are critical. All health care providers who care for older adults have an important role in promoting routine oral hygiene practices and identifying the need for referral and comprehensive oral health care.

Abdulsamet T, Mehmet SD, Faith D, Izzet Y. Polypharmacy and oral health among the elderly. *J Dent Oral Dis Ther.* 2016;4:1-5.

Chavez EM, Wong LM, Subar P, Young DA, Wong A. Dental care for geriatric and special needs populations. *Dent Clin North Am.* 2018;62(2):245-267.

Cole HA, Carlson CR. Mind-body considerations in orofacial pain. *Dent Clin North Am.* 2018;62(4):683-694.

Hyde S, Dupuis V, Boipelo M, Dartevelle S. Prevention of tooth loss and dental pain for reducing the global burden of oral diseases. *Int Dent J.* 2017;67(suppl 2):19-25.

Liu C, Cao Y, Lin J, et al. Oral care measures for preventing nursing home-acquired pneumonia. *Cochrane Database Syst Rev.* 2018;9:CD012416.

Nishimura RA, Otto CM, Bonow RO, et al. 2017 AHA/ACC focused update of the 2014 AHA/ACC guideline for the management of patients with valvular heart disease: a report of the American College of Cardiology/American Heart Association task force on clinical practice guidelines. *J Am Coll Cardiol.* 2017;70(2):252-289.

Pretty IA, Ellwood RP, Lo EC, et al. The Seattle care pathway for securing oral health in older patients. *Gerodontology.* 2014;31(suppl 1):77-87.

Sollecito TP, Elliot A, Peter B, et al. The use of prophylactic antibiotics prior to dental procedures in patients with prosthetic joints. Evidence practice guidelines for dental practitioners: a report of the American Dental Association Council on Scientific Affairs. *J Am Dent Assoc.* 2015;146(1):11-16.

Sroussi HY, Epstein JB, Bensadoun RJ, et al. Common oral complications of head and neck cancer radiation therapy: mucositis, infections, saliva change, fibrosis, sensory dysfunctions, dental caries, periodontal disease, and osteoradionecrosis. *Cancer Med.* 2017;6(12):2918-2931.

Wahl MJ, Pinto A, Kilham J, Lalla RV. Dental surgery in anticoagulated patients: stop the interruption. *Oral Surg Oral Med Oral Pathol Oral Radiol.* 2015;119(2):136-157.

USEFUL WEBSITES

American Association of Oral and Maxillofacial Surgeons. Medication-Related Osteonecrosis of the Jaw—2014 Update. https://www.aaoms.org/docs/govt_affairs/advocacy_white_papers/mronj_position_paper.pdf. Accessed April 9, 2020.

Appropriate use criteria for antibiotics prophylaxis. https://aaos.webauthor.com/go/auc/terms.cfm?auc_id=224965&actionxm=Terms. Accessed April 9, 2020.

Appropriate use criteria for the management of patients with orthopedic implants undergoing dental procedures. http://www.orthoguidelines.org/go/auc/default.cfm?auc_id=224995&actionxm=Terms. Accessed April 9, 2020.

Dimension of Dental Hygiene. National Oral Health Report: A State of Decay. https://dimensionsofdentalhygiene.com/national-oral-health-report-a-state-of-decay/. Accessed April 9, 2020.

Healthy People. https://www.healthypeople.gov. Accessed April 9, 2020.

Oral Health Assessment of Older Adults: The Kayser-Jones Brief Oral Health Status Examination (BOHSE). https://consultgeri.org/try-this/general-assessment/issue-18.pdf. Accessed April 9, 2020.

Smiles for Life. Oral cancers. http://smilesforlifeoralhealth.org. Accessed April 9, 2020.

58

Common Rheumatologic Disorders

Lisa Strano-Paul, MD

Asha Patnaik, MD

Gout, calcium pyrophosphate crystal disease (CPPD), and polymyalgia rheumatica are common conditions that can cause joint pain in geriatric patients. Erosive osteoarthritis is an uncommon cause of joint pain and all these conditions are discussed in this chapter. For a discussion of osteoarthritis, please see Chapter 34.

GOUT

▶ General Principles

Gout was first described thousands of years ago. Major risks for gout and hyperuricemia include obesity and age. One study suggests that the incidence of gout is increasing in older persons. The strongest predictor for the development of gout is an elevated uric acid level. Levels between 6 and 8.99 mg/dL predict a two-fold increase in gout flares, and a level >9 predicts a three-fold rise. Although gout more commonly affects men, male predominance is not seen in patients older than age 60 years, where the incidence of gout in men and women is about equal. Additional risks for gout include high-purine diet (red meat, shellfish), alcohol (beer and spirits), high-fructose drinks, chronic kidney disease, medications (thiazides), organ transplantation, lead exposure, and genetic factors. Certain diseases that are common in the elderly are also risk factors for gout and include hypertension, diabetes, hyperlipidemia, metabolic syndrome, and hematologic malignancies.

▶ Symptoms

Gout is characterized by episodic self-limited oligoarticular joint pain. The presence of erythema and swelling is characteristic. A history of podagra (first metatarsal joint attack) and or tophi, which are deposits of uric acid crystals around the ear helix or joints, further increases the specificity of diagnosis. Most gout attacks are monoarticular, although recurrent attacks can affect more than one joint. Patients may also present with fevers and constitutional symptoms. The ear and lower extremities are common sites of attacks because lower temperatures favor uric acid deposition. Periarticular structures such as bursa and tendons can also be involved. Gout often develops in previously damaged joints or after a trauma. Gout typically resolves in 3 to 14 days if untreated; however, crystals remain in affected joints and recurrent attacks are common, ranging from 60% in 1 year to up to 84% in 3 years.

▶ Findings

The gold standard for the diagnosis of gout is the finding of monosodium urate crystals from aspirated fluid from an inflamed joint or tophi. These crystals are needle shaped and seen inside of polymorphonuclear leukocytes from aspirated joint fluid. They are strongly birefringent when viewed under polarized microscopy. Crystals from tophi are seen alone because the tophus material is acellular. Joint fluid in gout is inflammatory, with elevated leukocyte counts, which can result in diagnostic confusion between septic arthritis and gout. Joint aspiration might not always be performed or be successful, and the American College of Rheumatology has developed additional criteria for diagnosis. Six of the following criteria are needed for diagnosis: recurrent acute arthritis; acute inflammation that develops over 1 day; monoarticular arthritis; redness of the joint; unilateral first metatarsal joint pain or swelling; unilateral tarsal joint swelling; suspected tophus; hyperuricemia; asymmetric swelling within a joint on x-ray; subcortical cysts without erosions on x-ray; and negative joint fluid culture during an attack. Additional tests that support the diagnosis of gout are elevated serum uric acid levels, complete blood count and differential, and serum creatinine. Radiography, although not typically helpful in diagnosing acute gout, can show characteristic changes with chronic gout, including subcortical cysts, proliferative bony reaction, and tophi-induced bone destruction away from the joint space.

Differential Diagnoses

CPDD can be confused with gout. The two diseases can be distinguished by crystal analysis from joint fluid as calcium pyrophosphate crystals are rhomboid shaped and weakly birefringent on polarized microscopy. CPDD results in cartilage calcification of the knee, symphysis pubis, glenoid and acetabular labrum, and wrist.

Rheumatoid arthritis (RA) presents as a symmetric polyarticular arthritis typically in the hands and feet. Gout, especially recurrent gout, may be polyarticular, but RA is more likely to involve the hands than gout. Rheumatoid synovitis may be confused with gout. Up to 20% of patients with RA will have rheumatoid nodules, but these do not occur in the same locations as gout tophi. Radiographs can distinguish RA from gout as RA results in diffuse joint space narrowing, osteopenia, and erosions of small joints.

Septic arthritis also presents as monoarticular or oligoarticular arthritis, associated with pain, swelling, and redness. Fever can be a common presenting sign with both conditions. The best way to distinguish these two conditions is with joint aspiration.

Osteoarthritis (OA) does not cause joint inflammation, but hallux valgus, or a bunion, is common and may be confused with podagra.

Psoriatic arthritis affects distal interphalangeal joints of the fingers and nail changes. These are not seen in gout.

However, patients with psoriasis can have elevated uric acid levels.

Treatment

Routine treatment of elevated uric acid levels is not recommended. Patients with elevated uric acid levels should be counseled on lifestyle changes, including dietary reduction of purines, weight loss, and reduction of alcohol intake. In addition, medications known to impair uric acid secretion should be avoided (Tables 58–1 and 58–2).

Nonsteroidal anti-inflammatory drugs (NSAIDs) are usually first-line treatment for acute gout. Patients should be treated with NSAIDs for 2 to 10 days. Nonprescription drugs, such as ibuprofen or naproxen, are as effective as indomethacin. If a patient is at increased risk for gastrointestinal complications, proton pump inhibitors can reduce the incidence of ulcers related to NSAIDs.

Colchicine is also a first-line agent for acute gout; however, its potential for side effects, especially diarrhea, can limit its effectiveness. The current recommendation is to treat with 0.6 mg two to three times a day.

Corticosteroids also can be used for acute gout and are preferred for patients with kidney disease. Intra-articular injections can be useful for monoarticular gout once infection has been ruled out.

Table 58–1. Gout medications.

Acute Gout	Chronic Gout
Nonsteroidal anti-inflammatory drugs (NSAIDs): All NSAIDs are equally effective; adverse effects include gastric bleeding and kidney injury. For patients older than 51 or those with GI risk, consider cyclooxygenase-2–specific NSAIDs or GI protection with misoprostol.	**Allopurinol (Lopurin, Zyloprim):** XOI that blocks the enzyme that breaks down purines into uric acid. It lowers uric acid levels, slows the production of uric acid, and helps dissolve uric acid crystals in tophi. It takes 3–6 months to take effect, and in that time, an acute attack can occur. It is the best option for those who overproduce uric acid versus those who under excrete it. Contraindicated in congestive heart failure, chronic kidney disease, or liver disease.
Indomethacin: The preferred NSAID of choice; however, there is no evidence that it is more effective than any other NSAID.	**Febuxostat (Uloric):** The mechanism of action is the same as allopurinol. It is safe in patients with mild to moderate kidney or liver disease. It has a higher risk of blood clots in comparison to allopurinol.
Avoid aspirin: Acts as an NSAID and a uricosuric agent at high doses. It can increase plasma uric acid levels and increase the risk of gout. Due to its short half-life, it is given every 4–6 hours.	**Probenecid (Benemid, Probalan):** Uricosuric agent that lowers uric acid in the body by increasing the amount excreted in the urine. Best for patients who have trouble excreting uric acid versus overproducing it. Contraindicated in kidney disease. Patients need to stay hydrated to avoid kidney stones.
Corticosteroids: Given by oral, intramuscular, or intra-articular routes. Preferred option when NSAIDs and colchicine are contraindicated. Taper to avoid rebound flares.	**Lesinurad (Zurampic):** Increases excretion of uric acid by inhibiting urate transporter 1 (URAT1), which is responsible for the majority of uric acid reabsorption by the kidneys. It is only used in addition to a XOI to enhance its effects. It is never used alone due to side effects including renal insufficiency and cardiovascular events. Patients need to stay hydrated to avoid kidney stones.
Colchicine: Has no analgesic properties; GI side effects are common; avoid in patients with renal and hepatic insufficiency.	**Pegloticase (Krystexxa):** Used in severe, chronic refractory gout. It is given every 2 weeks by intravenous infusion. It lowers uric acid quickly to lower levels when compared to all other medications, but it loses potency over time.

GI, gastrointestinal; XOI, xanthine oxidase inhibitor.

Table 58–2. American College of Rheumatology guidelines for the management of gout.

Patient Education	Consider Secondary Causes of Hyperuricemia	Eliminate Drugs That Induce Hyperuricemia	Evaluate Gout Disease Burden
Weight loss, healthy diet, exercise, smoking cessation, hydration	Obesity, metabolic syndrome, type 2 diabetes mellitus, excessive alcohol intake	Decreased urate excretion: cyclosporine, ethambutol, levodopa, tacrolimus, diazoxide, certain ACEIs (lisinopril, ramipril, trandolapril)	Tophus or tophi identified on clinical examination or imaging study
Avoid organ meats high in purine (liver, kidney), high-fructose corn syrup, alcohol overuse	Modifiable risk factors for CAD or stroke, HTN, HLD, smoking, physical inactivity, diet	Inhibition of renal tubular urate secretion: pyrazinamide, low-dose salicylates like aspirin, thiazide diuretic	Frequent attacks of acute gouty arthritis, ≥2 attacks per year
Limit serving sizes of beef, lamb, pork, seafood high in purine (sardines, shellfish), sugar, salt, and alcohol	Serum urate elevating drugs (thiazide and loop diuretics, niacin), urolithiasis, CKD, glomerular or interstitial renal disease	Increased uric acid production in the proximal tubule: acetazolamide, bumetanide, chlorthalidone, ethacrynic acid, furosemide, metolazone, torsemide, triamterene	CKD stage 2 or greater
Encourage low-fat or nonfat dairy products and vegetables	Genetic or acquired cause of excess uric acid (inborn error of purine metabolism or psoriasis, myeloproliferative or lymphoproliferative disease)	Miscellaneous: ethanol, fructose, didanosine, high doses of filgrastim, pancreatic enzymes, niacin, cytotoxic chemotherapy, glucocorticoids	Previous urolithiasis

ACEI, angiotensin-converting enzyme inhibitor; CAD, coronary artery disease; CKD, chronic kidney disease; HLD, hyperlipidemia; HTN, hypertension.

Long-term treatment directed at lowering uric acid levels is recommended for a patient who has had more than two or three acute gout attacks. It should also be given for tophaceous gout, severe attacks of polyarticular gout, joint damage seen on radiographs, and uric acid nephrolithiasis. Patients with known inborn errors of uric acid metabolism should also be treated. The goal of treatment is to maintain uric acid levels <6 mg/dL.

Xanthine oxidase inhibitors include allopurinol and febuxostat. These drugs should be started after the acute gout attack subsides. Concurrent treatment with colchicine reduces gout attacks initially. Dose range for allopurinol is usually 100 to 800 mg, with the average dose usually in the 400- to 600-mg/day range. The febuxostat dose range is 40 to 120 mg/day.

Probenecid is the only uricosuric drug available in the United States. To determine if a patient should be treated with probenecid, a 24-hour urine for uric acid and creatinine should be collected while consuming a low-purine diet and not during an acute flare. If the uric acid level is <600 to 700 mg/dL, then probenecid can be considered. Probenecid should not be used in patients with known uric acid nephrolithiasis. Probenecid can be combined with allopurinol in resistant patients.

Rasburicase is a recombinant form of urate oxidase that promotes the conversion of uric acid to allantoin. It is used for the prevention of tumor lysis syndrome.

Baker JF, Schumacher HR. Update on gout and hyperuricemia. *Int J Clin Pract*. 2010;64(3):371-377.

Malik A, Schumacher HR, Dinnella JE, Clayburne GM. Clinical diagnostic criteria for gout: comparison with the gold standard of synovial fluid crystal analysis. *J Clin Rheumatol*. 2009;15(1):22-24.

Mandell BF. Clinical manifestations of hyperuricemia and gout. *Cleve Clin J Med*. 2008;75(suppl 5):S5-S8.

Wallace KL, Riedel AA, Joseph-Ridge N, Wortmann R. Increasing prevalence of gout and hyperuricemia over 10 years among older adults in a managed care population. *J Rheumatol*. 2004;31(8):1582-1587.

Wallace SL, Robinson H, Masi AT, Decker JL, McCarty DJ, Yü TF. Preliminary criteria for the classification of the acute arthritis of primary gout. *Arthritis Rheum*. 1977;20(3):895-900.

Wilson JF. In the clinic. Gout. *Ann Intern Med*. 2010;152(3):ITC21.

CALCIUM PYROPHOSPHATE CRYSTAL DISEASE

▶ General Principles

CPPD is associated with aging. The average age of patients with CPPD is 72 years, with an incidence of >50% in patients older than age 85 years. The sex distribution for disease occurrence is roughly equal for men and women. CPPD may occur in previously traumatized joints or in joints that have required surgery. Some metabolic conditions, including hemochromatosis, hyperparathyroidism, hypophosphatasia, hypomagnesemia, and Gitelman syndrome, should be ruled out when younger patients present with CPPD. The European League Against Rheumatism (EULAR) recently established the following nomenclature for CPPD: pseudogout for acute attacks of crystal-induced synovitis resembling gout; chondrocalcinosis when calcification is seen in hyaline or fibrocartilage (this finding can also occur with crystal deposition); and pyrophosphate arthropathy to describe joint disease or radiographic abnormalities accompanying CPPD crystal disease.

Symptoms and Differential Diagnosis

Clinically, the disease may present in different ways. Asymptomatic disease is common with CPPD crystal deposition seen on radiographs. Pseudogout presents as self-limited acute attacks that resemble gout with acute inflammation and swelling. Fever and elevated leukocyte count can also be seen. These attacks, like gout, can be precipitated by trauma or medical illness, but can also be associated with fluctuations in calcium levels that can occur after parathyroidectomy. The joints that are affected by pseudogout differ from those affected by gout because the knee is the most commonly affected joint. Urate and CPPD crystal disease can occur together, and definitive diagnosis can only be made with joint aspiration. Pseudo-RA (chronic calcium pyrophosphate crystal inflammatory arthritis) should be suspected with more chronic symptoms of inflammatory arthritis in multiple joints associated with CPPD crystals in the joint fluid. The diagnosis can be difficult to distinguish from RA, as patients can experience morning stiffness and synovial thickness. Radiographs can be helpful, as the findings are more suggestive of OA than RA. Pseudo-OA (OA with CPPD) can occur with or without superimposed acute attacks. Half the patients with symptomatic CPPD will develop joint degeneration. The most common joint affected is the knee, which is often difficult to distinguish from OA. The diagnosis is more straightforward when the joints involved are less typical for OA, such as wrists, metacarpophalangeal joints, hips, shoulders, elbows, or spine. Pseudoneuropathic joint disease caused by CPPD crystal deposition can lead to joint degeneration and Charcot joint. Spinal involvement can be seen in CPPD and result in spine stiffness resembling ankylosing spondylitis or diffuse idiopathic skeletal hyperostosis.

Findings

Analysis of synovial fluid is the most important diagnostic criterion for CPPD. The presence of positively birefringent rhomboid crystals within leukocytes is pathognomonic for the disease. The synovial leukocyte count will also be elevated. A definitive diagnosis can be made when both weakly positive birefringent crystals are seen in synovial fluid or tissues and cartilage or joint capsule calcification is seen on radiographs.

Treatment

Acute pseudogout is managed in the same way as gout. Pseudogout should be treated with joint aspiration and NSAIDs. Intra-articular steroids can be used if infection has been ruled out. Colchicine and oral glucocorticoids are additional options. Patients with recurrent pseudogout attacks who present with three or more episodes should be treated with colchicine prophylaxis. The dose is 0.6 mg twice a day, although in elderly patients or patients unable to tolerate twice-a-day dosing, once daily can be considered.

Pseudo-RA can be treated with NSAIDs or colchicine. Second-line agents include low-dose glucocorticoid, methotrexate, and hydroxychloroquine.

For patients with OA with CPPD, treatment is determined by the presence or absence of intermittent episodes of pseudogout. If unaccompanied by acute episodes, then treatment is the same as that for OA.

McCarty DJ. Calcium pyrophosphate dihydrate crystal deposition disease. *Arthritis Rheum.* 1976;19(suppl 3):275-285.

Zhang W, Doherty M, Bardin T, et al. European League Against Rheumatism recommendations for calcium pyrophosphate deposition. Part I: terminology and diagnosis. *Ann Rheum Dis.* 2011;70(4):563-570.

EROSIVE OSTEOARTHRITIS

Erosive OA is an uncommon form of inflammatory OA of the hands seen in postmenopausal women. The median age of onset is 50 years. It presents as acute-onset pain, swelling, redness, and warmth of proximal interphalangeal joints and distal interphalangeal joints of the hands. It can result in instability of the interphalangeal joints with progressive loss of function.

Patients with erosive OA are likely to be positive for HLA-DRB*07. C-reactive protein can also be positive. X-rays of the hands show joint space narrowing and central erosions described as "gull wing and sawtooth deformities." This central bony erosion helps differentiate erosive hand OA from hand OA that does not have erosion.

Treatment is the same as that for OA of the hands, with topical NSAIDs, oral analgesics, and chondroitin sulfate to help control symptoms and reduce pain. Randomized clinical trials with conventional or biologic disease-modifying antirheumatic drugs did not show improvement in erosions.

Punzi L, Ramonda R, Oliviero F, et al. Value of C reactive protein in the assessment of erosive osteoarthritis of the hand. *Ann Rheum Dis.* 2005;64:955-957.

Punzi L, Ramonda R, Sfriso P. Erosive osteoarthritis. *Best Pract Res Clin Rheumatol.* 2004;18:739. 739-758.

Rovetta G, Monteforte P, Molfetta G. Balestra V. A two-year study of chondroitin sulfate in erosive osteoarthritis of the hands: behavior of erosions, osteophytes, pain and hands dysfunction. *Drugs Exp Clin Res.* 2004;30(1):11-16.

POLYMYALGIA RHEUMATICA

General Principles

Polymyalgia rheumatica (PMR) is a common condition affecting middle-age and older persons. The incidence of PMR increases after the age of 50 years and peaks between 70 and 80 years. It is more common in women than in men. It is related to temporal arteritis or giant cell arteritis in approximately 16% of cases. They may be different phases of the same disease.

Symptoms

PMR should be suspected when a patient older than 50 years presents with typical symptoms, which include at least 1 month of bilateral aching of the shoulders or proximal muscles of the arms and hips or proximal aspects of the thighs. Neck or torso stiffness might also be present. The stiffness is worse in the morning and lasts up to 1 hour. Muscular pain can interfere with activities of daily living. Patients may complain of discomfort with activities that use proximal muscles of the arms and legs such as grooming or stair climbing. Shoulder pain is the most typical presenting symptom, with the hip and neck less frequently involved.

Findings

On physical examination, both passive and active range of motion of the shoulders is reduced because of pain. Joint tenderness or swelling is not seen with PMR. Systemic symptoms, such as malaise, fever, fatigue, and weight loss, can be seen in up to one-third of patients. Erythrocyte sedimentation rate (ESR) will be >40 mm/h, and other inflammatory markers, such as C-reactive protein, will be elevated. Mild normocytic anemia can also be seen (Table 58–3).

Differential Diagnosis

Proximal pain and stiffness can be seen in many rheumatologic diseases that affect older people. Half the cases of PMR have distal symptoms, such as an asymmetric peripheral arthritis, that primarily affect the wrists and knees. Hand swelling with pitting edema of the dorsum of the hand and carpal tunnel syndrome can be seen. When these symptoms are present, it is difficult to differentiate between PMR and RA.

Table 58–3. 2012 EULAR/ACR provisional criteria for polymyalgia rheumatica (PMR).

Required: Age ≥50 Years, Bilateral Shoulder Aching, Abnormal CRP and/or ESR		
Feature	**Points Without USS[a]**	**Points With USS[b]**
Morning stiffness: duration >45 minutes	2	2
Hip pain or limited range of movement	1	1
Absence of RF or CCP	2	2
Absence of other joint involvement	1	1
• Ultrasound EITHER • ≥1 shoulder with subdeltoid bursitis and/or biceps tenosynovitis and/or glenohumeral synovitis and • ≥1 hip with synovitis and/or trochanteric bursitis	NA	1
OR		OR
BOTH shoulders with subdeltoid bursitis and/or biceps tenosynovitis and/or glenohumeral synovitis	NA	1

ACR, American College of Rheumatology; CPP, cyclic citrullinated peptide; CRP, C-reactive protein; ESR, erythrocyte sedimentation rate; EULAR, European League Against Rheumatism; NA, not applicable; RF, rheumatoid factor; USS, ultrasound score.

[a]Without USS, score ≥4 is categorized as PMR (sensitivity 68%, specificity 78%).

[b]With USS (optional), score ≥5 is categorized as PMR (sensitivity 66%, specificity 81%).

Data from Dasgupta B, Cimmino MA, Maradit-Kremers H, et al. 2012 provisional classification criteria for polymyalgia rheumatica: a European League Against Rheumatism/American College of Rheumatology collaborative initiative, *Ann Rheum Dis* 2012 Apr;71(4):484-92.

A negative rheumatoid factor and absence of joint erosions can distinguish the two conditions. The rare condition of remitting seronegative symmetric synovitis with pitting edema also causes pitting edema of the hands and feet and responds to steroids. Rheumatoid factor is negative in this condition, which may be part of the same disease spectrum as PMR.

Systemic lupus erythematosus can present in the elderly with symptoms that mimic PMR. The presence of additional findings such as pericarditis, pleuritis, leukopenia, or thrombocytopenia and a positive antinuclear antibody will distinguish these conditions.

Late-onset spondyloarthropathy can result in proximal symptoms, but the presence of peripheral enthesitis, anterior uveitis, and sacroiliitis differentiates these conditions.

Polymyositis presents with more muscle weakness and causes elevated muscle enzymes. Fibromyalgia patients experience painful trigger points and have a normal ESR.

Primary systemic amyloidosis may share symptoms with PMR, but these patients do not respond to steroids and have a monoclonal band on immunoelectrophoresis.

▶ Treatment

Corticosteroids are the drug of choice for PMR. The dose for prednisone is 10 to 20 mg, and the response to treatment is rapid. Symptoms typically resolve within days. Treatment with the initial dose should be continued for 2 to 4 weeks and gradually tapered every 1 to 2 weeks. Rapid taper can result in recurrent symptoms, and caution should be taken to ensure judicious tapering of steroid dose. Even with slow tapering, 30% to 50% of patients can have spontaneous recurrence of symptoms requiring increased steroid dose. Monitoring patients by assessment of symptoms and ESR is useful. Steroid dose should not be increased if ESR is increased without recurrent symptoms. Most patients require 1 to 2 years of treatment.

Methotrexate can be used as a steroid-sparing agent in patients with severe symptoms requiring high doses of steroids.

Dasgupta B, Cimmino MA, Maradit-Kremers H, et al. 2012 provisional classification criteria for polymyalgia rheumatica: a European League Against Rheumatism/American College of Rheumatology collaborative initiative. *Ann Rheum Dis.* 2012;71(4):484-492.

Salvarani C, Cantini F, Boiardi L, Hunder GG. Polymyalgia rheumatica and giant-cell arteritis. *N Engl J Med.* 2002;347(4):261-271.

Sleep Disorders

59

Diana V. Jao, MD

Cathy Alessi, MD

ESSENTIALS OF DIAGNOSIS

▶ Insomnia is a disorder involving difficulty falling asleep, difficulty staying asleep, and/or early morning awakening that is associated with daytime symptoms such as fatigue, irritability, or problems with concentration.

▶ Sleep apnea is common among older adults and may present with symptoms such as snoring, choking, fatigue, insomnia, or other signs and symptoms.

▶ Sleep disorders are common with certain neurologic disorders, such as dementia and Parkinson disease.

▶ Depending on the particular sleep disorder, diagnoses are made based on clinical presentation and/or by testing in a sleep laboratory or by home-based sleep testing.

General Principles

Sleep disturbance is common among older adults. The National Heart, Lung, and Blood Institute has highlighted the prevalence and associated deleterious health consequences of poor sleep with its statement of "one in three adults does not regularly get the recommended amount of uninterrupted sleep to protect their health." Sleep difficulties and several primary sleep disorders increase in prevalence with age. However, in older adults, sleep disturbance often coexists with other conditions, which can exacerbate or lead to additional medical and psychosocial conditions and may impact treatment. For these reasons, sleep disturbance in older adults might often be best approached as a geriatric syndrome as the causes and contributing factors are generally multifactorial.

The prevalence of sleep difficulties varies based on how these problems are identified and defined, but studies suggest that >50% of community-dwelling older adults and >65% of long-term care facility residents experience sleeping difficulties. In addition, many community-dwelling older adults use nonprescription or prescribed sleeping medications.

Sleep architecture can be described based on findings of polysomnography, which involves multiple channels (eg, electroencephalogram, electrooculogram, electromyogram) of physiologic recording during sleep. Based on polysomnography, sleep can be categorized into two states: nonrapid eye movement (NREM) and rapid eye movement (REM) sleep. NREM sleep is further divided into three stages, where N1 is the lightest sleep, N2 is where the majority of sleep time is spent, and N3 is deep sleep. N1 and N2 sleep increase with age, whereas N3 sleep decreases. Altered sleep patterns include decreased sleep efficiency (time asleep as a percentage of time in bed), decreased total sleep time, increased sleep latency (time to fall asleep), more arousals during the night, more daytime napping, and other changes.

Older adults may not report sleep complaints unless specifically asked. Presenting symptoms overlap significantly among common sleep disorders.

INSOMNIA

Clinical Findings

A. Symptoms & Signs

Occasional difficulty falling asleep or staying asleep is common. To diagnose insomnia, the *International Classification of Sleep Disorders*—3rd edition (ICSD 3) requires that the individual must have a sleep complaint (ie, difficulty initiating sleep, difficulty maintaining sleep, and/or waking up too early), the sleep complaint must occur despite adequate opportunity and circumstances for sleep, and there must be daytime impairment related to the nighttime sleeping difficulty (eg, fatigue or malaise, mood disturbance or irritability, daytime sleepiness). In addition, the sleep disturbance and associated daytime symptoms must occur at least three times per week. Chronic insomnia is diagnosed when these symptoms are present for at least 3 months.

B. Patient History

A detailed history is essential in determining the causes of insomnia. Key factors include recent stressors, symptoms of depression, anxiety, or other psychiatric conditions; medical and neurologic conditions; prescription and over-the-counter medications; and other issues.

C. Special Tests

Instruments that can be helpful in the evaluation of insomnia include sleep questionnaires, sleep logs, symptom checklists, psychological screening tests, and interviews of bed partners. Examples of self-administered questionnaires are the Insomnia Severity Index (specific to insomnia) and the Pittsburgh Sleep Quality Index (a general questionnaire of sleep problems). Polysomnography and/or wrist actigraphy (which estimates sleep and wakefulness based on wrist movements) are not indicated for the routine evaluation of insomnia unless suggested by signs and symptoms of comorbid sleep disorders. Laboratory tests should be similarly guided based on signs or symptoms of comorbid conditions that appear associated with the insomnia.

▶ Differential Diagnosis

In older adults, symptoms related to underlying medical or psychiatric illnesses and the effects of medications are common causes of insomnia. Often, multiple factors may coexist to contribute to insomnia in the older patient.

Diverse medical conditions can interfere with sleep, such as chronic pain, dyspnea, gastroesophageal reflux disease, and nocturia. Medications reportedly account for 10% to 15% of cases of insomnia. Table 59–1 lists common offending agents. Many other agents can disrupt sleep, including caffeine and nicotine. Caffeine is an ingredient frequently found in nonprescription medications and beverages, and consumers may not be aware that they are ingesting caffeine-containing products. Nighttime alcohol use, while causing initial drowsiness, can interfere with sleep architecture later in the night and worsen sleep. Long-term use and withdrawal from sedative-hypnotic agents can also lead to worsening insomnia.

▶ Treatment

A. Behavioral

All recent published guidelines recommend psychological and behavioral treatments as first-line therapy for the management of chronic insomnia in all adults. Cognitive-behavioral therapy for insomnia (CBT-I) for insomnia generally

Table 59–1. Examples of agents that can contribute to insomnia.

Cardiovascular Medications
Furosemide
β-Blockers
Respiratory Medications
Pseudoephedrine
β-Agonists
Theophylline
Antidepressants
Bupropion
Fluoxetine
Paroxetine
Sertraline
Venlafaxine
Others
Corticosteroids
Cimetidine
Phenytoin
Caffeine and caffeine-containing drugs
Nicotine
Alcohol

combines several treatments, including stimulus control, sleep restriction, and cognitive therapy; other treatments may also be involved. Stimulus control promotes behaviors such as establishing regular morning rising and bedtimes, using the bedroom exclusively for sleep and sexual activity, going to bed only when sleepy and getting out of bed if unable to fall asleep, and avoiding or limiting naps. Sleep restriction therapy seeks to improve sleep efficiency by causing modest sleep deprivation through limiting time in bed and then gradually increasing time in bed as sleep efficiency improves. Cognitive therapy focuses on correcting inaccurate ideas and thoughts about sleep. CBT-I for insomnia is generally provided by a psychologist with expertise in behavioral sleep medicine, but research has shown CBT-I can be successfully provided by nurses and other clinicians and by nonclinician sleep coaches. Brief behavioral therapy for insomnia, a shorter version of CBT-I, has been developed with demonstrated success. Mobile health tools and Internet-based methods to provide CBT-I have also been developed and shown to improve insomnia.

Sleep hygiene addresses lifestyle and environmental factors (Table 59–2) and is often included in CBT-I. However,

Table 59–2. Examples of measures to improve sleep hygiene.

1. Regular morning rising time.
2. Avoid daytime napping or limit to <1 hour in the morning or early afternoon.
3. Exercise during the day but not immediately before bedtime.
4. Avoid caffeine, nicotine, and alcohol in the evening.
5. Avoid excessive fluid intake at night to reduce nighttime urination.
6. Avoid large meals before bedtime, but a light snack may promote sleep.
7. Follow a nighttime routine of preparation for bedtime and wear comfortable bedclothes.
8. Ensure a tranquil nighttime environment, minimizing noise and light and keeping room temperature comfortable.
9. Avoid use of electronic devices before bedtime.

sleep hygiene alone is rarely effective in the patient with a longstanding, severe chronic insomnia. Other behavioral interventions may also be included, such as meditation and relaxation techniques to guide patients in recognizing and relieving tension and anxiety.

B. Pharmacologic

1. Prescription medications—Recent insomnia treatment guidelines suggest that sedative-hypnotic medications (Table 59–3) can be considered if behavioral interventions for chronic insomnia are not fully successful and a discussion with the patient about risks and benefits of these agents has occurred. These agents may also be considered in the patient with acute insomnia when the benefits appear to outweigh the risks of these medications. Thoughtful selection of agents to minimize adverse side effects and drug interactions is reached by evaluating symptom types (eg, problem with sleep onset vs awakening during the night), agent characteristics,

comorbid conditions, and cost. In older adults, the starting dose should be the lowest available. Patient self-adjustment of dose upward should be discouraged.

Benzodiazepines and related drugs are commonly prescribed for sleep. Long-acting benzodiazepines (eg, flurazepam) should not be used in older adults because of the risk of daytime carryover (sedation), falls, and fractures. Short- and intermediate-acting benzodiazepines can be used with caution due to the risk of tolerance to the hypnotic effects of the medication and the potential for rebound insomnia on withdrawal. These agents also result in an increased risk of falls, and their half-life can be longer in older adults.

Nonbenzodiazepine benzodiazepine (BZD) receptor agonists may have fewer side effects and less daytime carryover compared with benzodiazepines. Although structurally different from benzodiazepines, these agents also act at the γ-aminobutyric acid (GABA) benzodiazepine receptor, but perhaps with greater specificity for sedative effects. In the United States, available BZD receptor agonists include zolpidem, zaleplon, and eszopiclone (see Table 59–3). Unfortunately, evidence suggests these agents increase risk for falls and fracture, and caution is also warranted in the use of these sleeping medications for the management of chronic insomnia in older adults. The American Geriatrics Society (AGS) 2019 Updated Beers Criteria for Potentially Inappropriate Medication Use in Older Adults recommend against use of benzodiazepines and BZD receptor agonists (citing moderate quality of evidence and strong strength of recommendation against their use).

The melatonin receptor agonist ramelteon is approved for sleep-onset insomnia. It is not a scheduled agent. With a half-life of 2.6 hours, it has been shown to reduce sleep latency and to increase total sleep time without rebound or withdrawal effects. Suvorexant is the first US Food and Drug Administration (FDA)–approved dual orexin receptor antagonist for use in sleep onset and/or sleep maintenance treatment. It is a schedule IV controlled substance.

Table 59–3. Examples of prescription sleeping medications.

Generic Name	Class	Usual Dose Range in Older People	Half-Life
Temazepam	Intermediate-acting benzodiazepine	7.5–15 mg	3.5–18.4 h
Zolpidem	Benzodiazepine receptor agonist	5 mg	2–3 h
Zolpidem extended-release	Benzodiazepine receptor agonist	6.25 mg	1.5–5.5 h
Zaleplon	Benzodiazepine receptor agonist	5 mg	1 h
Eszopiclone	Benzodiazepine receptor agonist	1–2 mg	6 h
Doxepin (low-dose)	Sedating antidepressant	3–6 mg	15 h
Trazodone (off-label)	Sedating antidepressant	25–150 mg	2–4 h
Ramelteon	Melatonin receptor agonist	8 mg	2.6 h
Suvorexant	Orexin receptor antagonist	Up to 20 mg	12 h

There is some evidence for using a low-dose sedating antidepressant at night (with a more stimulating antidepressant during the day) for depressed patients who also report insomnia. Most published guidelines discourage use of a sedating antidepressant for insomnia unless the patient has failed other agents or has an indication for an antidepressant. Low-dose doxepin is the only antidepressant that has been FDA approved for insomnia. Use of sedating antipsychotic medications for insomnia is not appropriate unless the patient has a serious psychiatric disorder that warrants use of these agents.

2. Nonprescription medications—Nonprescription sleeping aids often contain a sedating antihistamine (eg, diphenhydramine) alone or in combination with an analgesic. Diphenhydramine and similar compounds are not recommended for older people because of potent anticholinergic effects and the development of tolerance to sedating effects over time. A bedtime dose of an analgesic agent alone (eg, acetaminophen) may be safe and helpful if pain disrupts sleep. The herbal product valerian does not have sufficient evidence to support routine use.

American Geriatrics Society. American Geriatrics Society 2019 updated AGS Beers criteria for potentially inappropriate medication use in older adults. *J Am Geriatr Soc.* 2019;67(4): 674-694.

Qaseem A, Kansagara D, Forciea MA, et al. Management of chronic insomnia disorder in adults: a clinical practice guideline from the American College of Physicians. *Ann Intern Med.* 2016;165:125-133.

Sateia MJ, Buysse DJ, Krystal AD, et al. Clinical practice guideline for the pharmacologic treatment of chronic insomnia in adults: an American Academy of Sleep Medicine clinical practice guideline. *J Clin Sleep Med.* 2017;13(2):307-349.

SLEEP APNEA

▶ General Principles

Sleep apnea is the repetitive cessation or marked decrease of airflow during sleep. In obstructive sleep apnea (OSA), the cessation or decrease in breathing is associated with continued ventilatory effort. Central sleep apnea is characterized by cessation or marked decrease of airflow during sleep, associated with absent or reduced ventilatory effort. The majority of patients with central sleep apnea have heart failure. The focus here will be on OSA.

▶ Clinical Findings

A. Symptoms & Signs

Increased body mass index is an important predictor of sleep apnea, although the relationship between obesity and OSA is not as strong in older adults, and many older adults with OSA are not obese. The prevalence of OSA is higher in men than women and in older age groups. Prevalence rates of OSA of up to 40% are reported in people age 65 years and older. There is also a higher prevalence of OSA among older adults with dementia. Although the traditional presentation of OSA includes excessive daytime sleepiness, unrecognized OSA is also common among older adults with insomnia. Other associated signs or symptoms include poorly controlled hypertension and morning headache. The bed partner or caregiver may be very helpful in reporting loud snoring, choking and gasping sounds, or apneic periods.

The clinical consequences of sleep apnea are likely related to sleep fragmentation, hypoxia, and hypercapnia. Sleep apnea, especially if untreated, is associated with cardiovascular diseases such as hypertension and coronary artery disease and increased mortality rates. Other adverse consequences include cognitive impairment and a higher rate of motor vehicle accidents.

B. Diagnosis

Along with diagnostic testing, a thorough sleep evaluation includes a detailed sleep history and physical exam. Polysomnography (PSG) in an overnight sleep laboratory remains the gold standard in diagnosing OSA. However, home sleep apnea testing (HSAT) is an acceptable alternative approach in many patients. The optimal patients for HSAT are those with high suspicion for OSA with no chronic conditions (eg, chronic obstructive pulmonary disease, congestive heart failure) who may warrant PSG testing in an overnight sleep laboratory. Limitations of HSAT may include the need for a repeat or in-laboratory PSG if initial HSAT results are negative in a patient with high risk for OSA or when the HSAT is technically inadequate (eg, the monitoring leads slipped off during sleep or suboptimal quality signals are obtained). Of note, HSAT does not screen for certain other sleep disorders such as abnormal nocturnal movements and REM sleep behavior disorder.

▶ Treatment

Positive airway pressure (PAP) is the treatment standard for moderate to severe OSA as defined by the apnea-hypopnea index (AHI), the sum of apneas and hypopneas per hour of sleep. PAP is an option in treatment of mild OSA, generally in patients with daytime symptoms or other consequences or conditions associated with OSA. One classification suggests that AHI >30 per hour denotes severe OSA, 16 to 30 per denotes moderate OSA, and 5 to 15 per hour denotes mild OSA. Consistent PAP use improves hypertension and congestive heart failure treatment responses and may also rectify some metabolic problems such as lipid abnormalities. The primary challenge with PAP usage is adherence. Initial experience with PAP is predictive of use as adherence is often established as early as the first week. Initial close follow-up to resolve issues interfering with regular use may promote long-term adherence. Subsequent periodic follow-ups are recommended as OSA should be managed as a chronic condition. Guidelines suggest standard treatment of OSA can include either continuous PAP (CPAP), which provides a constant and continuous flow of air, or auto-adjusting PAP (APAP), which sets airflow within a high and low range that titrates to the minimum pressure that will sustain airway patency. APAP generally does not require PAP titration in an overnight sleep laboratory, as is needed with CPAP therapy. Other treatments are available, such as bilevel PAP, which delivers two pressures, one for inspiration and another for expiration. The sleep specialist can determine the most appropriate treatment.

Patients with OSA should be advised to avoid alcohol and sedative use (particularly if OSA is untreated) and to lose weight if body mass index is elevated. Positional therapy, which keeps patients in the nonsupine position during sleep, can be an effective secondary treatment approach, particularly in patients with OSA that occurs primarily in the supine position. For those who fail or are unable to tolerate PAP treatment, other approaches may be considered. Oral-dental devices that reposition the jaw or tongue can be tried, particularly in patients with mild OSA. Surgical procedures such as laser-assisted uvuloplasty or mandibular-maxillary advancement offer mixed results, with little evidence for use in older adults. There is also evidence for use of a hypoglossal nerve stimulator (an implanted medical device) for selected cases of moderate to severe OSA, with recent evidence for use in older adults.

No medication is directly effective for OSA treatment. Medical cannabis and its synthetic extracts are not recommended for OSA since there is not sufficient evidence regarding effectiveness, tolerability, and safety.

Chowdhuri S, Patel P, Badr MS. Apnea in older adults. *Sleep Med Clin.* 2018;13(1):21-37.

Leng Y, McEvoy CT, Allen IE, et al. Association of sleep-disordered breathing with cognitive function and risk of cognitive impairment: a systematic review and meta-analysis. *JAMA Neurol.* 2017;74(10):1237-1245.

Ramar K, Dort LC, Katz SG, et al. Clinical practice guideline for the treatment of obstructive sleep apnea and snoring with oral appliance therapy: an update for 2015. *J Clin Sleep Med.* 2015;11(7):773-827.

PERIODIC LIMB MOVEMENT DURING SLEEP AND RESTLESS LEGS SYNDROME

▶ General Principles

Among older adults, the prevalence of periodic limb movements during sleep (PLMS) ranges from 20% to 60%; however, the clinical significance of many of these cases is unclear. The prevalence of restless legs syndrome (RLS) ranges from 2% to 15%. RLS may cause insomnia and nighttime restlessness and discomfort. RLS and PLMS often coexist, with PLMS present in 80% to 90% of patients with RLS. Prevalence of PLMS increases with age and appears to be higher in those of Northern and Western European descent and lower in Asians. The cause of both conditions is unknown, but increased age, family history, uremia, and low iron stores have been suggested as risk factors.

▶ Clinical Findings

A. Symptoms & Signs

PLMS is characterized by recurring episodes of stereotypic rhythmic movements during sleep, generally involving the legs. The diagnosis of PLM disorder (PLMD) is reserved for individuals with PLMS that causes a sleep disturbance that cannot be explained by the presence of another disorder. Many patients who exhibit PLMS-like movements are asymptomatic or may have another sleep disorder (eg, OSA), and specific treatment for the PLMS is not indicated.

RLS has four features that make up the mnemonic URGE: (1) an **u**ncontrollable urge to move the legs, usually accompanied or caused by uncomfortable and unpleasant sensations in the legs; (2) symptoms begin or worsen during periods of **r**est or inactivity; (3) symptoms are partially or entirely relieved with movement or **g**etting up; and (4) symptoms are worse in the **e**vening or night.

B. Special Tests

The diagnosis of PLMS, but not RLS, requires PSG. RLS is diagnosed clinically based on history. Subjective scales such as the International RLS Rating Scale may help evaluate RLS severity and assess treatment outcomes. Patients with RLS should be screened for iron deficiency with a serum ferritin test.

▶ Treatment

The treatment of PLMS depends on the severity of symptoms and their impact on the patient's general well-being. If another sleep disorder is present (eg, OSA), that disorder should be treated first because PLMS-like movements may improve with treatment of that disorder.

RLS may improve with leg stretching and avoidance of caffeine, alcohol, and medications that precipitate symptoms, such as antihistamines, antidepressants, and promotility agents. A low ferritin should prompt iron replacement and appropriate evaluation for the cause of iron deficiency as RLS symptoms may resolve after iron replacement.

Pharmacotherapy should be considered for RLS when these maneuvers are ineffective or when symptoms are severe. Medication choice should depend on evidence of effectiveness and comorbid conditions. Dopaminergic agents are the best studied agents for both RLS and PLMS and are considered to be the treatment of choice in older adults. Treatment near bedtime with a dopamine agonist (eg, pramipexole 0.125 mg or ropinirole 0.25 mg or higher) may be effective for both RLS and PLMS. Rotigotine, a nonergot dopamine agonist, is available as a 24-hour transdermal patch. It is a treatment option for moderate to severe RLS with effective dosing of up to 3 mg/day. Adverse effects of dopamine agonists include excessive daytime sleepiness, hallucinations, and compulsive behaviors (eg, uncontrolled shopping, gambling, eating, sexual urges). Carbidopa-levodopa (one-half to one full tablet of 25/100-mg tablets, or higher) has also been suggested. Rebound symptoms that occur as the medication wears off or augmentation (shift of symptoms to early in the day) can occur with treatment. Augmentation is more common with carbidopa-levodopa than with the dopamine agonists. Both rebound and augmentation may resolve with medication dose decrease or discontinuation.

There is also some evidence for use of gabapentin (and pregabalin) for RLS. Unlike the dopamine agonists, these agents do not cause augmentation. Opioids such as oxycodone and hydrocodone may help patients with severe symptoms unresponsive to other therapies, but the side effects of these agents limit their usefulness for RLS in the older adults. Clonazepam has also been used for RLS, but potential adverse effects in older adults limit its usefulness in many older adults.

Aurora RN, Kristo DA, Bista SR, et al. The treatment of restless legs syndrome and periodic limb movement disorder in adults—an update for 2012: practice parameters with an evidence-based systematic review and meta-analyses: an American Academy of Sleep Medicine Clinical Practice Guideline. *Sleep.* 2012;35(8):1039-1062.

Salminen AV, Winkelmann J. Restless legs syndrome and other movement disorders of sleep - treatment update. *Curr Treat Options Neurol.* 2018;20(12):55.

Trotti LM, Becker LA. Iron for the treatment of restless legs syndrome. *Cochrane Database Syst Rev.* 2019;1:CD007834.

NARCOLEPSY

General Principles

Narcolepsy is a disorder of recurrent, uncontrollable, brief episodes of sleep that interfere with wakefulness and that are often associated with hypnagogic hallucinations (which occur near the onset of sleep or awakening), cataplexy, and sleep paralysis. This disorder generally presents in adolescence or young adulthood, and only rarely presents for the first time in old age. Narcolepsy is a lifelong disorder, but it does not usually worsen with advanced age. A new diagnosis of narcolepsy in middle or older age may represent a previously missed diagnosis, but evaluation for an underlying neurologic abnormality should be considered.

Clinical Findings

A. Symptoms & Signs

The key clinical features of narcolepsy are excessive daytime sleepiness without cataplexy (a sudden and transient loss of muscle tone triggered by emotions). The excessive daytime sleepiness is described as an irrepressible need to sleep or daytime lapses into sleep that have been occurring for at least 3 months.

B. Special Tests

Testing involves the Multiple Sleep Latency Test (MSLT), a structured examination that is performed to determine the severity of daytime sleepiness and to identify sleep episodes with early onset of REM (ie, sleep-onset REM periods). True cataplexy is diagnostic of narcolepsy, but not all patients with narcolepsy will have cataplexy.

Differential Diagnosis

Narcolepsy can be complicated by other sleep disorders, including sleep apnea, periodic limb movements, and REM behavior disorder. These other disorders would generally be identified during overnight PSG, which is typically performed prior to MSLT.

Treatment

Nonpharmacologic interventions involve maximizing nighttime sleep, supplemented by scheduled daytime naps, and avoiding emotional situations that precipitate attacks. Various medications are available including wake-promoting agents such as modafinil, selective serotonin reuptake inhibitors (SSRIs), serotonin-norepinephrine reuptake inhibitors (SNRIs), tricyclic antidepressants, and sodium oxybate. Treatment of narcolepsy typically requires input from a sleep specialist.

Kovalska P, Kemlink P, Nevsimalova S, et al. Narcolepsy with cataplexy in patients aged over 60 years: a case-control study. *Sleep Med.* 2016;26:79-84.

Lammer GJ. Drugs used in narcolepsy and other hypersomnias. *Sleep Med Clin.* 2018;13(2):183-189.

CIRCADIAN RHYTHM SLEEP DISORDERS

General Principles

Circadian rhythm sleep disorders (CRSDs) may be primarily intrinsic (eg, advanced sleep-wake phase disorder, delayed sleep-wake phase disorder, irregular sleep-wake rhythm disorder, non–24-hour sleep-wake rhythm disorder) or extrinsic (eg, jet lag disorder, shift work disorder). Correlations have been made between changes in circadian rhythms and advancing age.

Clinical Findings

A. Symptoms & Signs

Commonly older adults experience an advanced sleep phase, which leads to a pattern of an early bedtime and early morning awakening. The alteration in circadian rhythm can be marked in people who are bed bound. When the internal clock is completely desynchronized, as may occur in severe neurodegenerative disorders, the sleep-wake cycles become irregular, with sleep occurring during the day and wakefulness at night or alternating periods of sleep and wakefulness throughout the 24-hour period. This irregular pattern is particularly common among nursing home residents.

B. Special Tests

Wrist actigraphy and/or sleep logs can be used for making a diagnosis and for monitoring treatment response. PSG is indicated when the diagnosis is unclear or another sleep disorder is suspected.

Treatment

Depending on the specific CRSD, treatments may include appropriately timed bright light exposure, appropriately timed melatonin use, prescribed sleep scheduling, and other treatments. Wake-promoting medications (eg, modafinil) have been used for shift workers during night shifts to increase wakefulness and in certain other conditions. Special expertise may be needed in the management of severe, chronic CRSDs, since inappropriately timed circadian rhythm treatments (eg, bright light, melatonin) can have limited or even adverse effects on the sleep-wake cycle.

Auger RR, Burgess HJ, Emens JS, et al. Clinical practice guideline for the treatment of intrinsic circadian rhythm sleep-wake disorders: advanced sleep-wake phase disorder (ASWPD), delayed sleep-wake phase disorder (DSWPD), non-24-hour sleep wake rhythm disorder (N24SWD), and irregular sleep-wake rhythm disorder (ISWRD). An update for 2015. *J Clin Sleep Med*. 2015;11(10):1199-1236.

Kim JH, Duffy JF. Circadian rhythm sleep-wake disorders in older adults. *Sleep Med Clin*. 2018;13:39-50.

REM SLEEP BEHAVIOR DISORDER

General Principles

REM sleep behavior disorder (RBD) usually presents in late life, more commonly in men than women. RBD is associated with certain neurodegenerative disorders, particularly

α-synucleinopathies (eg, Parkinson disease, Lewy body dementia, multiple-system atrophy). The RBD may present several years prior to the clinical presentation of the neurodegenerative disorder.

Clinical Findings

A. Symptoms & Signs

RBD presents with symptoms of dream enactment behavior along with the absence of the normal muscle atonia that should be present during REM sleep. Patients act out dreams with forceful movements and behaviors during sleep. They usually present for medical care as a result of injury to themselves or their bed partners; these injuries can be quite severe. Medications such as SSRIs, SNRIs, and tricyclic antidepressants can precipitate RBD. It has also been associated with brain disorders, including dementia and stroke. As mentioned earlier, RBD may be a prodrome for neurodegenerative disorders

B. Special Tests

PSG is required to confirm the diagnosis and to rule out other conditions.

Treatment

Environmental measures should be taken to make the sleeping environment safe for the patient and the bed partner. Clonazepam was traditionally used for this condition but should be used with caution in older adults, particularly in those with concurrent neurodegenerative disorders, frailty, or gait abnormalities. Melatonin is increasingly recognized as first-line therapy for RBD, particularly in older people with neurodegenerative disorders. A variety of agents have been described as second-line therapy when first-line treatment fails or inadequately controls symptoms.

Malhotra RK. Neurodegenerative disorders and sleep. *Sleep Med Clin*. 2018;13(1):63-70.

Postuma RB, Iranzo A, Hu M, et al. Risk and predictors of dementia and parkinsonism in idiopathic REM sleep behavior disorder: a multicentre study. Brain. 2019;142:744-759.

Rodriguez CL, Jaimchariyatam N, Budur K. Rapid eye movement sleep behavior disorder: a review of the literature and update on current concepts. *Chest*. 2017;152(3):650-662.

SLEEP PROBLEMS IN SPECIAL POPULATIONS

A. Sleep Patterns in Dementia

Most research on sleep problems with dementia has focused on Alzheimer disease. Compared with older adults without dementia, those with dementia have more sleep disruption, more arousals, lower sleep efficiency, and other problems. Sundowning, a worsening of confusion or agitated behaviors in late afternoon or evening or at night, may be present in up to two-thirds of patients with dementia. If the dementia patient is unable to voice their symptoms or actively participate in their care, this may further compound their sleep difficulties. The presence of sundowning warrants a search for potentially contributing factors such as pain, anxiety, or other causes of discomfort. Antipsychotic and sedative hypnotic agents have not been consistently effective in older adults with dementia and nighttime worsening of problematic behaviors; these agents also carry significant risks. Sensory interventions (aromatherapy, thermal bath, and calming music with hand massage) may be beneficial. PSG may be useful in select cases where primary sleep disorders (eg, OSA) are suspected and treatment might be warranted.

B. Sleep Disturbance in Long-Term Care Facility Residents

Superimposed on the multifactorial etiologies leading to sleep problems in older adults, long-term care residents also have other factors that may contribute to sleep disturbance. The common pattern of sleep disturbance among these residents involves frequent nighttime arousals and daytime sleeping. Many factors seem to affect quality of sleep, including multiple physical illnesses and medications that can interfere with sleep, debility and inactivity, increased prevalence of primary sleep disorders, minimal daytime sunlight exposure, and environmental factors, including frequent nighttime noise, light, and nursing care activities.

An increase in daytime physical activity levels to enhance daytime wakefulness may lead to improved nighttime sleep in nursing home residents. Exercise programs combined with socialization may also be helpful. Bright light therapy may also improve total nighttime sleep and decrease daytime sleeping, but effects may be modest. Reduction of nighttime noise and consistent sleep hygiene practices are also recommended. Application of multicomponent nonpharmacologic interventions to improve sleep-wake patterns in nursing home residents may have some modest effect, but results (in randomized controlled trials) have been mixed.

Hughes JM, Martin JL. Sleep characteristics of Veterans Affairs adult day health care participants. *Behav Sleep Med.* 2015;13(3):197-207.

Shang B, Yin H, Jia Y, et al. Nonpharmacological interventions to improve sleep in nursing home residents: a systematic review. *Geriatr Nurs.* 2019;40(4):405-416.

Ye L, Richards KC. Sleep and long-term care. *Sleep Med Clin.* 2018;13(1):117-125.

USEFUL WEBSITES

American Academy of Sleep Medicine. http://www.aasmnet.org. Accessed April 13, 2020.

National Institutes of Health National Center on Sleep Disorders Research. http://www.nhlbi.nih.gov/sleep. Accessed April 13, 2020.

National Sleep Foundation. http://www.sleepfoundation.org. Accessed April 13, 2020.

Sleep Research Society. http://www.sleepresearchsociety.org. Accessed April 13, 2020.

▶ Sleep Questionnaires

Insomnia Severity Index
International Restless Leg Rating Scale
Pittsburg Sleep Quality Index

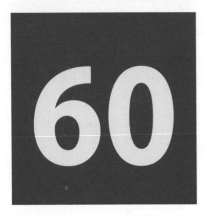

Confusion

Candace J. Kim, MD

Caroline Stephens, PhD, RN, GNP, FAAN

General Principles

Confusion is a symptom characterized by an altered state of awareness. It may be accompanied by disorientation, memory loss, altered perception, and/or behavioral change. It is a common presenting problem in many older adults and a frequent reason why families and caregivers seek medical attention. As part of normal aging, many adults experience some cognitive changes such as decreases in the speed of processing information, lessened spontaneous recall, and small decreases in executive skills. Confusion, however, is not a normal part of aging. Assessment of the onset and duration of symptoms is important to differentiate causes of confusion.

Confusion may be a feature of other acute or chronic medical illnesses. It is often unrecognized in older adults unless it interferes with their ability to perform their usual activities. Confusion in the acute care setting (often referred to using various terms such as delirium, altered mental status, or encephalopathy) is associated with longer hospital length of stay, increased health care costs, caregiver distress, and worse patient outcomes including higher mortality. Over time, confusion results in impaired functional status and a decreased quality of life.

Clinical Findings

When a patient presents with confusion, it is critical to perform a detailed history and in-depth physical exam, including a mental status exam, as well as laboratory and diagnostic tests. Interviewing the family and caregiver(s), as well as the patient, is necessary to determine an individual's baseline state as well as any changes that have occurred.

A. Symptoms & Signs

A thorough history should focus on understanding the specific cognitive, functional, and behavioral changes and how these symptoms have evolved over time. The interviewer must seek to identify any events such as a fall, focal pain, recent medical procedure, medication change, or environmental trigger and consider whether or not it was related to the development of confusion. It is also important to ask about substance use and screen for drug and/or alcohol overuse and potential risk factors for intoxication or withdrawal. Seeking a better understanding of any preexisting medical, neurologic, or psychiatric conditions is also potentially informative and relevant. Table 60–1 details key history domains to assess. The medical evaluation should incorporate data from the psychosocial assessment, a thorough and accurate review of medications (including nonprescription and complementary alternative therapies), and any barriers to taking medications as prescribed such as a misunderstanding about the purpose or dosing of the medication, access problem or cognitive impairment.

The physical exam often provides numerous diagnostic clues in the context of confusion. Vital sign abnormalities (including pain severity and location) must not be overlooked, and they should be further investigated. For example, a patient presenting with confusion and a respiratory rate of 40 breaths per minute needs to have imaging and laboratory studies directed at making a diagnosis related to their acute respiratory distress, whereas a patient with confusion and high fever requires an evaluation for infection.

Observation in a general medical examination can provide substantial insights into the nature of confusion. The presence of tremor, asterixis, or other abnormal movements may indicate renal or hepatic dysfunction or be due to an adverse drug reaction. Behavioral abnormalities, interactions with family members, and assessment of level of consciousness may lead the examiner to understand more about the neuropsychiatric aspects of the problem.

The examination of specific organ systems should be performed with attention to signs of systemic disease and organ dysfunction, as nearly any systemic process may produce confusion. For example, a new heart murmur and splinter

Table 60–1. Key history domains when evaluating confusion.

Medical History
- Active infection
- Family history of dementia
- Head trauma
- Medication review, recent medication changes
- Neurologic diseases, including Parkinson disease, seizures, or cerebrovascular disease
- Prior episodes of delirium
- Sleep quality or sleep disturbances
- Surgical history, response to anesthesia, and postoperative recovery
- Vascular risk factors

Psychiatric History
- Behavioral disturbances, such as problems with impulse control, physical or verbal aggression, wandering or disrobing inappropriately
- Family history of psychiatric disorders (especially depression)
- Past or current alcohol or drug use
- Previous psychiatric diagnoses
- Recent stressors and losses

Functional Status
- Change in ADLs and IADLs
- Falls/gait impairment
- Hearing loss
- Impaired vision
- Urinary incontinence

ADLs, activities of daily living; IADLs, instrumental activities of daily living.

Table 60–2. The Confusion Assessment Method (CAM) diagnostic algorithm.

The diagnosis of delirium using the CAM requires the presence of #1 and #2 and either #3 or #4:

Evidence	
#1: Acute onset and fluctuating course	Positive responses (usually obtained collaterally) to the following questions: "Is there evidence of acute change in mental status from the patient's baseline? Did the abnormal behavior fluctuate during the day, that is, tend to come and go or increase and decrease in severity?"
#2: Inattention	Positive response to the question: "Did the patient have difficulty focusing attention, for example, being easily distractible, or difficulty keeping track of what was being said?"
#3: Disorganized thinking	Positive response to the question: "Was the patient's thinking disorganized or incoherent, such as rambling or irrelevant conversation, unclear or illogical flows of ideas, or unpredictable switching from subject to subject?"
#4: Altered level of consciousness	An answer other than "alert" to the question: "Overall, how would you rate this patient's level of consciousness?" (Alert [normal], vigilant [hyperalert], lethargic [drowsy, easily aroused], stupor [difficult to arouse], or coma [unarousable])

Data from Inouye SK, van Dyck CH, Alessi CA, Balkin S, Siegal AP, Horwitz RI. Clarifying confusion: the confusion assessment method. A new method for detection of delirium, *Ann Intern Med* 1990 Dec 15;113(12):941-948.

hemorrhages in a patient with confusion and fever suggest possible endocarditis. Skin changes may be indicative of an adverse drug reaction, hepatic injury, or an acute infectious process. Other common cardiovascular conditions such as acute coronary syndrome or heart failure may present with confusion as a prominent symptom.

B. Mental Status Examination

Mental status should be assessed in the domains of memory, abstract thinking, judgment, mood and affect, orientation, attention or concentration, level of consciousness (wakefulness or sleepiness), communication or language abilities, and behavior and personality changes (eg, suspiciousness or loss of impulse control). Standardized mental status questionnaires, diagnostic rating scales, and symptom inventories can assist in this assessment process. Together with the history and physical examination, instruments such as the Montreal Cognitive Assessment (MoCA), Confusion Assessment Method (CAM; Table 60–2), and Geriatric Depression Scale (GDS) can aid the clinician in differentiating among dementia, delirium, and depression. Recognize, however, that the results of these tools cannot be interpreted in isolation. Findings must be interpreted within the context of an individual's

clinical presentation, socioeconomic status, cultural background, education and literacy level, current/previous occupation, and other psychosocial factors.

In addition, the way patients respond to these standardized assessment instruments can be just as informative as the score they achieve. For example, a patient with depression may score low on the MoCA as a result of poor effort, apathy, and frequent answers of "I don't know," whereas someone with dementia obtains the same score while putting forth great effort, attempting to rationalize mistakes, and/or feeling bad if they are unable to answer questions appropriately. Alternatively, someone with delirium may exhibit poor attention and concentration by being easily distracted and/or falling asleep during the assessment process.

▶ Diagnostic Approach

A. Laboratory Findings

There are no specific laboratory tests that in themselves establish the diagnosis of confusion. Instead, testing is directed by the details obtained from the history and physical examination to establish whether or not an underlying cause can be identified. Blood chemistries, including transaminases and ammonia, as well as a complete blood count are appropriate to screen for electrolyte disturbance, new or worsening organ dysfunction, or infection that may be causing confusion. Additional testing of thyroid function and vitamin B_{12} and methylmalonic acid levels is potentially useful if the initial screening exam and laboratory studies do not yield a diagnosis. Also, obtaining a urine and serum toxicology screen as well as drug levels (eg, digoxin, lithium) in patients taking medications that may produce confusion is appropriate and can be helpful.

B. Imaging Studies

Neuroimaging with head computed tomography (CT) or brain magnetic resonance imaging (MRI) identifies structural brain abnormalities that may cause confusion. Such imaging is especially important to obtain if there are any focal neurologic findings on examination or in the case of new-onset headaches. Characteristically, lesions such as tumor or subacute stroke involving one or both frontal lobes may result in confusion, sometimes without other obvious neurologic exam findings. There are also imaging findings associated with other causes of confusion such as severe hypoglycemia, thiamine deficiency, and obstructive hydrocephalus. Patients with head trauma, alcohol overuse, or unwitnessed falls need to have neuroimaging to assess for evidence of traumatic brain injury, since a subdural hematoma may present as confusion days to weeks after an injury.

C. Special Tests

An electroencephalogram (EEG) may be diagnostic if there is any clinical suggestion of seizure activity or if an individual remains confused without any alternative explanation for their symptoms. Nonconvulsive seizure activity may present with alteration of consciousness or confusion and is characterized by the absence of the tonic-clonic movements that are most often associated with seizure. EEG is also helpful in confirming a diagnosis of confusion due to a psychiatric disorder, as background EEG activity would show normal wakefulness in this setting.

▶ Differential Diagnosis

A. Delirium

Delirium, often presenting as acute confusion, is a highly prevalent, preventable, life-threatening clinical syndrome that may occur at any age, but it is especially prevalent in acutely ill older adults. It is characterized by an abrupt change and fluctuation in attention and awareness, with a disturbance in cognition that is not explained by an identified neurocognitive disorder. In contrast to dementia, which is a progressive confusional state that develops over months to years, delirium typically develops over a shorter period of time (hours to days), fluctuates in severity (often worsening at night), and is characterized by prominent inattention. Anxiety, irritability, and psychomotor restlessness with insomnia are common. These patients may pick at their intravenous lines, take off their oxygen, disconnect monitoring equipment, and exhibit poor impulse control and environmental awareness. Perceptual disturbances (often visual hallucinations) are commonly accompanied by paranoid delusional thinking, which exacerbates the patient's behavioral and emotional disturbance. Agitated behaviors commonly associated with delirium often lead to use of physical and chemical restraints, further compounding the risk of functional loss and serious complications.

Family and caregivers may report the patient was "fine" during the day but became confused, restless, and agitated during the middle of the night. Other times, the symptoms reported may be less apparent: "She isn't acting quite right." When family and caregivers observe such a subtle change over the course of a day or week, that symptom should be taken seriously by the medical team, and delirium should be actively considered and ruled out. Delirium is considered a medical emergency and should always be medically evaluated prior to assuming the patient has dementia or a psychiatric disorder. See Chapter 36 for details on delirium.

B. Dementia

Unlike delirium, dementia is more chronic in nature and develops insidiously over months to years. Specifically, dementia is a clinical syndrome characterized by difficulties in memory, disturbances in language, psychological and psychiatric changes, and impairments in activities of daily living. Unlike delirium, an individual's attention is generally intact in dementia. Although there are many different types of dementia (see Chapter 9, "Cognitive Impairment & Dementia"), the most common is Alzheimer disease, which accounts for 50% to 80% of all dementia cases.

Alzheimer dementia is typically noticed as forgetfulness of recent events or conversations. Family and loved ones may report that, over several months or longer, the patient has been increasingly getting lost in familiar areas; misplacing items; having language difficulties (eg, finding the name of familiar objects); having problems performing tasks that require some thought but that used to come easily (eg, balancing a checkbook, playing card games, learning new information or routines); and/or experiencing personality changes or a loss of social skills leading to inappropriate behaviors. As the dementia slowly progresses, these symptoms become much more apparent and severe and interfere with the patient's ability to care for self. The patient may also begin to exhibit psychosis, mood, and behavioral difficulties (eg, paranoid delusions, hallucinations, depression, physical and/or verbal aggression, social withdrawal), or sleep disturbances (eg, often waking at night), with increasingly poor insight and judgment. Many of these behaviors often present significant caregiving challenges and may become an escalating emotional, physical, and/or financial burden to families and caregivers. In the severe stages, patients are unable to perform basic self-care, recognize family members, understand language, speak, or ambulate independently.

It is important to note that confusion or a decline in cognitive functioning that is abnormal for age and education but does not meet criteria for dementia should *not* be attributed to normal aging. Mild cognitive impairment (MCI) is the intermediate-stage neurocognitive disorder between normal cognitive aging and dementia. MCI is associated with an increased lifetime risk for developing dementia. A person with MCI will have problems with memory, language, or another cognitive function severe enough to be noticeable to others and show up on testing, but not serious enough to interfere with daily life. Understanding the degree of functional impairment is a key component in determining whether the person has MCI or early dementia.

C. Psychiatric Disorder

Depression is the most common psychiatric disorder in the older adult population, primarily affecting those with chronic medical illnesses, cognitive impairment, and disability. It is clinically defined as a syndrome of either depressed mood or loss of interest or pleasure in most activities of the day. To establish the diagnosis, these symptoms must represent a change from the person's usual functioning and be present for at least 2 weeks. Personality changes (eg, social withdrawal, apathy, irritability), forgetfulness, and mood changes (eg, complaints of decreased ability to think, feelings of hopelessness and/or helplessness, changes in sleep or appetite, psychomotor slowing/agitation) may be signs of depression, dementia, or both. Patients with depression may recognize their feelings of sadness, experience somatic complaints, or simply exhibit decreased engagement in activities of daily living. The mnemonic "SIGECAPS" (Table 60–3) is an assessment of the eight major diagnostic symptoms of depression.

Unlike dementia, confusion in a patient with depression is more task specific than global. For example, the patient may have difficulties with certain activities, like paying bills, but remains capable of completing equally difficult tasks, such as doing a crossword puzzle. Similarly, the patient may not initiate or engage in conversation, but retains the ability to speak. A person with depression is also more likely to relate many themes of loss, as well as detail their cognitive complaints, whereas someone with dementia may be unaware of their cognitive difficulties and/or try to mask their deficits. Table 60–4 presents a comparison of the key diagnostic features to help differentiate delirium, dementia, and depression.

Table 60–3. The eight major diagnostic neurovegetative symptoms of depression (SIGECAPS).

S leep disturbance* (increased during day or decreased at night)
I nterest reduced (loss of interest in previously enjoyable activities)
G uilt (worthlessness*, hopelessness*, regret, self-blame)
E nergy loss or fatigue*
C oncentration impairment*
A ppetite change* (usually decreased; occasionally increased)
P sychomotor change (retardation/lethargy or agitation/anxiety)
S uicidal thoughts/preoccupation with death

Note: To meet the diagnosis of major depression, a patient must have 4 of the symptoms plus depressed mood or anhedonia, for at least 2 weeks. To meet the diagnosis of dysthymic disorder, a patient must have 2 of the 6 symptoms marked with an asterisk (*), plus depression, for at least 2 years.

Reproduced with permission from Carlat DJ. The psychiatric review of symptoms: a screening tool for family physicians, *Am Fam Physician* 1998 Nov 1;58(7):1617-24.

D. Overlapping Diagnoses

Finally, it is important to recognize that when evaluating confusion in an older adult the three common clinical syndromes (ie, dementia, delirium, depression) may overlap. For example, between 25% and 75% of patients with delirium have coexisting dementia, and the presence of dementia increases the risk of delirium up to five-fold. Depression also often coexists with dementia in approximately 20% of individuals with Alzheimer disease and is associated with higher levels of functional impairment and reduced enjoyment in activities. Late-life depressive symptoms may be an early manifestation of cognitive decline in older adults.

▶ Prevention

In addition to early identification, preventing confusion is a critical aspect of care and the most effective means to avoid the associated adverse outcomes. Educating families and caregivers about environmental or medical triggers and how to appropriately access early interventions to minimize the effects of confusion is important.

Some potential triggers are changes to an individual's medications, daily routine, or environment. Avoiding major environmental changes, optimizing sleep, and avoiding nighttime disruptions may help to prevent confusion. Minimizing emotional and physical stressors, maintaining and encouraging mobility and regular cardiovascular activity, and optimizing any sensory impairments that may be causing or contributing to confusion are all potentially effective preventative measures. For example, ensuring that a person has access to and is appropriately using corrective lenses, hearing

Table 60–4. Comparison of the clinical features of delirium, dementia, and depression.

Clinical Feature	Delirium	Dementia	Depression
Onset/course	Acute; onset within hours to days with diurnal fluctuations in symptoms (worse at night, in darkness, and on awakening)	Chronic; generally insidious or gradual onset; progressive symptoms yet relatively stable over time (depends on the type of dementia)	Fairly abrupt; may coincide with major life changes; diurnal effects typically worse in morning
Duration	Hours, days to weeks (or longer)	Months to years	At least 2 weeks; can be months to years
Awareness/alertness	Reduced; fluctuates; lethargic or hypervigilant	Generally clear or normal until more advanced stages	Generally clear or normal
Attention/concentration	Impaired; very short attention span; fluctuates	Generally normal, until more advanced	Minimal impairment but may have difficulty concentrating
Orientation	Disorientation early; severity varies	Disorientation later in the disease (usually after months to years)	Usually normal, but may have selective disorientation
Memory	Global impairment; ability to test may be limited due to severe inattention	First recent and then later remote impairment	Selective or "patchy" impairment; "islands" of intact memory
Thinking	Disorganized; fragmented, incoherent speech, either slow or accelerated; changes in consciousness	Word finding difficulties; difficulty with abstraction, calculation; agnosia; thoughts impoverished later in disease	Some difficulty with concentration; may have slowed processing and/or speech; themes of loss, hopelessness, or self-deprecation
Perception	Distorted; illusions, delusions, and hallucinations; difficulty distinguishing between reality and misperceptions	Variable depending on the type of dementia; paranoid delusions (eg, people stealing items) and visual hallucinations most common	Generally intact; may have paranoid ideation and/or hallucinations in severe cases
Psychomotor behavior	Marked changes (hyperactive, hypoactive, or mixed)	Generally normal until late stage; may have apraxia	Variable, psychomotor retardation or agitation
Sleep-wake cycle	Disturbed; reversed cycle; hour-to-hour variation	Fragmented with day-night reversal but not hour-to-hour variation	Insomnia common—may have difficulty with sleep onset and/or early morning awakening; also hypersomnia
Associated features	Variable affective changes; symptoms of autonomic hyperarousal; exaggeration of personality type; associated with acute physical illness	Affect tends to be superficial, inappropriate, and/or labile; attempts to conceal deficits in intellect; personality changes, aphasia, agnosia may be present; lacks insight	Affect depressed; dysphoric mood; exaggerated/detailed complaints, often many themes of loss; preoccupied with personal thoughts; insight present
Assessment	Failings highlighted by providers/family; distracted from task; numerous errors	Failings highlighted by family, caregiver, friend; frequent "near miss" answers; struggles with test; puts forth great effort to find an appropriate reply	Failings highlighted by individual; frequently answers "I don't know"; little/poor effort; frequently gives up; indifferent toward test

aids, and walking aids are all nonpharmacologic strategies that help to prevent confusion in the appropriate context. An ideal environment is one that is personalized to optimize safety, comfort, hydration, and sleep.

Fong TG, Davis D, Growdon ME, et al. The interface between delirium and dementia in elderly adults. *Lancet Neurol.* 2015;14:823-832.

Haigh EAP, Bogucki OE, Sigmon ST, et al. Depression among older adults: a 20-year update on five common myths and misconceptions. *Am J Geriatr Psychiatry.* 2018;26(1):107-122.

Han JH, Schnelle JS, Ely EW. The relationship between a chief complaint of "altered mental status" and delirium in older emergency department patients *Acad Emerg Med.* 2014;21(8):937-940.

Hasemann W, Tolson D, Godwin J, et al. A before and after study of a nurse led comprehensive delirium management programme (DemDel) for older acute care inpatients with cognitive impairment. *Int J Nurs Stud.* 2016;53:27-38.

Hshieh TT, Yue J, Oh E, et al. Effectiveness of multicomponent nonpharmacologic delirium interventions: a meta analysis. *JAMA Int Med.* 2015;175(4):512-520.

Inouye S, van Dyck C, Alessi C, et al. Clarifying confusion: the confusion assessment method. *Ann Intern Med.* 1990;113(12):941-948

Inouye SK, Westendorp RGJ, Saczynski JS. Delirium in elderly people. *Lancet.* 2014;383:911-922.

Kalisch Ellet LM, Pratt NL, Ramsey EN, et al. Central nervous system-acting medicines and risk of hospital admission for confusion, delirium or dementia. *J Am Med Dir Assoc.* 2016;17(6):530-534.

Lippmann S, Perugula ML. Delirium or dementia? *Innov Clin Neurosci.* 2016;13(9-10):56-57.

Meyer JD, Koltyn KF, Stegner JS, et al. Influence of exercise intensity for improving depressed mood in depression: a dose-response study. *Behav Ther.* 2016;47(4):527-537.

Zheng G, Xia R, Zhou W, et al. Aerobic exercise ameliorates cognitive function in older adults with mild cognitive impairment: a systematic review and meta-analysis of randomised controlled trials. *Br J Sports Med.* 2016;50:1443-1450.

Constipation

61

Myung Ko, MD
Sara Lewin, MD

▶ Constipation is common in older adults and requires careful assessment to rule out mechanical causes.

▶ May present with other abdominal complaints, such as pain, bloating, and/or gas.

▶ May involve infrequent defecation, difficulty passing stool, or incomplete evacuation of stool.

▶ A diagnosis of chronic constipation requires the presence of symptoms for at least 12 weeks.

General Principles

Chronic constipation is one of the most frequent gastrointestinal disorders encountered among older adults in clinical practice. Constipation may be caused by medications, as a manifestation of systemic disease, or due to psychosocial factors. It may involve difficulty in passing stool, infrequent stool passage, or incomplete evacuation of stool. Infrequent passage of stool is not a requirement to meet the diagnosis of constipation if difficulty with or incomplete evacuation of stool is present. For chronic constipation to be diagnosed, symptoms should be present for at least 12 weeks.

Chronic constipation is common in older adults. About one-third of adults age 60 years or older report at least occasional constipation, and more than half of nursing home residents experience constipation. Women are at increased risk, experiencing constipation two to three times more often than men. African Americans also exhibit increased risk. Many community-dwelling older adults commonly use nonprescription preparations, such as stimulant and bulking laxatives. Nearly 85% of physician visits for constipation result in a prescription for laxatives, and more than $1.6 billion dollars are spent on constipation-related emergency department visits.

Clinical Findings

A. Symptoms & Signs

Health care providers often regard constipation to mean infrequent bowel movements, but patient-reported symptoms of constipation are often more varied and associated with other abdominal complaints, including pain, bloating, fullness, gas, and incomplete evacuation. Straining is often the predominant symptom in older adults and occurs in up to 65% of community-based individuals older than 65 years of age. Hard stools are reported in approximately 40%.

B. Clinical Evaluation

In most cases, patients with chronic constipation do not warrant extensive diagnostic evaluation. Historical features are key, and specific questions should be asked, including what symptom the patient finds most distressing—infrequency, straining, hard stools, incomplete defecation, or symptoms unrelated to bowel habits (eg, bloating, pain, or malaise). The presence of bloating or abdominal pain may suggest underlying irritable bowel syndrome.

Additional questions should assess for "alarm symptoms," including symptoms of hematochezia, family history of colon cancer or inflammatory bowel disease, anemia, positive fecal occult blood test, unexplained weight loss ≥10 pounds, constipation that is refractory to treatment, and new-onset constipation without evidence of potential primary cause. Older patients who have "alarm" symptoms should consider the benefits and risks of doing further evaluation with colonoscopy or other invasive testing.

The clinical evaluation should consist of a thorough history containing the above questions and an appropriate physical examination and laboratory testing. Physical examination should include a rectal exam, palpating for hard stool and assessing for masses, anal fissures, sphincter tone, hemorrhoids, and prostatic hypertrophy in males. During simulated defecation, the anal verge should be observed for any patulous opening or prolapse of anorectal mucosa. The digital examination should evaluate resting tone of the sphincter segment and augmentation by a squeezing effort. Acute localized tenderness to palpation along the puborectalis is a feature of levator ani syndrome. The patient should also be instructed to "expel" the examiner's finger while the examiner evaluates for any evidence of paradoxical movement (eg, relaxation instead of contraction) of the anorectal muscles.

After the initial history and physical examination, focused testing should be considered to assess for disorders that are treatable or important to diagnose early. Laboratory testing should include a complete blood count, serum calcium, thyroid function tests, and fecal occult blood testing. Radiologic examination with abdominal plain films may also detect significant stool retention in the colon and suggest the diagnosis of megacolon. Marker studies or colonic transit studies can be used in patients with infrequent defecation. A marker study involves ingestion of radiopaque markers with a subsequent abdominal radiograph to detect the markers in the right, left, or rectosigmoid colon. Other forms of transit time evaluation with radioactive tracers and wireless motility capsule technologies that record data after ingestion are also available.

▶ Differential Diagnosis

The causes of constipation can be categorized as primary or secondary (eg, caused by a medical diagnosis or use of medications). Table 61–1 lists primary causes of constipation, and Table 61–2 lists secondary causes.

Many prescription drugs have constipation and slowed colonic motility as side effects. Table 61–3 lists constipation-inducing medications in older adults.

Table 61–1. Primary pathophysiologic causes of chronic constipation.

Type	Characteristics
1. Normal transit constipation	Most common subtype Transit and stool frequency are within normal ranges, but patients complain of constipation, bloating, and pain[a]
2. Slow-transit constipation	Increased intestinal transit time Reduced colonic motility
3. Dyssynergic defecation	More common in older adults and women Structural problems seen on anorectal manometry and defecography Pelvic floor dyssynergia (failure to relax or inappropriate contraction of puborectalis muscle and external anal sphincter during defecation)

[a]Presence of pain increases the likelihood of a diagnosis of constipation-predominant irritable bowel syndrome (IBS-C) instead of chronic constipation.

Table 61–2. Secondary causes of chronic constipation in older adults.

- Malignancy
- Medications/polypharmacy (prescription and nonprescription drugs, including opioids)
- Endocrine/metabolic (diabetes mellitus, hypothyroidism, hypercalcemia, hypokalemia)
- Neurologic disorders (Parkinson disease, diabetic autonomic neuropathy, spinal cord injury, dementia, stroke)
- Rheumatologic disorders (systemic sclerosis and other connective tissue disorders)
- Psychological disorders (depression or eating disorders)
- Anatomic dysfunction (strictures, postsurgical abnormalities, anal fissures, megacolon, hemorrhoids)
- Decreased mobility/sedentary lifestyle

▶ Treatment

Once secondary causes of constipation have been evaluated and addressed as possible, the management of constipation varies according to type. The treatment and prevention of slow-transit constipation include patient education about bowel habits, dietary changes, and drug therapies. Management of dyssynergic defecation involves biofeedback, relaxation exercises, and suppository programs. Patients with slow-transit and dyssynergic defecation should receive treatment for the dyssynergia first before other measures are started.

A. Nonpharmacologic Therapy

Nonpharmacologic treatment options or lifestyle modifications involve diet, exercise, and biofeedback (if dyssynergic defecation is diagnosed). There is limited evidence that

Table 61–3. Medications that cause constipation.

- Anabolic steroids
- Anticonvulsants (carbamazepine, oxcarbazepine, phenobarbital, phenytoin, valproic acid)
- Anticholinergic agents (atropine, dicyclomine, ipratropium, oxybutynin, scopolamine)
- Antidiarrheal agents
- Antihistamines
- Antihypertensive agents (calcium channel blockers)
- Antiparkinsonian agents (benztropine, trihexyphenidyl)
- Antipsychotics (clozapine)
- Diuretics
- Nonsteroidal anti-inflammatory medications
- Opioid pain relievers (morphine, codeine)
- Supplements (calcium, iron)
- Sympathomimetic agents
- Tricyclic antidepressants (amitriptyline, desipramine, doxepin, imipramine, nortriptyline)

lifestyle modifications resolve constipation, but it is generally accepted as a first-line approach. Studies assessing the effect of exercise on constipation in older adults were unable to show an improvement, although it has been shown to enhance the quality of life.

Dietary options include increasing fluid and fiber. It must be noted, however, that patients with confirmed slow-transit constipation or pelvic floor dyssynergia respond poorly to high-fiber diet and fiber supplementation. Such individuals should be encouraged to minimize dietary fiber. The studies on dietary fiber in older adults reported mixed results. Soluble fiber (eg, psyllium) has better evidence than insoluble fiber. The daily recommended amount of fiber is 20 to 35 g/day, but most Americans only consume 5 to 10 g/day. Increasing daily fiber intake through dietary measures is recommended. Information should be given on the fiber contained in common foods. Patients should increase fiber intake slowly—5 g/day at 1-week intervals—until the recommended intake is attained. Patients should be informed that an immediate response is not expected, and that flatus and bloating may occur, but are usually temporary. Increasing fiber intake gradually may help minimize some of these unwanted side effects.

Probiotics have also been studied for the treatment of constipation. *Lactobacillus* and *Bifidobacterium* are symbiotic flora in the large intestine that may promote colonic mucosal health. Low levels of both have been reported in individuals with chronic constipation. Probiotics have shown decreased intestinal transit time in older adults in randomized control trials. The optimal dose, probiotic strain, and duration of treatment have not been well established in studies to date.

Biofeedback is an effective treatment for dyssynergic defecation, which is characterized by paradoxical contraction or failure to relax the pelvic floor muscles during defecation. Biofeedback can involve both sensory training and muscle contraction/relaxation techniques. In patients with dyssynergic defecation, biofeedback was consistently found to be more effective than continuous use of polyethylene glycol (PEG, Miralax), standard therapy (other types of stool softeners and laxatives), sham therapy (therapy aimed at overall body relaxation), or the use of diazepam in four randomized controlled trials. However, trials are needed to determine the efficacy of biofeedback in older adults.

Preventing and treating constipation with nonpharmacologic and pharmacologic treatments may be needed for older adults in specific situations—that is, in the postoperative period, during hospitalization, or in other health care environments when decreased mobility is anticipated—and when using acute or chronic opioid medications.

B. Pharmacologic Therapy (Including Nonprescription Preparations)

The main categories of nonprescription medications for prevention of constipation are bulking agents, stool softeners/

Table 61–4. Evidence-based pharmacologic management options for chronic constipation.

Therapy	Recommendations
Bulking agents	
Psyllium	Grade A
Calcium polycarbophil	Grade B
Methylcellulose	Grade B
Stool softeners/emollients	
Docusate calcium/sodium	Grade B
Mineral oil (linked with aspiration in older adults)	Grade C
Osmotic laxatives	
Lactulose	Grade A
PEG (polyethylene glycol)	Grade A
Sorbitol	Grade B
Magnesium hydroxide	Grade C
Stimulants	
Senna	Grade A
Bisacodyl	Grade A
5-HT$_4$ (serotonin) agonists	
Prucalopride	Grade A
Chloride channel activator	
Lubiprostone	Grade A
Guanylate cyclase-C receptor antagonists	
Linaclotide	Grade A
Plecanatide	Grade A

Grade A: evidence from ≥2 randomized, controlled trials (RCTs) with adequate sample sizes, good design, and results at the *P* <.05 level.
Grade B: evidence from a single, high-quality RCT as defined for Grade A, or recommendations based on evidence from ≥2 RCTs with conflicting evidence or inadequate sample sizes.
Grade C: no RCT data.

emollients, and osmotic agents. The main categories for the treatment of chronic constipation are bulking agents, stool softeners/emollients, osmotic agents, stimulants, chloride change activators, 5-HT$_4$ receptor agonists, and guanylate cyclase-C receptor agonists. Table 61–4 lists the pharmacologic treatments for constipation based on existing evidence from the American College of Gastroenterology Chronic Constipation Task Force.

1. Bulking agents—Bulking agents are natural or synthetic polysaccharides or cellulose derivatives that absorb water and increase fecal mass, with the ultimate goal of achieving softer stool. They are considered to be first-line agents for constipation given minimal adverse effects. However, objective evidence regarding their effectiveness is inconsistent. A systematic review found evidence that psyllium increases stool frequency in patients with chronic constipation but found insufficient evidence of other forms of fiber including calcium polycarbophil, methylcellulose, and bran.

Bulking agents should also be increased slowly over weekly periods to avoid side effects, similar to increasing dietary fiber consumption. However, many older adults may not be good candidates for using a bulking agent. Some examples of when bulking agents should not be the first-line agent include older adults who are taking high doses of narcotic medications; who have difficulty with swallowing or dysphagia (because of the consistency of certain types of fiber when mixed with water); with a surgical resection of the majority of the colon; who have a suspected rectal mass or possible bowel obstruction; or who do not consume adequate amounts of fluid.

2. Stool softeners and emollients—While stool softeners and emollients are commonly prescribed due to their safety profile and detergent effect on stool consistency, these medications have limited evidence of efficacy in treating constipation. A systematic review concluded that stool softeners may be inferior to psyllium for improvement in stool frequency. Rare side effects include aspiration. Lipoid pneumonia is a known risk of using mineral oil in older adults.

3. Osmotic laxatives—Osmotic laxatives promote the secretion of water into the intestinal lumen by osmotic activity and the hyperosmolar nature of these medications. PEG has the best evidence of use and is now available over the counter as a treatment for occasional constipation. It improves stool frequency and consistency in patients with chronic constipation. Studies suggest that PEG can be dose adjusted or used every other day with efficacy. An open-label study with 117 participants, ≥65 years of age, using PEG over 12 months reported relatively few side effects and no serious adverse events related to the medication. A recent evidence-based review article concluded that PEG may be better for constipation symptoms than lactulose. Frequent use of PEG or magnesium hydroxide–containing preparations (milk of magnesia) in patients with congestive heart failure or chronic kidney disease should be done with extreme caution as they can cause electrolyte imbalances, such as hypokalemia and diarrhea, further worsening fluid-electrolyte balances. Osmotic agents are useful when first-line bulking agents and/or stool softeners are not effective.

4. Stimulants—Stimulants, such as senna and bisacodyl-containing compounds, increase intestinal motility by increasing peristaltic contractions. Stimulants also decrease water absorption from the lumen. Patients usually report more unfavorable side effects from these medications such as abdominal discomfort and cramping. Placebo-controlled studies support the use of bisacodyl or senna, although fewer clinical trials exist comparing senna to placebo than for bisacodyl. There is no evidence that long-term use of stimulant laxatives damages the enteric nervous system. Stimulant laxatives have been associated with melanosis coli. The presence of melanosis coli (which may be seen on colonoscopy) is a marker of chronic laxative use and may not indicate any other clinical consequences.

5. 5-HT$_4$ (serotonin) agonists—5-Hydroxytryptamine receptor subtype 4 (5-HT$_4$) receptors are found in the colon and mediate the release of other neurotransmitters that may initiate peristaltic action. These prokinetic agents enhance gastrointestinal motility by increasing intestinal contractions. Prucalopride was approved by the US Food and Drug Administration (FDA) in 2018. Prucalopride is a selective 5-HT$_4$ agent. In a study of nursing home patients with high rates of cardiovascular disease, use of prucalopride was not associated with significant hemodynamic or electrocardiographic changes, including QT prolongation or bradycardia, compared to placebo. Other less selective 5-HT$_4$ agents have been associated with increased cardiovascular events, including QT prolongation and bradycardia.

6. Colonic secretagogues (increase intestinal fluid secretion)

a. Chloride channel activators—Lubiprostone is a chloride channel activator that improves motility in the intestine by increasing intestinal fluid secretion without altering serum electrolyte concentrations. Retrospective data from three pooled clinical trials of lubiprostone in older patients without significant comorbidities showed improvement in stool frequency and stool consistency and decreased straining compared to patients taking placebo. The side effects of this medication include nausea, diarrhea, headache, abdominal distention, and abdominal pain.

b. Guanylate cyclase-C receptor antagonists—Linaclotide is another colonic secretagogue that stimulates intestinal fluid secretion and transit. In two large trials of individuals with chronic idiopathic constipation, the linaclotide-treated groups had significantly higher rates of three or more complete spontaneous bowel movements per week and an increase in one or more complete spontaneous bowel movements from baseline during at least 9 of 12 weeks compared with placebo. The most common adverse event was diarrhea, which led to discontinuation of treatment in approximately 4% of patients. Plecanatide is another colonic secretagogue that was approved by the FDA in 2017 for chronic idiopathic constipation. It has a similar efficacy and safety profile to linaclotide.

c. Opioid antagonists—Peripherally acting mu-opioid receptor antagonists may have some role in the treatment of opiate-induced constipation (methylnaltrexone and naloxegol) and for short-term treatment of paralytic ileus (alvimopan).

Data are currently lacking in older adults. These medications act peripherally and do not cross the blood-brain barrier; thus, they do not affect the analgesic properties of opioids.

▶ Fecal Impaction

Constipation is an important factor in the development of fecal impaction in older adults, especially in those who have limited mobility in the community and in long-term care settings. Fecal impaction results from an individual's lack of ability to sense and respond to the presence of stool in the rectum. Mobility and decreased rectal sensation contribute to fecal impaction in older adults. Fecal impaction can cause increases in intraluminal pressure, leading to rectal ulceration, colitis, ischemia, or even perforation. Sustained dilation of the colon may cause megacolon and increased colonic secretions, which, in combination with decreased sphincter tone seen in older adults, can lead to incontinence and diarrhea. The presence of diarrhea and incontinence may cause the diagnosis of fecal impaction and underlying constipation to be missed.

To diagnosis fecal impaction, a digital rectal examination is essential. Although impacted stool may not be a hard consistency, the key to diagnosis is finding a large amount of stool in the rectum. Fecal impaction can also occur in the proximal rectum or sigmoid colon, which would not be detected on digital rectal examination. If fecal impaction is suspected, obtaining an abdominal radiograph may help identify the area of impaction.

The management of fecal impaction involves disimpaction and colon evacuation, followed by a maintenance bowel regimen. Digital disimpaction can be used to fragment a large amount of fecal material in the rectum. Following digital disimpaction, a warm-water enema with or without mineral oil may be used to soften the impaction and assist with emptying the remaining stool from the impacted area. Proximal fecal impactions may be treated with oral PEG solutions. If conservative measures with digital disimpaction and enemas fail, local anesthesia to relax the anal canal along with abdominal massage may be useful. If abdominal tenderness or bleeding occurs at any time, which may indicate bowel perforation or ischemia, surgery may be necessary.

Camilleri M, Beyens G, Kerstens R, Robinson P, Vandeplassche L. Safety assessment of prucalopride in elderly patients with constipation: a double-blind, placebo-controlled study. *Neurogastroenterol Motil.* 2009;21(12):1256-e117.

Farmer AD, Holt CB, Downes TJ, Ruggeri E, Del Vecchio S, De Giorgio R. Pathophysiology, diagnosis, and management of opioid-induced constipation. *Lancet Gastroenterol Hepatol.* 2018;3(3):203-212.

Gallegos-Orozco JF, Foxx-Orenstein AE, Sterler SM, Stoa JM. Chronic constipation in the elderly. *Am J Gastroenterol.* 2012;107(1):18-25.

Hayat U, Dugum M, Garg S. Chronic constipation: update on management. *Cleve Clin J Med.* 2017;84(5):397-408.

Mearin F, Lacy BE, Chang L, et al. Bowel disorders. *Gastroenterology.* 2016;18:pii: S0016-5085(16)00222-5.

Miller LE, Ouwehand AC. Probiotic supplementation decreases intestinal transit time: meta-analysis of randomized controlled trials. *World J Gastroenterol.* 2013;19(29):4718-4725.

Rao SSC, Valestin JA, Xiang X, Hamdy S, Bradley CS, Zimmerman MB. Home-based versus office-based biofeedback therapy for constipation with dyssynergic defecation: a randomized controlled trial. *Lancet Gastroenterol Hepatol.* 2018;3(11):768-777.

Sbahi H, Cash BD. Chronic constipation: a review of current literature. *Curr Gastroenterol Rep.* 2015;17(12):47.

Sommers T, Corban C, Sengupta N, et al. Emergency department burden of constipation in the United States from 2006 to 2011. *Am J Gastroenterol.* 2015;110(4):572-579.

Wald A. Constipation: advances in diagnosis and treatment. *JAMA.* 2016;315(2):185-191.

Voelker R. New chronic constipation medication. *JAMA.* 2019;321(5):444.

Benign Prostatic Hyperplasia & Lower Urinary Tract Symptoms

62

Scott R. Bauer, MD, MSc

Lindsay A. Hampson, MD, MAS

Lower urinary tract symptoms (LUTS) are common in older women and men and can have a significant impact on quality of life. The diagnostic evaluation and treatment plan of such conditions can be challenging for the primary care clinician, who must align the patients' goals of care with the risks and benefits of the available testing and treatment options. This chapter discusses two common causes of LUTS that frequently occur in older adults: benign prostatic hyperplasia (BPH) in men and overactive bladder (OAB) in both men and women.

BENIGN PROSTATIC HYPERPLASIA

ESSENTIALS OF DIAGNOSIS

▶ Symptoms of obstruction while voiding in men.

▶ An elevated American Urologic Association Symptom Index score with bothersome obstructive symptoms; establish baseline symptoms to monitor symptom trajectory and treatment efficacy.

▶ Absence of other diagnoses that might cause symptoms (eg, prostatitis or urinary tract infection [UTI]) as determined through a urinalysis.

General Principles

BPH remains a common condition in older men that can lead to diminished quality of life. Based on physician office visits, BPH affects 70% of men over age 60 and 80% of those over age 70. Although not all men with BPH will develop bothersome symptoms, many older men who are symptomatic underreport their symptoms to their clinicians and, therefore, are less likely to receive treatment for bothersome complaints.

Pathogenesis

BPH is a histologic diagnosis in which smooth muscle and epithelial cell proliferation in the prostatic transition zone can lead to LUTS via bladder outlet obstruction and increased smooth muscle tone and resistance.

Prevention

Data from observational studies suggest that men who maintain a healthy weight and exercise regularly are less likely to develop BPH; however, no randomized studies have been conducted to confirm these associations.

Clinical Findings

A. Symptoms & Signs

When patients develop clinically significant BPH, they typically complain of LUTS such as increased urinary hesitancy, straining, a weak urinary stream, and incomplete bladder emptying. In addition to these symptoms, BPH often presents with concurrent symptoms of overactivity, such as urgency and nocturia. Dysuria and hematuria are not commonly associated with BPH and may be an indication that another disease process is present.

The American Urological Association Symptom Index (AUASI; referred to interchangeably as the International Prostate Symptom Score [IPSS]) is a seven-item tool that health care providers can use to screen for symptomatic BPH as well as to assess a patient's LUTS severity. Individual item scores range from 0 for "not at all" to 5 for "almost always," with a total maximum score of 35 (Table 62–1). Symptoms such as incomplete emptying, a weak urinary stream, and straining with urination are particularly specific for obstructive symptoms that could be due to BPH. Scores of 1 to 7 are

Table 62–1. The American Urological Association (AUA) Symptom Index for BPH.

Patient Name:_____ DOB:_____ ID:_____ Date of assessment:_____

Initial Assessment ( ) Monitor during:_____ Therapy ( ) after:_____ Therapy/surgery ( )_____

AUA BPH Symptom Score							
	Not at all	**Less than 1 time in 5**	**Less than half the time**	**About half the time**	**More than half the time**	**Almost always**	
1. Over the past month, how often have you had a sensation of not emptying your bladder completely after you finished urinating?	0	1	2	3	4	5	
2. Over the past month, how often have you had to urinate again less than two hours after you finished urinating?	0	1	2	3	4	5	
3. Over the past month how often have you found you stopped and started again several times when you urinated?	0	1	2	3	4	5	
4. Over the past month, how often have you found it difficult to postpone urination?	0	1	2	3	4	5	
5. Over the past month, how often have you had a weak urinary stream?	0	1	2	3	4	5	
6. Over the past month, how often have you had to push or strain to begin urination?	0	1	2	3	4	5	
	None	**1 time**	**2 times**	**3 times**	**4 times**	**5 or more times**	
7. Over the past month, how many times did you most typically get up to urinate from the time you went to bed at night until the time you got up in the morning?	0	1	2	3	4	5	
					Total Symptom Score		

considered mild, 8 to 19 considered moderate, and 20 to 35 considered severe.

It is important to ask patients if they are bothered by their BPH symptoms; the IPSS is a validated questionnaire that includes the same questions as the AUASI as well as an additional question about patients' quality of life related to their urinary symptoms ("If you were to spend the rest of your life with your urinary condition the way it is now, how would you feel about that?"). It is also important to ask patients about concurrent urinary incontinence, which could be a sign of overflow incontinence or OAB leading to urgency urinary incontinence.

On physical examination, a digital rectal examination (DRE) may sometimes reveal a symmetrically enlarged prostate gland with a smooth and rubbery consistency. However, BPH may not be apparent on DRE in up to 52% of cases, and prostate size on DRE does not correlate with the severity of symptoms related to BPH. The finding of a nodule or irregular prostate may be concerning for prostate cancer, and in these cases, shared decision making should be used to discuss whether a potential workup for prostate cancer is in line with the patient's goals. If significant urinary retention has resulted from a critically enlarged prostate gland, a distended and tender bladder may be found during palpation of the abdomen.

B. Laboratory Findings

Guidelines recommend a urinalysis for any patient with bothersome LUTS in order to rule out reversible etiologies such as infection. There are no blood tests that confirm the presence of BPH. The American Urologic Association (AUA) does not recommend obtaining a serum prostate-specific antigen (PSA) level when patients present with LUTS. LUTS are not a common symptom of prostate cancer, and a decision of whether or not to perform prostate cancer screening should be made independently of LUTS.

C. Adjunctive Testing

Select patients may benefit from additional in-office testing such as uroflowmetry, which provides information about the patient's urinary stream, or a postvoid residual (PVR), which can be obtained via an ultrasound bladder scanner or catheterization and provides information about how well the patient is emptying their bladder. Typically, a patient with BPH will have a decreased maximum flow rate (Q_{max} <15 mL/s) on uroflow.

Differential Diagnosis

BPH manifests clinically as bladder outlet obstruction; therefore, other causes of bladder outlet obstruction, such as bladder stones, strictures, or scarring in the urethra or bladder neck, should be considered in the differential diagnosis. Men may also have weak urinary stream or urinary retention due to detrusor muscle dysfunction and bladder underactivity, which can be caused by diabetes, spinal cord injury, stroke, multiple sclerosis, Parkinson disease, or even chronic untreated BPH.

Differentiating between obstructive symptoms (more likely related to BPH) and irritative/storage symptoms (more likely related to overactivity) can be very helpful in determining treatment. OAB is a commonly missed cause of LUTS, particularly among older men with irritative/storage urinary symptoms such as urgency, frequency, and nocturia. Nocturia may also be caused by patients' fluid intake prior to bedtime, as well as medications they have been instructed to take at night. Consequently, asking patients to keep a voiding diary, where they record what types of beverages they drink at what time of day, along with the times they urinate and estimates of urine volume with each void, can help providers both identify the etiology and make treatment recommendations.

Medications should be considered in the differential diagnosis, particularly if the patient is taking diuretics, medications with anticholinergic side effects that might lead to urinary retention (eg, diphenhydramine), and nonprescription sympathomimetic decongestants that might exacerbate prostatic smooth muscle contraction (eg, pseudoephedrine). Increased urinary frequency, urgency, and nocturia may be presenting symptoms of type 2 diabetes mellitus, particularly in the setting of family history of diabetes and concomitant symptoms of polydipsia, polyphagia, and weight change.

If patients complain of dysuria, hematuria, fever, and chills, in addition to those symptoms more commonly seen in BPH, obtain a urinalysis and urine culture to rule out UTI. Prostatitis should be considered if patients complain of pain on ejaculation, the prostate is painful and edematous on palpation during DRE, and leukocytosis is seen on urinalysis. Nephrolithiasis should be considered when patients present with concomitant unilateral flank pain and hematuria (gross or microscopic).

Certain historical factors, signs, symptoms, and testing results should trigger an immediate referral of the patient with LUTS to urology for further evaluation. These include a history of recurrent UTIs, prostate or bladder cancer, history or risk of urethral strictures, underlying neurologic disease that could be associated with a neurogenic bladder, persistent or recurrent urinary retention (PVR >150 mL in older adults), renal compromise due to urinary retention, a palpable bladder on exam, abnormal DRE findings that are suspicious for prostate cancer, and hematuria.

Complications

Bladder outlet obstruction due to BPH may lead to urinary retention, which is associated with the development of recurrent UTIs, bladder stones, bladder diverticuli, and chronic kidney disease if left untreated. Long-standing urinary retention can also lead to bladder dysfunction such as underactive or overactive bladder.

 ESSENTIALS OF TREATMENT

▶ Treatment decisions should be based on shared decision making with patients based on the level of bother and risk/benefit profile for all treatment options.

▶ Conservative therapies include modifying fluid intake as well as timed and double voiding.

▶ The two mainstays of BPH medical therapy includes α-adrenergic blockers and 5α-reductase inhibitors.

▶ Surgical interventions should be considered for patients who have bothersome symptoms that are refractory to other therapies or complications of BPH.

Treatment

Severity of LUTS due to BPH should guide treatment recommendations. Patients with mild symptoms (AUASI/IPSS score 0–7) or those who report minimal bother may experience improvement from conservative therapies alone, and there is no evidence to support the use of medications in this setting. Given that BPH is known to progress with age, patients should also be monitored for worsening of symptoms (ie, watchful waiting) that might warrant medical or surgical intervention. Patients with moderate to severe symptoms (AUASI/IPSS score 8–35) warrant additional treatment beyond conservative therapies to improve their symptoms. Primary care clinicians can initiate and manage medical therapy for BPH, although patients with symptoms refractory to medical management, with BPH complications, or who are interested in discussing surgical options should be referred to a urologist.

A. Conservative Therapies

Behavioral modifications are the first-line treatment for any patient with BPH. Patients should be counseled about minimizing intake of caffeinated and alcoholic beverages, reducing excessive daytime fluid intake, and eliminating nighttime fluid intake. Patients can also be instructed to urinate on a timed voiding schedule (every 3–4 hours, even if they do not have the sensation to urinate) and perform double voiding (void twice in a row to empty any residual urine that remains after a first void).

B. Herbal Therapy

Patients may inquire about using complementary and alternative medicines to treat BPH symptoms. Several products are currently available for over-the-counter purchase, including supplements containing saw palmetto (*Serenoa repens*), β-sitosterols, and stinging nettle (*Urtica dioica*). Many herbal remedies have been evaluated for use in treating BPH, but none have shown efficacy in clinical trials when compared to placebo. One of the most commonly used, saw palmetto, was found to have no benefit when compared to placebo in a Cochrane review evaluating 32 randomized clinical trials. It is important to note that these herbal supplements are not regulated by the US Food and Drug Administration (FDA) and may have significant variation in the active ingredients.

C. Medical Therapy

Two main classes of medications are used for BPH: α-adrenergic blockers and 5α-reductase inhibitors.

α-Adrenergic blockers have been found to improve BPH symptoms significantly when compared to placebo, largely through inhibition of prostatic smooth muscle contraction in the urethra and bladder neck that results in improved urine flow. Common side effects include orthostatic hypotension, headaches, retrograde ejaculation, rhinitis, and dizziness. First-generation formulations (eg, prazosin and phenoxybenzamine) are no longer recommended due to higher risks of adverse events. Second-generation agents (eg, terazosin and doxazosin) require titration to effect, starting at 1 mg and titrating upward as tolerated if needed for better symptom control. Third-generation agents (eg, tamsulosin, alfuzosin, and silodosin) are more selective for the α_1-receptors in the prostate, may cause fewer systemic side effects, and require less titration. However, comparative effectiveness studies of different α-blockers are limited. An association between α-blocker use and intraoperative floppy iris syndrome (IFIS) is reported in the literature, with the highest risk observed among patients taking tamsulosin as compared to other α-blockers. Therefore, initiation of α-blocker therapy should be postponed until after any planned cataract surgeries. IFIS is associated with prior use of α-blockers at any time; thus, discontinuing α-blocker therapy prior to cataract surgery is not effective in preventing IFIS.

5α-Reductase inhibitors have been shown in clinical trials to improve maximum urinary flow rates and reduce rates of urinary retention and BPH surgery. This class of medications works through blocking the conversion of testosterone to dihydrotestosterone, which results in prostate volume reduction. Importantly, patients should be counseled prior to initiating treatment that these medications take 3 to 6 months to reach full efficacy and, thus, should not be used for short-term symptom improvement. Two medications in this class are currently available—finasteride (dosed at 5 mg daily) and dutasteride (dosed at 0.5 mg daily)—and efficacy appears to be similar with both medications. Side effects include sexual dysfunction (particularly ejaculatory disorders), gynecomastia, breast tenderness, and rash. Of note, finasteride cannot be crushed and thus can only be given to patients who are able to swallow pills. Dutasteride has a half-life of 5 weeks, so associated adverse side effects may last longer compared to finasteride.

Combination therapy with both α-blockers and 5α-reductase inhibitors has been shown to result in larger improvements in AUASI/IPSS scores, as well as slightly reduced rates of composite outcomes including acute urinary retention, renal insufficiency, recurrent UTIs, and urinary incontinence.

In addition to α-blockers and 5α-reductase inhibitors, there are other medications that can be used to treat LUTS due to BPH. One newer class of FDA-approved medications to treat BPH is daily use of phosphodiesterase type 5 inhibitors, such as tadalafil (dosed at 5 mg daily). While these medications are typically used to treat erectile dysfunction, improvements in LUTS have been observed in patients with both BPH and erectile dysfunction. Studies have shown that improvement in AUASI/IPSS occurs within 4 weeks of initiating therapy. Common side effects include headache, dyspepsia, and flushing.

Lastly, medications such as anticholinergics and β_3-adrenoceptor agonists can be used to treat irritative/storage symptoms that can occur with BPH due to detrusor overactivity (see "Overactive Bladder" section later in this chapter).

D. Surgical Therapy

In the event that medical therapy does not improve patients' LUTS or patients want to discuss surgical interventions, they should be referred to a urologist. Surgical therapy is also indicated when patients have BPH-related complication, such as renal insufficiency, recurrent UTIs, and bladder stones or gross hematuria caused by BPH. Multiple surgical options exist, including open simple prostatectomy, transurethral resection of the prostate, transurethral incision of the prostate, transurethral vaporization of the prostate, photoselective vaporization of the prostate, prostatic urethral lift, transurethral microwave therapy, water vapor thermal therapy, and laser enucleation. The choice of surgical approach will depend on the patient's presentation, anatomy, and prostate size; the urologist's experience with the different surgical techniques; the patient's ability to tolerate the procedure based on the patient's preexisting comorbid conditions; and the patient's preferences based on the risk-to-benefit profiles of each individual surgical option. Urologists may determine prostate volume prior to surgical therapy via ultrasound (either transabdominal or transrectal), cystoscopy, or previous cross-sectional imaging; however, routine use of imaging studies to diagnose BPH is currently not recommended. Although there are some minimally invasive therapies now available that may have fewer side effects, such as UroLift (prostatic urethral lift procedure) and Rezum (water vapor thermal therapy procedure), data are not yet available on long-term outcomes and comparative effectiveness with existing therapies. Transurethral needle ablation and prostate artery embolization are not recommended for the treatment of BPH based on the AUA guidelines.

▶ Prognosis

Increased mortality associated with BPH occurs only when complications arise (eg, acute kidney failure or UTI), usually related to chronic urinary retention or severe adverse events related to medical or surgical therapies. The presence of BPH in itself is not associated with increased mortality.

OVERACTIVE BLADDER

 ESSENTIALS OF DIAGNOSIS

▶ Diagnosis based on presence of urinary urgency with or without frequency, nocturia, or incontinence.

▶ Absence of other diagnoses that might cause symptoms (eg, UTI, volume overload states, diabetes).

▶ Establish baseline symptoms with AUASI/IPSS or Overactive Bladder Symptom Score in order to monitor symptom trajectory and treatment efficacy.

▶ General Principles

OAB is a symptom-based diagnosis defined by urinary urgency in the absence of secondary causes such as UTI or other bladder pathology. Urgency is defined as a sudden desire to urinate with the sensation of difficulty postponing urination. Other common symptoms of OAB include urinary frequency, nocturia, and urge urinary incontinence ("wet OAB"; see Chapter 10, "Urinary Incontinence"). OAB affects 45% to 51% of women and 34% to 49% of men over age 65 and is associated with falls, psychiatric conditions such as anxiety and depression, social isolation, and poor quality of life.

▶ Pathogenesis

Age-related changes in bladder function include neurologic, anatomic, and biochemical alterations, which may cause OAB symptoms. These include heightened sensory perception, bladder ischemia leading to nerve and smooth muscle damage, neuronal signaling changes, inflammation, and hormonal effects. Detrusor muscle overactivity can cause OAB symptoms; however, not all patients with OAB have detrusor overactivity identified during invasive urodynamic testing.

▶ Prevention

Data from observational studies suggest that avoidance of excessive fluid and caffeine intake may prevent LUTS from OAB; however, no randomized studies have been conducted to confirm these associations.

▶ Clinical Findings

A. Symptoms & Signs

Patients with OAB will complain of LUTS, particularly urgency, frequency, or nocturia. Urinary incontinence, particularly urgency related (urine leakage associated with the symptom of urgency), may also be present and should be screened for. Dysuria and hematuria are not associated with OAB, and if present, more extensive workup for alternative diagnoses is indicated. Many chronic conditions can manifest as LUTS and mimic OAB; therefore, a comprehensive medical history is an important component of the evaluation. A genitourinary history should be collected to evaluate for history of recurrent UTIs, urinary retention, urologic surgery, or pelvic exposure to radiation. On physical examination, abdominal, genitourinary, pelvic, and rectal examination as well as a volume assessment should be completed for patients with new LUTS due to suspected OAB. Lower extremity edema or other signs of volume overload, neurologic deficits, stool impaction, distended bladder, atrophic vaginitis or urethritis, and pelvic organ prolapse are all potential exam findings that point toward alternative causes of irritative/storage LUTS.

B. Laboratory Findings

All patients with suspected OAB should be tested with a urinalysis to rule out infection or proteinuria. If symptoms or urinalysis are concerning for UTI, a urine culture should be sent.

C. Adjunctive Testing

If the diagnosis is uncertain, the AUASI/IPSS questionnaire (see earlier "Benign Prostate Hyperplasia" section) can be used to try to differentiate between obstructive and overactive symptoms. There are also several questionnaires that have been validated to assess baseline OAB symptoms and

Table 62–2. The Overactive Bladder Symptom Score (OABSS) for urinary storage symptoms.

| Patient Name:_____ DOB:_____ |
| ID:_____ Date of assessment:_____ |
| Initial Assessment ( ) Monitor during:_____ |
| Therapy ( ) after:_____ Therapy/surgery ( )_____ |

	Response	Score
1. How many times do you typically urinate from waking in the morning until sleeping at night?	≤7	0
	8–14	1
	≥15	2
2. How many times do you typically wake up to urinate from sleeping at night until waking in the morning?	0	0
	1	1
	2	2
	≥3	3
3. How often do you have a sudden desire to urinate, which is difficult to defer?	None	0
	Less than once a week	1
	Once a week or more	2
	About once a day	3
	2–4 times a day	4
	≥5 times a day	5
4. How often do you leak urine because you cannot defer the sudden desire to urinate?	None	0
	Less than once a week	1
	Once a week or more	2
	About once a day	3
	2–4 times a day	4
	≥5 times a day	5

Patients are instructed to circle the score that best applied to their urinary condition during the past week; the overall score is the sum of the four scores.

monitor response to therapy if a diagnosis of OAB is suspected, such as the four-item Overactive Bladder Symptom Score (OABSS) (Table 62–2). OABSS scores range from 0 to 15 and indicate mild (0–5), moderate (6–11), or severe (12–15) symptoms. Voiding diaries provide additional information regarding frequency and volume of voids, symptom triggers, fluid intake, and polyuria. We recommend patients fill out a voiding diary for three complete 24-hour periods and record hourly fluid intake (type, volume), volume voided, leakage, and urgency. An example voiding diary can be found at http://www.urologyhealth.org/educational-materials/bladder-diary. It is also important to assess patients' bother related to their OAB symptoms.

There are no imaging studies indicated for OAB workup. However, a PVR can be useful to assess for incomplete bladder emptying for patients with diabetes, spinal cord injury, and symptoms of retention or men with BPH, as well as to determine the safety of certain OAB treatments. Urodynamics, cystoscopy, and diagnostic bladder or renal ultrasounds should not be used in the initial workup of uncomplicated OAB.

D. Special Tests

Cognitive impairment is an important risk factor and mediator of LUTS due to OAB and will influence management decisions, particularly given that many of the medical therapies used for OAB have potential cognitive side effects. Therefore, screening for cognitive impairment in older adults with new OAB symptoms should be strongly considered.

▶ Differential Diagnosis

The differential diagnosis for irritative/storage LUTS includes many medical conditions in addition to OAB and overlaps with the conditions listed earlier for BPH. UTI is the most common mimicker of OAB and should be excluded in all patients before initiating treatment. Medications should be considered, including diuretics, cholinesterase inhibitors, and, when urinary retention is present, anticholinergics, opioids, and calcium channel blockers. Constipation is a common reversible cause of LUTS in older adults. Atrophic vaginitis or urethritis due to estrogen deficiency can exacerbate symptoms in older women. Among men, BPH should be considered for LUTS consistent with obstruction.

LUTS, particularly irritative/storage symptoms, can be caused by any disease that affects cognitive or sensory functions, such as stroke, dementia, multiple sclerosis, spinal stenosis or cord injury, and peripheral neuropathy. Diabetes is a particularly common cause of LUTS due to osmotic diuresis and polyuria directly from hyperglycemia as well as diabetic complications such as neuropathy and neurogenic bladder. Cardiovascular diseases, such as heart failure and venous insufficiency, can cause LUTS via volume overload, redistribution while supine, and diuretic therapy. Sleep apnea and other sleep disorders can cause nocturia. Psychiatric conditions, such as anxiety and depression, can both cause LUTS and exacerbate symptoms due to other causes.

Certain historical factors, signs, symptoms, and testing results should trigger an immediate referral of the patient with LUTS to urology for further evaluation. These include a history of recurrent UTIs, bladder cancer, bladder pain, underlying neurologic disease that could be associated with a neurogenic bladder, persistent or recurrent urinary retention (PVR >150 mL in adults), renal compromise suspected due to urinary retention, a palpable bladder on exam, and hematuria. In men, red flags include history of prostate cancer or abnormal DRE findings and elevated PSA levels that are suspicious for prostate cancer.

▶ Complications

OAB may progress to urgency urinary incontinence, which is associated with functional decline, loss of independence, and disability. However, most serious complications related to OAB are due to the impact of OAB on quality of life as well as adverse events related to medical or surgical treatments.

ESSENTIALS OF TREATMENT

► Treatment decisions should be based on shared decision making with patients based on the level of bother and risk/benefit profile for all treatment options.

► First-line treatments include behavioral (eg, bladder training, fluid management, and pelvic physical therapy) and lifestyle modification.

► Medical therapy for OAB includes antimuscarinics and β_3-adrenoreceptor agonists; however, these medications must be used carefully in older adults due to potential drug interactions and side effects.

► Surgical or procedural interventions should be considered for patients who have bothersome symptoms and who are refractory to or cannot receive other therapies due to side effects.

▶ Treatment

While receiving treatment for bothersome OAB, patients should be regularly monitored for efficacy using a standardized symptom questionnaire (eg, AUASI/IPSS or OABSS) and evaluated for adverse events related to treatment. For nonbothersome LUTS due to OAB, watchful waiting and reassessment is a reasonable approach since this is not a life-threatening, progressive, or irreversible disease, and delaying treatment can minimize the exposure to polypharmacy or therapies with potential side effects.

A. Behavioral Treatments (First Line)

First-line treatment for OAB includes patient education and behavioral and lifestyle modification. Patient education regarding normal lower urinary tract function, OAB natural history, and treatments can be helpful in determining necessity for treatment and setting treatment expectations. Behavioral interventions such as bladder training (timed voiding and urge suppression techniques), fluid management, and pelvic floor physical therapy, with or without biofeedback, are effective at reducing urgency symptoms, reducing urgency urinary incontinence episodes, and improving quality of life. Referral to a pelvic physical therapist experienced in pelvic floor muscle training can be helpful and typically starts with 8 to 12 sessions, assessing response, and continuing exercises at home if effective. The patient's functional and cognitive status, environment, and caregiver support should be considered prior to recommending these interventions.

Modest weight loss for women who are overweight or obese with "wet OAB" or urgency urinary incontinence and physical activity for sedentary older women are both effective treatments to reduce the number of urinary incontinence episodes, although it remains unknown whether these are effective treatments for older women with OAB without incontinence or men. Other lifestyle interventions, such as avoiding dietary bladder irritants (eg, spicy or acidic foods, alcohol, and caffeine), can be recommended for motivated patients, although high-quality evidence for these interventions is lacking. Fluid restriction is sometimes recommended for younger patients but may not be appropriate for frail older adults.

Comparative effectiveness randomized trials indicate that behavioral interventions are either equivalent or superior to medication for reducing urinary frequency, nocturia, and urgency urinary incontinence episodes, and improving quality of life. However, some patients do not obtain satisfactory symptom control from behavior therapy alone and require combination therapy with both behavioral modification and medication.

B. Pharmacotherapy (Second Line)

For patients who have failed behavioral therapy or with significantly bothersome symptoms, medication can be started immediately or added to existing therapies. However, given the significant side effect profile of most medications for OAB, cognitive impairment screening should be done prior to initiating therapy. Medications may not be appropriate for all patients. When starting medications for OAB in older adults, clinicians should prescribe the lowest dose possible, monitor closely for side effects, and up-titrate slowly.

Antimuscarinic therapy is the most common and well-studied medication for OAB and inhibits inappropriate bladder, or detrusor, muscle contractions via blockage of acetylcholine at the detrusor neuromuscular junctions. Compared to placebo, antimuscarinic therapy has been demonstrated to reduce urgency as well as number of daily voids and urinary incontinence episodes. Comparative effectiveness studies have shown no difference in efficacy between the antimuscarinic medications used to treat OAB, including oxybutynin, tolterodine, fesoterodine, solifenacin, darifenacin, and trospium. When considering antimuscarinic therapy, it is important to identify patients with contraindications such as other medications with antimuscarinic properties, which are common in older adults. Antimuscarinic load can be estimated using the Anticholinergic Burden Scale (example can be found at https://americandeliriumsociety.org/resources/tools); common contributors in older adults include warfarin, ranitidine, digoxin, codeine, and diazepam. Common side effects of antimuscarinic medications include dry eyes, dry mouth, constipation, blurry vision, dyspepsia, urinary retention, and impaired cognitive function. AUA guidelines currently recommended against prescribing medications for OAB to frail older adults due to risk of progressive cognitive impairment. Patients with pre-existing cognitive impairment or dementia should also avoid antimuscarinic therapy. The transdermal formulation of oxybutynin may have a lower risk of cognitive impairment and first-pass metabolism. Trospium is considered the least likely formulation to cause cognitive impairment due to hydrophilic properties that decrease blood-brain barrier crossing. Extended-release formulations are also less likely to cause some side effects, such as dry mouth. If patients experience poor symptom control or bothersome side effects related to the use of antimuscarinic medication, options include management of the side effect (eg, treatment of constipation or dry mouth), dose reduction, trial of another antimuscarinic medication, or switching to a β_3-adrenoreceptor agonist before abandoning oral therapy altogether. It is important to note that antimuscarinic medications should not be used in patients with narrow-angle glaucoma unless approved by an ophthalmologist and should be used with caution in patients with impaired gastric emptying or a history of urinary retention.

Oral β_3-adrenoreceptor agonists, of which mirabegron is the only current FDA-approved formulation, work through relaxation of the detrusor muscle of the bladder by decreasing the sensation for urination and by increasing bladder storage volumes, although the exact mechanism is not known. Studies have shown that patients randomized to β_3-adrenoreceptor agonist therapy are more likely to experience improvements in mean voided volume, urgency, nocturia, and number of incontinence episodes. However, achieving complete continence occurred in less than half of patients regardless of intervention arm (44%–46% in β_3-adrenoreceptor agonist group compared to 38% in placebo group). This class of medications has been found to have fewer antimuscarinic side effects, particularly dry mouth, but has not been evaluated specifically in older frail adults or those with cognitive impairment. Mild increases in blood pressure and heart rate are also reported side effects, β_3 receptors are also expressed in the vasculature and heart, although these physiologic changes appear small and can be monitored after initiation of β_3-adrenoreceptor agonist therapy.

AUA guidelines currently recommended using caution if prescribing any medication type for OAB to older adults with frailty, cognitive impairment, or dementia. OAB medications in this population may also have a lower therapeutic benefit and higher chance of adverse events, and typically these medications are not studied in frail older adults.

C. Procedures & Surgical Interventions (Third Line)

Patients with bothersome symptoms refractory to behavioral and medical therapy should be referred to a urologist for further evaluation. Procedural treatments for OAB should be performed by a specialist and include peripheral tibial nerve stimulation (PTNS), sacral neuromodulation (SNM), and intradetrusor botulinum toxin.

PTNS involves using an acupuncture-type needle along the posterior tibial nerve to create neuropathic feedback to the bladder. The posterior tibial nerve contains fibers from spinal roots L4–S3 and sacral nerves of the pelvic floor and bladder. PTNS is typically administered as an in-office treatment for 30 minutes once or twice a week for 12 weeks followed by maintenance treatments as indicated. Although limited studies have been conducted among older adults, PTNS generally has fewer side effects and a similar objective and subjective success rate to pharmacotherapy. The biggest barrier to PTNS for older, and particularly frail, adults is the frequency of treatments.

SNM involves electrical stimulation of the S3 nerve root through placement of a lead that contains electrodes in the sacrum during a short surgical procedure. The lead is then connected to an implantable pulse generator, which is permanently placed under the skin of the upper buttock if symptom improvement (>50% improvement in urgency, frequency, or urge incontinence) is noted. The exact mechanism of the feedback signaling is not known. Studies have shown that >50% symptomatic improvement with SNM is reported by 68% of patients with urgency urinary incontinence and 56% of patients with frequency and urgency. Patient satisfaction with this procedure is reportedly high (>90%). However, some small studies have suggested that older adults are less likely to achieve complete remission of urgency urinary incontinence after treatment compared to younger patients. Side effects include pain at lead or pulse generator site, lead migration, infection, and need for surgical revision. SNM does require participation from the patient (ie, the patient must have sufficient cognitive ability to optimize the device), requires special screening at airport security, and is not compatible with magnetic resonance imaging scans, which are factors that should be considered before pursuing this option based on patient characteristics. In addition, the device does require replacement periodically, which entails another short surgical procedure.

Lastly, intradetrusor botulinum toxin is another third-line treatment for OAB. In this procedure, onabotulinumtoxinA (100–300 units) is injected into the bladder detrusor muscle via cystoscopic injection; this can be done as an in-clinic procedure or under intravenous sedation in the operating room depending on patient and clinician preference. Botulinum toxin works through inhibition of calcium-mediated release of acetylcholine in peripheral nerve endings, resulting in muscle relaxation. The effects of botulinum toxin are temporary, typically lasting between 4 and 6 months. Studies have shown three- to four-fold reductions in urinary incontinence episodes with onabotulinumtoxinA compared to placebo. Side effects include UTI and urinary retention (~6%); all patients receiving onabotulinumtoxinA must be counseled about assessment of PVR after treatment to evaluate for urinary retention and the possible need for temporary clean intermittent catheterization after the procedure if severe urinary retention occurs. The effects of onabotulinumtoxinA wear off, so the complication of urinary retention is usually temporary; however, this also means that periodic injections (typically every 6 months) are needed to maintain efficacy for patients who find the treatment effective.

Other interventions for refractory OAB include an indwelling catheter (eg, a urethral foley catheter or suprapubic tube) or surgery, such as urinary diversion and augmentation cystoplasty. These interventions are typically considered as a last resort and are not recommended as a typical management strategy for OAB, particularly among older adults with frailty or multimorbidity.

▶ Prognosis

OAB is not associated with mortality. Follow-up should be conducted to monitor treatment compliance, symptom improvement, and side effects. Medications that do not improve symptoms and/or bother should be discontinued given their side effect profiles. Although OAB is persistent or progressive in most older adults, LUTS due to OAB spontaneously may resolve in approximately 10% to 30% of cases.

Berry SJ, Coffey DS, Walsh PC, Ewing LL. The development of human benign prostatic hyperplasia with age. *J Urol.* 1984;132(3):474-479.

Burton C, Sajja A, Latthe PM. Effectiveness of percutaneous posterior tibial nerve stimulation for overactive bladder: a systematic review and meta-analysis. *Neurourol Urodyn.* 2012;31(8):1206-1216.

Chapple C, Sievert KD, MacDiarmid S, et al. OnabotulinumtoxinA 100 U significantly improves all idiopathic overactive bladder symptoms and quality of life in patients with overactive bladder and urinary incontinence: a randomised, double-blind, placebo-controlled trial. *Eur Urol.* 2013;64(2):249-256.

Gormley EA, Lightner DJ, Faraday M, Vasavada SP. Diagnosis and treatment of overactive bladder (non-neurogenic) in adults: AUA/SUFU guideline amendment. *J Urol.* 2015;193(5):1572-1580.

Gray SL, Anderson ML, Dublin S, et al. Cumulative use of strong anticholinergics and incident dementia: a prospective cohort study. *JAMA Intern Med.* 2015;175(3):401-407.

Kadow BT, Tyagi P, Chermansky CJ. Neurogenic causes of detrusor underactivity. *Curr Bladder Dysfunct Rep.* 2015;10(4):325-331.

McVary KT, Roehrborn CG, Avins AL, et al. Update on AUA guideline on the management of benign prostatic hyperplasia. *J Urol.* 2011;185(5):1793-1803.

Pratt TS, Suskind AM. Management of overactive bladder in older women. *Curr Urol Rep.* 2018;19(11):92.

Tacklind J, Fink HA, MacDonald R, Rutks I, Wilt TJ. Finasteride for benign prostatic hyperplasia. *Cochrane Database Syst Rev.* 2010;10:CD006015.

Tacklind J, Macdonald R, Rutks I, Stanke JU, Wilt TJ. Serenoa repens for benign prostatic hyperplasia. *Cochrane Database Syst Rev.* 2012;12:CD001423.

Persistent Pain

Tessa Rife, PharmD, BCGP

Brook Calton, MD, MHS

► General Principles

Persistent pain is defined as pain that continues beyond the expected healing time, usually longer than 3 months. Persistent pain is widely prevalent in older adults. Up to 50% of community-dwelling older adults report pain that has a negative impact on function; a similar percentage of nursing home residents report experiencing daily pain. Pain from musculoskeletal disorders including back pain and arthritis, neuropathy, and pain related to chronic conditions such as congestive heart failure, chronic obstructive pulmonary disease, and end-stage renal disease are most common. Persistent pain may or may not be associated with identifiable underlying pathology or may be out of proportion to the pathology observed. Older adults are at risk for undertreatment of pain due to underreport of pain, variable presentations of pain, cognitive impairment, and unconscious bias.

Pain limits functional status in older adults, can amplify frailty, and can result in diminished quality of life or appetite, sleep disturbances, falls, social isolation, depression, delirium, and increased health care costs and resource utilization. Relief of suffering and promotion of patient dignity are primary tenets of the practice of medicine. Timely and effective assessment and management of persistent pain in older adults will help in alleviating their suffering, while maintaining and augmenting quality of life.

► Evaluation

A. Key Principles

A thorough assessment is a necessary first step. Any pain that affects function or quality of life should be evaluated. Specific goals of the pain assessment include determining the type and cause of the pain; understanding the impact of the pain on the patient's daily life including function, sleep, emotional well-being, and safety; identifying chronic conditions influencing pain; and reviewing patient and caregiver beliefs, attitudes, and expectations toward the pain.

B. History

The patient's and/or caregiver's description of pain is likely to be the highest yield information to formulate a treatment plan. During history taking, it is critical to attend to any communication deficits the patient may be experiencing, including hearing, vision, and cognition. Strategies include using a pocket-talker for those with decreased hearing, selecting appropriate pain assessment scales for those with decreased vision, observing for behaviors that may indicate pain, and relying more heavily on caregiver report for those with cognitive impairment. It is important to remember that older adults are more likely to underreport pain than their younger counterparts due to misconceptions that pain is a natural part of aging, a reluctance to burden their clinician or caregiver with a complaint of pain, or not wanting to detract from the clinician's attention on other medical concerns. Older adults may also use different descriptors for their pain than younger adults (eg, aching, soreness, or discomfort).

When discussing pain, clinicians should assess pain location(s), radiation, timing, onset, and quality; alleviating and exacerbating factors; and associated neurologic symptoms.

During the initial encounter and follow-up assessments, the importance of understanding the impact of the patient's pain on their function cannot be overstated. Function includes the patient's ability to attend to activities of daily living, as well as their energy, sleep, and ability to engage in pleasurable and social activities. Function can be used to inform the aggressiveness of initial interventions, to develop patient-centered treatment goals (eg, with improved pain control, the patient should be able to walk three more blocks than at present), and to monitor the effectiveness of interventions. Suggested questions listed in Table 63–1 can help

Table 63–1. Suggested questions about the impact of pain on function and quality of life.

Social and recreational functioning: How often do you participate in pleasurable activities, such as hobbies, going out to movies or concerts, socializing with friends, and travel? Over the past week, how often has pain interfered with these activities?

Mood, affect, and anxiety: Has pain interfered with your energy, mood, or personality? Are you readily tearful?

Relationships: Has pain affected relationships with family members/significant others/friends/colleagues?

Occupation: Has the pain required that you modify your work responsibilities and/or hours? When was the last time you worked, and (if applicable) why have you stopped working?

Sleep: Does pain interfere with your sleep? How often over the past week?

Exercise: How often do you do some sort of exercise? Over the past week, how often has pain interfered with your ability to exercise?

From Rosenquist EWK. Evaluation of chronic pain in older adults. Aronson MD, ed. UpToDate. Waltham, MA: UpToDate Inc. https://www.uptodate.com. Accessed on July 27, 2019.

clinicians determine the impact of pain on a patient's function and quality of life.

Standardized pain assessment tools can provide additional information beyond what is gathered by history and physical exam. Pain assessment scales can be unidimensional, typically a single item that relates to pain intensity, or multidimensional, attempting to measure pain in a variety of domains, including the intensity, location, and effect. Although more time intensive, multidimensional scales can provide a wealth of information about the patient's unique experience of pain. Choice of scale may depend on the presence of language or sensory impairment, patient health literacy, numeracy, and practical considerations such as time requirements. It is important to use the same assessment across visits with the patient to monitor trends over time.

Regarding unidimensional scales, the Numeric Rating Scale and the FACES Pain Scale are effective. The patient is asked to rate pain by assigning a numerical value (with zero indicating no pain and 10 representing the worst pain imaginable) or a facial expression corresponding to the pain. Older adults, especially those with limited English proficiency or with cognitive impairment, may be unable or unwilling to use numbers to describe their pain. The Wong-Baker FACES Pain Rating Scale with Foreign Translations is useful for both English- and non–English-speaking patients.

Regarding multidimensional scales, the Pain, Enjoyment, and General Activity (PEG) scale is a brief, multidimensional pain measurement tool with a focus on function (Figure 63–1). The PEG should be administered on initial assessment and then completed at each subsequent assessment. It has demonstrated reliability and validity in older adults with persistent pain.

Patients with limited verbal or cognitive abilities, including those with cognitive impairment, dementia, delirium, and some stroke syndromes, pose challenges to accurate pain assessment. Fortunately, data suggest that older adults with mild to moderate cognitive impairment can rate pain reliably and validly using a combination of history and the scales discussed earlier. For patients with more severe cognitive impairment and/or for those who are nonverbal, no pain scales have been reliably validated. However, the following techniques recommended by the American Society for Pain Management Nursing can be helpful: (1) obtain a self-report from the patient if at all possible; (2) investigate for possible pathologies that could produce pain; (3) observe for patient behaviors during the visit and through history from the patient's caregivers that may indicate pain (eg, agitation, restlessness, irritability); (4) obtain a history from the patient's caregiver whenever possible (data suggest caregivers have limited ability to accurately estimate pain intensity but can be an excellent source of information regarding patient behavior, medication history, and aggravating and alleviating factors); and (5) consider an analgesic trial to see if potentially associated behaviors diminish with pain management. Scheduling a medication several times per day (eg, low-dose acetaminophen), at a safe dose, will likely prove most effective.

C. Physical Exam

A physical exam should be conducted to inform the differential diagnosis, identify chronic conditions, and confirm treatment targets. Routine vital signs should be performed alongside a physical exam that focuses on the musculoskeletal and neurologic systems. Focal muscle weakness, abnormal reflexes, sensory impairment, or atrophy may represent damage to the central or peripheral nervous system. Mobility should be evaluated as part of the exam given the association between pain and fall risk. This assessment should include self-report and in-office assessments such as gait speed, tests of balance, and the timed up and go test (see Chapter 6, "Falls & Mobility Impairment").

D. Imaging

Diagnostic imaging is often overused, and when used inappropriately, it puts older adults at risk for incidental findings that trigger diagnostic cascades, unnecessary procedures, and significant expense. Informing patients of findings that may be benign can result in unintended harms related to labeling, often causing patients to experience increased anxiety and to focus on symptoms that may be minor, and ultimately may lead to avoidance of exercise or activities due to fear of worsening or causing structural damage. Furthermore, the severity of imaging findings does not always correlate to the degree of pain. In general, imaging should be considered when there is a high suspicion for a disease that would benefit

PEG Scale Assessing Pain Intensity and Interference (Pain, Enjoyment, General Activity)

1. What number best describes your <u>pain on average</u> in the past week?

0	1	2	3	4	5	6	7	8	9	10
No Pain							Pain as bad as you can imagine			

1. What number best describes how, during the past week, pain has interfered with your <u>enjoyment of life</u>?

0	1	2	3	4	5	6	7	8	9	10
Does not interfere									Completely interferes	

1. What number best describes how, during the past week, pain has interfered with your <u>general activity</u>?

0	1	2	3	4	5	6	7	8	9	10
Does not interfere									Completely interferes	

Computing the PEG Score.
Add the responses to the three questions, then divide by three to get a mean score (out of 10) on overall impact of points.

Using the PEG Score.
The score is best used to track an individual's changes over time. The initiation of therapy should result in the individual's score decreasing over time.

Source.
Krebs, E.E., Lorenz, K. A., Bair, M. J., Damush, T. M., Wu, J., Sutherland, J. M., Asch S, Kroenke, K. (2009). Development and Initial Validation of the PEG, a Three-item Scale Assessing Pain Intensity and Interference. Journal of General Internal Medicine, 24(6), 733-738. http://doi.org/10.1007/s11606-009-0981-1

▲ **Figure 63–1.** PEG (Pain, Enjoyment, General Activity) Scale assessing pain intensity and interference. (Data from US Department of Health and Human Services. Centers for Disease Control and Prevention. Checklist for prescribing opioids for chronic pain. https://www.cdc.gov/drugoverdose/pdf/pdo_checklist-a.pdf.)

from specialized intervention (eg, hip pain indicative of hip fracture) or there are red flag signs or symptoms such as fever, unexplained weight loss, or new pain in a patient with a history of cancer that may signal underlying pathology.

▶ Management

A. Key Principles

The United States is undergoing a major cultural shift in the way persistent pain is viewed and managed. The biomedical model of pain care, which was widely accepted during the 1990s and early 2000s, focused on fixing or numbing pain with medications, surgery, or other medical interventions.

Pain became the fifth vital sign, and opioids were used for the treatment of persistent pain. We now have data that opioids are associated with risks for harm and are unlikely to provide long-term relief in persistent pain. We have come to appreciate that persistent pain is a complex, multidimensional experience, often better treated with multimodal and integrated care approaches that attend to each individual patient's physical, social, cultural, and spiritual dimensions.

Clinicians should consider a patient-centric approach to managing persistent pain, incorporating each individual's capabilities, needs, goals, and preferences, as well as including input from family and/or caregiver(s) in the treatment plan. After a thorough baseline pain assessment, clinicians should provide education about persistent pain and appropriate

Table 63–2. Nonpharmacologic therapies for persistent pain.

Psychosocial Interventions	Complementary and Integrative Health Therapies[a]	Physical and Rehabilitation Therapies	Exercise Therapies[b]
Cognitive behavioral therapy	Acupuncture, acupressure	Patient education (neurophysiology) and self-management training	Stretching
Dialectical behavioral therapy	Massage therapy	Cognitive functional therapy for low back pain	Walking, hiking
Acceptance and commitment therapy	Chiropractic therapy		Swimming, aqua therapy
Progressive relaxation therapy	Meditation	Safe movement experiences	Yoga
Mindfulness-based and relaxation therapy	Aromatherapy	Spinal mobilization and manipulation	Pilates
Biofeedback	Music therapy	Graded motor imagery	Tai chi
Pain groups, classes	Pet therapy	Tactile acuity testing	Qigong
	Hot compress (caution to avoid skin burns)	Custom orthotics	Chair exercises
	Cold compress, ice packs	Lumbar supports for low back pain	

[a]See Chapter 71, "Integrative Geriatrics & Cannabis Use."
[b]See Chapter 72, "Encouraging Appropriate Exercise for Older Adults."

therapeutic treatment options. Together, the clinician can collaborate with the patient, family, and caregiver(s) and use shared decision making to develop a treatment plan. It is important to set explicit and specific pain management goals, such as improved muscle strength, endurance, function, and quality of life. Examples could include having pain well-enough managed that the patient can sleep, interact with grandchildren, or garden. Long-term follow-up should include ongoing assessment of pain; evaluation for risks, benefits, and adverse effects; and progress toward pain management goals. Patients with co-occurring conditions, such as depression, anxiety, insomnia, sleep apnea, and substance use disorders, should be considered for referral to appropriate specialists for treatment. An interdisciplinary team approach to treatment may be useful for patients with complex pain or who are poorly responsive to first-line treatments.

B. Patient Self-Management

Patients with persistent pain often experience significant impacts on psychological functioning, such as low mood, increased anxiety, stress, anger, hostility, and poor sleep. Patients often report lower self-esteem and may feel less confident exerting control over pain and functioning (self-efficacy). Management of persistent pain in older adults should begin with effective clinician communication, acknowledgement and empathy for the impact of psychological stressors, and a focus on strategies to promote patient self-efficacy. Exploring the patient's inner experience with pain and their fear of pain, as well as recognizing and supporting their self-coping strategies, can be helpful to reduce anxiety and distress around persistent pain. Support groups can be especially useful for patients to meet with peers with similar pain concerns, share personal experiences, and offer emotional support. Patients should be encouraged to engage in holistic health-promoting activities. These activities will vary by person depending on

what patients value most in life. Potential ideas include fostering relationships with family and friends, a mindfulness practice, and healthy eating habits. Additional strategies, such as sleep hygiene, tobacco cessation, anti-inflammatory diet, physical activity, and weight loss for low back pain and hip/knee osteoarthritis (see Chapter 34, "Osteoarthritis"), should also be encouraged when applicable.

C. Nonpharmacologic Therapies

For patients who continue to experience pain, nonpharmacologic therapies are the next step. Patients can be offered a variety of psychosocial interventions, complementary and integrative health therapies, physical and rehabilitation therapies, and exercise therapies based on individual care needs, preferences, cost, and access to services (Table 63–2). Patients often benefit from combining multiple types of therapies, thus promoting active learning of new coping skills, a better understanding of persistent pain, enhanced self-efficacy in lifestyle and functional goals, and incorporation of active movement and exercises into daily life. For patients with advanced illness who are bedbound, regular repositioning, passive range of motion exercises, and gentle massage are effective interventions (see Chapter 72, "Encouraging Appropriate Exercise for Older Adults").

D. Nonopioid Pharmacotherapies

When self-management and nonpharmacologic strategies are insufficient, patients should be offered topical (Table 63–3) and/or oral nonopioid pharmacotherapy (Table 63–4). Topical therapies have the lowest risk for adverse effects and can provide benefit in both reducing pain and improving function. Topicals may be especially useful in older adults with difficulty swallowing or taking oral medications. The choice of medication should depend on the indication, risks and benefits, chronic conditions, renal and hepatic function,

Table 63–3. Common topical nonopioid pharmacotherapies.

Drug	Formulations and Strengths	Dosing	FDA-Approved Indication(s)	Contraindications and Precautions	Clinical Pearls
Diclofenac	1% topical gel	Upper extremity (hand, wrist, elbow): apply 2 g 4 times daily. Max dose 8 g daily to any single joint. Lower extremity (foot, knee, ankle): apply 4 g 4 times daily. Max dose 16 g daily to any single joint.	Osteoarthritis	Avoid with oral NSAIDs. Not recommended in advanced renal impairment. Contraindicated for treating preoperative pain before coronary artery bypass graft and should be avoided for 14 days after surgery.	Produces a local anti-inflammatory effect. Evidence does not support use for lower back pain. Not evaluated for use on the hip, spine, or shoulder. Fewer systemic side effects compared to oral NSAIDs due to minimal systemic absorption. Risk of gastrointestinal bleeding is lower than oral diclofenac but can occur. Safer to use than oral NSAIDs in patients taking anticoagulants.
	1.5% topical solution	Apply 10 drops topically and spread around front, back, and sides of each affected knee. Repeat until 40 drops have been applied. Apply 4 times daily.			
	2% topical solution	Apply 40 mg (2 pump actuations) topically to affected knee 2 times daily.			
	1.3% (180 mg) patch, extended release	Apply 1 patch topically to the most painful site twice daily.	Acute pain due to minor strains, sprains, and contusions		
Lidocaine	5% extended release patch	Apply 1–3 patches once, for up to 12 hours within a 24-hour period. Smaller areas of treatment are recommended in patients with renal or hepatic impairment, geriatrics, or debilitated patients.	Postherpetic neuralgia, diabetic neuropathy	Use caution in patients with severe renal or hepatic disease due to increased risk of toxicity. Use caution in patients with cardiac issues (impaired conduction, impaired function, bradycardia). Avoid concurrent use with class I and III antiarrhythmics and other local anesthetics.	Blocks abnormal peripheral neuronal conduction to provide local analgesia. May cut patches to fit painful area. May consider using patches every 12 hours if pain responds to patch. Systemic absorption and toxicity can occur if used on irritated or broken skin. Application site reactions (blisters, bruising, burning sensation, depigmentation, dermatitis, discoloration, edema, erythema, exfoliation, irritation, papules, petechia, pruritus, vesicles) have been reported.
	0.5% aerosol spray, 4% topical cream, 4% topical gel	Apply topically to affected area no more than 3–4 times daily.	Topical local anesthetic to skin		
	5% topical ointment	Apply up to 6-inch length of ointment (5 g) from tube. Max 17–20 g/day.			
Methyl salicylate/ menthol	10%/15% cream, 16%/30% cream 10%/3% patches	Apply to affected area 3–4 times daily. Apply 1 patch every 8–12 hours. Max 2 patches daily.	Musculoskeletal pain[a]	Avoid use on open wounds, contact with eyes or mucous membranes, and with a heating pad.	Works as an irritant, causing mild topical inflammation and resulting in deeper pain relief.

(continued)

Table 63–3. Common topical nonopioid pharmacotherapies. (*continued*)

Drug	Formulations and Strengths	Dosing	FDA-Approved Indication(s)	Contraindications and Precautions	Clinical Pearls
Capsaicin	0.025% cream, 0.075% cream 8% patches	Apply thin film to affected area 3–4 times daily. Apply a single 60-minute application of up to 4 patches every 3 months as needed. Do not apply more frequently than every 3 months.	Arthritis pain, musculoskeletal pain, postherpetic neuralgia, neuropathy due to HIV or postoperative complications[a]	Avoid use on open wounds, contact with eyes or mucous membranes, or on face or scalp. May increase risk of cardiovascular adverse events in patients with recent history of cardiovascular or cerebrovascular events.	Wash hands after use or wear nitrile gloves to apply. Latex gloves do not provide adequate protection. Requires scheduled use. Aerosolization of capsaicin can occur when patches are rapidly removed. Inhalation can cause coughing, sneezing, or shortness of breath. Roll adhesive side of patch inward and remove gently and slowly. Hypertension associated with treatment-related increases in pain can occur. Treat acute pain with local cooling agents (ice pack).

FDA, US Food and Drug Administration; NSAIDs, nonsteroidal anti-inflammatory drugs; HIV, human immunodeficiency virus.
[a]Non–FDA-approved indication.

other concurrent medications, and cognition. In general, a "start low and go slow" approach should be followed to reduce risk for side effects in older adults. Many oral nonopioid pharmacotherapy options have increased risk for anticholinergic and central nervous system (CNS) effects in older adults. Clinicians should consider avoiding or minimizing use of anticholinergic medications and limiting to three or fewer total CNS-active drugs whenever possible. Once medications are started, the patient should be regularly monitored to evaluate for efficacy and side effects, with a low threshold to discontinue the medication if it is causing side effects.

E. Opioid Pharmacotherapy

1. Role of opioids in persistent pain management— Prior to the 1980s, opioids were rarely used for persistent pain management due to concerns for tolerance, dependence, and addiction. During the 1980s, hospice and palliative care initiatives advocated for aggressive treatment of pain in those with serious illness, and opioid use increased in these patients. These initiatives were followed by efforts to destigmatize opioid use in the primary care setting, which increased the use of opioids in patients with nonmalignant, persistent pain management. Despite lack of long-term efficacy and safety data, opioids continued to be used for persistent pain management. This increase in opioid use has run parallel to dramatic increases in opioid abuse, overdose, and associated morbidity and mortality.

Given the overwhelming evidence for opioid-related harms and emerging evidence for safer and more effective alternative treatments, opioid use should typically be reserved

for severe acute pain, postoperative pain (see Chapter 29, "Perioperative Care for Older Surgical Patients"), and pain in patients with terminal illnesses like cancer (see Chapter 22, "Geriatric Palliative Care"). For persistent pain management, clinicians should encourage patient self-management strategies, offer nonpharmacologic and nonopioid pharmacotherapies, and reserve opioids for use when the potential benefits clearly outweigh the risks.

2. Considerations in older adults—For a small, select group of patients, intermittent, nondaily opioid therapy may be a reasonable option. Clinicians should only consider opioid therapy when other modalities have been optimized and the expected benefits for pain and function are anticipated to outweigh the individual patient risks. Many older adults have reduced renal function and medication clearance, even in the absence of renal disease, as well as increased rates of acute illnesses, such as pneumonia, influenza, and urinary tract infections, which can also decrease medication clearance. Thus, older adults may be susceptible to accumulation of opioids and a smaller therapeutic window between safe opioid doses and those resulting in adverse effects. Older adults often have multiple chronic conditions, such as sleep apnea, chronic pulmonary disease, cognitive impairment, reduced bone density, falls, or fractures, or are prescribed concurrent CNS depressants, such as benzodiazepines, nonbenzodiazepine receptor agonists, or skeletal muscle relaxants, which increase opioid-related risks. Whenever possible, opioids should be avoided in patients with a history of falls or fractures or in combination with other CNS-active medications. Finally, other medical conditions, such as fibromyalgia

Table 63–4. Common oral nonopioid pharmacotherapies.

Drug	Formulations and Strengths	Dosing	Contraindications and Precautions	Clinical Pearls
Acetaminophen	325, 500 mg tablet; 650 mg extended-release tablet; 325 mg capsule	650 mg every 4–6 hours as needed. Max of 4000 mg/day (healthy patients) and consider limiting to 2000 mg/day (hepatic impairment).	Contraindicated in active and severe hepatic disease. Heavy alcohol use increases the risk for hepatic injury. Consider reducing the dose in severe renal impairment (CrCl ≤30 mL/min) to prevent hepatic injury.	FDA-approved for mild to moderate pain and moderate to severe pain in combination with opioids. Used off-label for migraine and osteoarthritis.
Nonsteroidal Anti-Inflammatory Drugs (NSAIDs)				
Diclofenac	25 mg capsule, 50 mg tablet, 75 mg enteric-coated tablet	Osteoarthritis: 50–150 mg/day in 2–3 divided doses. Rheumatoid arthritis: 150–200 mg/day in 2–4 divided doses. Mild to moderate pain: 25–50 mg 3–4 times daily. Initial dose of 100 mg may be used.	Beers criteria recommend avoiding chronic use unless other alternatives are not effective and patient can take a gastroprotective agent due to increased risk for gastrointestinal bleeding or peptic ulcer disease. Use with caution in renal and hepatic impairment, gastrointestinal disease, or in patients taking anticoagulants or lithium. Avoid in stage 4–5 kidney disease.	Consider using in conjunction with a proton pump inhibitor or misoprostol, especially for patients at high risk for upper gastrointestinal bleeding (history of gastric or duodenal ulcers, age >75, concurrent corticosteroids, anticoagulants, or antiplatelet agents). Most NSAIDs are FDA approved for osteoarthritis, rheumatoid arthritis, pain, headache, and/or migraine.
Etodolac	Immediate release: 200, 300 mg capsule; 400, 500 mg tablet Extended release: 400, 500, 600 mg tablet	Osteoarthritis and rheumatoid arthritis: Initial dose, 300 mg 2–3 times daily or 400–500 mg twice daily. Maintenance dose, 400–1000 mg extended release once daily or 600–1000 mg/day in 2–4 divided doses. Pain: 200–400 mg every 6–8 hours as needed Max of 1200 mg/day.		
Ibuprofen	200, 400, 600, 800 mg tablet; 200 mg capsule	Osteoarthritis and rheumatoid arthritis: 1200–3200 mg/day in 3–4 divided doses. Pain: 200–400 mg every 4–6 hours as needed. Max 1200 mg/day for up to 10 days. Headache: 200–400 mg every 4–6 hours as needed. Max 1200 mg/day. Migraine: 400 mg daily for up to 10 days.	Contraindicated for treating preoperative pain before coronary artery bypass graft and should be avoided for 14 days after surgery. Avoid in patients with asthma, urticaria, or allergic-type reaction following aspirin or other NSAIDs. Fluid retention or edema may occur. Caution in patients with CHF. Indomethacin is more likely than other NSAIDs to cause adverse CNS effects and is not recommended in older adults.	
Meloxicam	7.5, 15 mg tablet; 5, 10 mg capsule; 7.5 mg/5mL suspension	Osteoarthritis: 5–15 mg daily. Rheumatoid arthritis: 7.5–15 mg daily.		
Naproxen	250, 375, 500 mg oral tablet; 375, 500 mg enteric-coated tablet; 125 mg/5 mL, 25 mg/1 mL suspension	Osteoarthritis, rheumatoid arthritis: 250–500 mg twice daily. May be titrated up to 1500 mg/day for up to 6 months. Pain: initial dose, 500 mg, followed by 250 mg every 6–8 hours as needed. Max 1250 mg/day.		
Piroxicam	10, 20 mg capsule	Osteoarthritis, rheumatoid arthritis: 20 mg/day in a single or divided dose		
Salsalate	500, 750 mg tablet	Osteoarthritis, rheumatoid arthritis: 3000 mg daily in 2–3 divided doses		
Sulindac	150, 200 mg tablet	Osteoarthritis, rheumatoid arthritis: 150 mg twice daily. Max 400 mg/day. Shoulder pain: 200 mg twice daily for 7–14 days.		

(continued)

Table 63–4. Common oral nonopioid pharmacotherapies. (*continued*)

Drug	Formulations and Strengths	Dosing	Contraindications and Precautions	Clinical Pearls
Skeletal Muscle Relaxants and Antispasmodics				
Baclofen	5, 10, 20 mg tablet	5 mg 3 times daily. May increase in 15 mg/day increments every 3 days. Max of 80 mg/day in 3–4 divided doses. Reduce dose by one-third in mild to moderate renal impairment (CrCl 30–80 mL/min) and by two-thirds in severe renal impairment (CrCl ≤30 mL/min and not on dialysis).	Beers criteria recommend avoiding in older adults due to anticholinergic effects, sedation, increased risk of fractures, and questionable efficacy. Avoid in patients with sleep apnea and combining with other CNS depressant medications and alcohol due to risk for respiratory depression, overdose, and death. Drowsiness is common. Avoid driving or operating heavy machinery. Cyclobenzaprine contraindicated in cardiac conditions (acute recovery after MI, arrhythmia, conduction disturbances, CHF, heart block), hyperthyroidism, and within 14 days of MAOI treatment. Metaxalone contraindicated in renal and hepatic impairment.	Limit to short-term use of ≤7 days. Consider tapering off baclofen and tizanidine due to withdrawal symptoms. Baclofen and tizanidine FDA approved for spasticity. Others approved for skeletal muscle spasm. Cyclobenzaprine has the strongest anticholinergic effects.
Cyclobenzaprine	5, 7.5 mg tablet; 15, 30 mg extended-release capsule	5 mg 3 times daily. May increase to 10 mg 3 times daily for no more than 2–3 weeks. 15 mg extended release once daily. May increase to 30 mg daily for no more than 2–3 weeks. Start with 5 mg immediate-release tablets and titrate up slowly in mild hepatic impairment. Consider less frequent dosing in geriatrics.		
Metaxalone	400, 800 mg tablet	800 mg 3–4 times daily.		
Methocarbamol	500, 750 mg tablet	1500 mg 4 times daily for 48–72 hours. Then, 750 mg every 4 hours, 1500 mg 3 times daily, or 1000 mg 4 times daily up to 4 g/day.		
Tizanidine	2, 4, 6 mg capsule; 2, 4 mg tablet	2 mg initially; may repeat every 6–8 hours to a max of 3 doses in 24 hours. May increase 2–4 mg per dose at 1- to 4-day intervals. Max of 36 mg/day. Reduce individual doses during titration in renal impairment (CrCl ≤25 mL/min) and hepatic impairment. If higher doses are required, increase individual doses rather than frequency.		
Selective Norepinephrine Reuptake Inhibitors				
Venlafaxine	25, 37.5, 50, 75, 100 mg tablet; 37.5, 75, 150 mg oral extended-release tablet and capsule; 225 mg extended-release tablet	37.5–75 mg daily. May increase by 75 mg/day every 4 days to 225 mg/day in divided doses. Extended release may be dosed once daily. Reduce dose 25%–50% in mild to moderate renal impairment. Reduce dose 50% in dialysis and mild to moderate hepatic impairment.	Avoid use in older adults with falls or fractures (unless safer alternatives not available). Avoid use within 14 days of MAOI treatment. Nausea, constipation, diarrhea, dry mouth, loss of appetite, dizziness, headache, and sedation may occur when starting therapy. Monitor sodium level when starting or changing doses due to risk for exacerbating or causing inappropriate antidiuretic hormone secretion or hyponatremia.	Venlafaxine used off-label for neuropathic pain. Duloxetine FDA approved for musculoskeletal pain and some types of neuropathic pain. Monitor blood pressure when starting treatment. Venlafaxine may cause increase in blood pressure, and duloxetine may cause orthostatic hypotension or syncope. Taper off to prevent serious discontinuation symptoms.
Duloxetine	20, 30, 40, 60 mg delayed-release capsule	30 mg daily for 1 week. Increase to 60 mg based on tolerability. Max 60 mg/day unless generalized anxiety disorder or depressive disorder also present; may increase to max of 120 mg/day. In geriatrics, may continue initial dose of 30 mg daily for 2 weeks, then titrate the dose. Avoid duloxetine in severe renal impairment (CrCl ≤30 mL/min) and chronic hepatic disease or cirrhosis.		

(*continued*)

Table 63–4. Common oral nonopioid pharmacotherapies. (*continued*)

Drug	Formulations and Strengths	Dosing	Contraindications and Precautions	Clinical Pearls
Tricyclic Antidepressants				
Amitriptyline	10, 25, 50, 75, 100, 150 mg tablet	10 mg daily. May increase to 75 mg/day in single or divided doses.	Beers criteria recommend avoiding in older adults due to risk for anticholinergic effects, sedation, orthostatic hypotension, and risk for falls. Avoid use within 14 days of MAOI treatment, during the recovery period after MI and with concurrent cisapride. May cause QTc prolongation. Avoid if QTc >450 ms. Monitor sodium level when starting or changing doses due to risk for exacerbating or causing inappropriate antidiuretic hormone secretion or hyponatremia.	Used off-label for neuropathic pain and headache. Amitriptyline and imipramine have more anticholinergic effects. Consider limiting quantity prescribed, especially in patients with suicide risk. Monitor for anticholinergic effects and changes in mood.
Imipramine	10, 25, 50 mg tablet			
Nortriptyline	10, 25, 50, 75mg capsule; 10 mg/5 mL oral solution			
Desipramine	10, 25, 50, 75, 100, 150 mg tablet			
Antiepileptics				
Gabapentin	100, 300, 400 mg capsule; 300, 600, 800 mg tablet; 250 mg/5 mL oral solution	100 mg at bedtime titrated weekly to 300–900 mg every 8–12 hours. Max of 3600 mg/day. When CrCl 30–59 mL/min, limit to 400–1400 mg/day in 2 divided doses. When CrCl 15–29 mL/min, limit to 200–700 mg daily. In hemodialysis patients with CrCl 15 mL/min, limit to 100–300 mg daily. In hemodialysis patients with CrCl <15 mL/min, reduce daily dose in proportion to CrCl. After hemodialysis, give a supplemental dose of 125 mg per each maintenance dose of 100 mg.	Beers criteria recommend using caution or avoiding in older adults due to risk of syncope and falls. May cause peripheral edema. Caution in patients with CHF. Pregabalin may cause constipation, nausea, dry mouth, blurred vision, increased appetite, and weight gain.	FDA approved for neuropathic pain Monitor for fatigue, somnolence, dizziness, and changes in mood.
Pregabalin	25, 50, 75, 100, 150, 200, 225, 300 mg capsule; 82.5, 165, 330 mg extended-release capsule; 20 mg/1 mL solution	50–150 mg/day (divided doses for immediate release) with weekly titration up to 300 mg/day. When CrCl 30–60mL/min: reduce dose of extended release by 50%. Avoid extended release when CrCl <30 mL/min. When CrCl 15–30 mL/min limit to 25–150 mg once or twice daily. When CrCl <15 mL/min, limit to 25–75 mg daily. In hemodialysis, adjust dose similar to gabapentin and provide supplemental dose after each session.		

CHF, congestive heart failure; CNS, central nervous system; CrCl, creatinine clearance; FDA, US Food and Drug Administration; MAOI, monoamine oxidase inhibitor; MI, myocardial infarction.

or headache, can worsen with opioids, so appropriate evaluation is warranted prior to starting opioid therapy.

3. Prior to initiating opioid therapy—Evidence-based guidelines, such as the 2016 Centers for Disease Control and Prevention Guideline for Prescribing Opioids for Chronic Pain, recommend careful consideration and discussion of the risks and benefits of opioid therapy with the patient, family, and/or caregiver(s) prior to initiation. When opioids are used, clinicians should avoid managing persistent pain with opioids as the only treatment modality. Instead, opioids should be combined with other evidence-based, multimodal therapies. Prior to initiating opioid therapy, clinicians should establish realistic treatment goals for function and pain and discuss a plan to discontinue opioids if the benefits do not outweigh the risks.

When considering opioid therapy, clinicians should incorporate risk assessment and mitigation tools into treatment planning and monitoring. For example, the Opioid Risk Tool (ORT) and the Screener and Opioid Assessment for Patients with Pain–Revised (SOAPP-R) are quick, easy, and useful tools to assess risk for developing aberrant behaviors when patients are prescribed opioids for persistent pain. Prescription drug monitoring programs are electronic databases available in most states that track real-time data on outpatient controlled substance prescribing. Clinicians should review local prescription drug monitoring programs prior to prescribing controlled substances to assess for receipt of prescriptions from multiple prescribers. Urine drug screening should also be completed to screen for presence of prescribed drugs, detect use of nonprescribed drugs and substances, and monitor for potential drug diversion. Confirmatory urine drug screening should be considered when unexpected results are found, and serum testing can be used in anuric and dialysis patients.

Prior to initiating therapy with opioids, it is also important to assess for concurrent substance use disorders and mental health conditions, such as depression, anxiety, and insomnia, which can worsen with opioid therapy and pose increased risk for overdose and suicide. Clinicians should ensure that treatment of these conditions is optimized prior to initiating opioid therapy, consulting with behavioral specialists if needed (see Chapter 12, "Depression & Other Mental Health Issues"). Fall precautions should be proactively implemented in patients with a history of falls, fractures, or low bone density (see Chapter 6, "Falls & Mobility Impairment"). Risks of opioids should be very carefully considered in patients with past suicide attempts or history of accidental or intentional drug overdose, and access to lethal means (eg, firearms, medications, other avenues for self-harm) should be restricted in patients at moderate to high acute risk of suicide. All nonterminal patients with potential exposure to opioids other than tramadol should be offered opioid overdose education and naloxone, an opioid antagonist used for opioid overdose reversal. Finally, it is important to discuss safe storage of opioid medications, such as medication lock boxes, to prevent opioid diversion from those with access to the home and unintentional access by young children and adolescents.

4. When initiating opioid therapy—When starting opioid therapy for persistent pain, clinicians should reevaluate the benefits and harms of treatment within 1 to 4 weeks. Opioid therapy should only be continued if a meaningful improvement in function and pain outweighs the risk for harms and adverse effects. Immediate-release opioids are recommended as initial therapy and prescribed at the lowest possible dosage, and extended-release or long-acting opioids should be avoided whenever possible, as these formulations have increased risk for respiratory suppression and overdose. The risk for opioid overdose starts as low as 20 mg morphine equivalent daily dose (MEDD), increases at doses ≥50 mg MEDD, and dramatically increases at higher doses of ≥90 mg MEDD. Thus, clinicians should carefully assess the individual benefits and risks of doses ≥50 mg MEDD and avoid doses ≥90 mg MEDD.

5. Ongoing opioid therapy monitoring—When patients are prescribed ongoing therapy with opioids for persistent pain, clinicians should reevaluate the benefits and harms of treatment at least every 3 months. This includes management of opioid-related adverse effects, ongoing safety monitoring, and risk mitigation. Common opioid-related adverse effects include constipation, abdominal pain, nausea, vomiting, headache, dizziness, somnolence, fatigue, and pruritus. Tolerance develops to most common adverse effects, except for opioid-induced constipation (see management strategies in Chapter 61, "Constipation"). Serious opioid-related adverse effects include hypotension, orthostatic hypotension, prolonged QT interval with methadone (electrocardiogram monitoring recommended), adrenal insufficiency, anaphylaxis, dyspnea, hyperalgesia, respiratory depression, and drug dependence and withdrawal. When side effects develop, consider reducing the dose, tapering off if appropriate, and incorporating alternative pain management strategies.

Patients should be routinely monitored for falls and fractures. Given the association of both persistent pain and opioid therapy with suicide risk, clinicians should routinely assess for suicidality during treatment and intervene when needed. For added safety monitoring and risk mitigation, prescription drug monitoring programs should be queried at least every 3 months and more frequently as required by local state laws, facility guidelines, and when unexpected results are found. Urine drug screens should be monitored at least annually, with more frequent monitoring as needed and confirmatory testing when unexpected results are found (eg, positive for drug not prescribed, negative for prescribed drug). Other useful risk mitigation strategies may include pill counts and opioid treatment (or pain care) agreements. Concurrent use of substances such as alcohol and the presence of substance use disorders should be routinely monitored, as well as signs of nonadherence to the treatment plan or unsafe behaviors, such as frequent requests for early refills, increased doses, emergency department visits for opioids, lost or stolen prescriptions, buying or borrowing opioids, or refusal to provide a urine drug screen. Concurrent use of CNS depressants such as benzodiazepines, which greatly increase risk for respiratory depression and overdose, should be avoided. Finally, clinicians should routinely assess for overdose and naloxone use and offer naloxone renewal when used or expired.

6. Individualized opioid tapering—When the benefits of opioid therapy do not outweigh the harms, clinicians should consider a supported opioid taper in partnership with the patient, family, and caregiver(s). This may occur when patients have inadequate improvement in function or pain, have severe or unmanageable side effects, are prescribed high doses ≥50 mg MEDD, or demonstrate nonadherence; when concerning behaviors are noted that may indicate presence of an opioid use disorder or drug diversion; or when patients develop multiple medical chronic conditions or are prescribed or using medications or substances that increase risk, experience an overdose event, or express suicidality. When tapering opioids, it is important to discuss an end goal (dose reduction or discontinuation), speed of the taper, and supported treatment of withdrawal. A slow taper, reducing by 2% to 10% every 4 to 8 weeks, may be appropriate for patients taking opioids for many years with no new or immediate risks for harm. The most common taper schedule is a 5% to 20% reduction every 4 weeks, with pauses as needed. Slower tapers often allow patients time to engage in other pain management modalities and acquire new coping skills. For patients who require a more rapid taper over weeks, consider reducing 10% to 20% weekly. And finally, for those with immediate risk or who need rapid reversal (typically in the inpatient setting), consider reducing 20% to 50% for the first dose, then 10% to 20% daily. Adjunctive medications should be offered to treat opioid withdrawal symptoms as needed, especially for those with a more rapid taper plan (eg, antiemetics for nausea, antidiarrheals, clonidine for sympathetic arousal). When opioid use disorder is present, clinicians should offer evidence-based treatment, including medication-assisted therapy with buprenorphine, methadone, or naltrexone. When opioids are being diverted and not taken by the patient, they can be safely discontinued.

▶ Approach to Common Pain Conditions

A. Back Pain

Back pain is one of the top three reasons for health care provider visits by older adults. Of the 1037 surviving subjects from the original Framingham Heart Study cohort (ages 68–100 years), 22% had back pain on most days. In older individuals, there are several specific causes for back pain (eg, lumbar spinal stenosis, osteoporotic vertebral compression fractures, sacral fractures) that are less common in younger individuals. Systemic conditions, such as malignancy and infections, although rarely the cause of back pain, are also more common in older compared to younger age groups. In older adults, mechanical low back pain is most common.

One of the most challenging aspects of assessing and managing back pain is identifying the source(s) of pain in the older adult who often has multiple musculoskeletal conditions (eg, trochanteric bursitis, hip osteoarthritis, multilevel lumbar degenerative changes, and lumbar stenosis). These conditions rarely occur in isolation, and pinpointing which one contributes most to the patient's pain is not a trivial endeavor. Clinicians should complete a thorough history and physical, as described earlier, as well as screen for red flag symptoms that may indicate serious underlying pathology, such as malignancy, fracture, infection, cauda equina syndrome, or inflammatory disease. Symptoms may be rapidly progressive or associated with severe neurologic deficits and may require additional diagnostic workup and treatment. While laboratory tests are not specific for back pain (eg, complete blood count, erythrocyte sedimentation rate, C-reactive protein, serum protein electrophoresis), these can be useful for diagnosis when red flag symptoms are present.

For patients with acute (<3 months), localized, nonradiating lower back pain, imaging and invasive diagnostic tests are not routinely recommended. Many patients with low back pain, including lumbar disk herniation and radiculopathy, often improve within 4 weeks of noninvasive pain care. Evidence demonstrates that use of imaging, such as radiographs, computed tomography (CT), or magnetic resonance imaging (MRI), in patients without serious underlying pathology does not significantly improve outcomes. Diagnostic imaging can lead to unnecessary health care costs, and when benign findings are seen on imaging (eg, degeneration of the spine as expected with normal aging), patients may become fearful of movement, resulting in a cascade of further testing, and ultimately have worse outcomes.

Diagnostic imaging may be appropriate for patients with red flag symptoms or radiating back pain or in those with persistent back pain that is nonresponsive to initial treatments. According to the American College of Radiology, the following criteria should be used to determine who is at higher risk for systemic disease-related back pain and when it may be appropriate to obtain imaging: recent significant trauma or milder trauma (age >50 years); unexplained weight loss or fever; immunosuppression (including diagnoses such as diabetes mellitus); history of cancer; intravenous drug use; osteoporosis or prolonged use of glucocorticoids; age >70 years; focal neurologic deficits that are progressive or produce disabling symptoms; and, lastly, duration of 6 weeks or more (subacute or chronic). When used, plain radiographs can evaluate alignment, instability, and scoliosis, as well as postoperative evaluation of instrumentation and fusion. CT or MRI may be appropriate for evaluation of underlying pathology of red flag symptoms.

Similar to other persistent pain conditions, the most appropriate therapy for an older patient with back pain must be determined in the context of the individual's chronic conditions, potential interactions with other medications, and after discussing their preferences and goals of treatment. Treatment of back pain usually begins with patient education on expected duration of symptoms, self-care, and conservative, nonoperative, multimodal modalities (Table 63–2). Whenever possible, patients should be advised to remain active and limit bedrest. Once the acute symptoms subside, a gentle progressive exercise program (often with guidance from a pain physical therapist) should be started to strengthen the spinal and abdominal musculature. The goals of therapeutic exercises include increased flexibility by stretching, improved muscle strength by resistive exercise, and improved endurance with repetition. Heat or cold modalities may relieve pain and loosen muscles prior to physical therapy exercises; use of a medium-firm mattress may also be helpful. Nonopioid pharmacotherapies, such as topical methyl salicylate/menthol, nonsteroidal anti-inflammatory drugs, and acetaminophen, may also be useful in reducing pain and inflammation with back pain (Tables 63–3 and 63–4). Evidence for use of other interventions, such as transcutaneous electrical nerve stimulation, lumbar traction, and electrical muscle stimulation, is limited and should be considered alongside other evidence-based modalities on a case-by-case basis.

When considering nonsurgical invasive pharmacotherapies, epidural steroid injections may be used for short-term (≤2 weeks) treatment of radicular low back pain. Epidural steroid injections are not recommended for long-term use, and intra-articular facet joint steroid injections, medial branch blocks, and radiofrequency ablative denervation are not recommended for routine management of low back pain due to limited evidence. Clinicians may refer patients for consultation alongside a thorough discussion of the risks and benefits of these invasive procedures. For discussion on use of injections in the treatment of osteoarthritis, see Chapter 34, "Osteoarthritis."

In severe cases that have not responded to conservative therapy, surgical options may be considered. Indications for referral to a surgeon include cauda equina syndrome, suspected cord compression, and progressive or severe neurologic deficits. Most surgical interventions (eg, decompression, laminectomy, fusion) are elective, so it is imperative to work closely with a thoughtful, conservative surgeon who can take time to explain the procedure, risks, and benefits to the older adult.

B. Neuropathic Pain

Neuropathic pain is a chronic pain arising as a direct consequence of a lesion or disease affecting the somatosensory system. Neuropathic pain is disproportionately experienced by older adults, affecting an estimated 8% of older adults. Older people are at high risk for neuropathic pain because many of the diseases that are associated with neuropathy become more common with age, such as diabetes, herpes zoster (postherpetic neuralgia), spinal stenosis, cancer, and stroke. Neuropathic pain can worsen function and increase the risk of frailty, falls, and polypharmacy. These risks are heightened in patients who are already suffering from multimorbidity.

Similar to the approach to persistent pain described previously, the first step in evaluating neuropathy is to take a thorough history and perform a physical exam. History of diabetes and other past medical history, new medications, alcohol use, and family history of neuropathies and medical conditions associated with neuropathy can all be obtained on history. Symptoms may not be as consistent in older adults but could include pain, tingling, loss of vibration or temperature sense, loss of proprioception, and distal weakness. A focused neurologic exam should be performed, as well as looking for other signs of systemic disease.

If suspected based on history and exam, the neuropathy should be characterized as much as possible. Axonal versus demyelinating neuropathies can be distinguished by electromyogram. Typically, large-fiber neuropathy manifests with the loss of joint position and vibration sense and sensory ataxia, whereas small-fiber neuropathy manifests with the impairment of pain, temperature, and autonomic functions.

The American Academy of Neurology recommends fasting glucose/2-hour glucose tolerance testing, vitamin B_{12} testing with methylmalonic acid/homocysteine levels, and serum protein electrophoresis with immunofixation electrophoresis testing for initial lab workup of peripheral neuropathy. Clinicians should be thoughtful about whether to order other additional labs tests as they are unlikely to be high yield. It is important to remember that 20% to 25% of neuropathies remain unclassified, and most of these are seen in older patients.

Treatment of peripheral neuropathy should include attempts to control the underlying disease, whenever possible, and alleviating symptoms, including pain. Removing offending agents such as toxins and medications or correcting a nutritional deficiency can help treat the underlying disease and improve symptoms. Whenever possible, multimodal and integrated care approaches should be incorporated into the neuropathic pain management plan. As previously described, patients can benefit from a variety of self-management, nonpharmacologic (Table 63–2), and pharmacologic treatment strategies. Practical considerations such as shoe choice, orthotics, and inserts for neuropathy affecting the feet can provide benefit.

Pharmacologic treatment of neuropathy is particularly challenging in older adults because medications have shown limited efficacy in this population, and many of the medications pose risk to older adults. Topical medications, such as lidocaine and capsaicin, should be used for local painful neuropathies to minimize potential drug-drug and drug-disease interactions (Table 63–3). Available oral medications for neuropathic pain include selective norepinephrine reuptake inhibitors, tricyclic antidepressants, and antiepileptics (Table 63–4). When oral medication is needed, patients and caregivers should be counseled that no one medication works for everyone and that it may take time and several drug trials to find a drug that relieves the neuropathic pain (the number needed to treat for any of these medications is three to eight). Some patients may benefit from combining medications with different mechanisms of action, such as gabapentin plus nortriptyline.

C. Other Pain Conditions

Two of the other more common persistent pain conditions in older adults, osteoarthritis and headache, are covered in detail in Chapters 34 and 64, respectively, of this book.

Barrell K, Smith AG. Peripheral neuropathy. *Med Clin North Am.* 2019;103(2):383-397.

Bowering KJ, O'Connell NE, Tabor A, et al. The effects of graded motor imagery and its components on chronic pain: a systematic review and meta-analysis. *J Pain.* 2013;14(1):3-13.

By the 2019 American Geriatrics Society Beers Criteria Update Expert Panel. American Geriatrics Society 2019 Updated AGS Beers Criteria for potentially inappropriate medication use in older adults. *J Am Geriatr Soc.* 2019;67(4):674-694.

Catley MJ, O'Connell NE, Berryman C, Ayhan FF, Moseley GL. Is tactile acuity altered in people with chronic pain? A systematic review and meta-analysis. *J Pain.* 2014;15(10):985-1000.

Dowell D, Haegerich TM, Chou R. CDC guideline for prescribing opioids for chronic pain–United States, 2016. *MMWR Recomm Rep.* 2016;65(1):1-49.

Foster NE, Anema JR, Cherkin D, et al. Prevention and treatment of low back pain: evidence, challenges, and promising directions. *Lancet.* 2018;391(10137):2368-2383.

Horgas AL. Pain assessment in older adults. *Nurs Clin North Am.* 2017;52(3):375-385. P

Johnson SM, Shah LM. Imaging of acute low back pain. *Radiol Clin North Am.* 2019;57(2):397-413.

Micromedex (electronic version). Truven Health Analytics, Greenwood Village, CO. http://www.micromedexsolutions.com/. Accessed February 27, 2019.

O'Sullivan PB, Caneiro JP, O'Keeffe M, et al. Cognitive functional therapy: an integrated behavioral approach for the targeted management of disabling low back pain. *Phys Ther.* 2018;98(5):408-423.

Reid MC, Eccleston C, Pillemer K. Management of chronic pain in older adults. *BMJ.* 2015;350:h532.

Rubem MA, Meterko M, Bokhour BG. Do patient perceptions of provider communication relate to experiences of physical pain? *Patient Educ Couns.* 2018;101(2):209-213.

The Diagnosis and Treatment of Low Back Pain Work Group. *VA/DoD Clinical Practice Guideline for Diagnosis and Treatment of Low Back Pain.* Version 2.0. Washington, DC: Veterans Health Administration and Department of Defense; 2017.

The Opioid Therapy for Chronic Pain Work Group. *VA/DoD Clinical Practice Guideline for Opioid Therapy for Chronic Pain.* Version 3.0. Washington, DC: Veterans Health Administration and Department of Defense; 2017.

Veterans Health Administration Pharmacy Benefits Management Academic Detailing Service. Transforming the Treatment of Chronic Pain: Moving Beyond Opioids—A VA Clinician's Guide. Washington, DC: Department of Veterans Affairs; August 2017.

Veterans Health Administration Pharmacy Benefits Management Academic Detailing Service. Transforming the Treatment of Pain: A Quick Reference Guide. Washington, DC: Department of Veterans Affairs; July 2017.

Veterans Health Administration Pharmacy Benefits Management Academic Detailing Service. Opioid Decision Taper Tool: A VA Clinician's Guide. Washington, DC: Department of Veterans Affairs; October 2016.

Wáng YXJ, Wu AM, Ruiz Santiago F, Nogueira-Barbosa MH. Informed appropriate imaging for low back pain management: a narrative review. *J Orthop Translat.* 2018;15:21-34.

Headaches

Katherine Anderson, MD
Jana Wold, MD

General Principles

In the headache literature, the term *older adult* usually refers to patients age 50 years and older because of changes in presentation and types of headache that occur in patients older than age 50. Primary headaches tend to abate, whereas secondary headaches, that is, headaches caused by another disease or medical condition, become more common with age. Up to 30% of headache complaints in the older adult are caused by other etiologies, including medical conditions or their associated treatments. Essentials to consider when assessing headaches in older adults include the following:

- New-onset headaches are rare in older adults and necessitate evaluation.
- Temporal arteritis is an emergency.
- Headaches in older adults are frequently due to an underlying medical diagnosis or treatment.

General Evaluation

Development of a new headache in an older adult or a change in pattern of chronic headaches warrants a thorough medical evaluation. This should include a detailed clinical history with review for red flag symptoms (systemic symptoms such as fevers, chills, myalgias, weight loss; focal neurologic findings; onset >50 years old; thunderclap headache onset; papilledema; positional headache; headache precipitated by Valsalva maneuver or exertion; progressive headache and/or headache with pattern change), complete pharmacologic review, and comprehensive neurologic examination. Additional workup may be necessary in the older adult, as new headaches are more often a result of serious conditions or exacerbations of comorbid disorders. Such workup may include brain imaging with computed tomography (CT) and/or magnetic resonance imaging (MRI) to evaluate for space-occupying lesions; cervical spine radiography to evaluate for facet disease causing cervicogenic headache; arterial imaging in the setting of ischemic headache symptoms; laboratory testing, including a complete blood count, erythrocyte sedimentation rate (ESR), C-reactive protein (CRP), and a complete metabolic panel; overnight oximetry in cases of morning headaches or to evaluate for nonrestorative sleep; and/or referral to ophthalmology to evaluate for vision impairment, glaucoma, or other ocular causes of headache.

Differential Diagnoses

A. Primary Headache

The three most common primary headache types (migraine, tension, and cluster) usually have onset before age 45 years. Generally, the presentation and management of these headaches are similar in younger and older adults; however, some unique features found in headaches in older adults are outlined below.

1. Migraine

a. General considerations—Approximately 6% of adults older than the age of 50 years experience migraine type headaches, and new-onset migraine in older adults accounts for approximately 3% of all migraine sufferers. Typically, older adults with a history of migraine experience fewer and milder migraines as they age. Traditional migraine should be differentiated from aura without migraine, which used to be called late life migraine accompaniments. Only 40% to 50% of patients with aura without migraine will go on to develop a typical migraine headache.

b. Clinical findings—Migraine attacks in the older adult are less typical compared with younger individuals. They are more frequently bilateral and have fewer associated symptoms, such as photophobia, phonophobia, nausea, and vomiting; thus, they may be misdiagnosed as tension-type headache. Symptoms such as rhinorrhea and bilateral tearing may increase with age. Patients may complain of throbbing pain, aura, and traditional triggering and ameliorating factors. Attacks are also more often associated with vegetative symptoms, such as anorexia, dry mouth, and paleness.

Aura without migraine often begins after the age of 40 years and is more common in people with a history of migraine. It can follow a migraine-free period. The overall course is benign, and patients experience predominantly positive or negative visual symptoms. Scintillating scotoma (bright shimmering lights that enlarge and move across both visual fields) are the most common positive visual symptom. Negative visual symptoms include visual field deficits, central scotomas, tunnel vision, altitudinal visual defects, or complete blindness. Other symptoms include migrating paresthesia, speech disturbance, and progression of one neurologic symptom to another. Most patients experience two or more identical spells, each lasting 15 to 25 minutes. These symptoms may raise concern for a transient ischemic attack (TIA). However, in TIA, visual deficits tend to have an abrupt onset and be dark, dim, and static, lasting only a few minutes. Paresthesias from migraine usually move up and down the extremities, may be bilateral, and clear in the reverse order. Ischemic paresthesias tend to occur suddenly and clear in the same order as they developed, and 90% last <15 minutes.

Menopause has variable effects on migraine. Two-thirds of women with migraine will experience a marked improvement, or complete cessation, once they are completely menopausal. Women who require hormonal therapy may have an increase in headache frequency secondary to therapy. Reducing the dose of estrogen or changing the type of estrogen from a conjugated estrogen to pure estradiol may reduce the number of headaches. The favorable course of migraine after menopause is primarily attributed to the absence of variations in sex hormone levels.

c. Evaluation—Because of the clinical overlap between aura without migraine and TIA, stroke imaging, such as brain MRI, is warranted. Vessel imaging, such as a CT or magnetic resonance angiogram, may also be considered to evaluate vascular risk factors.

d. Treatment—Because of their vasoconstrictive effects, abortive agents, such as triptans and ergotamines, should be used cautiously in older adults. They are contraindicated in patients with uncontrolled hypertension or evidence of vascular disease. Effective abortive agents include the limited use of acetaminophen, caffeine, nonsteroidal anti-inflammatory drugs (NSAIDs), and opioid analgesics. Patients on NSAIDs chronically should be monitored for azotemia, hypertension, or worsening cerebral or coronary artery disease. New abortive treatments thought to not cause vasoconstriction are currently in phase III trials.

Biofeedback, botulinum toxin, nerve blocks, and neuromodulation therapies have been shown to be helpful in older adults and avoid unwanted medication side effects and drug-drug interactions. β-Blockers, angiotensin-converting enzyme inhibitors/angiotensin receptor blockers, and calcium channel blockers have been shown to be effective for prevention and are often effective at lower doses. Antidopaminergic medications may be helpful for addressing the nausea symptoms associated with migraine but should be used with caution as many of these agents have anticholinergic properties that are exacerbated in older adults. Tricyclic antidepressants (TCAs), such as amitriptyline and nortriptyline, are often used for migraine prevention; however, these are not a first-line choice in older individuals because of their anticholinergic side effects. Anti-calcitonin gene related peptides (anti-CGRP) are promising new injectable treatments recently approved for migraine prevention but have not been trialed in adults older than 65 years of age.

2. Tension headache

a. General considerations—Tension headaches typically begin before age 45 years and are most commonly caused by physical or psychological stress. Despite the decreased incidence associated with aging, approximately one-third of older adults experience a tension-type headache each year. New-onset tension headache later in life may be secondary to age-related musculoskeletal, visual, or dental changes.

b. Clinical findings—Classic symptoms of tension-type headache are common in the older adult and include a bilateral, diffuse headache described as pressure or squeezing without aggravation from exercise and may last from 30 minutes to 7 days. Some patients complain of spasms of the temporomandibular joint (TMJ) from teeth clenching, arthritis in the joint, or an abnormal bite. Cervical nerve root irritation can also occur, resulting in complaints of tenderness over the occipital neurovascular bundle, suggesting occipital nerve involvement.

c. Evaluation—Physical exam should include evaluation for muscle tension in the neck, scalp, and face and an assessment of the patient's posture. Attention to the patient's bite and screening for TMJ disorders should be performed. Imaging may be warranted if there are concerns for cervical arthritis.

d. Treatment—Nonpharmacologic therapies include physical therapy for posture, balance, and range of motion in patients with musculoskeletal causes; referral to optometry or ophthalmology in the setting of decreased vision or eye strain; and relaxation therapy when stress is identified as a primary trigger.

Acetaminophen can be used safely in older patients and should be considered prior to other agents. Caffeine may be helpful as well but may lead to sleep disturbances or anxiety. TCAs, muscle relaxants, and NSAIDs can also be used but should be used with caution in older adults because of the adverse side effect profile.

3. Cluster headache

a. General considerations—The typical onset of cluster headache is age 20 to 40 years; however, peak incidence has been reported at 40 to 49 years of age in men and 60 to 69 years of age in women. The etiology of these headaches is not completely understood; however, there appear to be genetic links. Frequently, patients are smokers.

b. Clinical findings—Cluster headaches consist of episodic, severe pain of the orbital, supraorbital, or temporal area. Associated autonomic symptoms include ptosis, miosis, lacrimation, conjunctival injection, rhinorrhea, and nasal congestion occurring ipsilateral to the side of pain. Characteristically, they are of short duration (15–180 minutes) and unilateral, yet symptoms may switch to the other side during a different cluster attack. Patients may describe feeling restless or the need to pace during an attack.

c. Evaluation—Cranial imaging is recommended with CT or MRI to exclude structural brain lesions, including pituitary abnormalities.

d. Treatment—Abortive therapy with oxygen is usually safe and effective. Oxygen therapy should be used cautiously in patients with severe chronic obstructive pulmonary disease given risk of severe hypercapnia and carbon dioxide narcosis. Vasoconstrictive drugs, such as triptans, have been shown to be effective but should be used cautiously in patients with vascular disease because of deleterious side effects. One should consider giving first doses in a monitored setting. Even though often effective, corticosteroids should be used cautiously because they can worsen other medical conditions, such as osteoporosis and diabetes. Preventative medications, such as verapamil, lithium, and antiepileptic drugs, can usually be safely used in older adults.

4. Hypnic headache

a. General considerations—Hypnic headache syndrome is a rare, benign, recurrent, sleep-related headache disorder that occurs almost exclusively in patients older than 50 years. Painful attacks awaken patients from sleep usually at a predictable time, can last from 15 minutes to 4 hours, and occur ≥10 to 15 nights per month.

b. Clinical findings—Patients describe the pain as a steady discomfort primarily in the frontal area similar to tension-type headaches, but there may be migraine-like features. Pain is most often described as bilateral, as opposed to the unilateral location of cluster headaches, and hypnic headaches are not accompanied by autonomic symptoms or restlessness.

c. Evaluation—Diagnosis is based on history and exclusion of secondary headache due to sleep apnea, nocturnal hypertension, hypoglycemia, and medication overuse. Brain imaging is usually indicated to rule out posterior fossa or brainstem lesions.

d. Treatment—Hypnic headaches are self-limited and may resolve after a few months. In cases in which medication therapy is needed, lithium carbonate has shown a favorable response; however, the side effect profile may limit its long-term use. TCAs, antiepileptics, indomethacin, or NSAIDs at bedtime may also be effective. In the older adult, caffeine and melatonin are often effective, safer options.

B. Secondary Headache

Primary headaches are more common than secondary headaches in older adults; however, the prevalence of secondary headache increases with age. Potential life-threatening headaches increase by 10-fold in patients over the age of 65, most of which are vascular-related events.

1. Temporal arteritis (giant cell arteritis)

a. General considerations—Also known as giant cell arteritis (GCA), temporal arteritis is a systemic necrotizing vasculitis occurring primarily in whites with a female predominance. It typically occurs in patients aged 70 to 80 years, but should always be considered in patients older than 50 with new-onset headache. It is a medical emergency and may result in permanent visual loss in 15% to 20% of patients due to ischemic optic neuropathy.

b. Clinical findings—The first symptom in 70% to 90% of patients is a steady or throbbing headache over the temples. Diagnostic criteria outlined by the American College of Rheumatology (ACR) include age of onset >50 years, new headache, decreased temporal artery pulsation or tenderness to palpation, and elevated ESR (>50 mm/h). Pain may involve any portion of the head or scalp and may come in waves, triggered by touching the face, laughing, or chewing. Visual symptoms such as amaurosis fugax, diplopia, and visual loss occur in 5% to 15% of patients. Symptoms consistent with polymyalgia rheumatica, such as pain and stiffness, are present in approximately 66% of patients. Nonspecific symptoms of fatigue, anorexia, low-grade fever, and weight loss may occur in up to 50% of patients. Jaw claudication, although uncommon, is highly specific for temporal arteritis.

c. Evaluation—Temporal artery biopsy remains the gold standard for diagnosis, with a sensitivity of 85%. Classic findings consistent with GCA, granulomatous inflammatory infiltrate with giant cells located at the intima-media junction, are only found in 50% of cases. Ideally, biopsy should be done within 48 hours of initiating treatment, which can be challenging to obtain. Research is currently underway to evaluate proposed revision of the ACR criteria that, if present, would warrant treatment without temporal artery biopsy. If elevated, CRP and ESR have 97% specificity in diagnosing GCA. A complete blood count may show findings consistent with thrombocytosis or a normochromic anemia. Pulses may be diminished, and palpation of carotid, brachial, radial, femoral, and pedal pulses is recommended. Funduscopic exam by an ophthalmologist is warranted.

d. Treatment—To prevent blindness, urgent treatment with systemic steroids is the standard of care. Even if temporal artery biopsy is not immediately available, treatment should be initiated because pathologic findings may be present for up to 2 weeks after steroid administration. Usual course includes 1 month of full-dose therapy, followed by a slow taper up to 1 to 2 years. Intravenous glucocorticoids may be recommended for patients at high risk of blindness.

2. Cerebral vascular disease

a. General considerations—Headache can be the heralding symptom in up to 50% of hemorrhagic strokes and 25% of ischemic strokes. In older adult patients with vascular risk factors and headache, cerebrovascular disease must be considered. See Chapter 38, "Cerebrovascular Disease," for clinical findings, evaluation, and treatment.

3. Trigeminal neuralgia

a. General considerations—Trigeminal neuralgia (TN) is one of the most common neuralgias seen in older adults, with the incidence increasing with age and a slight female predominance. Primary TN occurs in 80% to 90% of cases and is thought to be caused by compression of the trigeminal nerve root by an aberrant arterial or venous loop. Secondary TN may be a result of other causes, such as an acoustic neuroma, meningioma, epidermoid cyst, or, rarely, an aneurysm or arteriovenous malformation. This secondary form is more likely when the disorder presents prior to the fifth decade of life.

b. Clinical findings—The updated International Headache Society Diagnostic Criteria for Trigeminal Neuralgia are as follows:

1. Recurrent paroxysmal attacks of unilateral facial pain affect one or more divisions of the trigeminal nerve with no radiation beyond.
2. Pain that has all of the following characteristics: severe intensity that may become more severe over time; electric shock–like, sharp, stabbing, or shooting pain quality; and pain that lasts from a fraction of a second to 2 minutes. In rare cases, pain may last longer than 2 minutes.
3. Pain is precipitated from innocuous stimuli in the trigger area or by trigger factors.
4. No other attributing disorder is present.

Episodes may last for weeks to months and may be followed by pain-free intervals. Some patients develop a general dull ache in the distribution of the affected nerve and/or experience lacrimation or erythema of the ipsilateral eye.

c. Evaluation—TN is a clinical diagnosis. Attacks may be triggered during an examination by touching the "trigger zone," usually an area in the distribution of the affected nerve, often near the midline. Actions that may trigger an attack include chewing, talking, brushing one's teeth, cold air against the face, smiling, or grimacing; notably, patients are not usually awoken from sleep.

Secondary TN is often indistinguishable from primary TN. Imaging with CT or MRI is warranted to rule out secondary causes. Electrophysiologic tests may be useful in distinguishing primary from secondary causes of TN.

d. Treatment—Pharmacologic therapy is the initial treatment for patients with primary TN. Carbamazepine is the best studied treatment, and side effects may be manageable if it is started at low doses with slow titration. Oxcarbazepine is probably effective, along with baclofen, lamotrigine, and pimozide. There is less evidence for the effectiveness of clonazepam, gabapentin, phenytoin, tizanidine, and valproate. Periodic taper or withdrawal trials should be attempted. Secondary TN requires treatment of the underlying condition; however, medications used in treatment of classic TN may provide pain relief. In the 30% of patients who fail medical management, microvascular decompression or ablative surgical procedures may be considered.

4. Mass lesions

a. General considerations—Older adults have a higher incidence of intracranial tumors than younger adults, with an incidence peak between the ages of 65 and 79 years of age. Up to 50% of patients presenting with brain tumors complain of headache. Glioblastoma is the most common primary brain malignancy in adults, with older age known to be a negative clinical prognostic factor. Meningiomas are the most common nonmalignant brain tumor in adults, representing 20% of all brain tumors.

b. Clinical findings—Pain is usually generalized but may be localized over the tumor. The classic severe morning headache, associated with nausea and vomiting, occurs in approximately 17% of patients. More often, patients complain of symptoms similar to tension or migraine headache.

c. Evaluation—If a mass lesion is suspected, an MRI must be obtained and neurosurgical subspecialty referral pursued.

d. Treatment—Neurosurgical, medical, and/or palliative care options should be considered. For malignant brain tumors such as glioblastoma, surgery, radiation, and chemotherapy are necessary to increase survival times. Nonmalignant tumors, such as meningiomas, can be managed conservatively, if they are without mass effect, or surgically with radiation based on their size and location.

5. Cervicogenic headache

a. General considerations—Cervicogenic headache occurs because of referred pain from anatomic structures and soft tissues of the neck. This headache type may be overdiagnosed in the older adult secondary to the large number of geriatric patients with radiographic changes consistent with cervical spondylosis. It is also often mistaken for tension-type headache.

b. Clinical findings—Symptoms are elicited by neck movement, certain head positions, or when pressure is applied over cervical musculature. There may be occipital-nuchal pain, limited range of motion of the neck, or spasms of the cervical muscles; however, in some cases, there is no associated neck pain. There should be evidence that the neck is the causative factor for pain in order to make this diagnosis.

c. Evaluation—Successful anesthetic blockade of the cervical facet joint, nerve root, or occipital nerves is confirmatory.

d. Treatment—Nonpharmacologic therapies include neck massage, physical therapy, and biofeedback. Muscle relaxants and NSAIDs may be necessary but should be used with caution in the older adult. Procedural treatments include radiofrequency, facet joint rhizolysis, and occipital nerve cryorhizolysis.

6. Medication-induced headache—Medications and supplements should be reviewed as a cause of headache. Patient symptoms may appear similar to migraine or tension-type headaches, but a careful history regarding the timing of headaches in relation to starting or taking medications is advised. Common offenders include nitrates, calcium channel blockers, estrogens/progestins, histamine blockers, theophylline, and NSAIDs. Overuse, or abrupt discontinuation, of caffeine, analgesics, opiates, and serotonin antagonists may also lead to daily headache.

7. Headache caused by other medical conditions—Older adults often have medical conditions or treatments that may cause or worsen headaches. Cardiac cephalalgia is one such example occurring in patients with cardiac disease who present with an exertional-based headache that resolves with rest. Morning headaches may be indicative of untreated sleep apnea, and headaches that occur in low-light conditions may be indicative of a subacute glaucoma. These and other such causes of headache often improve or resolve with appropriate treatment of the underlying medical condition and should be considered in the differential diagnosis.

Berk T, Ashina S, Martin V, Newman L, Vij B. Diagnosis and treatment of primary headache disorders in older adults. *J Am Geriatr Soc.* 2018;66:2408-2416.

International Headache Society. International Classification of Headache, 3rd edition; Cephalalgia 2018. https://www.ichd-3.org. Accessed April 16, 2020.

Kunkel R. Headaches in older patients: special problems and concerns. *Cleve Clin J Med.* 2006;73(10):922-928.

Sait MR, et al. The 2016 revised ACR criteria for diagnosis of giant cell arteritis – Our case series: Can this avoid unnecessary temporal artery Biopsies? *International J Surgery Open* 2017;9: 19-23

Sharma TL. Common primary and secondary causes of headache in the elderly. *Headache.* 2018;58(3):479-484.

Starling AJ. Diagnosis and management of headache in older adults. *Mayo Clin Proc.* 2018;93(2):252-262.

Tanganelli P. Secondary headaches in the elderly. *Neurol Sci.* 2010;31(suppl 1):S73-S76.

65

Chest Pain

Alejandra Sanchez-Lopez, MD
Miguel Paniagua, MD, FACP

General Principles

Chest pain is the most common reason for emergency department visits in patients older than 65 years of age in the United States. The differential diagnosis encompasses both benign and life-threatening diseases. Although not all causes of chest pain in the older adult will lead to fatal events, timely diagnosis can improve a patient's health outcomes in the short term, as well as long term, including quality of life and functional status.

It is essential that clinicians take a thorough history, perform a targeted physical exam, and have a high level of suspicion in order to choose the most appropriate diagnostic laboratory tests and imaging studies to make the correct diagnosis in a timely manner.

Clinical Findings

A. Symptoms & Signs

The onset of chest pain should be clarified first, followed by a description and evolution of the symptom. Typical angina at any age presents as substernal chest pain, often described as "pressure like," with radiation to the jaw, neck, or arm. Clinicians should also ask about associated cardiopulmonary symptoms such as diaphoresis, cool clammy skin, new or progressive shortness of breath, and/or exertional shortness of breath. If a patient has a history of acute coronary syndrome (ACS) in the past, asking if the pain is similar to that experienced previously can be an important clue.

Descriptions of chest pain as radiating to the back, abrupt onset, severe in intensity, or tearing, stabbing, or sharp in quality may be more suggestive of aortic dissection. Pleuritic chest pain occurs with inspiration and is caused by inflammation of the pleural lining of the lung. If patients feel chest pain after eating or when lying flat and with a burning quality, one should consider a gastroesophageal etiology.

Older patients are typically more likely to delay seeking medical care or be more inclined to attribute their symptoms to "normal aging," which can lead to increased adverse outcomes or death if the etiology of the chest pain is serious in nature. Moreover, patients with delirium, severe depression, or cognitive impairment may have trouble communicating their symptoms accurately. In addition, given that older adults have a higher prevalence of chronic conditions, concurrent disease processes may cloud the presentation.

1. Physical examination—The first step should be to obtain vital signs to assess the clinical stability of the patient with special attention to heart rate, blood pressure in both arms, and oxygen saturation. Next, the clinician should assess the cardiovascular system. If heart sounds are muffled on cardiac auscultation, pulsus paradoxus is present (a decrease in systolic pressure of >10 mm Hg during inspiration), or there is hypotension, then cardiac tamponade should be considered. A loud new holosystolic murmur is suggestive of acute coronary pathology and possibly mitral valve papillary dysfunction. Elevated jugular venous pressure, hepatojugular reflux, and an S_3 gallop suggest congestive heart failure. Furthermore, in patients with acute chest pain, the finding of an S_3 increases by three-fold the likelihood of myocardial infarction. Lower extremity edema that is symmetric in both limbs and acute or subacute may be suggestive of right heart failure; however, if there is unilateral swelling, one must suspect venous thromboembolism and consider pulmonary thromboembolism, especially if hypoxia and tachycardia are present.

Lung auscultation would provide further information; for example, absence of breath sounds may indicate pneumothorax or a pleural effusion. Other lung findings such as rales, wheezes, or bronchophony can suggest other lung etiology.

Complete assessment of the chest includes observation of the skin in search for rashes, such as in the case of herpes zoster, or even ecchymosis that could indicate trauma, which would raise suspicion for physical abuse. Palpation of the chest wall with reproducible chest pain may indicate musculoskeletal etiology and decreases the likelihood of ACS but does not exclude it.

Further clues in the diagnosis can be obtained from abdominal examination, such as epigastric pain, which may point to a gastrointestinal etiology causing referred pain to the chest.

2. Laboratory findings—The standard cardiac panel includes creatinine kinase (CK) and troponin I and T. CK is leaked out of injured muscle cells and is not specific to myocardial injury. Troponin is more specific and sensitive to myocardial injury and appears within 6 hours of infarction and remains elevated for 4 to 8 days. Sensitivity is only 50% when measured within 4 hours of symptom onset; in contrast, CK has a shorter half-life, and in the case of recurrent injury in an acute setting, it would be a more reliable marker of repeat myocardial injury. It is important to keep in mind that elevated troponins should be interpreted within the clinical context, given that this can be seen not only in ACS, such in as non–ST-segment elevation myocardial infarction (NSTEMI) and ST-segment elevation myocardial infarction (STEMI) where there is a degree of blockage of coronary arteries, but also in demand ischemia where there is a mismatch between oxygen's blood supply and demand, as in tachyarrhythmias or sepsis and in other nonischemic conditions such as heart failure exacerbation, pulmonary embolism (PE), or renal failure. In addition, a negative troponin, does not rule out ACS because the patient could be having unstable angina.

Another diagnostic test commonly used is the D-dimer to rule out PE in patients with low and intermediate clinical probability. D-dimer levels increase with age, and even though the ADJUST-PE study showed that patients with a low age-adjusted D-dimer cutoff (defined as 10 times the age) in combination with pretest clinical probability assessment had a low likelihood of subsequent clinical thromboembolism, the use of age-adjust D-dimer is currently not part of standard practice.

3. Diagnostic tests and imaging studies—Electrocardiogram (ECG) is the first step in the chest pain workup of an older patient and preferably should happen in the first 10 minutes of an encounter. If available, the last ECG previous to the onset of chest pain should be used for comparison; in this age group, patients may already have significant cardiac history with baseline abnormalities on ECG further confounding acute findings. ST-segment elevations in a specific coronary territory raise concern for acute coronary plaque rupture and STEMI. Diffuse ST-segment elevations or depressions may be more suggestive of pericarditis in the appropriate clinical context. ECG findings of cardiac tamponade include blunting of the voltage of QRS complexes and the presence of electrical alternans—a beat-to-beat variation of QRS complexes in an alternating pattern.

On chest radiography, the presence of a widened mediastinum, if clinical history suggests, should raise suspicion of an aortic dissection, and this imaging modality can be useful to rule out a pneumonia or pleural effusion. Suspicion for pulmonary thromboembolism or aortic dissection should prompt the clinician to order a computed tomography (CT) of the chest with contrast for diagnostic purposes.

4. Special tests—Progressive dyspnea that accompanies chest pain with exertion (angina) should be evaluated with a stress test, such as an exercise stress test with an imaging modality such as stress echocardiogram, radionuclide myocardial perfusion imaging, or stress MRI. An imaging modality is necessary because baseline abnormalities on ECG can confound results. Frail older patients may be limited by their functional capacity and unable to complete an exercise stress test. In appropriate patients, using a bicycle instead of a treadmill can sometimes compensate for these functional deficits. For patients who are unable to reach the target heart rate with exercise, pharmacologic stress can be induced with dobutamine or vasodilators such as dipyridamole, adenosine, or regadenoson.

As noted previously, gastrointestinal causes of chest pain can be mistaken for angina, and if clinically indicated and after ruling out life-threatening diagnoses, an upper endoscopy may be helpful in the diagnosis of esophagitis, or a barium swallow exam may show multiple strictures in corkscrew pattern if the patient is suffering from esophageal spasm or other anatomic abnormalities. (See Chapter 47, "Gastrointestinal Disease," for further discussion of the workup for esophageal and other gastrointestinal disorders.)

▶ Differential Diagnosis

The differential diagnosis of chest pain in older patients is as broad as it is in younger adults, with the complexity of possible coexisting multimorbidity. Once established, chest pain should be assessed for its likelihood of being cardiac or noncardiac, followed by initial consideration of diagnoses associated with the highest mortality or complication rates, the so-called "can't miss diagnoses" (Figure 65–1).

A. Cardiac Diagnoses

Cardiac causes of chest pain include ACSs, such as STEMI, NSTEMI, and unstable angina, as well as aortic dissection, cardiac tamponade, and pericarditis. The incidence of myocardial infarction (MI) increases with age; the average age at first MI is 65 years for males and 72 years for females, and chest pain is the most frequent chief complaint of older patients with ACS. Therefore, ACS should be considered first when an older adult presents with chest pain due to its high incidence and mortality in this patient population. At the same time, older people are more likely than younger patients to have a cardiac event in the absence of chest pain or have an atypical presentation, such as nausea, abdominal pain, or delirium.

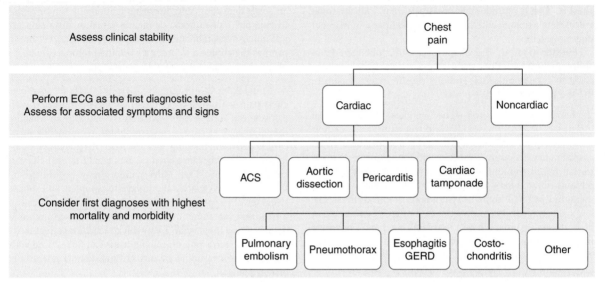

▲ **Figure 65–1.** Diagram to guide assessment of chest pain. The first step is to determine clinical stability by measuring vital signs and assessing level of consciousness. The second step includes taking an electrocardiogram (ECG) preferably within the first 10 minutes of arrival, especially to rule out ST-segment elevation myocardial infarction and recognize other electrical abnormalities. A detailed history of present illness considering past medical history and a thorough physical exam will guide the differential diagnosis, considering first diagnoses with highest mortality and increased morbidity if timely diagnosis is not made. This process will assist in selecting further testing. ACS, acute coronary syndrome; GERD, gastroesophageal reflux disease.

Features suggesting ACS include diaphoresis, cool clammy skin, new or progressive shortness of breath, and/or exertional shortness of breath. Doing a risk stratification can be helpful to assess the likelihood of a major adverse cardiac event and to guide next steps. There are different risk scores. A common score used in emergency departments is the HEART score, which takes into account elements from **h**istory, **E**CG, **a**ge, **r**isk factors, and **t**roponin and classifies patients in three groups (Table 65–1). The HEART score has been shown to outperform the Global Registry of Acute Coronary Events (GRACE) and Thrombolysis In Myocardial Infarction (TIMI) scores in discriminating between those with and without major adverse cardiac events in patients with chest pain and identified the largest group of low-risk patients at the same level of safety.

Aortic dissection is another life-threatening condition with peak incidence in the seventies, and hypertension is a major risk factor. Typical sudden-onset, tearing, stabbing, or sharp chest pain; a systolic blood pressure limb differential >20 mm Hg (without a history of vascular compromise in either limb); and a widened mediastinum on a chest x-ray should raise suspicion for aortic dissection.

Cardiac tamponade is more common in the setting of certain chronic illnesses including autoimmune disease, malignancy, or a recent history of acute trauma to the chest. If a cardiac rub is present, pericarditis should be entertained.

B. Noncardiac Diagnoses

Pulmonary causes of chest pain include acute PE, pneumothorax, and pleuritis. Pleuritic chest pain is a nonspecific symptom that can have a variety of causes including infectious, autoimmune, or other systemic illnesses; when associated with fever and/or sputum production, it may suggest pneumonia. A chest x-ray showing air space opacification in a lobar or segmental distribution will aid in the diagnosis of infectious diagnoses such as pneumonia.

Pleuritic chest pain is present in 40% to 48% of patients with PE, and when considering this diagnosis, using the Wells score or the revised Geneva score can help assess the probability of a PE. The Wells Score is more widely used; however, only the Geneva score uses age as a risk factor in the scoring system (Table 65–2).

The most common musculoskeletal cause of chest pain is costochondritis (swelling of the costal cartilages), and on exam, pain would be reproducible by palpation. However, it is always important to make sure other life-threatening causes are ruled out before making this diagnosis. Chest pain caused by gastrointestinal diseases is generally related to esophageal reflux, esophagitis, or esophageal motor disorders and should be considered in the presence of heartburn or burning pain related to food ingestion or that is worsened when lying flat. Chemical esophagitis (or pill esophagitis) related to medications such

Table 65–1. HEART score.

HEART Score	Points
History	
• Highly suspicious	2
• Moderately suspicious	1
• Slightly suspicious	0
ECG	
• Significant ST depression	2
• Nonspecific repolarization disturbance	1
• Normal	0
Age	
• ≥65 years	2
• 45–64 years	1
• ≤44 years	0
Risk factors: hypertension, hypercholesterolemia, diabetes, obesity, smoking (current or cessation ≤3 months), family history (first degree with CVD before age 65) or atherosclerotic disease	
• ≥3 risk factors or history of atherosclerotic disease	2
• 1 or 2 risk factors	1
• No risk factors known	0
Troponins	
• ≤3 × normal limit	2
• 1≥3 × normal limit	1
• ≤ normal limit	0

Scores:
0–3: 0.9%–1.7% risk of adverse cardiac event.
4–6: 12%–16.6% risk of adverse cardiac event.
≥7: 50%–65% risk of adverse cardiac event.

CVD, cardiovascular disease; ECG, electrocardiogram.
Reproduced with permission from Backus BE, Six AJ, Kelder JC, et al. A prospective validation of the HEART score for chest pain patients at the emergency department, *Int J Cardiol* 2013 Oct 3;168(3):2153-2158.

Table 65–2. Wells criteria and revised Geneva score.

Wells Criteria		Revised Geneva Score	
• Clinical signs and symptoms of DVT	3	• Age >65	1
• PE is the number 1 diagnosis or equally likely	3	• Previous DVT or PE	3
		• Surgery or lower limb fracture in past month	2
• Heart rate >100 beats/min	1.5	• Active malignant condition	2
• Immobilization at least 3 days or surgery in the previous 4 weeks	1.5		
		• Unilateral lower limb pain	3
• Previous PE or DVT	1.5	• Hemoptysis	2
• Hemoptysis	1	• Heart rate	0
• Malignancy within the last 6 months	1	• <75 beats/min	
		• 75–94 beats/min	3
		• ≥95 beats/min	5
		• Pain on lower limb palpation and unilateral edema	4
Risk stratification		**Risk stratification**	
Low: 0–1		Low: 0–3	
Moderate: 2–6		Intermediate: 4–10	
High: ≥6		High: ≥11	

DVT, deep vein thrombosis; PE, pulmonary embolism.

as bisphosphonates may be particularly prevalent in older patients, especially those with a high daily pill burden. Suspicion of pill esophagitis should prompt a close examination of the patient's medication list for possible contributors.

▶ Treatment

Treatment is specific to the underlying cause of chest pain. In the case of an STEMI, rapid diagnosis by ECG and clinical history can lead to prompt activation of the cardiac catheterization team. If no cardiac catheterization is available at the location of presentation and if the patient can be transported to a hospital with cardiac catheterization capabilities within 90 minutes of presentation, then arrangement for transfer should be made immediately. If catheterization is not possible, then pharmacologic thrombolysis can be considered (see Chapter 39, "Coronary Artery Disease").

At presentation, if clinical history of aortic dissection is confirmed by a CT scan, treatment depends on type of dissection. Type A involves the ascending aorta and is considered a surgical emergency. Type B dissections are localized to the descending aorta and are typically managed nonoperatively. The 2010 American College of Cardiology/American Heart Association guidelines recommend maintaining a heart rate goal of ≤60 beats/min and a systolic blood pressure of <120 mm Hg as part of the immediate management.

Pericarditis requires additional workup after diagnosis to establish the etiology. In addition to treatment of the underlying cause, most cases can be treated with nonsteroidal anti-inflammatory agents, colchicine, or aspirin, if there are no contraindications. In older adults, consider creatinine clearance, concurrent use with anticoagulation, and increasing pill burden prior to initiating nonsteroidal anti-inflammatory agents.

If the diagnosis of PE is definitively made with CT scan or with ventilation-perfusion scan, the patient should be started on anticoagulation therapy if no absolute contraindications are present. If the patient has contraindications for anticoagulation, consideration can be given to inferior vena cava filter placement; however, this is paradoxically prothrombotic and should be retrieved according to manufacturer guidelines when the contraindication is no longer present.

Inflammation and strain of the muscles of the rib cage can lead to chest pain causing significant distress. Once all life-threatening causes of chest pain are effectively ruled out and the physical exam is consistent with costochondritis, the patient can be reassured and pain relief can generally be achieved with an anti-inflammatory agent.

Gastrointestinal manifestations of chest pain such as gastroesophageal reflux disease and esophagitis can be managed with antihistamine-1 blockers or with proton pump inhibitors (see Chapter 47, "Gastrointestinal Disease"). If esophageal spasm is diagnosed, a calcium channel blocker and avoidance of triggers can effectively manage symptoms.

SUMMARY

Chest pain in the older adult is a common symptom, and its cause can potentially be life threatening or carry high risk for complications affecting a patient's quality of life. It is important for clinicians to think through cardiac and noncardiac causes of chest pain and risk stratify patients upon presentation so that appropriate treatment is not delayed. Ischemic heart disease is the first diagnosis to consider due to the high incidence and significant cause of morbidity and mortality in older adults. Atypical presentations of chest pain are frequent in this patient population, and providers need to have a high index of suspicion. Tools to accomplish this include a thorough history, physical exam, ECG, cardiac enzymes, and chest radiography on initial evaluation and tailored use of further testing in the appropriate clinical scenario.

Alexander KP, Newby KL, Cannon CP, et al; American Heart Association Council on Clinical Cardiology; Society of Geriatric Cardiology. Acute coronary care in the elderly part 1: non-ST-segment-elevation acute coronary syndromes: a scientific statement for healthcare professionals from the American Heart Association Council on Clinical Cardiology: in collaboration with the Society of Geriatric Cardiology. *Circulation.* 2007;115(19):2549-2569.

Benjamin EJ, Muntner P, Alonso A, et al. Heart disease and stroke statistics-2019 update: a report from the American Heart Association. *Circulation.* 2019;139:e56-e528.

Brieger D, Eagle KA, Goodman SG, et al. Acute coronary syndromes without chest pain, an underdiagnosed and undertreated high-risk group: insights from the Global Registry of Acute Coronary Events. *Chest.* 2004;126(2):461-469.

Canto JG, Fincher C, Kiefe CI, et al. Atypical presentations among Medicare beneficiaries with unstable angina pectoris. *Am J Cardiol.* 2002;90(3):248-253.

Chun AA, McGee SR. Bedside diagnosis of coronary artery disease: a systematic review. *Am J Med.* 2004;117(5):335-343.

Gupta, R, Munoz R. Evaluation and management of chest pain in the elderly. *Emerg Med Clin N Am.* 2016;34:523-542.

National Hospital Ambulatory Medical Care Survey: 2015 Emergency Department Summary Tables (Table 10). https://www.cdc.gov/nchs/data/nhamcs/web_tables/2015_ed_web_tables.pdf. Accessed April 16, 2020.

Righini M, Van Es J, Den Exter PL, et al. Age-adjusted D-dimer cutoff levels to rule out pulmonary embolism: the ADJUST-PE study. *JAMA.* 2014;311(11):1117-1124.

Dyspnea

Ashwin Kotwal, MD, MS

Rebecca Starr, MD

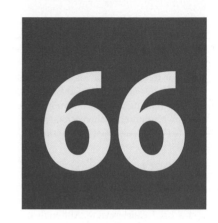

General Principles

Dyspnea is a common symptom affecting older adults, occurring in 17% to 62% of community-dwelling adults >65 years old, with the highest rates in those 80 years and older. According to Smith and colleagues (2016), "one in four adults aged 70 and older in the United States experiences breathlessness, which is associated with lack of well-being, greater health services use, and a 40% greater risk of worsened function and 60% greater risk of death over the next five years." The 2012 American Thoracic Society consensus statement defines dyspnea as "a subjective experience of breathing discomfort that consists of qualitatively distinct sensations that vary in intensity." Descriptions of dyspnea can be further classified into three domains: (1) sensory-perceptual experience (eg, what breathing "feels like" to the patient), (2) affective distress (eg, the perception of immediate unpleasantness), and (3) symptom impact or burden (eg, how breathing affects behaviors, function, or quality of life). Importantly, dyspnea is a *symptom* that is self-reported and should be distinguished from clinical signs of respiratory distress, such as tachypnea, the use of accessory muscles, or nasal flaring.

Dyspnea is often inadequately addressed in older adults. It may not be routinely assessed due to limited appointment time, a clinician's inappropriate presumption that the dyspnea is caused by a chronic condition and cannot be treated further, or underreporting among older adults. Consequently, older adults may experience dyspnea with minimal symptomatic management along with underdiagnosis of the underlying cause. Indeed, it is common for dyspnea to signal either a new significant medical problem or a worsening of one (or more) of the chronic cardiopulmonary diseases that are prevalent among older adults. Moreover, dyspnea is a distressing physical symptom, which, if left untreated, can impair mobility, social function, mood, and ability to perform activities of daily living (ADLs), all while independently increasing mortality risk. For these reasons, clinicians should consider routine assessment of dyspnea in the geriatric patient, and its presence should never be ignored.

Clinicians should be aware of the following key principles of geriatric care when evaluating and treating the older patient with shortness of breath: (1) recognize that dyspnea commonly arises from nonrespiratory mechanisms; (2) consider soliciting history from caregivers or other knowledgeable informants; (3) consider the possibility of alternative presentations or symptoms; (4) pay special attention to medications; (5) consider the benefits and burdens of diagnostic procedures and treatments; and (6) consider palliative care if the patient has advanced chronic cardiopulmonary illness.

Diagnostics

Evaluations of dyspnea in older adults often focus on cardiopulmonary diseases; however, recent literature suggests that dyspnea should be considered a multifactorial geriatric syndrome with potential contributors from multiple domains of health. Sarcopenia or deconditioning, chronic kidney disease, anemia, medication-related adverse events, and psychiatric illness can all contribute to the presence of dyspnea. Each factor on its own might not seem great enough to cause dyspnea, but combined, these factors can cause significant cumulative symptoms. A comprehensive history and physical may therefore identify multiple sources to be targeted by medical interventions. Patients and families often appreciate clinicians letting them know that more than one condition may be causing the dyspnea and that a degree of therapeutic trial and error may be required.

Although an initial office-based assessment for dyspnea can be completed in all older adult patients, more extensive testing (eg, pulmonary function tests, computed tomography [CT] scans, cardiac stress tests) can be burdensome for frail or cognitively impaired patients with limited life expectancy and often has limited additional diagnostic utility. For example, abnormal spirometry has a poor positive predictive value for dyspnea in older adults. Similarly, invasive treatments for dyspnea can be more burdensome for older adults than others. For these reasons, clinicians should consider benefits and burdens before referring patients for more extensive evaluations or treatments and should attempt to discuss benefits and burdens with patients and families as part of a shared decision-making process. For more on how to identify older adults with limited life expectancy, see Chapter 4, "Goals of Care & Consideration of Prognosis."

▶ History

Given the extensive differential diagnosis for dyspnea in older adults, clinicians should start with a thorough history and a brief chart review. Although many older adults are capable of providing an excellent history, others may be limited by cognitive problems, hearing impairments, or speech difficulties. Clinicians should therefore consider including a knowledgeable informant. Moreover, older adults may complain less of the sensation of affective distress from dyspnea due to adapting to a physiologic "new normal." Informants can provide collateral history on whether they observe sedentary behavior or dyspnea contributing to limited mobility, ADL impairment, or poor quality of life.

The goals of history taking are to:

- Determine whether the complaint is a new problem, a worsening of a chronic complaint, or an ongoing complaint that has failed to resolve
- Determine the duration, severity, frequency, temporal pattern, exacerbating/alleviating factors, and qualitative character
- Identify the impact on physical and psychological function
- Identify associated symptoms, such as peripheral edema, fever, chest pain or pressure, or pleuritic pain, which may point toward an underlying etiology
- Identify chronic conditions or previous conditions associated with dyspnea
- Check for the presence of environmental or occupational exposures that may provoke or aggravate dyspnea, such as cigarette smoking, cold air, and allergens such as pets, or poor air quality
- Review medication use, with special attention to (1) inhalers, which are often difficult to use correctly; (2) diuretics, which patients sometimes skip to reduce incontinence; and (3) psychoactive or sedating medications, which can lead to the development of dyspnea through sedentary behaviors and deconditioning

A. Quantitative & Qualitative Assessment of Dyspnea

The severity of dyspnea can be assessed by asking the patient to report using a visual analog scale or a numerical scale (ie, 0–10), with 0 corresponding to none, 1 to 4 corresponding to mild, 5 to 8 corresponding to moderate, and 9 to 10 corresponding to severe dyspnea. Patients should be encouraged to describe what the dyspnea "feels like" because certain qualitative sensations have been linked with underlying pathophysiologies. For example, descriptions of "work" and "effort" are associated with asthma, chronic obstructive pulmonary disease (COPD), or impaired conditioning. "Chest tightness" can be associated with acute bronchoconstriction in asthma. Cardiac deconditioning has been linked to the feeling of "heavy breathing." "Air hunger," or the sensation of not getting enough air or having an unpleasant urge to breathe, is common in asthma, COPD, and interstitial lung disease. Sensations of "suffocating" or "smothering" are nonspecific but have been associated with panic disorder and COPD.

B. Assessing Functional Impact

Assessing dyspnea's impact on physical, psychological, and social function is important in both acute and chronic presentations. The impact on physical function can be quickly assessed by asking the patient and caregiver questions such as, "How far can you walk? How does that compare to before?" or "What activities are you having difficulty with as a result of your shortness of breath?" Assessing mood is important in patients suffering from chronic dyspnea, such as those with COPD, given the association with anxiety and depression. This can be briefly assessed by asking questions such as, "How does your breathing difficulty make you feel?" or "How bothersome does your breathing feel to you?" For patients endorsing feelings of sadness, apathy, or anxiety, more detailed evaluation for depression or anxiety should be considered. Dyspnea can limit older patients' ability to participate in activities outside of the home or socialize. Consequently, patients should be evaluated for loneliness, social isolation, adequate social supports, and relevant social interventions (see Chapter 18, "The Social Context of Older Adults").

C. Associated Signs & Symptoms

Breathing problems in older adults may manifest as another complaint or symptom, such as fatigue, pain, depression, anxiety, chest discomfort, or decreased physical activity. Patients with moderate or severe dementia may no longer be able to clearly articulate a breathing complaint.

In addition, the presence or absence of certain signs and symptoms can help identify the underlying etiology of the dyspnea. In particular, clinicians should ask about:

- Cough and characteristics of sputum, if any
- Fever
- Nasal congestion
- Acute or chronic nonpleuritic chest pain or pressure
- Pleuritic pain
- Edema of the legs or elsewhere

D. Relevant Chronic or Past Medical Conditions

Clinicians should note the presence of any chronic medical conditions associated with dyspnea, as these provide an important context in which to consider the current complaint. Past conditions (eg, acute anemia) may have an increased chance of recurrence. The most common chronic conditions associated with dyspnea are the following:

- COPD
- Heart failure
- Coronary artery disease
- Deconditioning/obesity
- Asthma
- Interstitial lung disease
- Anemia
- Chronic kidney disease
- Frailty

▶ Physical Exam

All evaluations of dyspnea in the geriatric patient should include a focused physical exam. On exam, the clinician should note the following:

- Vital signs including respiratory rate and oxygen saturation; consider ambulatory oxygen saturation if dyspnea on exertion has been reported
- General appearance, including visible distress and work of breathing, as well as signs of anemia such as conjunctival pallor or palmar crease pallor
- Head and neck exam, with attention to signs of upper respiratory infection or obstruction, placement of the trachea, and use of accessory muscles in breathing
- Lung exam, focused on the presence of wheezing, crackles, or other abnormal sounds
- Cardiovascular exam, with attention to the cardiac rhythm, S_3 gallop, heart murmurs, jugular venous pressure, and leg edema
- Frailty assessment, with special attention to the chair stand as a measure of proximal muscle function, grip strength, and weight loss

▶ Additional Diagnostic Tests

Table 66–1 lists additional tests to consider. The appropriate test depends on the history, physical exam, and acuity of the complaint. For an acute complaint, CT of the chest is generally only indicated for high suspicion of pulmonary embolism. For chronic shortness of breath, CT of the chest

Table 66–1. Additional diagnostic tests for dyspnea

Test	Indication
Electrocardiogram	Suspicion of ongoing or recent cardiac ischemia, or if concern for atrial fibrillation or other symptomatic arrhythmia
Chest radiograph	Suspicion of pneumonia, pleural effusion, or pneumothorax
Laboratory testing	Complete blood count (CBC) if concern for anemia Brain natriuretic peptide (BNP) if concern for heart failure Consider D-dimer if suspicion of deep venous thrombosis (DVT)/pulmonary embolism (PE) (negative predictive value much higher than positive predictive value)
Peak flow	Suspicion of asthma exacerbation
Spirometry and pulmonary function tests	Evaluation of ongoing or chronic dyspnea (not usually performed for acute dyspnea)
Echocardiogram	Consider if concern for heart failure or valve disease
Cardiac stress testing	Consider if concern for coronary artery disease

is generally only considered for evaluation of interstitial lung disease.

▶ Differential Diagnosis

Table 66–2 details the differential diagnoses to consider for both acute (symptoms that have developed over hours to days) and chronic dyspnea (symptoms lasting >4 weeks). The differential diagnoses are strongly influenced by whether the dyspnea complaint appears to be new and acute versus chronic and ongoing. In older adults, clinicians should be aware of noncardiopulmonary contributors to dyspnea including chronic kidney disease, anxiety, depression, frailty, sarcopenia related to deconditioning or nutritional deficiencies, medications that impact the experience of dyspnea, or anemia. For subacute presentations (ie, development over days to weeks), both lists in Table 66–2 should be considered.

▶ Next Steps and Treatment

The approach to managing dyspnea includes optimizing treatments of the underlying illness and providing symptomatic support. Clinicians should tailor treatments to fit with the patient's preferences and goals of care and provide anticipatory guidance on the expected benefits and burdens when selecting among treatment options.

Table 66–2. Differential diagnoses for dyspnea in the geriatric patient.

Acute Dyspnea	Chronic Dyspnea
Pneumonia	COPD
Acute coronary syndrome	Heart failure
COPD or asthma exacerbation	Deconditioning
Heart failure exacerbation	Interstitial lung disease
Rapid atrial fibrillation or other tachyarrhythmia	Asthma
Aspiration	Anemia
Anemia	Valvular disease
Pulmonary embolism	Chronic kidney disease
Cardiac tamponade	Cancer
Pneumothorax	Psychiatric illness
Anaphylaxis	
Panic attack	

COPD, chronic obstructive pulmonary disease.

A. General Principles

Clinicians treating a complaint of dyspnea in the older adults should do the following:

- **Take an individualized and multicomponent approach.** Clinicians should examine medications to ensure proper adherence, reduce polypharmacy, and minimize sedating medications that can promote sedentary behaviors. Deconditioning and sarcopenia are key predictors of dyspnea in older adults, so clinicians should address gait instability, foot problems, nutritional deficiencies, and exercise habits. Environmental modifications to address stairs at home or excess clutter can reduce exertional workload. Clinicians should address coexisting symptoms such as pain, fatigue, or depression that can modify the experience of dyspnea.

- **Provide clear written instructions to patient and caregivers.** Older adults with cognitive impairment, especially when feeling unwell, may have difficulty remembering verbal instructions. Furthermore, caregivers who are involved in managing medications or other aspects of care may not be present during the clinical encounter. Clear written instructions reduce the chance of misunderstandings and facilitate sharing of the care plan with other caregivers or clinicians involved.

- **Realize that inhalers can be problematic for some older adults to use correctly.** Older adults may be at risk of using inhalers incorrectly and of misunderstanding instructions for use (especially if both short-acting and

long-acting inhalers are prescribed). Inhalers are often expensive for patients to obtain, causing many patients to decline to fill the prescription. Consequently, clinicians should be aware of potential financial strain interfering with adherence, and regimens should be simplified if possible. Clinicians should encourage patients and caregivers to obtain inhaler training, either in clinic, from pharmacists, or through free online videos provided by the COPD Foundation (see "Online Resources"). Older adults may benefit from prescriptions of spacers to improve efficacy of medication administration (eg, metered-dose inhalers) and to reduce the pressure of getting the timing of the press-inhale sequence correct. Clinicians should consider ordering a nebulizer for patients; both albuterol and ipratropium, for instance, are much less expensive as generic nebulizer solutions.

- **Arrange prompt follow-up of symptoms and medication adherence.** Clinicians should arrange prompt follow-up in order to ensure that the dyspnea is improving. This is especially important for more vulnerable patients, including those who live alone or with a frail spouse, or those with cognitive impairment. Patients and caregivers should be asked to bring all medications, including the ones newly prescribed, to the follow-up visit. Difficulty adhering to medication changes or recommendations is a common cause for dyspnea symptoms to persist or even worsen.

- **Regular and repeated documentation of dyspnea.** Clinicians should regularly document severity, impact on function, and distress from dyspnea because this allows clinicians to reassess the efficacy of the current dyspnea care plan and adjust as needed. This is particularly important in older adults who may need multiple trials of therapeutic strategies targeting different contributors. In addition, regular inquiry can provide reassurance and support to the patient and caregivers.

- **Consider palliative care if the patient has advanced chronic cardiopulmonary illness.** Older adults can experience persistent dyspnea in the context of advanced cardiopulmonary illness, such as stage 4 COPD or advanced heart failure, despite disease-directed therapies. In these cases, a palliative care approach, which combines a thoughtful discussion of prognosis and goals with an emphasis on symptom control and quality of life, should be considered. Clinicians should consider assessing the patient's and family's understanding of prognosis because treatment preferences regarding symptomatic management may be influenced by this information. For example, a patient and family may be more willing to consider low-dose opioids for treatment of refractory dyspnea in advanced COPD if the patient understands their poor prognosis and high likelihood of death in the coming year (see Chapter 4, "Goals of Care & Consideration of Prognosis," and Chapter 22, "Geriatric Palliative Care").

B. Symptomatic Management of Dyspnea in Older Adults

Even with optimal management of underlying contributors, older adults may experience significant symptomatic burden from dyspnea. In addition to managing cardiopulmonary impairment from conditions such as COPD or heart failure, clinicians should take an individualized multicomponent approach to address other underlying contributors. Concurrently, clinicians can consider the following approaches to symptom relief.

1. Oxygen, medical air, and fans—Specific guidelines exist for the provision of supplemental oxygen for treatment of lung disease (see Chapter 46, "Chronic Lung Disease"). Literature generally suggests a *symptomatic* benefit from supplemental oxygen for patients with demonstrated hypoxemia (SpO_2 <88%) either at rest or with ambulation. Supplemental oxygen in the absence of severe hypoxemia is generally not recommended given the lack of evidence for benefit. A randomized controlled trial comparing the use of oxygen versus room air delivered via nasal cannula in patients with chronic dyspnea found that oxygen was not superior. Interestingly, however, both groups reported improvements in dyspnea and quality of life, suggesting that in nonhypoxic patients, it may be air flow itself that palliates symptoms, rather than increased oxygen. Consequently, older patients may benefit from fans, either at bedside or hand-held, directed at the face to relieve dyspnea, a practice supported by recent randomized controlled trials.

2. Relaxation, psychosocial support, and cognitive-behavioral therapy—Formal counseling and therapy can help many patients develop positive ways to psychologically cope with chronic breathlessness. Such therapy can reduce anxiety and dyspnea-related distress, with resultant improvements in quality of life. In addition, patients can be asked what self-care strategies they use to manage dyspnea, and activities should be encouraged. Self-care strategies used by patients may include social activities (talking to friends or family), distractions (reading, music, TV, Internet, writing), and others (fresh air, cooking, prayer, meditation, yoga, self-talk). Patients can be taught behavioral techniques such as pursed lip breathing or abdominal breathing. The American Thoracic Society recommends the COMFORT seven-step plan be taught to patients who experience sudden breathlessness crises at home (see "Online Resources").

3. Pulmonary rehabilitation and exercise—Pulmonary rehabilitation has been shown to reduce dyspnea and improve quality of life in patients with limitations from cardiopulmonary illness, including patients with stages III and IV COPD or those who become breathless when hurrying on level ground or walking up a slight hill. It typically combines supervised exercise training with coaching in breathing technique and dyspnea self-management strategies and can include psychosocial support and nutrition support. Pulmonary rehabilitation is generally safe for older adults with stable chronic conditions. Therefore, although participation might be limited by cognitive impairment or overall frailty, it should be encouraged. In addition, exercise training, both aerobic and resistive, helps to reverse deconditioning and can improve well-being. Exercise has been shown to improve exercise tolerance and dyspnea in patients with chronic breathlessness, especially those with COPD.

4. Opioids and other pharmacotherapy—Growing evidence suggests that opioids are effective at relieving refractory dyspnea at low doses in patients with severe COPD and to some extent in those with restrictive pulmonary disease, cancer, or heart failure. The mechanism is thought to be through a central reduction in the effect of hypoxemia or hypercarbia on ventilation. A dose increment study found that 70% of enrolled patients experienced significant symptom improvement with 10 mg of sustained morphine daily (approximately half of the 85 participants had COPD, and the age ranged from 51 to 88 years old). In addition to improving symptoms, opioids may improve patients' ability to engage in exercise and social activities if there is a predictable pattern of symptoms. At this time, evidence suggests that, at low doses, opioids have a low risk for respiratory depression. Still, clinicians prescribing opioids for breathlessness should counsel patients and families regarding the prevention of overdose and of diversion, and should anticipate common side effects such as drowsiness, constipation, and nausea (see Chapter 63, "Persistent Pain," on pain management for dosing of opiates and treatment of side effects). Moreover, there are few data on the long-term effects of opioids for dyspnea, and a systematic review found that patients may have a reduced response to opioids for management of dyspnea with increasing age. Nevertheless, at this time, multiple expert groups recommend clinicians consider oral opioids to treat refractory dyspnea in patients with advanced disease. The "start low and go slow" principle should be used if considering this therapy in older adults, with dose titrations no faster than weekly and generally not exceeding 30 mg of oral morphine (or equivalent) for this indication.

In addition, benzodiazepines are often considered for the relief of chronic breathlessness. Evidence in support of this practice is weak: a Cochrane review concluded that "there is no evidence for a beneficial effect of benzodiazepines for the relief of breathlessness in patients with advanced cancer and COPD." However, many clinicians have noted anecdotal improvement, especially in patients suffering from anxiety related to breathlessness. Given the strong link between benzodiazepines and poor outcomes in older adults, including falls and delirium, clinicians should use caution in prescribing benzodiazepines to the older patient in the community setting with refractory breathlessness.

Dyspnea at the End of Life

Dyspnea is a common and distressing symptom among older adults at the end of life. A study of older adults (mean age 87 years old) found that the prevalence of breathlessness severe enough to restrict activity was approximately 30% in the last month of life. Consequently, dyspnea should be routinely assessed and managed in end-of-life care of older adults to ensure optimal symptom management. In the last days of life, breathing patterns can change to include Cheyne-Stokes breathing, agonal breathing, gurgling (the so-called "death rattle"), or an elevated respiratory rate. Clinicians can provide anticipatory guidance to caregivers and family members about expected changes in breathing patterns. Several nonpharmacologic strategies can be used. Sitting patients up with their arms elevated or supported or having the head of the bed elevated can provide relief by increasing vital capacity. A cold cloth can be placed on the face for symptomatic relief. Oxygen or cool air directed at the nose or mouth can be provided, with similar principles as those outlined in the general treatment section earlier. For patients experiencing gurgling or "death rattle," caused by pooling of secretions at the back of the throat, caregivers should be reassured that it is not dangerous, and patients can be repositioned on their side or semi-prone to reduce pooling. Pharmacologic management includes the use of low-dose opioids titrated to the patient's report of dyspnea or display of dyspnea behaviors. Less concentrated, liquid formulations of opioids can be used if patients have difficulty swallowing pills. There is no clear evidence for the use of benzodiazepines to relieve dyspnea at the end of life, although there may be a role to relieve anxiety or fear associated with dyspnea.

SUMMARY

Key points to remember in addressing dyspnea in older adults include:

- Dyspnea is common, affecting approximately one in four older adults over age 70.

- Dyspnea should never be ignored or dismissed as it is associated with a lack of well-being, greater health service use, worsened function, and increased mortality. New or worsened dyspnea should prompt a thorough history and physical examination often with assistance from a knowledgeable informant and special attention to medication adherence. Clinicians should evaluate the impact of dyspnea on functional health, mood, and social interactions.

- Goals of care and life expectancy should be considered before engaging in more complicated diagnostic or therapeutic procedures, as the burdens may outweigh the likely benefits in patients who are frail or prefer to have fewer interventions.

- Dyspnea is often a multifactorial geriatric syndrome. Consequently, clinicians should take an individualized and multicomponent approach to management, including attention to polypharmacy, deconditioning, environmental modifications, multimorbidity, and coexisting symptoms such as pain, fatigue, or depression.

- Chronic dyspnea caused by advanced incurable cardiopulmonary disease can often be successfully palliated through techniques such as oxygen or medical air, psychosocial support, pulmonary rehabilitation, or low-dose opioids. Palliative care referrals are often appropriate for those patients struggling with chronic dyspnea refractory to traditional treatments.

- Dyspnea occurs in approximately 30% of older adults in the last month of life. Clinicians can provide anticipatory guidance to caregivers on changes in breathing patterns, nonpharmacologic strategies to reduce dyspnea, and the use of low-dose opioids to reduce dyspnea or the display of dyspnea-related behaviors.

Clark N, Fan VS, Slatore CG, et al. Dyspnea and pain frequently co-occur among Medicare managed care recipients. *Ann Am Thorac Soc.* 2014;11(6):890-897.

Ekström MP, Abernethy AP, Currow DC. The management of chronic breathlessness in patients with advanced and terminal illness. *BMJ.* 2015;349:g7617.

Hegendörfer E, Vaes B, Matheï C, Van Pottelbergh G, Degryse J-M. Correlates of dyspnoea and its association with adverse outcomes in a cohort of adults aged 80 and over. *Age Ageing.* 2017;46(6):994-1000.

Johnson MJ, Bland JM, Gahbauer EA, et al. Breathlessness in elderly adults during the last year of life sufficient to restrict activity: prevalence, pattern, and associated factors. *J Am Geriatr Soc.* 2016;64(1):73-80.

Johnson MJ, Hui D, Currow DC. Opioids, exertion, and dyspnea: a review of the evidence. *Am J Hosp Palliat Med.* 2016;33(2):194-200.

Marcus BS, McAvay G, Gill TM, Vaz Fragoso CA. Respiratory symptoms, spirometric respiratory impairment, and respiratory disease in middle-aged and older persons. *J Am Geriatr Soc.* 2015;63(2):251-257.

Miner B, Tinetti ME, Van Ness PH, et al. Dyspnea in community-dwelling older persons: a multifactorial geriatric health condition. *J Am Geriatr Soc.* 2016;64(10):2042-2050.

Parshall MB, Schwartzstein RM, Adams L, et al. An official American Thoracic Society statement: update on the mechanisms, assessment, and management of dyspnea. *Am J Respir Crit Care Med.* 2012;185(4):435-452.

Petersen S, von Leupoldt A, Van den Bergh O. Geriatric dyspnea: doing worse, feeling better. *Ageing Res Rev.* 2014;15:94-99.

Smith AK, Currow DC, Abernethy AP, et al. Prevalence and outcomes of breathlessness in older adults: a national population study. *J Am Geriatr Soc.* 2016;64(10):2035-2041.

van Mourik Y, Rutten FH, Moons KG, Bertens LC, Hoes AW, Reitsma JB. Prevalence and underlying causes of dyspnoea in older people: a systematic review. *Age Ageing.* 2014;43(3):319-326.

Vaz Fragoso CA, Araujo K, Leo-Summers L, Van Ness PH. Lower extremity proximal muscle function and dyspnea in older persons. *J Am Geriatr Soc.* 2015;63(8):1628-1633.

Vaz Fragoso CA, Beavers DP, Hankinson JL, et al. Respiratory impairment and dyspnea and their associations with physical inactivity and mobility in sedentary community-dwelling older persons. *J Am Geriatr Soc.* 2014;62(4):622-628.

Wysham NG, Miriovsky BJ, Currow DC, et al. Practical dyspnea assessment: relationship between the 0–10 numerical rating scale and the four-level categorical verbal descriptor scale of dyspnea intensity. *J Pain Symptom Manage.* 2015;50(4):480-487.

ONLINE RESOURCES

American Thoracic Society. Management of sudden breathlessness crises. https://www.thoracic.org/patients/patient-resources/resources/sudden-breathlessness.pdf. Accessed April 16, 2020.

COPD Foundation. Free online inhaler training videos. https://www.copdfoundation.org/Learn-More/Educational-Materials-Resources/Educational-Video-Series.aspx. April 16, 2020.

Syncope

Natalie A. Sanders, DO, FACP

Mark A. Supiano, MD

"The incidence of syncope in older adults may overlap with falls, so it may be difficult to distinguish one from the other. The management of syncope in older adults is particularly challenging. The incidence is high; the differential diagnosis is broad; the diagnosis is imprecise . . ."

From the *ACC/AHA/HRS Guidelines for the Evaluation and Management of Patients with Syncope* (2017)

"Given that up to 70% of falls in older persons are not witnessed, these patients may present with a report of a fall rather than syncope."

From the *AGS/BGS Clinical Practice Guideline: Prevention of Falls in Older Persons* (2011)

▷ General Principles

Falls and syncope are commonly encountered syndromes in older adults, and both are associated with significant morbidity and mortality. It is often difficult to know when to consider syncope as the primary or a contributing cause to falls in older adults. In part, for this reason, current guidelines recommend evaluating patients with unexplained falls for syncope. This chapter provides some guidance for the clinician faced with the question, "Is this patient's fall caused by syncope?"

Most studies estimate that one-third of community-dwelling older adults fall each year. Falls are the leading cause of injury among patients age 65 years and older. Up to nearly 40% of falls among older adults result in injury or restricted activity. Falls are associated with functional decline, increased risk for nursing home placement, decreased quality of life, higher health care costs, and mortality.

Syncope is also common among older adults. Its prevalence in the general population has a trimodal distribution peaking in people at age 20 years, at age 60 years, and again in those age 80 and older. Almost half of emergency department visits for syncope are made by persons 65 years of age or older. Because of underlying multiple chronic conditions and increased prevalence of cardiovascular disease in older people, the morbidity and mortality associated with syncope are higher in older adults compared to younger adults.

▷ General Approach to the Patient with Falls or Syncope

A. Falls

The literature varies widely on the definition of falls, but typically falls are defined as unintentionally coming to rest on the ground or a lower surface. When evaluating a patient with falls, obtaining a detailed history of the fall from the patient and witnesses, if available, is imperative and a good starting point. This history should include the circumstances surrounding the fall; any preceding symptoms, such as dizziness or lightheadedness; whether the fall was witnessed or not; and whether there was loss of consciousness with the fall. A focused physical exam including a cognitive and functional assessment should also be completed. During the evaluation, it is important to remember that falls constitute a geriatric syndrome. As such, the cause of falling in an older patient is rarely the result of a single cause but instead the result of a complex interaction between intrinsic and extrinsic risk factors. In addition to a detailed history and physical exam, identifying and addressing these risk factors is at the core of a fall evaluation. Current guidelines emphasize assessing the following risk factors: (1) history of falls; (2) medications; (3) gait, balance, and mobility; (4) visual acuity; (5) neurologic impairments; (6) muscle strength; (7) heart rate and rhythm; (8) postural hypotension; (9) feet and footwear; and (10) assessment of environmental hazards (Table 67–1). Medication classes to specifically identify in older adults with falls include anticonvulsants, antipsychotics, benzodiazepines, nonbenzodiazepine hypnotics, tricyclic antidepressants, selective serotonin reuptake inhibitors, and opioids.

Table 67–1. Multifactorial fall risk assessment.

History of previous falls
Medications
Gait, balance, and mobility
Visual acuity
Presence of other neurologic impairments (ie, neuropathy)
Muscle strength
Heart rate and rhythm
Postural hypotension
Feet and footwear
Environmental hazards

Because of their propensity to worsen postural hypotension, diuretics, vasodilators, and other, particularly centrally acting, antihypertensive medications should also be evaluated. Interventions should initially focus on modifiable risk factors.

B. Syncope

Fainting is a common problem and encompasses any disorder associated with a real or perceived transient loss of consciousness. Nontraumatic transient loss of consciousness is further classified into syncope, epileptic disorders, psychogenic pseudosyncope, and rare miscellaneous causes, such as cataplexy or drop attacks. Syncope specifically refers to transient loss of consciousness caused by global hypoperfusion. Hallmark features of its presentation are sudden loss of consciousness with associated loss of postural tone and rapid spontaneous recovery. The causes of syncope can be classified into three broad categories: reflex-mediated syncope, syncope caused by orthostatic hypotension, and cardiac syncope (Table 67–2).

Table 67–2. Classification of syncope.

Reflex (neurally mediated) syncope
Vasovagal
Situational
Carotid sinus syndrome
Atypical forms
Syncope caused by orthostatic hypotension
Primary autonomic failure
Secondary autonomic failure
Drug-induced
Volume depletion
Cardiac syncope
Arrhythmia
Structural

Data from Task Force for the Diagnosis and Management of Syncope; European Society of Cardiology (ESC); European Heart Rhythm Association (EHRA); Guidelines for the diagnosis and management of syncope (version 2009), *Eur Heart J* 2009 Nov;30(21):2631-2671.

The initial goal of the evaluation of syncope is risk stratification, that is, to define those patients who warrant urgent cardiac evaluation because of the high short-term risk of recurrence of syncope. As with falls, the evaluation of the patient with syncope should start with obtaining a comprehensive history of the event and physical examination, including checking orthostatic vital signs. Historical questions should be targeted to try to identify which class of syncope is most likely. An electrocardiogram (ECG) may also be performed, keeping in mind the high pretest probability of an abnormal ECG in an older adult. Patients in whom the cause of syncope is uncertain may warrant additional tests. These tests include, but are not limited to, targeted blood testing, echocardiography, stress testing, short-term or long-term ECG monitoring, electrophysiology study, tilt-table testing, and supine and upright carotid sinus massage. While the short-term prognosis of patients with syncope is related to the underlying cause of syncope and the acute reversibility of this condition, the long-term prognosis of these patients is driven by underlying chronic conditions. Similar to falls, older adults frequently have more than one factor contributing to their syncope. Physiologic changes associated with aging, such as inability to preserve sodium and water, decreased baroreceptor responsiveness, autonomic dysfunction, multimorbidity, and frailty, all contribute to the older adult's increased vulnerability to syncope. The use of multiple medications that affect blood pressure, heart rate, and volume status, such as diuretics and β-blockers, also predisposes older adults to syncope. Lastly, patient preferences can help guide further evaluation. Specifically, presuming medical decision capacity is intact for the specific situation, when the treatment that is likely to be recommended based on the results of the testing is not one the patient would desire, it is reasonable to forego the testing needed to identify the problem and focus on the patient's preferences. An example of a clinical scenario in which this may be encountered is pursuing ambulatory ECG monitoring when a patient has indicated they would not desire placement of a pacemaker or defibrillator or to take medications for an arrhythmia were an arrhythmia to be found. All of these factors are particularly important to consider in older adults with syncope.

How Falls and Syncope Overlap

There is increasing evidence of an overlap between nonaccidental falls and syncope. The rates of serious adverse events for older adults presenting with a report of syncope compared to near syncope are similar. Furthermore, because of the lack of a witness account, history provided by the patient may be unreliable. In addition to patients not recalling the circumstances of their fall, several studies indicate patients do not accurately remember the number of falls they have. Individual patient factors that increase the risk of poor fall recall include older age, cognitive impairment, and occurrence of a noninjurious fall. Patients may also not recall loss of consciousness. Retrograde amnesia for loss of consciousness affects up to 30% of patients with syncope. Finally, in patients with gait or balance problems, hypotension and bradycardia may be less well tolerated, resulting in a fall. Both hypotension and bradycardia can decrease cardiac output enough to cause cerebral hypoperfusion and loss of postural tone without causing complete loss of consciousness. These patients may be misclassified as having only suffered a fall and not a syncopal event. Yet, the underlying physiology is the same (decreased global cerebral perfusion) and may be treatable. For these reasons, current guidelines recommend evaluating patients with unexplained falls for syncope.

▶ When to Consider Syncope as a Cause of Falls

Clinicians should consider evaluating patients for syncope when the following factors are present: (1) history of loss of consciousness with the fall, (2) unexplained nonaccidental fall, or (3) recurrent falls despite adherence to a multifactorial targeted treatment program (Table 67–3).

COMMON DIAGNOSTIC CATEGORIES

There are three diagnostic categories to consider in the differential diagnoses of these patients: orthostatic hypotension and its variants, carotid sinus syndrome, and cardiac syncope due to arrhythmia (see Table 67–3).

▶ Orthostatic Hypotension and Its Variants

A. Classical Orthostatic Hypotension

Classical orthostatic hypotension, defined as a drop in systolic blood pressure of ≥20 mm Hg within 3 minutes of standing, is common in older adults. However, it is often not tested by clinicians, or the symptoms may be simply disregarded by patients. In the Cardiovascular Health Study, the prevalence of orthostatic hypotension was 18% in subjects age 65 years or older, yet only 2% of these subjects reported symptoms with standing.

B. Delayed Orthostatic Hypotension

Delayed orthostatic hypotension is characterized by a drop in systolic blood pressure of ≥20 mm Hg after >3 minutes of standing. It should be considered in older adults with underlying neurologic disorders, which put them at risk for autonomic dysfunction. These include idiopathic Parkinson disease, multiple system atrophy, and diabetes. Because nearly 40% of patients with this condition will drop their blood pressure only after at least 10 minutes of upright posture, tilt-table testing is typically used to evaluate for delayed orthostatic hypotension.

C. Postprandial Hypotension

Postprandial hypotension is another diagnosis to consider when evaluating patients with falls for the possibility of syncope. Postprandial hypotension is defined as a fall in systolic blood pressure of ≥20 mm Hg within 2 hours of eating a meal. Nearly half of healthy older patients with unexplained syncope have been found to have postprandial hypotension. Patients with classical orthostatic hypotension or autonomic dysfunction are also at higher risk for postprandial hypotension. Obtaining a detailed history of events and their association with meals can help identify patients with possible postprandial hypotension. Some patients may require 24-hour ambulatory blood pressure monitoring to confirm the diagnosis.

▶ Carotid Sinus Syndrome

Carotid sinus hypersensitivity is caused by an exaggerated response to carotid sinus massage. In some studies, up to 70% of patients ≥65 years old with unexplained falls have carotid sinus hypersensitivity during supine and upright tilt-table testing. Carotid sinus syndrome is diagnosed when there is reproduction of a patient's symptoms associated with a systolic blood pressure drop of ≥50 mm Hg (vasodepressor response), an asystolic pause of ≥3 seconds (cardioinhibitory response), or both (mixed response) with carotid sinus massage. Carotid sinus syndrome has been reported to be the cause of unexplained falls in up to 40% of patients. Performing carotid sinus massage in the supine and upright positions increases the sensitivity. Permanent cardiac pacing may be helpful in reducing falls in select patients with a marked cardioinhibitory response to carotid sinus massage in the setting of associated symptoms and syncope of unexplained cause.

Table 67–3. Considering syncope as a cause of falls.

Clinical Situations
History of loss of consciousness
Unexplained nonaccidental fall
Recurrent falls despite adherence to multicomponent treatment program targeting risk factors
Common Diagnostic Categories Associated with Unexplained Falls
Orthostatic hypotension variants
Classical
Delayed
Postprandial
Carotid sinus syndrome
Vasodepressor response
Cardioinhibitory response
Mixed response
Cardiac syncope due to arrhythmia

Cardiac Syncope Caused by Arrhythmia

Cardiac syncope caused by arrhythmia may be responsible for up to 30% of syncope in older adults. Its high prevalence in older adults is thought to be related to the increased number of underlying cardiovascular chronic conditions older adults have as well as the increased prevalence of sinus node dysfunction seen with aging. Atrial fibrillation, one manifestation of sinus node dysfunction, has been found to be an independent risk factor for unexplained nonaccidental falls in older adults. Ambulatory ECG monitoring can be used to diagnose syncope caused by arrhythmia. The frequency of symptoms along with patient goals should dictate what type of ambulatory ECG monitoring is pursued. Clinical guidelines endorse the use of long-term ECG monitoring with implantable loop recorders for patients with unexplained syncope or unexplained falls.

SUMMARY

When evaluating an older adult who has fallen or with frequent falls, it is important to do the following: (1) conduct a multifactorial fall risk assessment (see Table 67–1); (2) consider clinical scenarios in which syncope may be the cause of falls, notably when no explanation for falls has been found (see Table 67–3); and (3) if syncope is the likely cause of the fall, classify syncope to determine next diagnostic and treatment steps (see Table 67–2).

American Geriatrics Society Beers Criteria Update Expert Panel. American Geriatrics Society 2019 Updated AGS Beers Criteria for potentially inappropriate medication use in older adults. *J Am Geriatr Soc*. 2019;67(4):674-694.

Bastani A, Su E, Adler DH, et al. Comparison of 30-day serious adverse clinical events for elderly patients presenting to the emergency department with near-syncope versus syncope. *Ann Emerg Med*. 2019;73(3):274-280.

Bhangu J, McMahon CG, Hall P, et al. Long-term cardiac monitoring in older adults with unexplained falls and syncope. *Heart*. 2016;102(9):681-686.

Fanciulli A, Jordan J, Biaggioni I, et al. Consensus statement on the definition of neurogenic supine hypertension in cardiovascular autonomic failure by the American Autonomic Society (AAS) and the European Federation of Autonomic Societies (EFAS): endorsed by the European Academy of Neurology (EAN) and the European Society of Hypertension (ESH). *Clin Auton Res*. 2018;28(4):355-362.

Heldeweg MLA, Jorge PJF, Ligtenberg JJM, Ter Maaten JC, Harms MPM. Orthostatic blood pressure measurements are often overlooked during the initial evaluation of syncope in the emergency department. *Blood Press Monit*. 2018;23(6):294-296.

Maggi R, Rafanelli M, Ceccofiglio A, Solari D, Brignole M, Ungar A. Additional diagnostic value of implantable loop recorder in patients with initial diagnosis of real or apparent transient loss of consciousness of uncertain origin [Europace 2014 16: 1226-1230]. *Europace*. 2015;17(12):1847.

Panel on Prevention of Falls in Older Persons, American Geriatrics Society/British Geriatrics Society. Summary of the Updated American Geriatrics Society/British Geriatrics Society clinical practice guideline for prevention of falls in older persons. *J Am Geriatr Soc*. 2011;59(1):148-157.

Shen WK, Sheldon RS, Benditt DG, et al. 2017 ACC/AHA/HRS guideline for the evaluation and management of patients with syncope: a report of the American College of Cardiology/American Heart Association Task Force on Clinical Practice Guidelines and the Heart Rhythm Society. *Circulation*. 2017;136(5):e60-e122.

Task Force for the Diagnosis and Management of Syncope, European Society of Cardiology (ESC). 2018 ESC Guidelines for the diagnosis and management of syncope. *Eur Heart J*. 2018;39:1883-1948.

US Preventive Services Task Force, Grossman DC, Curry SJ, et al. Interventions to prevent falls in community-dwelling older adults: US Preventive Services Task Force recommendation statement. *JAMA*. 2018;319(16):1696-1704.

Pressure Ulcers

Courtney K. Gordon, DNP, GNP-BC, MSN
David R. Thomas, MD, FACP, AGSF, GSAF

ESSENTIALS OF DIAGNOSIS

▶ Pressure ulcers are caused by pressure applied to susceptible tissues. Tissue susceptibility may be increased in the presence of maceration and by friction as well as shear forces.

▶ Chronic conditions, especially immobility and decreased tissue perfusion, increase the risk of pressure ulcers.

▶ Most pressure ulcers develop over bony prominences, most commonly the sacrum, heels, and trochanteric areas.

▶ Most pressure ulcers develop in acute hospitals; the risk is greatest in orthopedic and ICU patients.

▶ There are different stages and classifications of pressure ulcers. Pressure ulcers are classified as stage 1 to 4 depending on depth and severity of the wound.

▶ Pressure ulcers do not necessarily progress from stage 1 to 4.

▶ Treatment options differ depending on the type as well as stage of the wound and are often difficult to heal.

▶ Pressure ulcers have a significant impact on the quality of life of a patient as well as caregivers.

▶ Pressure ulcers have a significant cost to the health care system and have been associated with increased mortality rates in both acute and long-term care settings.

General Principles

In 2016, the National Pressure Ulcer Advisory Panel convened a task force to reexamine the literature and definitions of pressure ulcers. One of the recommendations of this task force was to shift from the term pressure *ulcer* to pressure *injury* to better reflect the pathophysiology and physical presentation of pressure-related injuries. As this publication comes at a time when the newer term of *pressure injury* is being adopted, we have chosen to continue using the more widely used and understood term *pressure ulcer* for now. Pressure ulcers are one of the leading hospital-acquired conditions and have a significant impact on health care quality for the patient as well as cost to the hospital for care. Age, incontinence, and body mass index (BMI) are all well-established risk factors, with older age and lower BMI of particular importance for pressure ulcer development. Prevention, treatment, and healing of pressure ulcers in older adults is difficult and depends on many factors.

A. Causes

Pressure ulcers are the visible evidence of pathologic changes in the blood supply to dermal tissues. Pressure ulcers are also referred to as bed sores and pressure injuries. The chief cause is extrinsic factor attributed to pressure, or force per unit area, applied to susceptible tissues. However, extrinsic and intrinsic factors combine to play an important role in pressure ulcer development. Intrinsic factors, such as peripheral arterial disease, congestive heart failure, hypoxia, and hypotension leading to derangement in tissue perfusion may account for the development of a pressure ulcer, despite the provision of common prevention measures that include pressure reduction. Both of these factors are beginning to be identified, but more research is needed.

Edsberg LE, Black JM, Goldberg M, McNichol L, Moore L, Sieggreen M. Revised national pressure ulcer advisory panel pressure injury staging system. J Wound Ostomy Continence Nurs. 2016;43(6):585-597.

Thomas DR. Does pressure cause pressure ulcers? An inquiry into the etiology of pressure ulcers. *J Am Med Dir Assoc.* 2010;11(6):397-405.

B. Incidence

Among patients who experience pressure ulcers, 57% to 60% do so in the acute hospital. Incidence in hospitalized patients ranges from 3% to 30%; common estimates range from 9% to 13%. The incidence differs by hospital location; intensive care unit (ICU) patients and orthopedic patients are at greatest risk. In patients with a hip fracture, 15% develop a pressure ulcer during hospital admission, and one-third develop a pressure ulcer in 1 month. Pressure ulcers develop early in the course of hospitalization, usually within the first week. The incidence of pressure ulcers in nursing homes is difficult to quantitate, and studies are lacking. After discharge from the hospital, pressure ulcers remain a major problem in community care settings.

C. Risk Assessment & Risk Factors

In theory, persons who are at high risk for pressure ulcers can be identified and an increased effort can be directed to preventing ulcers. The classical risk assessment scale is the Norton Score, developed in 1962 and still widely used. Patients are classified using five risk factors graded from 1 to 4. Scores range from 5 to 20; higher scores indicate lower risk. The generally accepted at-risk score is 14; patients with scores lower than 12 are at particularly high risk.

A commonly used risk assessment instrument in the United States is the Braden Scale. This instrument assesses six items: sensory perception, moisture exposure, physical activity, mobility, nutrition, and friction/shear force. Each item is ranked from 1 (least favorable) to 3 or 4 (most favorable), with a maximal total score of 23. A score of 16 indicates a high risk.

Both the Norton Score and the Braden Scale have good sensitivity (73%–92% and 83%–100%, respectively) and specificity (61%–94% and 64%–77%, respectively) but poor positive predictive value (approximately 37% at a pressure ulcer incidence of 20%). In populations with a lower incidence of pressure ulcers, such as those in nursing homes, the same sensitivity and specificity produce a positive predictive value of 2%. The net effect of poor positive predictive value means that many patients who will not develop pressure ulcers will receive expensive and unnecessary treatment.

A systematic review of 33 clinical trials of risk assessment found no decrease in pressure ulcer incidence that could be attributed to the use of an assessment scale. In long-term care settings, a Braden score had no predictive value for the development of a pressure ulcer. In two studies of pressure ulcer risk assessment tools in acute care hospitals, the incidence and severity of pressure ulcers was not different using the Braden Scale or other tools compared with clinical judgment plus clinical training or clinical judgment alone.

Because most pressure ulcers develop in the acute hospital, risk assessment in this setting is particularly important. In an ICU, five factors contribute to the risk of pressure ulcers after adjustment for confounders: norepinephrine infusion, Acute Physiology and Chronic Health Evaluation (APACHE) II score, fecal incontinence, anemia, and length of stay in the ICU. Additional independent risk factors for the development of a pressure ulcer after admission to a surgical service include emergency admission (which increased the risk 36-fold), age, days in bed, and days without nutrition.

In functionally limited (bed- or chair-confined) hospitalized patients, nine factors were associated with the development of pressure ulcers while hospitalized, including nonblanchable erythema (increasing the risk seven-fold), lymphopenia (increasing the risk almost five-fold), and immobility/functional impairment, dry skin, and decreased body weight (each of which increased the risk two-fold). Characteristics also associated with pressure ulcers in nonhospitalized individuals include recent institutional discharge and having had a previous ulcer.

Not surprisingly, risk factors in long-term care populations differ. In the long-term care setting, some factors associated with development of pressure ulcers include difficulty in ambulation, difficulty feeding oneself, and male gender, which were associated with a two- to four-fold risk of pressure ulcer. The risk of pressure ulcers increases with a history of cerebrovascular accident (five-fold increase), bed or chair confinement (3.8-fold increase), and impaired nutritional intake (2.8-fold increase). In data derived from the Minimal Data Set, logistic regression analysis determined that dependence in transfer or mobility, confinement to bed, history of diabetes mellitus, and a history of pressure ulcer were significantly associated with an existing stage 2 to 4 pressure ulcer. In community-dwelling persons age 55 to 75 years, the presence of a pressure ulcer was predicted by self-assessed poor health, current smoking, dry or scaly skin on examination, and decreased activity level.

The importance of these epidemiologic risk predictors lies in understanding which factors (Table 68–1) are amenable to correction or modifiable. Risk factors that are potentially

Table 68–1. Pressure ulcer risk factors.

Presence of a fracture
History of a previous pressure ulcer
Recent institutional discharge
Age
Incontinence
Immobility[a]
Functional impairment[a]
Decreased serum albumin level
Lymphopenia
Nonblanchable erythema
Dry skin[a]
Decreased body weight/lower body mass index[a]
Nutritional status[a]

[a]Indicates modifiable risk factors.

modifiable include immobility, dry skin, and nutritional factors. Efforts have centered on correction of these problems.

Prevention

A. Quality of Care

Pressure ulcers are increasingly used as indicators of quality of care. Whether or not pressure ulcers are preventable remains controversial. When aggressive measures for prevention of pressure ulcers have been applied, a "floor effect" for incidence has been noted. Pressure ulcers often occur in terminally ill patients, for whom the goals of care may not include prevention of pressure ulcers. Pressure ulcers also occur in severely ill patients, such as orthopedic patients or ICU patients, for whom the necessity for immobilization may preclude turning or the use of pressure-relieving devices.

Systematic efforts at education, heightened awareness, and specific interventions by interdisciplinary wound teams suggest that a high incidence of pressure ulcers can be reduced. Over time, reductions of 25% to 30% have been reported. The reduction may be transient, unstable over time, vary with changes in personnel, or occur as a result of random variation. Development of pressure ulcers can be, but is not always, a measure of quality of care.

Many hospitals, skilled nursing facilities, and nursing homes have used wound care teams, in particular wound care nurses who specialize in wound treatment, to attempt to reduce pressure ulcer development and help with healing and treatment options in those with pressure ulcers. Unfortunately, there are no data yet to support significant reduction in pressure ulcer development or faster healing times with wound care nurses and teams alone. One theory is that wound care specialist become involved too late when pressure ulcers have already developed and consultation would be much more beneficial early on for patients identified with significant risk factors for pressure ulcer development.

B. Pressure Relief

The first efforts toward prevention should be to improve mobility and reduce the effects of pressure, friction, and shear forces. It must be noted that even using a pressure-reducing surface might not relieve the need to position people frequently.

The most expedient method for reducing pressure is frequent turning and positioning. A 2-hour turning schedule for spinal injury patients was deduced empirically in 1946. However, turning the patient to relieve pressure may be difficult to achieve despite best nursing efforts and is very costly in terms of staffing. The exact interval for optimal turning in prevention is unknown. The interval may be shortened or lengthened by host factors. Despite commonsense approaches to turning, positioning, and improving passive

activity, no published data support the view that pressure ulcers can be prevented by passive positioning.

Consensus guidelines for turning and positioning have been developed by the European and US committees, but no single turning schedule has been adopted. A comparison between a 2- and 3-hour repositioning schedule using a standard hospital mattress was not different than a 4- or 6-hour repositioning schedule using a viscoelastic foam mattress. A similar study in at-risk nursing home residents showed no difference in pressure ulcer incidence over 3 weeks of observation among those turned at 2-, 3-, or 4-hour intervals using high-density foam mattresses, despite being consistently repositioned and skin frequently monitored.

Some pressure-reducing devices have been proven more effective than "standard" hospital foam mattresses in moderate- to high-risk patients. Pressure-relieving mattresses in the operating theater have reduced the incidence of pressure ulcers postoperatively. Limited evidence suggests that low-air-loss beds reduce the incidence of pressure sores in ICUs. The differences among devices are unclear and do not demonstrate a superior device compared with other devices. There is some evidence that air–fluid beds and low-air-loss beds improve healing rates.

Krapfl LA, Gray M. Does regular repositioning prevent pressure ulcers? *J Wound Ostomy Continence Nurs.* 2008;35(6):571-577.

McInnes E, Dumville JC, Jammali-Blasi A, Bell-Syer SE. Support surfaces for pressure ulcer prevention. *Cochrane Database Syst Rev.* 2011;12:CD009490.

C. Nutritional Interventions

One of the most important reversible factors contributing to wound healing is nutritional status. Of newly hospitalized patients with stage 3 or stage 4 pressure ulcers, most were below their usual body weight, had a low prealbumin level, and were not taking in enough nutrition to meet their needs. There is no single laboratory test that confirms undernutrition. Prealbumin (transthyretin) and albumin, among others, are inconsistent with nutritional status and more properly viewed as acute phase inflammatory reactants. A comprehensive dietary consultation is required to confirm nutritional status.

The results of nutrition trials to improve pressure ulcer healing have been disappointing. The effects of mixed nutritional supplements (seven trials), proteins (three trials), zinc (two trials), and ascorbic acid (two trials) have shown no clear evidence of improvement of pressure ulcer healing using nutritional supplements. Eleven trials evaluated several nutritional supplements in the prevention of pressure ulcers, and eight trials evaluated nutritional supplements with standard hospital diets. In addition, overnight supplemental enteral feeding has not been shown to affect development of pressure ulcers and severity. There was no clear evidence of an effect on pressure ulcer prevention.

Basal metabolic rate appears to be similar or slightly increased in persons with a pressure ulcer. Clinical judgment and prediction equations suggest a caloric intake of 30 kcal/kg per day. An optimum dietary protein intake in patients with pressure ulcers is unknown but may be much higher than current adult recommendations of 0.8 g/kg per day. Half of chronically ill older persons are unable to maintain nitrogen balance at this level. Increasing protein intake beyond 1.5 g/kg per day may not increase protein synthesis and may cause dehydration. A reasonable protein requirement is, therefore, between 1.2 and 1.5 g/kg per day.

The deficiency of several vitamins has significant effects on wound healing. However, supplementation of vitamins to accelerate wound healing is controversial. There is no substantial evidence to support use of a daily vitamin C supplement for healing pressure ulcers.

Zinc supplementation has not been shown to accelerate healing except in zinc-deficient patients. High serum zinc levels interfere with healing, and supplementation >150 mg/day may interfere with copper metabolism.

Immune function declines with age, which increases risk for infection and is thought to delay wound healing. Specific amino acids such as arginine and branched-chain amino acids have not demonstrated an effect on pressure ulcer healing.

Houston S, Haggard J, Williford J Jr, Meserve L, Shewokis P. Adverse effects of large-dose zinc supplementation in an institutionalized older population with pressure ulcers. *J Am Geriatr Soc.* 2001;9(8):1130-1132.

Langer G, Fink A. Nutritional intervention for preventing and treating pressure ulcers. *Cochrane Database Syst Rev.* 2014;6:CD003216.

▶ Clinical Findings

A. Signs & Symptoms

A pressure ulcer is localized damage to the skin and underlying soft tissue usually over a bony prominence or related to a medical or other device. The wound can present as intact skin or an open ulcer and may be painful. The wound occurs as a result of intense and/or prolonged pressure or pressure in combination with shear. The tolerance of soft tissue for pressure and shear may also be affected by microclimate, nutrition, perfusion, comorbidities, and condition of the soft tissue.

Several differing scales have been proposed for assessing the severity of pressure ulcers. The most common staging, recommended by the National Pressure Ulcer Task Force, is derived from a modification of the Shea Scale. Under this schematic, pressure ulcers are divided into six clinical stages.

The first response of the epidermis to pressure is hyperemia. Hyperemia is due to dilation of the capillaries due to excess pressure. Blanchable erythema occurs when capillary refilling occurs after gentle pressure is applied to the area. Nonblanchable erythema exists when pressure of a finger in the reddened area does not produce a blanching or capillary refilling.

B. Staging Pressure Ulcers

A stage 1 pressure ulcer is defined by nonblanchable erythema of intact skin. Nonblanchable erythema is believed to indicate extravasation of blood from the capillaries. A stage 1 pressure ulcer always understates the underlying damage because the epidermis is the last tissue to show ischemic injury. Color changes do not include purple or maroon discoloration; these may indicate deep tissue pressure injury or other concerns with the skin. Diagnosing stage 1 pressure ulcers in darkly pigmented skin can be problematic.

Stage 2 ulcers extend through the epidermis or dermis. The ulcer is superficial and presents clinically as an abrasion, laceration, blister, or shallow crater.

With stage 3 pressure ulcers, there is full-thickness skin loss involving damage or necrosis of subcutaneous tissue that may extend down to, but not through, underlying fascia. The ulcer presents clinically as a deep crater with or without undermining of adjacent tissue. Fascia, muscle, tendon, ligament, cartilage, and/or bone are not exposed. If slough or eschar obscures the extent of tissue loss, this is an unstageable pressure injury, rather than a stage 3 pressure ulcer.

Stage 4 pressure ulcers are full-thickness wounds with extensive destruction, tissue necrosis, or damage to muscle, bone, or supporting structures. Stage 4 pressure ulcers are considered full-thickness tissue loss with exposed bone, tendon, or muscle. Slough or eschar may be present on some parts of the wound bed, often include undermining and tunneling. The depth of a stage 4 pressure ulcer varies by anatomic location. The bridge of the nose, ear, occiput, and malleolus do not have subcutaneous tissue, and these ulcers can be shallow. Stage 4 ulcers can extend into muscle and/or supporting structures (eg, fascia, tendon, or joint capsule), making osteomyelitis possible. Exposed bone/tendon is visible or directly palpable. Undermining and sinus tracts are frequently associated with stage 4 pressure ulcers.

If slough or eschar obscures the extent of tissue loss, this is defined as an unstageable pressure injury. If the bottom of the wound is not visualized, you cannot assess the depth of the wound, and therefore, the wound is classified as unstageable.

Deep tissue pressure injury (DTPI) is defined as intact or nonintact skin with localized area of persistent nonblanchable deep red, maroon, or purple discoloration or epidermal separation revealing a dark wound bed. Pain and temperature change often precede skin color changes. Discoloration may appear differently in darkly pigmented skin. This injury results from intense and/or prolonged pressure and shear forces at the bone-muscle interface. The wound may evolve rapidly to reveal the actual extent of tissue injury or may resolve without tissue loss. If necrotic tissue, subcutaneous tissue, granulation tissue, fascia, muscle, or other underlying structures are visible, this indicates a full-thickness stage 4 pressure ulcer rather than a DTPI. Do not use DTPI to describe vascular, traumatic, neuropathic, or other dermatologic conditions.

Stage 1 pressure ulcers occur most frequently, accounting for 47% of pressure ulcers, followed by stage 2 ulcers (33%). Stage 3 and 4 ulcers compose the remaining 20%. The staging system for pressure ulcers has several limitations. The primary difficulty lies in the inability to distinguish progression between stages. Pressure ulcers do not progress absolutely through stage 1 to stage 4, but may appear to develop from the inside out as a result of the initial injury. Healing from stage 4 does not progress through stage 3 to stage 1; rather, the ulcer heals by contraction and scar tissue formation. Second, clinical staging is inaccurate unless all eschar is removed, because the staging system reflects only depth of the ulcer. Because the staging system is based only on the depth of an ulcer, when an ulcer is covered by eschar or when the depth is unable to be assessed, it is designated as "unstageable."

Muscle tissue, subcutaneous fat, and dermal tissue are differentially susceptible to injury, in that order. The differential effect of pressure on the tissue layers suggests that injury occurs first in muscle tissue before changes are observed in the skin. This is the basis for the so-called deep tissue pressure injury. In many cases, the changes visible at the surface of the tissue are minor compared to the damage seen at the deepest layers of tissue. The surface discoloration is often classified as a stage 1 pressure ulcer, which rapidly evolves into a deep stage 4 ulcer. This differential tissue susceptibility suggests that a number of factors are involved in the development of pressure ulcers, including the type of pressure load and biochemical changes in the tissue because of reperfusion injury or tissue compression.

Because pressure ulcers heal by contraction and scar formation, reverse staging is inaccurate in assessing healing. No single measure of wound characteristics has been useful in measuring healing. Several indexes of ulcer healing have been proposed but lack validation studies. The Pressure Ulcer Status for Healing (PUSH) tool (Figure 68–1) was developed and validated by the National Pressure Ulcer Advisory Panel to measure healing of pressure ulcers. The tool measures three components—size, exudate amount, and tissue type—to arrive at a numerical score for ulcer status. The PUSH tool adequately assesses ulcer status and is sensitive to change over time.

Stotts NA, Rodeheaver GT, Thomas DR, et al. An instrument to measure healing in pressure ulcers: development and validation of the pressure ulcer scale for healing (PUSH). *J Gerontol A Biol Sci Med Sci.* 2001;56(12):M795-M799.

Thomas DR. Does pressure cause pressure ulcers? An inquiry into the etiology of pressure ulcers. *J Am Med Dir Assoc.* 2010;11(6):397-405.

▶ Differential Diagnosis

Acute wounds proceed through an orderly and well-described process to produce healing with structural and functional integrity. Chronic wounds fail to proceed through this process and result in poorly healing wounds of long duration. There are four types of chronic wounds: peripheral arterial ulcers, diabetic ulcers, venous stasis ulcers, and pressure ulcers. Each of these wounds differs in their underlying pathophysiology and, more importantly, with respect to local wound treatment.

A. Arterial Ulcers

Arterial ulcers tend to occur over the distal part of the leg, especially the lateral malleoli, dorsum of the feet, and the toes. The clinical appearance is that of gangrene, which can be wet or dry. Arterial ulcers tend to be painful, and pain control features prominently in their management. Peripheral arterial disease results from atherosclerosis of the aorta and iliac and lower extremity arteries. Ischemic vascular ulcers are difficult to heal, and therapy is aimed at improving blood flow. A careful examination of arterial pulses may be useful but is dependent on the examiner's skill and may be misleading. An ankle-brachial pressure index is an inexpensive and accurate diagnostic test for peripheral arterial disease.

B. Diabetic Ulcers

The etiology of diabetic ulcers is multifactorial. Among these, the presence of neuropathy is the most important factor in the development of a diabetic ulcer, while inadequate vascular supply is the most important factor in healing. Diabetic ulcers typically occur in areas of repetitive trauma, producing a callus formation. Microvascular changes in blood flow lead to a deep crater-like appearance, especially in areas of foot deformity.

C. Venous Ulcers

The underlying pathophysiology of venous leg ulcers includes reflux, obstruction, or insufficiency of the calf muscle pump, involving the superficial venous system (greater and smaller saphenous vein), the deep venous system, or the veins that perforate between those systems. The etiology of chronic deep venous disease results from primary (often idiopathic) or secondary causes (postthrombotic obstruction), but most commonly represents a combination of both. The skin in chronic venous stasis disease demonstrates hyper- or hypopigmentation, lipodermatosclerosis, weeping of the skin, and ulceration. Edema is often present but not necessary for the diagnosis. A venous leg ulcer is irregularly shaped and shallow, but with well-defined borders. Location is usually from the malleolar area upward to the knee (the "gaiter" area, so-called because this area is covered by leggings known as gaiters). The ulcer bed is often exudative,

Patient name: _____ Patient ID#: _____

Ulcer location: _____ Date: _____

Directions: Observe and measure the pressure ulcer. Categorize the ulcer with respect to surface area, exudate, and type of wound tissue. Record a subscore for each of these ulcer characteristics. Add the subscore to obtain the total score. A comparison of total scores measured over time provides an indication of the improvement or deterioration in pressure ulcer healing.

Length	0 0 cm²	1 <0.3 cm²	2 0.3–0.6 cm²	3 0.7–1.0 cm²	4 1.1–2.0 cm²	5 2.1–3.0 cm²	
x Width		6 3.1–4.0 cm²	7 4.1–8.0 cm²	8 8.1–12.0 cm²	9 12.1–24.0 cm²	10 >24.0 cm²	Subscore
Exudate amount	0 None	1 Light	2 Moderate	3 Heavy			Subscore
Tissue type[a]	0 Closed	1 Epithelial tissue	2 Granulation tissue	3 Slough	4 Necrotic tissue		Subscore
							Total score

Length × Width: Measure the greatest length (head to toe) and the greatest width (side to side) using a centimeter ruler. Multiply these two measurements (length × width) to obtain an estimate of surface area in square centimeters (cm²). Caveat: Do not guess! Always use a centimeter ruler and always use the same method each time the ulcer is measured.

Exudate amount: Estimate the amount of exudate (drainage) present after removal of the dressing and before applying any topical agent to the ulcer. Estimate the exudate (drainage) as none, light, moderate, or heavy.

Tissue type: This refers to the types of tissue that are present in the wound (ulcer) bed. Score as a "4" if there is any necrotic tissue present. Score as a "3" if there is any amount of slough present and necrotic tissue is absent. Score as a "2" if the wound is clean and contains granulation tissue. A superficial wound that is reepitheliazing is scored as a "1". When the wound is closed, score as a "0".

[a]**Necrotic tissue (eschar):** black, brown, or tan tissue that adheres firmly to the wound bed or ulcer edges and may be either firmer or softer than surrounding skin. **Slough:** yellow or white tissue that adheres to the ulcer bed in strings or thick clumps or is mucinous. **Granulation tissue:** pink or beefy red tissue with a shiny, moist, granular appearance. **Epithelial tissue:** for superficial ulcers. New pink or shiny tissue (skin) that grows in from the edges or as islands on the ulcer surface. **Closed/resurfaced:** wound is completely covered with epithelium (new skin).

▲ **Figure 68–1.** Pressure Ulcer Status for Healing (PUSH) tool version 3.0. (Reproduced with permission from National Pressure Ulcer Advisory Panel.)

and bacterial and fungal overgrowth on the wound and surrounding skin surface is common.

D. Pressure Ulcers

Pressure ulcers are the visible evidence of pathologic changes in the blood supply to dermal tissues. Pressure ulcers usually occur over bony prominences, when the tissue is compressed to pressures above capillary closing pressure. However, patient-specific intrinsic factors may lessen the time or pressure amounts required to produce tissue damage. The most common site for the development of a pressure ulcer is the sacrococcygeal area, followed by the heels.

All of the four types of chronic wounds have in common some relationship to pressure. However, the classification of these wounds should be related to the underlying pathophysiology with respect to appropriate treatment.

▶ Complications

A. Wound Infections

Colonization of chronic wounds with bacteria is common and unavoidable. All chronic wounds become colonized, usually with skin organisms followed in 48 hours by gram-negative bacteria. Thus, routine wound cultures are not recommended. For suspected infection, a wound swab using the Levine technique is preferred over a surface swab. The Levine technique is done by rotating a swab over a 1-cm-square area with enough pressure to express fluid from within the wound tissue.

The presence of microorganisms alone (colonization) does not indicate an infection in pressure ulcers. The primary source of bacterial infections in chronic wounds appears to be the result of suprainfection resulting from contamination. Therefore, protection of the wound from secondary contamination is an important goal of treatment. Evidence suggests that occlusive dressings protect against clinical infection, although the wound may be colonized with bacteria. Occlusive dressings very rarely cause a clinical infection.

It is often difficult to determine the presence of an infection in chronic pressure ulcers. The diagnosis of infection in chronic wounds must be based on clinical signs: advancing erythema, presence of pain, edema, odor, fever, or purulent exudate. When there is evidence of clinical infection, topical or systemic antimicrobials are required. Topical treatment may be useful when the wound is failing to progress toward healing. Systemic antibiotics are indicated when the clinical condition suggests spread of the infection to the bloodstream or bone. Wounds with extensive undermining create pockets for infection with an increased likelihood of infection with anaerobic organisms. Obliteration of dead space reduces the possibility of infection.

Other complications include prolonged hospital or skilled nursing facility days due to wound care, financial cost on the health system, mental health impact on the patient, caregiver burden and strain from providing wound care, and injury to caregivers during repositioning. Longer hospital and skilled nursing facility stays due to pressure ulcers have a significant impact on the financial cost of the health care system. Prolonged stays also impact the patient who can become even more debilitated, depressed, and at risk for other hospital-acquired conditions. Most pressure ulcer treatment requires training of patient's family members or caregivers to provide appropriate wound care if patients are discharged home. This is burdensome on the caregiver and the patient. The patient is often completely dependent on others for care due to location of wounds and comorbidities. The caregiver can face challenges physically when it comes to frequent turning, repositioning, and providing wound care. Proper supplies, education, and support for family members and caregivers are important to promote healing and prevent further pressure ulcer development.

Thomas DR. When is a chronic wound infected? *J Am Med Dir Assoc.* 2012;13(1):5-7.

B. Lab Findings

Patients who develop pressure ulcers often exhibit comorbid conditions that affect laboratory findings. There are no specific laboratory findings for a pressure ulcer per se. Abnormal acute phase reactants (albumin, prealbumin) are frequent findings. Often a complete blood count with differential is obtained to monitor for signs of infection. An erythrocyte sedimentation rate and C-reactive protein can be obtained and are useful to detect osteomyelitis in which the parameters are elevated.

C. Imaging Studies

If osteomyelitis is suspected in a stage 4 pressure ulcer, magnetic resonance imaging is superior to plain x-rays.

D. Special Examinations

Bone biopsy is useful in defining organisms in osteomyelitis.

▶ Treatment

Recognition of risk, relief of pressure, and optimizing nutritional status are all components of both prevention and management guidelines for treatment of pressure ulcers. For persons with identified pressure ulcers, assessing the wound and implementing strategies for local wound care are paramount. Consideration can be made to place referrals to occupational therapy as well as physical therapy to help assess durable medical equipment needs that might reduce pressure points as well as attempts to improve functional mobility.

Maintaining a moist wound environment increases the rate of healing. Moist wound healing allows experimentally induced wounds to resurface up to 40% faster than air-exposed wounds. Any therapy that dehydrates the wound such as dry gauze, heat lamps, air exposure, or liquid antacids is detrimental to chronic wound healing. Dressings that maintain a moist wound environment are occlusive, describing the propensity of a dressing to transmit moisture vapor from the wound to the external atmosphere. The available dressings differ in their properties of permeability to water vapor.

A. Topical Dressings

Occlusive dressings can be divided into broad categories of polymer films, polymer foams, hydrogels, hydrocolloids, alginates, and biological membranes. Each has several advantages and disadvantages. The choice of a particular agent depends on the clinical presentation. The agents differ in the ease of application. This difference is important in pressure ulcers in unusual locations or when considering their use for home care. Dressings should be left in place until wound fluid is leaking from the sides, a period of days to up to 3 weeks.

1. Polymer films—Polymer films are impermeable to liquid but permeable to both gas and moisture vapor. Because of low permeability to water vapor, these dressings are not dehydrating to the wound. Nonpermeable polymers such as polyvinylidene and polyethylene can be macerating to normal skin. Polymer films are not absorptive and may leak, particularly when the wound is highly exudative. Most films have an adhesive backing that may remove epithelial cells when the dressing is changed. Polymer films do not eliminate dead space and do not absorb exudate. Therefore, films need to be placed on clean wound beds to promote effective healing. An absorptive dressing or hydrogel may be required in exudative wounds.

2. Hydrogels—Hydrogels are three-layer hydrophilic polymers that are insoluble in water but absorb aqueous solutions. They are poor bacterial barriers and do not adhere to the wound. Because of their high specific heat, these dressings are cooling to the skin, aiding in pain control and reducing inflammation. Most of these dressings require a secondary dressing to secure them to the wound.

3. Hydrocolloid dressings—Hydrocolloid dressings are complex dressings similar to ostomy barrier products. They are impermeable to moisture vapor and gases (their impermeability to oxygen is theoretically a disadvantage) and are highly adherent to the skin. In addition, they offer bacterial resistance. Their adhesiveness to surrounding skin is higher than some surgical tapes, but they do not adhere to wound tissue and do not damage epithelialization of the wound. The adhesive barrier is frequently overcome in highly exudative wounds. Hydrocolloid dressings cannot be used over tendons or on wounds with eschar formation. Several of these dressings include a foam padding layer that may reduce pressure to the wound and prevent further break down.

4. Alginates—Alginates are complex polysaccharide dressings that are highly absorbent in exudative wounds. This high absorbency is particularly suited to exudative wounds. Alginates do not adhere to the wound; however, if the wound is allowed to dry, damage to the epithelial tissue may occur with removal.

5. Biological membranes—Biological membranes offer bacterial resistance but are very expensive and not readily available. These dressings could be problematic in wounds contaminated by anaerobes, but this effect has not been demonstrated clinically.

6. Saline-soaked gauze—Saline-soaked gauze that is not allowed to dry is an effective wound dressing. Moist saline gauze and occlusive-type dressings have similar pressure ulcer–healing abilities. The use of occlusive-type dressings has been shown to be more cost-effective than traditional dressings primarily because of a decrease in nursing time for dressing changes. Saline-soaked dressings require a minimum of two or three dressing changes per day and a patient, caregiver, and/or nurse must be trained and available in providing adequate care.

Table 68–2 provides a comparison of dressing types.

Table 68–2. Dressings and topical agents for treating pressure ulcers—Network meta-analysis: Proportion with complete healing interventions versus saline gauze.

Dressing	Number of persons Healed per 1000 (comparator saline)	Confidence Limits
Alginate dressings	14 more	140 fewer to 1000 more
Sequential hydrocolloid alginate	79 fewer	138 fewer to 155 more
Basic wound contact	47 more	55 fewer to 250 more
Collagenase ointment	176 more	9 more to 506 more
Dextranomer	590	22 fewer to 1000 more
Foam dressings	82 more	5 more to 196 more
Hydrocolloid/alginate	35 more	148 fewer to 1000 more
Hydrocolloid	68 more	0 fewer to 165 more
Hydrogel	86 more	0 fewer to 165 more
Iodine dressing	13 more	66 fewer to 159 more
Phenytoin	42 more	66 fewer to 305 more
Protease-modulating	102 more	13 fewer to 305 more
Polyvinylpyrrolidone plus zinc	49 more	99 fewer to 575 more
Combination silicone foam	146	97 fewer to 1000 more
Soft polymer	55 more	71 fewer to 360 more
Tripeptide copper gel	455 more	6 more to 1000 more
Vapor-permeable	71 more	39 fewer to 283 more

Data from Westby MJ, Dumville JC, Soares MO, Stubbs N, Norman G. Dressings and topical agents for treating pressure ulcers, *Cochrane Database Syst Rev* 2017 Jun 22;6(6):CD011947.

B. Growth Factors

Acute wound healing proceeds in a carefully regulated fashion that is reproducible from wound to wound. A number of growth factors have been demonstrated to mediate the healing process, including transforming growth factor-α and -β, epidermal growth factor, platelet-derived growth factor, fibroblast growth factor, interleukin-1 and -2, and tumor necrosis factor-α. Accelerating healing in chronic wounds using these acute wound factors is attractive. Several of these factors have been favorable in animal models; however, they have not been as successful in human trials.

C. Adjunctive Therapies

Alternative or adjunctive therapies include electrical therapy, electromagnetic therapy, ultrasound therapy, low-level light therapy/laser therapy, and vacuum-assisted closure. None of these interventions has been clearly proven effective despite widespread clinical use.

Westby MJ, Dumville JC, Soares MO, Stubbs N, Norman G. Dressings and topical agents for treating pressure ulcers. *Cochrane Database Syst Rev.* 2017;6:CD011947.

D. Debridement

Necrotic debris increases the possibility of bacterial infection and delays wound healing. The preferred method of debriding pressure ulcers remains controversial. Options include mechanical debridement with dry gauze dressings, autolytic debridement with occlusive dressings, application of exogenous enzymes, or sharp surgical debridement.

Surgical sharp debridement produces the most rapid removal of necrotic debris and is required in the presence of infection. Sharp debridement can be done safely in the outpatient clinic and does not require advanced training by the provider. Limitations include provider competency in the procedure and patients' pain tolerance. Mechanical debridement can be easily accomplished by allowing a saline gauze dressing to dry before removal. Remoistening of gauze dressings in an attempt to reduce pain can defeat the debridement effect.

Both surgical and mechanical debridement can damage healthy tissue or fail to clean the wound completely. Debridement with a dry gauze should be stopped as soon as a clean wound bed is obtained because dry dressings have been associated with delayed healing.

Thin portions of eschar can be removed by occlusion under a semipermeable dressing. Both autolytic and enzymatic debridement require periods of several days to several weeks to achieve results. Enzymatic debridement can dissolve necrotic debris, but whether it harms healthy tissue is debated. Penetration of enzymatic agents is limited in eschar and requires either softening by autolysis or cross-hatching by sharp incision before application.

Only one enzyme preparation is currently available in the United States for debridement. Topical collagenase reduced necrosis, pus, and odor compared with inactivated control ointment and produced debridement in 82% of pressure ulcers at 4 weeks compared with petrolatum. Unfortunately, wound care products, in particular topical collagenase, can be quite expensive, and not all patients can afford treatment, nor will insurance necessarily provide prescription coverage for the products. Moist saline dressings may be the most cost-effective approach for some patients. The issues of when to debride and which method to use remain controversial. Whether debridement improves the rate of healing remains undetermined. A total of five trials have not shown that the use of enzymatic agents increased the rate of complete healing in chronic wounds compared with control treatment.

E. Surgical Therapy

Surgical closure of pressure ulcers results in a more rapid resolution of the wound. The chief problems are frequent recurrence of ulcers and inability of frail patients to tolerate the procedure. The efficacy of surgical repair of pressure ulcers is high in the short term; however, its long-term efficacy has been questioned. Problems with surgical repair include suture line dehiscence, nonhealing wounds, and recurrence as well as poor survival rate and lengthy hospital stays for frail older adults.

The proportion of pressure ulcers suitable for operation depends on the patient population, but normally only a low percentage are candidates for surgery. However, among selected groups of patients, such as those with spinal cord injury and deep stage 3 or 4 pressure ulcers, surgery may be indicated for the majority. If the factors contributing to the development of the pressure ulcer cannot be corrected, the chance of recurrence after surgery is very high.

▶ Prognosis

Pressure ulcers have been associated with increased mortality rates in both acute and long-term care settings. Death has been reported during acute hospitalization in 67% of patients who develop a pressure ulcer compared with 15% of at-risk patients without pressure ulcers. Patients who develop a new hospital-acquired pressure ulcer are 2.8 times as likely to die in the hospital compared to persons without a pressure ulcer. The odds ratio for mortality in 30 days is 1.7 times as high, and readmission within 30 days is 1.3 times as high. In long-term care settings, development of a pressure ulcer within 3 months among newly admitted patients was associated with a 92% mortality rate, compared with 4% among residents who did not subsequently develop a pressure ulcer. Residents in a skilled nursing facility who had pressure ulcers experienced a 6-month mortality rate of 77.3% compared with 18.3% in those without pressure ulcers. Patients whose pressure ulcers healed within 6 months had a significantly lower mortality rate (11% vs 64%) than those whose pressure ulcers did not heal.

Despite this association with death rates, it is not clear how pressure ulcers contribute to increased mortality. Patients with stage 2 pressure ulcers have been equally as likely to die as those with stage 4 pressure ulcers. In the absence of complications, it is difficult to imagine how stage 1 or 2 pressure ulcers contribute to death. Pressure ulcers may be associated with mortality because of their occurrence in otherwise frail, sick patients.

Thomas DR. Are all pressure ulcers avoidable? *J Am Med Dir Assoc.* 2001;2:297.

Driving & Older Adults

Annie C. Harmon, PhD
David B. Carr, MD

69

OLDER DRIVERS

In 2017, one out of every five licensed drivers in the United States was age 65 years or older. Concern about older drivers has grown along with the number of older drivers on the roads, reinforced by sensationalized media reports about rare but tragic fatalities caused by impaired older drivers. As a group, the 43.6 million older licensed drivers are very safe, with lower absolute yearly crash rates than younger counterparts and fewer aggressive driving behaviors. According to data from the Insurance Institute for Highway Safety, exposure-adjusted crash risk increases around age 75 years. However, chronologic age plays less of a role in older adults' driving outcomes than health issues that threaten the ability to continue driving safely.

Driving is not only a valued instrumental activity of daily living (IADL), but it also provides meaning and a sense of control over one's life. Former drivers consistently report serious physical, mental, and social consequences of driving cessation. Therefore, the importance of public safety should not automatically outweigh individual autonomy and the right to drive, especially based on age alone. The difficult question remains: How can we identify older drivers who are unsafe or at high risk before a serious event, without placing unnecessary restrictions on their driving?

As a direct contact with intimate understanding of patients' overall health, clinicians and, in particular, primary care providers remain one of the most trusted stakeholders in determining medical fitness to drive. Unfortunately, medical education contains little, if any, training on how to evaluate medical fitness to drive or communicate to patients when there is concern about their driving. Discussing driving with patients can be difficult and emotional, made more challenging because of time restrictions and competing medical priorities. Clinicians need the tools to navigate these situations, including clinical assessments to objectively evaluate patients' driving-related functional abilities and a broader understanding of the roles driving and transportation mobility play in quality of life at every age.

In this chapter, we will lay out the underlying skills and abilities necessary for driving safety at every age; describe age-related physiologic changes and how they impact driving safety; consider tools for clinical environments to assess driving risk; outline the process and impacts of driving cessation; and finally discuss developing technologies with the potential to improve transportation mobility across the life span.

American Geriatrics Society. *Clinician's Guide to Assessing and Counseling Older Drivers*. 4th ed. Washington, DC: National Highway Traffic Safety Administration. 2019. https://geriatricscareonline.org/ProductAbstract/clinicians-guide-to-assessing-and-counseling-older-drivers-4th-edition/B047_cliniciansguidetoolderdrivers.pdf. Accessed May 28, 2019.

Betz MEJ, Jones J, Petroff E, Schwartz R. "I wish we could normalize driving health:" a qualitative study of clinician discussions with older drivers. *J Gen Intern Med*. 2013;28(12):1573-1580.

Naumann RB, Dellinger AM, Kresnow MJ. Driving self-restriction in high-risk conditions: how do older drivers compare to others? *J Safety Res*. 2011;42:67-71.

Tefft BC. Driver license renewal policies and fatal crash involvement rates of older drivers, United States, 1986-2011. *Inj Epidemiol*. 2014;1(1):25.

FUNCTIONAL DEMANDS OF DRIVING

Clinicians have a unique overview of patient health and functioning, which can inform the discussions about driving continuation at any age. At baseline, drivers must be able to operate a vehicle and apply fundamental knowledge about the rules of the road, both easily observed driving behaviors. Accomplishing the task (ie, getting safely from point A to point B) relies on hidden coordination between the eyes, brain, and body. Any impairment, age-related or otherwise, that lowers a driver's capability to meet task demands increases driving risk.

Driving concerns can be among the first indicators of visual, cognitive, and motor declines. As with handling finances or medications, driving relies on higher-order reasoning and decision making that are more difficult to mask than with other common activities. However, driving is unique among IADLs in its sustained cognitive demands, as well as the potential danger to both the individual and other roadway users.

Fuller R. Towards a general theory of driver behaviour. *Accid Anal Prev.* 2005;37(3):461-472.

Michon JA. A critical view of driver behavior models. What do we know, what should we do? In: Evans L, Schwing RC (eds). *Human Behavior and Traffic Safety.* New York, NY: Plenum Press; 1985.

HOW AGING AFFECTS DRIVING

While age itself is a poor predictor of driving safety, age is a risk factor for physiologic changes and health conditions that are associated with medical fitness to drive. Up to a point, decrements in vision, slower cognition, and muscular weakness are part of the normal aging process. Cerebrovascular, cardiovascular, and pulmonary conditions commonly affect driving indirectly through symptoms, side effects, and treatment. However, not every adult experiences functional limitations in their later years. Among older adults who do experience declinations, they occur at different ages, to varying degrees of severity, and with different rates of progression. Therefore, it is important to recognize that individual functional abilities, and not age itself, are what determine medical fitness to drive.

▶ Vision

Receiving visual information from the roadway environment is essential to driving. Visual acuity; spatial relationships; and information from the on-road environment, including other vehicles, roadway and traffic signs, and pedestrians, affect driving safety in several ways. Age is a risk factor for several eye diseases, including cataracts, glaucoma, and macular degeneration, which limit a driver's ability to comprehensively view the driving environment. Older adults without disease still experience general declines in vision, including decreased visual acuity, contrast sensitivity, and slowed adaptation to low-light conditions. Difficulties seeing or loss of sight is one of the most common reasons people reduce or stop driving and one of the easiest for former drivers to accept.

In addition to sensory loss, the speed with which visual information is processed by the brain can slow in advanced age. Useful field of view (UFOV), a common test to assess visual processing speed, requires divided attention in the presence of distracting stimuli. Therefore, the decline in

UFOV associated with aging may also be related to impaired attention with inefficient visual search strategies, highlighting the difficulty of disentangling vision problems from underlying cognitive processes.

▶ Cognition

Because driving is both common and overlearned, it can be difficult to parse the numerous cognitive demands drivers face simultaneously. Basic vehicle operation includes speed regulation and lane maintenance. While maintaining the route and destination, drivers generally apply the rules of the road, adapting to local regulations such as speed limits. In addition, drivers are faced with dynamic on-road conditions with other vehicles and pedestrians operating independently, at varying speeds and various distances. Unfamiliar routes, inclement weather, and low light between dusk and dawn all add additional stress or risk to driving.

Understanding the demands faced by drivers can assist clinicians in determining the level of concern for patient safety. Be aware of other flags for functional decline, especially needing assistance or restrictions with other IADLs such as medication and financial management. If a patient exhibits cognitive difficulties with sustained attention, short- and long-term memory, spatial relationships, attention switching, visual information processing, reasoning, or decision making, driving should be addressed. This includes not only clinically significant cognitive impairment, but also functional decrements resulting from medication side effects, poor sleep, malnutrition, and psychological distress.

For patients with dementia, the question of driving cessation is a matter of timing. For as long as their cognition allows, discussions about driving continuation can and should involve patients as well as caregivers. If diagnosed in the early stages, there may not be an immediate need to stop driving, providing opportunity for planning and patient engagement before complete cessation. These discussions can center around a contract outlining when they will stop driving, based on on-road events, health markers, or a set time. Patients in moderate and severe stages are unsafe to drive and should cease immediately, even if they drive infrequently to familiar and nearby locations. Patients who struggle to remember they stopped driving may benefit from "prescriptions" or letters from clinicians for caregivers to use as reminders.

▶ Motor Function

Operating an automobile even in this day of power steering and driving does require adequate power, range of motion, and coordination in the upper and lower limbs, which can all be assessed by the interested clinician in the office. The upper extremity is usually relegated to the tasks of steering and other vehicle controls (eg, turn signals, lights), while the lower extremities are responsible for the brake and accelerator. A variety of conditions that afflict older adult drivers have the potential to impair these key motor abilities. Arthritis (eg, osteoarthritis, rheumatoid arthritis) can restrict power due to pain and/or weakness in the extremities and also limit range of motion. Cervical degenerative joint disease can limit neck range of motion and decrease the field of view. Parkinson disease, essential tremor, and/or cerebellar disease can cause difficulties with tremor, muscle rigidity, bradykinesia, and/or a decline in coordination. These conditions may result in slowness in speed of movement with a resultant delay in detecting oncoming vehicles, slow steering maneuvers, and/or diminished brake reaction time.

Frailty can decrease endurance and require modification or reduction of the duration of the driving task. Thankfully, vehicle modifications exist for loss of muscle weakness (eg, stroke, amputation) with implementation of steering knobs, hand controls, and left foot accelerators. Wide-angle mirrors may be able to overcome restrictions in neck range of motion. For patients with osteoporosis and increasingly short stature, portable stable elevated seats exist to enable adequate vision above the dashboard. Many of the newer cars now offer ergonomically adjustable seats that can assist older adults with proper positioning and comfort while driving.

Karthaus M, Falkenstein M. Functional changes and driving performance in older drivers: assessment and interventions. *Geriatrics (Basel)*. 2016;1(2):E12.

NTC Australia. Austroads. Assessing Fitness to Drive. 2016. https://austroads.com.au. Accessed January 20, 2020.

CHRONIC CONDITIONS AND MEDICATIONS ASSOCIATED WITH DRIVING RISK

With increased longevity and medical advancements to manage chronic conditions, older adults may accumulate several of these illnesses across their life span. Both the symptoms and treatment for comorbid conditions can affect driving ability. There are many medical conditions and medications that should be considered in medical fitness to drive evaluations. Although acute medical conditions may be a rare cause of motor vehicle crashes, their impact on driving if present may not be insignificant. However, the sheer presence of multiple medical conditions and/or drugs is unlikely to be a major predictor of unsafe driving.

The medical literature has many evidenced-based reviews on chronic conditions to guide clinicians in subspecialty areas. Most of these are in areas where there is a fair amount of literature such as dementia and mild cognitive impairment, Parkinson disease, brain injury, and stroke. Although some of the summaries may be several years old, many reviews are still relevant given they are based on solid evidence and there have not been many additions to the driving literature that would significantly alter the findings or recommendations.

Most of these consensus statements or meta-analyses are based on specific medical conditions and not focused on older adults in general.

Clinicians also need to be aware of which medication side effects most directly affect driving ability (eg, changes in vision, awareness, balance, muscle strength, and coordination). Benzodiazepines have been associated with increased risk for a motor vehicle crash. Opioids, sedative-hypnotic medications including over-the-counter medications, antidepressants, anxiolytics, antipsychotics, and cardiac medications, especially antihypertensives, can affect driving ability. Medications with anticholinergic side effects have the potential for causing daytime sedation and delayed reaction time. Thus, there may be opportunities to reduce the risk to safe driving, from alerting patients to potential driving impairment from medications to deprescribing.

Clinicians should be aware of how fatigue or sleepiness may impact patients' driving, whether caused by medication side effects and interactions or, increasingly in the adult population of all ages, sleep disorders. Drowsy driving is implicated in up to 6000 fatal motor vehicle crashes each year. Obstructive sleep apnea (OSA) is associated with an increased risk of motor vehicle crashes. Treating OSA has been shown to decrease motor vehicle crash risk. The Epworth Sleepiness Scale, a brief questionnaire, can be used to screen for hypersomnolence in the assessment of driving fitness.

Crizzle AM, Classen S, Uc EY. Parkinson disease and driving. An evidenced-based review. *Neurology*. 2012;79:2067-2074.

Devos H, Akinwuntan AE, Nieuwboer A, Truijen S, Tant M, De Weerdt W. Screening for fitness to drive after stroke: a systematic review and meta-analysis. *Neurology*. 2011;76(8):747-756.

Driving and Dementia Working Group. Driving with dementia or mild cognitive impairment: consensus guidelines for clinicians. 2018. United Kingdom. https://research.ncl.ac.uk/driving-and-dementia/consensusguidelinesforclinicians/. Accessed April 21, 2020.

Hetland A, Carr DB. Medications and impaired driving. *Ann Pharmacother*. 2014;48(4):494-506.

Palubiski L, Crizzle, A. Evidence based review of fitness-to-drive and return-to-driving following traumatic brain injury. *Geriatrics*. 2016;1(3):17.

EVALUATING FITNESS TO DRIVE

▶ Patient Driving History

The history should focus on those elements that may put older adults at risk and are evidenced based. For the potentially at-risk driver with cognitive impairment, collecting collateral history from a well-informed contact is important. History of a previous motor vehicle crash, moving violation, caregiver opinion of driving competency, and aggressive or impulsive driving can be clues to unsafe driving. Clinicians should not be reassured if the collateral informant states the patient's trips are infrequent, as low-mileage older adult drivers may be counterintuitively at greater risk per miles driven for a crash than high-mileage drivers. Checklists of abnormal driving behaviors, such as those from the Alzheimer's Association and the Hartford Foundation, may supply useful additional information but have not been well validated. Furthermore, these checklists often overlap with driving behaviors among healthy older adults, blurring the sensitivity to identify high-risk drivers.

Functional Screens

Functional screens can easily be administered in the office setting to flag patient impairment in the baseline abilities necessary to drive safely (Table 69–1). Several short tests can be used to identify marked difficulties with vision, cognition, motor skills, or multidomain functional performance. For instance, vision tests are common and easily completed in clinical settings and, when required for licensing, have been shown to reduce crash rates. Visual acuity alone is less predictive of vehicle crashes than other visual constructs, such as contrast sensitivity and visual field. Cognition can be gleaned through difficulties with IADLs (eg, cooking a hot meal or managing finances) because they require executive function skills, and difficulty performing these tasks might be a warning sign for impaired driving. The American Geriatrics Society/National Highway Traffic Safety Administration guidelines recommend that physicians check manual motor strength and joint range of motion, along with the rapid pace walk, which was validated in a large prospective study during license renewal. A history of falls has been associated with increased risk of a motor vehicle crash, although the findings are mixed and may be at least partly driven by confounding and bias in observational studies.

The most useful functional screens include cognitive elements, which may enable clinicians to classify with a modest degree of accuracy performance on a standardized road test.

Table 69–1. Screening tests associated with older adult driving impairment.

Visual acuity
Visual fields
Contrast sensitivity
Selective and divided attention (useful field of view)
Visual search (Trails Making Test Parts A, B)
Visuospatial skill (Clock Drawing Test)
Rapid pace walk
Joint range of motion
Manual muscle strength

Among samples with conditions that affect cognition, such as drivers with dementia, prediction of on-road safety is even greater. The Clock Drawing Test, Maze Test, and Trail Making Test Parts A and B tap into visual search, attention, visuospatial, and executive function skills, particularly those pertaining to planning and foresight. Performance on the UFOV, a computerized test that assesses selective and divided attention, allows for reliability of administration, and impairment on these tests has been associated with motor vehicle crash risk.

Limitations of Screens

There have been myriad efforts over the past few decades to develop individual screening tools or a combined testing battery to assist clinicians with fitness-to-drive decisions. Despite these determined efforts, no single screen, or group of screens, has emerged as a clear indicator of medical fitness to drive, in large part due to limitations in generalizability. Screens are most effective at identifying conditions or outcomes with a prevalence between 30% and 70%. However, the prevalence of adverse driving outcomes among general older adult samples is much lower, around 10%. This significantly decreases the utility of fitness-to-drive screens to solely guide decision making, and this is especially the case when tests are applied to a heterogeneous group of relatively healthy older adults, such as those who present for license renewal. Overall, screens can be useful for flagging risk but should be considered only one part of the larger assessment for individual patients.

Even disease-specific driving studies regularly use specific ratings of the disorder (eg, Clinical Dementia Rating scores for Alzheimer disease and related dementias), which may not be applicable, practical, or available to many clinicians in practice.

Finally, it is challenging for one test to have an acceptable cutoff using a dichotomous (pass/fail) approach. Published studies that do not include receiver operator curves or provide cutoffs with likelihood ratios make clinical decisions difficult. Studies that have adopted multidomain testing typically use discriminant analysis or regression equations to assist with predicting driving outcomes. Many investigators are using multiple tests and/or trichotomous outcomes where there is an intermediate group where uncertainty is accepted. These studies need to be validated in real-world clinical environments and in larger sample sizes to ensure that the results are generalizable.

Because of these limitations, brief screens should not be used as the only criteria for determining driving privileges. In reality, driving recommendations in regard to medical conditions are often based on general consensus from expert opinion rather than on evidence-based literature for several reasons. First, disease severity and its proportional impact on driving-related function are rarely measured in driving studies of specific medical conditions. While general associations can be drawn from this research, it does not allow clinicians to determine driving risk directly for individuals at different stages of a health condition. Alzheimer disease, where the level of dementia severity and its driving correlates have been reported, is a rare exception. Second, as disease severity increases, driving exposure typically decreases, making crash data harder to capture unless large sample sizes are studied. Third, hazard ratios for risk based on the presence or absence of the disease are typically modest.

Finally, proving causation, as opposed to association, becomes even more pertinent in older adults with polypharmacy and multimorbidity. For instance, studies have noted increased crash risk in older adults with the use of tricyclic antidepressants. However, it is not clear whether that association is due to the symptoms of depression, the presence of the drug, other unaccounted chronic conditions, or perhaps a combination of factors.

American Geriatrics Society, Pomidor A, ed. *Clinician's Guide to Assessing and Counseling Older Drivers*, 4th Edition. Washington, DC: National Highway Traffic Safety Administration. 2019. https://www.nhtsa.gov/sites/nhtsa.dot.gov/files/documents/812228-cliniciansguidetoolderdrivers.pdf. Accessed April 21, 2020.

Carr DB, Barco PP, Wallendorf MJ, Snellgrove CA, Ott BR. Predicting road test performance in drivers with dementia. *J Am Geriatr Soc*. 2011;59(11):2112-2117.

Orriols L, Salmi LR, Philip P, et al. The impact of medicinal drugs on traffic safety: a systematic review of epidemiological studies. *Pharmacoepidemiol Drug Saf*. 2009;18(8):647-658.

Papandonatos GD, Ott BR, Davis JD, Barco PP, Carr DB. Clinical utility of the trail-making test as a predictor of driving performance in older adults. *J Am Geriatr Soc*. 2015;63(11):2358-2364.

Staplin L, Gish KW, Wagner EK. MaryPODS revisited: updated crash analysis and implications for screening program implementation. *J Safety Res*. 2003;34(4):389-397.

DRIVING REDUCTION AND CESSATION

Older drivers prefer and rely on driving as much as younger drivers but have different demands than earlier in life. Driving patterns change in later life as people transition out of active parental and work roles, as well as in response to physiologic changes with age that make drivers more cautious to drive in low-light conditions, in inclement weather, or on higher-speed roadways. Eventually, full driving cessation is a reality for many older adults, who then are faced with meeting their transportation mobility needs and wants as a nondriver for their remaining years. On average, male former drivers live an additional 6 years after driving cessation. Older female drivers face 10 years as nondrivers as a result of generally retiring from driving at younger ages and living longer than their male counterparts.

While there are commonalities, the process of transitioning to nondriver is very personal, as not everyone over 65 has the same needs, wants, social situation, and/or resources. Holistically considering individual older adults and their resources is critically important when talking about a nondriving present or future. Older adults vary widely in terms of **functional abilities**, both physical and cognitive; **financial means** to pay for taxis or rideshare services such as Uber or Lyft (where available); **social resources**, including family, friends, and others who can provide rides, information, and emotional support; and **community characteristics**, including availability of public transportation, walkability, and perceived safety. By framing driving retirement within an individual older adult's broader contexts, the particular challenges nondrivers face become clearer, as do their assets to respond to such challenges in order to maintain community mobility.

Because older drivers do not generally plan directly for future mobility loss, probing for indirect markers of behavior change is an important tool for clinicians. Driving cessation is often the final decision in a longer process of strategic driving reduction, both in terms of self-regulation intended to extend driving time, as well as related to the older adult's lifestyle and preferences. Asking older patients about common ways they may be limiting their driving (eg, only driving during daylight, avoiding inclement weather, staying in nearby and/or familiar areas, reducing overall driving speed) can provide insight into the underlying functional decline (eg, reduced visual acuity and contrast sensitivity, executive cognition and attention, slowed overall response time). These and similar adaptations to extend safe driving time can be used as a marker to segue into discussing future mobility more broadly with older patients. However, older drivers may still be resistant to others broaching the topic with their physician.

▶ Preparation for Mobility Transitions

Given the centrality of driving in daily life, discussions about driving abilities or cessation are highly sensitive. Older drivers may discuss driving with trusted persons, such as clinicians, family members, and friends; however, the enormity of the potential loss can inhibit discussions. Older adults fear becoming a burden to family members and express concern about finding convenient alternative transportation. An older adult's general understanding of mobility limitations or options does not necessarily connect to action, intention, or even personal contemplation about their own situation. Given lifelong dependence on driving and limited or inaccessible public alternatives for transportation, some older drivers report feeling pressure to continue driving longer than safe because of a few perceived options.

Fortunately, there are growing efforts to promote early mobility planning, with the general goals of removing stigma by normalizing the process of driving cessation and avoiding sudden loss of mobility without emotional or logistical preparation. By starting these conversations earlier, prior to a crisis or other immediate threat of cessation, older drivers may be more likely to engage in planning. For example, Advance Driving Directives (ADDs) and other mobility planning tools assist older adults in planning for future transportation decisions. They can also help older drivers communicate expectations with family or others involved in order to avoid assumptions or miscommunication. Finally, mobility planning provides details about nondriving alternatives for times when rides are unavailable, both before and after complete driving cessation.

▶ Reporting Medically Unsafe Drivers

Unfortunately, there are instances when a driver is unable or unwilling to acknowledge that they are no longer safe to drive. In situations where an individual presents a clear and immediate danger to others on the road, reporting them to state licensing officials is the worst-case scenario, but at times necessary. States vary in terms of mandatory reporting laws for certain conditions, as well as protections (including anonymity) for those who report potentially unsafe drivers in good faith. Generally, reporting a driver flags them for medical examination and driving performance test in order to maintain their license. When faced with this option, some older drivers choose to cease driving voluntarily, trading in their license for a state identification card.

Foley DJ, Heimovitz HK, Guralnik JM, Brock DB. Driving life expectancy of persons aged 70 years and older in the United States. *Am J Public Health.* 2002;92(8):1284-1289.

King MD, Meuser TM, Berg-Weger M, Chibnall JT, Harmon AC, Yakimo R. Decoding the Miss Daisy syndrome: an examination of subjective responses to mobility change. *J Gerontol Soc Work.* 2011;54(1):29-52.

Molnar LJ, Eby DW, Charlton JL, et al. Driving avoidance by older adults: is it always self-regulation? *Accid Anal Prev.* 2013;57:96-104.

LIVING AS A NONDRIVER

The fear older drivers have about the impact driving cessation will have on their lives is not without merit. Former drivers report a variety of difficulties in meeting their transportation mobility needs after driving cessation. Without the freedom and flexibility driving provides, former drivers take fewer trips outside their homes compared to drivers. Many former drivers and caregivers prioritize asking for assistance to meet medical or household needs, choosing to limit or forgo "nonessential" trips such as visiting friends, enjoying nature, or going to social activities. While pragmatic, the decision to limit or cut out social engagement leads to increased social isolation and depression. In addition to social and mental health consequences, former older drivers experience physical health declines, higher risk for institutionalization, and higher rates of mortality compared to current older drivers.

Therefore, it is critical for older former drivers to identify nondriving transportation alternatives to maintain independence and quality of life.

▶ Five A's of Senior Transportation

When discussing nondriving options with older patients, it is important not to oversimplify the challenges nondrivers face in finding a driving alternative. Considering the main facets of transportation older adults find important provides context to identify the benefits and barriers of the options at hand. The Beverly Foundation's 5 A's of Senior Transportation provide a framework through which to assess the viability of any form of transportation, relative to the rider's individual needs. First is **availability**, meaning the transportation option exists and is available when needed, ideally including evenings and weekends. Options also range in **accessibility,** which affects how easily riders are able to get to the onboarding points (eg, bus stops or train stations) and navigate the vehicle (eg, climb steps to reach seating area). **Acceptability** includes standards relating to conditions such as cleanliness, safety, and user-friendliness. **Affordability** considers the out-of-pocket expenses for transportation, including fees for service or cost of owning and operating a personal vehicle. Finally, modes of transportation vary in their **adaptability** to functional limitations (eg, wheelchair accommodations) or other personal needs, such as allowing several destinations (trip chaining). It is valuable to note that few transportation modes, including driving, universally meet the 5 A's.

▶ Rides with Others

Former drivers strongly prefer and often expect to get rides from others. In fact, being a passenger in a personal vehicle is the most common way former drivers report getting around. However, the fear of becoming a burden on loved ones is significant and can become a source of tension internally as well as interpersonally. Even among former drivers who have social support available, the effort to ask for rides, coordinate transportation, and prioritize needs is significant. The dependence on personal vehicles is not only a personal choice for autonomy, freedom, and enjoyment, but it can also be a necessity because public, accessible, and acceptable alternatives to driving or riding in an automobile are simply limited in most of the United States.

▶ Public Transportation Alternatives

Since the 1950s, political interest and government funding have shifted from public transportation options to personal automobiles and interstate highways. Consequently, mass transportation is available primarily in large, population-dense cities, leaving non–urban living older adults who do not drive with few options. Efforts to aggregate local transportation options are growing through websites such as ITNAmerica/Regeneron's "Rides in Sight" (www .ridesinsight.org), which allows users to search for transportation by ZIP code. Even when buses or trains are available, older adults who have relied solely on personal automobiles for decades face a steep learning curve for navigating fixed schedules and routes, discomfort of sharing communal space, and having deep concerns about safety. In addition, older adults experiencing physical or cognitive decline may also struggle getting to pick-up points, getting on or off without assistance, or traveling from where they are dropped off to their ultimate destination. Personalized public transportation options, such as those focused on older adults and those with disabilities, still require coordination in advance and waiting but may be more flexible in meeting individual riders' needs.

▶ Private Transportation Alternative

For nondrivers without public transportation options but financial resources, private alternatives (eg, taxis, rideshare, volunteer-based services such as ITNAmerica) can supplement community mobility. One of the most recent significant changes in transportation is rideshare (also called e-hail or on-demand) services. Companies like Uber, Lyft, and Curb provide many of the advantages of a personal vehicle at relatively low cost. The benefits are similar to driving oneself, and advanced coordination or reservations are not required, reducing long wait times or advanced planning whenever leaving one's house. Compared to buses or other scheduled transportation systems that follow fixed routes, ridesharing allows riders to personalize pickup locations and destinations. This feature not only reduces wait time, but also the need for additional travel. For example, when using a bus, passengers have to get to a predetermined location to get on and then transport themselves from the closest stop to their final destination. Finally, although they are not driving, being a passenger in a personal automobile provides the familiar comfort of rides with family or friends without having to ask for favors or coordinate with others' schedules.

Despite the advantages rideshare services could provide older adults, the little research available shows that few older adults know about, much less use, app-based transportation services. While the exact reasons are still unknown, two likely explanations are discomfort with technology and concerns about safety. Demographic differences are clear in usage and comfort with e-hail technology, with younger adults (age 18–29) and college-educated individuals reporting the most use. Age is also inversely associated with technology use, making rideshare services' reliance on smart phone applications (apps) a significant barrier to older adults without the technology (smart phones) or technological savvy to use them.

Chihuri S, Mielenz TJ, DiMaggio CJ, et al. Driving cessation and health outcomes in older adults. *J Am Geriatr Soc.* 2016;64(2):332-341.

Dickerson AE, Molnar L, Bedard M, Eby DW, Classen S, Polgar J. Transportation and aging: an updated research agenda for advancing safe mobility. *J Appl Gerontol.* 2019;38(12):1643-1660.

King MD, Meuser TM, Berg-Weger M, Chibnall JT, Harmon AC, Yakimo R. Decoding the Miss Daisy syndrome: an examination of subjective responses to mobility change. *J Gerontol Soc Work.* 2011;54(1):29-52.

Transportation Research Board. Enhancing the visibility and image of transit in the United States and Canada (Transit Cooperative Research Program Report 63). Washington, DC: National Research Council; 2000.

Vivoda JM, Harmon AC, Babulal GM, Zikmund-Fisher BJ. E-hail (rideshare) knowledge, use, reliance, and future expectations among older adults. *Transp Res Part F Traffic Psychol Behav.* 2018;55:426-434.

DEVELOPING TRANSPORTATION TECHNOLOGY: AUTONOMOUS VEHICLES

The landscape of transportation is evolving across the globe for many reasons, including maximizing safety, increasing traffic and travel efficiency, and reducing the environmental consequences of hyperindividualized personal travel. Rideshare technology has already shifted how we think about and use personal vehicles. On the horizon is the advent of autonomous vehicles (AV), both partially and fully self-driving, hailed as the next great advancement in human travel. Older adults, along with persons with disabilities, are the groups poised to potentially benefit the most from developing transportation technologies that allow greater convenience and flexibility of travel without the onerous coordination of arranging for rides from others or the physical and cognitive demands of navigating public transportation options (where available). However, it is important to understand that AV technology, when commercially available, will not usher in immediate or quick fixes to the challenges nondrivers currently experience and will likely continue to face for decades to come.

Similar to rideshare technology, the people and groups who need it the most are likely not going to be first in line. Without thoughtful planning and intervention, these patterns could perpetuate social disparities instead of providing solutions to those who could most benefit from AVs. Older adults are slow to trust and adopt new technologies historically, a trend that has continued even with increased use of technology in our day-to-day lives. Trust in AVs is highest among people who are younger, white, male, and educated, although the level of trust varies with news about safety concerns. Lower educational attainment and other institutional inequalities in earlier generations among older persons of color, especially women, exacerbate fear and distrust; in addition, the associated lifetime of lower income results in a financial barrier to adoption, even for those interested.

In addition, AVs are not a safety catch-all. Reasons people stopped driving, especially dementia, can be barriers to safely riding in AVs, especially those with override features. For example, if a driver-passenger with dementia is riding alone, they may not be able to appropriately intercede in an emergency by taking manual control of the vehicle. Conversely, if the same rider-passenger becomes confused or concerned, they may attempt to regain control of the vehicle at inappropriate times, which can also be dangerous. Overall, AVs have great potential for benefits but are not likely to change how older adults or anyone else travels in the near future.

American Automobile Association (AAA). AAA finds partially automated vehicle systems struggle in real-world conditions. November 14, 2018. https://newsroom.aaa.com/2018/11/americans-misjudge-partially-automated-driving-systems-ability-based-upon-names/. Accessed April 21, 2020.

American Automobile Association (AAA). Three in four Americans remain afraid of fully self-driving cars. March 14, 2018. https://newsroom.aaa.com/2018/05/aaa-american-trust-autonomous-vehicles-slips/. Accessed April 21, 2020.

Anderson M, Perrin A. Tech adoption climbs among older adults. Washington, DC: Pew Research Center. 2017. http://www.pewinternet.org/2017/05/17/technology-use-among-seniors/. Accessed April 21, 2020.

Milakis D, Snelder M, van Arem B, Homem de Almeida Correia G, van Wee GP. Development and transport implications of automated vehicles in the Netherlands: scenarios for 2030 and 2050. *Eur J Transport Infrastructure Res.* 2017;17(1). https://repository.tudelft.nl/islandora/object/uuid:154a5dd5-3296-4939-99c7-776e3ba54745?collection=research. Accessed April 21, 2020.

FOR MORE INFORMATION

▶ Resources for Clinicians

Although laws, statutes, and practices may differ by state or country, the following guidelines are comprehensive, updated regularly, and cover a myriad of medical conditions that practitioners often face in day-to-day practice.

- *Clinicians' Guide to Assessing and Counseling Older Drivers*. AGS/NHTSA 2019. Available from geriatricscareonline.org/ProductAbstract/clinicians-guide-to-assessing-and-counseling-older-drivers-4th-edition/B047.

- *CMA Driver's Guide: Determining Medical Fitness to Operate Motor Vehicles* (ninth edition) by the Canadian Medical Association. Available from shop.cma.ca/products/dg9d.

- *Assessing Fitness to Drive for Commercial and Private Vehicle Drivers: Medical Standards for Licensing and Clinical Management Guidelines* by Austroads/National Transport Commission. Available from austroads.com.au/__data/assets/pdf_file/0022/104197/AP-G56-17_Assessing_fitness_to_drive_2016_amended_Aug2017.pdf.

- *Driving with Dementia or Mild Cognitive Impairment. Consensus Guidelines for Clinicians.* Available from research.ncl.ac.uk/driving-and-dementia/consensus-guidelinesforclinicians/Final%20Guideline.pdf.

▶ Resources for Patients and Families

- **Hartford Center for Mature Market Excellence** publications on aging, including "We Need to Talk: Family Conversations with Older Drivers" and the dementia-specific "At the Crossroads: Family Conversations about Alzheimer's disease, Dementia, & Driving." Available from www.thehartford.com/resources/mature-market-excellence/publications-on-aging.

- **AAA Senior Driving:** Helping seniors drive safer and longer through information on self-evaluation of driving ability, classes to improve or refresh driving skills, and more. Available at seniordriving.aaa.com.

- **Choices for Mobility Independence: Transportation Options for Older Adults.** Published through Eldercare locator (https://eldercare.acl.gov/Public/Index.aspx) and National Aging and Disability Transportation Center (https://www.nadtc.org/). Available at www.n4a.org/files/TransportationOptions.pdf.

- **Local transportation options by ZIP code** available at www.ridesinsight.org.

Unhealthy Alcohol Use

Esperanza Romero Rodríguez, MD, MSc
Richard Saitz, MD, MPH

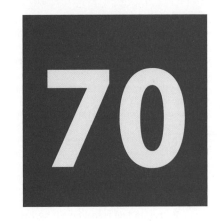

INTRODUCTION

Unhealthy alcohol use is a common but unrecognized problem in older persons, associated with substantial physical, psychological, social, and legal consequences. Older adults are particularly vulnerable to the adverse effects of alcohol, and as their numbers increase in the population, so too will the number of those with unhealthy alcohol use. Alcohol consumption leads to almost one-fifth of all hospitalizations in older adults.

Definitions

Alcohol use exists on a spectrum, from none, to lower risk use, to unhealthy alcohol use. Unhealthy alcohol use also includes a spectrum, from risky (use associated with important health risks in people without a diagnosis of alcohol use disorder) to alcohol use disorder (AUD).

Thresholds for Alcohol Use in Older Adults

Given that there are different definitions of older adults, we note that for adults who are 65 years old or younger, limits are no more than seven standard drinks per week for women and no more than three drinks on an occasion, and no more than 14 standard drinks per week for men and no more than four drinks on an occasion. The same circumstances that are associated with risks in older adults also apply here, with the addition of pregnancy or trying to conceive, which might be of relevance to the lowest ages of older adults.

A standard drink in the United States is 12 oz of beer, 5 oz of wine, or 1.5 oz of 80-proof spirits (~14 g of ethanol). Of note, alcoholic beverages vary greatly in alcohol content in part because there is variability in products (eg, 100-proof spirits, 14% ethanol wines, fortified wines, craft beers with double or more than usual strength) and in drink sizes at establishments (in many premises, a "martini" cocktail contains the alcohol of two to three standard drinks; a pint of beer is 16 oz and not 12 oz).

Lower Risk Use

Nonhazardous, lower, or low-risk use is alcohol use in someone who has not experienced consequences and use that is not known to be associated with a substantial increased risk of health consequences. For example, an older adult drinking less than seven standard drinks per week who has experienced no negative consequences from alcohol use would be considered low risk.

Unhealthy Alcohol Use

Unhealthy alcohol use is defined as the whole spectrum of use from risky use through AUD.

Hazardous Use or At-Risk or Risky Use

Hazardous or at-risk use is defined as use that increases the probability or risk of a negative consequence but has not necessarily yet resulted in one. For adults over age 65 years, the following are considered risky: more than seven standard drinks per week or more than three drinks on one occasion; any drinking in risky situations (eg, driving, climbing a ladder, taking medications that interact with alcohol); any drinking in the presence of a medication or comorbidity that contraindicates use; and any drinking in someone who has a family history of or past AUD.

Alcohol Use Disorder

According to the *Diagnostic and Statistical Manual of Mental Disorders*, fifth edition (DSM-5) a diagnosis of AUD can be made when a patient meets two or more criteria within a 12-month period. The diagnostic criteria for AUD are posted at the following website: https://www.drugabuse.gov/publications/media-guide/science-drug-use-addiction-basics.

Table 70–1. Questions to assess the DSM-5 criteria for the diagnosis of alcohol use disorder.

In the past year, have you:

1. Had times when you ended up drinking more, or longer, than you intended?
2. More than once wanted to cut down or stop drinking, or tried to, but couldn't?
3. Experienced craving—a strong need, or urge, to drink?
4. Spent a lot of time drinking? Or being sick or getting over other aftereffects?
5. Found that drinking—or being sick from drinking—often interfered with taking care of your home or family? Or caused job troubles? Or school problems?
6. Continued to drink even though it was causing trouble with your family or friends?
7. Given up or cut back on activities that were important or interesting to you, or gave you pleasure, in order to drink?
8. More than once gotten into situations while or after drinking that increased your chances of getting hurt (such as driving, swimming, using machinery, walking in a dangerous area, or having unsafe sex)?
9. Continued to drink even though it was making you feel depressed or anxious or adding to another health problem? Or after having had a memory blackout?
10. Had to drink much more than you once did to get the effect you want? Or found that your usual number of drinks had much less effect than before?
11. Found that when the effects of alcohol were wearing off, you had withdrawal symptoms, such as trouble sleeping, shakiness, restlessness, nausea, sweating, a racing heart, or a seizure? Or sensed things that were not there?

DSM-5, *Diagnostic and Statistical Manual of Mental Disorders*, fifth edition.

Reproduced with permission from National Institute on Alcohol Abuse and Alcoholism. Alcohol use disorder. Alcohol Use Disorder: A Comparison Between DSM–IV and DSM–5 https://www.niaaa.nih.gov/publications/brochures-and-fact-sheets/alcohol-use-disorder-comparison-between-dsm. Accessed June 15, 2020.

Questions to ask patients about the criteria appear in Table 70–1. If the answer is yes to any two or more questions, that is consistent with the diagnosis of AUD. In addition, to make a diagnosis of AUD, the symptoms must be causing clinically significant distress or impairment and not be largely due to another cause. The severity of the disorder can be classified as follows:

- Mild: The presence of two or three symptoms (criteria)
- Moderate: The presence of four or five symptoms (criteria)
- Severe: The presence of six or more symptoms (criteria)

Because research studies (such as those that determine which treatments are efficacious) and older documents use earlier versions of the DSM, one should be aware of older DSM (DSM-4, or fourth edition) terminology. Prior to 2013,

AUD was labeled using two terms, *alcohol abuse* and *alcohol dependence*. Although the cross-walk is inexact, dependence is similar to moderate to severe DSM-5 AUD and abuse is similar to mild AUD. The distinction was abandoned because of research suggesting the disorder is unitary and on a continuum (and because "abuse" is pejorative). Billing and health care claims sometimes use these older DSM terms, and they often use the International Classification of Diseases (ICD) system, which includes "harmful" use (similar to DSM-4 abuse) and "dependence" (similar to DSM-4 dependence). A disadvantage of the term *dependence* that had a role in the DSM-5 update to "disorder" is that it is often used to indicate physical dependence (tolerance and withdrawal), which alone is not indicative of a disorder (one can have dependence on an antihypertensive or other nonaddictive medications).

Older adults with AUD can be categorized as early onset (prior to the age of 40) or late onset. Early-onset AUD represents two-thirds of the older population who have AUD. In these individuals, the incidence of psychiatric and physical chronic conditions (often alcohol associated) and the prevalence of a family history of AUD tend to be higher than in those with late-onset AUD. Frequently, those with late-onset AUD have had a recent stressful life event, such as the loss of a partner and bereavement, retirement, loss of income, or a new serious illness or impairment affecting activities of daily life.

EPIDEMIOLOGY

Alcohol is the most commonly used substance in older adults. Although older adults report lower rates of alcohol use than younger adults, recent demographic trends show an increase in unhealthy alcohol use among older adults in the United States.

According to the National Epidemiologic Survey on Alcohol and Related Conditions III (NESARC-III), a nationally representative survey of the US adult population, the lifetime prevalence rates of mild, moderate, and severe AUD (DSM-5) and AUD overall (any severity) in adults aged 65 years or older were 5%, 3%, 6%, and 13%, respectively. Lifetime prevalence means they met criteria at some point (ever) but may not meet criteria for a current (past 12 months) disorder.

The prevalence of current, past-12-month high-risk drinking (defined in the NESARC-III report as drinking four or more standard drinks on any day for women and as drinking five or more standard drinks on any day for men at least weekly during the prior 12 months) in adults aged 65 years or older was 4%.

The NESARC-III survey revealed a substantial increase in high-risk drinking and DSM-4–defined AUDs between 2001–2002 and 2012–2013. The National Survey on Drug Use and Health (NSDUH), another US population-based survey, indicated that the prevalence of "binge" alcohol use and AUD increased significantly among adults aged ≥50 years from 2005–2006 to 2013–2014. "Binge" (often called a "heavy drinking episode" or "heavy episodic drinking") was defined as drinking five or more drinks on the same occasion on at least 1 day in the past 30 days for men and four or more drinks on the same occasion on at least 1 day in the past 30 days for women.

According to the 2017 NSDUH, 12% of people aged 65 or older reported "binge" alcohol use in the past month, 3% reported heavy alcohol use (defined as binge drinking on 5 or more days in the past 30 days based on the thresholds described previously), and 4% of individuals over 50 years old had a current AUD (DSM-4 abuse or dependence).

Only 21% of AUDs in people over age 65 years are identified by their health care providers. Older patients are less likely to be screened and more likely to have their symptoms attributed to aging or common diseases than suspected as an alcohol-related condition. The factors leading to low detection rates are less socialization, less awareness of drinking behaviors, underdiagnosis by health care providers, patients not accepting the diagnosis or concealing behaviors, family unwillingness to report, and less job or legal pressure to initiate treatment.

Project SHARE (Senior Health and Alcohol Risk Education) identified primary care patients 60 years of age and older at risk for harm from their alcohol use based on the combination of alcohol consumption with selected chronic conditions (eg, hepatitis, pancreatitis), use of medications that can interact with alcohol, or alcohol use–related behaviors (eg, driving under the influence of alcohol). Among those older adults, 62% had alcohol consumption in the context of high-risk chronic conditions, 61% had high-risk medication use, and 64% had high-risk alcohol behaviors.

▶ Etiology

Unhealthy alcohol use in older adults may be considered a complex entity influenced by genetic, environmental, and demographic factors.

A. Genetics

Hereditary factors play an important role in alcohol use among older adults. Alcohol dehydrogenase (ADH) and aldehyde dehydrogenase (ALDH) metabolize alcohol in the liver. When altered activity of these enzymes based on inheritance of genetic alleles coding for them allows accumulation of the intermediary acetaldehyde, adverse reactions to alcohol occur (eg, facial flushing, nausea). These reactions reduce the risk for AUD; conversely, with less accumulation of acetaldehyde, the risk for AUD is higher.

Furthermore, twin studies strongly suggest a genetic component to the risk for AUD. Although it is very unlikely that there will be a single specific gene associated with the risk for AUD, genome-wide association studies suggest that the genes and combinations of these genes will contribute to risk. There is no known specific genetic or hereditary risk

for late-onset AUD; nonetheless, the risks from earlier in life persist into older age.

B. Environment

Early exposure to alcohol is a strong risk factor for developing AUD. AUD is much less common among those whose first drink is not until age 21 or older. Stress and trauma in early childhood or adulthood are also risk factors.

In addition, psychosocial factors associated with aging, such as loneliness, isolation, and depression, contribute significantly as etiologic factors in the development of AUDs in older adults.

C. Demographic Risk Factors

There are several factors associated with a higher likelihood of unhealthy alcohol use in older adults:

- **Sex.** The prevalence of AUD among men is approximately twice as high as the prevalence among women. In addition, older women drink less often and are less likely to drink heavily compared to older men. Older men remain significantly more at risk for the development of AUD than women.

- **Race.** Asian or Polynesian heritage decreases risk for AUD, likely due to the higher prevalence of protective alcohol metabolism alleles in these groups. The prevalence is about half as common as it is among European or African descendants. Conversely, American Indians are at increased risk for developing AUD (>50% higher risk than European and African descendant groups).

- **Family history of AUD.** Having a positive family history only in second- or third-degree relatives increased odds of alcohol dependence (DSM-4) by 45% compared with those with a negative family history. The relative increase in odds is 86% for those with a positive family history in only first-degree relatives and 167% for those with a positive family history in both first- and second- or third-degree relatives.

- **Marital status.** Being single, separated, or divorced increases the risk for AUD among older adults.

ESSENTIALS OF DIAGNOSIS

The US Preventive Services Task Force recommends all adults be screened for unhealthy alcohol use. The Center for Substance Abuse Treatment (US Substance Abuse and Mental Health Services Administration) recommends that everyone age 60 and older be screened for alcohol use as part of regular health care services. Older adults should be screened annually, unless certain physical or mental health symptoms emerge during the year or during a period of major life changes or transitions, at which time screening should be done.

There are various validated tools for screening unhealthy alcohol use in older adults. These screening tests have different validity and feasibility. The details of each test are provided in this section. Although not perfect, the best validated tools that are feasible in primary care settings are the Alcohol Use Disorders Identification Test–Concise (AUDIT-C) and the single-item screening test.

Prior to detailing screening tools and their use, we consider here several clinical features related to alcohol use in older adults. First, older adults are more susceptible to the deleterious effects of alcohol as a result of physiologic changes and health conditions associated with aging. Decrease in lean body mass, with a concomitant increase in body fat and a reduction in total body water, increases the sensitivity to alcohol and the deleterious effects of its use. Second, aging is associated with decreased levels of ADH. Last, with aging comes an impaired ability to develop tolerance. Generally, older adults are more vulnerable to injury from vehicular crashes and even more so if they drink alcohol. Older adults are more susceptible to falls if alcohol is used, and consequently, there is an increased probability of suffering a hip fracture, a leading cause of death. Another consideration more common in older persons is the likelihood that there will be adverse alcohol-medication interactions, greater medication nonadherence, and worse control of conditions that are treated by these medications.

In addition, older adults exhibit a great deal of variability in drinking patterns. While aging, some older adults maintain drinking patterns, and others may increase their consumption in response to lack of social support or connections, health problems, and life transitions such as job loss, retirement, or the death of a family member. The incidence of medical and neurologic complications associated with unhealthy alcohol use in older adults is higher than in those without unhealthy use. The prevalence of dementia in older adults is almost five times higher than in those without unhealthy alcohol use, and approximately 25% of older patients with dementia have an AUD. Nearly one-third of adults aged 65 or older with selected chronic conditions (eg, hypertension, diabetes, Alzheimer disease, chronic obstructive pulmonary disease, or stroke) report alcohol use, and almost 7% report at-risk drinking (defined as more than seven drinks per week or more than three drinks on any single day). Older people with unhealthy alcohol use often have co-occurring psychiatric disorders. AUD is the third most common psychiatric disorder among older adults and is associated with other substance use disorders, major depression, bipolar disorder, and antisocial personality disorder.

The above clinical information provides context for screening. There are a number of validated screening tools. The easiest to use are a single item recommended by the National Institute on Alcohol Abuse and Alcoholism (NIAAA) and the AUDIT-C. We recommend these tools because they are brief and valid, even if not specifically designed for older adults.

We also discuss several other tools. A longer tool like the full AUDIT can provide more information for discussion. The CAGE questionnaire can be useful for assessing for AUD quickly but is not useful for screening for the spectrum of unhealthy use. The remaining validated tools of relevance were developed for older adults; they are more extensive but could be used in practices where the focus is the care of older adults and where there is sufficient time and expertise to use them.

The NIAAA recommends the single-item test for screening for unhealthy alcohol use in adults. The single-item screening test is sensitive and specific for detecting unhealthy alcohol use:

- How many times in the past year have you had five (four for women) or more drinks in a day?

The NIAAA suggests an optional prescreening question about any alcohol use, which can serve as an introduction:

- Do you sometimes drink beer, wine, or other alcoholic beverages?

The single-item screening is scored positive when the response is greater than zero or when the patient has difficulty thinking of the correct number (because it is therefore greater than zero).

Validation studies of the single-item screening test have included older adults but have not focused on them. Some suggest that the single-item screening test may be less useful in older adults because adverse effects can occur at lower amounts. While studies have not yet confirmed any worse operating characteristics of the single-item screening test in older adults, it is possible that the single-item screening may be less sensitive for lower levels of unhealthy use in older adults. Of note, most adults who exceed weekly alcohol risk limits also exceed the daily/per-occasion limits, which is why the single-item test that asks only about the latter is generally accurate.

An alternative approach to the single screening question is the administration of the AUDIT-C questionnaire, a screening test composed of three items asking about consumption from the Alcohol Use Disorders Identification Test (AUDIT). The AUDIT-C is briefer than the original 10-item test but still requires scoring.

- How often do you have a drink containing alcohol?
- How many drinks containing alcohol do you have on a typical day when you are drinking?
- How often do you have six or more drinks on one occasion?

In older adults, it is ideal (for sensitivity) to replace the "six" in the third item with "four." Scores considered positive for unhealthy drinking are three or more in women and four or more in men. Although the AUDIT-C contains no items specific to disorders, the score is associated with severity. A score of 7 to 10 or higher suggests DSM-4 alcohol dependence.

If the AUDIT-C or single-item test screening is positive, the next recommended step is to find out if the patient has an AUD.

The AUDIT is a 10-item screening tool developed by the World Health Organization to assess alcohol use, drinking behaviors, and alcohol consequences (Table 70–2). Its reliability and validity have been established in several clinical settings and in different nations, although studies specific to older adults are not available. A cutoff of 5+ for men or 3+ for women is sensitive and specific for unhealthy alcohol use. A cutoff of 15+ for men or 13+ for women is reasonable for identifying DSM-4 dependence with high specificity.

Another option for briefly assessing dependence among those who screen positive on other tests is the four-item CAGE questionnaire. Affirmative responses suggest a lifetime (ever) disorder in patients who screen positive with the single-item test or AUDIT-C. The CAGE questionnaire alone should not be used for screening because it is insensitive for detecting at-risk use.

Table 70–2. The Alcohol Use Disorders Identification Test (AUDIT).

1. How often do you have a drink containing alcohol?
   - ❐ 0 Never
   - ❐ 1 Monthly or less
   - ❐ 2 2 to 4 times a month
   - ❐ 3 2 to 3 times a month
   - ❐ 4 4 or more times a week
2. How many drinks containing alcohol do you have on a typical day when you are drinking?
   - ❐ 0 1 or 2
   - ❐ 1 3 or 4
   - ❐ 2 5 or 6
   - ❐ 3 7 or 9
   - ❐ 4 10 or more
3. How often do you have 6 or more drinks on one occasion?
   - ❐ 0 Never
   - ❐ 1 Less than monthly
   - ❐ 2 Monthly
   - ❐ 3 Weekly
   - ❐ 4 Daily or almost daily
4. How often during the last year have you found that you were not able to stop drinking once you had started?
   - ❐ 0 Never
   - ❐ 1 Less than monthly
   - ❐ 2 Monthly
   - ❐ 3 Weekly
   - ❐ 4 Daily or almost daily
5. How often during the last year have you failed to do what was normally expected from you because of drinking?
   - ❐ 0 Never
   - ❐ 1 Less than monthly
   - ❐ 2 Monthly
   - ❐ 3 Weekly
   - ❐ 4 Daily or almost daily
6. How often during the last year have you needed a first drink in the morning to get yourself going after a heavy drinking session?
   - ❐ 0 Never
   - ❐ 1 Less than monthly
   - ❐ 2 Monthly
   - ❐ 3 Weekly
   - ❐ 4 Daily or almost daily
7. How often during the last year have you had a feeling of guilt or remorse after drinking?
   - ❐ 0 Never
   - ❐ 1 Less than monthly
   - ❐ 2 Monthly
   - ❐ 3 Weekly
   - ❐ 4 Daily or almost daily
8. How often during the last year have you been unable to remember what happened the night before because of your drinking?
   - ❐ 0 Never
   - ❐ 1 Less than monthly
   - ❐ 2 Monthly
   - ❐ 3 Weekly
   - ❐ 4 Daily or almost daily
9. Have you or someone else been injured as a result of your drinking?
   - ❐ 0 No
   - ❐ 2 Yes, but not in the last year
   - ❐ 4 Yes, during the last year
10. Has a relative, friend, doctor or other health worker been concerned about your drinking or suggested you cut down?
    - ❐ 0 No
    - ❐ 2 Yes, but not in the last year
    - ❐ 4 Yes, during the last year

Record sum of individual item scores here: [   ]

The first three items constitute the AUDIT-C; when using the AUDIT-C it is best (for sensitivity) to replace the "six" with "four" in the third item.
A cutoff of 5+ for men, 3+ for women is sensitive and specific for unhealthy alcohol use. A score of 3 or more warrants additional assessment in the elderly.
A cutoff of 15+ for men or 13+ for women is reasonable for identifying DSM IV dependence with high specificity.

Several questionnaires have been designed specifically to screen for unhealthy alcohol use in older persons:

- The Michigan Alcoholism Screening Test–Geriatric Version (MAST-G) is an older adult–specific tool. The MAST-G consists of 24 questions with dichotomous responses (yes or no). In this instrument, each yes response has a 1-point value, and the cutoff is 5 points. The questionnaire was originally validated to detect DSM-3-R alcohol dependence. This questionnaire has the potential advantage of addressing perceptions about health and risk behaviors of older adults, as well as the damage caused by alcohol consumption. In addition, there is a 10-item short version available that is positive with two affirmative responses. However, subsequent studies have found that a major disadvantage of these screening tests is that, like the CAGE questionnaire, they are insensitive for at-risk drinking in people without an AUD.

- The Alcohol-Related Problem Scale (ARPS) was developed to detect the spectrum of unhealthy alcohol use in older patients. It performs better for this purpose than the CAGE, the Short MAST-G, and the AUDIT when compared to a reference standard consisting of medical record, clinical interview, physical examination, and interview with a collateral informant. The ARPS asks about alcohol consumption, medication use, common medical symptoms, physical and mental health function and symptoms, and health conditions. Its main limitation is that it consists of >50 items, which significantly limits its utility for universal screening in primary care settings.

- The Comorbidity Alcohol Risk Evaluation Tool (CARET) is a shorter version of the ARPS that takes 2 to 5 minutes (about 29 items) and assesses consumption (frequency and quantity), chronic conditions, and medication use to identify older adults at risk for alcohol consequences (unhealthy alcohol use). No validation study has been published, although it has moderate agreement with the AUDIT-C; many discrepant cases were those with alcohol use prior to driving identified by the CARET.

In summary, to screen for unhealthy alcohol use in older patients, while not perfect, the best validated tools that are feasible in primary care settings are the AUDIT-C and the single-item screening test. Clinicians should have a low threshold to supplement these with questions about medications, symptoms, behaviors, and health conditions that could be related to alcohol (eg, associated with risks, such as drinking and driving or medication interactions; or symptoms that could be worsened, such as gastroesophageal reflux or memory problems). Examples of such questions can be drawn from the ARPS (http://bit.ly/ARPS_inst) or the CARET.

Although lower-risk use is not the focus of this chapter, several points are warranted here. First, low amounts of alcohol can have substantial consequences in individual older persons who are susceptible. Second, because alcohol is a carcinogen even at low amounts (eg, one to six drinks per week increase the risk for breast cancer), it cannot be described as safe or as a particularly desirable chemopreventive (for cardiovascular disease or death, presumably) agent. Finally, scientific consensus is shifting from the notion that low amounts of alcohol can reduce cardiovascular disease and mortality to the understanding that such findings in observational studies are likely to have been incorrect (due to methodologic limitations). While there is no doubt that some older persons may consume low amounts of alcohol with little immediate risk, no professional organization or practice guidelines recommend starting consumption as a preventive health measure.

Any patient who screens positive should be assessed using clinical interviews or questionnaires to identify AUD. If the patient meets diagnostic criteria for AUD, then a more detailed alcohol history should be done:

- Drinking history timeline: age started drinking, first consequences of drinking alcohol
- Current situation: living situation, social support and isolation, legal issues
- Social history: family of origin, childhood, occupation, relationships, abuse and trauma history
- Current medications: particularly antidepressants, anxiolytics, benzodiazepines, opioid pain medications
- Past alcohol and other drug treatment history
- Past and recent use of other drugs and disorders, particularly tobacco use
- Current and past mental health symptoms, diagnoses, and treatment
- Suicidality, self-harm, aggression, and violence
- Drinking goals and readiness to change

Clinical examination should focus on signs and symptoms of potential alcohol use consequences and common chronic conditions in older adults such as:

- Mental health conditions, such as anxiety and depression, and cognitive dysfunction
- Neurologic conditions, such as neuropathy, seizures, delirium, and dementia
- Gastrointestinal disorders and symptoms, such as liver disease, gastritis, pancreatitis, and acid reflux
- Cardiovascular conditions, such as hypertension
- Other conditions, such as poor nutrition and coagulation disorders

To assess for these, the physical examination should include a mental status and psychiatric examination, neurologic examination, abdominal examination, cardiac examination with vital signs and check for edema, and a skin examination for signs of bruising and the stigmata of liver disease.

In addition to an alcohol history, a medical history, and a mental health and physical examination, it can be revealing to interview family members (or other collateral informants). Family members of patients with unhealthy alcohol use can provide important information such as that about the living situation, social circumstances, and daily activities and about current and past drinking and consequences.

Family members may also be able to assist with talking to the patient about drinking and encouraging them to seek medical attention. They may also notice any cognitive deterioration or diminution of the patient's self-care abilities and may be key to coordination of health care and community services.

Laboratory tests can be useful in the evaluation of AUD, although they are not as useful as questionnaires when screening for unhealthy alcohol use. Laboratory tests can be useful to confirm heavy drinking and to confirm reduced use in follow-up (when the tests were elevated during heavy use initially), as well as when the medical history is unreliable in dementia, delirium, coma, or injury. Some biomarkers can be detected in urine, breath, serum, and body fluids. Routine blood tests such as alanine aminotransferase (ALT), aspartate aminotransferase (AST), γ-glutamyl transpeptidase (or transferase) (GGT), and mean corpuscular volume (MCV), which are widely available, should be measured in people with AUD. They can be elevated with heavy drinking, but they are neither sensitive nor specific. For example, GGT is elevated in nonalcoholic liver disease, in hyperthyroidism, and with use of anticonvulsants.

An AST/ALT ratio >1 and significantly raised GGT are suggestive of alcohol-related liver damage and heavy drinking, respectively. Elevated bilirubin and liver enzymes suggests acute alcoholic hepatitis. Low albumin and abnormal coagulation tests may result from reduced liver production in the context of more severe and longer-term liver damage and cirrhosis.

The carbohydrate-deficient transferrin (CDT) has been used to detect and monitor heavy drinking but is not useful to detect risky use. It is sensitive and specific for daily recent heavy drinking (eg, for several weeks). The main advantage of CDT is its high specificity. Phosphatidylethanol (PEth) is also very specific because it is only produced in the body with alcohol exposure. It can detect recent heavy drinking but cannot rule out risky use. Heavy alcohol consumption also can lead to an elevated MCV, but most people with heavy drinking do not have elevated MCV, and macrocytosis is not specific for heavy drinking. The sensitivity of MCV and GGT in detecting heavy alcohol use may be higher in older than in younger populations, but sensitivity and specificity are still inadequate for diagnosis.

▶ Different Clinical Manifestations in Older Adults

Heavy drinking and AUD can be suggested by the presence of other health conditions and related circumstances common in older adults (Table 70–3).

▶ Challenges in the Diagnosis of AUD

Several physiologic, biologic, and psychosocial characteristics related to age pose unique challenges in the diagnosis and management of unhealthy alcohol use in older persons. These are some key elements of a more effective approach to diagnosis. First, amounts of alcohol use that are the same as or lower than in the past do not preclude unhealthy alcohol use; new alcohol-related symptoms and consequences can occur despite those amounts. Second, many symptoms and conditions could be due to alcohol, or not, and they should be considered for their possible relationship to drinking, rather than attributing them to age or other causes (eg, dementia, delirium). Third, many common conditions in older adults can be symptoms or signs of an AUD (eg, dementia, hypertension, functional decline, disrupted sleep, recurrent pneumonia, seizures, depression, fatigue, sexual dysfunction). Finally, excessive alcohol use should not be viewed as a "last remaining pleasure," a sleep aid, or a remedy for pain or psychological distress. In fact, excessive use can be leading to harm (worse sleep, worse psychological symptoms such as depression), and reducing use or abstaining can help improve quality of life, mental health symptoms, and sleep. More effective treatments for pain and psychological symptoms should be sought.

Table 70–3. Clinical manifestations of alcohol use in older adults.

Worsening of a chronic disease due to direct effects of alcohol or the effects of alcohol use on nonadherence to treatments (hypertension, diabetes mellitus, osteoporosis, macrocytic anemia, hypercholesterolemia, gastritis, Parkinson disease, and gout)

Onset of gastrointestinal disorders, urinary or fecal incontinence, accidental hypothermia, orthostatic hypotension, frequent falls, fainting, heart failure, aspiration pneumonia, dehydration, malnutrition, and injuries

Onset or deterioration of cognitive or psychiatric disorders (disorientation, acute confusion, memory impairment, anxiety-depression syndrome, persistent irritability, sleep disturbances, Alzheimer disease, and Wernicke-Korsakoff syndrome)

Social and behavioral changes such as withdrawal from usual social activities, estrangement from family, premature requests for refills of prescription medications, and evidence of self-neglect

Changes in medical utilization such as nonadherence with medical appointments and treatments and frequent visits to the emergency department

Table 70–4. Medical consequences of alcohol use in older adults.

Falls and fractures due to osteoporosis and gait and balance deficits
Co-occurring mental health conditions (eg, depression, anxiety, suicide)
Nutritional deficiencies
Neurologic consequences such as cognitive impairment, dementia, delirium, subdural hematoma, intracranial hemorrhage, hepatic encephalopathy, insomnia and other sleep disorders, Wernicke syndrome, Korsakoff dementia, seizures
Infectious diseases such as pneumonia, hepatitis C, tuberculosis, HIV, sexually transmitted diseases
Cardiovascular diseases such as hypertension, atrial fibrillation (holiday heart syndrome), dysrhythmia, cardiomyopathy, and coronary artery disease
Gastrointestinal problems and liver disorders including gastroesophageal reflux, gastritis, pancreatitis, steatosis, acute and chronic hepatitis, and cirrhosis
Cancers such as those of the oral cavity, pharynx, esophagus, larynx, liver, colon, rectum, and female breast, which are associated with heavy alcohol use
Pulmonary complications such as aspiration pneumonia and respiratory depression

MEDICAL CONSEQUENCES

There are many medical consequences of unhealthy alcohol use in older persons (Table 70–4).

PREVENTION

Unhealthy alcohol use has a substantial effect on public health and has been linked to multiple chronic health conditions among older adults. Public health strategies can aim to prevent and reduce the harms associated with risky use and address AUD when it arises. These efforts can be categorized into three types based on their targets: *universal or primary* (ie, applying to everyone), *selective or secondary* (ie, applying only to those identified as being at greater risk), and *indicated or tertiary* (ie, treatment targeted at preventing progression of the disorder for those already demonstrating symptoms).

One secondary approach to preventing unhealthy alcohol use is clinical prevention, a universal approach at the individual level. The approach is to identify and briefly counsel (selective) those with risky alcohol use or who have already had consequences of use or symptoms of AUD. This process is known as screening and brief intervention. If people are identified by screening and assessment as having AUD, then treatment in primary care or by referral can be offered if and when the patient is ready for such a step (indicated care).

Alcohol screening, followed by brief counseling for those who screen positive, is recommended by the US Preventive Services Task Force in primary care settings for all adults. They note that the accuracy of screening tests is similar regardless of age and that there is insufficient evidence for recommending a geriatric-specific test or a specific screening interval, although annually is appropriate. Screening serves a preventive purpose. However, in older adults, screening also informs differential diagnosis of symptoms (it is not possible to properly diagnose the etiology of anxiety or gastroesophageal reflux without knowing about alcohol use) and is useful prior to prescribing or recommending medications that might interact with alcohol (including acetaminophen or aspirin).

For patients being evaluated for symptoms that could be due to alcohol use, screening is no longer the relevant construct, and an assessment of alcohol use (which can begin with a screening tool but go further) is warranted (tertiary prevention). Examples of such symptoms or circumstances particularly relevant in older adults include:

- Health problems that could be adversely affected by any alcohol use

- Functional impairment with impaired daily activities or social/family/legal problems

- Medical conditions suggestive of heavy alcohol use (new-onset or poorly controlled hypertension, gastrointestinal symptoms, recurrent accidents/injuries/falls)

- Physical examination findings suggestive of heavy alcohol use

- Laboratory findings suggestive of heavy alcohol use (elevated MCV, GGT, or other liver transaminases)

- Mental status exam abnormalities, especially dysphoric or anxious affect, or cognitive deficits

When screening is positive for unhealthy use, assessment helps distinguish between risky use and disorder. For those with risky use, brief counseling, approximately 30 minutes, repeated several times, can help patients recognize their risks and reduce consumption or abstain. Such counseling is best proven efficacious when delivered in primary care settings. Clinicians other than the primary care clinician (eg, behavioral health specialists, nurses, or others) can deliver counseling to improve feasibility, as long as the clinician initially identifies the risk and opens the conversation. Counseling typically involves presenting feedback on risk (eg, alcohol amounts that exceed limits and associated risks, any laboratory abnormalities of relevance), normative feedback if possible (eg, that many people drink less or abstain), specific advice (to abstain or cut down), and discussion about the patient's perceptions regarding the importance of the risk and their confidence that they can make a change. The conversation includes goal setting, which could be to abstain (best choice for those with a disorder), to cut down (ideally below risky limits), or to discuss it again and gather more information. If the patient has AUD, then treatment should be considered, or if the patient is not ready, then further discussion to increase importance and confidence from the patient's perspective is warranted. Such discussions, as with all brief counseling, should be nonjudgmental and empathic and based on the principles of motivational interviewing.

Several studies support the efficacy of, and thus we recommend, screening and brief intervention (counseling) for reducing alcohol use. Data from randomized trials in older adults suggest that brief intervention reduces drinking by about two to five drinks per week >12 months later compared with control groups who do not receive brief intervention (from approximately 14–17 drinks per week). Of note, brief intervention appears to have efficacy for reducing self-reported drinking amounts, but findings regarding injury and other health consequences and health care utilization have been inconsistent and not definitive. In Project SHARE, older primary care patients (60 years and older) were identified using the CARET and then randomized to an intervention consisting of "personalized reports, educational materials, drinking diaries, physician advice during office visits, and telephone counseling delivered by a health educator." This intervention reduced at-risk drinking and emergency department visits.

However, most studies of brief interventions have excluded people with very heavy drinking or AUD. For those with AUD, or when there is other drug use or psychiatric comorbidity, brief counseling is less likely to have efficacy. For those with AUD, treatment is indicated. However, a meta-analysis of randomized controlled trials revealed that there was a lack of evidence to support the efficacy of brief interventions for increasing utilization of alcohol treatment. This means that people with AUD should be treated in the primary care setting where they are identified if possible. If not possible, referral remains the next best option, with follow-up to check whether the patient has received care and to continue to encourage it if they have not.

TREATMENT

The concept of treatment, as distinguished from brief interventions for risky use, generally applies to those with AUD. Most clinical trials of the efficacy of treatments for AUD have been done for people with (or with the rough equivalent of) moderate to severe DSM-5 AUD (eg, past studies based on older diagnostic criteria focused on DSM-3-R or DSM-4 dependence, and even older studies often included people with "alcoholism"). Medications are generally reserved and needed for those with moderate to severe AUD, as are other specialized treatments (eg, counseling and other specialized services).

The first step in treatment is to decide with the patient on their goals, which is usually abstinence but sometimes cutting down. Abstinence is the most likely successful course for those with AUD because it leads to the best health outcomes and because those who abstain are most likely not to relapse, but cutting down is an initial option for those not yet ready to abstain. In either case, patients should be asked about symptoms of tolerance and withdrawal. If they have had seizures or delirium, have had significant symptoms of withdrawal, or have concomitant acute illness or other drug use, they should have withdrawal managed with medication (benzodiazepines, preferably lorazepam doses repeated until symptoms resolve) often in a supervised setting. The majority of patients, however, can cut down on their own (eg, at home with no medication). A significant other should be present to note any symptoms that the patient might not notice that would require contact with the clinician, such as confusion.

Treatment itself involves medication, counseling, and attention to social circumstances. In addition to treatment for AUD, co-occurring conditions should be addressed in part because they can interfere with successful AUD treatment if they are ignored. Much treatment and monitoring/follow-up can be done in the primary care setting by a clinician/prescriber, ideally the primary care clinician, and an integrated behavioral health team that includes a social worker or other counselor. Referral to specialized settings will also be needed for those with severe or complex AUD, particularly if there is a coexisting significant mental health condition and if residential or hospital care is needed.

In addition to diagnostic challenges presented regarding AUD in older adults addressed previously in this chapter, there are additional issues that need to be considered when starting treatment. In older adults, loss, loneliness, and new challenges in family or personal relationships can be precursors to a new AUD or recurrence of a past AUD. Life transitions such as retirement can trigger unfamiliar and stressful social circumstances. Changes in employment and income may lead to new poverty and even inadequate access to food, shelter, or medical care.

Treatment for early-onset AUD may be complicated by limited social support, poor emotional skills, long-term denial, and cognitive impairment. However, patients with late-onset alcohol use have more family support and are more likely to complete treatment and to have a successful outcome than early-onset cases.

Most treatments can be delivered in an outpatient setting. Inpatient settings are useful for patients with significant acute comorbid health conditions and for those in dire social circumstances such as homelessness; situations in which patients are surrounded by others drinking, which makes it difficult to abstain; or patients with mental health conditions that need simultaneous attention. Counseling may be in the form of individual counseling, group therapy, and family therapy. Involving the family in treatment can be a critical support facilitating recovery.

In addition to treatment with counseling and/or medication, it is important to address the common circumstances of a limited social network, loneliness, and depression in older adults. Group therapy and senior day programs or centers can help, as can AUD-relevant social support and mutual help groups and networks such as Alcoholics Anonymous (AA) and SMART (Self-Management and Recovery Training) Recovery. Although these have different fundamental approaches (AA is a 12-step approach; SMART is a cognitive-behavioral approach), they can both support AUD treatment goals.

▶ Counseling/Behavioral Therapy

The following approaches to counseling/behavioral therapy are evidence-based strategies that have demonstrated their effectiveness in treating AUD. Few except cognitive-behavioral therapies have been studied in older adults specifically, although generally older adults have not been excluded.

A. Twelve-Step Facilitation

The 12-step facilitation (TSF) is a highly structured manual-guided approach delivered over the course of 12 to 24 weeks. It consists of a set of elective topics (assessment and overview, acceptance, surrender, and getting active) that can be selected to tailor the treatment of patients individually or jointly with family members. The main focus of TSF is connecting patients with 12-step groups, facilitating their involvement so that they benefit maximally, and following up over time to monitor and add any additional treatments if needed. The main adaptation for older adults is to assure linkage to a 12-step group that has suitable membership.

B. Motivational Interviewing

Motivational interviewing (MI) has also not been specifically studied in older adults. It is a nonconfrontational, patient-centered treatment. It is most useful initially for patients in precontemplation or contemplation stages of change (who do not perceive alcohol use to be important to change or who are very ambivalent about the importance of their use and consequences of their use) with the goal of moving the patient along the motivational continuum. It includes aspects such as empathy, working with ambivalence, assessing a patient's readiness for change, assessing strengths and barriers to change, eliciting motivational responses, and placing the responsibility of change directly with the patient. It can be used alone or to support adding other types of treatments.

C. Cognitive-Behavioral Therapy

Cognitive-behavioral therapy (CBT) is effective for AUD in older adults. CBT helps patients become aware of inaccurate or negative thinking, so that they can respond to situations and circumstances more effectively. However, one common comorbidity in older adults with AUD can interfere with the effectiveness of CBT—cognitive dysfunction. For those

with significant cognitive dysfunction, the sayings (eg, "one day at a time"), routine, and repetitive consistency of 12-step approaches can be helpful.

▶ Medications

There are currently three US Food and Drug Administration (FDA)–approved pharmacotherapies (four products) for the treatment of AUD: acamprosate, naltrexone (oral and injectable), and disulfiram. Topiramate, a medication approved for the treatment of epilepsy, also has proven efficacy for treating AUD, although it is not currently FDA approved for this indication.

All four medications are available in daily oral form, although one challenge to this form is adherence to medication. Naltrexone is also available as an extended-release monthly injection, which may help with adherence (at least initially), since its effects last almost 1 month. All four have been shown in some clinical trials to modestly increase abstinence and decrease heavy drinking. None have been studied specifically in older adults, although studies have generally not excluded older adults. In general, naltrexone is considered first-line treatment. Dementia precludes use of disulfiram, and topiramate can have significant adverse effects in older adults.

A. Naltrexone

Naltrexone blocks opioid receptors, reducing craving for alcohol and the euphoric sensation (reward) associated with drinking. The oral form is a daily tablet, and injectable naltrexone is monthly. Naltrexone's main side effects are nausea, dizziness, and dysphoria. It cannot be used in people who are taking opioids, and it precludes treatment with opioids. Low muscle mass, which may be seen in older persons, may preclude use of the injectable form, which is high volume.

B. Acamprosate

Acamprosate acts on the γ-aminobutyric acid (GABA) and glutamate neurotransmitter systems; however, its exact mechanism of action is unclear. It is believed to decrease return to drinking by mitigating the symptoms of the protracted abstinence syndrome, including insomnia, anxiety, and dysphoria. Its main side effect is diarrhea, which resolves with continued use of the medication. Three-time-a-day dosing makes adherence challenging.

C. Disulfiram

Taking disulfiram makes drinking alcohol very unpleasant. The medication interferes with the metabolism of alcohol, allowing acetaldehyde to accumulate, which produces severe reactions that include nausea, flushing, and palpitations. A notable drawback of disulfiram is that adherence (and therefore effectiveness) is generally poor, except in controlled environments or in circumstances where supervised administration is possible (directly observed by a clinician or significant other). A main side effect is idiosyncratic liver damage and neuropathy. For older adults, the idea of having a significant other administer the medication daily can help address limited social connections. Age-related reasons to avoid disulfiram are that the disulfiram-ethanol reaction can be severe and harmful to those with significant coronary artery disease, and substantial cognitive dysfunction precludes its use since one must be aware of the consequences of drinking for the medication to prevent drinking.

D. Topiramate

Topiramate, an anticonvulsant, has been shown in some trials to decrease heavy drinking days and to increase abstinence. Topiramate's mechanism of action in treatment of AUD is not well understood, and symptomatic side effects are substantial (eg, anorexia, difficulty concentrating).

Although unhealthy alcohol use is common, including among older persons, only a few studies have analyzed the treatment outcomes specifically among older adults.

Aalto M, Alho H, Halme JT, Seppä K. The alcohol use disorders identification test (AUDIT) and its derivatives in screening for heavy drinking among the elderly. *Int J Geriatr Psychiatry.* 2011;26(9):881-885.

American Psychiatric Association. *Diagnostic and Statistical Manual of Mental Disorders.* 5th ed. Arlington, VA: American Psychiatric Association; 2013.

Breslow RA, Castle IP, Chen CM, Graubard BI. Trends in alcohol consumption among older Americans: National Health Interview Surveys, 1997 to 2014. *Alcohol Clin Exp Res.* 2017;41:976-986.

Caputo F, Vignoli T, Leggio L, Addolorato G, Zoli G, Bernardi M. Alcohol use disorders in the elderly: a brief overview from epidemiology to treatment options. *Exp Gerontol.* 2012;47:411-416.

Ettner SL, Xu H, Duru OK, et al. The effect of an educational intervention on alcohol consumption, at-risk drinking, and health care utilization in older adults: the Project SHARE study. *J Stud Alcohol Drugs.* 2014;75(3):447-457.

Grant BF, Chou SP, Saha TD, et al. Prevalence of 12-month alcohol use, high-risk drinking, and DSM-IV alcohol use disorder in the United States, 2001-2002 to 2012-2013: results from the National Epidemiologic Survey on Alcohol and Related Conditions. *JAMA Psychiatry.* 2017;74(9):911-923.

Grant BF, Goldstein RB, Saha TD, et al. Epidemiology of DSM-5 alcohol use disorder: results from the National Epidemiologic Survey on Alcohol and Related Conditions III. *JAMA Psychiatry.* 2015;72(8):757-766.

Han BH, Moore AA, Sherman S, Keyes KM, Palamar JJ. Demographic trends of binge alcohol use and alcohol use disorders among older adults in the United States, 2005-2014. *Drug Alcohol Depend.* 2017;170:198-207.

Kelly S, Olanrewaju O, Cowan A, Brayne C, Lafortune L. Alcohol and older people: a systematic review of barriers, facilitators and context of drinking in older people and implications for intervention design. *Plos One.* 2018;13(1):e0191189.

Kuerbis A, Sacco P. A review of existing treatments for substance abuse among the elderly and recommendations for future directions. *Subst Abuse.* 2013;7:13-37.

Lehmann SW, Fingerhood M. Substance-use disorders in later life. *N Engl J Med.* 2018;379(24):2351-2360.

National Institute on Alcohol Abuse and Alcoholism (NIAAA). Older adults. https://www.niaaa.nih.gov/older-adults. Accessed March 3, 2019.

Ryan M, Merrick EL, Hodgkin D, et al. Drinking patterns of older adults with chronic medical conditions. *J Gen Intern Med.* 2013;28(10):1326-1332.

Schonfeld L, Hazlett RW, Hedgecock DK, Duchene DM, Burns LV, Gum AM. Screening, brief intervention, and referral to treatment for older adults with substance misuse. *Am J Public Health.* 2015;105:205-211.

Substance Abuse and Mental Health Services Administration. Results and detailed tables from the 2017 National Survey on Drug Use and Health (NSDUH). https://www.samhsa.gov/data/nsduh/reports-detailed-tables-2017-NSDUH. Accessed March 3, 2019.

US Preventive Services Task Force. Screening and behavioral counseling interventions to reduce unhealthy alcohol use in adolescents and adults: US Preventive Services Task Force recommendation statement [published November 13, 2018]. *JAMA.* 2018;320(18):1899-1909.

Wilson SR, Knowles SB, Huang Q, Fink A. The prevalence of harmful and hazardous alcohol consumption in older U.S. adults: data from the 2005-2008 National Health and Nutrition Examination Survey (NHANES). *J Gen Intern Med.* 2014;29:312-319.

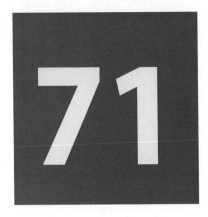

71

Integrative Geriatrics & Cannabis Use

Louise Aronson, MD, MFA

Salomeh Keyhani, MD, MPH

INTEGRATIVE GERIATRICS

General Principles

Forty percent of older adults regularly use integrative medicine, and growing numbers are turning to strategies variably known as healthy aging, restorative aging, functional medicine, antiaging medicine, lifestyle medicine, and age management medicine. Usage rates by older adults in particular are expected to increase in coming decades since baby boomers are more likely to question convention, seek alternative care, and use multiple modalities than earlier generations.

The popularity of alternative and wellness approaches to health care reveals significant gaps in mainstream medicine's ability to adequately address patient concerns and belief systems. The most common reasons older adults go beyond conventional medicine include symptom management, disease prevention, wellness, forestalling aging, and treatment of chronic conditions. Clinicians who can discuss complementary modalities with patients in educated, collaborative, evidence-based ways may find that they not only are better able to identify their patients' unmet care needs and health goals but also have a larger toolbox with which to address them. Equally important, they will have the knowledge to direct patients toward useful modalities and counsel them away from the people and organizations profiting from sales of unproven and potentially harmful therapies.

Background, Definitions, and Usage Patterns

Integrative medicine is defined as care and research that attends to social, psychological, spiritual, behavioral, environmental, and biological determinants of health; emphasizes the clinician-patient relationship and patient empowerment; and brings together conventional and nonmainstream therapies in a coordinated, evidence-informed way to foster healing. Nonmainstream therapies are called "alternative" when

used instead of conventional medicine and "complementary" when used with conventional medicine. Integrative medicine takes an evidence-based approach to these diverse practices and treatments, drawing from all traditions and considering the patient's mind-body-spirit needs and sociocultural contexts to optimize health, wellness, and disease management (Table 71–1).

Current data on integrative medicine usage by older adults are limited. In periodic surveys through 2012, the most recent comprehensive data on complementary medicine use were collected, and the National Health Interview Survey (NHIS) consistently found that nonvitamin, nonmineral dietary supplements were the most frequently used approach among adults, although which ones top the list change in this unregulated $8 billion market. In 2002, echinacea, ginseng, and gingko were most popular; in 2012, it was fish oil and probiotics. In 2017, turmeric/curcumin was the top seller, while cannabidiol (CBD) and Ashwagandha showed the biggest increases in use.

NHIS 2017 examined only three mind-body modalities. It found that among people aged 65 years and older, >13% used meditation, 9.5% used chiropractic, and nearly 7% did yoga. These usage patterns differed from those in adults <65 years old, who used yoga most often and chiropractic least.

Patients using complementary and alternative medicine (CAM) therapies often do not report their use to their physicians. Some therapeutics, such as herbs, may have side effects or interactions with conventional medications. Physicians should ask specifically whether older patients are using CAM treatments or seeing CAM practitioners. Questions about CAM interest and use can help identify unmet care needs, strengthen the physician-patient relationship, provide clinicians with opportunities to learn about useful evidence-based nonconventional therapies, and facilitate exploration of a patient's health beliefs and values.

Geriatrics and integrative medicine are natural allies. The two fields share a broad, person- and values-centered approach to patient care. In the conventional medicine

Table 71–1. Classifications of diagnostic and treatment approaches in integrative geriatrics.

Domain	Definition	Example Interventions
Conventional		
Biomedical	Biology and organ systems-based approach to the diagnosis and management of disease	Prescription medications, procedures
Geriatric	Life stage–specific health care focused on function, geriatric syndromes, and care systems informed by patient goals, health, and life expectancy	Functional assessment, medication reconciliation and deprescribing, home safety assessment
Integrative	Evidence-informed focus on health and healing, a holistic approach in partnership with an empowered patient	Nutrition, physical activity and exercise, motivational interviewing
Complementary/alternative[a]		
Natural products	The use of herbs, dietary manipulation, vitamins, minerals, supplements, or mixtures prepared from biologic sources to enhance health or treat disease	Herbal remedies (eg, ginseng and ginkgo), supplements (eg, glucosamine and vitamin E), and mixtures (eg, shark cartilage), as well as natural products previously classified as recreational drugs (eg, cannabis and plant-based hallucinogens)
Mind-body practices	Therapies that target the potential for the mind to affect the body's basic function and reaction to disease; manipulative and body-based therapies that use a relationship between form and function to treat disease	Mindfulness-based stress relaxation (MBSR), meditation, prayer and mental healing, hypnosis, guided imagery Massage, chiropractic manipulation, osteopathy
Other	Whole medical systems: Complete systems of theory and practice that are completely independent of a biomedical approach Energy therapies: Modify internal sources or flow of energy or alternately apply external sources of energy to modify body function or health	Ayurvedic medicine, homeopathy, naturopathic medicine, and traditional Chinese medicine including acupuncture and cupping, and traditional healers Use of magnets or electromagnetic fields, which involve external sources of energy, or the practice of Qi Gong or therapeutic touch, which involve manipulating the internal balance or flow of energy

[a]National Center for Complementary and Integrative Health (NCCIH) Classification system.

tradition, however, geriatrics focuses primarily on disfunction, disease, diagnostic testing, prescription medications, and medical care settings. Two of the fundamental principles that distinguish integrative medicine are (1) the elevation of prevention and wellness alongside disease diagnosis and treatment and (2) identification of the simplest, least invasive "medical" intervention with the maximum positive impact that emphasizes lifestyle behavior change. Since geriatrics has historically focused on frailty and other conditions of advanced old age and integrative medicine on health and prevention, integrative geriatrics offers a means of expanding both fields for the good of all patients across all the substages of old age.

AARP, National Center for Complementary and Alternative Medicine. Complementary and alternative medicine: what people aged 50 and older discuss with their health care providers. *Consumer Survey Report*; April 13, 2010. https://www.aarp.org/health/alternative-medicine/info-04-2011/complementary-alternative-medicine-nccam.html. Accessed April 21, 2020.

Friedman SM, Mulhausen P, Cleveland ML, et al. Healthy aging: American Geriatrics Society white paper executive summary. *J Am Geriatr Soc*. 2019;67:17-20.

Friedman SM, Shah K, Hall WJ. Failing to focus on healthy aging: a frailty of our discipline? *J Am Geriatr Soc*. 2015;63:1459-1462.

Groden SR, Woodward AT, Chatters LM, et al. Use of complementary and alternative medicine among older adults: differences between baby boomers and pre-boomers. *Am J Geriatr Psychiatry*. 2017;25(12):1393-1401.

Nahin RL, Barnes PM, Stussman PJ. Expenditures on complementary health approaches United States, 2012. *Natl Health Stat Report*. 2016;95:1-11.

National Institutes of Health, National Center for Complementary and Integrative Health. https://nccih.nih.gov. Accessed April 21, 2020.

Clinical Fundamentals

The integrative medicine (IM) patient history focuses on health and health behaviors in addition to symptoms and disease. Key areas include nutrition and daily eating habits, physical activity and exercise, sources of strength and stress, emotional state, social supports, spiritual beliefs and practices, use of medications of all kinds (prescription, over-the-counter, herbs, supplements, caffeine, alcohol, cannabis, and other substances), and use of CAMs. The IM history also asks questions designed to help people achieve insights and recognize whether their behaviors are consistent or inconsistent with their stated health goals. Some questions that might enable geriatrics clinicians to optimally support their patients include asking about key life events, sources of stress, support, strength and joy, and exploration of their beliefs and feelings about aging and old age (Table 71–2).

Table 71–2. Select integrative geriatrics additions to the patient history.

Beginning
My goal is to get a sense of who you are as a person, to understand the important relationships and events in your life in addition to the medical conditions that bring you in today.
What have been pivotal events in your life?

Social History
What are important features of your background I should know about?
Who are the important people in your life today? Who do you consider to be your family?
Tell me about a typical day in your life now.

Physical History
What time of day or what activities make you feel energized? What time of day or activities tire you out?
What illnesses, if any, most affect your life?
What sorts of physical activity do you do? How do you feel about the word "exercise"?
What are the sources of stress in your life?
How do you relax?

Spiritual History
Where do you get your strength in difficult times?
How often do you feel lonely?
What brings you joy?
What gives your life purpose and meaning?

Aging History
What impact has aging had on your life?
Do you think of old age as positive, negative, or something else?
Can you think of someone you think aged well? How about someone whose aging didn't go so well?
What are your hopes for the future?

Adapted with permission from Maizes V, Koffler K, Fleishman S. Revisiting the health history: an integrative medicine approach, *Adv Mind Body Med* Winter 2002;18(2):31-34.

Integrative geriatrics differs from conventional care by putting more emphasis on patient wellness. Three areas best illustrate the potential of the integrative approach. (The first two are covered from conventional medicine approaches in greater detail in Chapters 72 and 13.)

A. Exercise

Regardless of functional status, no conventional intervention does more to prevent and treat multiple diseases while improving health, well-being, and longevity than exercise. Older adults can build muscle mass at all ages, yet clinicians, including physical therapists and geriatricians, often focus on basic function rather than health-transforming potential. As a result, integrative geriatrics always includes an assessment of activity and exercise, motivational interviewing to promote behavior change, and a "FIT ABS" prescription specifying **f**requency, **i**ntensity, and **t**ime each week for **a**erobic, **b**alance, and **s**trength exercises, including the mind-body practices discussed later.

B. Nutrition

In integrative geriatrics, food is medicine. Abundant evidence demonstrates that health-promoting diets delay age-related illnesses and death. Since most chronic diseases are at least exacerbated by inflammation, anti-inflammatory diets are essential interventions for clinicians caring for older adults. Additionally, while nutritional deficiencies are clearly related to disease and accelerated aging, scant evidence exists for supplements, whereas population-based studies show significant associations between dietary patterns, the microbiome, and disease. All healthy diets emphasize fruits, vegetables, clean proteins, healthy fats, and whole grains, whereas disease-causing diets include large amounts of refined sugars and processed foods. Clinicians caring for older adults should be informed about the Mediterranean, DASH (Dietary Approaches to Stop Hypertension), and MIND (Mediterranean-DASH Intervention for Neurodegenerative Delay) diets, each of which can be adapted to Asian, African, and Latin American dietary preferences. Familiarity with the basics of dietary elimination diets is also useful as patients may ask about the impacts of gluten, dairy, nightshades, and other food groups on their health, symptoms, and chronic diseases or about low FODMAP (fermentable oligo-, di-, and monosaccharides and polyols) and Paleo diets, intermittent fasting, and other dietary therapeutic interventions.

C. Attitude About Aging

Positive or negative age stereotypes predict health status and willingness to engage in healthy behaviors from exercise and sex to work and rehabilitation after illness. While there are no data on whether addressing a patient's age stereotypes can improve health, the strong correlations of negative stereotypes to poor health outcomes suggest this is a fruitful area for geriatrics research and clinical exploration.

Integrating CAM and Conventional Treatment

Approaches to management and integration of CAM and conventional therapeutics should consider patient priorities, potential harms, and potential benefits. Patient trust increases when practitioners discuss the evidence (or lack thereof) for the safety and efficacy of both conventional and alternative options. In the absence of evidence, individualized risk-benefit assessment empowers patients. For example, improvement that might well represent the placebo effect might be a good outcome if the cost is manageable, there is low toxicity, and the patient is not rejecting other appropriate treatments. Finally, it is recommended that physicians get to know licensed integrative, complementary, and alternative practitioners and develop a referral base. Patients are more likely to disclose and discuss complementary therapies and unmet needs with a clinician who is interested in the full spectrum of potentially useful therapeutics.

Estruch R, Ros E, Salas-Salvadó J, et al; PREDIMED Study Investigators. Primary prevention of cardiovascular disease with a Mediterranean diet. *N Engl J Med*. 2013;368(14):1279-1290.

Knowles LM, Skeath P, Jia M. New and future directions in integrative medicine research methods with a focus on aging populations: a review. *Gerontology*. 2016;62(4):467-476.

Levy BR. Mind matters: cognitive and physical effects of aging self-stereotypes. *J Gerontol B Psychol Sci Soc Sci*. 2003;58(4):P203-P211.

Maizes V, Kiffler K, Fleishman S. Revisiting the health history: an integrative medicine approach. *Adv Mind Body Med*. 2002;18(2):31-34.

Rozanski A. Behavioral cardiology: current advances and future directions. *J Am Coll Cardiol*. 2014;64(1):100-110.

Sullivan DH, Johnson LE. Chapter 38. Nutrition and aging. In: Halter JB, Ouslander JG, Tinetti ME, Studenski S, High KP, Asthana S, eds. *Hazzard's Geriatric Medicine and Gerontology*. 6th ed. New York, NY: McGraw-Hill; 2009.

Taylor D. Physical activity is medicine for older adults. *Postgrad Med J*. 2014;90:26-32.

Tittikpina NK, Issa A, Yerima M, et al. Aging and nutrition: theories, consequences, and impact of nutrients. *Curr Pharmacol*. 2019;5:232-243.

Valdes AM, Walter J, Segal E, Spector TD. Role of the gut microbiota in nutrition and health. *BMJ*. 2018;361:k2179.

Complementary Treatments

The National Center for Complementary and Integrative Health divides treatment modalities into the following three major domains: (1) natural products, including food, botanicals (herbs), vitamins, minerals, probiotics, and other plant- or animal-derived supplements; (2) mind-body practices, such as meditation, yoga, tai chi, relaxation and breathing techniques, chiropractic, osteopathic manipulation, acupuncture, and massage; and (3) "other," which serves as a catch-all for alternate whole systems of medicine including homeopathy, naturopathic medicine, Ayurveda, and traditional Chinese medicine, as well as treatments such as aromatherapy and energy medicine (Table 71–1). This classification system is recent, and integrative institutions and practitioners use a variety of taxonomies to classify integrative treatment modalities. Furthermore, some therapies could easily be placed in more than one category. For example, acupuncture is both manual medicine and traditional Chinese medicine, music therapy is both a mind-body practice and a form of energy healing, and Qi Gong involves both movement and meditation.

A. Natural Products

Herbs and supplements (vitamins, minerals, botanicals, and dietary substances) are the most common CAM therapies used by older persons, and usage is increasing. They are most commonly used for pain, arthritis, bone health, heart health, cognition, and healthy aging, with older adults more likely than younger adults to report site-specific reasons for use. Because herbs and supplements are pharmacologically active, clinicians must not only understand their usage but consider drug-herb, drug-supplement, herb-supplement, supplement-supplement, and herb-herb interactions, including up- or downregulation of cytochrome P450 isoenzymes. To further complicate the issue, in contrast to pharmaceuticals, the production, marketing, and sale of herbs and supplements is only partially regulated. The Dietary Supplement Health and Education Act gave the US Food and Drug Administration (FDA) authority to prohibit unsafe and mislabeled products. However, there is no premarket requirement to prove efficacy and minimal regulation of the purity, quality, or standardization of preparations. As a result, active ingredients can vary among manufacturers and even from lot to lot for a given manufacturer. In addition, most herbs and supplements are not routinely covered by insurance and, as such, may be cost prohibitive for people with low and fixed incomes.

Clinicians should advise patients to select suppliers with regular product turnover and supply chain oversight and products from companies that specify the amounts of ingredients, dose, directions, and where appropriate, plant part used and extraction method. Products from more reliable manufacturers will be certified by one or more nonprofits. The US Pharmacopeia (USP) verification program evaluates voluntarily submitted product against scientific standards of quality, purity, potency, performance, and consistency. The National Sanitation Foundation (NSF) certifies contents, checks label accuracy, and checks for contaminants but does not check all product or continuous verification. Other organizations that provide oversight include ConsumerLab.com, which conducts tests of potency and heavy metal contamination. Industry-led Emerson Ecologics does site audits and product testing. The National Institutes of Health's Office of Dietary Supplements is a good source of information for patients.

Table 71–3 lists the typical doses, uses, evidence, and key interactions and adverse effects of herbs and supplements

Table 71–3. Herbs and supplements: doses and use.

Herb/Supplement	Dose	Uses	Evidence	Notes/Interactions/Cautions
Ashwagandha	300–500 mg QHS or BID (lower AM dose)	Insomnia Anxiety Chronic stress	IE IE PE	Higher doses may cause nausea and diarrhea
Chondroitin	1000–1500 mg QD or divided BID	Osteoarthritis	PE/IE	Anti-inflammatory properties Increases warfarin effect
Cinnamon	120 mg–6 g QD	Diabetes (type 2)	IE	Possible increased risk hypoglycemia
CoQ10	30–600 mg BID	Congestive heart failure Immune function Parkinson disease	IE I	Given with statins to minimize myalgia, hypertension Fish oil aids absorption Possible warfarin interaction
Garlic	600–900 mg QD	Hypercholesterolemia Hypertension Cancer prevention	IE PE PE	Dietary intake associated with reductions in gastrointestinal cancers Slight lowering blood pressure; mixed results on lipids
Ginger	0.5–1.0 g QD	Vertigo Postoperative nausea Osteoarthritis	PE IE IE	Increased risk toxicity from antidepressants, benzodiazepines, antipsychotics, quinidine, anticoagulants
Gingko	40 mg TID	Cognition/dementia Cerebral insufficiency Tinnitus Peripheral artery disease	I I PE	Caution with blood thinners, seizure medications Increased risk of serotonin syndrome in patients on SSRI, SNRI Headache, gastrointestinal distress, skin reactions
Ginseng	200–600 mg QD or divided BID	Physical performance Psychomotor performance Immune system function	IE IE IE	Side effects: headache, insomnia, gastrointestinal Blocks estrogen Warfarin interaction
Glucosamine	1500–2000 mg QD or divided BID	Osteoarthritis	PE	More effective than chondroitin Increases intraocular pressure
Green tea		Mental alertness Cancer prevention Cardiovascular disease Parkinson disease	IE IE PE PE	Lowers total and LDL cholesterol, no effect on HDL Caffeine may cause insomnia, jitteriness Increased risk of side effects from theophylline, anticoagulants, antiandrogens
Magnesium	100–600 mg QHS (divide higher doses BID, TID)	Hypertension Diabetes type 2 Leg cramps	PE PE I	Calcium increases magnesium requirements, add if on calcium Oxide form cheap; chloride salts best with diuretics Loose stools
Melatonin	1–5 mg QHS (30-min $T_{1/2}$ so take just before sleep)	Insomnia (especially sleep latency) β-Blocker insomnia	E PE	Increases non-REM sleep, may produce vivid dreams Hangover sedation Higher doses may cause hypothermia
Omega-3 fatty acids	1–3 g/day	AD, CAD, CVD, DM Congestive heart failure Depression (EPA only) Hypertension Hypertriglyceridemia After CABG/angioplasty	I PE IE PE E PE	Diet best: counsel to increase fish consumption and ALA-increasing oils (flax, hemp, walnut, canola) May be most effective for secondary CVD prevention and cardioprotection in patients not on statins Loose stools, diarrhea, "fish burps" May exacerbate iron deficiency
Probiotics	5–10 billion CFUs taken with food	Diarrhea, antibiotic, *Clostridium difficile* Respiratory infections Functional constipation	E PE PE	Only certain strains have proven efficacy Allergic reactions, anaphylaxis, bacteremia Avoid in immunocompromised patients
S-Adenosyl methionine	400–1600 mg divided BID to QID	Depression Osteoarthritis	PE E	Contraindicated with MAOI; caution with SSRI, SNRI Stop before surgery Higher doses can cause insomnia, anxiety, gastrointestinal distress

(continued)

Table 71–3. Herbs and supplements: doses and use. (*continued*)

Herb/Supplement	Dose	Uses	Evidence	Notes/Interactions/Cautions
Saw palmetto	320 mg divided BID to TID	BPH Pre-TURP	I PE	No drug interactions Mild headache or gastrointestinal distress possible
St. John's wort	300 mg TID	Anxiety Depression (mild to moderate)	IE E	Caution with SSRI/risk of serotonin syndrome Upregulates CYP3A4, so interferes with irinotecan
Turmeric/curcumin	500–1000 mg QD	Allergic rhinitis Alzheimer disease Osteoarthritis	PE I PE	Absorption increased by fats and black pepper
Valerian root	300–900 mg 30–60 min before bed 200–250 mg AM, noon	Anxiety Insomnia	I PE	Best for middle of night awakening No adverse effects on sleep cycle Few side effects

AD, arterial disease; ALA, α-linoleic acid; BPH, benign prostatic hyperplasia; BID, twice a day; CABG, coronary artery bypass graft; CAD, coronary artery disease; CFU, colony-forming units; CVD, cardiovascular disease; DM, diabetes mellitus; E, sufficient evidence to suggest efficacy; EPA, eicosapentaenoic acid; HDL, high-density lipoprotein; I, ineffective based on adequate study; IE, insufficient or conflicting evidence; LDL, low-density lipoprotein; MAOI, monoamine oxidase inhibitor; PE, possibly effective; QD, every day; QHS, every night at bedtime; QID, four times a day; REM, rapid eye movement; SNRI, serotonin-norepinephrine reuptake inhibitor; SSRI, selective serotonin reuptake inhibitor; $T_{1/2}$, half-life; TID, three times a day; TURP, transurethral resection of the prostate.

used for common health concerns and conditions in old age. Other supplements to become familiar with include CBD, which became the top selling herbal supplement in the United States in 2018 and is covered in depth in the second half of this chapter, and functional mushrooms, marketed as "superfoods" with antioxidant, immune-boosting, and cancer prevention properties despite few human trials and many mushroom types. While single herb supplements remain the most popular, patients are increasingly turning to combination supplements targeting a disease or symptoms through multiple mechanisms. Patients are also likely to inquire about vitamins given associations of cardiovascular disease and death with inadequate vitamin intake. Most do not realize that lowered risk of death is generally associated with intake through the diet, not from supplements, or that high doses of various vitamins have been associated with poor health outcomes, such as the association of high levels of vitamins B_6 and B_{12} with fractures.

B. Mind-Body Practices

There are many types of mind-body practices with health applications, including (1) manual and movement therapies; (2) mindfulness and meditation; (3) clinical hypnosis and guided imagery; and (4) self-control techniques. All combine mental focus, breathing, and movement to foster health, manage symptoms, or treat disease.

1. Manual & movement therapies—Manual and movement therapies is an umbrella term for a broad range of modalities with distinct origins and professional training but similar techniques. Included in this diverse category are acupuncture, Qi Gong, and tai chi from traditional Chinese

medicine (TCM); chiropractic and osteopathic manipulative treatment (OMT), both of which began in the United States in the 1800s; massage, which has been used across cultures for millennia; yoga from Ayurvedic medicine; and additional exercise therapies such as Feldenkrais and the Alexander Technique.

Acupuncture is a >2000-year-old therapeutic modality that involves the use of sterile, disposable, stainless-steel needles to stimulate points on the surface of the body along vital energy meridians. In the United States, acupuncture is often used independent of TCM, with usage tripling from 1997 to 2007 and continuing to grow. Treatments consist of weekly to biweekly sessions involving the insertion of up to 20 needles of varying thickness at selected points for times ranging from several seconds to 30 minutes. Inserted needles can be stimulated manually or with electricity, heat, or burning herbs. Adverse effects are typically mild and include pain, bleeding, fatigue, nausea, and dizziness. Serious events (pneumothorax or vascular injuries) are rare.

Although acupuncture's mechanism of action remains unclear, neurochemical, immunologic, and functional magnetic resonance imaging studies reveal both local and distal biologic responses, including alterations in endorphins, epinephrine, serotonin, prostaglandins, and tumor necrosis factor-α, as well as upregulation of gene expression. Few studies focus on an exclusively geriatric population, and research is limited by the lack of an effective sham comparison. In adults generally, acupuncture has been shown to be efficacious in the treatment of postoperative and dental pain and fibromyalgia and for the management of nausea and vomiting resulting from a wide variety of causes. Acupuncture has also been shown to be possibly efficacious for or noninferior to conventional treatment of postherpetic neuralgia, migraines, tension headaches, peripheral joint osteoarthritis, Parkinson disease, stroke rehabilitation, depression, and insomnia. It is also commonly used for chronic pain, hypertension, gastroesophageal reflux disease, Bell palsy, and back pain, but its efficacy in treating these conditions has not been established.

Tai chi and *Qi Gong* are ancient Chinese forms of coordinated body movements meant to cultivate, build, and manipulate internal energy called "chi" or "qi." In the United States, tai chi is more common, with nearly 4 million Americans practicing it in 2017, including many at senior centers and as part of fall prevention programs. Although distinct practices, both tai chi and Qi Gong involve slow movements combined with breathing to increase physical and mental wellness. In older adults, both practices can increase functional abilities, flexibility, strength, balance, and range of motion. A 2016 systematic review of tai chi found the strongest evidence of benefits for hypertension, falls in noninstitutionalized older adults, pain, osteoarthritis, depression, chronic obstructive pulmonary disease, and balance confidence. Studies of Qi Gong are less rigorous in proving health benefits, although a geriatrician watching the practice will note the dominance of movements that will assist in the maintenance or renewal of functional positions essential to completing activities of daily living and instrumental activities of daily living.

Chiropractic medicine has spinal manipulation as the core clinical activity. The vast majority of patients seek chiropractic care for back, neck, or head pain. Treatment involves spinal manipulation with or without adjunctive treatments such as heat, cold, traction, electricity, and counseling about exercise, fitness, nutrition, weight loss, smoking cessation, and relaxation techniques. Several systematic reviews have found sufficient evidence to support the beneficial use of chiropractic therapy for acute and chronic back pain. Spinal manipulation and mobilization have also shown benefit for mechanical neck pain, migraines, cervicogenic headaches, cervicogenic dizziness, and painful conditions in some extremity joints. Chiropractic treatment has not been shown to be effective treatment of nonmusculoskeletal illnesses, such as hypertension, dysmenorrhea, or asthma. As with most research, older persons make up a small minority of subjects in manipulation research trials.

Doctors of *osteopathy* also provide manual medicine, called OMT, although their overall training and practice closely resembles that of allopathic physicians with greater focus on health and wellness. Evidence for the efficacy of OMT is largely poor and of low quality with high risk of bias. Common side effects of both chiropractic and OMT are usually mild and transient and include localized pain, headache, and fatigue. More serious side effects are very rare. The risk of serious complications from lumbar manipulation has been estimated to be 1 in 100 million manipulations. The risk of stroke from cervical manipulation is also low, estimated at between 1 in 400,000 and 1 in 2 million manipulations. A large, case-control study found no increased risk of vertebrobasilar stroke with cervical manipulation.

Massage is manual manipulation of soft tissues. Swedish, deep tissue, Trager method, and reflexology are the most commonly used types of massage in the United States. Studies have consistently found benefit for massage therapy in the treatment of pain, including back pain, fibromyalgia, and headaches. Massage has also been found to be of benefit in the palliative care of patients with HIV, breast cancer, and terminal cancer pain. The improvements include decreases in pain, anxiety, and depression, along with improved sleep.

Yoga encompasses a large number of different practices, from ones that more closely resemble mindfulness meditation (Vedic, Kundalini) to other forms that focus more on physical training (Hatha, Ashtanga). In the United States, most yoga emphasizes asanas or stretching and holding of body positions in concert with breathing techniques. Recent reviews suggest that yoga helps with mild to moderate depression; is likely to be helpful with functional fitness, bone density, and mental and social well-being in physically inactive elders; and might help with back pain, glycemic control, and blood pressure. Additional exercise therapies often aimed at aging and older adults include *Feldenkrais*, which uses gentle movements and directed attention, and the *Alexander Technique*, which places emphasis on correct anatomic posture and movements. Both aim to correct self-damaging postural, functional, and movement habits. Evidence is scant for both.

2. Meditation & mindfulness—Meditation and mindfulness are overlapping practices that also often intersect with spirituality. Both involve the act of paying purposeful, nonjudgmental, nonreactive attention to the present moment. In the United States, the most popular form of mindfulness practice is mindfulness-based stress reduction, which can be learned via classes, online, or through an app. Participants learn calmer and more productive responses to life stress. Meta-analyses of randomized controlled trials support the benefits of mindfulness in hypertension, coronary artery disease progression, coping with cancer, chronic pain, diabetes, anxiety, depression, and caregiver stress, although not all positive trials included older adults.

3. Clinical hypnosis & guided imagery—Hypnosis is a state of altered consciousness, inner absorption, and focused attention. Clinical hypnotists present ideas to the patient for subconscious exploration. Training programs vary widely in length and rigor. Guided imagery is a subset of hypnosis that can be done by a clinician in person or via audio recording. The patient is guided through a visual and sensory journey of music and words aimed at creating a state of deliberate, directed daydreaming. Significant research demonstrated the benefits of hypnosis alone or as an adjunct for common conditions including insomnia, stress, anger, smoking cessation, and weight loss, and in preparing for medical procedures.

4. Self-control techniques—Self-control techniques including *breathwork* and *progressive muscle relaxation (PMR)* are easily taught procedures patients can use to calm and focus themselves. *Breathwork* seeks to connect mind and body, conscious and unconscious, by focused, repetitive breathing exercises, such as breath counting and 4-7-8 breathing where the patient breathes in for 4 seconds, holds for 7 seconds, and breathes out for 8 seconds. PMR involves isolating one muscle group, tensing it for 8 to 10 seconds, and then relaxing it. PMR can be used on a particular painful body region or more generally by beginning at one end of the body and moving sequentially to the other end. The evidence base for both techniques includes data showing neurochemical changes with breathing and small studies demonstrating possible improvement in quality of life, physical functioning, pain, and stress relief from PMR.

Biofeedback therapists teach patients how to use breathing and PMR to modulate their physical and emotional responses by controlling usually involuntary bodily processes. The most common forms are heart rate variability, electromyography, thermal, and electroencephalography, although balance sensors are increasingly used with older adults. Electrodes attached to the skin or scalp measure and display responses such as heart rate, blood pressure, muscle tension, or skin temperature. Biofeedback is primarily used for balance, headaches, stress, hypertension, chronic pain, and incontinence (both female stress urinary incontinence and after prostatectomy in males). Effect sizes are often small. Preliminary evidence also suggests benefits for cardiac remodeling in heart failure patients.

C. Other CAM Treatments

The words *alternative medicine* apply most aptly to therapies in this category. Although patients and clinicians may combine these modalities with conventional care, each relies on a paradigm that differs substantially from conventional medicine.

1. Whole medical systems—*Homeopathy* is an alternative medical system based on the vitalistic theory that illness results from imbalances in the patient's vital force. The goal of homeopathy is to use medications to restore the balance and then to rely on the self-healing potential of the body to lead to a cure. A practitioner selects a remedy, after a thorough history and physical exam, by matching symptoms and findings to remedies. Homeopathic remedies have been shown to be effective but are limited by methodologic flaws (eg, small numbers, lack of control groups or randomization, selection bias) and publication bias. Studies of better methodologic quality were more likely to report negative results. Until rigorous studies have validated the use of specific remedies, it would be prudent to approach their use with caution.

TCM and *Ayurveda* from the Indian subcontinent are comprehensive medical systems with their own understandings of physiology, pathology, diagnosis, and treatment. Both pay attention to health fundamentals including nutrition, sleep, appetite, digestion, excretion, activity, function, and pain. Both focus on energy balance as the basis of health and healthy aging.

Naturopathic medicine emphasizes prevention, supporting the body's ability to heal itself, and the healing power of nature. It focuses less on symptoms and diagnoses and more on the foundational aspects of health, including physiological, biochemical, structural, and psychospiritual contributors and whole-person health. It also views doctors first and foremost as teachers and empowers patients to be active in their own health maintenance.

2. Aromatherapy—Aromatherapy consists of using volatile essential oils extracted from plants for the relief of anxiety and agitation. Essential oils can be topically applied, aerosolized, or used in massage. Side effects are rare and typically mild, making aromatherapy a useful therapeutic adjunct. A systematic review found evidence of a mild anxiolytic effect and improvement in quality of life with essential oils combined with massage in several populations, including terminal cancer patients receiving palliative care and hospitalized dementia patients. Aromatherapy has been safely used in the treatment of behavioral disturbances in people with dementia; however, benefit in clinical dementia trials is short term and most pronounced when combined with other individualized nonpharmacologic modalities.

3. Energy medicine—Many cultures have longstanding beliefs in subtle energy or "biofields" that are present in all animate life. In 2012 in the United States, adults spent >$400 million on bioenergetic healing. In elders, the most common usage was for pain, anxiety, mood, wound healing, immune restoration, supportive cancer care, and palliative care. Practitioners use intention and their hands on or over patients to unblock and rebalance the patient's energy fields, although some techniques can also be practiced at a distance. Common therapies include therapeutic touch, reiki, spiritual healing, chakra balancing, and music therapy. Most research in this area is preclinical or involves small pilot studies. Systematic reviews sometimes support benefit but more often call for better evidence quality.

Agbabiaka TB, Wider B, Watson LK, Goodman C. Concurrent use of prescription drugs and herbal medicinal products in older adults: a systematic review. *Drugs Aging.* 2017;34(12):891-905.

Balk EM, Rofeberg VN, Adam GP, et al. Pharmacologic and nonpharmacologic treatments for urinary incontinence in women: a systematic review and network meta-analysis of clinical outcomes. *Ann Intern Med.* 2019;170:465-479.

Brown AC. An overview of herb and dietary supplement efficacy, safety and government regulations in the United States with suggested improvements. *Food Chem Toxicol.* 2017;107(A): 449-471.

Buhr G, Bales CW. Nutritional supplements for older adults: review and recommendations—part II. *J Nutr Elder.* 2010;29(1): 42-71.

Clarke TC, Black LI, Stussman BJ, et al. Trends in the use of complementary health approaches among adults: United States, 2002–2012. National Health Statistics Reports; no 79. Hyattsville, MD: National Center for Health Statistics; 2015.

Guillaud A, Darbois N, Monvoisin R, Pinsault N. Reliability of diagnosis and clinical efficacy of cranial osteopathy: a systematic review. *PLoS One.* 2016;11(12):e0167823.

Kogan M (ed). *Integrative Geriatric Medicine.* Oxford, United Kingdom: Oxford University Press; 2017.

Lee MS, Earnst E. Acupuncture for pain: an overview of Cochrane reviews. *Chin J Integr Med.* 2011;17(3):187-189.

Lemon R. Acupuncture for pain. *J Fam Pract.* 2018;67(4):224-226, 228-230

Meyer HE, Willett WC, Fung TT, Holvik K, Feskanich D. Association of high intakes of vitamins B_6 and B_{12} from food and supplements with risk of hip fracture among postmenopausal women in the Nurses' Health Study. *JAMA Netw Open.* 2019;2(5):e193591.

National Institutes of Health, Office of Dietary Supplements. https://ods.od.nih.gov. Accessed April 21, 2020.

Newberg AB, Serruya M, Wintering N, Moss AS, Reibel D, Monti DA. Meditation and neurodegenerative diseases. *Ann NY Acad Sci.* 2014;1307:112-123.

Solloway MR, Taylor SL, Shekelle PG, et al. An evidence map of the effect of Tai Chi on health outcomes. *Syst Rev.* 2016;5(1):126.

Wayne PM, Walsh JN, Taylor-Piliae RE, et al. Effect of tai chi on cognitive performance in older adults: systematic review and meta-analysis. *J Am Geriatr Soc.* 2014;62(1):25-39.

Yeh VM, Schnur JB, Montgomery GH. Disseminating hypnosis to health care settings. *Psychol Conscious (Wash DC).* 2014;1(2): 213-228.

SUMMARY

IM provides tools and strategies that can enhance geriatric care with greater attention to health, prevention, lifestyle, and behavior. Since a majority of older adults use natural health products, mind-body practices, or alternative whole medical system approaches to health and disease, clinicians should specifically ask about use and adopt an integrative approach to care to deepen the therapeutic alliance. Learning which modalities are supported by the best evidence and which have been shown to not be effective is also important when discussing the pros and cons of using complementary therapies.

CANNABIS

Cannabis and Health in Older Adults

National surveys suggest older adults are using plant-based cannabis to treat a variety of conditions. Counseling patients on use of cannabis is challenging given the paucity of data available with which to make a recommendation. Geriatricians and primary care providers should discuss cannabis use with older patients given the rising prevalence of use in older adults. Given the known toxic effects of smoke on human health, physicians can counsel users to avoid smoking or vaping marijuana, avoid compounds with high concentrations

of delta-9-tetrahydrocannabinol (THC), avoid daily or prolonged use, and preferably use CBD-containing products given their more favorable safety profile. In addition, physicians should counsel patients with family history of psychosis to completely avoid use of cannabis and especially forms with high THC content given the potential earlier onset of psychotic disorders among individuals with a family history. In the sections that follow, more detail is provided on cannabinoid compounds, the known therapeutic benefits, the epidemiology of use and use disorders, dosing, safety, and risks associated with use.

Cannabinoid Compounds

The cannabis plant contains >100 different compounds. The most commonly used cannabinoid compounds are THC and CBD. THC produces the high associated with cannabis. CBD does not have an intoxicating effect.

Therapeutic Benefits of Cannabinoid Compounds

THC-based pharmaceuticals are currently approved for the treatment of chemotherapy-induced nausea and vomiting and the treatment of HIV-induced wasting. A systematic review found some low-quality evidence for the use of cannabinoids in the treatment of neuropathic pain. The meta-analysis was heterogeneous and included both different forms of cannabinoids. A meta-analysis examining the effect of cannabinoids (predominantly THC-based pharmaceuticals) on the treatment of several conditions including pain and spasticity of multiple sclerosis suggested that cannabis may also be effective in the treatment of these conditions, although studies were generally of poor quality. The American Academy of Neurology (AAN) has also endorsed use of oral cannabis extract for the treatment of pain and spasticity associated with multiple sclerosis, although the AAN guidelines point out that the risks and benefits of cannabis oils compared to other standard treatments are unknown. The CBD component of cannabis has been approved by the FDA for the management of Dravet syndrome, a refractory form of childhood epilepsy. It is important to note that the majority of studies that found a benefit from cannabinoids have been based on pharmaceuticals. The available data for any benefit from plant-based cannabis is limited. There are multiple ongoing studies registered at ClinicalTrials.gov examining the effects of CBD. Table 71–4 summarizes current trial-based evidence.

Epidemiology

Use of cannabis among older adults in the United States is rising. In 2002, the prevalence of cannabis use among those

Table 71–4. Therapeutic benefits associated with cannabinoids.

Targeted Symptom or Disorder	Study Types	Strength of Evidence	Comments/Limitations
Nausea and vomiting due to chemotherapy	21 crossover randomized controlled trials 7 parallel-group randomized controlled trials	Low	0 with low risk of bias 23 with high risk of bias 5 with unclear risk of bias
Appetite stimulation in HIV/AIDS	1 crossover randomized controlled trial 3 parallel-group randomized controlled trials	Insufficient evidence	All 4 studies at high risk of bias
Chronic pain	14 crossover randomized controlled trials 14 parallel-group randomized controlled trials	Low	Low-strength evidence that marijuana may have a role in management of pain; 2 with low risk of bias, 17 with high risk of bias 9 with unclear risk of bias
Spasticity in multiple sclerosis and paraplegia	5 crossover randomized controlled trials 9 parallel-group randomized controlled trials	Low	Low-strength evidence that marijuana may improve patient-centered outcomes in the management of multiple sclerosis; 2 studies were with low risk of bias 7 with high risk of bias, 5 with unclear risk of bias
Sleep disorder	1 crossover randomized controlled trial 1 parallel-group randomized controlled trial	Insufficient evidence	1 with low risk of bias 1 with high risk of bias 0 with unclear risk of bias
Glaucoma	1 crossover randomized controlled trial	Insufficient evidence	Insufficient evidence; study at unclear risk of bias
Depression	No included studies; results are from other indications that reported data for this outcome	No evidence	No evidence
Anxiety disorder	1 parallel-group randomized controlled trial	Insufficient evidence	Insufficient evidence; study at high risk of bias
Psychosis	1 crossover randomized controlled trial 1 parallel-group randomized controlled trial	Insufficient evidence	Insufficient evidence; 2 studies at high risk of bias
Posttraumatic stress disorder	3 observational studies	Insufficient evidence	1 study at medium risk of bias; 2 studies at high risk of bias

Data from O'Neil ME, Nugent SM, Morasco BJ, et al. Benefits and harms of plant-based cannabis for posttraumatic stress disorder: a systematic review. *Ann Intern Med.* 2017;167(5):332-340; Nugent SM, Morasco BJ, O'Neil ME, et al. The effects of cannabis among adults with chronic pain and an overview of general harms: a systematic review. *Ann Intern Med.* 2017;167(5):319-331; and Whiting PF, Wolff RF, Deshpande S, et al. Cannabinoids for medical use: a systematic review and meta-analysis. *JAMA.* 2015;313(24):2456–2473.

aged 65 years and older barely registered (0%) in national surveys. Past-year cannabis use among adults aged ≥50 years increased significantly from 2006 to 2013, with a 250% relative increase for those aged 65 years and older (0.4%–1.4%). More recent data indicate that the prevalence of cannabis use among older adults has risen from 1.4% in 2013 to 5.7% in 2017, suggesting use in this group is increasing by 1% per year. Specifically, among this same group, prevalence of past-year use of smoked cannabis has reached 4.6%, prevalence of past-year use of edibles has reached 2.2%, and prevalence of past-year use of multiple forms of cannabis has reached 2.1%. Despite this increase in use and despite aggressive marketing of cannabis to the public, little is known about its health effects in older adults.

Media Coverage and Messages Directed at Older Adults

High-profile media outlets have covered stories of retirees and caregivers using cannabis recreationally. Despite insufficient evidence on the health effects of cannabis in older adults, it is being promoted as a treatment for insomnia, a sedative to be used in nursing homes, a remedy for caregiver fatigue, and as a harmless recreational activity for older adults. The coverage is similar to the popularization of benzodiazepines in the 1960s as a safer alternative compared to barbiturates for multiple conditions before research demonstrated the harms associated with these drugs in the elderly. There are very few data available on the health effects of THC in elderly populations.

▶ Types of Products Available to the Public

The commercial market for novel medical and recreational cannabis products has grown significantly amid expanding legalization, with a recent study identifying 2264 unique products. Slightly less than half of all products were in the form of an edible, among which a quarter were a candy, 22.7% were a sublingual (capsule/pill, lozenge, tincture, spray), 14.8% were a baked good, 10% were a drink, 3.7% were a spread (butter, jam, peanut butter, honey), and 3.6% were in another form (gum, nut, sugar cube). Just less than a third of all products were in the form of bud or flower, whereas 20.8% were in the form of extracts (also known as concentrates), 6% were in the form of topicals (lotions, balms, oils), and <1% were in the form of a vaginal or rectal suppository.

Slightly more than half of all products listed THC content. While the majority of products adhered to the most commonly mandated THC thresholds of 10 mg of THC per serving and 100 mg of THC per package, extracts were found to have a median THC level 10 times that limit with a median of 100 mg of THC per serving and 1000 mg of THC per package. Moreover, a fifth of products advertised therapeutic benefit for which there exists no research, such as alleviation from symptoms associated with depression and anxiety.

▶ Cannabis Dosing and Safety

A pooled analysis of 79 trials examining the efficacy of cannabinoids for several conditions reported severe adverse events including vomiting, diarrhea, disorientation, anxiety, confusion, dyspnea, seizures, psychosis, hallucination, and paranoia. The median dose of THC in cannabinoid pharmaceuticals in these trials was 8 mg. The side effect profile of THC may cause adverse events in the elderly and may have interactions with other sedating drugs. The THC concentrations of currently available cannabis products are much higher than cannabinoid pharmaceutical tests in trial and in cannabis used by participants in observational studies. Pre-rolled cannabis cigarettes available for purchase in cannabis dispensaries contain THC concentrations often exceeding 18% and reaching as high as 35%. There are no safety data available on use of high-concentration forms of THC among the elderly.

The FDA's approval of Epidiolex for the management of some forms of refractory epilepsy in children paved the way for the US Drug Enforcement Administration to reclassify cannabinoid compounds with <0.1% THC as Schedule 5 drugs. This action may result in more testing and evaluation of CBD products containing therapeutics. However, there are significant inconsistencies between labs tasked with assessing the content of commercially available marijuana products, resulting in little guarantee that the commercially available compounds are pure formulations (<0.1 THC).

▶ Risks Associated with Cannabis Use

A. Cannabis Use Disorder

The *Diagnostic and Statistical Manual of Mental Disorders*, fifth edition (DSM-5) includes cannabis use disorder (CUD). CUD occurs when the brain adapts to large amounts of the drug by reducing production of and sensitivity to its own *endocannabinoid* neurotransmitters. Around 20% of lifetime cannabis users develop CUD. Cannabis use is associated with an increased risk of alcohol use disorder or any substance use disorder. It is also associated with mood disorders and anxiety disorders. The DSM-5 criteria for the diagnosis of CUD include a problematic pattern of cannabis use leading to impairment and distress with at least two of the following criteria within a 12-month period: (1) using a larger quantity or over a longer duration than intended; (2) unsuccessful attempts to limit/quit; (3) significant amount of time spent obtaining cannabis; (4) cravings; (5) school/occupational impairment; (6) social/interpersonal impairment; (7) reduction of social/occupational/recreational activities; (8) recurrent use in physically harmful situations; (9) continued use despite recurrent physical or psychological harms; (10) tolerance; and (11) withdrawal. Mild CUD is diagnosed based on presence of two to three criteria, moderate based on four to five criteria, and severe based on six or more criteria.

B. Cannabis Withdrawal Syndrome

Cannabis withdrawal is reported by a third of regular users. Symptoms of withdrawal peak within 1 week of cessation of use and can persist for up to a month. Symptoms include anxiety, restlessness, depression, irritability, insomnia, odd dreams, tremors, and decreased appetite. Cannabis withdrawal is defined as three or more of these symptoms after a long duration of use. Many patients mistake withdrawal for the symptoms they are trying to treat with cannabis because the symptoms overlap with symptoms of anxiety and depression. Individuals with symptoms of severe cannabis withdrawal, such as severe anxiety and irritability, can be treated with dronabinol and gabapentin. Both dronabinol and gabapentin have been found to reduce withdrawal symptoms in clinical trials.

C. Cannabis Hyperemesis Syndrome

Cannabis hyperemesis syndrome is an increasingly recognized form of cyclic vomiting syndrome associated with cannabis use that can be accompanied by abdominal pain. It is seen in those using cannabis on a regular basis. The hallmark of this syndrome is improved symptoms with hot showers. However, this symptom is not present in all individuals. The cyclic vomiting may take up to a month to resolve after cessation of use.

D. Adverse Neurocognitive Effects

Cannabis use is associated with impairments in cognitive functioning, both acutely during intoxication and days after use. There is an increasing body of evidence showing that the cognitive impairment from marijuana use may persist far beyond days. Regular marijuana use has been linked with reduced neural connectivity in brain regions associated with memory and learning, and it appears that the functional connectivity is more prominently disrupted with earlier age of regular use. On imaging studies, regular cannabis users have reduced activity of the prefrontal regions of the brain and decreased hippocampal volume compared to controls. In the Coronary Artery Risk Development in Young Adults (CARDIA) study, lifetime cannabis use was associated with verbal memory impairment. Older adults, given existing deficits in cognition and function, may be at higher risk of adverse neurocognitive outcomes.

E. Adverse Mental Health Effects

Acute effects also include impaired judgment, paranoia, and psychosis. Longer-term use is associated with altered brain development, poor educational outcomes, and increased risk of psychotic disorders. High-potency cannabis has also been linked to psychosis and paranoid delusions. These adverse effects are especially concerning given the rising THC concentrations in commercial cannabis products. Cannabis use has been associated with poor outcomes in patients being treated for anxiety and depression, although for each of these disorders, there are also studies that did not show an association.

F. Other Adverse Health Effects

Few studies have examined cannabis use in older populations and especially older individuals with underlying chronic conditions. Currently available evidence suggests that marijuana use (once to twice weekly) is associated with cough, wheezing, and sputum production. There is insufficient evidence on the effects of chronic marijuana use on pulmonary function. Most studies include too few participants with long-term daily exposure. Therefore, the results of such studies should be viewed with caution. Cannabis use is associated with tachycardia. The data examining the effects of marijuana use on cancer are limited but suggest there may be an association between marijuana use and different types of cancer, including testicular and lung cancer. There are very few data on the association of marijuana use with cardiovascular events.

There is an emerging body of literature using animal studies and studies in humans suggesting that marijuana smoke may be toxic. In addition, exposure to particulate matter is associated with cardiovascular and respiratory risks.

▶ Screening Patients for Use

There are a variety of CUD assessment tools, although they have not been as broadly tested in clinical practice as tools for other substance use disorders. The Cannabis Use Disorder Identification Test–Short Form (CUDIT-SF) is a short three-question screen proposed for practice tested in both American medical cannabis users and in Australian users. Health care providers can incorporate simple screening using the CUDIT-SF in medical practice to identify individuals who may need mental health follow-up and further evaluation.

▶ Treatment of Cannabis Use Disorders

Psychological treatments such as cognitive-behavioral therapy are the main treatment strategies. Both motivational interviewing and cognitive-behavioral therapy have been tested in trials and have reduced mean days of cannabis use in follow-up. No medication has been approved by the FDA for the management of CUD; however, N-acetylcysteine (over the counter) has demonstrated positive effects in one trial and negative results in another trial. It is generally safe with limited side effects and is available over the counter. Gabapentin has also been found to decrease cannabis withdrawal symptoms and improve cognitive tests.

Bonn-Miller MO, Heinz AJ, Smith EV, Bruno R, Adamson S. Preliminary development of a grief cannabis use disorder screening tool: the cannabis use disorder identification test short-form. *Cannabis Cannabinoid Res.* 2016;1(1):252-261.

Ghasemiesfe M, Ravi D, Vali M, et al. Marijuana use, respiratory symptoms, and pulmonary function: a systematic review and meta-analysis. *Ann Intern Med.* 2018;169(2):106-115.

Keyhani S, Steigerwald S, Ishida J, et al. Risks and benefits of marijuana use: a national survey of U.S. adults. *Ann Intern Med.* 2018;169(5):282-290.

Moore TH, Zammit S, Lingford-Hughes A, et al. Cannabis use and risk of psychotic or affective mental health outcomes: a systematic review. *Lancet.* 2007;370(9584):319-328.

Nugent SM, Morasco BJ, O'Neil ME, et al. The effects of cannabis among adults with chronic pain and an overview of general harms: a systematic review. *Ann Intern Med.* 2017;167(5):319-331.

Park S, Myung SK. Cannabis smoking and risk of cancer: a meta-analysis of observational studies. https://ascopubs.org/doi/abs/10.1200/jgo.18.79302. Accessed April 21, 2020.

Ravi D, Ghasemiesfe M, Korenstein D, Cascino T, Keyhani S. Associations between marijuana use and cardiovascular risk factors and outcomes: a systematic review. *Ann Intern Med.* 2018;168(3):187-194.

Steigerwald S, Wong PO, Cohen BE, et al. Smoking, vaping, and use of edibles and other forms of marijuana among U.S. adults. *Ann Intern Med.* 2018;169(12):890-892.

Whiting PF, Wolff RF, Deshpande S, et al. Cannabinoids for medical use: a systematic review and meta-analysis. *JAMA.* 2015;313(24):2456-2473.

Wright S, Yadav V, Bever C Jr, et al. Summary of evidence-based guideline: complementary and alternative medicine in multiple sclerosis: report of the Guideline Development Subcommittee of the American Academy of Neurology. *Neurology.* 2014;83(16):1484-1486.

Encouraging Appropriate Exercise for Older Adults

72

Ellen F. Binder, MD

► General Principles

Physical activity has a profound positive impact on health, chronic disease prevention, function, and fall prevention, especially for older adults; higher levels of physical activity have been linked to reduced morbidity and mortality. New evidence has emerged indicating the positive impact of physical activity on cognition and psychological health. Although physical activity has clear benefits to health and function, most older adults are not physically active or do not engage in activity at high enough intensities to obtain the noted health benefits. In fact, <10% of older adults meet the recommended guidelines for physical activity (ie, 30–60 minutes of moderate-to-vigorous physical activity per day, 5 or more days a week), accumulating only 5 to 10 minutes of moderate-to-vigorous physical activity per day.

Physical activity is not synonymous with exercise. *Physical activity*, as defined by the American College of Sports Medicine, is "any bodily movement produced by skeletal muscles that results in energy expenditure," whereas *exercise*, a subset of physical activity, is "planned, structured, and repetitive bodily movement done to improve or maintain one or more components of physical fitness." Physical activity may not achieve the increased fitness levels that are often expected with exercise; however, physical activity can reduce the risks and complications of many chronic conditions and increase well-being if it is of sufficient intensity.

► Before an Older Adult Begins an Exercise Program

A. Education

Many older adults do not understand the importance of exercise for health promotion or have beliefs that their age or health conditions will limit the benefits of exercise and/or their ability to perform exercises. Most people perceive barriers to starting or continuing an exercise program. It is important for the health provider to explain to the patient how exercise can mitigate the effects of age-associated decrements in physical function, chronic diseases, and "disuse" syndromes and discuss this information in the context of each patient's limitations and goals for independence, mobility, and quality of life. A discussion of perceived barriers and suggestions about how to manage issues such as access, costs, and time can be extremely helpful for overcoming such barriers.

Several websites exist for both the patient and the clinician to use as resources (Table 72–1).

B. Screening

The extent to which an older adult should be screened prior to becoming physically active is controversial. Most exercise screening guidelines focus on recognizing conditions that require modifications to activities (Table 72–2) and determining safety during exercise (specifically cardiac screening and contraindications to exercise); however, cardiac screening (ie, exercise stress testing) is difficult to perform for many older adults and uncovers a huge reservoir of silent cardiac disease of unclear clinical significance. Many older adults do not plan to undertake a vigorous activity program, and moderate activity may be associated with negligible accumulated cardiac risk because of the associated cardiac risk reductions. For healthy and asymptomatic older adults, standard recommendations and precautions are appropriate with no need for cardiac screening. Cardiac screening is also not necessary for sedentary older adults beginning a low- to moderate-intensity activity program, especially considering the risks associated with being sedentary are worse than the risks of being physically active. Sedentary patients should undergo a pre-participation history and physical exam that focuses on cardiovascular risk factors and other conditions that could limit participation in exercise. Discussion of the symptoms during exercise that may indicate an inappropriate response to activity (eg, chest/jaw/arm pain, excessive dyspnea, syncope

Table 72–1. Physical activity/exercise web resources for the patient and the clinician.

Patient Resource	Clinician Resource	Website Information and URL
X	X	Centers for Disease Control and Prevention Physical Activity website. http://www.cdc.gov/physicalactivity/index.html
		Information about many different topics related to physical activity.
X	X	Exercise is Medicine. http://exerciseismedicine.org/
		Website designed to increase the discussion of physical activity between physicians and patients; includes handouts and fliers for both the clinician and the patient; includes a template for an exercise prescription.
X	X	Go4Life. http://go4life.nia.nih.gov/
		Provides information about exercise, including health benefits, safety information, motivation, exercise instruction, and tracking tools.
X		President's Council on Fitness, Sports, and Nutrition—Be Active website. http://www.fitness.gov/be-active/
		Information on why physical activity is important, how to be physically active, physical activity guidelines; provides links to other resources and also provides links to information on eating healthy.

or presyncope, palpitations) is sufficient for these groups. Individuals with known cardiovascular disease or possible ischemic symptoms are at risk for symptoms during activity and would benefit from cardiac screening prior to beginning an activity program.

The few *contraindications* to physical activity include the following conditions: recent myocardial infarction, unstable angina, uncompensated congestive heart failure, severe valvular heart disease, resting systolic blood pressure >160 mm Hg, resting diastolic blood pressure >100 mm Hg, and significant or unstable abdominal, thoracic or cerebral aneurysm. Some acute conditions may *transiently limit activity*, such as major bone fracture, nonhealing lesion on a weight-bearing extremity, acute change in mental status including delirium

Table 72–2. Modifications of exercise prescription for selected conditions.

Condition	Modification
Back pain	Moderate-intensity activities, water activities; low-resistance, low-repetition strength training; flexibility exercises; modified abdominal strengthening activities
Chronic obstructive lung disease	Moderate-intensity activities using interval or intermittent approach; low-resistance, low-repetition strength training; modified flexibility and stretching exercises
Coronary artery disease	Symptom-limited activities: moderate-intensity activities (eg, walking, cycling); more vigorous activities at clinician's discretion; low-resistance, high-repetition strength training
Degenerative joint disease	Non–weight-bearing activities: stationary cycling, water exercises, chair exercises; low-resistance, low-repetition strength training
Diabetes mellitus	Daily, moderate-intensity activities; low-resistance, high-repetition strength training; flexibility exercises
Dizziness, ataxia	Chair exercises; low-resistance, low-repetition strength training; moderate flexibility activities with minimal movement from supine or prone to standing
Hypertension	Dynamic large-muscle aerobic activities; minimize isometric work and focus on low-resistance, high-repetition isotonic strength training
Orthostatic hypotension	Minimize movements from standing to supine and supine to standing; sustained moderate-intensity activities with short rest intervals
Osteoporosis	Weight-bearing activities with intermittent bouts of activity spaced throughout the day; low-resistance, low-repetition strength training; chair-level flexibility activities

Data from American College of Sports Medicine, Chodzko-Zajko WJ, Proctor DN, et al. American College of Sports Medicine position stand. Exercise and physical activity for older adults. *Med Sci Sports Exerc.* 2009;41(7):1510-1530; Whaley MH, ed. *ACSM's Guidelines for Exercise Testing and Prescription.* 7th ed. Philadelphia, PA: Lippincott Williams & Wilkins; 2006; and Bryant CX, Green DJ, eds. *Exercise for Older Adults: ACE's Guide for Fitness Professionals.* 2nd ed. San Diego, CA: American Council on Exercise; 2005.

or psychosis, active suicidal ideation, cerebral hemorrhage, acute myocardial infarction, deep venous thrombosis, pulmonary embolus within 3 months, eye surgery within 2 weeks, proliferative diabetic retinopathy or severe nonproliferative retinopathy, uncontrolled malignant cardiac arrhythmias, symptomatic hernia (abdominal or inguinal), bleeding hemorrhoids, systemic infection, or febrile illness.

Exercise Prescription

The exercise prescription is based on the individual's current health and physical activity level. The prescription includes frequency, intensity, duration, and progression, as well as inclusion of warm-up, cool-down, different types of exercise (eg, aerobic, strength), stretching, and safety precautions. Exercise frequency, intensity, and duration may also vary depending on the type of exercise.

Multiple methods exist to identify the level of intensity of an activity. One method compares the energy cost of the activity to the energy cost at rest, assigning metabolic equivalent (MET) values to different activities. Estimates of the MET values are summarized in the *Compendium of Physical Activities* (https://sites.google.com/site/compendiumofphysicalactivities/corrected-mets), and the level of intensity of an activity is based on its MET value. However, the *Compendium* was developed based on data from healthy adults. Because energy use may be more inefficient in older adults, the intensity based on the MET value may underestimate the intensity at which the older adult is working. For this reason, the best use of the *Compendium* in the older adult population is to create a hierarchy of activities that can be used to select gradually increasing energy-demanding activities, rather than using it to define the exact intensity of an activity.

Because MET levels may not be the best method to determine the intensity of an activity, other methods should be used to estimate how hard the older adult is working, such as heart rate, rating of perceived exertion (RPE), or the talk test. Using a percentage of the estimated maximum heart rate, traditionally calculated by subtracting the person's age from 220, is a simple way to determine intensity. Moderate intensity is defined as 40% to 59% of estimated maximum, and 60% to 85% of estimated maximum is considered vigorous intensity. Using heart rate methods is not appropriate in the presence of conditions that alter the heart rate response to exercise, such as the use of β-blockers, some pacemakers, and many atrial arrhythmias.

Another option is the Borg RPE scale. While participating in an activity, a person rates how hard he or she is working on a scale from 6 to 20. Moderate-intensity activity would be rated in the 12 to 13 range.

Another simple, although informal, method for determining intensity level is the talk test. While exercising at moderate intensity, a person should be able to talk, but not sing. If the person can sing, the activity is light intensity; if the person can only respond with a couple of words before needing to take a breath, the activity is vigorous intensity.

The health care provider should assess medical safety for exercise and recommend modifications for different conditions. Most older adults have at least one medical condition that requires consideration when prescribing a physical activity program. Activities can be adapted to benefit specific needs or to avoid problems based on the condition (see Table 72–2). Many resources are available that provide specific guidelines and tips on how exercise prescription will differ for various diagnoses. Some older adults may appear independent in activities of daily living but have subclinical disability, demonstrated by reduced physical performance, requiring modifications to the exercise prescription.

The provider should also give the older adult key recommendations for safe, unsupervised exercise and be involved in improving patient adherence to exercise programs. The challenge for the clinician is to prescribe activity that is appropriate and feasible based on the individual needs, motivation, and resources of the patient.

Moderate intensity is often recommended; however, not all older adults will be able to perform moderate levels of intensity. An activity that is light intensity for one older adult may be vigorous activity for another older adult. The recommended duration of 30 minutes or more for aerobic exercise may be intolerable for more deconditioned older adults. Brief episodes of activity (ie, stopping before fatigued) several times per day can help build toward more sustained activity.

All programs should progress over time with the goal to induce a level of stress on the body that results in change to the tissues. Duration should be progressed toward bouts of activity that last 20 to 30 minutes before intensity is progressed. It can take weeks or even months to reach this goal in the older adult population. All activity should begin with a warm-up of somewhat easy activities that slightly increase energy demands to prepare the body for exercise. The cool-down after exercise is also important as it is the transition phase for heart rate and oxygen consumption to return to resting levels. Slower walking and biking are examples of appropriate activities for warm-up and cool-down. Stretching should be performed after the warm-up and/or during the cool-down. General safety guidelines (Table 72–3) should also be included in the exercise prescription.

Exercise can be performed in the community, within the health care system, or at home, and can be supervised or unsupervised. Advantages and disadvantages exist for each situation, and the best fit for each patient depends on the needs of that patient.

Physical Activity

The current public health recommendation for older adults is to accumulate 30 minutes of moderate-intensity physical

Table 72–3. General patient instructions for exercise.

1. Start slowly and increase gradually.
2. Avoid holding your breath.
3. If you are on a medication or have a heart condition that changes your natural heart rate, do not use your pulse rate to judge how hard you should exercise.
4. Use safety equipment as recommended for the activity.
5. Drink plenty of fluids if performing activities that make you sweat unless your doctor has asked you to limit fluids.
6. Bend from the hips, not the waist, when bending forward.
7. Warm up muscles before stretching.
8. No exercise should be painful.
9. You can find the right amount of effort using the guideline, "If you can talk without any trouble at all, your activity is probably too easy. If you cannot talk at all, it is too hard."
10. Always include a warm-up and cool-down that moves your body but doesn't tire you.

Data from Bryant CX, Green DJ: Exercise for Older Adults: ACE's Guide for Fitness Professionals, 2nd ed. San Diego, CA: American Council on Exercise; 2005 and the National Institute on Aging.

activity on most days of the week; recommendations for the other types of exercise (strength, flexibility, and balance) are in addition to this recommendation. Physical activity can be easily incorporated into daily life—simple ideas, such as taking the stairs instead of the elevator or parking further from the entrance to a building, can increase physical activity. Cross-training promotes variability in an activity program, reduces boredom, and decreases risk for injury. Activities such as swimming and use of exercise equipment that requires upper extremity effort can complement lower extremity activities such as walking or bicycling.

Types of Exercise

Exercise is a subset of physical activity. Multiple types of exercise exist, including, but not limited to, aerobic, strength, flexibility, and balance. The recommendations for aerobic exercise are typically considered to be the primary physical activity recommendations (ie, 30–60 minutes 5 or more days a week). Strength training to all major muscle groups is recommended 2 or more days per week, but not on consecutive days to allow for muscle recovery. Flexibility exercises should also be performed at least 2 days per week and can be incorporated into an aerobic or strength program. For those older adults at risk for falls, balance exercises should be performed three times per week. Examples of the different types of activities or exercises for each of the categories are provided later in this chapter.

Older adults benefit from a prescription that includes all types of exercise, as all types are important for mobility and function. Major constraints on combined programs are time and fatigue; it is unrealistic for most older adults to undertake a program that demands hours of exercise each day. Some programs combine a mix of aerobic, strength, and balance activities into an hour-long session 3 days a week. The individual's preferences and current level of health should dictate the details of the prescription (Table 72–4).

Table 72–4. Physical activity prescription by patient type.[a]

Patient Type	Duration (minutes)	Frequency	Examples of Exercise
Overt Disability			
Recently bed bound	5–10	Several times per day	Sitting ADL, passive and active range of motion, progress to standing and walking
Nonambulatory	5–10	Several times per day	Self-propel wheelchair, seated self-care, upper extremity games and activities individually and in groups
Subclinical Disability			
Very sedentary	5–10	Several times per day	Slow walking program, group recreation
Inactive	20 or more	Most days of the week	Walking, gardening, housework, bicycling
Usual aging	30	Most days of the week	Brisk walking, stair climbing, moderate endurance recreation
Fit	30 or more	Most days	Moderate-to-high intensity: very brisk walks on uneven surfaces and hills, brisk stair climbing, moderate-to-vigorous sports

ADL, activity of daily living.

[a]Prescribing activity: (1) Let the patient select the preferred mode of activity; (2) start with an intensity and duration that is well tolerated; (3) initial exercise sessions should be observed if there has been no recent moderate activity; (4) initial sessions of moderate activity should include assessment of blood pressure and heart rate; (5) increase duration to a target training level (20–30 minutes or a set of 10 reps) before increasing intensity; (6) teach about self-monitoring of effort (eg, percentage of maximum heart rate, rating of perceived exertion, talk test).

A. Aerobic

Aging limits peak performance of aerobic exercise, but not the ability to benefit from training. Unsupervised aerobic exercise is appropriate for healthy older adults who are able to walk steadily at a brisk pace. Supervised aerobic exercise is appropriate for persons who have clinical or subclinical disability and cannot exercise continuously at moderate intensity.

Some examples of aerobic activity include walking, jogging/running, biking, and swimming. Other activities can be considered aerobic exercise if done at a high enough intensity; activities such as dancing, golfing, gardening, vacuuming, cleaning windows, and mowing the lawn are just a few examples.

The major risk associated with aerobic exercise is a cardiac event, such as myocardial infarction or death; however, this risk has been described after participation in *vigorous* exercise. Participating in *regular* aerobic exercise improves many cardiac risk factors and subsequently reduces the risk of cardiac events during activity.

B. Strength

Aging is associated with loss of muscle mass and power, but both are responsive to strength training in older adults. Strength training can be performed with weight machines, free weights, or using body weight for resistance. Weight machines offer safe ways to lift heavier weights and provide complex systems to control the rate of muscle contraction. Using free weights such as wrist or ankle weights, low-tech items such as elastic bands, or household items like milk jugs or tin cans will work for strength training. Bearing the weight of the whole body in standing, transfers, and walking or performing active range-of-motion exercises can be a strength training activity for many frail older adults. Examples of body weight exercises include repeated chair stands, wall squats, and step ups.

Strength training should be performed for all major muscle groups, including, but not limited to, the shoulders, arms, hips, legs, ankles, back, and trunk. The lower extremity muscle groups are larger and more important for functional mobility and independence; however, upper extremity exercises will induce a higher heart rate response. Initial durations may be much briefer than with lower extremity exercise, as many people tend to have more deconditioned arms than legs.

The major risks with strength training include muscle soreness and musculoskeletal injury. Completing the exercise in good form by moving in a smooth, controlled manner rather than shaking or jerking through the movement will reduce the risk of injury. To prevent injury and learn to perform exercises correctly, patients should be counseled to receive instruction in proper technique, preferably by a certified exercise trainer. Most gyms have someone on site who, at minimum, is available to provide guidance about appropriate use of the machines and equipment at that facility. Starting with a low number of repetitions and a low amount of resistance will also reduce the risk of injury. It is also very important to avoid holding one's breath during strength training as it induces increased blood pressure. Key breathing guidelines are to start by taking a breath before lifting, exhale during lifting, and inhale during controlled release.

C. Flexibility

Flexibility decreases with age and can become significantly restricted with disease or disuse. Loss of range of motion affects mobility and function and, in the worst case, can result in contractures that limit standing, walking, and reaching. Stretches should last 30 to 60 seconds and involve all major joints of the upper and lower extremity and trunk. The stretch should cause a sensation of pulling but not acute pain. To prevent injury, light to moderate activity to warm up the muscle before stretching for flexibility is advised. Contraindications to flexibility exercises include acutely inflamed joints, fused joints, and recent fracture.

D. Balance

Balance training is recommended for those older adults at risk for falls. The types of exercises and activities included in "balance training" are rarely defined in the literature, and there is little to no consensus on the frequency, intensity, and duration needed to induce benefits. Healthy older adults can improve balance through recreational activities that require displacement and recovery, such as dancing or tennis. Balance training for the very frail person involves movement practice in a seated position that requires displacement of the trunk and arms. Balance training in water allows patients to explore the margins of their ability to displace and recover without fear of injury, as falls are cushioned by the water.

Balance training requires progression of difficulty, making it inherently more dangerous than other types of exercise due to the increased risk of falling. Therefore, to reduce this risk, an older adult should only begin a balance training program after proper instruction by a health professional. Such patients may require supervised exercise with a physical therapist prior to starting a balance training program on their own.

▶ Interactions of Exercise with Medications

Many older adults take medications that can affect their ability to tolerate exercise. For example, those prescribed antihypertensive or cardiac medications are at risk for hypotension during or after a bout of aerobic or resistance exercises. Since both types of exercise can evoke an acute drop in blood pressure or reductions in blood pressure in response to physiologic adaptations to exercise over time, it is important to counsel older adults about the risk of transient orthostasis that can lead to imbalance and fall risk and ways to mitigate the risk, such as adequate hydration during exercise and breaks between exercises. Those who experience symptoms should be advised to notify their health care provider so that appropriate measures can be taken to continue exercise safely.

▶ Gaps in Current Exercise Recommendations

Recommendations exist for physical activity/aerobic exercise, strength, flexibility, and balance; however, these recommendations leave out an important aspect of physical activity in older adults—the timing and coordination of movement. Aging and disease can alter the timing and coordination of walking and subsequently reduce gait efficiency, resulting in older adults working harder to walk than they should be. Performing exercises to improve the timing and coordination of walking (ie, stepping and walking patterns with progression of difficulty) results in improved gait efficiency and subsequently improved walking ability. While the evidence for the benefits of this type of exercise is emerging, it should be considered as part of an exercise prescription.

Common barriers to exercise include the lack of motivation to participate in regular activity and the often boring and repetitive nature of many types of activity (eg, walking, jogging, bicycling). Providing the older adult with examples of ways to make exercise fun and a social activity, such as listening to music while performing the exercise, joining an exercise class or gym, exercising with a partner, or doing interactive fitness activities (eg, dance, golf, video-based classes), may be one way to increase participation and adherence.

▶ Continuing an Exercise Program

Convincing an older person to exercise can be a formidable challenge. Modern civilization has created a living environment that, although immeasurably beneficial, reduces the need for physical activity in daily life. How to begin and adhere to an exercise program is an important aspect of prescribing an activity plan that should be discussed with all patients.

Prior experience, knowledge, and beliefs about exercise will influence attitudes and expectations toward exercise. An older adult is more likely to participate in physical activity if the person feels confident in one's ability to succeed and that the activity is safe and enjoyable. For many older adults, the opportunity to socialize during exercise is a key motivating factor. Identifying these important contributors to participation and adherence for each older adult will encourage the initiation and maintenance of an exercise program.

A. Progression

All exercise requires a minimum frequency, intensity, and duration to achieve gain by inducing moderate physiologic stress; thus, exercise must include a plan for progression over time. Many sedentary older adults are unable to sustain a moderate-intensity activity for more than a few minutes. For this reason, the exercise program often must begin with a gradual increase in duration before any effort to increase intensity is considered. A necessary and important part of the exercise prescription includes checking with the older adult as to how the program is going and if the frequency, intensity, or duration of the activities needs to be adjusted.

B. Adherence

Adherence to an activity program improves when an individual commits to personally meaningful and measurable goals, uses a self-monitoring plan such as a calendar to record exercise, receives specific feedback, and has access to support as desired from others. A clinician's formal recommendation to exercise, delivered as a prescription based on individualized risks and needs, increases motivation and adherence.

Case Vignette

Ethel, your 75-year-old patient, comes into your office inquiring about starting an exercise program. Some of her friends participate in an exercise group and have been talking about the benefits of exercise. Ethel asks for your advice about starting her own exercise program. She has arthritis and hypertension, for which she takes a β-blocker; otherwise, Ethel is in good health.

You discuss with Ethel her goals and interests with an activity program. You find that she loves to walk and dance, but she is concerned about falling. You recommend that Ethel start an exercise program in which she performs aerobic exercise 4 to 5 days a week, starting with walking for as long as she can tolerate before needing a rest break. Given that Ethel is relatively healthy, you would expect her to be able to walk for about 15 to 20 minutes continuously. However, if Ethel can only tolerate about 5 to 10 minutes of walking, she should walk for that long, take a short rest break, then walk again, repeating this a few times (for 20–30 minutes of total walking time). You tell her to gradually increase the amount of time she walks until she is able to tolerate 30 minutes continuously. Because of her use of β-blockers, you explain the RPE scale and the talk test as ways to measure her level of intensity. You encourage Ethel to find dancing classes that she can attend with her husband and educate her about swimming or group exercise classes at the local gym. You also advise Ethel about the importance of strength training, giving her a few exercises to perform at home. You schedule a follow-up appointment with Ethel in 3 months to check her progress with her short- and long-term goals and to address any barriers she has noticed, as well as discuss how to progress her current activity program.

SUMMARY

Physical activity positively impacts multiple aspects of life and is beneficial to almost all older adults. Very few instances exist in which physical activity is contraindicated. Depending on the needs and preferences of the individual, physical activity programs can be performed in a supervised setting or unsupervised, incorporating all types of exercise. Providing an exercise prescription that is tailored to the individual, sets reasonable and attainable goals, and monitors the individual's maintenance and progression of the activity program is key for initiation and adherence.

Ainsworth BE, Haskell WL, Herrmann SD, et al. 2011 Compendium of Physical Activities: a second update of codes and MET values. *Med Sci Sports Exerc.* 2011;43(8):1575-1581. American College of Sports Medicine, Chodzko-Zajko WJ, Proctor DN, et al. American College of Sports Medicine position stand. Exercise and physical activity for older adults. *Med Sci Sports Exerc.* 2009;41(7):1510-1530.

Centers for Disease Control and Prevention. *Measuring Physical Activity Intensity.* http://www.cdc.gov/physicalactivity/everyone/measuring/index.html. Accessed August 2, 2012.

Centers for Disease Control and Prevention. *Perceived Exertion (Borg Rating of Perceived Exertion Scale).* http://www.cdc.gov/physicalactivity/everyone/measuring/exertion.html. Accessed August 2, 2012.

Centers for Disease Control and Prevention. *Target Heart Rate and Estimated Maximum Heart Rate.* http://www.cdc.gov/physicalactivity/everyone/measuring/heartrate.html. Accessed August 2, 2012.

de Labra C, Guimaraes-Pinheiro C, Maseda A, Lorenzo T, Millán-Calenti JC. Effects of physical exercise interventions in frail older adults: a systematic review of randomized controlled trials. *BMC Geriatr.* 2015;15:154.

Exercise Is Medicine. Your Prescription for Health series. https://fcymca.org/programs/health-wellness/exercise-is-medicine/. Accessed April 21, 2020.

Garber CE, Blissmer B, Deschenes MR, et al. American College of Sports Medicine position stand. Quantity and quality of exercise for developing and maintaining cardiorespiratory, musculoskeletal, and neuromotor fitness in apparently healthy adults: guidance for prescribing exercise. *Med Sci Sports Exerc.* 2011;43(7):1334-1359.

Gill TM, DiPietro L, Krumholz HM. Role of exercise stress testing and safety monitoring for older persons starting an exercise program. *JAMA.* 2000;284(3):342-349.

National Institute on Aging. *Exercise & Physical Activity: Your Everyday Guide from the National Institute on Aging.* 2011. http://www.nia.nih.gov/sites/default/files/exercise_guide.pdf. Accessed August 15, 2012.

Sherrington C, Michaleff ZA, Fairhall N, et al. Exercise to prevent falls in older adults: an updated systematic review and meta-analysis. *Br J Sports Med.* 2017;51(24):1750-1758.

Swain DP, ed. *American College of Sports Medicine Resource Manual for Guidelines for Exercise Testing and Prescription.* Philadelphia, PA: Wolters Kluwer Health/Lippincott Williams & Wilkens; 2014

Tyndall AV, Clark CM, Anderson TJ, et al. Protective effects of exercise on cognition and brain health in older adults. *Exerc Sport Sci Rev.* 2018;4:215-223.

Van Norman KA. *Exercise and Wellness for Older Adults: Practical Programming Strategies.* 2nd ed. Champaign, IL: Human Kinetics; 2010.

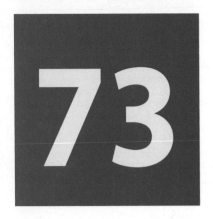

Meeting the Unique Needs of LGBT Older Adults

Jeffrey de Castro Mariano, MD, AGSF

Aleksandr Lewicki, MD

▶ Overview

The 2011 Institute of Medicine (IOM) report, Health of LGBT People: Building a Foundation for Better Understanding, highlighted both the health disparities and diversity of the lesbian, gay, bisexual, and transgender (LGBT) population.

This chapter describes specific health concerns related to LGBT aging and the impact of historical context and institutional and social stigma on medical, psychological, and social outcomes that confer both vulnerability and resilience. A heightened awareness of these disparities and the heterogeneity of the population can allow for optimal and culturally appropriate care to all older LGBT patients.

DEFINITIONS

Table 73–1 defines terms used to define sexual and gender minorities. In general, sexual orientation describes a person's emotional and/or physical attraction to people of the same and/or different gender. Most identify as lesbian, gay, bisexual, or heterosexual. However, it is also important to appreciate how factors including life course and historical context affect the diversity of gender identity and expression, in addition to sexual orientation. Older generations in particular often felt the need to hide their sexual orientation or conform to their gender of birth to avoid rejection and discrimination, thus "staying in the closet," and giving rise to a mix of diverse family structures.

▶ Demographics

Given the legal and social status of LGBT persons globally, few official estimates exist. In the United States, approximately 11.3 million people (4.5% of the population) identify as LGBT, and it is estimated that there are 2.7 million LGBT people over age 50. Although self-identified LGBT individuals

more frequently live in urban areas, US census data from 2000 and 2010 showed that same-sex–headed households existed in >90% of all counties and that more than 1 in 10 same-sex couples included a partner older than age 65 years. One-third of LGBT individuals over 50 years live at or below 200% of the federal poverty level, while nearly one-half of bisexuals and transgender individuals live at or below this level. Racial and ethnic composition of the LGBT population is roughly identical to that of the general population.

▶ History of Stigma and Prejudice Linked to Disparities and Health Equity

Studies on minority stress theory and health equity reveal that there is a direct relationship between stigma, discrimination, and health. This cascade involves the interaction of interpersonal stigma (between people) and structural stigma (institutional laws, religion) contributing to intrapersonal stigma (internal alienation), which then worsens stress/anxiety and depression (minority stress theory). This cascade can lead to health disparities and inequities (exclusion or avoidance).

There are three LGBT older adult cohorts in the United States. Those born between 1910 and 1925, the "Greatest Generation," grew up in a world where same-sex behavior led to imprisonment and nondisclosure of sexual orientation was self-protective. Those born between 1926 and 1945, the "Silent Generation," came of age in that same repressive environment, including World War II and McCarthyism. Thus, they are much more likely to have kept, and continue to keep, their sexual orientation hidden. The Stonewall Riots of 1969, considered the beginning of the gay civil rights movement in the United States, marked the "Proud Generation." This cohort born between 1946 and 1964 are more partially or completely out. However, studies show that one-third to one-half of baby boomers have not disclosed their sexual orientation with their primary care physician or at their place of

Table 73–1. Terms and definitions for gender and sexual minorities.

Gay and lesbian	Sexual orientation and physical and/or emotional attraction toward members of the same gender (men = gay and women = lesbian).
Bisexual	Have an orientation toward people of both genders.
Transgender	People whose gender identity and expression do not match. It was not until 1980 in the DSM-III that sexual orientation was differentiated from gender identity.
Gender nonconformity	Refers to the extent to which a person's gender identity, role, or expression differs from the cultural norms prescribed for people of a particular sex (Institute of Medicine, 2011).
Gender identity	Defined as a personal conception (self-identification) of oneself as male or female (or rarely, both or neither); result of a combination of inherent and extrinsic or environmental factors.
Coming out of the closet	The unique, individualized, and often difficult lifelong process of disclosing one's identity as LGBT. Affected by generational and historical realities and further influenced by personal history, ethnic, cultural, and religious background; experiences of victimization; family and societal messages; and presence or absence of community support.
Intersectionality	Defined as the intersection of multiple identities and experiences of exclusion. The relationship of a person's many identities (sexual, racial, economic, geographic) that coexist into a "new" whole. This process can lead to stress and stigma in marginalized communities, especially older ethnic minority communities.
Heterosexism	System of attitudes, bias, and discrimination in favor of opposite-sex sexuality and relationships.
Homophobia	System of negative attitudes and feelings toward homosexuality or people who are identified or perceived as being lesbian, gay, bisexual, or transgender.
Cultural competence in health care	The skills, knowledge, and attitudes in the assessment and care of a minority cultural group. Although considered important as a starting point, cultural competence itself may bias the assessment and management of someone from the minority group.
Cultural humility in health care	Recommended to supplement cultural competence as a nonjudgmental recognition that one's own experiences or identities may not project onto the experiences or identities of others. Requires acknowledgment of the social, cultural, and historical context that affect the individual. Through a lens of social justice, it also focuses on the dignity and autonomy of the individual as well as delivery of high-quality medical care to all members regardless of race, gender, sexual orientation or gender identity, or socioeconomic background.

DSM-III, *Diagnostic and Statistical Manual of Mental Disorders*, third edition.

employment. These findings are worse for nonwhite older adults, who face additional stigma as a double minority with even less levels of disclosure and less visibility.

Nondisclosure has been implicated in health disparity, contributing to worse mental health outcomes by exacerbating internalized heterosexism and homophobia. Studies suggest that discrimination and stigma can be associated with lower life satisfaction, lower self-esteem, depression, suicide, substance abuse, and unhealthy and risky behavior. Nondisclosure of sexual orientation and gender identity may also lead to delay in care and inappropriate care and may prevent the development of a trusting patient-provider relationship.

▶ Patient-Provider Communication

Health care providers should provide culturally competent care that creates an environment of respect for LGBT older adults. Because sexual orientation and gender identity can be hidden characteristics, it is important for health care providers to create a safe space to allow individuals to disclose these aspects of their identity if they choose. The importance of using open language without forcing labels is magnified among older adults, who may have cumulative life experience that leads to higher levels of resistance to LGBT labels and disclosure of sexual and gender minority status. Data shows that LGBT individuals, including baby boomers, have low confidence that health care providers will treat them with respect, and this leads to reluctance to seek care. Local LGBT centers of the clearinghouse at Services and Advocacy for LGBT Elders (http://www.lgbtagingcenter.org) and the Gay and Lesbian Medical Association website (http://www.glma.org) are good sources of information in finding welcoming providers. Individual health care organizations may have their own lists of such providers. Table 73–2 lists examples of open language that can be used to address sexuality. Table 73–3 lists factors that help to create a welcoming environment.

Table 73-2. Factors that help create a welcoming environment.

Having LGBT-friendly symbols, signs, and fliers visible in the office
Ensuring privacy and confidentiality
Using inclusive forms and encouraging all providers and staff to use inclusive language
Avoiding a heteronormative or gender-normative stance toward older adults, including if they are parents or grandparents
Using patient-requested names and pronouns
Having transgender and gender-nonconforming inclusive bathrooms

HEALTH ISSUES FOR LGBT OLDER ADULTS

Although research on health maintenance and medical issues for older LGBT adults is often limited, there are certain mental and physical health disparities that affect these groups (Table 73-4). In addition, there is evidence that successful aging in older LGBT people is negatively affected by lifetime discrimination, identity nondisclosure, and specific health conditions.

▶ Health Issues for Older Gay and Bisexual Men

A. Sexual Health

Sexual health (function, activity, and safer sex methods) should be discussed with older gay and bisexual men to assess for and reduce the risk of sexually transmitted diseases. This acknowledges that 48% of older LGBT adults do not use condoms regularly, and 9% never do. Screening for HIV, gonorrhea, chlamydia, and syphilis should be a part of routine preventive health for sexually active older men who

Table 73-3. Examples of inclusive and open language.

How do you like to be called? What is your preferred name?
What is your preferred pronoun?
Who are the important people in your life?
Who lives with you at home?
How do you refer to your loved ones?
What is your relationship status (eg, single, partnered, married, open)?
Who are your sexual partners?
Do you use any kind of protection against STIs/STDs?
Have you been tested for HIV or other STIs/STDs?
Are you comfortable with your sexuality?
Are you comfortable with me documenting this information in the chart?

STD, sexually transmitted disease; STI, sexually transmitted infection.

Table 73-4. Overview of specific health care issues to address in older LGBT adults.

Gay and Bisexual Men	Lesbian and Bisexual Women	Transgender
HIV/AIDs	Prevention/screening	HIV/AIDs
Sexually transmitted diseases/sexual health	Sexually transmitted diseases/sexual health	Sexually transmitted diseases/sexual health
Anal papilloma/anal cancer	Breast cancer/gynecologic cancer	Preventive care/access to health care
Substance abuse	Substance abuse	Substance abuse
Cardiovascular disease	Cardiovascular disease	Hormone therapy
Mental health	Mental health	Mental health
Psychosocial issues	Psychosocial issues	Psychosocial issues

have sex with men, and vaccinations for hepatitis A and B should be offered. Recommendations for human papillomavirus (HPV) vaccination currently extend only to age 26.

B. Cardiovascular Health

Younger gay and bisexual men are more likely to smoke cigarettes. While older gay men appear to have similar rates of smoking as compared to heterosexuals, the effects of previously higher rates of smoking in this group may continue to be a risk factor for cardiovascular disease, including stroke and heart attacks. Smoking cessation should be advised and treatments offered among this population.

C. Cancer

There are several cancers that may be more common among gay and bisexual men: anal cancer, caused by the HPV; lung cancer, caused by smoking; colon cancer, perhaps attributable to reduced rates of screening; and liver cancer, related to an increase in hepatitis B and C infections. Treatment of prostate cancer, anal cancer, and colon cancer may have different psychosocial effects, and effects on sexual behavior among men who have sex with men should be reviewed and explored as part of shared decision making.

Anal Pap screening for anal dysplasia is a validated technique with sensitivity and specificity comparable to that of cervical cytology screening techniques. The incidence of anal cancer is comparable to that used to justify colorectal cancer screening and mammography only among men who have sex with men who have with AIDS beginning at age 30 and those with HIV beginning at age 45. Although there are no guidelines available from the US Preventive Services Task Force, there are guidelines from smaller state agencies and organizations, such as the New York State Department of Health AIDS Institute, which recommends screening annually with anal Pap smears among the following HIV-positive populations: men who have sex with men, patients with a history of anogenital condylomas, and women with abnormal cervical and/or vulvar histology. Incidence rates of HPV-associated cancers are a moving target, given that current younger generations now have significant vaccination rates against HPV, so guidelines for both cervical cancer and anal cancer screening will likely change.

Older Lesbian and Bisexual Women's Health

There is good evidence that lesbians receive less preventive care, access health care services less often, and enter the health care system later than heterosexual women. Most of the health disparities are related to nonrecognition of same-sex partnerships and employer-based insurance and lack of culturally competent providers.

A. Sexual Health

Sexual health (function, activity, and safer sex methods) should be routinely discussed. See Chapter 11, "Sexual Health & Dysfunction." Studies show that sexual minority women, especially lesbians, frequently underestimate their risk of acquiring or being capable of transmitting sexual disease, especially HPV.

Clinicians should avoid assuming heterosexuality of older patients. It is important to use nonheteronormative and inclusive language. Some women are or have been sexually active with both men and women, which studies show is more often true for ethnic minority lesbian women.

B. Cardiovascular Disease

Several studies including combined national data show that lesbian women are more likely to report moderate psychologic distress, have poor or fair health, have higher body mass index (BMI), and be heavy smokers and drinkers, a finding very similar to that in bisexual women. Since cardiovascular disease is a leading cause of death in women in the United States, the focus should be on identifying modifiable risk factors such as smoking and obesity.

C. Cancer

Cancer risks in lesbian and bisexual groups are, for the most part, related to screening and lifestyle risks. Lesbians have lower rates of Pap screening (43%–71% vs 73%) and mammograms as compared to heterosexuals. Unfortunately, although national surveys for sexual minority women are lacking, epidemiologic studies from California show a possible increased risk for breast cancer given risk factors such as nulliparity, alcohol use, smoking, and obesity and increased risk of cervical cancer including sexual contact with men, smoking, and obesity. Because of increased smoking rates, lesbian and

bisexual women may also have a greater risk of lung cancer, although lung cancer screening recommendations in this group do not differ compared to the general population.

As with other women, older lesbian and bisexual women should be screened for exercise, intimate partner violence, and other geriatric syndromes that may be affected by access to health care and institutional stigma.

Older Transgender Health

Studies show that transgender older adults are the most stigmatized of the LGBT population, suffering from discrimination within and outside the LGBT community. This has resulted in less access to health care; an increase in smoking, alcohol use, and substance use; and higher rates of depression and violence.

A. Transgender Medicine

Transgender medicine and decisions on transitions and hormone use are individualized. There are four steps, including diagnosis by a mental health professional (psychotherapy, counseling), lifestyle assumption of desired gender role, hormonal and drug therapy, and surgical treatment. Studies show that up to 70% of transgender adults aged 54 years and older admit to delaying transitions to await milestone events such as divorce, growth of their children, and retirement to avoid discrimination.

B. Sexual Health

Transgender older adults have higher rates of HIV and viral hepatitis infections, often a result of lack of access to preventative health care and fear of discrimination.

C. Cardiovascular Disease

Heart disease is also a significant issue in the transgender population due to the higher rates of modifiable risk factors such as smoking, hormone use (especially estrogen), and obesity; hence, addressing these risk factors is important.

D. Cancer

Prevention guidelines and health screenings should be geared toward birth gender and should be recorded in the electronic health records (an "organ inventory"). Examples of such issues include breast cancer screening and dysfunctional uterine bleeding in female-to-male transitions as well as osteoporosis and prostate screening in male-to-female transitions.

E. Hormone Use

It is important to assess goals and risks and benefits of hormonal treatment, other medical conditions (coronary artery disease [CAD], hypertension [HTN], deep vein thrombosis

[DVT]), social and economic issues, and whether hormonal treatment is being obtained through the health system or illicit market.

Female-to-male transitions involve the use of testosterone. Testosterone can lead to cardiovascular effects, venous thromboembolism (VTE), elevated hematocrit, and HTN. Absolute contraindications to testosterone are similar to those in hypogonadal men, including unstable CAD and polycythemia with hematocrit of 55%. It is important to monitor for breast cancer, osteoporosis, mood changes, and increased libido. Bone mineral density screening is recommended for those aged 60 and older who have been on testosterone for >5 to 10 years.

Male-to-female transitions involve the use of estrogen, with absolute contraindications including VTE, history of estrogen-sensitive neoplasm, and end-stage chronic liver disease. These risks are increased with smoking and obesity. Studies show that nonoral modalities (especially transdermal) are preferred. Studies are conflicting on cardiovascular disease risk with oral versus transdermal estrogen.

It is important to note that patients who undergo male-to-female transition should be counseled on the need for regular vaginal dilation or penetrative intercourse and the impact of anatomic dimensions in the neovagina that can affect intercourse. There is also increased urinary tract infection risk due to a shortened urethra, increased bladder dysfunction, and change in the position of the bladder itself. A dysfunctional bladder that results in stress or urge in urinary incontinence is common.

F. Antiandrogen Therapy

Spironolactone and gonadotropin-releasing hormone agonists that can lead to less estrogen use are options in male-to-female transitions, although they have a higher risk for osteoporosis.

The University of California San Francisco's Center of Excellence for Transgender Health offers a resource for a primary care protocol, including recommendations for general prevention and screening. For example, it recommends routine mammogram screening in trans women (male-to-female transgender persons) older than age 50 years with additional risk factors (estrogen and progestin use >5 years, positive family history, or BMI >35). Trans men pelvic exams are recommended every 1 to 3 years for those >50 years old.

► Mental Health and Resilience

There is a link between mental health and health disparities. Communities that suffer health disparities are more likely to have higher rates of mental health issues, particularly depression and anxiety. Furthermore, all LGBT adults experience one common developmental challenge: deciding if, when, and how to reveal to others their gender identity and/or sexual orientation. Older LGBT people who have lived in the closet for much of their lives can have significant stress, loss of self-esteem, and less-fulfilled lives. Trying to manage stigma, marginalization, and identity can lead to higher rates of depression, suicide, risky sexual behavior, and substance abuse. In addition, coming out or returning into the closet can be influenced by changing social situations like moving to an assisted living facility or into a child's home.

Recent studies show prevalence rates of depression for LGBT older adults of 31%, which is two times higher than Centers for Disease Control and Prevention estimates. Transgender depression rates are even higher at 48%, related to both gender dysphoria (emotional distress from "a marked incongruence between expressed and assigned gender") and a history of victimization and discrimination. Evaluating for suicide is important. Studies have shown that of the 40% who have contemplated suicide, a minority of reasons (39%) were due to sexual orientation.

Providers should also screen for substance use disorder (alcohol and others) given studies showing an increased risk due to stigma/minority status, decreased social support, internalized homophobia, and the importance of bars as social venues in LGBT neighborhoods. For example, recent surveys showed a higher prevalence of moderate alcohol use among LGBT people, with an incidence of five or more drinks at least one time per year of 14.5%, versus 6.7% in the general population.

► HIV in Older Adults

A. Demographics

Although the topic of HIV is covered in Chapter 55, "HIV & AIDS," it is worth noting that there is increasing prevalence of older adults living longer with HIV. Gay and bisexual men are the population most affected by HIV in the United States, accounting for 67% of new HIV diagnoses in 2016. The incidence of HIV among gay men older than 55 has remained stable in recent years, at around 6.5% of all diagnoses among gay men. Minorities with HIV/AIDS have higher mortality rates: the death rates are five times higher among older Hispanics, and 12 times higher in older blacks. Additionally, HIV-positive individuals are one of the subgroups among LGBT persons with the greatest risk of economic insecurity.

B. Prevention

Preexposure prophylaxis (PrEP) for HIV has been approved by the US Food and Drug Administration since 2012 as an effective HIV prevention measure. Attitudes toward PrEP are generally positive among men who identify as gay or bisexual who are familiar with PrEP. However, familiarity is low among older men who were young adults during the height of the AIDS epidemic, as well as those who are currently young adults.

C. Frailty & Effects of Antiretroviral Therapy

HIV/AIDS has been associated with an "early aging" phenomenon, including early emergence of the frailty phenotype. Although antiretroviral therapy (ART) medication adherence tends to be higher in older adults, the resulting low viral load does not automatically confer high CD4 counts, consistent with overall less resilient immunity in older adults. The use of ART is a predictor of frailty and has paralleled the rising proportion of non–AIDS-related morbidity and mortality in HIV-positive individuals. This is partly due to better control of HIV and the prevalence of chronic illness, but also partially due to the deleterious effects of ART itself, including metabolic (CAD, diabetes, bone loss), renal, hepatic, and central nervous system toxicities. Among LGBT individuals who are at increased risk of CAD, perhaps partially due to increased smoking rates, ART may confer a disproportionate burden of negative cardiovascular outcomes.

D. Anal Cancer

Anal cancer occurs at higher rates among HIV-positive individuals, regardless of sexual practices. However, the burden is again disproportionately high among certain LGBT groups, with incidence of anal cancer ranging from a low of 18.6 per 100,000 HIV-positive heterosexual females to a high of 89.0 per 100,000 HIV-positive men who have sex with men. See section titled "Health Issues for Older Gay and Bisexual Men" for a discussion on screening for anal cancer.

BIOPSYCHOSOCIAL ASPECTS OF CARE

▶ Social Supports and Family Structure

The definition of "family" should be expanded and inclusive of those who maintain an ongoing emotional relationship with a person, regardless of their legal or biological relationship. Given the realities of social exclusion, the social support structures of LGBT older adults tend to be different from those of older adults in the general population. Whereas older adults in the general population tend to rely on spouses and adult children as part of a network of support that can meet an older individual's psychosocial and caregiving needs, LGBT older adults are more frequently socially isolated and may rely on informal networks for their social needs. Studies highlight the importance of social networks in fostering resilience and enhancing physical and mental quality of life.

There are several reasons for this social isolation: LGBT older adults are less likely to be partnered, less likely to have children, and more likely to live alone. The lack of societal acceptance can lead to estrangement from biologic family members, like former spouses or adult children. One study found that 40% of children have no communication with their transgender parents. Furthermore, there is a cohort of LGBT older adults whose partners/friends succumbed to the AIDS epidemic.

Due to these factors, LGBT older adults are more likely (some studies showing as high as 65%–70%) to rely on informal "families of choice," composed of extensive networks of friends. Because of these informal networks, it is imperative that clinicians carefully document patient choices for surrogate decision makers, who may often be a person that is not the legal default next of kin (see later section on advance care planning). These surrogates are even more important for patients with dementia as there were an estimated >200,000 LGBT individuals living with the disease in the United States as of 2018 (Alzheimer's Association and National Institute on Aging). Legal issues affecting surrogacy with the next of kin versus family of choice may become a challenge, especially if family is not supportive of the individual's choices, identity, and values.

The abuse of an older LGBT person can be broken down into three subcategories: abuse of older people who are also LGBT; homophobic, biphobic, and/or transphobic abuse toward older LGBT people; and abuse that is associated with the intersections of older age and LGBT status. Overall, the literature on the abuse of older LGBT people is scant. However, small epidemiologic studies reveal that as many as 25% of LGBT individuals have knowledge of others who have encountered abuse (sexual, financial, physical, or emotional abuse or neglect by caregivers).

It is important to stress that there are resilient members of the community, and it is important to evaluate and support protective factors that research has found to foster resilience and mitigate depression in LGBT older adults, including social support and network size, more active religious and spiritual life, and a more positive sense and disclosure of sexual identity. These factors should be considered along with those that are protective in all older adults, including mobility, physical activity, self-reliance, and social support.

▶ Housing and Long-Term Care

Antidiscrimination laws in housing do not extend themselves to sexual orientation or gender identity status. Unmarried partners, or those in domestic partnerships, may not enjoy the same benefits of inheritance laws as partnerships of marriage. In these situations, legal planning is necessary to secure housing for a surviving partner.

Entering a long-term care (LTC) facility is a particularly vulnerable time for this population. Discrimination is the greatest concern of aging for 32% of gay men and 26% of lesbians. There is a significant amount of real or feared discrimination in LTC, from both the staff and other residents. It is important that LGBT individuals are not coerced (overtly or inadvertently) into hiding their identities or key relationships when moving into a nursing home. In the LTC system, unmarried residents are typically paired with other residents in same-sex rooms, and facilities are not required to allow consenting adults to choose to share rooms. There are no federal policies for how to house transgender and gender nonconforming individuals, and access to gender-inclusive restrooms may be limited, especially for those who have mobility challenges and thus rely on caregivers with different gender identities than their own. States, including New York and California, are passing legislation to protect LGBT individuals in the LTC setting.

There are multiple models for how to address issues of LGBT inclusivity in senior housing and LTC. Some housing options are designed specifically for LGBT seniors, such as the Los Angeles LGBT Center's Triangle Square, the nation's largest affordable housing development specifically for LGBT seniors. Within LTC, where specific LGBT options are usually not available, one model has explored utilizing local LGBT "community advisors" to run focus groups with LTC staff that address knowledge gaps and personal views and beliefs among staff to attempt to improve cultural competency in caring for LGBT individuals. Some organizations provide outreach and training in the community, such as Fenway Health through the LGBT Aging Project, and an equality index for LTC is under development through a collaboration between the Human Rights Campaign and Services and Advocacy for LGBT Elders. Additionally, curricula, such as the Health Education About LGBT Elders (HEALE) curriculum for LGBT cultural competency, have been used in various health care settings, including in nursing homes. Finally, harnessing the resilience that LGBT elders have developed by overcoming a lifetime of discrimination is another tool that is being increasingly investigated.

▶ Policy Issues Affecting LGBT Older Adults

Social attitudes toward LGBT people began to evolve in the early 2000s. In 2003, the US Supreme Court struck down the remaining laws that criminalized male same-sex behaviors in 14 states (Lawrence v Texas). The rapid shift in attitudes toward same-sex marriage resulted in landmark decisions by the US Supreme Court in 2013 (USA v Windsor) and 2015 (Obergefell v Hodges), which made same-sex marriage legal throughout the United States. However, these recent events cannot reverse the laws and regulations that have contributed to inequality. Medicare did not cover unmarried partners and did not recognize married same-sex couples until 2015. Institutional policies affecting retirement/pensions and government programs such as Social Security have impacted the financial well-being of LGBT older persons. Eighty-five percent of nonprofit assisted living facilities in the United States are religiously affiliated, and some states have laws that protect religious freedom that may enable the creation of a stigmatized unwelcoming environment.

At the time of publication, 12 US states do not prohibit employment discrimination on the basis of sexual orientation and gender identity. In 2019, the US House of Representatives held hearings on the Equality Act, federal legislation that would expressly prohibit discrimination on the basis of sex, gender identity, and sexual orientation in employment, housing, public accommodations, jury service, and other settings. This legislation was approved by the House of Representatives and is being debated in the Senate. As in other global political bodies, legislation and laws to protect from discrimination based on sexual orientation and gender identity are variable and mostly nonexistent.

The American College of Physicians, American Medical Association, American Geriatrics Society, and other professional organizations support data collection of sexual orientation and gender identity (through electronic health records) and research into understanding the demographics of the LGBT population, potential causes of LGBT health disparities, and best practices in reducing these disparities.

▶ Advance Care Planning, Palliative Medicine, and Hospice Care

The factors that contribute to health care disparities experienced by LGBT persons also impact them during serious and terminal illness. Current health practice places the responsibility of disclosing one's minority status on the patient, who may fear discrimination at the very time they feel vulnerable due to illness. This may lead to fears of disclosure to family, incorrect assumptions regarding surrogate decision making, higher levels of disease-associated distress, the experience of bias, and delayed access to care, especially pastoral care resources. Furthermore, disenfranchised grief is a significant problem, where the partner may not be recognized by the family, legal system, or health care system either during critical illness or after death.

As a result, a recent consensus panel of 60 members, including experts in palliative medicine, oncology, and public health and LGBT cancer patients and survivors, made the following recommendations:

1. Collect (sexual orientation and gender identity (SOGI) data for all patients at initial encounters and create individualized plans about disclosure or nondisclosure of SOGI to others.

2. Acknowledge that reconciliation with families of origin may or may not be welcome or needed and should be discussed and pursued as per patients' wishes.

3. The lack of specific guidelines and standards of care for transgender patients in palliative and hospice settings should be acknowledged. Patients' wishes regarding burial rights and when to discontinue hormones should be discussed and addressed. Physicians can help balance risks and benefits (eg, taking into consideration risks of DVT or hormone-mediated cancer).

4. Address the increased risk of mental health problems and unique psychosocial barriers that exist for some older

LGBT patients. In addition to pain and symptom management, consider psychosocial distress, suicide risk, financial planning, and relationship with family of origin and family of choice when performing screening and intake.

5. Discuss and formalize surrogate decision making during initial patient encounters, including medical proxy documentation, formalization of custody of dependent children, burial rights forms, and hospital visitation. It is a patient's legal right to involve their family of choice. Discussions should reflect changing laws and regulations on a national, state, and local/institutional level

6. Documenting advance health directives with the designated family of choice is one strategy that older LGBT adults can pursue to ensure that their wishes are respected in the health care setting. This includes an advance directive where one can legally safeguard their choice of decision maker ("health care proxy" or "durable power of attorney for health care") and the orders for life-sustaining treatments by which a person can declare their specific instructions for their end-of-life care. Both documents can ensure that LGBT families' preferences will be respected and validated. See Chapter 21, "Ethics & Informed Decision Making," for more information.

CONCLUSION

There are millions of American older adults who identify as LGBT, and this population will continue to grow as the baby boomer generation ages. Education, awareness, knowledge, and skill are essential to a culturally competent practice that promotes the well-being of LGBT older adults.

The Health Equity Promotion Model (Figure 73–1) illustrates the heterogeneity and intersectionality within LGBT communities. It shows the influence of structural and environmental contexts and their impact on health-promoting and adverse pathways that encompass behavioral, social, psychological, and biological processes.

Providers must be aware of the historical contexts in which LGBT older adults lived and the impact it had in creating health disparities (medical, psychological, and social). By practicing cultural humility, using an affirmative inclusive communication approach, and documenting sexual orientation and gender identity, we can support and mobilize prevention and intervention services for this diverse, vulnerable, and resilient group.

For additional resources to aid the provider in caring for older LGBT patients, including topics on caregiving, housing, and advocacy, see Table 73–5.

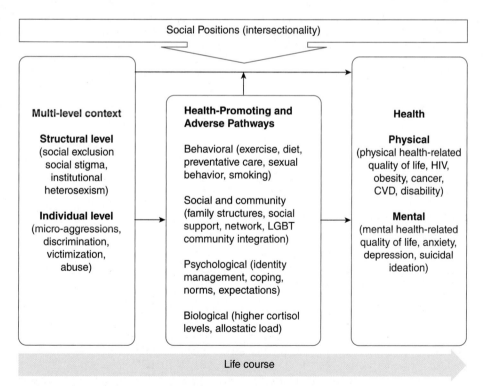

▲ **Figure 73–1.** Health Equity Promotion Model. CVD, cardiovascular disease. (Reproduced with permission from Fredriksen-Goldsen KI, Simoni JM, Kim HJ, et al. The health equity promotion model: Reconceptualization of lesbian, gay, bisexual, and transgender (LGBT) health disparities, *Am J Orthopsychiatry* 2014 Nov;84(6):653-663.)

Table 73–5. Resources for LGBT health and aging.

Name	Website
National Resource Center on LGBT Aging	https://www.lgbtagingcenter.org/
Services and Advocacy for Gay, Lesbian, Bisexual & Transgender Elders (SAGE)	http://www.sageusa.org
American Society on Aging (ASA): The LGBT Aging Issues Network (LAIN)	http://www.asaging.org/lain
National LGBT Health Education: Fenway Institute	https://www.lgbthealtheducation.org/
World Professional Association for Transgender Health (WPATH)	https://www.wpath.org/publications/soc
American Academy of HIV Medicine: HIV and Aging	https://aahivm.org/hiv-and-aging/

All websites accessed April 26, 2020.

American Geriatrics Society Ethics Committee. American Geriatrics Society care of lesbian, gay, bisexual, and transgender older adults position statement: American Geriatrics Society Ethics Committee. *J Am Geriatr Soc.* 2015;63(3):423-426.

Baptiste-Roberts K, Oranuba E, Werts N, Edwards LV. Addressing health care disparities among sexual minorities. *Obstet Gynecol Clin North Am.* 2017;44(1):71-80.

Braun H, Nash R, Tangpricha V, Brockman J, Ward K, Goodman M. Cancer in transgender people: evidence and methodological considerations. *Epidemiol Rev.* 2018;39(1):93-107.

Center of Excellence for Transgender Health UCSF. https://prevention.ucsf.edu/transhealth. Accessed April 26, 2020.

Colón-López V, Shiels MS, Machin M, et al. Anal cancer risk among people with HIV infection in the United States. *J Clin Oncol.* 2018;36(1):68-75.

Croghan CF, Moone RP, Olson AM. Factors that signal a welcoming service environment to LGBT baby boomer and older adults. *J Gerontol Social Work.* 2015;58(6):637-651.

Daniel H, Butkus R; Health and Public Policy Committee of American College of Physicians. Lesbian, gay, bisexual, and transgender health disparities: executive summary of a policy position paper from the American College of Physicians. *Ann Intern Med.* 2015;163(2):135-137.

Gates GJ. Social, economic, and health disparities among LGBT older adults. https://escholarship.org/uc/item/0kr784fx. Published 2014. Accessed April 26, 2019.

Gooren LJ, T'Sjoen G. Endocrine treatment of aging transgender people. *Rev Endocr Metab Disord.* 2018;19(3):253-262.

Griggs J, Maingi S, Rowland JH. American Society of Clinical Oncology position statement: strategies for reducing cancer health disparities among sexual and gender minority populations. *J Clin Oncol.* 2017;35(19):2203-2208.

Hafford-Letchfield T, Simpson P, Willis PB, Almack K. Developing inclusive residential care for older lesbian, gay, bisexual and trans (LGBT) people: an evaluation of the Care Home Challenge action research project. *Health & Social Care in the Community.* 2017;26(2):12521.

Hammack PL, Meyer IH, Krueger EA, Lightfoot M, Frost DM. HIV testing and pre-exposure prophylaxis (PrEP) use, familiarity, and attitudes among gay and bisexual men in the United States: a national probability sample of three birth cohorts. *Plos One.* 2018;13(9):0202806.

Hardacker CT, Rubinstein B, Hotton A, Houlberg M. Adding silver to the rainbow: the development of the nurses Health Education About LGBT Elders (HEALE) cultural competency curriculum. *J Nurs Manage.* 2013;22(2):257-266.

Hoy-Ellis CP, Fredriksen-Goldsen KI. Lesbian, gay, & bisexual older adults: linking internal minority stressors, chronic health conditions, and depression. *Aging Ment Health.* 2016;20(11):1119-1130.

Kim HJ, Jen S, Fredriksen-Goldsen KI. Race/ethnicity and health-related quality of life among LGBT older adults. *Gerontologist.* 2017;57(suppl 1):S30-S39.

Leeds IL, Fang SH. Anal cancer and intraepithelial neoplasia screening: a review. *World J Gastrointest Surg.* 2016;8:41-51.

Mahan RJ, Bailey TA, Bibb TJ, Fenney M, Williams T. Drug therapy for gender transitions and health screenings in transgender older adults. *J Am Geriatr Soc.* 2016;64(12):2554-2559

Maingi S, Bagabag AE, O'Mahony S. Current best practices for sexual and gender minorities in hospice and palliative care settings. *J Pain Symptom Manage.* 2018;55(5):1420-1427.

Nurses HEALE. www.nurseheale.org. Accessed April 26, 2020.

Westwood S. Abuse and older lesbian, gay bisexual, and trans (LGBT) people: a commentary and research agenda. *J Elder Abuse Neglect.* 2019;31:97-114.

World Professional Association for Transgender Health. Standards of care version 7 https://www.wpath.org/publications/soc. Accessed April 2019.

Yarns BC, Abrams JM, Meeks TW, Sewell DD. The mental health of older LGBT adults. *Curr Psychiatry Rep.* 2016;18(6):60.

Optimizing Care of Older Adults with Limited Health Literacy

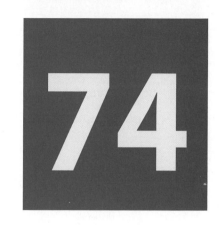

74

Leah B. Rorvig, MD, MS

Anna H. Chodos, MD, MPH

Rebecca L. Sudore, MD

General Principles

Health literacy is defined as "the degree to which individuals have the capacity to obtain, process, and understand basic health information and services to make appropriate health decisions." The construct of health literacy is complex. Limited health literacy (LHL) is thought to occur at or below an eighth-grade reading level. However, health literacy not only involves reading and writing skills, but also listening and verbal communication skills and computational or numeracy skills required for such tasks as pill counting or insulin dosing. Language barriers also contribute to LHL, and the number of foreign-born, older adults in the United States who have limited English proficiency is growing (see Chapter 78, "Unique Needs of Older Immigrants"). Health literacy is also affected by the health care environment, which places a heavy burden on patients to manage their own complex disease processes and health care benefits.

Close to half of US adults have LHL, and up to 90% report difficulty with routine health information. The prevalence of LHL increases among older age groups, with the prevalence reported to be as high as 60% among older populations. Although the average adult in the United States reads at an eighth-grade level, the average adult age 65 years or older reads at a fifth-grade level. Older adults with LHL have been shown to have significant difficulty weighing the risks and benefits of complex treatment options and reading and completing medical forms. Yet, most health care materials are written at or beyond a college reading level. LHL also results in worse clinical outcomes for older adults, including poor functional status, disparities in health care access and the receipt of preventative services, worse chronic disease management, increased hospitalization, and a two-fold increase in mortality. By universally adopting clear health communication techniques outlined in this chapter, clinicians can ensure informed medical decision making and patient safety for all patients and especially for older adults with LHL.

UNIQUE HEALTH LITERACY CONSIDERATIONS IN OLDER ADULTS

For all age groups, LHL has been found to be more common among persons of lower socioeconomic status, limited education, nonwhite race, and limited English proficiency. However, many unique, patient-related factors contribute to LHL in older populations (Figure 74–1), including a high prevalence of impairments in hearing, vision, and cognition, as well as a high burden of chronic disease and polypharmacy. A caregiver's LHL may also affect a patient's medical care and safety.

Hearing and Vision Impairment

Hearing impairment, a significant contributor to LHL, is common among older adults, with estimates as high as 66% among adults older than age 70. Clinicians and patients often miss a diagnosis of hearing loss. Up-to-date audiology evaluations and access to hearing aids are the first step. For patients whose hearing is undercorrected with hearing aids or who cannot access hearing aids due to cost, small portable sound amplifiers (eg, Pocket Talkers) can be used and even worn over hearing aids. Portable amplifiers, which belong to a growing category of assistive devices called personal sound amplification products, can be used in the outpatient clinic, inpatient hospital wards, and at home, to ensure patient understanding of medical information. Compared to hearing aids, personal amplification products are affordable, can be purchased over the counter, and can be used with minimal training in use of hearing-related equipment. Telephone amplifiers, often available through state-supported programs (Table 74–1), can also improve comprehension of medical information relayed by phone. For more information, please refer to Chapter 8, "Managing Hearing Impairment."

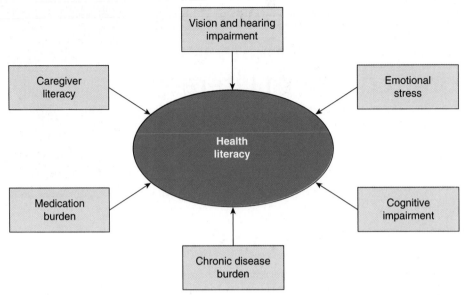

▲ **Figure 74–1.** Unique health literacy considerations in older adults.

Table 74–1. Health literacy resources.

Informational Websites and General Resources
Centers for Disease Control and Prevention (CDC) health literacy facts and resources: http://www.cdc.gov/healthliteracy/ Department of Health and Human Resources, Office of Disease Prevention and Health Promotion, health literacy facts and resources: https://health.gov/our-work/health-literacy
Provider Training and Self-Assessment Tools
Harvard School of Public Health, literacy resources and provider/clinic assessment tools: http://www.hsph.harvard.edu/healthliteracy/ Health Resources and Services Administration's (HRSA) course in health literacy training for providers: https://www.hrsa.gov/about/organization/bureaus/ohe/health-literacy/index.html
Literacy-Appropriate Written Materials
CDC Healthy Literacy guide: http://www.cdc.gov/healthliteracy/ CDC Health Literacy training courses for health professionals: https://www.cdc.gov/healthliteracy/gettraining.html Arizona Health Literacy Coalition: https://azhealthliteracy.org/ PREPARE for Your Care, Low-literacy Advance Healthcare Directive (multiple languages): https://prepareforyourcare.org/welcome Plain Language Action and Information Network, examples of plain language and health literacy information to customize materials: http://www.plainlanguage.gov/populartopics/health_literacy/index.cfm
Resources for Hearing Impairment
Telecommunications Equipment Distribution Program Association: http://www.tedpa.org/ National Institute on Aging: Hearing Loss in Older Adults: https://www.nia.nih.gov/health/hearing-loss-common-problem-older-adults
Resources for Vision Impairment
American Foundation for the Blind Directory of Services for People Who are Blind or Visually Impaired: http://www.afb.org/directory.aspx American Printing House for the Blind: VisionAware for Independent Living with Vision Loss: https://www.visionaware.org/info/for-seniors/1

Websites accessed April 26, 2020.

Visual impairment, which also contributes to LHL, increases with age as a consequence of the high prevalence of macular degeneration, cataracts, and glaucoma. Up-to-date vision evaluations, access to digital or manual magnification and adequate corrective lenses, and use of prescribed medications for ophthalmic-related conditions can help mitigate visual barriers to adequate health literacy. Community-based organizations offer blind and low-vision skills training that can help older adults with vision loss to maintain their independence and quality of life (Table 74–1). For more information, please refer to Chapter 7, "Managing Vision Impairment."

Cognitive Impairment

Cognitive impairment contributes significantly to LHL in older adults. Twenty-one percent of older adults have mild cognitive impairment, and close to 9% of US adults over age 65 have dementia. It is estimated that by 2050 there will be 13.8 million adults living with Alzheimer disease in the United States.

LHL is highly correlated with cognitive impairment, and therefore, screening for cognitive impairment is crucial. The three-item Mini-Cog is a quick screening test (79% sensitive and 90% specific for cognitive impairment), and the Montreal Cognitive Assessment (MoCA) is a more thorough assessment shown to detect cognitive impairment even in early stages (90% sensitive and 87% specific for mild cognitive impairment). After ruling out reversible causes, detecting cognitive impairment early allows clinicians to maximize vascular risk reduction measures such as increased exercise and optimizing blood pressure management. The diagnosis of cognitive impairment also signals the need to identify caregivers who can help interpret medical information for the patient and should serve as an impetus to address advance care planning. For more information about cognitive impairment, please refer to Chapter 9.

Multimorbidity and Polypharmacy

Many older adults have multiple chronic conditions resulting in a high volume and burden of medical information, a large number of medications and disease management tasks, and often many doctors and specialists. Conditions or procedures associated with multimorbidity, such as prior strokes, chronic pain, surgery, or acute hospitalization, also impair cognition, influence patients' ability to understand discharge instructions, and have a negative impact on patients' ability to manage their medical conditions.

Polypharmacy also plays a significant role in LHL, particularly psychoactive medications, such as antidepressants and pain medications. In addition, patients with LHL have difficulty reading and interpreting medication labels and are often nonadherent as a result of poor understanding. The risk of nonadherence increases with increased medication burden and recent hospitalization.

Emotional Stress of Illness

Emotional stress related to serious illness can also affect LHL. For example, older adults are more likely to be widowed, obtain a new diagnosis of cancer, endure new disabilities or chronic pain, and encounter new surroundings during a hospitalization or institutionalization. Stress is associated with impaired memory, poor medication adherence, and inadequate disease self-management. It is important to inquire about how patients are coping with new diagnoses as well as cumulative disability and to screen for depression and anxiety. If needed, counseling and/or pharmacologic treatment may improve health information processing.

Caregivers and LHL

Paid and unpaid caregivers are often an important part of older adults' health care. Caregivers may be responsible for health-related tasks, such as medication management, and for obtaining health care instructions from clinicians on behalf of the patient. However, up to 53% of caregivers may themselves have LHL. Two studies of caregivers found an association between lower caregiver health literacy and worse patient health, including increased frequency and duration of hospital admissions. The person responsible for critical health tasks, if not the patient, should be identified, and clear health communication techniques should be used for both the patient and the caregiver.

Limited English Proficiency and LHL

Limited English proficiency is strongly associated with LHL. As of 2017, more than one in five US residents speaks a language other than English at home. When possible, access to a clinician who is language concordant with the patient may improve care and health outcomes. Health care facilities receiving federal funding must provide language assistance to patients with limited English proficiency. In addition, all clinicians should use in-person professional medical interpreters or video or telephone interpretation whenever available. When able, clinicians should provide patients with health information not only in an easy-to-read format, but also in their preferred language. Emerging online translation technology shows preliminary evidence for accurate medical translation. However, caring for older adults with limited English proficiency presents special challenges. For example, patients with cognitive impairment may struggle to understand the function of video interpreters, or there may be limitations in providing written materials that are language concordant for patients when only telephone and video interpreters are available.

SCREENING

The patient's social history may alert the clinician to potential LHL, such as a history of limited education; almost half of adults who did not graduate from high school had LHL in one study. Limited English proficiency, lack of social engagement, or lower socioeconomic status may also raise concern for LHL. However, providers should have a broad approach to screening and evaluating patients from all backgrounds. Other clues include noncompliance with medical instructions or difficulty completing medical forms, such as reporting they forgot their glasses or that they prefer to review materials at home. A powerful screening tool for LHL is the medication review. This involves asking patients to bring all medications to a medical visit, including nonprescription medications; to list the name of each medication; to describe what each medication is for; and to describe how the medication is taken. Any confusion likely indicates LHL and may raise concern for cognitive impairment.

Formal screening tools to identify patients with LHL, such as the Rapid Estimate of Adult Literacy in Medicine (REALM) and the Test of Functional Health Literacy in Adults (TOHFLA), are generally used for research purposes. Quick three-item and one-item screening questions are also available (eg, "How confident are you filling out medical forms by yourself?"). However, formal screening is generally not needed if clinicians use clear health communication best practices for all older patients.

CLEAR HEALTH COMMUNICATION STRATEGIES

Adults with LHL experience shame and feel less empowered in their interactions with health care providers than patients with adequate health literacy, often leading to a breakdown in communication. Clear health communication techniques are one way to ensure patients are more engaged and empowered.

▶ Clear Verbal Communication

Clear verbal communication techniques are helpful for all patients (Table 74–2). Before offering a recommendation or providing teaching, it is important to tailor communication to the individual. First, assess what patients already know (eg, "What do you already know or believe about . . . ?"). The answer to this question can help clinicians detect misunderstandings and focus their instructions. Next, attempt to learn and then to match instructions to the patient's regular, day-to-day routine. This may help elicit barriers and enhance compliance.

Table 74–2. Clear health communication.

Setting up the discussion:
- Ensure hearing aids and amplification are available.
- Determine the patient's preferred language and ensure medical interpretation is available in that language, either in-person or by phone or video.
- Face the patient.
- Involve the caregiver.

Tailor communication:
- Ask, *"What do you already know about . . . ?"*
- Ask patients about their day-to-day routine to tailor instructions.

Clear communication techniques
- Speak slowly.
- Avoid medical jargon; for example, say "not cancer" instead of "benign."
- Keep number of points to three or less.

Confirm understanding (teach-back)
- Encourage questions by asking:
  - "What questions do you have?"
- Put onus on clinicians by saying:
  - "We have just talked about a lot of things. To make sure I did a good job and explained things clearly, can you tell me in your own words/show me . . . ?"

Reinforce instructions
- Offer pictures, graphs, and written information in the patient's preferred language to reinforce verbal communication.

When discussing health-related topics, providers should attempt to slow their speech, use lay language, and avoid jargon. For instance, clinicians can say "high blood pressure" instead of "hypertension." Clinicians should limit information to three topics or less and focus the discussion on concrete instructions about what the patient needs to do when they go home. To improve patient understanding and health outcomes, every effort should be made to provide information to patients in their preferred language and to offer interpreters.

Importantly, if a patient is known to be hearing impaired, before beginning a discussion, ensure the patient has working hearing aids or is using a personal assistive hearing device. With all patients, the clinician should face the patient to allow for lip reading, which may assist in understanding.

▶ Teach-Back

We recommend that all verbal communication is followed by a confirmation of understanding, often called the "teach-back" or "teach-to-goal strategy." Asking, "Do you understand?" or "Do you have any questions?" often conveys to the patient that they should understand. Instead, we recommend clinicians ask, "What questions do you have?" After questions are answered, clinicians can ask patients or caregivers to restate in their own words what was just discussed or to demonstrate what skill was just taught (eg, insulin dosing). We recommend placing the onus of clear communication on the clinician: "We have just talked about a lot of things. To make sure I did a good job and explained things clearly, can you tell me in your own words/show me . . . ?" Teach-back has been associated with better chronic disease management and informed medical decision making, yet has not been shown to increase the length of a medical visit.

Reinforcing Verbal Communication

Verbal communication can be reinforced with written materials, pictures, or graphs. Using written materials to reinforce verbal instructions has been shown to increase knowledge and improve patients' satisfaction with communication. In addition, literacy-appropriate written materials can improve the completion rate of medical forms and can help with chronic disease management (see Table 74–1). Patients with LHL have been shown to have difficulty accessing information through standard electronic patient portals. Older adults may need help from family or friends, may need written information rather than online information, and may need tailored instructions to be able to use such portals.

When looking for appropriate written information for older patients, the target grade level should be the fifth-grade reading level or lower and should include clear headings, bright contrasting colors, a font size of 14 points or larger, and a combination of both upper- and lowercase letters (ie, not all capital letters). Because of the high prevalence of ophthalmic-related conditions in older adults, non-serif (sans serif) fonts, such as Arial or Helvetica, and nonglossy, matte materials are recommended because they are easier to see. Sentences should contain one topic, be no more than six to eight words in length, and be written in an active "how to" voice. Written materials should also have a high white-space-to-text ratio and include carefully chosen pictures that explain the text and put written material into context. Particular attention should be paid to ensuring that after-visit summaries and hospital discharge instructions adhere to these guidelines. Specifically, for older adults with limited English proficiency, newer tools, such as Google Translate, have been shown to have adequate accuracy for translations and should be considered when preparing after-visit summaries and hospital discharge instructions when no formal translation services are available.

When creating health care materials, several resources can be used to ensure the materials are literacy appropriate. The Suitability Assessment of Materials uses criteria standards in six categories—content; literacy demand; graphics; layout and typography; learning stimulation/motivation; and cultural appropriateness—to help assess if the literacy level is appropriate. The Lexile Framework and the Lexile Analyzer (http://www.lexile.com) can also be used to assess the readability of written materials based on sentence length and word frequency. It is important to include the target population in the design and pilot testing of materials to ensure proper understanding and to improve the material's acceptability.

Strategies for Medically Complex Patients

Patients with multiple medical conditions can benefit from disease management programs that incorporate strategies for LHL patients. Disease management programs for heart failure and diabetes that include literacy-appropriate verbal communication, literacy-appropriate written materials with pictures, automated telephone calls, and/or nurse follow-up calls have been shown to improve disease management, decrease hospitalizations, and decrease mortality. Telehealth interventions, some of which include remote monitoring with feedback and action plans, have shown improved glycemic control in patients with type 2 diabetes and mortality benefit for patients with heart failure. New technology, such as tailored, computerized, discharge instructions from virtual nurses, also shows promise for older adults with LHL. These computer technologies allow patients to repeat the information as often as needed.

Creative use of interprofessional teams may improve medical care and patient understanding for all older adults with multimorbidity and especially for older adults with LHL. Some examples include group medical visits, collaborating with pharmacists to help review medications and fill pill boxes, and asking social workers to help complete advance directive or informed consent forms. The use of health care navigators and community health workers may also help patients navigate the health care system and manage their disease processes.

SYSTEMS APPROACHES

The health care environment often places a heavy burden on patients to manage their disease and to navigate the health care system. For health literacy to improve on a public health level, health systems need to be modified. At the clinic and system levels, signs should include large font and pictures. Standard forms, such as intake forms, informed consent forms, and advance directives, should be written at or below a fifth-grade reading level and should be concordant with a patient's preferred language when possible. Medication labeling should be consistent and should match written instructions to improve patient safety. In addition, all staff should have training in communication techniques for patients with LHL and limited English proficiency. Phone triage and menu systems should be carefully designed with no more than two to three options at a time. By universally adopting these clear health communication techniques, clinicians can help ensure informed medical decision making and patient safety for all patients, and especially for older adults with LHL.

Berkman ND, Sheridan SL, Donahue KE, Halpern DJ, Crotty K. Low health literacy and health outcomes: an updated systematic review. *Ann Intern Med*. 2011;155(2):97-107.

Chesser AK, Keene Woods N, Smothers K, Rogers N. Health literacy and older adults: a systematic review. *Gerontol Geriatr Med*. 2016;2:2333721416630492.

Institute of Medicine. *Health literacy: A Prescription to End Confusion*. Washington, DC: National Academic Press; 2004.

Jacobs B, Ryan AM, Henrichs KS, Weiss BD. Medical interpreters in outpatient practice. *Ann Fam Med*. 2018;16(1):70-76.

Paasche-Orlow MK, Parker RM, Gazmararian JA, Nielsen-Bohlman LT, Rudd RR. The prevalence of limited health literacy. *J Gen Intern Med*. 2005;20(2):175-184.

Pacala JT, Yueh B. Hearing deficits in the older patient: "I didn't notice anything." *JAMA*. 2012;307(11):1185-1194.

Pignone M, DeWalt DA, Sheridan S, Berkman N, Lohr KN. Interventions to improve health outcomes for patients with low literacy. A systematic review. *J Gen Intern Med*. 2005;20(2):185-192.

Reed NS, Betz J, Kendig N, Korczak M, Lin FR. Personal sound amplification products vs a conventional hearing aid for speech understanding in noise. *JAMA*. 2017;318(1):89-90.

Sudore RL, Schillinger D. Interventions to improve care for patients with limited health literacy. *J Clin Outcomes Manag*. 2009;16(1):20-29.

Taira BR. Improving communication with patients with limited English proficiency. *JAMA Intern Med*. 2018;178(5):605-606.

Effects of Homelessness & Housing Instability on Older Adults

75

Rebecca Brown, MD, MPH

Margot Kushel, MD

HOMELESSNESS AND HOUSING INSTABILITY IN OLDER ADULTS

Homelessness and housing instability are common in the United States and increasingly affect the health and welfare of many older adults. In the past three decades, the proportion of the homeless population in the United States aged 50 years or older has increased dramatically. Approximately half of single homeless adults are now aged 50 years or older, compared to only 11% in 1990. The aging of the homeless population is thought to be the result of a cohort effect: individuals born in the second half of the "baby boom" generation (1954–1964) have an increased risk of homelessness compared to other age groups. As this cohort ages, the median age of the homeless population is expected to continue to increase. In the wake of the foreclosure crisis and with rising housing costs in many areas of the United States, the number of adults experiencing housing instability is also increasing. To provide appropriate clinical care to the growing population of older adults experiencing homelessness and housing instability, clinicians need to understand how housing problems interact with health.

DEFINITIONS OF HOMELESSNESS AND HOUSING INSTABILITY

Although definitions of homelessness vary, the most commonly used definition in the United States comes from Congress's 1987 McKinney-Vento Homeless Assistance Act. The McKinney Act defines homeless individuals or families as lacking "a fixed, regular, and adequate nighttime residence," including persons in emergency shelters and places not meant for human habitation. In 2009, Congress expanded the definition of homelessness to include people facing imminent loss of housing (eg, within 14 days after their application for homeless assistance) (Table 75–1).

Most individuals who become homeless have a preceding period of housing instability. *Housing instability* is defined by varying criteria, including difficulty paying a mortgage, rent, or utilities; spending >50% of household income on housing; moving frequently; living in overcrowded conditions; and "doubling up" (ie, living temporarily with family or friends).

PATHWAYS TO HOMELESSNESS AMONG OLDER ADULTS

Homelessness is not a monolithic experience; it has different manifestations and trajectories and requires different solutions. A common schema divides homeless people into three broad groups: first time/crisis homelessness, episodic homelessness, and chronic homelessness (Table 75–2).

Older adults arrive at homelessness by different paths. Some older adults have experienced a long history of personal challenges, such as severe mental illness, imprisonment, substance use disorders, low educational attainment, and poor job histories. These individuals tend to become homeless as younger adults and then remain chronically homeless for many years as they age. Older adults who have been chronically homeless are likely to benefit from permanent supportive housing.

Other older adults have led lives that are relatively conventional, although economically vulnerable, and become homeless for the first time following a crisis late in life. Crises may include the death of a partner or parent, divorce, or disabling illness. Most people who become homeless do so after a period of housing instability; those with fewer social supports are at higher risk of homelessness. These individuals may benefit from rapid rehousing after the initial episode of homelessness or from efforts to prevent homelessness before it occurs. Interventions to prevent homelessness are critical in this group, because adults who become homeless late in life are at increased risk for becoming chronically homeless and experiencing poor health outcomes.

Clinicians can play an important role in recognizing patients at risk of becoming homeless and working to prevent

Table 75–1. Definition of homelessness, US Department of Housing and Urban Development.

1. An individual or family who lacks a fixed, regular, and adequate nighttime residence. Includes persons residing in an emergency shelter, a place not meant for human habitation, or an institution where the person temporarily resided
2. An individual or family who will imminently lose their housing (eg, within 14 days after the date of their application for homeless assistance)
3. An unaccompanied youth (defined as <25 years of age) and families with children and youth defined as homeless under other federal statutes
4. An individual or family who is fleeing, or attempting to flee, domestic violence, dating violence, sexual assault, stalking, or other dangerous or life-threatening conditions

Data from the US Congress, Homeless Emergency Assistance and Rapid Transition to Housing (HEARTH) Act. 111th Congress, 1st session. S 896. Washington: US Government Printing Office, 2009.

a first episode of homelessness. If a patient becomes homeless, clinicians can help prevent chronic homelessness by helping to connect patients to the resources needed to regain housing.

RISK FACTORS FOR HOMELESSNESS AMONG OLDER ADULTS

Although the causes of homelessness are complex, they can be understood in three broad categories as defined by Dr. Martha Burt: predisposing personal vulnerabilities (eg, poverty and social isolation); structural factors (eg, availability of low-cost housing); and the absence of a safety net (eg, lack of social insurance).

Older adults at risk for homelessness have financial, social, and medical vulnerabilities (Table 75–3). Poverty is nearly universal among older adults at risk for homelessness; financial problems rank first on self-reported causes of homelessness among older adults. One-third of older adults reported that difficulty paying a rent or a mortgage triggered

Table 75–2. Categories of homelessness.

1. First time/crisis homelessness: individuals who are homeless for the first time, often following a catastrophic life event
2. Intermittent homelessness: individuals who experience one or more periods of homelessness of less than a year in total duration
3. Chronic homelessness: individuals with a disabling condition who have either been continually homeless for a year or more or who have had at least four episodes of homelessness in the past 3 years

Table 75–3. Risk factors for becoming homeless after age 50.

Personal factors
Death of a relative or close friend
Breakdown of a marital or cohabiting relationship
Disputes with a landlord, cotenant, or neighbor
Domestic or elder abuse
Lack of children, relatives, or friends willing to provide temporary housing
Release from prison

Economic factors
Job loss
Difficulty paying a mortgage, rent, or utilities
Spending >50% of household income on housing
Loss of home (due to foreclosure of one's own home or a home one is renting, sale or conversion of a home one is renting, not having one's name on a lease, falling behind on rent, precipitous rise in rent)

Medical factors
New onset or increased severity of mental illness
New onset or increased severity of cognitive impairment

Data from Brown RT, Goodman L, Guzman D, Tieu L, Ponath C, Kushel MB. Pathways to homelessness among older homeless adults: results from the HOPE HOME Study. *PLoS One.* 2016;11(5):e0155065; Shinn M, Gottlieb J, Wett JL, Bahl A, Cohen A, Baron Ellis D. Predictors of homelessness among older adults in New York City: disability, economic, human and social capital and stressful events. *J Health Psychol.* 2007;12(5):696-708; Crane M, Byrne K, Fu R, et al. The causes of homelessness in later life: findings from a 3-nation study. *J Gerontol B Psychol Sci Soc Sci.* 2005;60(3):S152-S159; and Williams BA, McGuire J, Lindsay RG, et al. Coming home: health status and homelessness risk of older pre-release prisoners. *J Gen Intern Med.* 2010;25(10):1038-1044.

their homelessness, and one-fifth became homeless after losing their housing as a result of external factors (eg, sale by the landlord). Spending >50% of household income on rent increases the risk of homelessness, as does not having one's name on a lease.

Social vulnerabilities also increase the risk of homelessness, including social isolation. Older adults who lack children, relatives, or friends willing to house them are at increased risk for homelessness. Breakdown or loss of interpersonal relationships may also precipitate homelessness, such as death of a spouse or relative, divorce or breakdown of a cohabiting relationship, or disputes with landlords, cotenants, or neighbors. It is suspected that elder abuse increases the risk of homelessness, and domestic violence is a well-recognized risk factor for homelessness. Conditions that are common among older adults at risk of homelessness increase the risk of elder abuse, including shared living situations and social isolation. Imprisonment also contributes to homelessness; older prisoners are at risk for homelessness following release (see Chapter 76, "Helping Older Persons in the Criminal Justice System"), and imprisonment of a partner may precipitate homelessness through loss of social or economic support.

Medical vulnerabilities can cause homelessness, including new onset or increasing severity of a chronic illness, mental health condition, or substance use disorder. These problems can lead to significant medical debt, job loss, or the inability to work, with consequent inability to pay rent or a mortgage. The role of cognitive impairment as a risk factor for homelessness is not known, but cognitive impairment could lead to homelessness if impaired cognition causes difficulty holding a job or managing money.

STRATEGIES TO PREVENT HOMELESSNESS AMONG OLDER ADULTS

To identify these risk factors for homelessness among older adults, clinicians should perform a detailed social history, including financial resources, ability to manage finances, social supports, substance use, and current housing situation. As part of the housing history, clinicians should ask if patients are living in market rate versus subsidized housing and ascertain whether patients are behind on rent, mortgage payments, or utilities. If patients are renting, ask if their name is on the lease or sublease, and determine the proportion of their household income that is being spent on rent. People who spend >50% of income on rent are considered severely cost burdened, which is a risk factor for homelessness. Ask if patients are living temporarily ("doubling up") with friends or relatives and, if so, with whom they are living and how long they will be able to stay. If a patient has risk factors for homelessness including being behind on rent or mortgage payments, paying >50% of their income on rent, or living doubled-up, help prevent a first episode of homelessness by referring the patient to social work, legal services, or community resources.

A social work referral may also be appropriate to determine eligibility for benefits such as Supplemental Security Income (SSI), Social Security Disability Insurance (SSDI), or the Supplemental Nutrition Assistance Program (SNAP). Although the availability of benefits differs by state, homeless older patients who are indigent and have disabilities that qualify them for SSI are usually eligible for Medicaid. Under the Affordable Care Act, in states that have accepted Medicaid expansion, Medicaid benefits are available to Americans earning <133% of the federal poverty level, with or without disabling conditions. This makes Medicaid available to most homeless individuals.

Individuals facing imminent loss of housing are defined as homeless by Congress and are therefore eligible for housing relocation and stabilization services, including rental assistance, mediation with property owners, and legal services. To access these services, clinicians can refer to social work or can refer patients directly to local housing counseling agencies; a list of counseling agencies approved by the US Department of Housing and Urban Development is available on their website.

HEALTH STATUS OF HOMELESS OLDER ADULTS

Most homeless older adults are 50 to 64 years of age; adults age 65 and older currently make up <5% of the total homeless population, although this proportion appears to be increasing as the baby boom cohort ages. Homeless adults in their 50s experience chronic illnesses and geriatric syndromes at rates similar to those of housed adults 15 to 20 years older. Approximately 75% of homeless adults age 50 years and older reported at least one chronic medical condition, and half reported two or more chronic conditions. The most common chronic illnesses were hypertension, arthritis, and asthma or chronic obstructive pulmonary disease. Because these studies relied on self-report by adults experiencing homelessness, who often have poor access to medical care and may have undiagnosed medical conditions, reported prevalences are likely to be underestimates.

Homeless older adults have high rates of geriatric syndromes. Several cohort studies show that despite a median age of just 55 to 56 years, the prevalence of geriatric conditions among homeless older adults is as high or higher than that of adults in the general population with a median age close to 80 years. One-third of homeless adults age 50 years and older reported difficulty performing activities of daily living (ADLs), and nearly 60% had difficulty performing instrumental activities of daily living (IADLs). Half of older homeless adults fell in the past year. Cognitive impairment, measured as a Mini-Mental Status Examination (MMSE) score <24, was present in about one-quarter of homeless older adults. Between one-third and one-half of homeless older adults reported hearing impairment, and approximately 20% had impaired vision, defined as acuity >20/40. Nearly 50% reported urinary incontinence.

Early onset of chronic illnesses and geriatric syndromes in homeless older adults may result from the high prevalence of risk factors for poor health in this population, including poorly controlled chronic illnesses, mental health conditions, traumatic brain injury, and substance use disorders. Several factors contribute to poor control of chronic illnesses, including competing priorities for obtaining health care and lack of health insurance. Nearly three-quarters of homeless older adults experiencing homelessness reported one or more psychiatric conditions, including depression (34%–60%), anxiety disorder (19%), and posttraumatic stress disorder (12%–34%). Although homeless adults age 50 years and older have lower rates of both lifetime and current substance use disorders compared to their younger homeless counterparts, rates of alcohol and drug use are significantly higher than in the general population.

Because homeless older adults have early onset of chronic illnesses and geriatric syndromes, many experts consider homeless adults to be "older" at age 50 years, 15 years earlier than in the general population. This so-called accelerated aging in homeless older adults has important implications for screening and clinical care in this population. Compared to older adults who have housing, homeless older adults have limited ability to modify their environment to match their personal abilities. This mismatch between environmental demands and personal abilities puts homeless older adults at increased risk for adverse outcomes.

INTERACTION BETWEEN HEALTH STATUS AND ENVIRONMENT

Homeless older adults must cope with high rates of chronic conditions in the chaotic setting of homeless shelters or the street. Living in a shelter or on the street is hazardous at any age but poses special hazards for older adults (Table 75–4). Most shelters are group living spaces, with bunk beds and shared bathing facilities. These features may increase the risk of falling. Older adults also encounter risks outside of the shelter. Many shelters require occupants to vacate each morning and return in the evening to wait in line for a bed. On the street during the day, homeless adults are exposed to the elements and at risk for victimization. They must navigate a complex web of social services to obtain meals or shelter. Homeless older adults with impaired function, mobility, or cognition may be unable to safely perform these activities, resulting in falls, injuries, or inability to obtain food or shelter. Other hazards include difficulty toileting because of limited public bathroom facilities and inability to safely store personal items, leading to lost or stolen medications, canes, and glasses.

APPROACH TO CLINICAL CARE FOR HOMELESS OLDER ADULTS

Although clinicians face many challenges in caring for homeless older adults, several measures may improve care for these vulnerable older patients. These measures include screening for geriatric syndromes, mental health problems, and substance use disorders. As noted earlier, clinicians should work with other members of the health care team to determine eligibility for benefits and to refer to available community resources.

Most screening tools for geriatric syndromes are not validated in homeless adults, and there are no evidence-based guidelines for when to screen homeless patients for geriatric syndromes. The American Geriatrics Society recommends comprehensive assessment for geriatric syndromes in frail, older patients who are at risk for functional decline, hospitalization, or nursing home placement. Because homeless older adults have rates of geriatric syndromes and hospitalizations similar to housed adults 15 to 20 years older, we recommend assessing homeless adults age 50 years and older for geriatric

Table 75–4. Environmental hazards for homeless older adults.

Environmental Hazard	Associated Risk
Homeless shelter	
Bunk beds	Falls, injuries
Lack of refrigeration	Inability to properly store medications (eg, insulin)
Lack of secure storage	Stolen/lost medications Stolen/lost adaptive equipment (eg, glasses, hearing aids, canes)
Loud environment	Disrupted sleep
Group living environment	Victimization, lack of privacy, falls, injuries
Group showers	Victimization, lack of privacy, falls, injuries
Bathing and toileting facilities without adaptive equipment (ie, raised toilet seats, grab bars)	Falls, injuries
Institutional meals, often with high starch and salt content	Limited ability to modify diet to accommodate health conditions
Street	
Lack of public toilet facilities	Urinary incontinence, inability to maintain hygiene
Need to walk long distances between services, requiring higher functional status	Falls, injuries
Need to navigate complex web of social services to obtain food and shelter, requiring intact cognition and executive function	Food insecurity
Exposure to elements	Falls, injuries

syndromes; most screening instruments have been validated in these age groups, despite the lack of specific evidence in the homeless population. Based on the prevalence of geriatric syndromes among homeless older adults, we recommend screening for functional and mobility impairment, falls, cognitive impairment, and urinary incontinence.

Although the Katz ADL Scale has not been validated in homeless adults, it has been widely used in younger patients with a range of chronic conditions. One-third of homeless older adults have difficulty performing ADLs, yet treatment options are limited because of the difficulty of modifying the environment of the shelter or street. Public or shared bathing facilities may lack modifications like grab bars and raised toilet seats. Informal caregiving by partners or friends is often not possible in the shelter, because shelters are segregated by sex, which may separate individuals from their caregivers. In addition, many adults experiencing homelessness are socially isolated. Furthermore, referrals for formal caregiving services such as home health aides are impractical in a shelter. A physical therapist may be able to recommend portable adaptive equipment for use in the shelter, such as canes, walkers, and dressing aids, but these materials are often stolen or lost.

Standard IADL scales include items that may not apply to homeless adults living in shelters or on the street, such as food preparation and housekeeping. The Brief Instrumental Functioning Scale (BIFS) was developed and validated for homeless adults and asks about ability to perform the following activities independently or with help: fill out an application for benefits, budget money, use public transportation, set up a job interview, find an attorney to help with a legal problem, and take medications as prescribed by a physician. Homeless patients who are unable to perform these activities independently should be referred to social work and/or case managers.

Taking medications as prescribed poses special challenges in the shelter or on the street, where loss or theft of medications is common. Clinicians should ask if patients have a secure location to store medication, such as a storage locker at a shelter. If they do not, consider other strategies, such as dispensing medications 1 week at a time. Standard measures that improve medication adherence in older adults may also be helpful (see Chapter 14, "Principles of Prescribing & Adherence").

The American Geriatrics Society recommends screening for falls beginning at age 65 years. However, homeless adults age 50 years and older fall at rates higher than the general older population and may benefit from earlier screening. A combination of factors may contribute to high rates of falls among homeless older adults, including environmental hazards (see Table 75-4), functional and mobility impairment, and substance use disorders. Clinicians may be able to decrease the risk of falls among homeless older patients by ensuring that patients have a pass to sleep on the lower bunk, referring patients with impaired function or mobility to physical therapy, and providing counseling for substance use disorders.

Although screening tests for cognitive impairment have not been validated among homeless adults, most have been widely used in younger patients. Patients who screen positive for cognitive impairment should undergo standard medical assessment for reversible causes (see Chapter 9, "Cognitive Impairment & Dementia"). Assess patients with cognitive impairment for decision-making capacity, and refer patients who lack decision-making capacity to social work.

Most screening tests for urinary incontinence have been validated in younger patients, such as the International Consultation on Incontinence Questionnaire (ICIQ). Managing urinary incontinence in shelters and on the street is challenging because of limited access to public toilets and use of shared toileting facilities. Where feasible, consider a trial of standard behavioral interventions, such as bladder training and pelvic muscle exercises (see Chapter 10, "Urinary Incontinence").

To screen for depression in homeless older adults, we recommend using a screening tool validated in patients younger than age 65 years, such as the Patient Health Questionnaire 9. Also consider screening for anxiety and posttraumatic stress disorder, as the prevalence of these conditions among homeless older adults appears to be much higher than in the general population.

Substance use disorders are often underrecognized in older adults. However, screening for substance use disorders in older adults is particularly important because older adults are at higher risk for adverse effects of substance use as a result of changes in body composition with aging, higher rates of prescription medication use, and impairments in function, gait, and balance, among other factors (see Chapter 70, "Unhealthy Alcohol Use"). The risk for adverse effects of substance use may be even more acute in homeless older adults, who have higher rates of substance use disorders and geriatric syndromes compared to the general older population.

RESOURCES FOR HOMELESS OLDER ADULTS

Clinicians caring for homeless older patients should be aware of several resources for homeless individuals, including rapid rehousing, permanent supportive housing, medical respite, and intensive case management (see Table 75-5).

Rapid rehousing provides rental assistance and services and is most appropriate for individuals who experience

Table 75-5. Resources for homeless older adults.

Resource	Definition and Population Who May Benefit
Rapid rehousing	Rental assistance and services. Most appropriate for individuals who experience barriers to housing but have the potential to sustain housing after rental subsidy ends.
Permanent supportive housing	Permanent, subsidized housing with closely linked supportive services (eg, medical, psychiatric, case management, substance use). For chronically homeless individuals.
Medical respite	Temporary posthospitalization care with medically oriented supportive services. For homeless people discharged from acute care hospitals who are not medically ready to return to a shelter or the street.
Intensive case management	Wraparound services delivered by highly trained case managers whose low case load allows for intensive follow-up with clients. Available in shelters and homeless assistance programs for people experiencing homelessness.

barriers to housing but have the potential to sustain housing after the rental subsidy ends. *Permanent supportive housing* is defined as permanent, subsidized housing with onsite or closely linked supportive services (eg, medical, psychiatric, case management, vocational, and substance use services) for chronically homeless individuals. Because permanent supportive housing programs help chronically homeless adults maintain housing and may decrease use of acute health services, the federal government has identified such programs as a priority intervention for people experiencing chronic homelessness. Permanent supportive housing units are available in an increasing number of communities, funded by a combination of resident income, rent subsidies, tax credits, grants, and service-linked funding, such as Department of Mental Health benefits.

Medical respite is also recognized by the federal government as a strategy to decrease the negative impacts of homelessness on health. Medical respite programs provide temporary posthospitalization care with medically oriented supportive services to homeless people discharged from acute care hospitals, but who are not medically ready to return to a shelter or the street. These services may be less costly compared to longer-term hospitalizations or stays in skilled nursing facilities or nursing homes. Moreover, patients discharged to medical respite instead of directly to shelters or to the street have fewer hospital readmissions. Medical respite services exist in a growing number of cities.

Intensive case management refers to a set of wraparound services delivered by highly trained case managers whose low case load allows for intensive follow-up with clients. Intensive case management programs were originally developed for patients with severe mental illness and were later adapted to support individuals who used health services frequently, many of whom were homeless. Intensive case management differs from case management, a general term used to describe a range of programs, from peer support to medically oriented services. Many shelters and homeless assistance programs offer case management programs to help individuals experiencing homelessness to identify and access appropriate services.

As in general geriatric medicine, interprofessional teams may help improve care for homeless older adults (see Chapter 3, "The Interprofessional Team"). An interprofessional team for a homeless older patient might include a case manager working to obtain permanent supportive housing, clinicians providing medical and psychiatric care, a social worker, and a substance use counselor.

CONCLUSIONS AND NEXT STEPS

Homelessness and housing instability are associated with poor health. As a result of demographic shifts and rising housing costs, these problems affect a growing proportion of older adults. Although clinicians face challenges in caring for adults experiencing homelessness and housing instability, understanding the unique health problems among homeless adults age 50 years and older and identifying risk factors for homelessness may improve care for this vulnerable group. Furthermore, a growing number of federal programs provide resources to prevent new homelessness and to end chronic and crisis homelessness.

Brown RT, Goodman L, Guzman D, Tieu L, Ponath C, Kushel MB. Pathways to homelessness among older homeless adults: results from the HOPE HOME study. *PLoS One.* 2016;11(5):e0155065.

Brown RT, Hemati K, Riley ED, et al. Geriatric conditions in a population-based sample of older homeless adults. *Gerontologist.* 2017;57(4):757-766.

Brown RT, Kiely DK, Bharel M, Mitchell SL. Geriatric syndromes in older homeless adults. *J Gen Intern Med.* 2012;27(1):16-22.

Burt M, Aron LY, Lee E, Valente J. *Helping America's Homeless: Emergency Shelter or Affordable Housing?* Washington, DC: Urban Institute Press; 2001.

Caton CL, Dominguez B, Schanzer B, et al. Risk factors for long-term homelessness: findings from a longitudinal study of first-time homeless single adults. *Am J Public Health.* 2005;95(10):1753-1759.

Crane M, Byrne K, Fu R, et al. The causes of homelessness in later life: findings from a 3-nation study. *J Gerontol B Psychol Sci Soc Sci.* 2005;60(3):S152-S159.

Culhane DP, Metraux S, Byrne T, Stino M, Bainbridge J. The age structure of contemporary homelessness: evidence and implications for public policy. *Anal Soc Issues Public Policy.* 2013:13(1):228-244.

Hahn JA, Kushel MB, Bangsberg DR, Riley E, Moss AR. Brief report: the aging of the homeless population: fourteen-year trends in San Francisco. *J Gen Intern Med.* 2006;21(7):775-778.

Shinn M, Gottlieb J, Wett JL, Bahl A, Cohen A, Baron Ellis D. Predictors of homelessness among older adults in New York City: disability, economic, human and social capital and stressful events. *J Health Psychol.* 2007;12(5):696-708.

Sullivan G, Dumenci L, Burnam A, Koegel P. Validation of the brief instrumental functioning scale in a homeless population. *Psychiatr Serv.* 2001;52(8):1097-1099.

US Congress, Homeless Emergency Assistance and Rapid Transition to Housing (HEARTH) Act. 111th congress, 1st session. S 896. https://www.hudexchange.info/resources/documents/S896_HEARTHAct.pdf. Accessed March 11, 2019.

US Interagency Council on Homelessness. Opening doors: federal strategic plan to prevent and end homelessness. https://www.usich.gov/resources/uploads/asset_library/USICH_OpeningDoors_Amendment2015_FINAL.pdf. Accessed March 11, 2019.

Helping Older Persons in the Criminal Justice System

76

Lisa C. Barry, PhD, MPH

Brie A. Williams, MD, MS

General Principles

Health care providers are increasingly managing the health of older persons who are currently or recently involved in the criminal justice system. These interactions occur in a variety of clinical arenas. Many correctional systems contract with community clinics to provide patients in their custody with specialty services, such as cardiology, neurology, and dialysis. When acute care is required that extends beyond the capacity of the correctional health care service in their prison or jail, patients are triaged to hospitals with prison/jail health care contracts or to the nearest appropriate community facility. As a result, people who are currently incarcerated are seen daily at community clinics, specialty clinics, hospitals, and emergency departments around the country. In addition, the number of older adults who are arrested, incarcerated, and released has increased markedly over the past decades. Consequently, community primary care providers are increasingly providing care to older adults who have been arrested for the first time and to older adults who have been released from jail or prison and are returning to the community.

Increased attention from the press, nonprofit advocacy groups, and policymakers has spurred a growing literature in health and criminal justice research aimed at addressing the rapid aging of the US correctional population. Studies have shown that currently and recently incarcerated older adults are a medically vulnerable group and that having a history of incarceration is an important life event for health care practitioners to consider when caring for older patients.

EPIDEMIOLOGY

Prisoners age 55 years or older ("older prisoners") are the fastest growing segment of the criminal justice population, both as a result of a wave of strict sentencing policies in the 1980s and 1990s and an increasing number of older adult arrests. Between 1993 and 2016, the number of sentenced prisoners age 55 or older increased nearly 300%, from 3% of the total state prison population in 1993 to 11.3% in 2016, and it has been estimated that older adults could compose up to one-third of the total US prison population by 2030 if current sentencing and release policies remain unchanged. Approximately 10% of individuals incarcerated in local jails are age 55 or older.

The percentage of new parolees who are older has also grown substantially. Between 1991 and 2012, the percentage of state prisoners released to the community on parole increased from 1.5% to approximately 6%. Patients transitioning from incarceration to the community in later life may experience severed relationships with family and friends and termination of housing and employment. In addition, reinstatement of government entitlement programs that are suspended during incarceration, including Medicare, Medicaid, Social Security Insurance, and Veterans Health Administration benefits, may take several months, causing considerable stress for many patients upon their return to the community. "Prisonization," or excessive dependence on the institutional routines of prison life, is also common among older adults who have spent much of their lives in prison, increasing the difficulty experienced when navigating life outside of prison.

Physical Health

In general, older adults who are incarcerated develop the onset of medical conditions and disability at relatively young age. This is commonly referred to as "premature" or "accelerated" aging. It has been asserted that the physiologic age of many incarcerated older adults appears about 10 to 15 years older than their chronologic age. This accelerated aging can result from multiple factors, including unhealthy experiences prior to incarceration (eg, substance use disorders, risky sexual encounters, homelessness, limited lifetime access to preventive health care) and during incarceration (eg, poor diet, minimal exercise, poor engagement in medical care due to mistrust of the medical profession, chronic stress) and substandard health care both prior to and (sometimes) during incarceration.

On average, older adults who are incarcerated tend to have high rates, and early onset, of multimorbidity, geriatric syndromes, and functional impairments. Many have considerably higher rates of chronic illnesses, such as diabetes, hepatitis C, hypertension, and chronic obstructive pulmonary disease as compared with younger prisoners and their age-matched contemporaries living in the community. As a consequence, many take multiple medications. Geriatric syndromes, including vision and hearing impairment, falls, chronic pain, and urinary incontinence, are also common in this population and may lead to unique challenges. For example, older prisoners with hearing loss may be at heightened risk for physical confrontation if they fail to respond to another resident or if malodorous consequences of incontinence aggravate their cellmates. The prevalence of disability in traditional activities of daily living (eg, bathing, dressing) is higher in incarcerated older adults than in older adults of similar ages in the community. Additionally, the day-to-day experience of disability in this population increases even more dramatically when considering the unique activities that are necessary for independence in prison. These activities of daily living for prison include, for example, being able to drop to the floor for alarms, climb on and off one's assigned bunk, and stand in line for medications. The inability to keep up with the fast pace of prison life because of disability may make older adults vulnerable to victimization from other prisoners and leave them at greater risk of disciplinary action from correctional staff.

▶ Mental Health

The prevalence of mental health conditions is considerably higher among prisoners compared to the general population, regardless of age. Compared with younger adults, older adults in prison have a higher likelihood of previous alcohol use disorders and higher rates of depression, the most common mental health condition in this population. Similar to older persons living in the community, depression among older adults in prison is often undertreated and frequently goes undetected. Depression may be misdiagnosed as a seemingly appropriate response to a medical illness or medication or to the general process of aging, and it may be difficult to disentangle from conditions such as bereavement, fatigue, or cognitive impairment. Mirroring trends seen in older community-dwelling individuals, older adults in prison and jail also have the highest rates of suicide among incarcerated persons.

Emerging evidence also suggests that the prevalence of cognitive impairment among incarcerated older adults is considerably higher than in the community. Histories of substance use disorders, posttraumatic stress disorder, and traumatic brain injury may contribute to higher rates of cognitive impairment in older prisoners. Yet, early stages of cognitive impairment and dementia may be difficult to detect in the structured prison or jail environment as a consequence of limited opportunities for prisoners to make decisions, make plans, or engage in complex tasks such as using transportation.

THE CLINICAL ENCOUNTER

With the aging of the population, an increasing number of older adults are coming into contact with the criminal justice system as arrestees, detainees in jail, incarcerated in prison, or as recently released members of the community. Clinicians should consider a recent history of criminal justice contact as a potential warning for underlying cognitive impairment, substance use disorders, or psychiatric illness. In addition, given the health risks of incarceration, clinicians should screen those recently released from prison or jail for a history of physical and sexual victimization, depression/suicidality, and infectious diseases such as hepatitis B and C and HIV. Recognition of the medical vulnerabilities of older adults involved in the criminal justice system is critical to maintaining the health and safety of this growing population. Table 76–1 details specific considerations that should guide the clinical encounter when a criminal justice history is identified. These considerations are further discussed in the following sections.

▶ Care of a Patient in Custody

In 2014, >641,000 US arrests occurred among persons age 55 years and older. These individuals include both first-time arrestees and those who are returning to jail or prison in later life, although many have been in the criminal justice system sporadically throughout their lives. Many of the myriad physical and mental health factors that are common in this population (eg, cognitive impairment, substance use disorder, hearing impairment, or mental health conditions) can adversely affect an older adult's ability to meaningfully participate in the legal process or obtain appropriate legal counsel and can also put them at risk for incarceration and associated decreased safety and worse health. Particularly for individuals arrested for the first time as an older adult, the event leading to the arrest may be indicative of an underlying medical condition or behavioral health risk factor. Clinicians can play a key role in evaluating for diagnoses such as alcohol or drug use, cognitive impairment, dementia, or delirium that may have compromised a patient's executive function and contributed to criminal justice involvement. Such diagnoses may have critical implications for sentencing and/or safety during incarceration.

Table 76–1. Considerations for the primary care physician whose patient has come in contact with the criminal justice system.

Clinical Encounter	Consideration	What to Do
Acute care of prisoners (eg, hospital, emergency department, specialty clinic)	Patients may have untreated or undertreated medical conditions resulting from suboptimal health care during incarceration. Conditions of incarceration (eg, overcrowding) are risk factors for poor health.	Optimize clinical care and evaluate for history of victimization during detainment including rape; screen for depression/suicidality and infectious diseases including tuberculosis (TB), HIV, methicillin-resistant *Staphylococcus aureus* (MRSA), and hepatitis B and C.
Outpatient care of persons who are recently arrested	A first arrest may be indicative of underlying medical condition.	Rule out medical conditions (eg, dementia, alcohol or drug abuse/dependence) that may have led to the illegal behavior. Evaluate for common conditions in the criminal justice population including risky sexual encounters, infectious diseases, alcohol or drug abuse/dependence, and homelessness.
	Poor health may compromise ability to obtain appropriate legal counsel and increase safety risks during jail detainment.	If patient is detained, consider contacting the jail chief medical officer (CMO) or patient's legal counsel if there are concerns about patient's ability to participate meaningfully in the legal process or to be safe while in detainment.
	Clinicians working in the prison system may have difficulty accessing prisoners' prior medical records and/or reconciling prisoners' medications.	Contact physician at the correctional facility to confirm receipt of important clinical records.
Outpatient care for persons reintegrating into the community after incarceration	Patients may have untreated or undertreated medical conditions resulting from suboptimal health care during incarceration.	Obtain clinical records from correctional facility and optimize clinical care.
	Conditions of incarceration (eg, overcrowding) are risk factors for poor health upon community reentry.	Evaluate patient for history of victimization during detainment including rape; screen for depression/suicidality and infectious diseases including TB, HIV, MRSA (skin), and hepatitis B and C.
	Barriers may hinder appropriate health care management.	Evaluate living situation (eg, homelessness, living with adult child); determine availability of social support.

▶ Care of a Patient Returning to the Community from Incarceration

A growing number of persons transitioning from incarceration to the community are older adults. Older adults are far less likely to be reincarcerated than younger adults. Yet, the transition from prison or jail to the community in later life may be particularly difficult given high rates of chronic health conditions requiring self-care, estrangement from family and friends, and challenges navigating the process necessary to reinstate suspended government entitlement programs.

Furthermore, regardless of the length of incarceration, health problems, which may be exacerbated by the stresses of community reentry, can pose additional difficulties securing employment and housing. Such difficulties can jeopardize patients' abilities to avoid reincarceration. For example, older parolees with dementia could violate parole unintentionally simply by forgetting to meet their parole officer at a designated time and place. In general, health care practitioners should know that older adults who are recently released from a jail or prison are at risk for adverse health outcomes including hospitalization, disproportionately high rates of all-cause mortality, suicide attempt, and death by suicide or drug overdose. These risks, particularly high in the immediate postrelease period, persist to several years following return to the community.

Ideally, clinicians who provide medical care to older adults who have been released from a jail or prison will have been contacted by a correctional clinician during their prerelease planning phase. However, this often does not occur. Even patients who have experienced serious illness in prison and have a documented Advance Care Plan may not leave with their records in hand. Therefore, it is critically important that clinicians ask new patients about a recent or remote history of arrest, detainment, or incarceration.

SUMMARY

The number of older persons who are incarcerated or who are being released from incarceration in later life is growing. This population is often medically complex. Those who have recently reentered our communities are often simultaneously contending with significant social stressors such as lack of housing, poverty, the demands of their postrelease probation or parole instructions, a history of abuse, and low health literacy. Increasing numbers of community agencies offer health and social service assistance to formerly incarcerated persons. Screening patients for criminal justice involvement is the first critical step in identifying this medically vulnerable and rapidly growing population of older adults so that they can receive the specialized help they need to reintegrate successfully into the community.

Ahalt C, Stijacic-Cenzer I, Miller BL, Rosen HJ, Barnes DE, Williams BA. Cognition and incarceration: cognitive impairment and its associated outcomes in older adults in jail. *J Am Geriatr Soc.* 2018;66(1):2065-2071.

Barry LC. Mass incarceration in an aging America: implications for geriatric care and aging research. *J Am Geriatrics Soc.* 2018;66(11):2048-2049.

Barry LC, Steffens DC, Covinsky KE, Conwell Y, Li Y, Byers AL. Increased risk of suicide attempts and unintended death among those transitioning from prison to community in later life. *Am J Geriatric Psychiatry.* 2018;26(11):1165-1174.

Barry LC, Wakefield DB, Trestman RL, Conwell Y. Disability in prison activities of daily living and likelihood of depression and suicidal ideation in older prisoners. *Int J Geriatric Psychiatry.* 2017;32(10):1141-1149.

Ekaireb R, Ahalt C, Sudore R, Metzger L, Williams B. "We take care of patients, but we don't advocate for them": advance care planning in prison or jail. *J Am Geriatr Soc.* 2018;66(12):2382-2388.

Green M, Ahalt C, Stijacic-Cenzer I, Metzger L, Williams B. Older adults in jail: high rates and early onset of geriatric conditions. *Health Justice.* 2018;6(3):1-9.

Human Rights Watch. *Old Behind Bars: The Aging Prison Population in the United States.* New York, NY: Human Rights Watch; 2012.

Williams B, Abraldes R. Growing older: challenges of prison and reentry for the aging population. In: Greifinger RB, ed. *Public Health Behind Bars: From Prisons to Communities.* New York, NY: Springer-Verlag; 2007;56-72.

Williams BA, Lindquist K, Sudore RL, Strupp HM, Willmott DJ, Walter LC. Being old and doing time: functional impairment and adverse experiences of geriatric female prisoners. *J Am Geriatr Soc.* 2006;54(4):702-707.

Williams BA, McGuire J, Lindsay RG, et al. Coming home: health status and homelessness risk of older pre-release prisoners. *J Gen Intern Med.* 2010;25(10):1038-1044.

Older Travelers

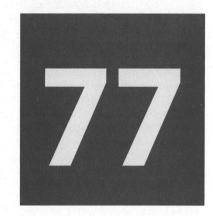

Leah Witt, MD

Megan Rau, MD, MPH

▶ General Principles

1. Some older adults may face barriers to safe travel due to multimorbidity, functional issues, cognitive impairment, or medication management difficulties.

2. While older adults and their caregivers often seek pre-travel advice from physicians and other health professionals, most clinicians have received no formal training about preparing patients for travel.

3. Exacerbation of chronic illness is a major risk for any traveler, and older travelers are particularly vulnerable to this phenomenon. Clinicians should provide anticipatory guidance to help travelers prepare, with advice focused on projected challenges based on health conditions and function.

4. Health professionals should learn about resources that can help with clinical decision making, if assisting in medical emergencies during travel.

▶ Overview of Travel Challenges

Travel, for leisure and social connection, is aspirational for many older adults, particularly with an increase in flexible time during retirement. For even the most experienced traveler, travel requires significant preparation. For older adults with multimorbidity, functional challenges, or cognitive impairment, travel preparation may be extensive and overwhelming. Unfortunately, medical education does not train clinicians to prepare older adults for safe travel, and little data exist about the best methods to prepare older adults for travel in order to mitigate risks or health hazards.

Booking travel and navigating technology for trip planning are just the first of several hurdles faced by travelers. Older adults may have to consider additional trip preparation steps that include securing accommodations for disabilities, organizing medical management needs during the trip, gathering and packing all necessary equipment (eg, walker, oxygen, medications, medical documents), accessing hubs of transit (eg, airports, train stations, cruise docks), and considering destination challenges (eg, unfamiliar medical systems, limited access to health care, limited accessibility for those with disabilities, climate differences, food safety issues, time zone changes).

Most people have experienced the stress of navigating a busy airport, transporting luggage, and finding a gate on time. For people with cognitive impairment, travel is particularly challenging, as unfamiliar environments and jet lag can precipitate delirium. For people with extra equipment needs, such as walkers, portable oxygen, and medical devices, travel can feel particularly burdensome, as they arrange for transport of these devices and navigate unfamiliar environments. For many older adults, travel preparation is far more complicated, and their health risks can be amplified.

▶ Resources for Travel Preparation

Resources for travelers and clinicians lack guidance for most geriatric issues but are useful for preparing for country-specific risks, such as pretravel vaccinations or possible safety issues. In the United States, the Department of State maintains a helpful international travel resource (http://www.travel.state.gov), in which travelers can search information by destination country and seek information on international health care coverage. Additionally, US citizens and nationals can sign up for the Smart Traveler Enrollment Program (STEP) to receive updates about the destination country and to identify oneself to an embassy in case of an emergency.

Internationally, the World Health Organization provides useful information on infectious disease risk by country along with pretravel vaccination guidance (https://www.who.int/ith). In the United States, the Centers for Disease Control and Prevention (CDC) website (http://wwwnc.cdc.gov/travel) is an important resource for clinicians seeking guidance for recommended vaccinations by destination country. The CDC also maintains the "Green Sheet" report from the Vessel Sanitation Program, which lists most international cruise ships and the results of sanitary inspections of those ships (http://wwwn.cdc.gov/inspectionquerytool/inspectiongreensheetrpt.aspx).

For travelers departing from the United States, the Transportation Security Administration (TSA) offers a resource for travelers with medical conditions to get advice on travel through their TSA Cares hotline or website (1-855-787-2227, https://www.tsa.gov/travel/passenger-support). Most mass transportation websites (eg, airports, cruise lines, local and national train companies) have created accessibility web pages with guidance specific to their travel hub and means of transportation, which can be useful in pretravel preparation.

To date, there are no evidence-based guidelines for clinicians to prepare older adults for travel. Our expert opinion is that clinicians should actively engage older adults in preparing for travel and provide anticipatory guidance to medical-related challenges. Health professionals should encourage older adults to carry lists of active medical problems, current medications, and emergency contact information (Table 77–1). This information is useful in the event of an emergency during travel and particularly important for any traveler with cognitive impairment. Older travelers should bring an adequate supply of medications and identify a means to obtain additional medications at their destination, should medications get lost.

Finally, older travelers should consider health coverage and costs when traveling. For US travelers insured by Medicare, there is typically no health care coverage outside of the United States except for certain emergency situations. For example, Medicare Part B may cover services on cruises within US territorial waters near US land. Medicare medication plans do not cover medications purchased outside of the United States. Medigap (supplemental) plans can provide coverage outside of the United States, and other travel insurance plans can be purchased before travel. Visit the Medicare travel website (https://www.medicare.gov/coverage/travel) for additional exceptions and details. A proposed "travel checklist" for clinicians is shown in Table 77–1.

▶ **Ship Travel**

Travel by cruise is a very popular vacation mode for older adults. According to the Cruise Line International Association, a record 25.8 million passengers cruised globally in 2017. Ship travel as a mode of transportation carries minimal risk short of gross navigational miscalculation. Events such as collisions, running aground, or pirate attacks are highly publicized but actually relatively infrequent. The principal risks to ship travelers involve the hazards of shore travel (eg, vehicle accidents,

Table 77–1. Travel checklist for clinicians.

1. Solicit trip information.
- ✔ Ask about destination, length of trip, and mode of travel.
- ✔ Refer to http://www.travel.state.gov for country-specific advice.
- ✔ If travelling by air, advise airport preparation by visiting the airport accessibility page.
- ✔ US travelers: consider seeking travel advice from TSA Cares (1-855-787-2227) or visit https://www.tsa.gov/travel/passenger-support for airport services.

2. Prepare health information.
- ✔ Advise patient to understand medical coverage during travel, and consider supplemental travel insurance programs if travelling internationally.

Medications:
- ✔ Ensure patients will have adequate medication supply for length of trip (may need to contact pharmacy, initiate prior authorization for early refill).
- ✔ Identify emergency pharmacy at destination.
- ✔ Recommend carrying medications in "carry on" luggage.
- ✔ Advise about any dose/timing adjustments (eg, related to time change).

Recommend items to carry:
- ✔ Active medical problem list
- ✔ Medication list
- ✔ Emergency contact information
- ✔ Clinic and provider contact information, including fax number
- ✔ Copy of recent ECG (if known coronary artery disease/arrhythmia)
- ✔ Insurance cards
- ✔ Advance directives (including health care proxy and code status)
- ✔ US travelers: consider completing a TSA notification card: https://www.tsa.gov/sites/default/files/disability_notification_card_508.pdf

3. Travel-specific anticipatory guidance
- ✔ Pretravel immunizations: Search by destination country http://wwwnc.cdc.gov/travel/page/vaccinations.htm
- ✔ Venous thromboembolism prevention
- ✔ Oxygen needs (portable oxygen concentrator)
- ✔ Assistive devices (walker, cane, wheelchair request)
- ✔ Cognitive impairment (advice for caregivers, safety plan)
- ✔ Urinary issues (incontinence, urinary frequency, retention)

ECG, electrocardiogram; TSA, Transportation Security Administration

pedestrian accidents, falls), which account for the vast majority of the traumatic medical problems while "cruising."

In preparation for ship travel, older adults should take steps to prevent illness by ensuring they are up to date on immunizations, especially the influenza vaccine. Caution should be taken when prescribing chemoprophylaxis for motion sickness, such as anticholinergics and antihistamines, due to the risk of urinary retention and delirium. Although shipboard epidemics attributable to viral gastroenteritis or viral upper respiratory infections are relatively uncommon, illness spread on a ship will be amplified by the contained environment. Older adults are particularly at risk from complications, such as dehydration from gastroenteritis.

An effective strategy to prevent viral outbreaks (eg, from norovirus, the most common cause of gastroenteritis) is good hand hygiene by washing with soap and water especially before eating and after using the toilet. Good hand hygiene, along with good epidemiologic surveillance, is effective in limiting shipboard epidemics.

Ships registered in countries with rigorous public health standards enforced by government agencies (eg, the United States and the United Kingdom) may be less likely to present infectious disease risks to travelers. Data about individual cruise lines and individual ships are readily available from the CDC in the form of the Green Sheet (http://wwwn.cdc.gov/inspectionquerytool/inspectiongreensheetrpt.aspx). Most larger cruise ships have a medical department aboard that can provide initial care for minor illness or injury and can help in arranging medical evacuation in more serious situations.

▶ Air Travel

"If there is a physician on board, could you please identify yourself to a flight attendant?" Some estimates suggest that 60% to 70% of physicians have been involved in management of an in-flight medical emergency. As there is no mandatory reporting system, in-flight medical emergencies are haphazardly recorded with little or no follow-up among the airlines. It is estimated that in-flight medical emergencies occur in 1 of every 604 flights, which is likely a gross underestimate. One study of in-flight emergencies showed approximately 0.3% were a cardiac arrest, and cardiac arrest was responsible for 86% of in-flight events resulting in death.

The nature and estimated frequencies of in-flight emergencies are shown in Table 77–2. It is clear that older adults are at greatest risk of in-flight emergencies. Older adults are more likely to have coronary artery disease, chronic obstructive pulmonary disease, syncope because of autonomic dysregulation, or underlying cognitive impairment, or to experience adverse medication side effects. Because a health professional managing an in-flight emergency does not have the diagnostic support to make more than a "best guess" assessment, consideration must be given to the illness frequencies shown in Table 77–2 that might account for the observed problem.

Health professionals should learn what resources are available to them in the event of an in-flight emergency.

1. Flight attendants are trained in emergency procedures and have some training in emergency first aid. Ask attendants for resources to aid in diagnosis and treatment of an ill passenger.

2. Most US carriers have contracted with a medical resource on the ground, staffed by an experienced physician trained in emergency medicine and aerospace medicine. These physicians are available for consultation by air-to-ground communication. As a general rule, a medical volunteer provider should advise the crew of the medical issue, including severity, urgency for treatment, and possible outcomes if a diversion plan is not pursued. Ultimately, the decision to divert an aircraft for an unscheduled landing lies solely with the captain.

3. All commercial airliners based in the United States are required by the Federal Aviation Administration (FAA) to have a medical kit on board. This kit contains diagnostic equipment (eg, blood pressure cuff, stethoscope), oropharyngeal airways, intravenous infusion equipment, medications (oral, intravenous, intramuscular), inhalers, and resuscitation equipment. Table 77–3 provides an enumeration of the requirements by the FAA.

Table 77–2. Nature of in-flight emergencies.

Category	% of All Emergencies
Syncope/presyncope	37%
Respiratory	12%
Gastrointestinal	10.9%
Cardiac	8%
Psychiatric	3.5%
Stroke	2%
Diabetes or complications	1.6%
Other[a] (ENT, trauma)	28.9%

ENT, ear, nose and throat

[a]Other: no clear diagnosis determined, likely cause included pain, dizziness, syncope, etc.

Table 77–3. Contents of on-board emergency medical kits required by FAA on all commercial airlines based in the United States.

Medications	Supplies
Analgesic tablets (nonopioid)	500 mL saline solution
Antihistamine, injectable	IV tubing
Antihistamine, tablets	IV catheter
Aspirin tablets	Bag-valve masks (3 sizes)
Atropine, injectable	CPR masks (3 sizes)
Bronchodilator inhaler	Oropharyngeal airways
Dextrose, 50%	Gloves, sponges, tape
Epinephrine 1:1,000 solution	Syringes and needles
Epinephrine 1:10,000 solution	**Monitoring**
Lidocaine IV	Sphygmomanometer
Nitroglycerin tablets	Stethoscope

CPR, cardiopulmonary resuscitation; FAA, Federal Aviation Administration; IV, intravenous.

4. All US aircraft with one or more flight attendants will have an automatic external defibrillator (AED) on board. An AED can indicate the cardiac rhythm and will not administer a shock unless the rhythm is one that may respond to the shock. The FAA mandates that flight attendants be trained yearly in the use of AEDs and cardiopulmonary resuscitation (CPR).

5. Larger aircrafts carry medical oxygen in "walk around" tanks, and the number of tanks varies with the size of the aircraft. This oxygen is intended for emergency use only. Each tank supplies approximately 30 minutes of oxygen, so extended hours of oxygen support are not possible. "Commuter airlines" aircraft are not required to carry medical oxygen. Passengers with known chronic lung disease and hypoxia should prepare for travel by securing an individual portable oxygen concentrator for use onboard prior to the flight.

In the United States, Canada, and the United Kingdom, medical professionals have no legal obligation to volunteer to provide care in an emergency. However, many European countries and Australia do impose a legal obligation to assist. Enforcement of the "must volunteer" provision may be problematic, as there will be uncertainty about legal jurisdiction in international flights.

In 1998, passage of the Aviation Medical Assistance Act (AMAA) (Public Law 105-170) provided clarity about liability for providers responding to on-board medical emergencies in the United States. The law protects health professionals rendering aid in a medical emergency in flight, if care is rendered in good faith and the professional is medically qualified. The care rendered "must be similar to the care that others with similar training would provide under such circumstances." Providers are not exempt from liability. If the treated passenger can establish the provider was "grossly negligent" or intentionally caused the alleged harm, the AMAA does allow for liability of providers.

In-flight emergencies are best handled if the provider is aware of the treatment resources available on board the aircraft, is prepared to render care in the face of considerable uncertainty, provides care only within their own professional scope of practice, and understands that clinical decisions made at 35,000 feet are often a "best guess." After assisting in a medical emergency, the provider should document the care provided and should not discuss the patient's treatment without proper authorization from the patient.

▶ Travel-Related Medical Considerations

A. Contraindications to Travel

Some older adults have medical problems that are contraindications to air travel. Many of these conditions are relative contraindications that can be mitigated by delaying travel or

Table 77–4. Suggested travel delay intervals after medical diagnosis and/or treatment before flying.

Travel Contraindicated	2- to 3-Week Travel Delay
Unstable angina	Uncomplicated MI
Severe decompensated heart failure	Resolution of pneumothorax
HTN urgency/emergency	Stroke
Uncontrolled arrhythmias	Recent surgery
Eisenmenger syndrome	
Severe symptomatic valvular heart disease	**24-Hour Travel Delay**
Seizure within 24 hours	Endoscopic procedures (eg, colonoscopy)
Cerebrospinal fluid leak	Scuba diving trip
Intracranial hemorrhage[a]	
PaO$_2$ <70 mm Hg	
Severe anemia (hemoglobin <8 g/dL)	
Acute sinusitis	
Acute otitis media	

HTN, hypertension; MI, myocardial infarction; PaO$_2$, partial pressure of arterial oxygen.

[a]Until cleared by neurologist/neurosurgeon.

preparing adequately. Air travel is contraindicated if patients have unstable coronary disease, a recent myocardial infarction (delay travel approximately 2 weeks), recent surgery (delay travel approximately 2 weeks for ear, nose, and throat [ENT], ocular, or gastrointestinal surgery, and several more weeks for orthopedic surgery where deep vein thrombosis [DVT] risk is increased), significant neurologic disability, a recent stroke (delay travel approximately 2 weeks), and behavioral issues caused by cognitive impairment or psychiatric problems. Table 77–4 provides proposed time periods one should delay travel after diagnosis, exacerbation, and/or treatment.

B. Infectious Disease

Most travel guidance for patients centers on infectious disease prevention and management. There are limited robust data regarding the prevalence of medical issues that arise during travel, and there is a lack of rigorous anticipatory guidance for older adults with multimorbidity and functional impairment. For older adults, the available data indicate that infections (upper respiratory infections and gastroenteritis) are most common. The principle that "common things occur commonly" pertains to travel. Surveillance systems, such as the GeoSentinel Surveillance Network (https://www.istm.org/geosentinel), aggregate data about infectious diseases worldwide from a network of travel medicine clinics in six continents. This network may be useful in assessing the likely causes of febrile illness in a returning traveler or understanding infectious disease risks based on travel destination.

C. Thrombosis

Venous thromboembolism (VTE) is a highly morbid and common condition, and immobility from travel, particularly air or car travel, is a recognized risk factor for VTE. Many of the recognized risk factors for VTE are more prevalent in older adults, including hypercoagulable states, cancer, and orthopedic problems. Advancing age is an *independent* risk factor for DVT and VTE. Preventing travel-related VTE should be an important consideration in preparing an older adult for travel. Although it has been recognized for some time, the increased risk of VTE due to travel has been somewhat difficult to quantify. Clinicians should assess the magnitude of VTE risk in individual patients in order to determine if a pretravel risk-reduction intervention is warranted. All older travelers should attempt to attenuate the modifiable risks of travel such as avoiding dehydration, addressing immobility, and combating lower extremity venous stasis. Treatment with VTE prophylaxis may be considered for those at greatest risk, including those with recurrent VTE, known hypercoagulable state, malignancy, or immobility.

D. Respiratory Conditions

Chronic lung disease, such as chronic obstructive pulmonary disease, is a common medical condition that presents challenges to travel. Pressurized aircraft typically maintain a cabin pressure that mimics the partial pressure of oxygen at 6000 to 8000 feet. Therefore, patients with chronic lung disease may experience more hypoxia with air travel. A PaO_2 (partial pressure of arterial oxygen) of <70 mm Hg at rest or a pulse oxygen saturation <89% is usually a contraindication to air travel, unless supplemental oxygen is arranged for the flight. Metal oxygen tanks are not allowed on board, but the TSA maintains a list of approved portable oxygen concentrator devices allowed onboard by the FAA (https://www.faa.gov/about/initiatives/cabin_safety/portable_oxygen/). Passengers may rent or purchase these devices for use, and prescriptions must be secured by their physician prior to travel. Passengers should not rely on onboard medical oxygen, as this may be used only in the event of a medical emergency, not for routine use.

Guidelines for managing other medical equipment (eg, walkers, medications, diabetic testing supplies) when traveling within the United States are outlined by the TSA (https://www.tsa.gov/travel/security-screening/whatcanibring/medical).

E. Urinary Incontinence

Urinary incontinence is common in older adults and can be challenging during periods of travel. Urinary incontinence, defined as the involuntary leakage of urine, should be addressed prior to travel, and travelers should be guided in managing this condition during the trip. First-line treatments include behavioral modifications with scheduled toileting, fluid manipulation, and pelvic floor exercises if able. Second-line treatments with medications to reduce bladder contractions and delay desire to void (eg, oxybutynin and tolterodine) should be avoided due to the risk of anticholinergic-induced adverse effects on cognition and function in the older adult. Travelers should consider purchasing aisle seats on airplanes for improved access to the bathroom. If there is limited access to toilets, incontinence products such as briefs and pads are useful to prevent soiling of clothing and property but are typically an out-of-pocket cost. Travelers and their caregivers should be instructed to change these products when soiled and use barrier cream if the traveler is immobile to prevent skin breakdown.

CONCLUSION

Travel is aspirational for many older adults and an important means for social connection and well-being. Older adults may face barriers to safe travel due to multimorbidity, functional issues, cognitive impairment, or medication management difficulties. Physicians and other health professionals should be equipped with information to help their patients mitigate the potential risks of travel and provide anticipatory guidance focused on projected challenges based on their health conditions and function. If called to assist in a medical emergency during travel, clinicians should be aware of their duties and understand the resources that can assist with decision making.

Butterfield S. A pre-flight check for patients. *ACP Internist.* 2019;39(5):8.

Chandra D, Parisini E, Mozaffarian D. Meta-analysis: travel and risk for venous thromboembolism. *Ann Intern Med.* 2009;151(3):180-190.

Flaherty GT, Rossanese A, Steffen R, Torresi J. A golden age of travel: advancing the interests of older travellers. *J Travel Med.* 2018;25(1). doi:10.1093/jtm/tay088.

Gendreau MA, DeJohn C. Responding to medical events during commercial airline flights. *N Engl J Med.* 2002;346(14):1067-1073.

Ko Y, Lin SJ, Salmon JW, Bron MS. The impact of urinary incontinence on quality of life of the elderly. *Am J Manag Care.* 2005;11:S103-S111.

Leder K, Torresi J, Libman MD, et al. GeoSentinal surveillance of illness in returned travelers, 2007-2011. *Ann Intern Med.* 2013;150(6):456-468.

Lee TK, Hutter JN, Masel J, Joya C, Whitman TJ. Guidelines for the prevention of travel-associated illness in older adults. *Trop Dis Travel Med Vaccines.* 2017;3(1):10.

Leung DT, Larocque RC, Ryan ET. Travel medicine. *Ann Intern Med.* 2018;168(1):ITC1-ITC16.

Marshall CA, Morris E, Unwin N. An epidemiological study of rates of illness in passengers and crew at a busy Caribbean cruise port. *BMC Public Health*. 2016;16(1):314.

McCabe T. "Doc, can I fly to Australia?" A case report and review of delirium following long-haul flight. *BJPsych Bull*. 2017;41(1):30-32.

Nable JV, Tupe CL, Gehle BD, Brady WJ. In-flight medical emergencies during commercial travel. *N Engl J Med*. 2015;373(10):939-945.

Pavli A, Maltezou HC, Papadakis A, et al. Respiratory infections and gastrointestinal illness on a cruise ship: a three-year prospective study. *Travel Med Infect Dis*. 2016;14(4):389-397.

Peterson DC, Martin-Gill C, Guyette FX, et al. Outcomes of medical emergencies on commercial airline flights. *N Engl J Med*. 2013;368(22):2075-2083.

Ross AGP, Olds GR, Cripps AW, et al. Enteropathogens and chronic illness in returning travelers. *N Engl J Med*. 2013;368(19):1817-1825.

Unique Needs of Older Immigrants

78

Pei Chen, MD

▶ Overview and General Principles

Immigration and immigrant population have gained increasing attention in the public health research and policy domains in recent years in the United States, and immigration is a global phenomenon. Although immigration is often the consequence of the push and pull of economic, environmental, sociopolitical, and safety factors, it is also a social determinant of health that plays an important role in the care of an older immigrant due to related health inequities and disparities. However, there is little written on immigration as a social determinant of health for older adults. The lack of high-quality studies examining immigration as a social determinant of health has a serious impact on health policies for older immigrants. To provide comprehensive care to older adults, it is important to look at immigration from the context of structural, cultural, and behavioral frameworks. To be inclusive of diverse older persons, the American Geriatrics Society (AGS) Ethnogeriatrics Committee developed a positional statement in 2016 that outlined health care disparities in the United States and provided guidance on quality indicators to promote high-quality multicultural geriatric care. This chapter provides an overview of the definitions commonly used to describe immigrants, the demographics of older immigrants in the United States, health insurance and access to care for older immigrants in the United States, common barriers and their impact on the care of older immigrants, interventions and resources, and the future steps to improve the care of older immigrants.

American Geriatrics Society Ethnogeriatrics Committee. Achieving high-quality multicultural geriatric care. *J Am Geriatri Soc.* 2016; 64(2):255-260.

Castaneda H, Holmes SM, Madrigal DS, Young ME, Beyeler N, Quesada J. Immigration as a social determinant of health. *Annu Rev Public Health.* 2015;36:375-392.

▶ Definitions

Clarity in definitions could aid in the understanding of immigrant communities and characteristics that may contribute to health-related behaviors and risks. However, there is a lack of formal consensus on the definitions, concepts, and categories of migrants. The United Nations International Organization for Migration defines a migrant broadly as a person who has moved across an international border or within a state away from the original place of residence, regardless of the legal status, whether the move is voluntary or involuntary, what the causes for the movements are, and what the length of stay is. *Migrant* is a neutral term regardless of the direction of movement. Based on the US Immigration and Nationality Act and for the purpose of this chapter, an *immigrant* refers to a foreign-born person who migrated across an international border into a destination country.

From the legal perspective, there are different categories of immigrants in the United States (Figure 78-1). These immigrants are categorized as authorized and unauthorized based on the legal status of whether they have been granted the rights to stay in the United States. Among the authorized lawful immigrants, some reside in the United States temporarily with temporary visas for tourism, academic learning and training, work, and so on, or with temporary protected status (TPS), whereas others reside permanently. There are two types of permanent residents: conditional permanent residents and lawful permanent residents (LPRs, also known as "green card" holders). Both conditional permanent residents and LPRs have the potential to become naturalized citizens depending on their individual situations and time spent in the United States. The permanent residents can legally come into the United States through family relationship, employment sponsorship, humanitarian protection (eg, refugee and asylees), and the Diversity Visa lottery.

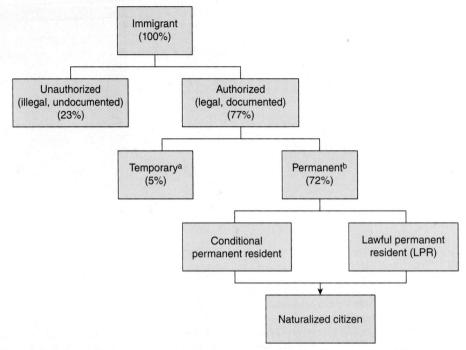

▲ Figure 78–1. Types of migrants in the United States. Percentage of the legal status is based on 2017 US Census Bureau data. [a]Temporary refers to shorter stay, such as for tourism, business, and so on, or special status, and generally without the intention of living in the United States permanently. [b]Permanent refers to longer stay, with the intention to ultimately live and work permanently in the United States.

From the social and cultural perspectives, there are two types of older immigrants: (1) those who immigrated at a younger age and are growing older in the foreign country and (2) those who immigrated at an older age and are "aging out of place" in a new foreign country. The older immigrants who immigrated early in life have had the time and opportunities to acculturate through education and work and accumulate more economic resources. Whereas the late-life immigrants tend to have more confined social networks, often living in multigenerational households and relying on families, and have more limited financial stability given lack of employment and limited public assistance. These different types of older immigrants face different types of challenges as they get older.

Douglas P, Cetron M, Spiegel P. Definitions matter: migrants, immigrants, asylum seekers and refugees. *J Travel Med.* 2019;26(2):taz005.

Sadarangani TR, Jun J. Newly arrived elderly immigrants: a concept analysis of "aging out of place." *J Transcult Nurs.* 2015;26(2):110-117.

USA.gov. Immigration and citizenship. https://www.usa.gov/immigration-and-citizenship. Accessed April 21, 2019.

▶ Demographics

As of 2016, the United States has 43.7 million immigrants, accounting for about one-fifth of the world's migrants, the greatest proportion of any country in the world. The immigrant population represents about 13.5% of the population in the United States. Among all immigrants, almost 45% are naturalized citizens; 27% are LPRs; 23% are unauthorized; and the rest are authorized immigrants. Since the 1960s, there has been a shift of immigrant populations from Europe and Canada to Latin America and Asia with almost 50% of the immigrants coming from Central and South America and 27% from South and East Asia. Although the proportion of older immigrants (age 65 and older) among all immigrants in the United States has decreased from 32.6% in the 1960 to about 16% in 2016 and the median age of the immigrants decreased from 57.2 years in 1960 to 44.8 years in 2017, the median age of the immigrant population is older than that of the general population born in the United States, which is 36.2 years. As of 2016, there are almost 7 million older immigrants, age 65 years and older, in the United States, and these older immigrants, along with the rest of the immigrant population, are expected to stay and age in the United States.

Batalova J, Blizzard B, Boltar J. Frequently requested statistics on immigrants and immigration in the United States. 2019. https://www.migrationpolicy.org/article/frequently-requested-statistics-immigrants-and-immigration-united-states#Demographic. Accessed April 21, 2019.

Radford J, Budiman A. Facts on U.S. immigrants, 2016: statistical portrait of the foreign-born population in the United States. 2018. https://www.pewhispanic.org/2018/09/14/facts-on-u-s-immigrants. Accessed April 21, 2019.

United Nations Department of Economic and Social Affairs, Population Division. *International Migration Report 2017: Highlight.* New York, NY: United Nations; 2017.

US Census Bureau. Foreign born. https://www.census.gov/topics/population/foreign-born/about.html#par_textimage. Accessed August 11, 2019.

▶ Health Insurance for Older Immigrants

Having health insurance is one of the first steps for an older immigrant to access health services in the new country. In the United States, Medicare is a federal health insurance for people who are aged 65 and older, younger people with disabilities, and people with end-stage renal disease requiring dialysis. The Social Security Administration determines eligibility of two core Medicare benefits, which include (1) Part A for the hospital for acute care, skilled nursing facility for postacute care, home health care, and hospice care; and (2) Part B for ambulatory care, mental health care, specific types of outpatient prescription medications, specific types of vaccinations, and specific types of durable medical equipment. The Centers for Medicare and Medicaid Services (CMS) manages Medicare Part D, which is the prescription drug benefit through private insurance companies. There are private insurance companies approved by CMS that may offer Medicare Part C, or Medicare Advantage Plans, which provide Medicare Parts A and B, most of the times Part D, and sometimes other extra coverages, such as vision, hearing, and dental. To join Part C, an individual must have Medicare Parts A and B.

Older immigrants in the United States can face challenges in obtaining health insurance. In order to be eligible for Medicare Parts A and B, the individual must be a citizen of the United States or an LPR in the United States with 5 years of continuous residence in the country. Medicare Part A premium is generally covered if there are adequate work credits, generally 40 quarters or 10 years, by the individual or the spouse. For those who do not have adequate work hours, they will need to pay a high premium. Medicare Part B also requires premium payment, and Medicare Parts C and D have variable premiums depending on the plans. While there is no citizenship or length of residency requirement for Part C or Part D on the insurance plan side, CMS requires the plans to disenroll unauthorized immigrants. In other words, unauthorized immigrants are ineligible to receive Medicare coverage. Even though authorized immigrants, such as a citizen or LPR with 5 year of residence, are technically eligible to receive Medicare, they may not actually be able to use this benefit due to limited or lack of financial capacity to pay high premiums in the setting of limited or no work credits.

In the United States, Medicaid programs, funded by the federal and state governments and administered by the state government, provide health coverage to those with disabilities and low-income individuals, including low-income immigrants. Each state has its own income and asset limits for the Aged and Disabled (A&D) Medicaid, which includes payment of Medicare Part B premium. Individual states may choose to participate in the expansion of Medicaid eligibility to cover more low-income individuals. For those who may not be able to afford the Medicare premiums and do not qualify for A&D Medicaid, Medicare Savings Programs (MSPs) operated by the state Medicaid agencies offer Medicare premium relief for those with higher income and asset limits. These state Medicaid programs have immigration status and length of residency requirements that vary by state. For A&D Medicaid and MSP, individuals must be qualified immigrants, including LPRs (but not TPS). This means that a Medicare-eligible immigrant with TPS cannot benefit from Medicaid with Part B premium or co-insurance.

There are other alternative health insurance coverage options for immigrants who do not qualify for premium free Medicare Part A. One option for those who do not qualify for Medicaid is a Qualified Health Plan (QHP) purchased from the marketplace along with the application for financial assistance in the form of premium tax credits and cost-sharing reductions. QHPs are available to LPRs and individuals with nonimmigrant visas (eg, visas for workers, students, victims of crimes or human trafficking) and with other status, such as many temporary status categories. There are no length of residency requirement for QHPs. Alternatively, some may choose to only have Medicare Part B and forgo Medicare Part A. Having Medicare Part B will allow them to enroll in Medicare Part D.

Health insurance options for older unauthorized immigrants are limited, since they are not eligible for Medicare or Medicaid. They could buy private insurance, but the premium is usually cost prohibitive. Emergency services may be provided and covered depending on available resources on the local and state levels.

Lack of adequate health insurance is one of the major structural barriers to health care utilization among older immigrants. Because of the eligibility criteria for Medicare, late-life immigrants are much less likely to have Medicare, more likely to have Medicaid, and less likely to have a regular source of care compared to their native-born and early-life immigrant counterparts. However, over time, these late-life immigrants may be able to qualify for Medicare by becoming citizens or residing in the country for 5 years or more, gain access to care, and establish a regular source of care, such as from primary care.

Burke G, Kean N. Justice in aging issue brief: older immigrants and Medicare. 2019. https://www.justiceinaging.org/wp-content/uploads/2019/04/FINAL_Older-Immigrants-and-Medicare.pdf. Accessed May 1, 2019.

Choi S. Longitudinal changes in access to health care by immigrant status among older adults: the importance of health insurance as a mediator. *Gerontologist.* 2011;51(2):156-169.

Migration Policy Institute. State immigration data profile: United States demographics and social. 2017. https://www.migrationpolicy.org/data/state-profiles/state/demographics/US. Accessed May 1, 2019.

Research and Analytic Studies Division. Medi-Cal's non-citizen population: a brief overview of eligibility, coverage, funding, and enrollment. Medi-Cal Statistical Brief. California Department of Health Care Services. 2015;2015-0142015:1-19.

▶ Common Barriers and Impact on Care

There are extrinsic and intrinsic of barriers that older immigrants face (Table 78–1) as they receive care. Immigration policies, insurance eligibility and access, and costs to care pose extrinsic barriers. As older immigrants gain access to and receive care, they can face additional challenges from the health services delivery system. A fragmented health services delivery system is difficult for any patient to navigate, but it can be more challenging for older immigrants when resources are in unfamiliar languages or are culturally insensitive. A well-integrated patient-centered health services delivery system incorporates resources in the older immigrants' native languages and in a culturally sensitive way. Other extrinsic barriers include transportation to and from social activities and care sites, especially in more suburban and rural areas, and limited human resources, such as interpreter services and caregivers who are bilingual or multilingual and trained to provide care in culturally sensitive ways. In addition to these extrinsic barriers, there are also intrinsic barriers that older immigrants encounter as

Table 78–1. Common barriers to care encountered by older immigrants.

Extrinsic	Intrinsic
• Costs	• Age-related physiologic changes
• Health insurance and related policies	• Cultural beliefs and practices
• Health services delivery systems	• Geriatric syndromes
• Immigration policies	• Health beliefs
• Limited language and culturally sensitive resources	• Health literacy
• Limited human resources	• Language proficiency
• Transportation	• Multimorbidities

they access health services. Intrinsic barriers, such as language proficiency, health literacy, culture, and health beliefs, can further widen the health disparities between native-born patients and immigrants and affect the access to care and quality of the care received by older immigrants. Furthermore, these barriers, along with age-related physiologic changes, geriatric syndromes, and multimorbidities generally experienced by many older adults, can further complicate their care. An understanding of these barriers by health care providers has the potential to result in improved care for older immigrants.

While language proficiency and health literacy are distinct concepts, they are related and are the most commonly cited barriers to access needed health services by older immigrants. Only about 50% of the immigrants in the United States report being proficient in English, which means that only half speak only English at home or can speak English very well if they speak a non-English language at home. Late-life immigrants generally have fewer opportunities to learn and become proficient in English. In addition to language proficiency, the immigrant population in the United States has fewer years of education as compared with native-born Americans. Both language proficiency and education attainment can affect health literacy, which is defined as the degree to which an individual has the capacity to obtain, process, and understand the basic health information and services needed to make appropriate health decisions. Sentell and Braun found that low health literacy was prevalent among those with limited English proficiency (LEP) and that those with both LEP and low health literacy have poorer self-perceived health status among different racial and ethnic groups. When older immigrants have limited language proficiency, it is more difficult for them to obtain health information, access primary care and mental health, and use screening services.

Immigrants bring rich cultural practices and associated health beliefs with them. The recent late-life immigrants bring their living arrangement preferences and gender role practices from their country of origin, and these preferences and practices can affect the social support and acculturation of the older immigrants. For example, late-life immigrants from Central and South America and Asia may prefer multigenerational households and strong intergenerational interaction, differing from early-life immigrants from northwestern Europe. Because of the multigenerational households and lower level of acculturation, family members may take on additional caregiver roles to care for the late-life immigrants, or vice versa. Aside from living arrangements, different immigrant groups may bring different health beliefs. For example, older Chinese immigrants may describe their symptoms and health beliefs based on their understanding of the tenets of traditional Chinese medicine, and they may try herbs, acupuncture, tui na (a type of massage therapy), qigong (a type of exercises incorporating body movements, breathing, and meditation), or other practices concurrently with Western medicine. Furthermore, the older immigrants' culture and health beliefs may also affect their utilization of medical and mental health services. Therefore, it is important to explore the cultural practices and health beliefs of older immigrants before the discussion of the care plans.

With the complex interplay between extrinsic and intrinsic barriers, older immigrants, when compared to the native-born population, are more likely to delay medical care, prescriptions, and preventive care; they also perceive worse overall health and mental health. Furthermore, older immigrants, especially late-life immigrants who are more dependent on others due to language and cultural barriers, may have less diverse social networks, increasing susceptibility to social isolation, loneliness, and depressive symptoms. At the end of life, older immigrants, especially those from Asia, Africa, and Central and South America, and those who have lived in the new country for less time are more likely to receive aggressive care and to die in an intensive care unit than those who were native born or have lived in the new country for a prolonged period of time. For the unauthorized immigrants in the United States, end-of-life care can be especially challenging due to limited access to routine care and hospice services.

The care of an older immigrant with dementia is an example that demonstrates the complexity of the barriers that older immigrants face. An older immigrant may receive a delayed dementia diagnosis due to the belief that symptoms and signs are related to normal aging, bad karma, or God's will. The delayed dementia diagnosis may also be from shame, lack of continuity of care from health professionals, low confidence of the health professionals in making the diagnosis given limited experience working with older immigrants, and perceived logistical challenges by health professionals in working with older immigrants. While family members may support and compensate for the symptoms of dementia, thus delaying the diagnosis, there are also older immigrants who have delayed diagnosis because of limited family support from family separation, social isolation, and limited interaction with the health care system. Furthermore, screening and diagnostic tools are not always designed or adjusted to accommodate the culture, language, and education, such as for those who are illiterate or have gone through different education systems, making diagnosis more challenging. There is also an added layer of challenge in that interpreters may be used for screening and diagnostic tests and the interpreters may modify the wording of the screening and diagnostic tests and results to facilitate translation, which can introduce errors.

Du Y, Xu Q. Health disparities and delayed health care among older adults in California: a perspective from race, ethnicity, and immigration. *Public Health Nurs.* 2016;33(5):383-394.

Garcia C, Garcia MA, Chiu CT, Rivera FI, Raji M. Life expectancies with depression by age of migration and gender among older Mexican Americans. *Gerontologist.* 2019;59(5):877-885.

Sagbakken M, Spilker RS, Nielsen TR. Dementia and immigrant groups: a qualitative study of challenges related to identifying, assessing, and diagnosing dementia. *BMC Health Serv Res.* 2018;18(1):910.

Sentell T, Braun KL. Low health literacy, limited English proficiency, and health status in Asians, Latinos, and other racial/ethnic groups in California. *J Health Commun.* 2012;17(suppl 3):82-99.

Wang L, Guruge S, Montana G. Older immigrants' access to primary health care in Canada: a scoping review. *Can J Aging.* 2019;38(2):193-209.

Wilmoth JM. Living arrangements among older immigrants in the United States. *Gerontologist.* 2001;41(2):228-238.

Yarnell CJ, Fu L, Manuel D, et al. Association between immigrant status and end-of-life care in Ontario, Canada. *JAMA.* 2017;318(15):1479-1488.

► Interventions and Resources

In 2016, the World Health Organization (WHO) adopted the Global Strategy and Action Plan on Aging and Health to provide guidance to different levels of governments on creating age-friendly environments, promote knowledge translation and exchange as related to aging, and change people's perspectives and actions toward aging. The WHO set up the Global Network of Age-Friendly Cities and Communities to improve the physical and social environments, such as accessibility to transportation and creation of public spaces for social interactions, in which people can age well. To become a member of the network, cities and communities must share and promote respect for diversity and equity, as well as value older adults' participation, contribution, and rights. The WHO encourages the engagement from the government and the people to design and create age-friendly environments that are responsive and adaptable to the needs of diverse older populations, including older immigrants. To achieve age-friendly environments, it is necessary to collect information on race, ethnicity, language, other demographics, and determinants of health to aid in the identification of gaps in services, development of new policies and interventions, linkage to social and health services, and reduction of health inequities faced by minorities and older immigrants. At the same time, in 2016, a white paper from the Institute for Healthcare Improvement (IHI) provided a conceptual framework that guides health care organizations in reducing health disparities in populations that have historically been linked to discrimination or exclusion, offers practical advice, and proposes steps to achieve health equity. The framework for health care organizations included steps to (1) prioritize health equity, (2) develop structures and processes to support the health equity work, (3) implement strategies to address the myriad determinants of health, (4) decrease racism within the organization, and (5) partner with the communities. Together, these guides from the WHO and IHI provide global directions to policymakers, social services, and health services to improve the lives of older adults from diverse backgrounds.

There are several key interventions and resources that health care professionals should be aware of as they work with older immigrants. While it is impossible to become familiar with all possible cultural beliefs, practices, and traditions, it is important for health care professionals to recognize the impact of older immigrants' backgrounds on their health beliefs and health-related behaviors. Health care professionals should explore older immigrants' beliefs, values, goals, and expectations about their medical concerns and treatments. Furthermore, it is imperative for health care professionals to learn and recognize their individual conscious and unconscious biases as they work with older immigrants. The unconscious biases can lead to unintentional behaviors that can have a negative impact on the therapeutic relationship between the older immigrants and their health care professionals. A publicly available resource, Project Implicit (https://implicit.harvard.edu/implicit/index.jsp), offers different Implicit Association Tests to individuals who are interested in learning about their own unconscious biases regarding race, ethnicity, religion, age, and so on, and tools to use this knowledge to improve one's own understanding of diversity and inclusion. In addition to learning about one's own biases, cultural competence and cultural humility trainings are important aspects of preparing health care professionals to work with older immigrants. In 2014, the AGS published the Doorway Thoughts series aimed to address issues and concerns regarding cultural beliefs, traditions, and customs that would apply to clinical encounters with older adults from 15 different ethnically diverse populations.

Because language proficiency is one of the major barriers for older immigrants to access and receive quality care, it is important to identify older immigrants' primary languages, offer trained professional medical interpreters, and incorporate trained professional medical interpreters when interacting with older immigrants instead of using untrained interpreters, such as family members or friends. Depending on the availability of resources in the local environment and the individual's needs and preferences, trained professional interpreters can meet the older immigrants in person, on the phone, or through video conference. When using phone or video interpreters, it is important to consider any hearing and/or visual impairments experienced by the older immigrant. It is also important to brief the trained professional medical interpreter prior to the encounter with an older immigrant on the topics to be covered, the time available for the encounter, the communication strategies, and the foreseeable challenges that may arise from the topics, especially topics that are emotionally laden. At the beginning of the encounter, it is important to acknowledge the older immigrant's sensory issues, such as vision and hearing impairments, and cognitive issues. The encounter should also include introduction of all the different members in the encounter and their

roles or relationships. During the encounter, it is important to speak in short sentences directly to and while facing the older immigrant and take pauses to provide opportunities for the trained professional medical interpreter to interpret. Be mindful and ask the trained medical interpreter to turn away or sometimes step out during the physical exam to protect the privacy of the older immigrant. The teach-back technique is an important tool to use to confirm the older immigrant's understanding of the encounter. Written materials, if available, should be provided to the older immigrant in his or her own language with the appropriate reading level.

Similar barriers that have an impact on the access to care and quality of care in older immigrants can also limit the participation of older immigrants in community activities. In the United States, the Area Agency on Aging (AAA), which is a state-designated public or private nonprofit agency, addresses the needs of older adults at the local or regional level, such as at the city, county, or multicounty district level, and tackles the issue of social exclusion, which is the inability to participate in social relationships and activities that occur within the community. The AAA coordinates a wide array of services to older adults and adults with disability at the community level. Some of these services may include, but are not limited to, aging and disability resource centers; senior and activity centers; community ambassador programs for seniors that train resource specialists to offer information, referrals, and counseling to older immigrants; and adult day and day care programs. These services may be tailored to specific ethnogeriatric populations, and the AAA can often provide additional guidance on the specifics of these services to older immigrants.

Brangman S, Periyakoil V. *Doorway Thoughts: Cross Cultural Health Care for Older Adults*. 2nd ed. New York, NY: American Geriatrics Society; 2014.

Neville S, Wright-St Clair V, Montayre J, Adams J, Larmer P. promoting age-friendly communities: an integrative review of inclusion for older immigrants. *J Cross Cult Gerontol*. 2018;33(4):427-440.

Periyakoil VS. Building a culturally competent workforce to care for diverse older adults: scope of the problem and potential solutions. *J Am Geriatr Soc*. 2019;67(S2):S423-S432.

Wyatt R, Laderman M, Botwinick L, Mate K, Whittington J. *Achieving Health Equity: A Guide for Health Care Organization*. Cambridge, MA: Institute for Healthcare Improvement; 2016.

▶ Conclusion and Future Direction

Today, more people than ever are migrating and aging in new host countries, and different countries are becoming more heterogeneous. While older immigrants face many extrinsic and intrinsic barriers that can contribute to the health disparities seen in this population, these barriers are increasingly being recognized and addressed by integrating policy changes, social services, and health care delivery. As a society seeks to be more inclusive of older immigrants as part of the natural makeup of the communities, it is important to address social exclusion by providing adequate social support and opportunities for social participation. Older immigrants have the potential to experience social inclusion—develop new social networks, improve social status, and gain connection within the community—when they become an integral part of the community. Active engagement of the community such as advocacy, research on culturally sensitive assessment tools and interventions, education on cultural competency and humility, diversity and inclusion, and support from local government are necessary to meet the unique needs of older immigrants.

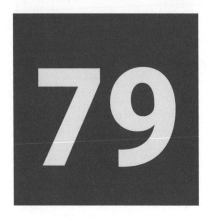

Age-Friendly Health Systems

Stephanie E. Rogers, MD, MS, MPH

Leslie Pelton, MPA

▶ General Principles

According to the US Census, the number of people in the United States aged 65 and older will nearly double between 2012 and 2050. Today, 46 million Americans are over the age of 65, making up 13% of the total population. With 10,000 people turning 65 every day, there are unique challenges changing the health care environment. Proportionally, there will be more adults living in the oldest ages (age 85+), as well as a shift in the ethnic and racial composition, with an increase in the proportion of Hispanic and nonwhite older adults. Consequently, there is expected to be a 200% rise in the demand for health care services, with an estimated 70% of older adults likely needing long-term care at some point. This changing landscape presents an urgent opportunity to redesign health systems to meet the complex needs affecting patients, families, and society.

▶ Unique Factors That Offer Opportunities to Improve Care for Older Adults

A. Individuals

Multimorbidity is common in older patients, with over half of older patients having three or more chronic diseases. Having multiple chronic conditions increases an individual's risk of disability and health care utilization, which leads to a disproportionate amount of spending for caregiving and higher levels of care like hospitals or nursing homes. Older adults have a lot of heterogeneity in not only disease presentation, but also in risk of harm, prognosis, and care preferences. This heterogeneity includes a diverse range of functional, cognitive, and sensory abilities, including varying degrees of social support or isolation. Older adults may prefer health care in a more assessable setting (like home) or need increased streamlining and simplification of information, medications, or transitions. A health system designed to care for older adults must have the flexibility to account for and adjust to this multiplicity.

B. Health Systems

There are many evidence-based models of care for older adults (eg, Acute Care of the Elderly [ACE] and Program of All-Inclusive Care for the Elderly [PACE]). However, for various reasons, health systems have found it difficult to scale up these models. Therefore, only a small portion of older adults are cared for in this way.

Many health systems do participate in quality assurance tactics to reduce variation in clinical care and to ensure adherence to guidelines. However, given that older adults have more multimorbidity, medications, and unique challenges, as described earlier, it becomes harder to account for patient preferences and cumulative disease burden complexities as a system. Current strategies often promote small changes in cumulative reduction of relative risk of a disease, with less focus on the cumulative risk of harm, which may be more important for older patients.

Although there are some health systems with well-integrated system-wide approaches for care coordination, the majority of care that older adults receive is fragmented and burdensome. Health systems continue to grow larger hospitals (where the majority of acute disease management is focused), while the number of nursing home beds is declining. Often, personal health information in one setting is not easily available in postacute settings or even to the patients and caregivers themselves. There is little attention paid to where patients and families spend the majority of their time, in regard to safety and mobility in the home. However, there is a trend to consolidate hospitals into health systems that include postacute care facilities, primary care, social services, home health, and hospice. This provides opportunities for systems to implement the wide array of evidence-based models of care for older adults across settings.

C. Society

Federal and state health policies are in need of serious reformations in order to promote the quality of life, independence, and health of older adults and their caregivers. Changing incentives from volume-based care to value-based care allows for better health outcomes, less waste, streamlined coordination, and prevention of harm—all improvements that will benefit older adults. Recent reform improves reimbursement for chronic care management, transitional care, comprehensive geriatric assessments, and assessment and care planning for cognitive impairment. Many gaps remain, including the need for improved policies to strengthen preventative care and care coordination, the need for improved options to promote independence and health care in the home, insufficient coverage of long-term care costs, and Medicare and Medicaid reform.

Approximately 75% of older Americans strongly agree that "what I'd like to do is stay in my current residence for as long as possible." Many communities are ill-equipped to provide what aging adults want: easy access to their destinations with personal significance, such as churches, stores, and recreation centers, as well as physical proximity to friends and family. Public transportation, housing to support physical and cognitive limitations, and enhanced social services and policies are greatly needed and are driving the initiative of making communities age-friendly.

Addressing These Challenges with Age-Friendly Health Systems

Age-friendly health systems aspire to "keep healthy older adults healthy, be proactive in addressing potential health needs, prevent avoidable harms, improve care of those with serious illness and at the end of life, and support family caregivers throughout." Age-friendly health systems should ensure that care for every older adult, their families, and caregivers is guided by an essential set of evidence-based practices, causes no harms, and is consistent with what matters to the older adult and their family. This is a national initiative of The John A. Hartford Foundation and the Institute for Healthcare Improvement (IHI) in partnership with the American Hospital Association (AHA) and the Catholic Health Association of the United States (CHA) and has the bold aim of reaching 20% of US hospitals by the end of 2020. Equally important is the focus on addressing the social influencers of health, such as food insecurity and housing, by the integration of community-based organizations with health systems.

Given that the first aspect of being an age-friendly health system is reliable delivery of care guided by an essential set of evidence-based practices, IHI's first step was to synthesize current knowledge by analyzing 17 evidence-based geriatric care models from which 90 core features were identified. There was considerable overlap in the features, and they could be further clustered into 13 distinct core features. IHI then engaged health systems, geriatric research experts, and clinical geriatric specialists and further refined the 13 core

features to the core features of age-friendly health systems, known as the "4Ms":

What Matters: Know and align care with each older adult's specific health outcome goals and care preferences including, but not limited to, end of life, and across settings of care.

Medication: If medication is necessary, use age-friendly medication that does not interfere with what matters to the older adult, mobility, or mentation.

Mentation: Prevent, identify, treat, and manage dementia, depression, and delirium across care settings of care.

Mobility: Ensure that each older adult moves safely every day in order to maintain function and do what matters.

These four components were selected because each represents an essential aspect in caring for older adults. Given there is obvious overlap and relationship between each one, they are pursued together to amplify the outcomes and effects in an age-friendly health system. For instance, changing a medication may improve mentation and mobility, which could be what matters to an older adult to maintain independence. Some systems may choose to implement the 4Ms condition by condition, whereas others may try to embed these within strategic initiatives. Often, the best way to bundle these four elements is by implementing an evidenced-based model of geriatric care.

In 2017, five pilot sites (Anne Arundel Medical Center, Ascension, Providence Health and Services, Trinity Health, and Kaiser Permanente) began testing ideas on how to make health systems more age-friendly. The initiative used implementation science and change theories to ensure that evidenced-based care is consistently applied throughout the continuum, from the hospital and into the community. Health systems were encouraged to use quality improvement principles, such as process mapping and small tests of change, before implementing changes more broadly. They determined data measurement goals (eg, numbers of days the older adult spent at home and free of institutional care or percentage of patients who reported receiving care that matched their goals) to help determine if their changes were leading to age-friendly change. Using what they learned, an Age-Friendly Action Community formed from an additional 70 health systems to share in a virtual community for collaboration, data sharing, and learning.

How to Build an Age-Friendly Health System

There is a large gap between the availability of evidence-based models of care for older adults and the care many health systems currently provide. The goal of implementing an age-friendly health system should be to eliminate that gap so that the 4Ms are integrated into care with every older adult in every setting. The following data measures are offered to help health systems known if they are age-friendly:

- Increasing number of days the older adult spends at home and free of institutional care
- Percentage of patients who are discharged from the hospital and postacute care setting to home or their community
- Percentage of patients and families in the community, the hospital, and the postacute setting who report receiving care that matched their goals

A health system can also learn much about how age-friendly it is by stratifying its standard outcome measures by age to learn whether these are improving over time for older adults:

- Thirty-day readmissions
- Emergency department visit rate
- Patient satisfaction scores (eg, Hospital Consumer Assessment of Healthcare Providers and Systems [HCAHPS])
- Length of stay

Health systems that have the capability should consider three additional measures:

- Thirty-day readmissions stratified by race/ethnicity
- Goal-concordant care
- Delirium

Five components are essential to implementing an age-friendly health system. First, there must be executive support and commitment to this realignment of care. Second, this realignment must be integrated into the health system's strategic plan and executive dashboard measures. The third component is the implementation of evidence-based clinical models (guided by the 4Ms) into front-line clinical practice. Additionally, the fourth component includes patient, family, and caregiver participation in advisory councils and governing committees. Finally, formal partnerships with community organizations should be formed.

▶ Social Movement and Dissemination

In 2018, the age-friendly health system model of care was tested in five health systems with a focus on learning replicable and scalable tactics in implementation and dissemination.

In 2019, the initiative adds an additional 70 hospitals or health systems in an action community who work to rapidly scale up the 4Ms in their institution. By 2020, the goal is for 20% of health systems to begin implementation of their age-friendly health system. The need to create an age-friendly health system has never been more important, and this movement is just the beginning.

Allen K, Ouslander JG. Age-friendly health systems: their time has come. *J Am Geriatr Soc.* 2018;66(1):19-21.

Fulmer T, Mate KS, Berman A. The age-friendly health system imperative. *J Am Geriatr Soc.* 2018;66(1):22-24.

Guiding principles for the care of older adults with multimorbidity: an approach for clinicians. *J Am Geriatr Soc.* 2012;60(10):E1-E25.

Harrington C, Carrillo H. Nursing facilities, staffing, residents and facility deficiencies, 2009 through 2016. https://www.kff.org/medicaid/report/nursing-facilities-staffing-residents-and-facility-deficiencies-2009-through-2016/. Accessed April 27, 2020.

Hollmann PA, Zorowitz RA, Lundebjerg NE, Goldstein AC, Lazaroff AE. Hard work, big changes: American Geriatrics Society efforts to improve payment for geriatrics care. *J Am Geriatr Soc.* 2018;66(11):2059-2064.

Keenan TA. Home and community preferences of the 45+ population. AARP. http://www.aarp.org/research/topics/community/info-2014/home-community-services-10.html. Accessed February 7, 2019.

Lundebjerg NE, Hollmann P, Malone ML. American Geriatrics Society policy priorities for new administration and 115th Congress. *J Am Geriatr Soc.* 2017;65(3):466-469.

Mate KS, Berman A, Laderman M, Kabcenell A, Fulmer T. Creating age-friendly health systems: a vision for better care of older adults. *Healthcare.* 2018;6(1):4-6.

Ortman JM, Velkoff VA, Hogan H. An aging nation: the older population in the United States. Population estimates and projections. *Current Population Reports.* Issued May 2014. https://www.census.gov/library/publications/2014/demo/p25-1140.html. Accessed April 27, 2020.

Pew Research Center. Baby boomers retire. http://www.pewresearch.org/fact-tank/2010/12/29/baby-boomers-retire/. Accessed February 5, 2019.

Robert Wood Johnson Foundation. Chronic Care: making the case for ongoing care. Published January 1, 2010. https://www.rwjf.org/en/library/research/2010/01/chronic-care.html. Accessed February 6, 2019.

Scharlach A. Creating aging-friendly communities in the United States. *Ageing Int.* 2012;37(1):25-38.

Tinetti ME, Bogardus ST Jr, Agostini JV. Potential pitfalls of disease-specific guidelines for patients with multiple conditions. *N Engl J Med.* 2004;351:2870-2874.

Index